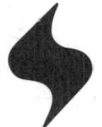

Stedman's

Cardiovascular &
Pulmonary

WORDS

INCLUDES
RESPIRATORY
FIFTH EDITION

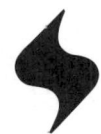

Stedman's
Cardiovascular &
Pulmonary
WORDS

INCLUDES
RESPIRATORY

FIFTH EDITION

Wolters Kluwer
Health

Lippincott
Williams & Wilkins

Publisher: Julie K. Stegman
Series Managing Editor: Eric Branger
Associate Managing Editor: H. Rae Gibbons
Manufacturing Coordinator: Margie Orzech
Typesetter: Susan Appler de los Rios
Printer & Binder: Data Reproductions Corporation

Printed in the United States of America

2007

Library of Congress Cataloging-in-Publication Data

Stedman's cardiovascular & pulmonary words: includes respiratory. — 5th ed.
   p. ; cm.
  Includes bibliographical references.
  ISBN-13: 978-0-7817-7611-0
  ISBN-10: 0-7817-7611-2
  1. Cardiopulmonary system—Diseases—Terminology. 2. Cardiopulmonary system—
Terminology. 3. Cardiology—Terminology. I. Stedman, Thomas Lathrop,
1853–1938. II. Title: Stedman's cardiovascular and pulmonary words. III. Title:
Cardiovascular & pulmonary words.
  [DNLM: 1. Cardiovascular Diseases—Terminology--English. 2. Cardiology—
Terminology—English. 3. Pulmonary Disease (Specialty)—Terminology—English.
WG 15 S8124 2007]
  RC702.S74 2007
  616.1001'4—dc22

2007017200

2 3 4 5 6 7 8 9 10

Contents

Acknowledgments

An important part of our editorial process is the involvement of medical transcriptionists — as advisors, reviewers, and/or editors.

We extend special thanks to Nicole Peck, CMT and Sue Dickinson, CMT, for editing the manuscript, helping resolve many difficult questions, and remaining dedicated to this project. We are grateful to our Editorial Advisory Board members, including Julie Conlon; Ulana Decyk, BSBA; Robin Hall; Kathy Hess, CMT; Deborah Hoplight; Andrea Kopitsky; Velta Jo Reider; Corey Russell, RMT; Suzanne Taubert, CMT, FAAMT; and Tina Whitecotton, RMT, FAAMT, who were instrumental in the development of this reference. They recommended sources and shared their valuable judgment, insight, and perspective.

We also extend thanks to Janet West for her exemplary work in researching and compiling the appendix. Additional thanks to Helen Littrell for performing the final prepublication review. Other important contributors to this edition include Sue Bartolucci, CMT, FAMMT; Susan Caldwell; RuthAnne Darr, CMT, FAAMT; Janice Deal, RN, ELS; Robin Koza; Heather Little; Lori Mongrella, CMT; Twila K. Neeld, CMT; Beth Pessetto; Rhonda Schlecht; Judi Walls; and Stephanie Wilcoxson.

Special thanks goes to Kathy Cadle for her precise and attentive work in reviewing the content files for format, updating the content, and serving as quality control contact for the content.

As with all our Stedman's word references, this resource incorporates the suggestions and expertise of our many contacts in the medical transcriptionist community. Thanks to all of our advisory board participants, reviewers, and editors; AAMT meeting attendees; and others who have written us with requests and comments — keep talking, and we'll keep listening.

Editor's Preface

Breathe in, breathe out, breathe in, breathe out — a simple thing really. Most of us don't even have to tell our bodies to do it; it just comes naturally. There are times when that simple act of bringing oxygen into our lungs becomes difficult though. It could be due to pregnancy, where the organs in a woman's body shift, giving the lungs a little less room and making it harder for her to breathe. Or it could be due to a child who is afflicted with asthma, struggling with an asthma attack or the type of harsh cough that accompanies this affliction which frightens the child, their loved ones, and others around them. There are also the chronic conditions of old age, where the simple, inevitable fact of aging means our bodies are deteriorating and, thus, not functioning quite as well as they used to, whether from chronic obstructive pulmonary disease, congestive heart failure, emphysema, or other ailments.

Our hearts are affected in the same way. Whether from old age, afflictions, wear and tear, or habitual misuse of our bodies, our hearts function less well as we age. Plaques build up, making it harder for blood to pass through our arteries, potentially leading to a heart attack, a stroke, and even death. We are blessed to live in a time when medical science has advanced well beyond the medicine practiced in the Middle Ages and continues to advance every day, so that we are better able to care for and treat these conditions.

Cardiology & Pulmonary Words, 5th edition, is a word book dedicated to the terms related to the conditions and treatment of the heart and lungs. We have strived to make this the most complete, accurate, up-to-date reference book we could. We checked medical journals, textbooks, manufacturers' websites, and other medical websites to find current terminology and equipment related to the care of the heart and lungs. You will find thousands of accurate terms in this book to help make your medical reports as precise as possible. However, as medicine is an ever-changing field of study, there are bound to be new terms we were unable to include or equipment that is no longer used but is still listed in this word book.

I would like to thank the entire Stedman's team for their work on this book, especially Rae Gibbons for her unending patience on this project. I would also like to thank Kathy Cadle, Sue Dickinson, CMT, and Jeanne Bock, CSR, MT, for their hard work and help in creating the final product you hold in your hands today. I also cannot forget the Editorial Advisory Board for their feedback, as well as the research contributors for their time and efforts spent culling new terms for inclusion in this word book. And last, but not least, you, as you are the reason we publish these books.

Nicole G. Peck, CMT
April 2007

Publisher's Preface

Stedman's Cardiovascular & Pulmonary Words, Fifth Edition, offers an authoritative assurance of quality and exactness to the wordsmiths of the healthcare professions — medical transcriptionists, medical editors and copyeditors, health information management personnel, court reporters, and the many other users and producers of medical documentation.

In *Stedman's Cardiovascular & Pulmonary Words, Fifth Edition,* users will find protocols, diagnoses, therapeutic procedures, new techniques, lab tests, and clinical research terms, as well as abbreviations with their expansions pertinent to cardiology, pulmonary, and respiratory medicine. The appendix sections, substantially enhanced over the previous edition, provide illustrations with useful captions and labels; a pulmonary function test table and lab values; pulmonary function terms; ventilation terms; sample reports; common terms by procedure; drugs by indication; and an exhaustive listing of cardiology-related trial and study names.

This new edition, including more than 5,000 new entries, includes the Stedman's Word Book Series trademarks: fully cross-indexed terms by first and last word, an A–Z format with main entries and subentries, and appendix material for additional comprehension and application of the terminology.

We at Lippincott Williams & Wilkins strive to provide you with the most up-to-date and accurate word references available. Your use of this Word Book will prompt new editions, which we will publish as often as updates and revisions justify. We welcome your suggestions for improvements, changes, corrections, and additions — whatever will make this Stedman's product more useful to you. Please complete the postage-paid card in this book for future suggestions and recommendations, or visit us online at www.stedmans.com.

Explanatory Notes

Medical transcription is an art as well as a science. Both approaches are needed to correctly interpret the dictation of a physician, whose language is a product of education, training, and experience. This variety in medical language means that there are several acceptable ways to express certain terms, including jargon. *Stedman's Cardiovascular & Pulmonary Words, Fifth Edition,* provides variant spellings and phrasings for many terms. These elements, in addition to complete cross-indexing, make *Stedman's Cardiovascular & Pulmonary Words, Fifth Edition,* a valuable resource for determining the validity of terms as they are encountered.

Alphabetical Organization

Alphabetization of main entries is letter by letter as spelled, ignoring punctuation, spaces, prefixed numbers, or other characters. For example:

echoreflective
echoreflectivity
egophony

Terms beginning or ending with Greek letters show the Greek letters spelled out and listed alphabetically. For example:

alpha
    a. adrenoreceptor
    a. agonist
    a. blocking agent

In subentry alphabetization, the abbreviated singular form or the spelled-out plural form of the noun main entry word is ignored.

Format and Style

All main entries are in **boldface** to expedite locating a sought-after term, to enhance distinction between main entries and subentries, and to relieve the textual density of the pages.

Irregular plurals and variant spellings are shown on the same line as the singular or preferred form of the word. For example:

dextra, pl. **dextrae**
anular, annular

Hyphenation

As a rule of style, multiple eponyms (e.g., Virchow-Robin space) are hyphenated. Some eponyms are actually first and last names, thus not hyphenated: Pierre Robin syndrome. Also, hyphens have been added between a manufacturer and one or more eponyms (e.g., Storz-Duredge steel cataract knife). Please note that in many cases, hyphenation is a question of style, not of accuracy, and thus is a matter of choice.

Possessives

Possessive forms have been dropped in this reference for the sake of consistency and conformance with the guidelines of the American Association for Medical Transcription (AAMT) and other groups. Please note, however, that in many cases, retaining the possessive, like hyphenating, is a question of style, not of accuracy, and thus is a matter of choice. To form the possessive of a word, simply add the apostrophe or apostrophe "s" to the end of the word.

Cross-indexing

The word list is in an index-like main entry-subentry format that contains two combined alphabetical listings:

(1) A *noun* main entry-subentry organization, which is typical of the A–Z section of medical dictionaries like Stedman's:

macrophage	magnesium
alveolar m.	m. deficiency
foamy m.	intracellular m.
hemosiderin-laden m.	m. oxide

(2) An *adjective* main entry-subentry organization, which lists words and phrases as you hear them. The main entries are the adjectives or modifiers in a multiword term. The subentries are the nouns around which the terms are constructed and to which the adjectives or modifiers pertain:

diastolic
  d. hump
  d. hypertension
  d. lumen

cholesterol
  c. embolism
  c. emboli syndrome
  c. embolization

This format provides the user with more than one way to locate and identify a multiword term. For example:

sleep
  s. apnea
  endovascular
  e. treatment

apnea
  sleep a.
  treatment
  endovascular t.

It also allows the user to see together all terms that contain a particular descriptor, as well as all types, kinds, or variations of a noun entity. For example:

murmur
  accidental m.
  bellows m.
  decrescendo m.

blood
  artificial b.
  b. clot
  b. expander

Wherever possible, abbreviations are separately defined and cross-referenced. For example:

ECLS
  extracorporeal lift support
  extracorporeal
  e. life support (ECLS)
  support
  extracorporeal life s. (ECLS)

References

In addition to the manufacturers' literature we gather at various medical meetings, scientific reports from hospitals, and the lists created by our MT Editorial Advisory Board members from their daily transcription work, we used the following sources for new terms and images in *Stedman's Cardiovascular & Pulmonary Words, Fifth Edition:*

Books

Alpert JS, Ewy GA. Manual of Cardiovascular Diagnosis and Therapy, 5th Edition. Philadelphia: Lippincott Williams & Wilkins, 2002.

Baim DS, Grossman's Cardiac Catheterization, Angiography, and Intervention, 7th edition. Philadelphia: Lippincott Williams & Wilkins, 2006.

Bordow RA, Ries AL, Morris TA, eds. Manual of Clinical Problems in Pulmonary Medicine, 6th edition. Philadelphia: Lippincott Williams & Wilkins, 2005.

Drake E. Sloane's Medical Word Book, 4th Edition. Philadelphia: Elsevier, 2001.

Hillis LD. Manual of Clinical Problems in Cardiology, 6th Edition. Philadelphia: Lippincott Williams & Wilkins, 2002.

Hoekstra JW, ed. Handbook of Cardiovascular Emergencies, 2nd Edition. Philadelphia: Lippincott Williams & Wilkins, 2001.

Jablonski S. Cardiology Acronyms & Abbreviations, 4th Edition. Philadelphia: Lippincott Williams & Wilkins, 2003.

Lance LL. Quick Look Drug Book 2007. Baltimore: Lippincott Williams & Wilkins, 2007.

Mandel J, Taichman D. Pulmonary Vascular Disease. Philadelphia: Saunders Elsevier, 2006.

Rao PS, Kern MJ, eds. Catheter Based Device: for the Treatment of Non-Coronary Cardiovascular Disease in Adults and Children. Philadelphia: Lippincott Williams & Wilkins, 2003.

Rhodes SB, David M, eds. Dorland's Cardiology Word Book for Medical Transcriptionists. Philadelphia: Elsevier, 2000.

Sharis PJ, Cannon CP, ed. Evidence-Based Cardiology, 2nd Edition. Philadelphia: Lippincott Williams & Wilkins, 2003.

Shifren A, ed. The Washington Manual Pulmonary Medicine Subspecialty Consult. Philadelphia: Lippincott Williams & Wilkins, 2006.

Stedman's Medical Dictionary, 28th Edition. Baltimore: Lippincott Williams & Wilkins, 2006.

Topol EJ. Textbook of Cardiovascular Medicine, 2nd Edition. Philadelphia: Lippincott Williams & Wilkins, 2002.

Vera Pyle's Current Medical Terminology, 10th Edition. Modesto, CA: Health Professions Institute, 2005.

Images

Agur, AMR, Lee, MJ. Grant's Atlas of Anatomy, 10th Edition. Baltimore: Lippincott Williams & Wilkins, 1999.

Anatomical Chart Company. Atlas of Pathophysiology. Philadelphia: Lippincott Williams & Wilkins, 2001.

Caldwell S. Pikesville, MD. Stedman's Medical Dictionary, 27th edition. Baltimore: Lippincott Williams & Wilkins, 2000.

Cohen BJ. Medical Terminology, 4th Ed. Philadelphia: Lippincott Williams & Wilkins 2003.

Hardy NO. Westport, CT. Stedman's Medical Dictionary, 27th Edition. Baltimore: Lippincott Williams & Wilkins, 2000.

Kandarpa, K, Aruny, JE. Handbook of Interventional Radiologic Procedures, 3rd Edition. Philadelphia: Lippincott Williams & Wilkins, 2002.

LifeART Super Anatomy Collection 1, CD-ROM. Baltimore: Lippincott Williams & Wilkins.

LifeART Super Anatomy Collection 2, CD-ROM. Baltimore: Lippincott Williams & Wilkins.

LifeART Super Anatomy Collection 5, CD-ROM. Baltimore: Lippincott Williams & Wilkins.

LifeART Super Anatomy Collection 7, CD-ROM. Baltimore: Lippincott Williams & Wilkins.

MediClip Clinical Cardiopulmonary Images, CD-ROM. Baltimore: Lippincott Williams & Wilkins.

Moore KL, PhD, FRSM, FIAC & Dalley AF II, PhD. Clinical Oriented Anatomy, 4th Ed. Baltimore: Lippincott Williams & Wilkins, 1999.

Nettina, Sandra M. The Lippincott Manual of Nursing Practice, 7th Ed. Philadelphia: Lippincott, Williams & Wilkins, 2001.

Smeltzer SC, Bare BG. Textbook of Medical-Surgical Nursing, 9th Ed. Philadelphia: Lippincott Williams & Wilkins, 2000.

Journals

The American Journal of Cardiology. Belle Mead, NJ: Excerpta Medica, 2005–2006.

Cardiology in Review. Baltimore: Lippincott Williams & Wilkins, 2005–2006.

Circulation. Baltimore: Lippincott Williams & Wilkins, 2006.

Chest. Northbrook, IL: American College of Chest Physicians, 2005–2006.

Clinical Pulmonary Medicine. Baltimore: Lippincott Williams & Wilkins, 2005–2006.

Current Opinion in Cardiology. Baltimore: Lippincott Williams & Wilkins, 2005.

Current Opinion in Pulmonary Medicine. Baltimore: Lippincott Williams & Wilkins, 2005–2006.

Journal of Cardiovascular Medicine. Baltimore: Lippincott Williams & Wilkins, 2006

The American College of Cardiology. New York: Elsevier Science, 2005–2006.

The Latest Word. Philadelphia: Elsevier, 2005-2006.

Websites

http://www.acc.org

http://www.bedfont.com

http://www.cardima.com/

http://www.cardiologyonline.com

http://www.cardiologytoday.com

http://www.cardiosource.com

http://www.centerwatch.com

http://www.chronolog.com

http://www.escardio.org

http://www.fda.gov/search/databases.html

http://www.healthcentral.com/ency/408/003371.html

http://www.hpisum.com

http://www.health.ucsd.edu/labref

http://www.medscape.com/cardiologyhome?LID=5762837

http://www.musc.edu/perfusion/glossary.htm

http://www.nhlbi.nih.gov

http://www2.umdnj.edu/~shindler/abc.html

http://www.ventworld.com/equipment/equipment.asp

A
  apical
  atrium
    avian influenza A
    A band
    biochanin A
    A greater than E
    A larger than V wave
    A 67 lead
    lipid A
    A mode
    neurokinin A (NKA)
    peptidase A (PEPA)
    A point
    A wave

a
  arterial
  arterial blood
  artery
    a dip
    a priori
    a wave

A1
  angiotensin I
  aortic first sound

A-I
  angiotensin I

A-II
  angiotensin II
    A-II receptor

A2
  angiotensin II
    apoprotein A1, A2
    A2 multipurpose catheter

A_2
    A_2 incisural interval
    A_2 to opening snap interval
    thromboxane A_2

A_{2A} adenosine receptor
A2C, A4C view
A_4
    leukotriene A_4

AA
  abdominal aorta
  African American
  alveoloarterial
  amino acid
  aortic arch
  arachidonate
  arachidonic acid
  arteries
  ascending aorta
    AA atheroma
    AA cascade

aa
  arteries
AAA
  abdominal aortic aneurysm
  aneurysm of ascending aorta
  angiography of abdominal aorta
  arrest after arrival
A-a
  alveolar-arterial
  alveolar-atrial
    A-a gradient
AACD
  abdominal aortic counterpulsation device
Aachen Aphasia Test (AAT)
AACP
  American Academy of Cardiology
    Perfusion
AACVPR
  American Association of Cardiovascular
    and Pulmonary Rehabilitation
AAD
  acute aortic dissection
  adaptive aerosol delivery
  antiarrhythmic drug
AAE
  anuloaortic ectasia
AAF
  aortic arch flush
AAG
  alveolar-arterial gradient
AAI
  activating adjusting instrument
  atrial demand inhibited
  atrial inhibited
    AAI pacemaker
    AAI pacing
    AAI rate-responsive mode
AAI/AAIR pacemaker
A-A interval
A_1-A_2 interval
AAI-RR pacing
AAL
  anterior axillary line
AAO
  ascending aorta
A-aO_2
  alveolar-arterial oxygen gradient
  alveolar-arterial oxygen tension
AAPF
  antiarteriosclerosis polysaccharide factor
AaPO_2
  alveolar-arterial PO_2 difference
AARC
  American Association for Respiratory
    Care

AAS
aneurysm of atrial septum
aortic arch syndrome
AASP
ascending aorta synchronized pulsation
AAST
American Association for the Surgery of Trauma
AAT
Aachen Aphasia Test
alpha-1 antitrypsin
atrial demand triggered
automatic atrial tachycardia
human pooled AAT
AAT mode
AAT pacemaker
AAT pacing
AAV
adeno-associated virus
AAV-CF therapy
AAVNRT
atypical atrioventricular nodal reentrant tachycardia
AAW
anterior aortic wall
AB
apex beat
A&B
apnea and bradycardia
ABA
arrest before arrival
ABAb
anti-beta-1 adrenoreceptor antibody
abacavir
abacterial
a. thrombosis
a. thrombotic endocarditis
ABAD
acute type B aortic dissection
abandonment of in-vein ablation
Abbe
A. flap
A. operation
Abbokinase
A. injection
A. Open-Cath
Abbott
A. infusion pump
A. TriMaxx drug-eluting stent
A. ZoMaxx drug-eluting stent
Abbreviated Injury Scale (AIS)
ABC
airway, breathing, circulation
ascending balloon cannula
aspiration biopsy cytology
ABC lead
ABC protocol
ABCD
airway, breathing, circulation, defibrillate

ABCDE
airway, breathing, circulation, disability, exposure
ABCDE in trauma patient
ABCIC
airway, breathing, circulation, intravenous crystalloid
abciximab (ABX)
ABD
automated border detection
automatic boundary detection
abdomen
abdominal
a. angina
a. aorta (AA, AO)
a. aortic aneurysm (AAA)
a. aortic aneurysmectomy
a. aortic counterpulsation device (AACD)
a. aortic endarterectomy
a. aortography
a. asthma
a. belt
a. bruit
a. compartment syndrome (ACS)
a. heart
a. jugular test
a. left ventricular assist device (ALVAD)
a. paradox breathing pattern
a. part
a. part of descending aorta
a. part of esophagus
a. pocket
a. pulse
a. respiration
a. vascular retractor
abdominalis
aorta a.
aortismus a.
ectopia cordis a.
abdominocardiac reflex
abdominojugular reflux
abdominothoracic
a. arch
a. pump
abductor spasmodic dysphonia
ABE
acute bacterial endocarditis
ABECB
acute bacterial exacerbation of chronic bronchitis
Abee support
Abelcet
Abell-Kendall equivalent
Abelson cannula
aberrancy
acceleration-dependent a.
atrial trigeminy with a.

bradycardia-dependent a.
deceleration-dependent a.
paradoxical a.
paroxysmal atrial tachycardia
   with a.
postextrasystolic a.
tachycardia-dependent a.

aberrant
a. condition of supraventricular
   beat (rSR)
a. innominate artery
a. obturator artery
a. QRS complex
a. subclavian artery
a. thyroid
a. ventricular conduction (AVC)

aberrantly conducted beat
aberration
intraventricular a.
nonspecific T-wave a.
ventricular a.

abetalipoproteinemia
Bassen-Kornzweig a.
familial a.

ABF
aortic blood flow
aortobifemoral

ABG
arterial blood gas
ABG point-of-care test

ABG PCT
arterial blood gas point-of-care test

abhesive
ABI
ankle-brachial index
atherothrombotic brain infarction
ABI Vest Airway Clearance system

ability, pl. **abilities**
conductive a.
Illinois Test of Psycholinguistic
   Abilities
torquing a.

AbioCor
A. implantable replacement heart
A. mechanical heart

Abiomed
A. biventricular support system
A. implantable heart-replacement
   device

ABL
ABL 555 analyzer
ABL 520 blood gas measurement
   system
ABL 625 system

ablation
abandonment of in-vein a.
accessory conduction a. (ACA)
alcohol septal a.
atrial flutter a.

atrial isthmus a.
atrioventricular junctional a.
atrioventricular nodal a.
A-V junction a.
a. catheter
catheter a.
catheter-induced a.
chemical a.
continuous-wave laser a.
coronary rotational a.
direct-current shock a.
electrical catheter a.
endocardial catheter a.
endovascular radiofrequency
   catheter a.
epicardial radiofrequency catheter a.
fast-pathway radiofrequency
   catheter a.
fluoroscopic isthmus a.
His bundle a.
in-vein a.
irrigated catheter a.
irrigated-tip a.
Kent bundle a.
laser a.
left atrial circumferential a.
linear atrial a.
linear-phased radiofrequency
   catheter a.
maze a.
percutaneous radiofrequency
   catheter a.
percutaneous transluminal coronary
   rotational a. (PTCRA)
percutaneous transluminal septal
   myocardial a. (PTSMA)
pulsed laser a.
radiofrequency a. (RFA)
radiofrequency catheter a.
radiofrequency energy a.
radiofrequency tissue a. (RFTA)
Revelation Tx microcatheter for
   RF a.
RF catheter a.
rotational a.
segmental ostial pulmonary vein a.
septal a.
slow-pathway a.
superior pulmonary vein a.
surgical a.
tissue a.
transcatheter a.
transcoronary alcohol a. (TAA)
transcoronary chemical a.
transvenous a.
a. treatment

ablative
a. cardiac surgery
a. device

3

ablative (*continued*)
    a. laser angioplasty
    a. technique
ablator
    radiofrequency a.
Ablaza-Blanco aortic wall retractor
ABLC
    amphotericin B lipid complex
abluminal elution
abnormal
    a. cleavage
    a. cleavage of cardiac valve
    a. coronary artery (ACA)
    a. ECG rhythm of small R, bigger R of QRS (rSR′, rsr prime)
    a. left axis deviation (ALAD)
    a. rhythm on ECG (rSR)
    a. right axis deviation (ARAD)
    a. ST segment
    a. vasopressin (AVP)
    a. wall motion (AWM)
abnormality, pl. **abnormalities**
    angiographically occult a.
    arterial compliance a.
    atrioventricular conduction a.
    baseline ST-segment a.
    brisk wall motion a.
    clotting a.
    coloboma, heart anomaly, ichthyosis, mental retardation, ear a. (CHIME)
    conotruncal a.
    electrical activation a.
    electrolyte a.
    familial congenital cardiac a. (FCCA)
    fibrinolytic a.
    figure-of-8 a.
    focal motion a.
    functional pacing a.
    hemodynamic a.
    high-risk repolarization a.
    immunochemical a.
    left atrial a.
    left ventricular wall motion a.
    lusitropic a.
    neurogenic a.
    nonspecific T-wave a.
    pleuroparenchymal a.
    regional wall motion a. (RWMA)
    sinus node/AV conduction a.
    snowman a.
    transient wall motion a.
    ventricular depolarization a.
    wall motion a. (WMA)
ABO blood group system
aborted
    a. sudden death
    a. systole

abortive pneumonia
abouchement
ABP
    ambulatory blood pressure
    arterial blood pressure
    automated boundary protection
    automatic systolic blood pressure measurement
aBP
    arterial blood pressure
ABPA
    allergic bronchopulmonary aspergillosis
ABPM
    ambulatory blood pressure monitoring
ABR
    arterial baroreflex
Abrahams sign
Abrams
    A. heart reflex
    A. needle
    A. pleural biopsy punch
Abrams-Lucas flap heart valve
abrasion
    pleural a.
abreugraphy
abrupt
    a. closure
    a. closure of arteries
    a. pulse
ABS
    acrylonitrile-butadiene-styrene
AB-SAAP
    autologous blood selective aortic arch perfusion
abscess
    anular a.
    aortic root a.
    apical a.
    Brodie a.
    caseous a.
    cold a.
    distal pyogenic a.
    embolic a.
    lung a.
    myocardial a.
    papillary muscle a.
    periaortic a.
    periprosthetic valve a.
    retropharyngeal a.
    ring a.
    subdiaphragmatic a.
    subphrenic a.
abscessus
    Mycobacterium a.
abscissa
absence
    congenital a.
absent
    a. breath sounds

a. pericardium
a. pulmonary valve
a. respiration
Absidia corymbifera
absolute
a. alcohol
atmosphere a. (ata)
a. cardiac dullness (ACD)
a. dullness (M3)
a. humidity
a. measurement
a. pressure
a. refractory period (ARP)
a. risk reduction (ARR)
A. self-expanding stent
absorbable
a. gelatin
a. gelatin film
a. gelatin sponge
a. suture
absorbance
time of flight and a. (TOFA)
absorbent vessel
absorptiometry
absorption
a. atelectasis
a. collapse
a., distribution, metabolism, excretion (ADME)
fluorescent treponemal antibody a. (FTA-ABS)
net a.
abuse
alcohol a.
cocaine a.
drug a.
ABX
abciximab
ABx, ABX, abx
antibiotic
AC
adenylyl cyclase
alternating current
anterior chamber
anterior circulation
anticoagulant
aortic closure
aortic compliance
aortocoronary
assist-control
atrial contraction
atriocarotid
Mytussin AC
Robafen AC
A-C
aortocoronary bypass
AC137
human analog amylin AC137

a.c.
ante cibum
ACA
abnormal coronary artery
accessory conduction ablation
anterior cerebral artery
anterior communicating aneurysm
anterior communicating artery
anticentromere antibody
arrhythmic cardiac arrest
asthma care algorithm
acacia
gum a.
ACAD
asymptomatic coronary artery disease
atherosclerotic coronary artery disease
acadesine
Acanthamoeba
A. *astronyxis*
A. *castellanii*
A. *culbertsoni*
A. *glebae*
A. *hatchetti*
A. *palestinensis*
A. *polyphaga*
A. *rhysodes*
acanthocytosis
Acanthosis nigricans
acapella chest physical therapy device
acapnia
acapnial alkalosis
acarbia
acarbose
acardia
acardiac
acardiotrophia
acardius
acarian asthma
acaricidal chemical
Acarosan dust mite powder
acaryote
Acat 1 intraaortic balloon pump
ACB
albumin cobalt binding
aortocoronary bypass
arterialized capillary blood
asymptomatic carotid bruit
ACB test
ACBG
aortocoronary bypass graft
ACC
American College of Cardiology
anodal closure contraction
ACCA
American College of Cardiovascular Administrators
ACC/AHA
American College of Cardiology/American Heart Association

ACC/AHA *(continued)*
> ACC/AHA heart failure (stage A-D)
> ACC/AHA pacemaker implantation guidelines

ACC-CathKIT
accelerans
accelerated
> a. atrioventricular junctional rhythm
> a. A-V junctional rhythm
> a. A-V node conduction
> a. hypertension
> a. idioventricular rhythm (AIVR)
> a. idioventricular tachycardia
> a. respiration
> a. silicosis
> a. ventricular rhythm (AVR)

acceleration
> flow a.
> isovolumic a. (IVA)
> a. time

acceleration-dependent aberrancy
acceleration-guided activity pacing
accelerator
> a. fiber
> a. globin (AcG)
> a. globin blood coagulation factor
> a. nerve
> proconvertin prothrombin conversion a.
> serum prothrombin conversion a. (SPCA)
> serum thrombotic a. (STA)

accelerometer
> Caltrac a.
> intracardiac a.
> multiaxis a.
> Stayhealthy RT3 triaxial a.
> triaxial a.
> TriTrac-R3D a.
> uniaxial a.

accelerometry
> triaxial a.

Accent balloon angioplasty catheter
Accent-DG balloon
accentuated antagonism
access
> A. AccuTnI troponin I test
> A-Port vascular a.
> Check-Flo performer introducer set for radial artery a.
> a. device
> echo record a. (ERA)
> Low Profile Port vascular a.
> A. MV system
> percutaneous a.
> a. by radial artery multilink stent (ARMS)

> Rapidpoint a.
> side-entry a. (SEA)
> venous a.
> venovenous a.

Access-9 large-bore hemostasis valve
accessory, pl. **accessories**
> a. arteriovenous connection
> a. atrium
> a. conduction ablation (ACA)
> a. cusp
> a. inspiratory muscle
> a. meningeal branch
> a. meningeal branch of middle meningeal artery
> a. muscles of respiration
> N95-Companion a.
> a. obturator artery
> a. pathway (AP)
> a. pathway effective refractory period (APERP)
> a. pathway mediated tachycardia
> a. pulmonary blood flow (APBF)
> a. saphenous vein
> a. thyroid

accident
> cardiac a.
> cardiovascular a. (CVA)
> cerebrovascular a. (CVA)
> right cerebrovascular a. (RCVA)

accidental murmur
Accolate
accommodation
> period of a.

accompanying
> a. artery
> a. artery of ischiadic nerve
> a. artery of median nerve

ACCP
> American College of Chest Physicians

accretio cordis
accrochage
Accucap CO_2/O_2 monitor
Accu-Chek II Freedom
Accucom cardiac output monitor
Accudynamic adjustable damping
Accufix
> A. II DEC pacing lead
> A. pacemaker
> A. pacemaker lead

AccuGage vessel calipers
Accuhaler
Acculink self-expanding stent
AccuMark calibrated infant feeding tube
AccuMeter theophylline test
accumulation
> lipid a.
> phytanic acid a.

A

Accunet
    A. embolic protection system
    A. filter
Accupril
Accurbron
Accuretic
Accurox mask
Accustaple
AccuTnI troponin I test
Accutorr
    A. multiparameter monitor
    A. oscillometric device
Accutracker
    A. blood pressure device
    A. II ambulatory blood pressure
      monitor
Accu-Vu catheter
ACD
    absolute cardiac dullness
    active compression-decompression
    alveolar capillary dysplasia
    area of cardiac dullness
    arrhythmia control device
      StarClose ACD
ACDA
    Alveolar Capillary Dysplasia Association
ACD-CPR
    active compression-decompression
    cardiopulmonary resuscitation
ACE
    acute coronary event
    Adriamycin, cyclophosphamide,
      etoposide
    aerosol cloud enhancer
    angiotensin-converting enzyme
      ACE antisense gene therapy
      ACE deletion/insertion
        polymorphism
      ACE detachable mask
      ACE fixed-wire balloon catheter
      ACE inhibitor
      ACE kit
      ACE MDI spacer
      universal ACE
ACE-II
    angiotensin-converting enzyme II
      ACE-II genotype
ACE-ID
    angiotensin-converting enzyme ID
      ACE-ID genotype
acebutolol hydrochloride
acecainide hydrochloride
acedapsone
ACE-DD
    angiotensin-converting enzyme DD
      ACE-DD genotype
ACEI, ACEi
    angiotensin-converting enzyme inhibitor
Acel-Imune

acenocoumarol
Aceon
acepifylline
ace of spades sign
acetabular
    a. artery
    a. branch
acetabuli
    protrusio a.
acetaldehyde
acetaminophen
    a. and dextromethorphan
    a., dextromethorphan,
      pseudoephedrine
    hydrocodone and a.
acetarsone
acetate
    anaritide a.
    carbon-11 a.
    caspofungin a.
    cortisone a.
    Cortone A.
    desmopressin a. (DDAVP, dDAVP)
    Florinef A.
    fludrocortisone a.
    guanabenz a.
    guanfacine a.
    leuprolide a.
    medroxyprogesterone a. (MPA)
    megestrol a.
    methylprednisolone a.
    paramethasone a.
    PET with C-11 a.
    pirbuterol a.
    sodium a.
acetazolamide
acetic acid
acetohexamide
acetonide
    triamcinolone a. (TAA)
acetoorcein stain
acetylcarnitine
acetylcholinesterase deficiency
acetylcholine test
acetyl-CoA
N-**acetylcysteine**
acetyldigitoxin
acetyldigoxin
acetylglucosaminyltransferase
acetylhydrolase
N-**acetylprocainamide**
acetylsalicylate
    lysine a.
acetylsalicylic acid (ASA)
acetylstrophanthidin (AcS)
ACG
    angiocardiogram
    angiocardiography
    aortocoronary graft

ACG *(continued)*
  apexcardiogram
  apexcardiography
AcG
  accelerator globin
    AcG blood coagulation factor
AChA
  anterior choroidal artery
achalasia
    esophageal a.
ACHD
  adult congenital heart disease
Achieve Off-Pump system
achiever
    A. balloon dilation catheter
    A. balloon dilator
Acholeplasma laidlawii
achondroplasia
achromatic mass
achromatin, achromin
achromatolysis
Achromobacter xylosoxidans
Achromycin V Oral
ACI
  acute cardiac ischemia
  acute coronary infarction
  acute coronary insufficiency
  asymptomatic cardiac ischemia
acid
    acetic a.
    N-acetylneuraminic a.
    acetylsalicylic a. (ASA)
    all-trans-retinoic a. (ATRA)
    alpha-linolenic a. (ALA)
    amino a. (AA)
    aminocaproic a.
    5-aminolevulinic a.
    aminosalicylic a.
    p-aminosalicylic a.
    amoxicillin and clavulanic a.
    arachidonic a. (AA)
    ascorbic a.
    aspartic a.
    betamethyliodophenyl
      pentadecanoic a. (BMIPP)
    carbon-11-labeled fatty a.'s
    clavulanic a.
    deoxyribonucleic a. (DNA)
    diethylenetriaminepentaacetic a.
      (DPTA, DTPA)
    docosahexaenoic a.
    EET a.
    eicosapentaenoic a. (EPA)
    enalaprilic a.
    endomethylene tetrahydrophthalic a.
      (EMTA)
    epoxyeicosatrienoic a.
    ethacrynic a.

    ethylenediaminetetraacetic a.
      (EDTA)
    fatty a.
    ferrous salt and ascorbic a.
    ferrous sulfate, ascorbic a., vitamin
      B complex, folic a.
    fibric a.
    folic a.
    free fatty a. (FFA)
    fusidic a.
    gadolinium-diethylenetriamine
      pentaacetic a. (Gd-DTPA)
    gamma-aminobutyric a. (GABA)
    gamma-linolenic a.
    glycyrrhizinic a.
    5-HPETE a.
    hyaluronic a.
    hydrobromic a.
    hydrochloric a.
    hydrocyanic a.
    hydrofluoric a.
    20-hydroxyeicosatetraenoic a. (20-
      HETE)
    hydroxyethyl piperazine-
      ethanesulfonic a. (HEPES)
    a. infusion test
    inorganic a.
    iodophenyl pentadecanoic a.
    lactic a.
    linoleic a.
    lysophosphatidic a.
    a. maltase deficiency
    mefenamic a.
    messenger ribonucleic a. (mRNA)
    mevalonate a.
    monosaturated fatty a.
    monounsaturated fatty a. (MUFA)
    a. mucopolysaccharide (AMP)
    nalidixic a.
    n-3 fatty a.
    n-6 fatty a.
    nicotinic a.
    nitric a.
    nonesterified fatty a.
    omega-3 unsaturated fatty a.
    osteopontin messenger
      ribonucleic a.
    palmitic a.
    paraaminobenzoic a.
    paraaminosalicylic a. (PAS, PASA)
    peracetic a.
    perchloric a.
    a. phosphatase
    phosphinic a.
    plicatic a.
    polyglycolic a.
    poly-L-lactic a. (PLLA)
    polyunsaturated fatty a. (PUFA)
    potassium citrate and citric a.

pyruvic a.
recombinant deoxyribonucleic a. (rDNA)
retinoic a.
ribonucleic a. (RNA)
saturated fatty a. (SFA)
sialic a.
sulfosalicylic a.
Tc-diethylenetriamine pentaacetic a.
ticarcillin and clavulanic a.
tranexamic a.
trans fatty a. (TFA)
triglyceride fatty a. (TGFA)
unesterified fatty a. (UFA)
uric a.
urocanic a.
valproic a.
very long chain fatty a. (VLCFA)
volatile fatty a. (VFA)
zofenoprilic a.

acid-base
a.-b. balance
a.-b. determination
a.-b. disorder
a.-b. imbalance

acidemia
acid-fast bacillus (AFB)
acidic fibroblast growth factor (aFGF)
acidity
total a.

acidominimus
Streptococcus a.

acidopnea
acidosis
acute respiratory a.
chronic metabolic a.
hypercapnic a.
hyperchloremic a.
ischemia-induced intracellular a.
lactic a.
metabolic a.
respiratory a.

acid-reactive
thiobarbituric a.-r.

aciduria
acinar
a. adenocarcinoma
a. nodule
a. rosette

Acinetobacter
A. anitratus
A. baumannii
A. calcoaceticus
A. calcoaceticus-baumannii complex
A. lwoffi

a-c interval
acinus, pl. **acini**
lung a.
pulmonary a.

acipimox
ACIST
angiographic contrast injection system technology
ACIST contrast delivery system
ACIST contrast injection system
ACIST CVi device

acitretin
ACLA, aCLa
anticardiolipin antibody
ACLA IgG
ACLA IgM

Acland-Banis arteriotomy set
Acland-Buncke counterpressor
acleistocardia
ACLS
advanced cardiac life support
ACLS protocol
ACLS protocol resuscitation

ACM
anticardiac myosin
automated cardiac flow measurement

ACMT
artificial circus movement tachycardia

acnes
Propionibacterium a.

ACO
acute coronary occlusion
anomalous coronary origin

ACoA, AcomA
anterior communicating artery

ACOM
automated cardiac output measurement

aconitine
acorn
A. CorCap
A. CorCap cardiac support device
A. II nebulizer

Acosta disease
Acoustascope esophageal stethoscope
acoustic
a. densitometry
a. imaging
a. impedance
a. impedance probe
a. microscope
a. pharyngometer
a. quantification (AQ)
a. quantification signal averaging
a. shadow
a. shadowing
a. window

ACPE
acute cardiogenic pulmonary edema

acquired
a. atelectasis
a. immunodeficiency syndrome (AIDS)
a. pulmonary hypertension

acquired *(continued)*
    a. valvular heart disease (AVHD)
    a. valvular heart syndrome (AVHS)
    a. ventricular septal defect (AVSD)
acquisition
    fast imaging employing steady-state a. (FIESTA)
    a. gate
    gated equilibrium ventriculography, frame-mode a.
    gated equilibrium ventriculography, list-mode a.
    multiple gated a. (MUGA)
    tagged a.
    a. time
    a. zoom (AZ)
    a. zoom technology
Acra-Cut Spiral craniotome blade
Acremonium
acridinium ester labeled nucleic acid probe
acrivastine and pseudoephedrine
acroasphyxia
acrocephalopolysyndactyly
acrocyanosis
acrocyanotic
Acrodisc unit
acrohypothermy
acromegalic heart disease
acromegaloid facial appearance (AFA)
acromegaly
acromelalgia
acromial
    a. anastomosis of thoracoacromial artery
    a. arterial network
    a. articular facies of clavicle
    a. articular surface of clavicle
    a. branch of suprascapular artery
    a. branch of thoracoacromial artery
    a. plexus
acromiothoracic artery
acrosclerosis
acrotic
acrotism
acrylate
acrylonitrile-butadiene-styrene (ABS)
ACS
    abdominal compartment syndrome
    acute chest syndrome
    acute confusional state
    acute coronary syndrome
    Advanced Cardiovascular Systems
    American Cancer Society
    anodal closure sound
    ascending aorta
        ACS Alpha balloon
        ACS Amplatz guidewire

ACS anchor exchange device
ACS Concorde over-the-wire catheter system
ACS Endura coronary dilation catheter
ACS Enhanced Torque 8/7.5-F Taper Tip catheter
ACS exchange guidewire
ACS extra-support guidewire
ACS Hi-Torque Balance middleweight guidewire
ACS LIMA guide
ACS LIMA guidewire
ACS Mini catheter
ACS Monorail catheter
ACS Multi-Link coronary system
ACS Multi-Link Duet coronary stent
ACS Multi-Link RX Ultra coronary stent system
ACS Multi-Link RX Ultra stent
ACS Multi-Link Tristar coronary stent system
ACS Multi-Link Tristar stent
ACS OTW Lifestream coronary dilation catheter
ACS OTW Photon coronary dilation catheter
ACS OTW Solaris coronary dilation catheter
ACS Photon coronary dilation catheter
ACS RX Comet angioplasty catheter
ACS RX Comet VP coronary dilation catheter
ACS RX Lifestream coronary dilation catheter
ACS RX perfusion balloon catheter
ACS RX Solaris coronary dilation catheter
AcS
    acetylstrophanthidin
ACSM
    American College of Sports Medicine
    ACSM regression equation
ACSV
    aortocoronary saphenous vein
ACSVBG
    aortocoronary saphenous vein bypass graft
ACT
    activated clotting time
    activated coagulation time
    adaptive current tomography
    anticoagulant therapy
    axial computed tomography
        ACT MicroCoil delivery system

act
emergency medical treatment and active labor a. (EMTALA)
Health Insurance Portability and Accountability A. of 1996 (HIPAA)
Prescription Drug User Fee A. (PDUFA)

ACTA
American Cardiology Technologists Association

ACTe
anodal closure tetanus

ACTH
adrenocorticotropic hormone

Acthar

ActHIB vaccine

Actigraph
Mini-Motionlogger A.

Actilyse

Actimmune

actin
alpha-cardiac a.
alpha-smooth muscle a.
a. cytoskeleton
a. fiber
a. filament
filamentous a. (F-actin)
a. gene
a. monomer
smooth muscle a. (SMA)

acting
long a. (LA, L.A.)

actin-myosin crossbridge

Actinobacillus
A. *actinomycetemcomitans*
A. *equuli*
A. *hominis*
A. *suis*
A. *ureae*

Actinomadura

Actinomyces
A. *bovis*
A. *israelii*
A. *naeslundii*

actinomycetemcomitans
Actinobacillus a.

actinomycetes
thermophilic a.

actinomycetoma

actinomycosis
pulmonary a.
thoracic a.

action
beating a.
catecholamine a.
girdle-like a.
mechanism of a.
a. potential

a. potential duration (APD)
purinergic a.
A. Research Arm Test
respiratory depressant a.
thoracic expanding a.

Actiq Oral Transmucosal

Actis VFC

Activase
Cathflo A.
A. injection

activated
a. balloon expandable intravascular stent
a. clotting time (ACT)
a. coagulation time (ACT)
eptacog alfa a.
a. factor VII (FVIIa)
a. graft
a. Jurkat T cell
a. partial thromboplastin time (APTT, aPTT)

activating
a. adjusting instrument (AAI)
a. transcription factor (ATF)

activation
complement a.
eccentric atrial a.
endothelial cell a.
eNOS a.
focal a.
granulocyte a.
heparin-induced platelet a. (HIPA)
length-dependent a.
a. map-guided surgical resection
myofilament contractile a.
platelet a.
right ventricle a. (RVA)
a. sequence
a. sequence mapping
thrombosis a.

activator
2-chain urokinase plasminogen a. (tcu-PA)
plasminogen a.
a. protein (AP)
recombinant tissue plasminogen a. (rt-PA)
recombinant tissue-type plasminogen a.
single chain urokinase-type plasminogen a.
tissue plasminogen a. (t-PA, tPA)
tissue-type plasminogen a.
urokinase plasminogen a. (uPA)
vampire bat salivary plasminogen a. (DSPA)

active
A. Can defibrillator lead system

active *(continued)*
    a. compression-decompression (ACD)
    a. compression-decompression cardiopulmonary resuscitation (ACD-CPR)
    a. compression-decompression resuscitator
    a. congestion
    a. dynamic stiffness
    a. fixation pacemaker lead
    a. hyperemia
    a. pressure (AP)
    A. Response Catheter (ARC)
    a. transport
    a. tuberculosis
active-site inhibited factor VIIa
Activitrax
    A. II pacemaker
    A. single-chamber responsive pacemaker
    A. variable rate pacemaker
activity, pl. **activities**
    antiacetylcholine receptor antibody a.
    antifactor Xa a.
    anti-FXa a.
    anti-Xa a.
    cardiac adrenergic a.
    cholesterol-esterifying a. (CEA)
    coagulation a.
    activities of daily living
    dehydrogenase a.
    early return to normal activities (ERNA)
    electrical a.
    eNOS a.
    heparin neutralizing a. (HNA)
    hyperadrenergic a.
    intrinsic sympathomimetic a.
    leisure time physical a. (LTPA)
    lipoprotein lipase a. (LPLA)
    matrix metalloproteinase a.
    mean daily physical a. (MDPA)
    melanoma inhibitory a. (MIA)
    membrane-stabilizing a.
    Motor Club Assessment test of motor a.
    muscle sympathetic nerve a. (MSNA)
    myocyte metabolic a.
    plasma renin a. (PRA)
    platelet a.
    postheparin lipolytic a. (PHLA)
    prothrombin a. (PTA)
    pulseless electrical a. (PEA)
    respiratory a.
    a. scale
    a. sensor
    sinoaortic baroreflex a.
    snooze-induced excitation of sympathetic triggered a. (SIESTA)
    spike a.
    sympathetic nerve a. (SNA)
    sympathetic nervous system a.
    triggered a.
    ventricular ectopic a. (VEA)
activity-guided
    a.-g. pacemaker
    a.-g. pacing
activity-sensing pacemaker
ACT-One stent
Actos
Actothil
Actron
Actros pacemaker
actuarial survival curve
actuation
    direct mechanical ventricular a. (DMVA)
AcuNav ultrasound catheter
acupuncture
Acuseal cardiovascular patch
Acuson
    A. cardiovascular system
    A. computed sonography
    A. echocardiograph
    A. V5M multiplane transesophageal echocardiographic transducer
    A. V5M transesophageal echocardiographic monitor
    A. XP-5 ultrasonoscope
    A. XP-10 ultrasonoscope
    A. XP-128 ultrasonoscope
acute
    a. allograft rejection
    a. aortic dissection (AAD)
    a. bacterial endocarditis (ABE)
    a. bacterial exacerbation
    a. bacterial exacerbation of chronic bronchitis (ABECB)
    a. brain syndrome
    a. cardiac ischemia (ACI)
    a. cardiogenic pulmonary edema (ACPE)
    a. cardiovascular (ACV)
    a. cardiovascular disease (ACVD)
    a. caudate stroke
    a. cellular xenograft rejection
    a. chemical injury
    a. chest syndrome (ACS)
    a. compression triad
    a. confusional state (ACS)
    a. congestive heart failure
    a. coronary care unit
    a. coronary event (ACE)
    a. coronary infarction (ACI)
    a. coronary insufficiency (ACI)

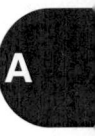

a. coronary occlusion (ACO)
a. coronary syndrome (ACS)
a. cor pulmonale
a. decompensated heart failure (ADHF)
A. Decompensated Heart Failure National Registry (ADHERE)
a. diaphragmatic myocardial infarction
a. dissecting aneurysm
a. endothelial dysfunction
a. eosinophilic pneumonia
a. exacerbation of chronic bronchitis (AECB)
a. exacerbation of chronic obstructive pulmonary disease
a. fibrinous pericarditis
a. glomerulonephritis (AGN)
a. heart disease (AHD)
a. hemispheric stroke
a. hemorrhagic bronchopneumonia
a. hypercapnic respiratory failure
a. hypoxemic respiratory failure
a. hypoxic respiratory failure
a. idiopathic pericarditis (AIP)
a. infective endocarditis (AIE)
a. intermittent porphyria (AIP)
a. interstitial pneumonia (AIP)
a. interstitial pneumonitis (AIP)
a. invasive aspergillosis
a. ischemic coronary syndrome (AICS)
a. ischemic stroke (AIS)
a. isolated myocarditis
a. laryngotracheal bronchitis
a. left ventricular failure (ALVF)
a. limb ischemia
a. lower respiratory tract infection (ALRI)
a. lung injury (ALI)
a. lung rejection
a. lupus pericarditis (ALP)
a. lupus pneumonitis (ALP)
a. lymphocytic leukemia (ALL)
a. margin of heart
a. mediastinitis
a. miliary tuberculosis
a. mitral stenosis (AMS)
a. mountain sickness (AMS)
a. multiple brain infarcts (AMBI)
a. myelocytic leukemia (AML)
a. myocardial infarction (AMI)
a. noncardiogenic pulmonary edema
a. obliterating bronchiolitis
a. occlusive thrombosis (AOT)
a. occlusive thrombus (AOT)
a. pharyngitis
A. Physiology, Age, Chronic Health Evaluation (APACHE)
A. Physiology and Chronic Health Evaluation score
a. pleurisy
a. preload alteration
a. pulmonary alveolitis
a. pulmonary edema (APE)
a. pulmonary embolism
a. pulmonary histoplasmosis
a. radiation pneumonitis
a. rejection (AR)
a. renal failure
a. respiratory acidosis
a. respiratory disease (ARD)
a. respiratory distress syndrome (ARDS)
a. respiratory failure (ARF)
a. response
a. retroviral syndrome
a. rheumatic arthritis
a. rheumatic fever (ARF)
a. right heart syndrome (ARHS)
a. severe hypotension
a. sickle cell chest syndrome
a. sickle chest syndrome (ASCS)
a. silicosis
a. tamponade
a. thrombosis (AT)
a. type B aortic dissection (ABAD)
a. ventricular assist device (AVAD)

acutely
a. decompensated congestive heart failure (ADCHF, AD-CHF)
a. decompensated cor pulmonale

acute-on-chronic
a.-o.-c. hypercapnic respiratory failure
a.-o.-c. status

Acutronic
A. Mistral ventilator
A. Monsoon ventilator

ACV
acute cardiovascular
assist-control ventilation
atrial carotid ventricular
ACV disease

ACVB
aortocoronary venous bypass

ACVD
acute cardiovascular disease
atherosclerotic cardiovascular disease

ACx
anomalous circumflex

acyanotic heart disease
acyclovir
acylcarnitine
acyl-CoA
acyl-coenzyme A

acyl-CoA:cholesterol acyltransferase inhibitor
acyl-coenzyme A (acyl-CoA)
acyltransferase
    lecithin cholesterol a. (LCAT)
AD
    aerosol bolus dispersion
    anodal duration
    autogenic drainage
        Stanford type B AD
Ad
    adenovirus
Ad5FGF-4 gene therapy product
ADA
    adenosine deaminase
    anterior descending artery
        ADA deficiency
Adagen
Adalat CC, PA
adalimumab
ADAM
    aerosol-derived airway morphometry
Adam circuit
Adamkiewicz artery
Adams-DeWeese
    A.-D. device
    A.-D. vena caval serrated clip
Adams disease
Adams-Stokes (AS)
    A.-S. attack
    A.-S. disease
    A.-S. syncope
    A.-S. syndrome
adaptation
    microcirculatory a.
adapter
    Bodai a.
    catheter a.
    Harris a.
    large-bore Tuohy-Borst side-arm a.
    Passy-Muir O2 A.
    Protex swivel a.
    side-arm a.
    Tuohy-Borst a.
    Venturi jet a.
adaptive
    a. aerosol delivery (AAD)
    a. current tomography (ACT)
    a. support ventilation (ASV)
adaptive-rate pacemaker
ADC
    anodal duration contraction
    apparent diffusion coefficient
        ADC imaging
ADCHF, AD-CHF
    acutely decompensated congestive heart failure
Adcon-C resorbable liquid patch
added support (AS)

Addison
    A. disease
    A. maneuver
    A. plane
    A. point
adducin polymorphism
adduction
    paradoxical vocal cord a.
    vocal cord a.
adductor canal
AddVent atrioventricular pacemaker
adefovir
adenine nucleotide translocator (ANT)
adeno-associated
    a.-a. viral vector
    a.-a. virus (AAV)
    a.-a. virus for cystic fibrosis
adenocarcinoma
    acinar a.
    adenosquamous a.
    alveolar a.
    bronchiolar a.
    bronchioloalveolar a.
    bronchogenic a.
    mucinous a.
    nonbronchioalveolar a.
    papillary a.
    pneumonic-type a.
Adenocard injection
adenochondroma
adenoid
    a. cystic carcinoma
    hypertrophic a.
adenoma
    adrenal a.
    bronchial mucous gland a.
    parathyroid a.
    pleomorphic a.
adenomatoid tumor
adenomatosis
    pulmonary a.
adenopathy
    hilar a.
    mediastinal a.
    perihilar a.
    retrocrural a.
Adenoscan
    A. contrast medium
    A. infusion
adenosine
    a. airways responsiveness
    a. deaminase (ADA)
    a. deaminase deficiency
    a. diphosphate (ADP)
    a. echocardiography
    a. monophosphate (AMP)
    a. nuclear perfusion imaging
    a. radionuclide perfusion imaging
    a. stress

A

a. ⁹⁹ᵐTc sestamibi SPECT
a. thallium test
a. triphosphatase (ATPase)
a. triphosphate (ATP)
a. triphosphate disodium
a. triphosphate-sensitive potassium channel opener
a. triphosphate single-photon emission computed tomography (ATP-SPECT)
adenosine-induced
a.-i. hyperemia
a.-i. mast cell degranulation
adenosine-supplemented blood cardioplegia
adenosquamous
a. adenocarcinoma
a. carcinoma
adenotonsillar hypertrophy
adenoviral
a. pneumonia
a. vector
Adenoviridae
adenovirus (Ad)
a. type 40/41 infection
adenovirus-based phospholamban-antisense expression
adenovirus-mediated gene transfer
adenylate
a. cyclase
a. cyclase stimulator forskolin
a. cyclase toxin
adenylyl cyclase (AC)
adequate
a. blood flow
a. blood supply
a. collateral
a. hemostasis maintained
ADG
atrial diastolic gallop
ADH
antidiuretic hormone
ADHERE
Acute Decompensated Heart Failure National Registry
ADHERE heart failure registry
adherence assay
adherens junction
adherent
a. leaflet
a. mobile thrombus
a. mural thrombus
a. pericardium
adhesin
adhesin-receptor interaction
adhesiolysis
adhesion
band of a.

chest wall a.
fibrinous a.
freeing up of a.
heterotypic a.
homotypic a.
inflammatory a.
pleural a.
adhesive
a. atelectasis
Biobrane a.
BioGlue protein-based surgical a.
Histoacryl Blue tissue a.
a. inflammation
a. pericarditis
a. phlebitis
a. pleurisy
adhesiveness
ADHF
acute decompensated heart failure
ad hoc procedure
adiabatic fast passage
adiaspiromycosis
adiastole
adiemorrhysis
adipocyte
adiponectin
adipose
a. fold
a. folds of pleura
a. tissue
adiposis
a. cardiaca
a. universalis
adipositas cordis
adiposity
intraabdominal a. (IAA)
adiposum
cor a.
adjudication
event a.
adjunctive
a. balloon angioplasty
a. measure
a. medical therapy
adjustable dilation pressure
adjustment
Bonferroni a.
ADL scale
ADMA
asymmetric dimethylarginine
ADME
absorption, distribution, metabolism, excretion
administration
bronchodilator a.
closed-loop sedative a.
sedative a.
Veterans A. (VA)

administration *(continued)*
 viability identification with
  dipyridamole-dobutamine a.
  (VIDA)
administrator
 American College of
  Cardiovascular A.'s (ACCA)
admixture
 venous a.
ADN
 aortic depressor nerve
ADP
 adenosine diphosphate
 area diastolic pressure
ADR
 adrenergic receptor
ADRA2
 alpha-2-adrenergic receptor
ADRA1A
 alpha-1A adrenergic receptor
ADRA1B
 beta-1B adrenergic receptor
ADRA2C
 alpha-2C adrenergic receptor
ADRC
 automatic dose rate control
adrenal
 a. adenoma
 a. cortex
 a. gland
 a. hyperplasia
 a. hypertension
 a. medulla
 a. medullary implant
Adrenalin Chloride
adrenaline
adrenergic
 a. antagonist
 a. nervous system
 a. receptor (ADR, AR)
 a. receptor kinase (ARK)
 a. receptor kinase 1 (ARK-1)
 a. stimulant
adrenoceptor
 alpha a.
 beta a.
 a. blocker
adrenocorticotropic hormone (ACTH)
adrenogenital syndrome
adrenomedullary triad
adrenomedullin (AM)
 a. infusion
 a. peptide
adrenoreceptor
Adriamycin
 A. cardiotoxicity
 A., cyclophosphamide, etoposide
  (ACE)
 A. PFS, RDF

Adrucil injection
Adson
 A. aneurysm needle
 A. hook
 A. maneuver
 A. retractor
 A. test
Adson-Coffey scalenotomy
ADTe
 anodal duration tetanus
ADU
 arbitrary densitometric unit
adult
 A. Congenital Heart Association
 a. congenital heart disease (ACHD)
 a. respiratory distress syndrome
  (ARDS)
 A. Star 2000 ventilator
 a. tuberculosis
adult-onset asthma
adultorum
 scleredema a.
Advair Diskus
advanced
 a. cardiac life support (ACLS)
 a. cardiac mapping
 A. Cardiovascular Systems (ACS)
 A. Care cholesterol test
 a. heart failure
 a. heart failure shared clinical
  experience network (AHF SCENE)
 a. life support (ALS)
 a. sleep phase syndrome
 A. Technology Laboratories, Inc.
  (ATL)
 a. trauma life support (ATLS)
 a. venous access device
advancement
 elastic mandibular a. (EMA)
 genioglossal a.
 maxillomandibular a. (MMA)
Advantx LC+ cardiovascular imaging
 system
adventitial
 a. bed
 a. cell
 a. fibroblast
 a. layer
 a. vasa vasorum
adventitious
 a. breath sounds
 a. heart sounds
 a. membrane
adverse
 a. cardiac effects
 a. event
 a. ventricular remodeling
Advicor
Advil Cold & Sinus Caplets

AE
air embolism
atrial ectopic
AE heartbeat
AE-60-I-2 implantable pronged unipolar electrode
AE-60-K-10 implantable unipolar endocardial electrode
AE-60-KB implantable unipolar endocardial electrode
AE-60-KS-10 implantable unipolar endocardial electrode
AE-85-I-2 implantable pronged unipolar electrode
AE-85-K-10 implantable unipolar endocardial electrode
AE-85-KB implantable unipolar endocardial electrode
AE-85-KS-10 implantable unipolar endocardial electrode
AECB
acute exacerbation of chronic bronchitis
AECD
automatic external cardioverter-defibrillator
Powerheart AECD
AECG
ambulatory electrocardiogram
AED
automated external defibrillator
automatic external defibrillator
Heartstream FR2 AED
Powerheart AED
AEF
aortoenteric fistula
AEG
atrial electrogram
Aegis
A. aortic cannula
A. ICD system
AEI
atrial emptying index
AEM
ambulatory electrocardiographic monitoring
Aequitron
A. Medical LP-6 ventilator
A. pacemaker
aequorin
AER
agranular endoplasmic reticulum
aerated lung
aeremia
aerendocardia
aeroallergen
Aerobacter aerogenes
aerobic
a. capacity (VO$_2$max)
a. exercise (AEX, AEx)

a. exercise stress test
a. metabolism
a. respiration
a. threshold
AerobiCycle
AeroBid-M
AeroBid Oral Aerosol Inhaler
AeroChamber
A. mask
A. Plus valved holding chamber
A. spacing device
A. VHC
aerodermectasia
aerodigestive tract mucosal inflammation
Aerodose insulin inhaler
aerodynamic
a. mass diameter
a. size
Aerodyne stationary bicycle
AeroEclipse breath actuated nebulizer
aeroembolism
aeroemphysema
AeroGear
A. asthma action kit
A. fanny pack
aerogenes
Aerobacter a.
Pasteurella a.
aerogenic tuberculosis
aerogenosum
sputum a.
aerogenous
Aerolate
A. III
A. JR, SR
Aerolizer
Foradil A.
Aeromonas
A. caviae
A. hydrophila biovar sobria
A. veronii
AeroNeb
A. InLine nebulizer
A. portable nebulizer
AeroNOx
A. nitric oxide delivery and analysis system
A. nitric oxide transport system
Aeropent
aerophagia
aerosol
albuterol sulfate inhalation a.
alcohol a.
a. bolus dispersion (AD)
Brethaire Inhalation A.
a. challenge test
a. cloud enhancer (ACE)
a. deposition
Flovent a.

aerosol *(continued)*
    a. inhalation monitor (AIM)
    a. mask
    Maxair Inhalation A.
    Nasalide Nasal A.
    a. nebulizer
    pirbuterol acetate inhalation a.
    respirable a.
    Sclerosol intrapleural a.
    sterile saline a.
    steroid a.
    Tilade Inhalation A.
    Virazole A.
aerosol-derived airway morphometry
(ADAM)
aerosolization
aerosolized
    a. antibiotic
    a. bronchodilator
    a. pentamidine
    a. pentamidine isethionate
    a. surfactant
    a. virus
Aerosomes drug delivery device
AeroSonic personal ultrasonic nebulizer
Aerospan
AeroTech II nebulizer
aerotherapy
aerothorax
AeroView optical intubation system
AERP
    atrial effective refractory period
aeruginosa
    Pseudomonas a.
AERx
    AERx drug delivery device
    AERx inhaler
AES
    aortic ejection sound
Aescula
    A. left ventricular lead
    A. LV lead
AET
    atrial ectopic tachycardia
AEX, AEx
    aerobic exercise
AF
    aortic flow
    atrial fibrillation
    atrial flutter
    atrial fusion
        nonrheumatic AF
        rheumatic AF
AF0150 contrast agent
AFA
    acromegaloid facial appearance
    AFA syndrome

AFB
    acid-fast bacillus
    aortofemoral bypass
AFBG
    aortofemoral bypass graft
AFCL
    atrial fibrillation cycle length
AFE
    amnionic fluid embolism
    amniotic fluid embolism
AfeCTA immunoassay
AFF
    atrial fibrillation-flutter
    atrial filling fraction
afferent
    a. arteriole
    a. artery
    a. impulse
    a. nerve fiber
    a. vessel
afferentia
    vasa a.
affinity
    A. blood pump
    a. chromatography
    a. maturation
    A. oxygenator
    A. pacemaker
afflux, affluxion
aFGF
    acidic fibroblast growth factor
AFL
    atrial flutter
AFm
    atrial fibrillation monitor
        Vitatron Selection AFm
AFO
    ankle-foot orthosis
AFocus steerable diagnostic catheter
AFORMED
    alternating failure of response,
        mechanical, to electrical depolarization
        AFORMED phenomenon
AFP
    alpha-fetoprotein
    doxorubicin, 5-fluorouracil, cisplatin
        AFP II pacemaker
AFR
    atrial flutter response
        AFR algorithm
African
    A. American (AA)
    A. Burkitt lymphoma
    A. cardiomyopathy
    A. endomyocardial
    A. endomyocardial fibrosis
    A. histoplasmosis
    A. sleeping sickness
    A. tick typhus

africanum
  Mycobacterium a.
Afrin Tablet
afterdepolarization
  delayed a. (DAD)
  early a. (EAD)
  late a.
  monophasic action potential
    early a. (mEAD)
afterload
  increased a.
  a. matching
  a. mismatching
  reduced a.
  a. reduction
  a. resistance
  right ventricle a.
  ventricular a.
afterloader
  MicroSelectron-HDR a.
afterloading
  a. catheter
  a. screw
afterload-reducing agent
afterpotential
  depolarizing a. (DAP)
  diastolic a.
  oscillatory a.
  a. oversensing
  pacemaker a.
  positive a.
  a. sensing
afterspike hyperpolarization (AHP)
AFV
  aortic flow velocity
AG
  angular gyrus
  atrial gallop
Ag
  antigen
  silver
Ag-AgCl₂ electrode bipolar catheter
agalactiae
  Streptococcus a.
agammaglobulinemia
agar
  brain-heart infusion a. (BHIA)
  brain-heart infusion blood a.
    (BHIBA)
  a. diffusion assay
agarose
  a. gel
  a. gel electrophoresis
  MetaPhor a.
Agatston score
AGE
  arterial gas embolism
age
  mean a.

age-dependent apnea
agency, pl. **agencies**
  A. for Health Care Policy and
    Research (AHCPR)
  South Carolina Organ
    Procurement A. (SCOPA)
Agenerase
agenesis
  pulmonary a.
AGENT
  angiogenic gene therapy agent
agent
  AF0150 contrast a.
  afterload-reducing a.
  Albunex contrast a.
  alpha-1-adrenergic blocking a.
  alpha blocking a.
  AlphaNine clotting a.
  angiogenic gene therapy a.
    (AGENT)
  AngioMARK contrast a.
  antianginal a.
  antiarrhythmic a.
  anticholinergic a.
  antidiabetic a.
  antifoaming a.
  antihypertensive a.
  antiinflammatory a.
  antimicrotubule a.
  antimycobacterial a.
  antiplatelet a.
  aquaretic a.
  bacteriostatic a.
  beta-adrenergic blocking a.
  beta-adrenoceptor blocking a.
  beta blocking a.
  bioterrorism threat a.
  blood-borne infectious a.
  bronchodilating a.
  calcium channel blocking a.
  calcium-sensitizing a.
  capsid binding a.
  chemoattracting a.
  chemotherapeutic a.
  cholinergic a.
  contrast a.
  cytoprotective a.
  demethylating a.
  diagnostic imaging a.
  diuretic a.
  dopaminergic a.
  Eaton a.
  EP-2104R injectable MRI a.
  Fibrimage diagnostic imaging a.
  fibrinolytic a.
  FS-069 contrast a.
  histocompatibility a. B27
  hydrophilic a.
  hypertensive a.

A

agent *(continued)*
    hypoglycemic a.
    hypotensive a.
    Imagent contrast a.
    imaging a.
    inhalation a.
    inotropic a.
    Levovist echocontrast a.
    lipid-lowering a.
    long-acting quaternary ammonium
      antimuscarinic a.
    macrolide antimicrobial a.
    mucoregulatory a.
    multiple antimycobacterial a.'s
    NeoTect imaging a.
    neuromuscular blocking a. (NMBA)
    neuroprotective a.
    nonglycoside inotropic a.
    nonsteroidal antiinflammatory a.
    Norwalk a.
    Optison contrast a.
    perfluoropolyether a.
    Pittsburgh pneumonia a.
    progestational a.
    prothrombin time fixing a. (PTFA)
    provoking a.
    psychotropic a.
    putative a.
    Quantison contrast a.
    saluretic a.
    sclerosing a.
    sonicated contrast a.
    steroid-sparing a.
    thrombolytic a.
    toxic a.
    TWAR a.
    type III antiarrhythmic a.
    ultrasound contrast a. (UCA)
    vagolytic a.
    vasodilator a. (VA)
age-related
    a.-r. apnea
    a.-r. bone loss
    a.-r. endothelial dysfunction
age-undetermined myocardial infarction
agger valvae venae
agglutinating antibody
agglutination
agglutinative thrombus
agglutinin
    cold a.
    a. febrile
Aggrastat
aggregate
    intravascular a.
aggregation
    ex vivo a.
    platelet a.

aggregometer
    Chrono-log optical a.
    Chrono-log platelet a.
    Model 700 a.
    optical a.
    whole blood a.
aggregometry
    Born a.
    impedance a.
Aggrenox
aggrephore
aggressive platelet blockade
Agiltrac 0.018, 0.035 peripheral dilation catheter
aging
agitated saline solution
agitation
    echocardiogram with saline a.
    a. syndrome
aglycon
AGN
    acute glomerulonephritis
agonal
    a. beat
    a. breathing
    a. clot
    a. respiration
    a. rhythm
    a. thrombosis
    a. thrombus
agonist
    alpha a.
    alpha-adrenoreceptor a.
    beta a.
    beta-adrenergic a.
    beta-adrenoceptor a.
    calcium channel a.
    imidazoline receptor a.
    inhaled beta a.
    muscarinic a.
    PD 123319 AT receptor a.
agony clot
agranular endoplasmic reticulum (AER)
agranulocytosis
agricultural anthrax
Agrobacterium tumefaciens
Agrylin
AH
    arterial hypertension
    artificial heart
    ataxic hemiparesis
    atrium-His
        AH bundle
        AH conduction time
        AH curve
        AH interval
A-H
    atrio-His

A

AHA
American Heart Association
antiheart antibody
AHA type I diet
AHA.SOC
American Heart Association Stroke
Outcome Classification
AHCPR
Agency for Health Care Policy and
Research
AHD
acute heart disease
arteriosclerotic heart disease
atherosclerotic heart disease
AHES
artificial heart energy system
AHF SCENE
advanced heart failure shared clinical
experience network
AH:HA ratio
AHI
apnea-hypopnea index
AHM
ambulatory Holter monitoring
AHMA
antiheart muscle autoantibody
Ahn thrombectomy catheter
AHP
afterspike hyperpolarization
AHR
airway hyperreactivity
airway hyperresponsiveness
atrial heart rate
AHTECAB
arrested heart totally endoscopic coronary
artery bypass grafting
A-hydroCort Injection
3a-hydroxy-dihydroprogesterone
AI
aortic incompetence
aortic insufficiency
apical impulse
apnea index
atherogenic index
atrial insufficiency
AIA
aspirin-induced asthma
AICA
anterior inferior cerebellar artery
anterior inferior communicating artery
AICA riboside
AICD, A-ICD
atrial implantable cardioverter-
defibrillator
automatic implantable cardioverter-
defibrillator
automatic internal cardioverter-
defibrillator

Guardian AICD
Ventak AICD
AICS
acute ischemic coronary syndrome
AID
automatic implantable defibrillator
AID-Check monitor
AIDS
acquired immunodeficiency syndrome
AIDS-related
AIDS-r. lymphoma (ARL)
AIDS-r. lymphoma of lung
(ARLL)
AIE
acute infective endocarditis
AIH
aortic intramural hematoma
aortic intramural hemorrhage
AIM
aerosol inhalation monitor
AIMO
anterior inferior mandibular osteotomy
AIOD
aortoiliac obstructive disease
AIP
acute idiopathic pericarditis
acute intermittent porphyria
acute interstitial pneumonia
acute interstitial pneumonitis
air
alveolar a.
ambient a.
a. bronchiologram
a. bronchogram
a. bronchogram sign
a. cell
a. clamp inflatable vessel occluder
complemental a.
complementary a.
a. conditioner lung
a. crescent sign
a. embolism (AE)
a. embolization
a. embolus
a. entrainment mask
a. entry
a. exchange
expiratory trapping of a.
extrapleural a.
a. flow
functional residual a.
high-efficiency particulate a.
(HEPA)
a. hunger
a. kerma exposure
a. leak
a. medical transportation (AMT)
a. movement
a. plethysmograph

air *(continued)*
    a. pollution
    a. pulmonary embolism
    reserve a.
    residual a.
    a. sac
    a. space
    supplemental a.
    A. Supply wearable air purifier
    tidal a.
    a. trapping
    a. tube
    a. vesicle
    vitiated a.
    A. Viva
    A. Wise program
airborne
    a. allergen
    a. fiber level
    a. transmission
air-driven artificial heart
Aire-Cuf tracheostomy tube
airflow
    a. cessation
    expiratory a.
    inspiratory a.
    a. limitation
    a. obstruction
    a. velocity
air-fluid level
Airlie House criteria
Air-Lon tracheal tube brush
AirMax external nasal dilator
AirMed
    A. mask
    A. ventilator
Airox Home 1, 2 ventilator
Airozin nutritional supplement
air-powered nebulizer
air-puff tonometer
AirSep
    A. CPAP
    A. OxiScan Oximetry recording, reporting, and archiving system
    A. Ultimate nasal seal gel insert
airspace
    a. consolidation
    a. disease
    peripheral a.
airspace-filling pattern
air-trapping
airway
    anatomic a.
    a. bacterial colonization
    Berman a.
    a. branching
    a., breathing, circulation (ABC)
    a., breathing, circulation, defibrillate (ABCD)

    a., breathing, circulation, differential diagnosis
    a., breathing, circulation, disability, exposure (ABCDE)
    a., breathing, circulation, intravenous crystalloid (ABCIC)
    a. clearance
    a. closure
    Combitube a.
    a. compromise
    conducting a.
    Connell a.
    difficult a.
    a. edema
    esophageal obturator a. (EOA)
    esophagogastric tube a. (EGTA)
    flabby a.'s
    a. hyperreactivity (AHR)
    hyperresponsive a.'s
    a. hyperresponsiveness (AHR)
    a. hypersecretion
    a. hysteresis
    laryngeal mask a. (LMA)
    lower a.
    a. lumen
    a. morphometry
    a. mucosa
    nasal a.'s
    a.'s obstruction (AO)
    a. occlusion technique
    a. pattern
    a. permeability
    pharyngotracheal lumen a. (PTLA)
    a. pressure
    a. pressure disconnect (APD)
    a. pressure release ventilation (APRV)
    a. protection
    PtL a.
    a.'s reactivity index (ARI)
    a. remodeling
    a.'s resistance (Raw)
    a. resistance
    resistance, a. (RAW)
    respiratory a.
    retropalatal a.'s
    a. secretion
    a.'s smooth muscle (ASM)
    steepling of glottic a.
    a. stenosis
    a. stenting
    a. submucosa
    a. tapering
    upper a.
    upstream a.'s
airway-esophageal balloon pressure
airway-parenchymal dysanapsis
AirZone peak flowmeter

AIS
  Abbreviated Injury Scale
  acute ischemic stroke
    AIS model
    AIS model of a beating ventricle
AITD
  autoimmune thyroid disease
AIV
  avian influenza virus
    AIV H5N1
AIV H5N1
  avian influenza virus strain H5N1
AIVR
  accelerated idioventricular rhythm
AJCC
  American Joint Committee on Cancer
    AJCC staging station
Ajellomyces dermatitidis
ajmaline test
Akaike information criteria
A-K diamond knife
A-kinase
akinesia, akinesis
    distal a.
    psychic a.
    septal a.
akinesic
akinetic segment
Akron tilt table
Akt gene transfer
Akutsu III total artificial heart
AL
  angiographic area of lateral projection
  anterior leaflet
    AL I, II guiding catheter
Al
  aluminum
ALA
  alpha-linolenic acid
ALAD
  abnormal left axis deviation
Aladdin
    A. Infant Flow system
    A. nasal CPAP system
Aladdin^II NCPAP
Alagille
    A. syndrome
    A. Syndrome Alliance
ala nasi
alanine
    a. aminotransferase (ALT)
    a. exchange
alanine/valine (A/V)
alanyl-tRNA synthetase
ALAO
  angiographic area of left anterior oblique
    projection
alar
    a. artery

    a. artery of nose
    a. chest
    a. flaring
alaryngeal speech
AlaSTAT latex allergy test
Alatest Latex-specific IgE allergen test kit
alatrofloxacin
alba
    pneumonia a.
albendazole sulfoxide
Albert
    A. Grass Heritage EEG system
    A. Grass Heritage PSG system
Albertini treatment
albicans
    Candida a.
    Monilia a.
albida
    macula a.
albidus
    Cryptococcus a.
Albini nodule
Albright syndrome
albumin
    a. cobalt binding (ACB)
    a. cobalt binding test
    macroaggregated a. (MAA)
    a. microspheres sonicated
    perfluorocarbon-exposed sonicated
      dextrose a. (PESDA)
    radioactive iodinated serum a.
      (RISA)
    a. resuscitation
    serum a.
    sonicated dextrose a.
albumin-coated vascular graft
albuminoid sputum
albuminuria
Albunex contrast agent
albuterol
    ipratropium and a.
    a. nebulizer updraft
    a. sulfate inhalation aerosol
    a. sulfate inhalation solution
    a. sulfate syrup
ALCA
  anomalous left coronary artery
Alcaligenes
    A. bookeri
    A. dentrificans
    A. faecalis
    A. odorans
    A. piechaudii
    A. xylosoxidans
ALCAPA
  anomalous left coronary artery arising
    from pulmonary artery

ALCAPA *(continued)*
  anomalous origin of left coronary artery
    from pulmonary artery
      ALCAPA syndrome
Alcatel pacemaker
Alcian blue-PAS stain
alcohol
  absolute a.
  a. abuse
  a. aerosol
  amino a.
  ethyl a.
  a. intoxication
  polyvinyl a. (PVA)
  a. septal ablation
  a. septal reduction
alcoholic
  a. cardiomyopathy
  a. heart muscle disease
  a. malnutrition
  a. myocardiopathy
  a. pneumonia
alcoholism, leukopenia, pneumococcal
  sepsis (ALPS)
Alcon Closure System
Aldactazide
Aldactone
aldehyde-tanned bovine carotid artery
  graft
aldesleukin
Aldoril
aldosterone
  a. antagonist
  a. depression
  plasma a.
  a. synthase
aldosterone-receptor blocker
aldosteronism
aldosteronoma
Aldrete needle
Aldrich ST elevation score
ALEC
  artificial lung-expanding compound
alemtuzumab
AlereNet system
ALERT
  atrial low energy reversion therapy
alert
  A. catheter
  A. Companion II biphasic
    defibrillator
alertness test
aleuronoid granule
Alexander-Farabeuf periosteotome
Alexander rib stripper
alexandrite laser
alexithymia
Alexithymia Provoked Response
  Interview

alexithymic personality features
alfa
  dornase a.
alfa-2a
  interferon a.-2a
alfa-2b
  interferon a.-2b
alfentanil hydrochloride
Alfieri
  A. method
  A. procedure
  A. repair
alfimeprase
ALG
  antilymphocyte globulin
algiovascular
alglucerase
algorithm
  AFR a.
  AMS a.
  Artrek automated edge-detection a.
  asthma care a. (ACA)
  atrial flutter response a.
  atrial tachycardic response a.
  automatic mode conversion a.
  automatic mode-switching a.
  AZTEC a.
  closed-loop a. (CLA)
  detection a.
  diagnostic a.
  Levenberg-Marquardt a.
  MAR a.
  mean atrial rate a.
  trilinear cylindric interpolation a.
algovascular
ALI
  acute lung injury
aliasing
  a. artifact
  a. flow
  image a.
Alice 3, 5 diagnostic sleep system
alignment
  a. catheter
  a. mark
alimentary habits
alimentation
Alimta
A-line
  arterial line
alinidine
aliphatic
  a. amines asthma
  a. polyamine
aliquot
Alkaban-AQ
alkalemia
alkaline
  a. phosphatase (AP)

a. phosphatase antialkaline
phosphatase (APAAP)
alkaloid
ergot a.
Rauwolfia a.
a. tylophorine
unsaturated pyrrolizidine a. (UPA)
vinca a.
alkaloidal cocaine
alkalosis
acapnial a.
altitude a.
hypochloremic metabolic a.
metabolic a.
respiratory a.
alkaptonuria
**Alka-Seltzer Plus Flu & Body Aches
Non-Drowsy Liqui-Gels**
alkavervir
Alkeran
**Alkermes AIR pulmonary drug delivery
technology**
ALKK
Arbeitsgemeinschaft Leitende
Kardiologische Krankenhausarzte
alkylxanthine
ALL
acute lymphocytic leukemia
antihypertensive and lipid lowering
all
a. or none
a. or none law
a. track wire (ATW)
Allain method
allantoic
a. circulation
a. vein
Allcarbon monodisc valve
Allegiance nasal prongs
Allegra
allele
AT1 receptor C a.
D, I a.
mutant a.
prothrombin G20210A mutated a.
S2 a.
TNF2 a.
tumor necrosis factor-2 a.
allele-specific T-cell response
allelic deletion
Allen
A. and Davis classification
A. test
Allen-Brown
A.-B. criteria
A.-B. shunt
Allerbiocid
Aller-Chlor Oral
Allerdryl

Allerest Maximum Strength
allergen
airborne a.
environmental a.
a. exposure
HDM a.
house dust mite a.
indoor inhalant a.
inhalant a.
Rattus norvegicus a.
urban a.
allergen-induced
a.-i. asthma
a.-i. mediator release
allergic
a. alveolitis
a. angiitis and granulomatosis
a. asthma
a. bronchopulmonary aspergillosis
(ABPA)
a. bronchospasm
a. diathesis
a. granulomatous angiitis
a. reaction
a. rhinitis
a. salute
a. shiner
a. vasculitis
allergically induced bronchospasm
allergy, pl. **allergies**
bronchial a.
IgE-mediated food a.
a. purpura
respiratory a.
seasonal a.
AllerMax Oral
Allernix
Allerphed Syrup
allescheriosis
allethrin
allethrolone
alliance
Alagille Syndrome A.
A. catheter delivery system
alligator clip
Allis clamp
Allison
A. hiatal hernia repair
A. lung retractor
alloantibody
allogeneic transplant
allogenic-blood transfusion
allograft
a. arteriosclerosis
cardiac a.
cryopreserved heart valve a.
cryopreserved human aortic a.
cryopreserved valved a.

allograft *(continued)*
    a. rejection
    a. vasculopathy
allometric
allorhythmia
allorhythmic
allosteric modification of enzyme
alloy
    cobalt chromium a.
Allport-Babcock searcher
all-purpose
    low energy a.-p. (LEAP)
all-trans-retinoic acid (ATRA)
ALMCA
    anomalous left main coronary artery
ALMI
    anterior lateral myocardial infarct
almokalant
ALMV
    anterior leaflet of mitral valve
Aloka
    A. color Doppler
    A. model SSD-830 2.5- and 3.5-
    MHz transducer
    A. ultrasound
ALP
    acute lupus pericarditis
    acute lupus pneumonitis
alpha
    a. adrenoceptor
    a. agonist
    a. blocking agent
    estrogen receptor a. (ER alpha)
    a. Gal antibody
    heavy chain cardiac myosin a.
    (MYHCA)
    lecithin cholesterol
    acyltransferase a. (LCATA)
    a. lipoprotein
    prostaglandin 2 a. (PGF2-alpha)
    a. receptor
    a. variable (Valpha)
alpha-1
    a.-1 adrenoceptor blockade
    a.-1 antitrypsin (AAT)
    a.-1 antitrypsin deficiency
    a.-1 proteinase inhibitor
alpha-2-adrenergic receptor (ADRA2)
alpha-2C adrenergic receptor (ADRA2C)
alpha-2 macroglobulin
alpha-2-plasmin inhibitor
alpha-1A adrenergic receptor (ADRA1A)
alpha-actinin
alpha-adrenergic
    a.-a. blocker
    a.-a. stimulation
alpha-1-adrenergic
    a.-1-a. blocking agent
    a.-1-a. receptor

alpha-adrenoreceptor
    a.-a. agonist
    a.-a. blocker
alpha-alpha homodimer
alpha-B-crystallin protein
alpha-cardiac actin
alpha-fetoprotein (AFP)
alpha-hydroxybutyrate dehydrogenase
alpha-interferon
alpha-linolenic acid (ALA)
alpha-methyldopa
alpha-MHC
    alpha-myosin heavy chain
alpha-myosin heavy chain (alpha-MHC)
AlphaNine clotting agent
alpha-smooth muscle actin
alpha-stat
Alpha-Tamoxifen
AlphaTest kit
alpha-tocopherol
Alphavirus
Alport syndrome
alprazolam
alprenolol hydrochloride
alprostadil
ALPS
    alcoholism, leukopenia, pneumococcal
    sepsis
        ALPS syndrome
ALRI
    acute lower respiratory tract infection
ALS
    advanced life support
    amyotrophic lateral sclerosis
Alstrom syndrome
ALT
    alanine aminotransferase
Altace Oral
ALTE
    apparent life-threatening event
alteplase (TPA)
    recombinant a.
alteration
    acute preload a.
    coexistent cardiac a.'s
    ST a.
altered airway secretion
alternans
    auditory a.
    auscultatory a.
    concordant a.
    cycle length a.
    discordant a.
    electrical a.
    microvolt T-wave a. (MTWA)
    pulsus a.
    QRS a.
    respiratory a.
    ST-segment a.

systole a.
a. test
total a.
T-wave a. (TWA)
U-wave a.
Alternaria tenuis
alternating
a. bidirectional tachycardia
a. current (AC)
a. failure of response, mechanical, to electrical depolarization (AFORMED)
a. pulse
alternation
cardiac a.
concordant a.
cycle length a.
discordant a.
electrical a.
mechanical a.
alternative
Cardia Salt a.
Citrol Smoking a.
alternobaric exposure
altitude
a. alkalosis
a. hypoxia
a. sickness
altretamine
aluminosis
aluminum (Al)
a. carbide
a. hydroxide gel
a. lung
a. nicotinate
a. oxide fibrosis
a. oxygen regulator
a. potroom asthma
Alupent
ALVAD
abdominal left ventricular assist device
Alvarez prosthesis
alvei
Bacillus a.
alveobronchiolitis
Alveofact
alveolar
a. adenocarcinoma
a. air
a. asthma
a. basement membrane
a. bronchiole
a. capillary dysplasia (ACD)
A. Capillary Dysplasia Association (ACDA)
a. carbon dioxide pressure
a. carbon dioxide tension
a. cell
a. cell carcinoma

a. dead space
a. destruction
a. duct
a. duct emphysema
a. ectasia
a. edema
a. flooding
a. gas
a. hemorrhage
a. hyaline membrane
a. hypertension
a. hyperventilation
a. hypoventilation
a. hypoxia
a. infiltrate
a. leak
a. macrophage
a. microlithiasis
a. opacification
a. overdistention
a. oxygen partial pressure (PAO_2)
a. oxygen tension
a. pattern
a. period
a. permeability (AP)
a. phospholipidosis
a. pore
a. pressure (Palv)
a. proteinosis
a. sac
a. sarcoidosis
a. septum
a. ventilation
a. ventilation/perfusion (Va/Q)
a. ventilation per minute (V_A)
a. volume (VA)
a. volume recruitment
alveolar-air equation
alveolar-arterial (A-a)
a.-a. gradient (AAG)
a.-a. oxygen gradient ($A-aO_2$)
a.-a. oxygen tension ($A-aO_2$)
a.-a. PO_2 difference ($AaPO_2$)
alveolar-atrial (A-a)
alveolar-capillary
a.-c. block
a.-c. intravascular pressure
a.-c. membrane
alveolares
sacculus a.
alveolar-filling pattern
alveolaris
sacculus a.
alveolarization
alveolar-pleural fistula
alveolar-septal amyloidosis
alveoli (*pl. of* alveolus)
alveolitis
acute pulmonary a.

alveolitis *(continued)*
    allergic a.
    chronic fibrosing a.
    cryptogenic fibrosing a. (CFA)
    desquamative a.
    diffuse sclerosing a.
    extrinsic allergic a.
    fibrosing a.
    lymphocytic a.
    lymphoid a.
    mononuclear a.
alveoloarterial (AA)
alveolocapillary
    a. membrane
    a. partial pressure gradient
alveoloclasia
alveolus, pl. **alveoli**
    pulmonary a.
    alveoli pulmonis
    A. stent
    A. stent technology system
    ventilated alveoli
Alvesco
ALVF
    acute left ventricular failure
ALVT
    aortic and left ventricular tunnel
ALWMI
    anterolateral wall myocardial infarct
AM
    adrenomedullin
AM-50 portable air compressor
AMA-Fab
    antimyosin monoclonal antibody with
      Fab fragment
      AMA-Fab scintigraphy
amalonatica
    Citrobacter a.
amantadine hydrochloride
Amapari virus
amaurosis partialis fugax
amaurotic
amazon thorax
Amazr ablation catheter
Amba
ambasilide
Ambenyl Cough Syrup
Amberlite particles
AMBI
    acute multiple brain infarcts
Ambien
ambient
    a. air
    a. gas
    a. ozone
    a. pressure
ambiguus
    situs a.
    visceroatrial situs a.

AmBisome
Amblyomma americanum
ambrisentan
Ambrose
    A. classification
    A. plaque type
ambroxol
Ambu
    A. bag
    A. CardioPump
    A. Res-Cue mask
    A. Spur disposable resuscitator
ambulance
    basic life support a.
ambulatory
    a. blood pressure (ABP)
    a. blood pressure monitoring
      (ABPM)
    a. electrocardiogram (AECG)
    a. electrocardiographic monitoring
      (AEM)
    a. electrocardiography
    a. Holter monitor
    a. Holter monitoring (AHM)
    a. monitoring
    a. nuclear detector
    a. O_2
    a. oximetry monitoring (AOM)
    a. pulse oximetry
    a. venous pressure (AVP)
    a. ventricular function probe
ambuphylline
Amcath catheter
AMD3100 stem cell mobilizer
amdinocillin
amebiasis
    pulmonary a.
amebic
    a. pericarditis
    a. pneumonia
ameboid
    a. cell
    a. movement
ameboma
A-MED percutaneous ventricular assist device
America
    Heart Failure Society of A.
      (HFSA)
    Infectious Diseases Society of A.
Americaine
American
    A. Academy of Cardiology
      Perfusion (AACP)
    African A. (AA)
    A. Association of Cardiovascular
      and Pulmonary Rehabilitation
      (AACVPR)

A. Association for Respiratory Care (AARC)
A. Association for the Surgery of Trauma (AAST)
A. Cancer Society (ACS)
A. Cardiology Technologists Association (ACTA)
A. College of Allergy, Asthma and Immunology
A. College of Cardiology (ACC)
A. College of Cardiology/American Heart Association (ACC/AHA)
A. College of Cardiology/American Heart Association Task Force on Practice guidelines
A. College of Cardiovascular Administrators (ACCA)
A. College of Chest Physicians (ACCP)
A. College of Physicians
A. College of Rheumatology
A. College of Sports Medicine (ACSM)
A. College of Sports Medicine regression equation
A. Heart Association (AHA)
A. Heart Association classification
A. Heart Association guidelines
A. Heart Association No-Fad Diet
A. Heart Association Nutrition Committee
A. Heart Association Stroke Outcome Classification (AHA.SOC)
A. Heart Association type I diet Hispanic A. (HA)
A. Joint Committee on Cancer (AJCC)
A. Joint Committee on Cancer staging station
A. Pacemaker Corporation lead
A. Roentgen Ray Society
A. Sleep Disorders Association (ASDA)
A. Society of Echocardiography
A. Society of Electrocardiography (ASE)
A. Society of Extra-Corporeal Technology (AmSECT)
A. Thoracic Society (ATS)
A. Thoracic Society classification of dyspnea
A. tracheotomy tube
A. trypanosomiasis
americanum
   Amblyomma a.
americanus
   Necator a.

Amesec
A-methaPred injection
AME tongue retaining device
Amgenal Cough Syrup
AMI
   acute myocardial infarction
      AMI infant apnea monitor
Amicar
Amidate
amifloxacin
amifostine
amikacin sulfate
Amikin injection
amiloride
   a. hydrochloride
   a. and hydrochlorothiazide
amine
   sympathomimetic a.
amino
   a. acid (AA)
   a. alcohol
aminoacyl-tRNA synthetase
aminocaproate
aminocaproic acid
aminoethylethanolamine
aminoglutethimide
aminoglycoside
aminoguanidine
aminolevulinic
   5-a. acid
aminopenicillin
aminopenicillins
aminophylline, amobarbital, ephedrine
Aminorex
aminosalicylate
   phenyl a.
   potassium a.
   a. sodium
   sodium a.
aminosalicylic
   a. acid
   a. acid hypersensitivity
aminoterminal propeptide
aminotransferase
   alanine a. (ALT)
   arginine a.
   aspartate a. (AST)
amiodarone
   a. hydrochloride
   a. pulmonary fibrosis
   a. therapy
amiodarone-induced hyperthyroidism
Amipaque contrast medium
Amiscan
Amis 2000 respiratory mass spectrometer
Ami-Tex LA
amitriptyline

AML
    acute myelocytic leukemia
    anterior mitral leaflet
amlodipine
    a. and benazepril
    a. besylate
AMM
    antibody to murine cardiac myosin
ammonia
    anhydrous a.
    aromatic a. spirit
    N-13 a.
    nitrogen-13 a.
ammonium
    a. carbonate
    a. chloride
ammunition
    beanbag shotgun round a.
amnesia
    global a.
    retrograde a.
    verbal a.
    visual a.
amniocentesis
amnionic fluid embolism (AFE)
amniotic
    a. fluid embolism (AFE)
    a. fluid syndrome
A-mode
    A-m. echocardiography
    A-m. echo-tracking device
Amorolfine
amorphous
    a. hydrogenated silicon carbide (a-SiC:H)
    a. parenchymal opacification
    a. plaque
    a. silica
amosite
amount of use (AOU)
amoxapine
amoxicillin
    a. and clavulanate potassium
    a. and clavulanic acid
Amoxil
AMP
    acid mucopolysaccharide
    adenosine monophosphate
    average mean pressure
    CAR AMP
ampere
amphetamine
    a. sulfate
    a. toxicity
amphibole asbestos
amphibolite
amphipathic helix
Amphojel

amphoric
    a. echo
    a. murmur
    a. rale
    a. resonance
    a. respiration
    a. voice
    a. voice sound
amphoriloquy
amphorophony
Amphotec
amphotericin
    a. B
    a. B cholesteryl sulfate complex
    a. B (conventional)
    a. B desoxycholate
    a. B lipid complex (ABLC)
    a. B (liposomal)
ampicillin and sulbactam
Ampicin
Amplatz
    A. dilator
    A. gooseneck microsnare
    A. left I, II catheter
    A. right coronary catheter
    A. right I, II catheter
    A. Super Stiff guidewire
    A. tapered extra stiff wire guide
    A. tapered movable core wire
    A. technique
    A. thrombectomy device (ATD)
    A. torque wire
    A. tube guide
    A. ultra stiff wire guide
    A. ventricular septal defect device
Amplatzer
    A. device
    A. duct occluder
    A. PFO occluder
    A. septal occluder (ASO)
Amplicor
    A. assay
    A. assay for *Mycobacterium tuberculosis*
    A. *Mycobacterium tuberculosis* test
amplification
    nucleic acid a. (NAA)
amplified *Mycobacterium tuberculosis* direct test (AMTDT)
amplifier
    endocardiographic a. (EA)
amplifying myocyte
amplitude
    apical interventricular septal a.
    atrial pulse a.
    carotid pulse a. (CAR AMP)
    contractile a.
    C-to-E a.
    D-to-E a.

A

a. image
a. linearity
pulse a.
a. of pulse
P-wave a.
R-wave a.
signal a.
ventricular pulse a.
wall a.
wave a.
zero a.
a. zone time epoch coding (AZTEC)
amprenavir
amprolium hydrochloride
ampulla, pl. **ampullae**
Bryant a.
Thoma a.
ampullary aneurysm
amrinone lactate
AMS
acute mitral stenosis
acute mountain sickness
automatic mode switching
AMS algorithm
amsacrine
AmSECT
American Society of Extra-Corporeal Technology
AMT
air medical transportation
AMTDT
amplified *Mycobacterium tuberculosis* direct test
AMV
assisted mechanical ventilation
aMVL
anterior mitral valve leaflet
amygdala
amyl
a. nitrite
A. Nitrite Aspirols
amylase
serum a.
amyloid
a. A protein
a. deposition
a. heart disease
a. polyneuropathy
a. precursor protein (APP)
amyloidogenic transthyretin (ATTR)
amyloidoma
amyloidosis
alveolar-septal a.
cardiac a.
familial a.
mediastinal a.
nodular pulmonary a.
parenchymal a.

pleural a.
primary systemic a.
pseudotumoral mediastinal a.
pulmonary a.
senile a.
senile systemic a. (SSA)
tracheobronchial a.
amyocardia
amyotrophic
a. chorea
a. lateral sclerosis (ALS)
amyotrophy
neuralgic a.
AN
anodal
atrionodal
AN interval
AN region
ANA
antinuclear antibody
anabolic steroid
Anaconda
A. device
A. device and delivery system
anacrotic
a. limb
a. notch
a. pulse
anacrotism
anadicrotic pulse
anadicrotism
anadicrotus
pulsus a.
anaerobe
anaerobic
a. empyema
a. metabolism
a. pneumonia
a. Pulsator syringe
a. respiration
a. threshold (AT)
anaerobiosis
Anaerobiospirillum
anaerobius
Peptostreptococcus a.
anagrelide HCl
analgesia
epidural a.
extrapleural catheter a.
intrapleural catheter a.
intravenous a.
patient-controlled a. (PCA)
percutaneous extrapleural a.
analgesic
a. nephropathy
patient-controlled a. (PCA)
analog, analogue
F2-alpha prostaglandin a.

analog *(continued)*
    human amylin a.
    a. video acquisition station
analog-to-digital conversion
analysis, pl. **analyses**
    arterial blood gas a.
    backscatter a.
    beat-to-beat a.
    body density a.
    breath a.
    centerline method of wall
      motion a.
    computerized texture a.
    Doppler flow a.
    Doppler spectral a.
    Doppler waveform a.
    electron microprobe a.
    fast Fourier spectral a.
    forced vital capacity a. (FVCA)
    Fourier series a.
    Fourier transform a.
    frequency-domain a.
    gas exchange a.
    hemodynamic a.
    hydroxyproline a.
    image a.
    immunoprecipitin a.
    isotime a.
    longitudinal a.
    microarray a.
    multivariate regression a.
    myocardial ischemia dynamic a.
      (MIDA)
    neutron activation a.
    NMR LipoProfile a.
    Northern hybridization a.
    phase image a.
    point-of-care a.
    post hoc a.
    power spectral a.
    pressure-volume a.
    quantitative coronary a. (QCA)
    quantitative coronary
      angiographic a.
    respiratory gas a.
    segmental wall motion a. (SWMA)
    sensitivity a.
    Southern blot a.
    spectral a.
    sputum a.
    time-domain a.
    univariate a.
    videodensitometric myocardial
      textural a.
    wall motion a. (WMA)
    x-ray energy microprobe a.
analyzer
    ABL 555 a.
    AVL Omni blood gas a.
    AVL Opti Critical Care A.
    AVL Opti 1 portable blood gas a.
    Beckman O_2 a.
    840 blood gas a.
    1620 blood gas a.
    breath gas a.
    BVA-100 blood volume a.
    Cat-a-Kit a.
    Cobas Fara centrifugal a.
    CO Sleuth handheld carbon
      monoxide a.
    Coulter RapidVUE particle shape
      and size a.
    DMI a.
    ERA 300 dual-chamber pacing
      system a.
    $ETCO_2$ multigas a.
    Gem Premier Plus blood
      gas/electrolyte a.
    Handi oxygen a.
    IL Synthesis a.
    i-STAT handheld a.
    Keystone PF a.
    Marquette Series 8000 Holter a.
    Maxtec Handi oxygen a.
    Medigraphics 2000 a.
    MiniOX IA oxygen a.
    MiniOX 1000 oxygen a.
    nitric oxide a. (NOA)
    Omni a.
    Opti 1 pH/blood gas a.
    Opti 1 portable blood a.
    pacing system a.
    platelet function a. (PFA)
    PrinterNOx nitric oxide with
      MKII a.
    PulmoTrack respiratory sound a.
    pulse-height a.
    Rapidpoint Coag A.
    RapidVUE particle shape and
      size a.
    Roche a.
    Shimadzu DAR-2400 coronary
      arteriographic a.
    Sievers model 280 nitric oxide a.
    UltraSom computerized sleep a.
    Vitros a.
    wave a.
Anandron
anangioplasia
anangioplastic
anaphase arrest
anaphylactic
    a. antibody
    a. crisis
anaphylactoid
    a. purpura
    a. reaction

a. syndrome
a. syndrome of pregnancy
anaphylatoxin
chemotactic a.
anaphylaxis
eosinophil chemotactic factors of a. (ECF-A)
slow-reacting substance of a. (SRS-A)
anaplastic
a. carcinoma
a. tumor
anaplerosis
anaplerotic sequence
anapnea
anapneic
anapnotherapy
Anaprox
anaritide acetate
anasarca
AnastaFlo shunt
anastomose
anastomosis, pl. **anastomoses**
aortic a.
aortopulmonary a.
arterial a.
arteriolovenular a.
a. arteriolovenularis
a. arteriovenosa
arteriovenous a. (AVA)
Béclard a.
biatrial a.
bidirectional cavopulmonary a. (BCA)
bidirectional superior cavopulmonary a. (BSCA)
bronchial a.
cavoatrial a.
cavopulmonary a.
Clado a.
a. clamp
cobra-head a.
Cooley intrapericardial a.
Cooley modification of Waterston a.
cruciate a.
curved end-to-end a. (CEEA)
distal a.
end-to-end a.
extracardiac cavopulmonary a.
Fontan atriopulmonary a.
Glenn a.
Hoyer a.
intermesenteric arterial a.
Kugel a.
Nakayama a.
portacaval a. (PCA)
portoportal a.
portosystemic a.

Potts a.
Potts-Smith a.
precapillary a.
pulmonary artery a.
RA-RV a.
a. of Riolan
Sucquet a.
Sucquet-Hoyer a.
sutureless a.
systemic to pulmonary artery a.
total cavopulmonary a.
Waterston a.
anastomotic
a. branch
a. branch of middle meningeal artery with lacrimal artery
a. stricture
a. vein
a. vessel
anastomotica
arteria a.
anastrozole
anatomic
a. airway
a. assessment
a. block
a. dead space
a. localization
a. pulmonary atresia
anatomical reentry
anatomy, pl. **anatomies**
aortic arch a.
coronary a.
designed after natural a.
native coronary a.
natural a.
anatricrotic
anatricrotism
Anatuss DM
ANCA
antineutrophil cytoplasmic antibody
AnCC
anodal closure contraction
Ancef
anchor
Harpoon suture a.
anchovy paste sputum
ancillary measure
Ancobon
Ancor imaging system
Ancotil
ancrod
Ancure
A. abdominal aortic aneurysm system
A. stent-graft
Ancylostoma
A. *braziiiense*

Ancylostoma (continued)
    A. caninum
    A. duodenale
Andersen
    A. syndrome
    A. triad
Anderson
    A. phasing score
    A. procedure
    A. test
Anderson-Fabry disease
Anderson-Keys method
Anderson-Wilkins (AW)
    A.-W. acuteness score
Andes virus
Andral decubitus position
Andrews-Pynchon tube
Andrews retractor
Androcur Depot
Androderm Transdermal system
Android
android obesity
Androsov vascular stapler
AnDTe
    anodal duration tetanus
anechoic
Anectine Chloride
Anel operation
anemia
    angiopathic hemolytic a.
    aplastic a.
    chronic hemolytic a.
    Cooley a.
    hemodilutional a.
    hemolytic a.
    Mediterranean a.
    megaloblastic a.
    microangiopathic a.
    sickle cell a.
    splenic a.
anemic
    a. anoxia
    a. hypoxia
    a. murmur
anemometer
    hot-wire a.
    mass-flow a.
anergy
    skin test a.
aneroid manometer
anesthesia
    Bier block a.
    inhalational a.
    nonsurgical bypass without a.
    topical a.
anesthetic
    eutectic mixture of local a.'s
     (EMLA)
    halogenated a.

    inhalational a.
    local a.
aneuploid
AneuRx
    A. DTA stent graft system
    A. fully supported modular system
    A. IDS delivery system
    A. stent
    A. stent graft
aneurysm
    abdominal aortic a. (AAA)
    acute dissecting a.
    ampullary a.
    anterior communicating a. (ACA)
    aortic sinus a.
    aortoiliac a.
    apical a.
    arterial a.
    arteriosclerotic a.
    arteriovenous pulmonary a.
    a. of ascending aorta (AAA)
    ascending thoracic aortic a.
     (ATAA)
    atherosclerotic a.
    atrial septal a. (ASA)
    a. of atrial septum (AAS)
    axial a.
    basilar artery fusiform a.
    Berard a.
    berry a.
    bilobed a.
    brain a.
    cardiac a.
    cerebral a.
    Charcot-Bouchard a.
    chronic fusiform a.
    cirsoid a.
    congenital aortic a.
    coronary a.
    Crisp a.
    cylindroid a.
    descending thoracic a.
    dissecting aortic a.
    dolichoectatic a.
    ectatic a.
    embolic a.
    embolomycotic a.
    endoluminal reconstruction of
     basilar artery fusiform a.
    extremity-artery a.
    false aortic a.
    familial intracranial a.
    fusiform aortic a.
    giant a.
    infected a.
    infective a.
    inflammatory abdominal aortic a.
     (IAAA)
    infrarenal abdominal aortic a.

A

innominate a.
interatrial septal a. (IASA)
interventricular septum a.
intracranial fusiform a.
left ventricular a. (LVA)
luetic a.
mitral valve a.
mixed a.
mouth of a.
mural a.
mycotic aortic a.
Park a.
phantom a.
popliteal a.
Pott a.
racemose a.
Rasmussen a.
Richet a.
a. of right ventricle or right
  ventricular outflow tract
Rodriguez a.
ruptured aortic a.
ruptured sinus of Valsalva a.
  (RSVA)
saccular false a.
Salmonella mycotic a.
serpentine a.
Shekelton a.
sinus of Valsalva a.
a. of sinus of Valsalva
spurious a.
stent-assisted coiling of basilar
  fusiform a.
suprasellar a.
syphilitic aortic a.
thoracic aortic a. (TAA)
thoracoabdominal aortic a.
traction a.
traumatic aortic a.
true aortic a.
tuberculous mycotic a.
ventricular a. (VA)
a. of ventricular portion of
  membranous septum
verminous a.
wide-necked a.
windsock a.
a. wrapping
wrapping of abdominal aortic a.

aneurysmal, aneurysmatic
a. bone cyst
a. bruit
a. cough
a. dilation
a. hematoma
a. murmur
a. phthisis
a. sac

a. thrill
a. varix
aneurysmectomy
abdominal aortic a.
Matas a.
aneurysmography
aneurysmoplasty
aneurysmorrhaphy
aneurysmotomy
Anexsia
ANF
atrial natriuretic factor
ANG
angiogenin
angiogram
angiography
angiotensin
Angeflex defibrillation lead
Angeion 2000 ICD generator
AngeLase combined mapping-laser
  probe
Angelchik antireflux prosthesis
Angell-Shiley
A.-S. bioprosthetic valve
A.-S. xenograft prosthetic valve
angel's trumpet
Anger scintillation camera
Angestat hemostasis introducer
Angetear tearaway introducer
angialgia
angiasthenia
angiectasia
angiectasis, angiectasia
angiectatic
angiectopia
ANG I
angiotensin I
ANG II
angiotensin II
ANG III
angiotensin III
angiitis
allergic granulomatous a.
Churg-Strauss a.
hypersensitivity a.
leukocytoclastic a.
necrotizing a.
nonnecrotizing a.
angina
abdominal a.
antecedent a.
anxiety a.
bandlike a.
benign croupous a.
Bretonneau a.
Canadian class I–IV a.
chronic stable a.
classic a.
cold-induced a.

angina *(continued)*
    a. cordis
    coronary spastic a.
    crescendo a.
    a. crouposa
    a. cruris
    a. decubitus
    decubitus a.
    diet and stress management in a. (DSMA)
    a. dyspeptica
    a. of effort
    effort a.
    ergonovine maleate provocation a.
    esophageal a.
    exercise-induced a.
    exertional a.
    false a.
    first-effort a.
    food a.
    a. gangrenosa
    Heberden a.
    hippocratic a.
    hypercyanotic a.
    hysteric a.
    a. index score
    a. inversa
    ischemic rest a.
    lacunar a.
    a. laryngea
    Ludwig a.
    a. membranacea
    microvascular a.
    mixed a.
    neutropenic a.
    nocturnal a.
    nonexertional a.
    a. notha
    office a.
    pacing-induced a.
    a. pectoris (AP)
    a. pectoris decubitus
    a. pectoris sine dolore
    a. pectoris vasomotoria
    a. phlegmonosa
    postinfarction a.
    postprandial a.
    preinfarction a. (PIA)
    Prinzmetal variant a.
    pseudomembranous a.
    Randomized Intervention Treatment of A. (RITA)
    rate-dependent a.
    rebound a.
    reflex a.
    rest a.
    a. rheumatica
    a. scarlatinosa
    Schultz a.
    second-wind a.
    sexual a.
    silent a.
    a. simplex
    a. sine dolore
    smoking-induced a.
    a. spuria
    stable a. (SA)
    toilet-seat a.
    a. tonsillaris
    a. trachealis
    treadmill-induced a.
    a. ulcerosa
    unstable a. (UA)
    variable threshold a.
    variant a. (VA)
    vasomotor a.
    vasospastic a. (VSA)
    vasotonic a.
    Vincent a.
    walk-through a.
    warmup a.
    white-coat a.
    A. with Extremely Serious Operative Mortality Evaluation (AWESOME)

anginae
    Saccharomyces a.
angina-guided therapy
anginal
    a. equivalent
    a. pain
    a. perceptual threshold
anginiform
anginoid
anginophobia
anginosa
    syncope a.
anginose, anginous
anginosus
    status a.
    Streptococcus a.
anginosus-constellatus
    Streptococcus a.-c.
anginous *(var. of* anginose)
angioarchitecture
angioblast
angiocardiogram (ACG)
angiocardiography (ACG)
    equilibrium radionuclide a. (ERNA)
    first-pass radionuclide a.
    radionuclide a.
    transseptal a.
angiocardiokinetic
angiocardiopathy
angiocarditis
Angiocath catheter
angiocatheter
    large-bore a.

Angio-Conray contrast medium
Angiocor rotational thrombolizer
angiodermatitis
AngioDynamics SOS Omni selective
  catheter
angiodynia
angiodynography
angiodysplasia of colon
angiodystrophy
angioedema
angioendotheliomatosis
angiofibrosis
Angioflow high-flow catheter
angiofollicular lymph node hyperplasia
angiogenesis
    a. factor
    myocardial a.
    therapeutic a.
    transplant-related a.
angiogenic
    a. gene therapy agent (AGENT)
    a. squamous dysplasia
angiogenin (ANG)
angiogliomatosis
angiogliosis
Angiografin
angiogram (ANG)
    aortic root a. (ARA)
    ECG-synchronized digital
      subtraction a.
    gated nuclear a.
    pulmonary a.
    venous digital a.
    wedge a.
angiograph
angiographer
angiographic
    a. area of lateral projection (AL)
    a. area of left anterior oblique
      projection (ALAO)
    a. area of right anterior oblique
      projection (ARAO)
    a. assessment
    a. catheter
    a. contrast
    a. contrast injection system
      technology (ACIST)
    a. instrumentation
    a. measurement
angiographically
    a. occult abnormality
    a. occult intracranial vascular
      malformation (AOIVM)
    a. significant CAD
angiography (ANG)
    a. of abdominal aorta (AAA)
    aortography a.
    balloon-occlusion pulmonary a.
    biplane orthogonal a.

black blood a.
cardiac a.
carotid a.
cerebral a.
color power a.
computed tomography a. (CTA)
contrast a.
contrast-enhanced magnetic
  resonance a. (CEMRA, CE-MRA)
coronary a. (CAG)
coronary magnetic resonance a.
CT a.
digital a. (DA)
digital subtraction a. (DSA)
3-dimensional time-of-flight
  magnetic resonance a.
directional color a. (DCA)
3D TF magnetic resonance a.
elective a.
electron beam a.
electronic beam a. (EBA)
equilibrium radionuclide a. (ERNA)
first-pass radionuclide a.
fluorescein a.
FluoroPlus a.
free-breathing coronary magnetic
  resonance a.
gated blood-pool a.
gated radionuclide a.
general a. (GA)
indocyanine green a.
internal mammary artery graft a.
intraarterial digital subtraction a.
  (IADSA, IA-DSA)
intraoperative digital subtraction a.
  (IDISA)
intraoperative vascular a. (IVA)
intravenous digital subtraction a.
  (IVDSA)
left aortic a.
left atrial a.
left ventricular a.
magnetic resonance a. (MRA)
magnetic resonance coronary a.
  (MRCA)
mesenteric a.
multigated a.
noncardiac a.
nonselective coronary a.
Parodi catheter for a. (ParCA)
phase-contrast magnetic
  resonance a. (PC-MRA)
pulmonary a. (PA, PAG)
pulmonary wedge a.
quantitative coronary a. (QCA)
quantitative edge-detection a.
radionuclide a. (RNA)
renal a.
renovascular a.

angiography *(continued)*
   rest and exercise gated nuclear a.
   rest radionuclide a.
   saphenous vein bypass graft a.
   selective a.
   single breathhold cardiac-
      synchronized a.
   subtraction a.
   surveillance a.
   synchrotron-based transvenous a.
   thermal a.
   time-of-flight magnetic resonance a.
   total absence of circulation on 4-
      vessel a.
   ultrasound a.
   ventricular a.
   wedge pulmonary a.
AngioGuard
   A. catheter device
   A. embolic protection device
   A. filter
   A. filter device
   saphenous vein graft intervention
      using A. (GUARD)
   A. XP emboli capture guidewire
   A. XP emboli protection device
angiohyalinosis
angiohypertonia
angiohypotonia
angioid
angioinvasive
Angioject syringe
AngioJet
   Possis A.
   A. rapid thrombectomy system
   A. rheolytic thrombectomy system
   A. saline jet/vacuum device
      catheter
   A. thrombectomy catheter
   A. Xpeedior device
angiokeratoma corporis diffusum
angiokinesis
Angio-Kit catheter
angioleiomyoma
Angiolink staple-mediated closure
angiolipofibroma
angiolipoma
angiolith
angiolithic degeneration
angiologia
angiology
**angiolymphoid hyperplasia with
   eosinophilia**
angiolysis
angioma
   cavernous a.
   cherry a.
   a. serpiginosum

   spider a.
   a. venosum racemosum
AngioMARK contrast agent
**Angiomat Illumena contrast delivery
   system**
angiomatoid
angiomatosis
   bacillary a.
angiomatous
Angiomax
Angiomedics catheter
angiomegaly
angiomyocardiac
angiomyofibroma
angiomyolipoma
angiomyoma
angiomyopathy
angiomyosarcoma
angiomyxoma
angionecrosis
angioneuropathy
angioneurotic edema
angioosteohypertrophy syndrome
Angiopac
angioparalysis
angioparesis
angiopathic
   a. hemolytic anemia
   a. neuropathy
angiopathy
   cerebral amyloid a. (CAA)
   congophilic a.
   microvascular a. (MVA)
angiopeptin-eluting stent
angiophacomatosis
angioplany
angioplasia
angioplasty
   ablative laser a.
   adjunctive balloon a.
   balloon catheter a. (BCA)
   balloon coarctation a.
   balloon coronary a.
   balloon dilation a. (BDA)
   balloon laser a.
   bootstrap 2-vessel a.
   brachiocephalic vessel a.
   carotid patch a.
   carotid stent-supported a. (CSSA)
   complementary balloon a.
   a. complication
   coronary artery a.
   culprit lesion a.
   culprit vessel a.
   cutting balloon a. (CBA)
   direct acute myocardial
      infarction a. (DAMIA)
   direct coronary a.
   directional coronary a. (DCA)

Dotter-Judkins percutaneous transluminal a.
emergent a.
excimer laser-assisted a. (ELA)
excimer laser coronary a. (ECLA, ELCA)
facilitated a.
failed rescue a.
Grüntzig balloon catheter a.
a. guiding catheter
high-pressure adjunctive percutaneous transluminal coronary a.
high-risk a.
Ho:YAG laser a.
IVUS-guided balloon a.
Kinsey rotation atherectomy extrusion a.
kissing balloon a.
laser-assisted balloon a. (LABA)
laser balloon a. (LBA)
laser thermal a.
multilesion a.
new device a. (NDA)
Osypka rotational a.
patch a.
patch-graft a.
percutaneous balloon a.
percutaneous excimer laser coronary a. (PELCA)
percutaneous laser a.
percutaneous transluminal a. (PTA)
percutaneous transluminal balloon a. (PTBA)
percutaneous transluminal coronary a. (PTCA)
percutaneous transluminal renal a. (PTRA)
peripheral excimer laser a. (PELA)
peripheral laser a. (PLA)
peripheral transluminal a.
plain old balloon a. (POBA)
precoronary a.
primary percutaneous transluminal coronary a. (pPTCA)
rescue a.
salvage a. (SA)
salvage balloon a.
smooth excimer laser coronary a. (SELCA)
staged a.
stand-alone balloon a.
supported a.
thulium:YAG laser a.
tibioperoneal vessel a.
transluminal a. (TAP, TLA)
transluminal coronary a.
transradial coronary a.

1-vessel a.
vibrational a.
angioplasty-related vessel occlusion
angiopneumography
angiopoietin 1, 2
AngioRad
    A. Afterloader system
    A. radiation system
angiorrhaphy
angiosarcoma
angioscintigraphy
angiosclerotic gangrene
angioscope
angioscopic
    a. assessment
    a. valvulotome
angioscopy
    coronary a.
    intracoronary a.
    percutaneous intracoronary a.
    percutaneous transluminal a. (PTAS)
    pulmonary a.
AngioSculpt scoring balloon
Angio-Seal
    6-French A.-S.
    A.-S. hemostatic puncture closure device
    A.-S. vascular closure device
angiosis
Angioskop-D
angiospasm
Angiostar Plus vascular imaging equipment
angiostenosis
AngioStent
angiostomy
angiotensin (ANG, AT, At)
    a. I (A-I, A1, ANG I, AT I)
    a. I-converting enzyme
    a. II (A2, A-II, ANG II, AT II)
    a. III (ANG III)
    a. II-independent pathway
    a. II receptor blockade
    a. II receptor blocker (ARB)
    a. II type 1 (AT1)
    a. receptor blocker
    renin a.
    a. sensitivity test (AST)
angiotensinase
angiotensin-converting
    a.-c. enzyme (ACE)
    a.-c. enzyme antisense gene therapy
    a.-c. enzyme DD (ACE-DD)
    a.-c. enzyme DD, ID, II genotype
    a.-c. enzyme deletion/insertion polymorphism
    a.-c. enzyme ID (ACE-ID)

angiotensin-converting *(continued)*
    a.-c. enzyme II (ACE-II)
    a.-c. enzyme inhibitor (ACEI, ACEi)
angiotensinogen gene
angiotomy
Angiovist
angle
    aortomitral a.
    a. between QRS and T vectors
    blunted costophrenic a.
    cardiodiaphragmatic a.
    cardiophrenic a.
    Cobb a.
    costophrenic a.
    costovertebral a. (CVA)
    Ebstein a.
    flip a.
    a. of insonation
    intercept a.
    leaflet a.
    Louis a.
    Ludwig a.
    nail-to-nail bed a.
    phase a.
    Pirogoff a.
    QRS-T a.
    sternoclavicular a.
    tracheobronchial a.
    xiphoid a.
angled
    a. balloon catheter
    a. pigtail catheter
angle-tipped catheter
angor
    a. animi
    a. pectoris
Ang-O-Span
Angstrom
    A. II ICD
    A. MD ICD
    A. MD implantable single-lead cardioverter-defibrillator
angular
    a. artery
    a. gyrus (AG)
    a. vein
angulated
    a. coarctation
    a. multipurpose catheter
angulation
    caudal plane a.
    cranial a.
    RAO a.
angusta
    aorta a.
Angus technique
anhydrase

anhydride
    a. asthma
    coumaric a.
    hexahydrophthalic a. (HHPA)
    trimellitic a.
Anhydron
anhydrous ammonia
Anichkov *(var. of* Anitschkow)
animal dander
animi
    angor a.
anion
    a. exchange resin
    a. gap
    organic a.
    superoxide a.
anisa
    Legionella a.
anisindione
anisopiesis
anisorrhythmia
anisosphygmia
anisotropic
    a. conduction
    a. reentry
anisotropy
anisoylated plasminogen streptokinase activator complex (APSAC)
anistreplase
anitplatelet therapy
anitratum
    Bacterium a.
anitratus
    Acinetobacter a.
Anitschkow, Anichkov
    A. cell
    A. myocyte
ankle
    a. edema
    a. exercise
ankle-arm index
ankle-brachial
    a.-b. blood pressure ratio
    a.-b. index (ABI)
    a.-b. index test
ankle-foot orthosis (AFO)
ankylosing spondylitis
anlagen
annexin V
    technetium-99m-labeled a. V
annihilation photon
annotation
    marker a.
annular *(var. of* anular)
annuli *(var. of* anuli)
annuloaortic *(var. of* anuloaortic)
AnnuloFlex flexible annuloplasty ring

AnnuloFlo
    A. annuloplasty ring
    A. annuloplasty ring system
annuloplasty
    a. band
    Carpentier a.
    DeVega tricuspid valve a.
    Gerbode a.
    Kay a.
    mitral ring a.
    percutaneous transverse mitral a.
      (PTMA)
    prosthetic ring a.
    a. ring
    septal a.
    tricuspid valve a.
    Wooler-type a.
annulus (*var. of* anulus)
AnOC, AOC
    anodal opening contraction
anodal (AN)
    a. closure contraction (ACC,
      AnCC)
    a. closure sound (ACS)
    a. closure tetanus (ACTe)
    a. duration (AD)
    a. duration contraction (ADC)
    a. duration tetanus (ADTe, AnDTe)
    a. excitation
    a. opening (AO)
    a. opening clonus
    a. opening contraction (AnOC,
      AOC)
    a. opening order (AOO)
    a. opening picture (AOP)
    a. opening sound (AOS)
    a. opening tetanus (AOT, AOTe)
anode
anomalous
    a. atrioventricular
    a. atrioventricular excitation
    a. bronchus
    a. circumflex (ACx)
    a. complex
    a. conduction
    a. coronary origin (ACO)
    a. first rib thoracic syndrome
    a. left coronary artery (ALCA)
    a. left coronary artery arising from
      pulmonary artery (ALCAPA)
    a. left main coronary artery
      (ALMCA)
    a. mitral arcade
    a. movement
    a. origin
    a. origin of left coronary artery
      from pulmonary artery (ALCAPA)
    a. origin of left coronary artery
      from pulmonary artery syndrome

    a. pulmonary vein
    a. pulmonary venous connection
      (APVC)
    a. pulmonary venous connections,
      total or partial
    a. pulmonary venous drainage
      (APVD)
    a. pulmonary venous return
    a. rectification
anomaly, pl. **anomalies**
    aortic arch a.
    asplenia with cardiovascular
      anomalies
    atrioventricular connection a.
    coloboma, heart anomaly, choanal
      atresia, retardation, genital and
      ear anomalies (CHARGE)
    congenital conotruncal a.
    conotruncal a.
    coronary artery a.
    DiGeorge a. (DGA)
    Ebstein a.
    Freund a.
    LI single coronary artery a.
    pulmonary valve a.
    pulmonary venous connection a.
    pulmonary venous return a.
    Shone a.
    Taussig-Bing a.
    Uhl a.
    ventricular inflow a.
    vertebral, vascular, anal, cardiac,
      tracheoesophageal, renal, limb
      anomalies (VACTERL)
    viscerobronchial cardiovascular a.
Anopheles
anorexia nervosa
anorexigenic
anoxemia test
anoxia
    anemic a.
    anoxic a.
    cerebral a.
    diffusion a.
    myocardial a.
    a. neonatorum
    stagnant a.
anoxic anoxia
ANP
    atrial natriuretic peptide
    atrial natriuretic polypeptide
ANP-A
    atrial natriuretic peptide A
ANP-B
    atrial natriuretic peptide B
ANP-C
    atrial natriuretic peptide C

Anrep
>A. effect
>A. phenomenon

ANRL
>antihypertensive neutral renomedullary lipid

ANS
>autonomic nervous system

ansa cervicalis
ansamycin
Ansel Flexor introducer sheath
ANT
>adenine nucleotide translocator

antacid
antagonism
>accentuated a.

antagonist
>adrenergic a.
>aldosterone a.
>beta a.
>beta-1 a.
>beta-2 a.
>calcium a.
>calcium channel a. (CCA)
>dihydropyridine calcium a.
>dopamine a.
>endothelin a.
>glycoprotein IIb/IIIa a.
>interleukin receptor a.
>leukotriene receptor a.
>mediator receptor a.
>tachykinin receptor a.
>thromboxane receptor a.
>TNF-alpha a.
>vitamin K a.

Antarth
antasthmatic
antecedent
>a. angina
>plasma thromboplastin a. (PTA)

ante cibum (a.c.)
antecubital
>a. approach
>a. fossa
>a. space
>a. vein
>a. venipuncture

Ante-Flo
>Gelweave A.-F.

antegrade
>a. aortogram
>a. aortography
>a. approach
>a. block
>a. block cycle length
>a. brain perfusion
>a. cardioplegia
>a. collateral
>a. conduction

>a. diastolic flow
>a. double balloon/double wire technique
>a. internodal pathway
>a. refractory period

antegrade/retrograde cardioplegia technique
antemortem
>a. clot
>a. thrombus

antepartum monitor (APM)
anterior
>a. aortic wall (AAW)
>a. approach
>a. axillary line (AAL)
>a. border
>a. border of lung
>carpal arch a.
>a. cerebral artery (ACA)
>a. chamber (AC)
>a. choroidal artery (AChA)
>a. circulation (AC)
>a. circumflex humeral
>a. clear space
>a. communicating aneurysm (ACA)
>a. communicating artery (ACA, ACoA, AcomA)
>a. cusp
>a. cusp of mitral valve
>a. cusp of right atrioventricular valve
>a. cusp of tricuspid valve
>a. dentis
>a. descending artery (ADA)
>a. descending coronary artery
>a. descending segmental artery
>a. descending segmental artery of right lung
>a. fibrous trigone
>a. flail chest
>glandula lingualis a.
>a. inferior cerebellar artery (AICA)
>a. inferior communicating artery (AICA)
>a. inferior mandibular osteotomy (AIMO)
>a. internodal pathway
>a. internodal tract
>a. internodal tract of Bachmann
>a. junction line
>a. lateral myocardial infarct (ALMI)
>a. leaflet (AL)
>a. leaflet of mitral valve (ALMV)
>a. mediastinoscopy
>a. mediastinotomy
>a. mitral leaflet (AML)
>a. mitral leaflet extension
>a. mitral valve leaflet (aMVL)

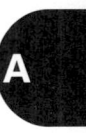

a. myocardial infarction
a. oblique (AO)
a. oblique projection
a. papillary muscle (APM)
a. papillary muscle of left
   ventricle
a. pulmonary leaflet
regio cruris a.
a. rib fracture
a. right ventricle (ARV)
a. sandwich patch technique
a. surface of heart
a. table
a. thoracic compression
a. thoracotomy
a. tracking of pML
a. tricuspid leaflet (ATL)
vena circumflexa humeri a.
a. wall (AW)
a. wall of aortic root (AWAR)
a. wall dyskinesis
a. wall infarction (AWI)
a. wall myocardial infarction
   (AWMI)
anteriores
venae cardiacae a.
anteriorly directed jet
anterius
segmentum bronchopulmonale
   basale a.
anteroapical dyskinesis
anterobasal wall
anterograde
a. APERP
a. block
a. conduction
a. flow
a. transseptal technique
anterogradely
anteroinferior myocardial infarction
anterolateral
a. flail chest
a. myocardial infarction
a. segment
a. wall myocardial infarct
   (ALWMI)
anteromesial hypokinesis
anteroposterior (AP)
a. dimension
a. paddle
a. paddle configuration
a. paddle location
a. paddle placement
a. paddle position
a. paddle positioning
a. projection
a. thoracic compression
a. thoracic diameter

anteroseptal
a. myocardial infarction (ASMI)
a. segment
anteroventral third ventricle (Av3V)
antesystole
anthopleurin-A
anthracis
Bacillus a.
anthraconecrosis
anthracosilicosis
anthracosis
anthracotic tuberculosis
anthracycline-induced cardiomyopathy
anthracycline toxicity
anthraquinone
anthrax
agricultural a.
cerebral a.
cutaneous a.
industrial a.
inhalational a.
intestinal a.
a. meningitis
a. pneumonia
pulmonary a.
a. septicemia
Anthron
A. heparinized antithrombogenic
   catheter
A. II catheter
anthropi
Ochrobactrum a.
anthropometric evaluation
**antiacetylcholine receptor antibody
   activity**
antiadhesion
a. antibody
a. clone
a. molecule
antiadrenergic
antiaggregant therapy
antialdosterone therapy
antialiasing technique
antianginal
a. agent
a. treatment
antiapoptosis
antiapoptotic effect
antiarrhythmic
a. agent
a. challenge
a. drug (AAD)
a. drug classification (Ia, Ib, Ic,
   II, III, IV)
a. medication
a. surgery
a. therapy
**antiarteriosclerosis polysaccharide factor
   (AAPF)**

antiasthmatic
antiatherogenic effect
antiatherosclerotic
antibacterial
antibasement membrane
anti-beta-1 adrenoreceptor antibody (ABAb)
antibiotic (ABx, ABX, abx)
    aerosolized a.
    antipseudomonal a.
    azalide class of a.'s
    a. class rotation
    a. efflux pump
    inhaled a.
    macrolide a.
    nonquinolone a.
    perioperative a.
    preoperative a.
    prophylactic a.
    a. sterilized aortic valve homograft (ASAH)
    streptogramin a.
antibody, pl. **antibodies**
    agglutinating a.
    alpha Gal a.
    anaphylactic a.
    antiadhesion a.
    anti-beta-1 adrenoreceptor a. (ABAb)
    anti-CagA serum a.
    anticardiolipin a. (ACLA, aCLa)
    anti-CD3 a.
    anti-CD11a a.
    anti-CD18 a.
    anti-CD31 a.
    anti-CD146 a.
    anticentromere a. (ACA)
    antidesmin a.
    anti-DNA a.
    antidystrophin a.
    antiglomerular basement membrane a.
    anti-GPIb a.
    antiheart a. (AHA)
    anti-IgE a.
    anti-Jo-1 a.
    anti-La a.
    antilactoferrin ANCA a.
    anti-MPO a.
    antimyosin a.
    antineutrophil cytoplasmic a. (ANCA)
    antinuclear a. (ANA)
    anti-omalizumab a.
    antiphospholipid a.
    antireceptor a.
    antiribonucleoprotein a.
    anti-Ro SSA a.
    anti-scl-70 a.
    anti-Sm a.
    anti-SSA/Ro a.
    anti-SSB/La a.
    B cell a.
    beta-adrenoceptor a.
    CD18 a.
    circulating antineutrophil cytoplasmic a. (cANCA)
    cross-reactive a.
    digitalis-specific a.
    direct fluorescent a. (DFA)
    7E3 glycoprotein IIb/IIIa platelet a.
    7E3 monoclonal Fab a.
    fibrin-specific a.
    fluorescence antimembrane a. (FAMA, FAMAT)
    fluorescent antimembrane a. (FAMA, FAMAT)
    glycolipid a.
    HMB45 a.
    huN901-DM1 a.
    IDEC-Y2B8 a.
    laminin a.
    monoclonal antifibronectin a.
    monoclonal anti-IgE a.
    monoclonal antimyosin a.
    monoclonal a. 3G4
    a. to murine cardiac myosin (AMM)
    myosin-specific a.
    OKT3 a.
    panel of reactive antibodies (PRA)
    panel-reactive a. (PRA)
    perinuclear antineutrophil cytoplasmic a. (pANCA)
    platelet a.
    Rh a.
    sheep antidigoxin Fab a.
    Sjögren syndrome A and B a. (SSA/SSB)
    streptococcal a.
    streptokinase a.
    teichoic acid a.
    thyroid a.
    tissue-specific a.
    treponemal a.
antibradycardia
anti-CagA serum antibody
anticardiac myosin (ACM)
anticardiolipin antibody (ACLA, aCLa)
anti-CD3 antibody
anti-CD11a antibody
anti-CD18 antibody
anti-CD31 antibody
anti-CD146 antibody
anticentromere antibody (ACA)
anticholinergic
    a. agent
    a. bronchodilator

anticipated systole
anticlot therapy
anticoagulant (AC)
    bridging a.
    circulating a. (CAC)
    lupus a.
    a. therapy (ACT)
anticoagulant-related hemorrhage
anticoagulation
    duration of a. (DURAC)
    a. regimen of aspirin
anticytokine therapy
antideoxyribonuclease B
antidepressant
    tricyclic a.
antidesmin antibody
antidiabetic agent
antidiuresis
    syndrome of inappropriate a.
     (SIAD)
antidiuretic
    a. hormone (ADH)
    a. hormone secretion
anti-DNA antibody
anti-DNase B
antidromic
    a. circus movement tachycardia
    a. conduction
    a. reciprocating tachycardia
antidysrhythmic
antidystrophin antibody
antielastase
antiendotoxin therapy
antiestrogen
antifactor
    a. Xa activity
    a. Xa inhibition
antifibrillatory
antifibrin antibody imaging
antifibrosis
antifilarial
antifoaming
    a. agent
    a. inhalant
antifolate
    multitargeted a.
antifungal
    azole a.
anti-FXa activity
antigen (Ag)
    Australia a.
    avian a.
    a. binding
    a. binding diversity
    bovine serum a.
    CagA a.
    carcinoembryonic a. (CEA)
    cephalin cholesterol a. (CCA)
    circulating anodic a. (CAA)

    cryptococcal capsular a.
    Epstein-Barr nuclear a. (EBNA)
    extractable nuclear a. (ENA)
    factor VII a. (FVIIag)
    heart shock protein a.
    Histoplasma polysaccharide a.
    HSP a.
    human leukocyte a. (HLA)
    inhalant a.
    KI a.
    KL-6 protein a.
    Legionella urinary a.
    Legionella urine a.
    O a.
    p24 a.
    PLA-I platelet a.
    platelet a. (PlA)
    proliferating cell nuclear a.
     (PCNA)
    recall a.
    serum cryptococcal a. (sCRAG)
    TF a.
    Thomsen-Friedenreich a.
    viral capsid a. (VCA)
    viral-free a. (VFA)
antigen-driven inflammatory reaction
antigenic
    a. drift
    a. shift
antigenicity
antigen-specific adaptive immune
  response
antiglomerular
    a. basement membrane antibody
    a. basement membrane disease
anti-GPIb antibody
antigravity suit
anti-G suit
antiheart
    a. antibody (AHA)
    a. antibody titer
    a. muscle autoantibody (AHMA)
antihemophilic
    a. factor (human)
    a. factor (recombinant)
antihistamine
antihypertensive
    a. agent
    a. diuretic therapy
    a. and lipid lowering (ALL)
    a. neutral renomedullary lipid
     (ANRL)
antihypotensive
anti-IgE antibody
antiinflammatory agent
antiinhibitor coagulant complex
antiischemic therapy
anti-Jo-1 antibody

anti-Jo-1-negative amyopathic dermatomyositis
anti-La antibody
antilactoferrin ANCA antibody
antileukotriene
antilipemic drug
antilymphocyte
    a. antibody preparation
    a. globulin (ALG)
    a. serum
antimalarial
    primaquine phosphate a.
antimetabolite
antimicrobial
    a. catheter cuff
    macrolide a.
    a. polymer material
    a. therapy
antimicrobial-resistant hospital-acquired pneumonia
antimicrotubule agent
antimitotic
antimony
    a. compound
    a. pentachloride
    a. pneumoconiosis
    a. potassium tartrate
    a. toxicity
    a. trichloride
    a. trioxide
anti-MPO antibody
antimuscarinic
antimycobacterial
    a. agent
    a. chemotherapy
antimycotic
antimyosin
    a. antibody
    a. antibody imaging
    a. autoantibody
    a. Fab fragment
    a. infarct-avid scintigraphy
    a. monoclonal antibody with Fab fragment (AMA-Fab)
antinatriuretic
antineoplastic effect
antineutrophil cytoplasmic antibody (ANCA)
antinuclear antibody (ANA)
anti-omalizumab antibody
antioncogene
antioxidant
antioxidative
antiparasitic
antiphospholipid (APL)
    a. antibody
    a. syndrome
antiphosphotyrosine immunoblot
antiplasmin

antiplatelet
    a. agent
    a. therapy
    A. Trialists' Collaboration (ATC)
antipneumococcal
antipodal
antipode
antiport
antiporter
antipressor
antiprotease
antiproteinase
antiproteolytic defense
antipseudomonal antibiotic
antipyrine salicylate
antireceptor antibody
antireflux
    a. prosthesis
    a. therapy
antirestenotic stent
antiretroviral therapy
anti-Rho(D) titer
antiribonucleoprotein antibody
anti-Ro SSA antibody
anti-scl-70 antibody
antisense oligodeoxynucleotide
antiseptic-impregnated central venous catheter
antishock garment
antisialagogue
anti-Sm antibody
antisnoring
anti-SSA/Ro antibody
anti-SSB/La antibody
antistasin
antistreptokinase
antistreptolysin O (ASO)
antistreptozyme test
antitachycardia
    a. pacemaker (ATP)
    a. pacing (ATP)
    a. pacing therapy
antitemplate
antithrombin (AT, At)
    a. III (AT-III)
    a. III deficiency
    recombinant human a. III (rhATIII)
antithromboplastin
antithrombotic
    a. factor
    a. prophylaxis
    a. regimen
antithymocyte globulin
antitopoisomerase
    a. I, II
    a. I, II antibody
antitoxin
    diphtheria a.

antitrypsin
    alpha-1 a. (AAT)
    a. deficiency
    M-type alpha-1 a.
    plasma alpha-1 a. (pAAT)
    recombinant alpha-1 a. (rAAT)
antituberculin
antituberculous
    a. chemotherapy
    a. drug
    a. therapy
antitubulin
antitussive
anti-VEGF
anti-Xa
    a.-Xa activity
    a.-Xa level
antler sign
antra (*pl. of* antrum)
antrectomy
Antrin
antrum, pl. **antra**
    cardiac a.
Antyllus method
anular, annular
    a. abscess
    a. array transducer
    a. calcification
    a. cartilage
    a. constriction
    a. dehiscence
    a. dilation
    a. flow
    a. ligament
    a. ligament of trachea
    a. phased array system (APAS)
    a. plane
    a. thrombus
anuloaortic, annuloaortic a. ectasia (AAE)
anulus, annulus, pl. **anuli**
    aortic a.
    aortic valve a. (AVA)
    atrioventricular a.
    a. fibrosus
    a. fibrosus dexter/sinister cordis
    mitral valve a.
    a. ovalis
    tricuspid valve a.
anxiety
    a. angina
    a. attack
    a. neurosis
anxiolysis
anxiolytic
any-plane echocardiography
AO
    abdominal aorta
    airways obstruction

    anodal opening
    anterior oblique
    aorta
    aortic opening
    atrioventricular valve opening
Ao
    aorta
AOA
    aortic orifice area
AoBP
    aortic blood pressure
AOC (*var. of* AnOC)
    anodal opening contraction
AOD
    arterial occlusive disease
    arterial oxygen desaturation
    arteriosclerotic occlusive disease
AOIVM
    angiographically occult intracranial
      vascular malformation
AOM
    ambulatory oximetry monitoring
AOMP, AoMP
    aortic mean pressure
AOO
    anodal opening order
    atrial asynchronous
      AOO pacemaker
      AOO pacing
AOP
    anodal opening picture
    aortic pressure
AoP
    aortic pressure
AOPW, AoPW
    aortic posterior wall
aorta, pl. **aortae (AO, Ao)**
    abdominal a. (AA, AO)
    a. abdominalis
    abdominal part of descending a.
    aneurysm of ascending a. (AAA)
    angiography of abdominal a.
      (AAA)
    a. angusta
    arch of a.
    arcus aortae
    a. ascendens
    ascending a. (AA, AAO, ACS,
      AsAo)
    bifurcation of a.
    buckled a.
    buckling of a.
    bulb of a.
    button of a.
    a. chlorotica
    coarctation of a. (CoA)
    cross-clamping of a.
    cystic medial necrosis of
      ascending a. (CMN-AA)

aorta *(continued)*
    a. descendens
    descending a. (DA, DAo)
    descending thoracic a. (DTA)
    dextropositioned a.
    dissecting a.
    dissection of a.
    double-barreled a.
    dynamic a.
    eggshell a.
    Erdheim cystic medial necrosis
      of a.
    esophageal branch of thoracic a.
    kinked a.
    medionecrosis aortae
    medionecrosis of a.
    overriding a.
    porcelain a.
    primitive a.
    pseudocoarctation of a.
    a. to pulmonary artery shunt
    recoarctation of a.
    retroesophageal a.
    sacrococcygeal a.
    straddling a.
    terminal a.
    a. thoracalis
    thoracic a. (ThA)
    a. thoracica
    transposition of a. (TA)
    tuberculous mycotic aneurysm of a.
    valvula coronaria dextra valvae
      aortae
aortal
aorta-left atrium ratio
aortalgia
aortarctia
aortartia
aortectasis, aortectasia
aortectomy
aortic
    a. anastomosis
    a. aneurysmal disease
    a. aneurysm clamp
    a. anulus
    a. arch (AA)
    a. arch anatomy
    a. arch anomaly
    a. arch arteriogram
    a. arch atheroma
    a. arch cannula
    a. arch epinephrine
    a. arch flush (AAF)
    a. arch interruption
    a. arch replacement
    a. arch syndrome (AAS)
    a. arch vessel
    a. arch vessel obstruction
    a. area

    a. area of auscultation
    a. arteritis syndrome
    a. assist balloon introducer
    a. atherosclerosis
    a. atresia
    a. bifurcation
    a. bioprosthesis stentless pericardial
      aortic heart valve replacement
    a. bioprosthetic valve
    a. blood flow (ABF)
    a. blood pressure (AoBP)
    a. body
    a. bulb
    a. catheter
    a. closure (AC)
    a. closure sound
    a. coarctation
    a. commissure
    a. compliance (AC)
    A. Connector system
    a. contour
    a. counterpulsation
    a. cross-clamp
    a. cross-sectional area/height ratio
      timing
    a. cuff
    a. cusp
    a. cusp separation
    a. degradation
    a. depressor nerve (ADN)
    a. dicrotic notch pressure
    a. dilation
    a. dissection (type A, B)
    a. distensibility
    a. ductal flow
    a. dwarfism
    a. ejection sound (AES)
    a. embolism
    a. endocarditis
    a. endograft
    a. end pulmonic
    a. envelope
    a. facies
    a. first sound (A1)
    a. flow (AF)
    a. flow velocity (AFV)
    a. hiatus
    a. homograft
    a. impedance
    a. incompetence (AI)
    a. injury
    a. insufficiency (AI)
    a. intramural hematoma (AIH)
    a. intramural hemorrhage (AIH)
    a. isthmus
    a. jet velocity
    a. knob
    a. knuckle
    left atrial to a.

a. and left ventricular tunnel (ALVT)
a. lumen
a. mean pressure (AOMP, AoMP)
a. nerve
a. nipple
a. notch
a. obscuration
a. opening (AO)
a. orifice
a. orifice area (AOA)
a. override
a. perfusion cannula
a. posterior wall (AOPW, AoPW)
a. pressure (AOP, AoP, AP)
a. pressure gradient
a. prosthesis
a. pullback
a. pullback pressure
a. pulse-wave velocity
a. reconstruction
a. reflex
a. regurgitation (AR)
a. regurgitation murmur
a. remodeling
a. ring
a. root
a. root abscess
a. root angiogram (ARA)
a. root compression
a. root dimension
a. root ratio
a. root replacement (ARR)
a. rupture
a. sac
a. sclerotic murmur
a. second sound opening snap (A2-OS)
a. second sound, pulmonary second sound (A2P2)
a. septal defect
a. sinus
a. sinus aneurysm
a. sinus cusp
a. sinus of Valsalva (ASOV)
a. sound (AS)
a. spindle
a. stenosis
a. stenosis jet
a. stenosis murmur
a. stiffness index
a. systolic pressure (ASP)
a. thrill
a. thromboembolic disease
a. thrombosis
a. triangle
a. tube graft
a. tunica adventitious breath sounds

a. tunica intima
a. tunica media
a. valve (AOV, AoV, AV)
a. valve anulus (AVA)
a. valve area (AVA)
a. valve atresia (AVA)
a. valve closure (AVC)
a. valve disease
a. valve echocardiogram (AVE)
a. valve gradient (AVG)
a. valve leaflet
a. valve opening (AVO)
a. valve orifice (AVO)
a. valve prolapse
a. valve regurgitation
a. valve replacement (AVR)
a. valve resistance
a. valve restenosis
a. valve rongeur
a. valve sclerosis
a. valve stenosis (AVS)
a. valve stroke volume (AVSV)
a. valve vegetation
a. valve velocity profile
a. valvoplasty
a. valvotomy
a. valvular disease (AVD)
a. valvular insufficiency
a. valvulitis
a. vasa vasorum
a. window
aortic-femoral-femoral
    descending thoracic a.-f.-f. (DTAF-F)
aortic-left ventricular tunnel murmur
aortic-mitral combined disease murmur
aorticopulmonary (*var. of* aortopulmonary)
aorticorenal
aortic-time-velocity integral
aorticus
    hiatus a.
    torus a.
aortismus abdominalis
aortitis
    arthritis-associated a.
    Döhle-Heller a.
    giant cell a.
    luetic a.
    nummular a.
    rheumatic a.
    syphilitic a.
    Takayasu a.
aortoannular ectasia
aortobifemoral (ABF)
aortobiiliac bypass
aortobronchopulmonary fistula
aortocarotid bypass

aortocaval
    a. compression syndrome
    a. fistula
aortocoronary (AC)
    a. bypass (A-C, ACB)
    a. bypass graft (ACBG)
    a. graft (ACG)
    a. saphenous vein (ACSV)
    a. saphenous vein bypass
    a. saphenous vein bypass graft
     (ACSVBG)
    a. snake graft
    a. venous bypass (ACVB)
aortoenteric fistula (AEF)
aortofemoral
    a. arterial runoff
    a. arteriography
    a. artery shunt
    a. bypass (AFB)
    a. bypass graft (AFBG)
aortogram
    antegrade a.
    digital subtraction supravalvular a.
    end-on a.
    flush a.
    rotational a.
    translumbar a. (TLA)
    a. with distal runoff
aortography
    abdominal a.
    a. angiography
    antegrade a.
    arch a.
    ascending a.
    atherosclerotic a.
    biplane a.
    caudally angled balloon
     occlusion a.
    digital subtraction supravalvular a.
    flush a.
    laid-back balloon occlusion a.
    mycotic a.
    retrograde a.
    selective a.
    single-plane a.
    sinus of Valsalva a.
    supravalvar a.
    thoracic arch a.
    transbrachial a.
    translumbar a.
    traumatic a.
    true versus false aneurysm a.
aortoiliac
    a. aneurysm
    a. bypass
    a. bypass graft
    a. obstructive disease (AIOD)
    a. occlusive disease
    a. thrombosis

aortoiliofemoral
    a. bypass
    a. circuit
    a. endarterectomy
aortolith
aortomalacia
aortomitral angle
aortomonoiliac graft
aortomyoplasty
aorto-ostial
    a.-o. junction
    a.-o. lesion
aortopathy
aortoplasty
    subclavian flap a. (SFA)
aortoptosia, aortoptosis
aortopulmonary, aorticopulmonary (AP)
    a. anastomosis
    a. collateral
    a. collateral artery (APC)
    a. fenestration
    a. septal defect (APSD)
    a. shunt
    a. window (APW)
aortorenal bypass
aortorrhaphy
aortosclerosis
aortostenosis
aortosubclavian bypass
aortosubclavian-carotid-axilloaxillary
  bypass
aortotomy
aortovelography
    transvenous a. (TAV)
AOS
    anodal opening sound
A2-OS
    aortic second sound opening snap
AOT
    acute occlusive thrombosis
    acute occlusive thrombus
AOT, AOTe
    anodal opening tetanus
AOU
    amount of use
AOV, AoV
    aortic valve
AP
    accessory pathway
    activator protein
    active pressure
    alkaline phosphatase
    alveolar permeability
    angina pectoris
    anteroposterior
    aortic pressure
    aortopulmonary
    apical pulse
    arterial pressure

atherosclerotic plaque
atrial pacing
atrioventricular pathway
    AP projection
A&P
    auscultation and percussion
AP-1 complex
A2P2
    aortic second sound, pulmonary second
      sound
APAAP
    alkaline phosphatase antialkaline
      phosphatase
APACHE
    Acute Physiology, Age, Chronic Health
      Evaluation
      APACHE II, III
      APACHE CV Risk Predictor
      APACHE score
apallic syndrome
APAP
    automatic positive airway pressure
APAS
    anular phased array system
apathetic hyperthyroidism
APB
    atrial premature beat
APBF
    accessory pulmonary blood flow
APC
    aortopulmonary collateral artery
    argon plasma coagulation
    argon plasma coagulator
    aspirin, phenacetin, caffeine
    atrial premature contraction
      blocked APC
APCG
    apexcardiogram
Ap4CH
    apical 4-chamber plane
APD
    action potential duration
    airway pressure disconnect
    atrial premature depolarization
APE
    acute pulmonary edema
A-peak velocity
ApEn
    approximate entropy
APERP
    accessory pathway effective refractory
      period
      anterograde APERP
Apert syndrome
aperture
    laryngeal a.
    transducer a.
apex, pl. **apices**
    a. beat (AB)

cardiac a.
a. cordis
false a.
hypertrophied a.
a. impulse
left ventricular a.
a. of lung
a. murmur
a. pneumonia
a. pulmonis
right ventricular a. (RVA)
ventricular a.
apexcardiogram (ACG, APCG)
apexcardiography (ACG)
aphasia
    ataxic a.
    expressive a.
    global a.
    nonfluent a.
    receptive a.
    Wernicke a.
aphasic
apheresis
    lipoprotein a.
    low-density lipoprotein a. (LDLA)
aphonic pectoriloquy
aphrophilus
    Haemophilus a.
API
    arterial pressure index
apical (A)
    a. abscess
    a. aneurysm
    a. blunting
    a. bronchopulmonary segment
    a. bronchus
    a. cap
    a. 2-chamber
    a. 4-chamber
    a. 4-chamber plane (Ap4CH)
    a. 2-chamber view
    a. 4-chamber view
    a. 2-chamber view echocardiogram
    a. 4-chamber view echocardiogram
    a. 5-chamber view echocardiogram
    a. diverticulum
    a. hematoma
    a. hypertrophy
    a. hypoperfusion
    a. hypoperfusion on thallium scan
    a. impulse (AI)
    a. infarction
    a. interventricular septal amplitude
    a. left ventricular puncture
    a. lordotic roentgenogram
    a. mid diastolic heart murmur
    a. pleural bleb
    a. pleural thickening
    a. pneumonia

A

apical *(continued)*
>   a. pseudoaneurysm
>   a. pulse (AP)
>   a. scarring
>   a. shelf
>   a. systolic heart murmur
>   a. tailoring
>   a. tailoring thoracoplasty

apicale
>   segmentum bronchopulmonale a.

apicalis

apices (*pl. of* apex)

apicobasal gradient

apicolysis
>   extrapleural a.
>   Semb a.

apicoposterior
>   a. branch of left
>   a. bronchopulmonary segment

apiospermum
>   *Scedosporium a.*

apista
>   *Pandoraea a.*

APIVR
>   artificial pacemaker-induced ventricular rhythm

APL
>   antiphospholipid

aplasia
>   bone marrow a.
>   focal media a.
>   pulmonary a.

aplastic anemia

apleuria

Aplisol

APM
>   antepartum monitor
>   anterior papillary muscle
>   Nicolet VersaLab APM

APM-2000 vital signs monitor

apnea
>   age-dependent a.
>   age-related a.
>   a. and bradycardia (A&B)
>   central a.
>   central sleep a. (CSA)
>   deglutition a.
>   end-expiratory a.
>   idiopathic central sleep a.
>   a. index (AI)
>   initial a.
>   late a.
>   mixed a. (MA)
>   a. monitor
>   a. neonatorum
>   obstructive sleep a. (OSA)
>   posthyperventilation a.

>   sleep a.
>   traumatic a.

apnea-hypopnea index (AHI)

apneic
>   a. oxygenation
>   a. pause

apneumatosis

apneumia

apneusis

apneustic
>   a. breathing
>   a. respiration

apo
>   apolipoprotein

apoA
>   apolipoprotein A

Apo-Amoxi

Apo-Ampi

Apo-ASA

Apo-Atenol

apoB
>   apolipoprotein B

apoC
>   apolipoprotein C

Apo-Capto

Apo-Cephalex

Apo-Chlorpromazine

Apo-Chlorthalidone

Apo-Clonidine

Apo-Cloxi

Apocynum venetum leaf extract

apoD
>   apolipoprotein D

Apo-Diltiaz

Apo-Dipyridamole FC

apoE
>   apolipoprotein E
>   apoE test

Apo E3 isoform

Apo-Enalapril

Apo-Erythro E-C

Apo-Furosemide

Apo-Gain

Apogee CX 100 Interspec ultrasound machine

Apo-Guanethidine

Apo-Hydralazine

Apo-Hydro

Apo-Hydroxyzine

Apo-ISDN

apoJ
>   apolipoprotein J

apolipoprotein (apo)
>   a. A (apoA)
>   a. AI
>   a. AI deficiency
>   a. AII
>   a. AIV
>   a. B (apoB)

a. B48
a. B100
a. C (apoC)
a. CI-CIII
a. D (apoD)
a. E (apoE)
familial defective a. B (FDB)
a. J (apoJ)
a. regulatory protein (ARP)
Apollo Light Systems
Apo-Methyldopa
Apo-Metoprolol
Apo-Nadol
aponeurosis
Sibson a.
aponeurotic
Apo-Nifed
Apo-Pen VK
Apo-Pindol
apoplectic
a. coma
a. cyst
apoplexy
asthenic a.
capillary a.
cerebral a.
ingravescent a.
Apo-Prazo
Apo-Prednisone
Apo-Procainamide
Apo-Propranolol
apoprotein
a. A1, A2
surfactant a. B
ApopTag kit
apoptosis
cardiac myocyte a.
cardiomyocyte a.
cellular a.
cortical neuronal a.
endothelial cell a.
hippocampal neuronal a.
ischemia/reperfusion-induced a.
myocyte a.
apoptotic
a. cell
a. cell death
a. change
a. destruction
a. endothelial microparticle
a. nucleus
a. pathway
A-Port vascular access
Apo-Salvent
aposthematosa
pneumonia a.
Apo-Sulfatrim
Apo-Tamox
Apo-Timol

Apo-Timop
Apo-Triazide
Apo-Verap
Apo-Zidovudine
APP
amyloid precursor protein
apparatus
Benedict-Roth a.
Fell-O'Dwyer a.
Jacquet a.
Langendorff a.
mitral a.
Nakayama anastomosis a.
a. respiratorius
respiratory a.
subvalvar a.
V-Vac suction a.
apparent
a. diffusion coefficient (ADC)
a. diffusion coefficient imaging
a. life-threatening event (ALTE)
appearance
acromegaloid facial a. (AFA)
bunch-of-grapes a.
cluster-of-grapes a.
cottage-loaf a.
dirty lung a.
finger-in-glove a.
ground-glass a.
hazy a.
saddle-backed a.
salt and pepper a.
tree-in-winter a.
appendage
atrial a.
auricular a.
left atrial a. (LAA)
right atrial a. (RAA)
appendectomy
atrial a.
auricular a.
applanation tonometry
apple picker's disease
applesauce sign
appliance
EMA a.
mandibular advancement a. (MAA)
oral a. (OA)
OSAP a.
SNOAR open airway a.
Snore-Ezzer oral a.
TheraSnore oral a.
application
MCAS modular clip a.
applicator
RapidMist metered dose spray a.
apposition
mitral-septal a.

apposition *(continued)*
    pleural-pleural a.
    stent a.
approach
    antecubital a.
    antegrade a.
    anterior a.
    Biosense revascularization a.
    Bobath physiotherapy a.
    brachial artery a.
    central a.
    cephalic a.
    dietary a.
    external jugular a.
    femoral a.
    groin a.
    Lortat-Jacob a.
    MIDCAB saloon door a.
    open lung a.
    percutaneous a.
    posterior a.
    radial a.
    retrograde femoral a.
    revascularization a.
    saloon door parasternal a.
    segmented K-space a.
    selective transvenous a.
    stepped bur a.
    tandem needle a.
    transradial a.
    transseptal a.
    transxiphoid a.
    trapdoor a.
approximate entropy (ApEn)
approximation
    Friedewald a.
    leaflet a.
approximator
    rib a.
apraxia
    buccolingual a.
    ideational a.
    ideomotor a.
    limb-kinetic a.
Apresoline
    A. injection
    A. Oral
aprindine
Aprinox
Aprodine
    A. Syrup
    A. Tablet
    A. w/C
aprotinin
APRV
    airway pressure release ventilation
APSAC
    anisoylated plasminogen streptokinase
    activator complex

APSD
    aortopulmonary septal defect
APSP
    assisted peak systolic pressure
APSS
    Associations of Professional Sleep
      Societies
Aptaer heliox delivery system
aptiganel
APT program
APTT, aPTT
    activated partial thromboplastin time
Apt test
APV
    average peak velocity
APVC
    anomalous pulmonary venous connection
APVD
    anomalous pulmonary venous drainage
APW
    aortopulmonary window
AQ
    acoustic quantification
      Nasacort AQ
AQLQ
    Asthma Quality of Life Questionnaire
aqua
      Rhinocort A.
Aquacare topical
aquae
aquagenic urticaria
Aquapheresis advance ultrafiltration
  procedure
aquaporin
aquaretic agent
Aqua-Seal chest drainage unit
AquaShield
Aquatherm radiant heat device
Aquazide
aqueductal stenosis
aqueous
      a. epinephrine
      a. oxygen
      a. solution for nebulization
      a. vasopressin (AVP)
AR
    acute rejection
    adrenergic receptor
    aortic regurgitation
    atrial rate
    atrial reversal
      beta-1 AR
      beta-2 AR
      AR jet height
AR-1 catheter
ARA
    aortic root angiogram

arachidic bronchitis
arachidonate (AA)
    a. metabolism
arachidonic
    a. acid (AA)
    a. acid cascade
    a. acid metabolite
arachidonylethanolamide
arachnodactyly
arachnophlebectomy
    a. needle
    a. procedure
    a. surgical device
ARAD
    abnormal right axis deviation
Aralast
Aralen Phosphate
Aramine
araneus
    nevus a.
arantii
    ductus a.
Arantius
    A. body
    body of A.
    canal of A.
    A. nodule
ARAO
    angiographic area of right anterior
    oblique projection
ARB
    angiotensin II receptor blocker
Arbeitsgemeinschaft Leitende
    Kardiologische Krankenhausarzte
    (ALKK)
arbitrary densitometric unit (ADU)
arborization block
arbovirus
arbutamine
ARC
    Active Response Catheter
arc
    a. of calcium
    hiccup reflex a.
    a. of Vieussens
    a. welder's pneumoconiosis
ARC-22 coronary balloon angioplasty
    catheter
arcade
    anomalous mitral a.
    arterial a.
    a. collateral
    mitral a.
    polygonal a.
    septal a.
arcanobacterial pharyngitis
arch
    abdominothoracic a.
    a. of aorta

aortic a. (AA)
    a. aortography
    a. arteriography
    axillary a.
    azygos a.
    carotid a.
    cervical aortic a.
    circumflex aortic a.
    congenital interrupted aortic a.
    double aortic a.
    interrupted aortic a. (IAA)
    jugular venous a.
    Langer axillary a.
    palmar a.
    pharyngeal a.
    pulmonary a.
    right aortic a.
    transverse aortic a. (TAA)
    Zimmermann a.
arch-first technique
Architect CTSTAT myoglobin assay
architecture
    lung a.
    sleep a.
    ventricular a.
arcus
    a. aortae
    corneal a.
    a. cornealis
    a. costarum
    a. lipoices
    a. senilis
ARD
    acute respiratory disease
ardeparin sodium
ARDS
    acute respiratory distress syndrome
    adult respiratory distress syndrome
    posttraumatic ARDS
Ardystil syndrome
area, pl. areae, areas
    aortic a.
    aortic orifice a. (AOA)
    aortic valve a. (AVA)
    Bamberger a.
    body surface a. (BSA)
    Brodmann a. 7, 9, 24, 40
    a. of cardiac dullness (ACD)
    cross-sectional a. (CSA)
    a. diastolic pressure (ADP)
    echo-spared a.
    EEL a.
    effective balloon-dilated a. (EBDA)
    effective orifice a. (EOA)
    end-diastolic a. (EDA)
    endocardial surface a. (ESA)
    Erb a.
    external elastic lamina a.
    geometric orifice a. (GOA)

area *(continued)*
    Head a.
    intrastent minimal lumen cross-sectional a. (ISMLCSA)
    in vitro effective orifice a.
    Killian-Jamieson a.
    Krönig a.
    left atrial a. (LAA)
    left atrial appendage a.
    left ventricular end-diastolic a. (LVEDA)
    local organ procurement a.
    mitral anular a.
    mitral valve a. (MVA)
    mitral valve orifice a. (MVOA)
    mounting a. (MA)
    noncontractile a. (NCA)
    occluded a.
    plaque a.
    precoronary care a. (PCA)
    proximal isovelocity surface a. (PISA)
    pulmonary valve a.
    pulmonic a.
    radiofrequency energy a.
    regurgitant jet a.
    regurgitant orifice a. (ROA)
    secondary aortic a.
    sewing ring a. (SRA)
    stenosed a.
    a. of stenosis (AS)
    subxiphoid a.
    supplemental motor a. (SMA)
    a. systolic pressure (ASP)
    targeted a.
    tricuspid valve a.
    truncoconal a.
    valve orifice a.
area-length
    a.-l. method
    a.-l. method for ejection
areflexia
    flaccid a.
Arelix
Arenaviridae virus
ARF
    acute respiratory failure
    acute rheumatic fever
ArF excimer laser
argatroban
Argesic-SA
arginine
    a. aminotransferase
    a. tolerance test (ATT)
    a. vasopressin (ARVP, AVP)
    a. vasotocin (AVT)
argipressin
argon
    a. beam coagulator

    a. ion laser
    a. needle
    a. plasma coagulation (APC)
    a. plasma coagulator (APC)
    a. plasma emission spectroscope
    a. plasma emission spectroscopy
    a. pumped tuneable dye laser
Argyle
    A. catheter
    A. CPAP nasal cannula
Argyle-Turkel thoracentesis
Argyll Robertson pupils
ARHS
    acute right heart syndrome
ARI
    airways reactivity index
aria
    A. coronary artery bypass graft
    A. LX CPAP system
Ariflo
Arimidex
Aristocort
    A. Forte
    A. Forte Injection
    A. Intralesional Injection
    A. Intralesional Suspension
    A. Oral
    A. Tablet
Aristospan
    A. Intraarticular Injection
    A. Intralesional Injection
Arixtra subcutaneous injection
arjuna
    Terminalia a.
ARK
    adrenergic receptor kinase
    beta ARK
ARK-1
    adrenergic receptor kinase 1
    beta ARK-1
Arkin-Z
ARL
    AIDS-related lymphoma
ARLL
    AIDS-related lymphoma of lung
Arloing-Courmont test
arm
    blood pressure, left a. (BPLA)
    blood pressure, right a. (BPRA)
    a. cranking
    a. cycle ergometry
    a. ergometry treadmill
    a. exercise stress test
Arm-a-Med endotracheal tube
armamentarium
arm-ankle indices
armed long sheath
arm-leg gradient
armored heart

armor heart
Armour Thyroid
ARMS
   access by radial artery multilink stent
Armstrong handheld pulse oximeter
arm-tongue
   a.-t. time
   a.-t. time test
arnica
aromatic
   A. Ammonia Aspirols
   a. ammonia spirit
arousal
   a. index
   mini a.
   respiratory effort-related a. (RERA)
ARP
   absolute refractory period
   apolipoprotein regulatory protein
ARR
   absolute risk reduction
   aortic root replacement
array
   convex linear a.
   multielement linear a.
   sock a.
   symmetrical phased a.
arrest
   a. after arrival (AAA)
   anaphase a.
   arrhythmic cardiac a. (ACA)
   asphyxial cardiac a.
   asystolic a.
   a. before arrival (ABA)
   blunt chest impact-induced
      cardiac a.
   bradyarrhythmic a.
   bradyasystolic a.
   cardiac a. (CA)
   cardioplegic a.
   cardiopulmonary a. (CPA)
   cardiorespiratory a.
   chronic sinus a.
   circulatory a.
   cold ischemic a.
   deep hypothermia circulatory a.
      (DHCA)
   dysrhythmic cardiac a.
   fatal cardiac a.
   heart a.
   hypothermic fibrillating a.
   intermittent sinus a.
   nonprimary cardiac a.
   out-of-hospital cardiac a. (OHCA,
      OOH/CA)
   prehospital cardiac a. (PCA)
   respiratory a.
   secondary a. (SA)
   sinuatrial a.

sinus a. (SA)
sudden cardiac a. (SCA)
total circulatory a. (TCA)
ventricular fibrillation a.
arrest-and-reversal treatment
arrested
   a. heart totally endoscopic coronary
      artery bypass grafting
      (AHTECAB)
   a. tuberculosis
Arrhigi
   point of A.
arrhythmia
   atrial a.
   atrioventricular junctional a.
   A-V nodal Wenckebach a.
   baseline a.
   burst of a.
   cardiac a.
   a. circuit
   a. circuit cryoablation
   continuous a.
   a. control device (ACD)
   cyanotic congenital heart disease a.
   exercise-induced a.
   a. focus
   hypokalemia-induced a.
   inducible a.
   inotropic a.
   juvenile a.
   lethal a.
   long QT a.
   Lown a.
   malignant a. (MA)
   malignant ventricular a. (MVA)
   a. mapping system
   Mönckeberg a.
   A. Net arrhythmia monitor
   nodal a.
   nonphasic sinus a.
   nonsuppressible a.
   paroxysmal supraventricular a.
   pause-dependent a.
   perpetual a.
   phasic sinus a.
   postperfusion a.
   primary cardiac a.
   reentrant ventricular a. (RVA)
   reperfusion a.
   respiratory a.
   respiratory sinus a. (RSA)
   senile a.
   sinus a. (SA)
   stress-related a.
   suppression of a.
   supraventricular a.
   tachybrady a.
   trigger of ventricular a. (TOVA)
   vagus a.

arrhythmia *(continued)*
    ventricular a. (VA)
    warning a.
arrhythmia-insensitive flow-sensitive
  alternating inversion recovery imaging
arrhythmic
    a. cardiac arrest (ACA)
    a. death
arrhythmogenesis
arrhythmogenic
    a. disorder
    a. pulmonary vein
    a. right ventricular cardiomyopathy
    (ARVC)
    a. right ventricular disease
    a. right ventricular dysplasia
    (ARVD)
    a. site
    a. substrate
    a. ventricular cardiomyopathy
arrhythmogenicity
arrhythmokinesis
arrhythmology
arrival
    arrest after a. (AAA)
    arrest before a. (ABA)
    chest pain onset to hospital a.
    (CPOTHA)
arrow
    A. balloon wedge catheter
    A. Berman angiographic balloon
    A. Flex intraaortic balloon catheter
    A. Hi-flow infusion set
    A. LionHeart heart assist device
    A. LionHeart left ventricular assist
    device
    A. pneumothorax kit
    A. Pullback atherectomy catheter
    A. QuadPolar electrode catheter
    A. QuadPolar pulmonary artery
    catheter
    A. sheath
Arrow-Clarke thoracentesis device
ARROWgard
    A. Blue antiseptic-coated catheter
    A. Blue Line catheter
    A. central venous catheter
Arrow-Howes multilumen catheter
arsenic (As)
    a. poisoning
    a. trioxide
arsine gas poisoning
Artegraft natural collagen vascular
  graft
Artemisin
arteria, pl. **arteriae** *(See* artery)
    a. anastomotica
    a. anastomotica auricularis magna
    a. femoris profunda

    a. genus superior lateralis
    a. genus superior medialis
    a. glutealis inferior
    a. glutealis superior
    a. laryngea
    a. laryngea superior
    a. lingualis
    a. pericardiacophrenica
    a. pharyngea
    a. pulmonalis
    a. pulmonalis dextra
    a. pulmonalis sinistra
arterial (a)
    a. access site
    a. anastomosis
    a. aneurysm
    a. arcade
    a. baroreflex (ABR)
    a. bleeding
    a. blockage
    a. blood (a)
    a. blood flow
    a. blood gas (ABG)
    a. blood gas analysis
    a. blood gas point-of-care test
    (ABG PCT)
    a. blood pressure (ABP, aBP)
    a. calcification
    a. carbon dioxide pressure
    a. carbon dioxide tension (PaCO$_2$)
    a. circulation
    a. compliance abnormality
    a. cone
    a. constriction
    a. coupling
    a. cutdown
    a. decortication
    a. desaturation
    a. dicrotic notch pressure
    a. dissection
    a. distensibility
    a. embolectomy catheter
    a. embolism
    a. entry site
    a. filter
    a. fluid
    a. gas bubble
    a. gas embolism (AGE)
    a. groove
    a. hyperemia
    a. hypertension (AH)
    a. hypotension
    a. hypoxemia
    a. impedance
    a. insufficiency
    a. line (A-line)
    a. line transducer
    a. mean
    a. mean line

mean pulmonary a. (MPA)
a. media
a. mesocardium
a. murmur
a. needle
a. occlusion
a. occlusive disease (AOD)
a. oxygen content (CAO₂)
a. oxygen desaturation (AOD)
a. oxygen partial pressure (PaO₂)
a. oxygen saturation (SaO₂)
a. oxygen tension (PaO₂)
a. partial pressure of CO₂ (PaCO₂)
a. portography
a. pressure (AP)
a. pressure of arterial fluid (P_A)
a. pressure index (API)
a. pseudoaneurysm
pulmonary a. (PA, Pa)
a. pulsatile volume change
a. pulse
a. pyemia
a. reconstruction
a. remodeling
a. runoff
a. saturation
a. sclerosis
a. sheath
a. shrinkage
a. spasm
a. spider
a. stem
a. stick
a. stiffness
a. switch operation
a. switch procedure
a. tension (TA)
a. thoracic outlet syndrome
a. thrill
a. thrombosis
A. Vascular Engineering, Inc. (AVE)
a. vein of Soemmerring
a. wave
a. wedge
arterialization
    percutaneous in situ coronary venous a. (PICVA)
arterialized capillary blood (ACB)
arteriectasis, arteriectasia
arteriectomy
arteries (*pl. of* artery) **(AA, aa)**
arterioatony
arteriocapillary sclerosis
arteriogenesis
arteriogram
    aortic arch a.
    brachial a.
    runoff a.

arteriograph
arteriographic regression
arteriography
    aortofemoral a.
    arch a.
    biplane pelvic a.
    biplane quantitative coronary a.
    bronchial a.
    carotid a.
    catheter a.
    coronary a. (CAG)
    cut-film a.
    digital subtraction a.
    femoral a.
    Judkins selective coronary a.
    longitudinal a.
    quantitative a.
    quantitative coronary a. (QCA)
    renal a.
    selective a.
    Sones selective coronary a.
    ultrasonic a. (UA)
arteriohepatic dysplasia syndrome
arteriolar
    a. hyalinosis
    a. nephrosclerosis
    a. sclerosis
arteriole
    afferent a.
    efferent a.
    ellipsoid a.
    Isaacs-Ludwig a.
    precapillary a.
arteriolith
arteriolitis
    necrotizing a.
arteriology
arteriolonecrosis
arteriolonephrosclerosis
arteriolosclerosis
arteriolosclerotic kidney
arteriolovenous
arteriolovenular
    a. anastomosis
    a. bridge
arteriolovenularis
    anastomosis a.
arteriomalacia
arteriomegaly
arteriometer
arteriomotor
arteriomyomatosis
arterionecrosis
    hyaline a.
arterionephrosclerosis
arteriopalmus
arteriopathy
    hypertensive a.
    plexogenic pulmonary a.

arterioplania
arterioplasty
    pulmonary a.
arteriopressor
arteriorrhaphy
arteriorrhexis
arteriosclerosis (AS, ATS) (*See also* atherosclerosis)
    allograft a.
    cerebral a.
    coronary a.
    decrudescent a.
    generalized a. (GAS)
    hyaline a.
    hypertensive a.
    Mönckeberg a.
    nodose a.
    nodular a.
    nonatheromatous a.
    a. obliterans
    peripheral a.
    senile a.
arteriosclerotic (*See also* atherosclerotic)
    a. aneurysm
    a. cardiovascular disease (ASCVD)
    a. gangrene
    a. heart disease (AHD, ASHD)
    a. kidney
    a. occlusive disease (AOD)
    a. peripheral vascular disease (ASPVD)
    a. retinopathy
    a. vascular disease (ASVD)
arteriospasm
arteriostenosis
arteriosum
    cor a.
    ligamentum a.
arteriosus
    conus a.
    ductus a. (DA)
    papillary muscle of conus a.
    patent ductus a. (PDA)
    persistent ductus a.
    persistent truncus a. (PTA)
    pseudotruncus a.
    reversed ductus a.
    truncus a. (TA)
arteriotomy
    brachial a.
arteriotony
arteriovenosa
    anastomosis a.
arteriovenous (A-V, AV)
    a. anastomosis (AVA)
    a. communication (AVC)
    congenital pulmonary a.
    a. crossing change
    a. fistula (AVF)

    a. malformation (AVM)
    a. nicking
    a. oxygen difference (AVDO$_2$)
    a. passage time (AVP)
    a. pulmonary aneurysm
    a. shunt (AVS)
arteritis, pl. **arteritides**
    brachiocephalic a.
    coronary a.
    cranial a.
    a. deformans
    fibrinoid a.
    giant cell a.
    granulomatous a.
    Horton a. (HA)
    a. hyperplastica
    infantile a.
    mesenteric a.
    a. nodosa
    a. obliterans
    pulmonary arteritides
    rheumatic a.
    rheumatoid a.
    syphilitic a.
    Takayasu a.
    temporal a.
    tuberculous a.
    a. umbilicalis
    a. verrucosa
artery, pl. **arteries (a)**
    aberrant innominate a.
    aberrant obturator a.
    aberrant subclavian a.
    abnormal coronary a. (ACA)
    abrupt closure of arteries
    accessory meningeal branch of middle meningeal a.
    accessory obturator a.
    accompanying a.
    acetabular a.
    acromial anastomosis of thoracoacromial a.
    acromial branch of suprascapular a.
    acromial branch of thoracoacromial a.
    acromiothoracic a.
    Adamkiewicz a.
    afferent a.
    alar a.
    anastomotic branch of middle meningeal artery with lacrimal a.
    angular a.
    anomalous left coronary a. (ALCA)
    anomalous left coronary artery arising from pulmonary a. (ALCAPA)
    anomalous left main coronary a. (ALMCA)

anomalous origin of left coronary artery from pulmonary a. (ALCAPA)
anterior cerebral a. (ACA)
anterior choroidal a. (AChA)
anterior communicating a. (ACA, ACoA, AcomA)
anterior descending a. (ADA)
anterior descending coronary a.
anterior descending segmental a.
anterior inferior cerebellar a. (AICA)
anterior inferior communicating a. (AICA)
aortopulmonary collateral a. (APC)
ascending ileocolic a.
ascending pharyngeal a.
atrioventricular node a.
A-V nodal a.
axillary a.
banding of pulmonary a.
basal collateral a.
basilar a. (BA)
beading of arteries
a. of Bernasconi and Cassinari
bilateral internal mammary a. (BIMA)
bilateral internal thoracic a. (BITA)
blocked heart a.
brachial a.
brachiocephalic a.
bronchial a.
bronchial arteries
bronchopulmonary segmental a. (BPSA)
callosomarginal a.
caroticotympanic a.
carotid a.
celiac a.
cephalic a.
circumflex a. (CX)
circumflex coronary a. (CCA, CFX)
coarctation of pulmonary a.
common carotid a.
common femoral a.
common hepatic a.
common iliac a.
common internal iliac a. (CIIA)
complete transposition of great arteries (CTGA)
congenitally corrected transposition of great arteries (CC-TGA)
copper-wire a.
corkscrew a.
coronary a.
cricothyroid a.
crural a.
deep lingual a.

descending thoracic aorta-to-femoral a. (DTAFA)
dextroposed transposition of great arteries
diagonal coronary a.
diaphragmatic a.
direct stenting of coronary a.
dorsal lingual branches of lingual a.
Drummond marginal a.
D-transposition of great arteries (D-TGA, dTGA)
EC a.
a. ectasia
efferent a.
end a.
epicardial coronary a.
esophageal branch of left gastric a.
external carotid a. (ECA)
external mammary a.
femoral a. (FA)
fetal-type posterior cerebral a.
first obtuse marginal a.
gastroepiploic a. (GEA)
great a.
hepatic a.
Heubner recurrent a.
ileal a.
ileocolic a.
iliac a.
iliofemoral a.
IM a.
infarct a.
infarct-related a. (IRA)
inferior epigastric a. (IEA)
inferior laryngeal a.
inferior mesenteric a. (IMA)
inferior temporal a. (ITA)
inferior thyroid a.
innominate a.
1,2 intercompartmental supraretinacular a.
intermediate circumflex a. (ICXA)
internal carotid a. (ICA)
internal mammary a. (IMA)
internal maxillary a. (IMAX)
internal thoracic a. (ITA)
intersegmental a.
intramural coronary a.
jejunal a.
Kugel anastomotic a.
LAC a.
LAD coronary a.
LADD coronary a.
lateral basal segmental a.
LC a.
LCC a.
LCF coronary a.
LCX coronary a.

artery *(continued)*

left anterior descending a. (LADA)

left anterior descending coronary a. (LADCA)

left circumflex a. (LCA, LCX)

left circumflex coronary a. (LCX)

left common carotid a. (LCCA)

left coronary a. (LCA)

left gastric a.

left internal mammary a. (LIMA)

left internal thoracic a. (LITA)

left main a. (LMA)

left main coronary a. (LMCA)

left pulmonary a. (LPA)

left subclavian a. (LSCA)

left vertebral a. (LVA)

lenticulostriate a.

LIC a.

lingual a.

LMC a.

LM coronary a.

LMS coronary a.

lumen of a.

lysed a.

main pulmonary a. (MPA)

mainstem coronary a.

major aortopulmonary collateral a. (MAPCA)

major coronary a. (MCA)

malposition of great arteries (MGA)

mammary a.

marginal branch of circumflex a.

medial basal branch of pulmonary a.

medial inferior a.

medial superior a.

mesenteric a.

midcoronary a.

middle capsular a.

middle cerebral a. (MCA)

native coronary a.

Neubauer a.

nodal a.

nonatheromatous a.

normal coronary arteries (NCA)

obtuse marginal a. (OMA)

obtuse marginal coronary a.

occipital a. (OA)

occluded a.

OM coronary a.

Palmaz balloon-expandable stent for renal arteries

parietooccipital a.

a. patency

penetrator a.

perforating a.

pericardiophrenic a.

perineal a.

peripheral a.

peroneal a.

pharyngeal branch of descending palatine a.

pharyngeal branch of inferior thyroid a.

phrenic a.

PLCx coronary a.

popliteal a.

porcine coronary a.

posterior basal segmental a.

posterior cerebral a. (PCA)

posterior circumflex a. (PC)

posterior communicating a. (PcomA)

posterior descending a. (PDA)

posterior inferior cerebellar a. (PICA)

posterior inferior communicating a. (PICA)

posterior margin of pulmonary a. (PPA)

posterior pulmonary a. (PPA)

posterior right coronary a. (pRCA)

posterolateral segment a. (PLSA)

posterolateral segment [coronary] a. (PLSA)

profunda femoris a., arteria femoris a. (PFA)

pulmonary a. (PA)

a. puncture site

radial a.

ramus intermedius a.

ranine a.

renal a.

retinal a.

RIC a.

right atrium to pulmonary a. (RA-PA)

right brachial a. (RBA)

right common carotid a. (RCCA)

right coronary a. (RCA)

right descending pulmonary a. (RDPA)

right gastroepiploic a. (RGEA)

right internal mammary a. (RIMA)

right internal thoracic a. (RITA)

right middle cerebral a. (R-MCA)

right pulmonary a. (RPA)

right vertebral a. (RVA)

second obtuse marginal a.

septal perforating a.

silver-wiring of retinal a.

single internal mammary a. (SIMA)

single internal thoracic a. (SITA)

sinuatrial nodal a.

sinus node a.

smooth coronary a.

stenting in small arteries (SISA)

sternocleidomastoid a.
subclavian a.
sublingual a.
superdominant a.
superficial external pudendal a.
superficial femoral a. (SFA)
superior carotid a.
superior cerebellar a. (SCA)
superior femoral a. (SFA)
superior laryngeal a.
superior mesenteric a. (SMA)
superior thyroid a.
terminal internal carotid a. (TICA)
thoracodorsal a.
threatened closure of arteries
tibial a.
tortuous right coronary a.
transposition of great arteries
  (TGA)
transverse cervical a.
umbilical a.
unilateral absence of pulmonary a.
  (UAPA)
unprotected a.
vertebral a. (VA)
a. waveform
arthritis, pl. **arthritides**
acute rheumatic a.
arytenoid joint a.
cricoarytenoid a.
A. Foundation Pain Reliever
juvenile rheumatoid a.
rheumatoid a. (RA)
arthritis-associated aortitis
arthrogenic diet
arthrogryposis multiplex congenita
arthropod venom
ArthroWand
Arthus-type reaction
articular
a. surface
a. surface of arytenoid cartilage
articularis
facies a.
articulation
artifact
aliasing a.
attenuation a.
bang a.
baseline a.
beam width a.
blooming a.
breast a.
catheter impact a.
catheter whip a.
chemical shift a.
coin a.
crush a.
cupping a.

end-pressure a.
flow a.
ghosting a.
mitral regurgitation a.
motion a.
muscle a.
N/2 a.
pacemaker stimulus a.
phantom flow a.
respiratory a.
reverberation a.
side lobe a.
smearing a.
susceptibility a.
T a.
view-aliasing a.
wrap-around ghosting a.
zebra a.
artifactual bradycardia
artificial
a. blood
a. body
a. cardiac valve
a. circus movement tachycardia
  (ACMT)
a. heart (AH)
a. heart energy system (AHES)
a. larynx
a. lung
a. lung-expanding compound
  (ALEC)
a. pacemaker
a. pacemaker-induced ventricular
  rhythm (APIVR)
a. pneumothorax
a. respiration
a. ventilation
Artrek automated edge-detection
  algorithm
ARV
anterior right ventricle
ARVC
arrhythmogenic right ventricular
  cardiomyopathy
ARVD
arrhythmogenic right ventricular
  dysplasia
Arvidsson dimension-length method
Arvin
ARVP
arginine vasopressin
arylesterase
arylsulfatase
arytenoid
a. cartilage
a. gland
a. joint arthritis
arytenoidea cricoideae
Arzbaecher pill electrode

Arzco
  A. pacemaker
  A. preamplifier
  A. Tapsul pill electrode
AS
  Adams-Stokes
  added support
  aortic sound
  area of stenosis
  arteriosclerosis
  atherosclerosis
  atrial septum
  atrial stenosis
    AS disease
As
  arsenic
ASA
  acetylsalicylic acid
  aspirin
  atrial septal aneurysm
    MSD Enteric Coated ASA
asaccharolyticus
  Peptostreptococcus a.
ASAH
  antibiotic sterilized aortic valve
    homograft
Asahi
  A. Light wire
  A. Prowater guidewire
  A. Soft guidewire
  A. Tornus specialty catheter
asahii
  Trichosporon a.
AsAo
  ascending aorta
Asaphen
Asasantine
asbestiform
asbestos
  amphibole a.
  a. bodies
  chrysotile a.
  a. pleural effusion
  a. pneumoconiosis
asbestosis
  parenchymal a.
Asbron G
ASCAD
  atherosclerotic coronary artery disease
A-scan echography
ascariasis
Ascaris lumbricoides
ascendens
  aorta a.
ascendentis
  plexus periarterialis arteriae
    pharyngeae a.
ascending
  a. aorta (AA, AAO, ACS, AsAo)

  a. aorta dilation
  a. aorta to pulmonary artery shunt
  a. aorta synchronized pulsation
    (AASP)
  a. aortic blood pressure
  a. aortic pressure (PAo)
  a. aortography
  a. balloon cannula (ABC)
  a. ileocolic artery
  a. loop of Henle
  a. pharyngeal artery
  a. pharyngeal plexus
  a. polyneuropathy
  a. thoracic aortic aneurysm
    (ATAA)
ascent
  barotrauma of a.
  A. guiding catheter
Aschner
  A. phenomenon
  A. reflex
  A. sign
Aschner-Dagnini reflex
Aschoff
  A. body
  A. cell
  A. nodule
Aschoff-Tawara node
ascites
  chylous a.
  a. praecox
ascorbate
  a. dilution curve
  sodium a.
ascorbic acid
Ascriptin
ASCS
  acute sickle chest syndrome
ASCVD
  arteriosclerotic cardiovascular disease
  atherosclerotic cardiovascular disease
ASCVP
  Australasian Society of Cardiology
    Perfusionists
ASD
  atrial septal defect
    ASD closure device
ASD2
  secundum atrial septal defect
ASDA
  American Sleep Disorders Association
ASDOS
  atrial septal defect occlusion system
  atrial septum defect occluder system
    ASDOS umbrella
    ASDOS umbrella occluder
ASE
  American Society of Electrocardiography
asequence

ASH
  asymmetric septal hypertrophy
ash
  fly a.
  A. Split Cath
  A. Split Cath II
ASHCVD
  atherosclerotic hypertensive
    cardiovascular disease
ASHD
  arteriosclerotic heart disease
  atrioseptal heart disease
Asherman chest seal
Asherson syndrome
Ashley phenomenon
Ashman
  A. beat
  A. phenomenon
Ashworth Scale
Asian influenza
a-SiC:H
  amorphous hydrogenated silicon carbide
Askin tumor
Ask-Upmark syndrome
ASM
  airways smooth muscle
Asmanex Twisthaler
asmaPLAN+ peak flowmeter
ASMI
  anteroseptal myocardial infarction
ASO
  Amplatzer septal occluder
  antistreptolysin O
ASOV
  aortic sinus of Valsalva
ASP
  aortic systolic pressure
  area systolic pressure
asparaginase
asparagine
aspartate aminotransferase (AST)
aspartic acid
aspergilloma formation
aspergillosis
  acute invasive a.
  allergic bronchopulmonary a.
    (ABPA)
  bronchopulmonary a.
  chronic invasive pulmonary a.
  chronic necrotizing a. (CNA)
  disseminated a.
  invasive pulmonary a. (IPA)
  necrotizing a.
  parenchymal a.
  pleural a.
  primary pleural a.
  pseudomembranous
    tracheobronchial a.
  pulmonary a.

  semiinvasive a.
  suppurative necrotizing a.
  tracheobronchial a.
Aspergillus
  A. avenaceus
  A. caesiellus
  A. candidus
  A. carneus
  A. empyema
  A. flavus
  A. fumigatus
  A. nidulans
  A. niger
  A. oryzae
  A. restrictus
  A. skin prick test
  A. sydowi
  A. terreus
  A. toxicosis
  A. tracheobronchitis
  A. ustus
  A. versicolor
asphygmia
asphyxia
  blue a.
  a. carbonica
  cyanotic a.
  a. cyanotica
  a. livida
  local a.
  a. neonatorum
  a. pallida
  secondary a.
  symmetric a.
  traumatic a.
  white a.
asphyxial cardiac arrest
asphyxiant
asphyxiate
asphyxiating thoracic dystrophy (ATD)
asphyxiation
aspirate
  bronchotracheal a.
  endotracheal a. (EA)
  needle a.
  tracheal a.
  tracheobronchial a.
aspirated and flushed
aspirating needle
aspiration
  a. biopsy
  a. biopsy cytology (ABC)
  bronchoscopic needle a. (BNA)
  a. catheter
  continuous a.
  diagnostic a.
  endobronchial ultrasound-guided
    needle a. (EBUS-NA)

aspiration *(continued)*
    endobronchial ultrasound-guided transbronchial needle a. (EBUS-TBNA)
    endoscopic ultrasound-guided fine-needle a. (EUS-FNA)
    fine-needle a. (FNA)
    fluid a.
    foreign body a.
    a. of foreign body
    gastric a.
    hydrocarbon a.
    intractable a.
    large-volume a.
    a. lung injury
    massive a.
    meconium a.
    nosocomial a.
    a. pneumonia
    a. pneumonitis
    real-time endobronchial ultrasound-guided transbronchial needle a.
    small-volume a.
    thoracic percutaneous needle a. (TPNA)
    transbronchial needle a. (TBNA)
    transthoracic needle a. (TTNA)
    transtracheal a.

aspiration-induced respiratory disease

aspirator
    Cavitron ultrasonic surgical a. (CUSA)
    Cook County a.
    Schueler Model 200 A.
    Ultra-Lite portable a.
    Vac-Pak-II ultra-lite portable a.
    Vacu-Aide home-use a.

aSpire
    a. controlled expansion delivery system
    a. covered stent
    a. covered stent and Controlled Release delivery system

Aspirex PE catheter

aspirin (ASA)
    anticoagulation regimen of a.
    Bayer Buffered A.
    buffered a.
    dipyridamole and a.
    enteric-coated a.
    Extra Strength Bayer Enteric 500 A.
    a., phenacetin, caffeine (APC)
    St. Joseph Adult Chewable A.
    ticlopidine plus a. (T + A)
    a. tolerance time (ATT)

aspirin/extended-release dipyridamole

aspirin-induced asthma (AIA)

Aspirols
    Amyl Nitrite A.
    Aromatic Ammonia A.

asplenia with cardiovascular anomalies

Asprimox

ASPVD
    arteriosclerotic peripheral vascular disease
    atherosclerotic peripheral vascular disease

ASS
    asthma severity score

assay
    adherence a.
    agar diffusion a.
    Amplicor a.
    Architect CTSTAT myoglobin a.
    Asserachrom D-DI ELISA a.
    Asserachrom tPA immunologic a.
    automated BNP a.
    biochemical enzyme a.
    Bioclot protein S a.
    Cardiac STATus rapid a.
    Cardiac T rapid a.
    cardiac troponin I a.
    Clauss a.
    CoA-set fibrin monomer a.
    cTnI a.
    Cushman a.
    D-dimer enzyme-linked immunosorbent a.
    Enzygnost TAT ELISA a.
    enzyme-linked immunosorbent a. (ELISA)
    FastPlaqueTB a.
    ferricytochrome a.
    GenoType MTBDR a.
    Hemochron high-dose thrombin time a.
    hemoSTATUS a.
    Heptest clotting a.
    Hybritech immunoradiometric a.
    immune adherence immunosorbent a. (IAIA)
    immunofluorescence a.
    immunoradiometric a. (IRMA)
    immunoturbidimetric a.
    INNO-LiPA Rif.TB a.
    Line Probe A.
    lipoprotein (a) a.
    lucigenin chemiluminescence a.
    matrix metalloproteinase-9 a.
    MonoClone immunoenzymetric a.
    MTBC LightCycler a.
    multimer a.
    myoglobin a.
    N High Sensitivity CRP a.
    nitrate reductase a. (NRA)
    Opus cardiac troponin I a.
    PCR a.

A

platelet-derived growth factor-AB a.
P2y12 Plavix a.
radioligand binding a.
rapid platelet function a. (RPFA)
restriction endonuclease a.
sandwich enzyme-linked
  immunosorbent a.
S-Mgb a.
soluble TREM-1 a.
Stachrom PAI chromogenic a.
thyrotoxin radioisotope a.
Tina-quant immunoturbidimetric a.
TRAP a.
TUNEL a.
Ultegra rapid platelet function a.
Velogene rapid TB a.
VerifyNow aspirin a.
Vidas D-dimer exclusion a.
viral antigen a.

assembly, pl. assemblies
blood pressure a. (BPA)
Collins SurveyTach with
  MicroTach a.
infant nasal cannula a. (INCA)

Asserachrom
A. D-DI ELISA assay
A. tPA immunologic assay

assessment
anatomic a.
angiographic a.
angioscopic a.
cardiovascular function a.
causality a.
Chedoke-McMaster Stroke A.
echocardiographic a.
functional a.
hemodynamic a.
invasive a.
jugular bulb catheter placement a.
noninvasive a.
sepsis-related organ failure a.
  (SOFA)
sequential organ failure a. (SOFA)
transposition a.
transthoracic echocardiographic
  Doppler a.

Assess peak flowmeter
assist
A. device
percutaneous transseptal
  ventricular A. (PTVA)
Venturi exhalation A.

assistance
external pressure circulatory a.
  (EPCA)
intraaortic balloon a. (IABA)
mechanical ventricular a. (MVA)
ventilatory a.

assist-control (AC)

a.-c. mode ventilation
a.-c. ventilation (ACV)

assist/control
assisted
a. circulation
a. mechanical ventilation (AMV)
a. peak systolic pressure (APSP)
a. respiration

Assmann
A. focus
A. tuberculous infiltrate

association
Adult Congenital Heart A.
Alveolar Capillary Dysplasia A.
  (ACDA)
American Cardiology
  Technologists A. (ACTA)
American College of
  Cardiology/American Heart A.
  (ACC/AHA)
American Heart A. (AHA)
American Sleep Disorders A.
  (ASDA)
atrioventricular a.
CHARGE a.
Kennedy's Disease A. (KDA)
National Cholesterol Education
  Program of the American
  Heart A.
National Home Oxygen Patients A.
New York Heart A. (NYHA)
A.'s of Professional Sleep Societies
  (APSS)
VACTERL a.

AST
angiotensin sensitivity test
aspartate aminotransferase
atrial overdrive stimulation rate

Astech peak flowmeter
Astelin nasal spray
astemizole
asterixis
asteroid body
asteroides
  Nocardia a.
asthenia
neurocirculatory a.
postinfluenza a.
vasoregulatory a.

asthenic apoplexy
asthenicus
thorax a.

asthma
abdominal a.
acarian a.
adult-onset a.
aliphatic amines a.
allergen-induced a.
allergic a.

asthma *(continued)*
  aluminum potroom a.
  alveolar a.
  anhydride a.
  aspirin-induced a. (AIA)
  atopic a.
  bacterial a.
  baker's a.
  benzalkonium chloride a.
  brittle a.
  bronchial a.
  bronchitic a.
  cacoon seed a.
  cardiac a.
  a. care algorithm (ACA)
  casein a.
  castor bean a.
  cat a.
  catarrhal a.
  A. Check peak flowmeter
  Cheyne-Stokes a.
  chlorella a.
  chronic a.
  cobalt a.
  cobalt-related a.
  cockroach a.
  coffee bean a.
  cold dry air-induced a.
  cotton-dust a.
  cough variant a.
  cough-variant a.
  a. crystal
  cutaneous a.
  daytime a. (DA)
  diisocyanate a.
  dust a.
  Elsner a.
  emphysematous a.
  essential a.
  exercise-induced a. (EIA)
  extrinsic a.
  factitious a.
  food a.
  gestational a.
  Global Initiative for A. (GIA, GINA)
  Global Institute for A. (GIA)
  grinder's a.
  Heberden a.
  horse a.
  humid a.
  hyperventilation-induced a. (HIA)
  idiosyncratic a.
  IgE-independent occupational a.
  IgE-mediated a.
  infective a.
  inner city a.
  intrinsic a.
  irritant-induced a.

  isocyanate-induced a.
  kapok a.
  karaya a.
  Kopp a.
  lycopodium a.
  mall a.
  meat-wrapper's a.
  methylene diphenyl diisocyanate a.
  Mexican bean weevil a.
  Millar a.
  miller's a.
  miner's a.
  mixed a.
  nacre dust a.
  nasal a.
  near-fatal a. (NFA)
  nervous a.
  nocturnal a.
  nonatopic a.
  noneosinophilic atopic a.
  nonwheezing bronchial a.
  occupational a. (OA)
  occupational formalin a.
  oil mist a.
  osmotically induced a. (OIA)
  pancreatin a.
  a. paper
  phthalic anhydride irritant-induced a.
  pollen a.
  polyether alcohol a.
  poorly reversible a.
  postcoital a.
  potter's a.
  prawn a.
  pseudo-steroid-resistant a.
  A. Quality of Life Questionnaire (AQLQ)
  red cedar a.
  red soft coral a.
  reflex a.
  rose hips a.
  Rostan a.
  royal jelly-induced a.
  a. severity score (ASS)
  sexual a.
  sheep blowfly a.
  shellfish a.
  soybean lecithin a.
  spasmodic a.
  steam-fitter's a.
  steroid-dependent a.
  steroid-resistant a. (SRA)
  stone stripper's a.
  styrene a.
  subclinical a.
  sunflower a.
  symptomatic a.
  tall oil a.

tartrazine a.
TDI-induced a.
thymic a.
toluene diisocyanate-induced a.
tragacanth a.
triad a.
a. trigger
trimellitic anhydride a.
true a.
tylosin tartrate a.
urban a.
Vicia sativa a.
weeping fig a.
Wichmann a.
work-aggravated a.
work-related a.
zardaverine a.
AsthmaMentor peak flowmeter
AsthmaPACK personal asthma care kit
Asthmastik
asthmatic
brittle a.
a. bronchitis
chronic stable a.
corticosteroid-dependent a.
steroid-dependent a.
tight a.
asthmaticus
status a.
asthmatiform
asthmatoid wheeze
asthmogen
hydrosoluble a.
occupational a.
asthmogenic
asthmoid
a. respiration
a. wheeze
Astler-Coller classification
Astra
A. profile
A. T4, T6 pacemaker
Astrand bicycle exercise stress test
Astrand-Rhyming protocol
astriction
astrocyte
astronyxis
Acanthamoeba a.
Astropulse cuff
Astro-Trace Universal adapter clip
Astroviridae virus
Astrup blood gas value
ASV
adaptive support ventilation
autogenous saphenous vein
autologous saphenous vein
ASVD
arteriosclerotic vascular disease

asymmetric
a. dimethylarginine (ADMA)
a. septal hypertrophy (ASH)
asymmetrical
bilateral a. (BA)
asymptomatic
a. cardiac ischemia (ACI)
a. carotid bruit (ACB)
a. complex ectopy
a. coronary artery disease (ACAD)
a. left ventricular dysfunction
a. myocarditis
asynchronous
atrial a. (AOO)
a. pacing
a. pulse generator
ventricular a. (VOO)
asynchrony
global a.
a. index
asynergy
asystole
atrial a.
Beau a.
transient a.
asystolia
asystolic arrest
AT
acute thrombosis
anaerobic threshold
angiotensin
antithrombin
atrial tachycardia
atropine
AT1
angiotensin II type 1
AT1 receptor C allele
At
angiotensin
antithrombin
atrial
atrium
AT I
angiotensin I
ata
atmosphere absolute
ATAA
ascending thoracic aortic aneurysm
Atacand
A. HCT
A. Plus tablet
atactic hemiparesis
Atakr II RF ablation system
Atarax Oral
AT-atropine stress echocardiography
ATA unit
ataxia
a. cordis
Friedreich a.

ataxia *(continued)*
    hereditary a.
    spinocerebellar a.
    a. telangiectasia
    a. telangiectasia syndrome
ataxia-telangiectasia
ataxic
    a. aphasia
    a. breathing
    a. gait
    a. hemiparesis (AH)
ATB
    atrial tachycardia with block
ATC
    Antiplatelet Trialists' Collaboration
ATD
    Amplatz thrombectomy device
    asphyxiating thoracic dystrophy
ATDR
    atrial tachycardia detection rate
atelectasia
atelectasis
    absorption a.
    acquired a.
    adhesive a.
    bibasilar a.
    cicatrization a.
    compression a.
    congenital a.
    lobar a.
    nonobstructive a.
    obstructive a.
    patchy a.
    platelike a.
    postobstructive a.
    primary a.
    relaxation a.
    resorption a.
    rounded a.
    secondary a.
    segmental a.
    subsegmental a.
    tricuspid a.
atelectatic
    a. band
    a. rale
atelocardia
Aten
atenolol and chlorthalidone
ATF
    activating transcription factor
Atgam
atherectomy
    Auth a.
    a. catheter
    coronary a.
    coronary rotational a. (CRA)
    directional a.
    excimer laser coronary a.

    excisional a.
    extraction a.
    high-speed directional coronary a.
    high-speed rotational a. (HSRA)
    a. index
    Kinsey a.
    percutaneous coronary rotational a. (PCRA)
    percutaneous transluminal rotational a. (PTRA)
    Rotablator a. (ROTA)
    rotational a. (RA)
    rotational coronary a. (RCA)
    transluminal extraction a. (TEA)
    transluminal extraction coronary a.
atheroablation
AtheroCath
    A. Bantam coronary atherectomy catheter
    A. GTO coronary atherectomy catheter
    Simpson peripheral A.
atheroemboli (*pl. of* atheroembolus)
atheroembolic stroke
atheroembolism
atheroembolus, pl. **atheroemboli**
atherogenesis
    monoclonal theory of a.
    response-to-injury hypothesis of a.
atherogenic
    a. dyslipidemia
    a. index (AI)
    a. lipid
    a. metabolic triad
atherogenicity index
atherolytic reperfusion guidewire
atheroma
    AA a.
    aortic arch a.
    a. burden
    complex a.
    core of a.
    coronary a.
    intimal a.
    protruding a.
atheromatous
    a. cap
    a. core
    a. debris
    a. degeneration
    a. embolism
    a. gruel
    a. plaque
atheroprotection
atherosclerosis (AS, ATS) *(See also* arteriosclerosis)
    aortic a.
    cardiac allograft a. (CAA)
    coronary artery a.

de novo a.
encrustation theory of a.
lipogenic theory of a.
a. obliterans
premature a.
a. prevention and treatment
radiation-induced a.
atherosclerotic (*See also* arteriosclerosis)
   a. aneurysm
   a. aortic disease
   a. aortography
   a. cardiovascular disease (ACVD, ASCVD)
   a. carotid artery disease
   a. coronary artery disease (ACAD, ASCAD)
   a. debris
   a. heart disease (AHD)
   a. hypertensive cardiovascular disease (ASHCVD)
   a. narrowing
   a. occlusive disease
   a. peripheral vascular disease (ASPVD)
   a. plaque (AP)
   a. plaque burden
   a. vascular disease (AVD)
atherosis
atherothrombosis
atherothrombotic
   a. brain infarction (ABI)
   a. cardiovascular disease
   a. stroke
atherotome
Atherotome microsurgical blade
athlete
   A. guidewire
   a.'s heart
athletic heart
AT II
   angiotensin II
AT-III
   antithrombin III
Ativan
Atkins-Cannard tracheal tube
Atkins diet
ATL
   Advanced Technology Laboratories, Inc.
   anterior tricuspid leaflet
   ATL UltraMark 7 colorflow ultrasound
   ATL UltraMark 4 ultrasound
   ATL Ultramark 9 ultrasound system
atlantis
   fovea articularis inferior a.
   fovea articularis superior a.
   fovea dentis a.

A. SR PRO coronary imaging catheter
atlas
   A. DG balloon angioplasty catheter
   A. DR ICD
   A. DR implantable cardioverter-defibrillator
   A. ICD
   superior articular facet of a.
   A. ULP balloon dilation catheter
   A. VR ICD
   A. VR implantable cardioverter-defibrillator
Atlee clamp
ATLS
   advanced trauma life support
atm
   atmosphere
atmosphere (atm)
   a. absolute (ata)
   ICAO standard a.
   a.'s of pressure
   standard a.
atmospheric pressure (P_{atm})
atmospherization
atmotherapy
ATnativ
atomic absorption spectrometry
atomizer
atopic asthma
atopy
atorvastatin calcium
atovaquone
ATP
   adenosine triphosphate
   antitachycardia pacemaker
   antitachycardia pacing
   ATP hydrolysis
ATPase
   adenosine triphosphatase
   myofibrillar ATPase
   SR calcium ATPase
ATP-SPECT
   adenosine triphosphate single-photon emission computed tomography
ATRA
   all-trans-retinoic acid
atra
   Stachybotrys a.
ATRAC-II double-balloon catheter
ATRAC multipurpose balloon catheter
atracurium
Atraloc needle
Atrauclip hemostatic clip
atraumatic needle
atresia
   anatomic pulmonary a.
   aortic a.
   aortic valve a. (AVA)

atresia *(continued)*

atrioventricular valve a.
bronchial a.
congenital bronchial a. (CBA)
esophageal a.
functional pulmonary a.
glottic a.
gross tracheoesophageal a.
infundibular a.
laryngeal a.
membranous pulmonary a.
mitral a.
pulmonary a. (PA)
pulmonary artery a.
pure pulmonary a. (PPA)
tricuspid a. (TA)
ventricular a.

atretic pulmonary valve

atria (*pl. of* atrium)

atrial (At)

a. activation mapping
a. anomalous band
a. appendage
a. appendectomy
a. arrhythmia
a. asynchronous (AOO)
a. asynchronous pacemaker
a. asystole
a. baffle
a. baffle operation
a. balloon septostomy
a. bigeminy
a. bolus dynamic computer tomography
a. bradycardia
a. capture
a. capture beat
a. capture threshold
a. carotid ventricular (ACV)
a. chaotic tachycardia
a. complex
a. contraction (AC)
a. cuff
a. defibrillation shock
a. defibrillation threshold
a. deflection
a. demand inhibited (AAI)
a. demand inhibited pacemaker
a. demand triggered (AAT)
a. demand triggered pacemaker
a. diastole
a. diastolic gallop (ADG)
a. disc
a. dissociation
a. echo
a. ectopic (AE)
a. ectopic beat
a. ectopic tachycardia (AET)
a. ectopy

a. effective refractory period (AERP)
a. ejection force
a. electrogram (AEG)
a. emptying index (AEI)
a. escape interval
a. escape rhythm
a. extrastimulus method
a. extrasystole
a. fibrillation (AF)
a. fibrillation cycle length (AFCL)
a. fibrillation detection
a. fibrillation-flutter (AFF)
a. fibrillation investigators
a. fibrillation monitor (AFm)
a. fibrillation threshold
a. filling fraction (AFF)
a. filling peak
a. filling pressure
a. fistula
a. flutter (AF, AFL)
a. flutter ablation
a. flutter response (AFR)
a. flutter response algorithm
a. fusion (AF)
a. fusion beat
a. gallop (AG)
a. heart rate (AHR)
a. implantable cardioverter-defibrillator (AICD, A-ICD)
a. incremental pacing
a. inhibited (AAI)
a. insufficiency (AI)
a. isomerism
a. isthmus ablation
a. kick
a. lead impedance
a. liver pulse
a. low energy reversion therapy (ALERT)
a. maze procedure
a. myocardial infarction
a. myocarditis
a. myxoma
a. natriuretic factor (ANF)
a. natriuretic peptide (ANP)
a. natriuretic peptide A (ANP-A)
a. natriuretic peptide B (ANP-B)
a. natriuretic peptide C (ANP-C)
a. natriuretic polypeptide (ANP)
a. noncavotricuspid isthmus-dependent flutter
a. nonsensing
a. notch
a. ostium primum defect
a. overdrive pacing
a. overdrive stimulation rate (AST)
a. pacing (AP)
a. pacing stress test

a. pacing wire
a. parasystole
a. paroxysmal tachycardia
a. partition
a. premature beat (APB)
a. premature complex
a. premature contraction (APC)
a. premature depolarization (APD)
a. pressure (PA)
pulmonary venous a. (PVa)
a. pulse amplitude
a. pulse width
a. rate (AR)
a. reentry
a. refractory period
a. relaxation
a. repolarization
a. repolarization wave
a. reversal (AR)
a. reverse remodeling
a. ring
a. sensing configuration
a. sensitivity
a. septal aneurysm (ASA)
a. septal defect (ASD)
a. septal defect occlusion system (ASDOS)
a. septal defect patch
a. septal defect umbrella
a. septal resection
a. septectomy
a. septum (AS)
a. septum defect occluder system (ASDOS)
a. septum septal pacing
a. shear
a. situs inversus
a. sound
a. spike
a. standstill
a. stasis index
a. stenosis (AS)
a. stimulation
a. stretch
a. stunning
a. switch
a. switch procedure
a. synchronous noncompetitive pacemaker
a. synchronous pulse generator
a. synchronous ventricular inhibited (VDD)
a. synchronous ventricular inhibited pacemaker
a. synchrony
a. systole
a. tachyarrhythmia
a. tachycardia (AT)

a. tachycardia detection rate (ATDR)
a. tachycardia with block (ATB)
a. tachycardic response
a. tachycardic response algorithm
a. thrombus
a. train pacing
a. transport function
a. trigeminy with aberrancy
a. triggered
a. triggered noncompetitive pacemaker
a. triggered pulse generator
a. undersensing
a. valve
a. vector loop
a. venous pulse
a. ventricular canal defect
a. and ventricular implantable cardioverter-defibrillator (AV-ICD)
a. ventricular nodal reentry tachycardia
a. ventricular reciprocating tachycardia (AVRT)
a. ventricular shunt
a. volume constant (Vak)
a. VOO pacemaker
atrial/aortic
left a./a. (LA/Ao)
atrial-axis discontinuity
atrial-based
a.-b. pacemaker
a.-b. pacing
atrial-femoral artery bypass
atrialized
a. chamber
a. ventricle
atrial-paced cycle length
atrial-to-pulmonary venous gradient
atrial-well technique
atriobiventricular pacemaker
atriocarotid (AC)
a. interval
atriocommissuropexy
atriocyte
atriodextrofascicular tract
atriodigital dysplasia
atrioesophageal fistula
atriofascicular
a. Mahaim reentrant tachycardia
a. tract
atriography
atrio-His (A-H)
a.-H. bypass tract
a.-H. fiber
a.-H. pathway
atrionodal (AN)
a. bypass tract
atriopeptidase inhibitor

atriopressor reflex
atriopulmonary shunt
atrioseptal
    a. heart disease (ASHD)
    a. sign
atrioseptostomy
    balloon a.
atriosystolic murmur
atriotomy
atrioventricular (A-V, AV)
    anomalous a.
    a. anulus
    a. association
    a. block (AVB)
    a. bundle
    a. canal (AVC)
    a. canal cushion
    a. canal defect
    a. circumflex branch (AVCx)
    complete a.
    a. conduction (AVC)
    a. conduction abnormality
    a. conduction defect
    a. conduction system (AVCS)
    a. conduction tissue
    a. connection anomaly
    a. delay (AVD)
    a. discordance
    a. dissociation (AVD)
    a. extrasystole (AVE)
    a. flow rumbling murmur
    a. furrow
    a. gradient
    a. groove
    a. interval
    a. junction (AVJ)
    a. junctional
    a. junctional ablation
    a. junctional arrhythmia
    a. junctional bigeminy
    a. junctional escape beat
    a. junctional escape complex
    a. junctional escape extrasystole
    a. junctional heart block
    a. junctional pacemaker augmentor
    a. junctional reciprocating
      tachycardia
    a. junctional rhythm (AVJR)
    a. junction motion
    a. junction rhythm
    a. malformation (AVM)
    a. nodal ablation
    a. nodal bigeminy
    a. nodal conduction (AVN)
    a. nodal extrasystole
    a. nodal reentrant tachycardia
      (AVNRT)
    a. nodal reentry (AVNR)

    a. nodal reentry tachycardia
      (AVNRT)
    a. nodal rhythm
    a. nodal tachycardia (AVNT)
    a. node (AVN)
    a. node artery
    a. node block
    a. node dysfunction (AVND)
    a. node functional refractory period
      (AVNFRP)
    a. node pathway
    a. opening (AVO)
    a. orifice
    a. pathway (AP)
    a. reciprocating tachycardia (AVRT)
    a. reentrant tachycardia (AVRT)
    a. refractory period (AVRP)
    a. septal defect (AVSD)
    sequential a. (SAV)
    a. sequential pacemaker
    a. sequential pacing
    a. situs concordance
    a. sulcus
    a. synchronous pacing
    a. synchrony
    a. time
    a. valve (AVV)
    a. valve atresia
    a. valve insufficiency
    a. valve opening (AO)
    a. valve regurgitation
    a. valve ring
atrioventricularis
    crus dextrum fasciculi a.
    crus sinistrum fasciculi a.
    crux dextrum fasciculi a.
    crux sinistrum fasciculi a.
    nodus a.
    truncus fascicularis a.
Atrioverter
    A. implantable atrial defibrillator
    A. implantable defibrillator device
    Metrix A.
atrium, pl. **atria (A, At)**
    accessory a.
    auricles of atria
    common a.
    congenital single a.
    a. cordis
    a. cordis sinistrum
    a. dextrum
    electrocardiographic wave
     corresponding to wave of
     depolarization crossing A. (P)
    Fontan right a.
    a. glottidis
    a. of heart
    high right a.
    left a. (LA)

low right a. (LRA)
low septal a.
low septal right a. (LSRA)
a. of lung
a. pulmonale
pulmonary venous a.
right a. (RA)
roof of left a.
single a.
stunned a.
systemic venous a.
atrium-His (AH)
a.-H. bundle
atrophic
a. cardiomyopathy
a. catarrh
a. emphysema
a. laryngitis
a. papulosis
a. pharyngitis
a. thrombosis
atrophy
brown a.
cardiac a.
cyanotic a.
Erb a.
multiple system a.
olivopontocerebellar a.
optic a.
peroneal muscular a.
red a.
atropine (AT)
Isopto A.
a. sulfate
a. test
Atropine-Care
Atropisol
Atrostim phrenic nerve stimulator
Atrovent
A. Aerosol Inhalation
A. Inhalation Solution
ATryn
ATS
American Thoracic Society
arteriosclerosis
atherosclerosis
autotransfusion system
ATS Open Pivot bileaflet heart
valve
ATS standard aortic valve
ATS standard mitral valve
ATT
arginine tolerance test
aspirin tolerance time
attachment
endpoint a.
epithelial-mucus a.
attack
Adams-Stokes a.

anxiety a.
drop a.
heart a.
nonfatal heart a.
odor-triggered panic a.
Stokes-Adams a.
transient ischemic a. (TIA)
vagal a.
vasovagal a.
Attain Select 6238 TEL guide catheter
attended polysomnography
attenuation
a. artifact
broadband ultrasound a. (BUA)
ground-glass a. (GGA)
heterogeneous parenchymal a.
vascular a.
attenuator
ATTR
amyloidogenic transthyretin
attraction sphere
attrition murmur
ATW
all track wire
ATW marker wire
ATW steerable guidewire
atypical
a. alveolar hyperplasia
a. atrioventricular nodal reentrant
tachycardia (AAVNRT)
a. chest pain
a. flutter
a. mycobacterial colonization
a. pneumonia
a. tamponade
a. tuberculosis
a. verrucous endocarditis
Au
gold
audiometry
heart rate a. (HRA)
auditory
a. alternans
a. fremitus
Auenbrugger sign
Auer body
Aufrecht sign
Aufricht elevator
augmentation
conduit a.
flow a.
pressure a. (PA)
a. therapy
augmented
a. lead
a. V wave
Augmentin

augmentor
> atrioventricular junctional
>   pacemaker a.
> pacemaker a.

auramine smear microscopy

auranofin

aureomycin sensitivity

aureus
> *Staphylococcus a.*

auricle
> a.'s of atria
> left a. (LA)
> right a. (RA)

auricular
> a. appendage
> a. appendectomy
> a. complex
> a. extrasystole
> a. fibrillation
> a. flutter
> a. premature beat
> a. standstill
> a. systole
> a. tachycardia

auricularis magna

Auriculin

auriculopressor reflex

auriculoventricular
> a. extrasystole
> a. groove
> a. interval

aurothiomalate

Aurous
> A. centimeter sizing catheter
> A. graduate sizing catheter

ausculatory triangle

auscultate

auscultation
> aortic area of a.
> cardiac a.
> Korányi a.
> percussion and a. (P&A)
> a. and percussion (A&P)

auscultatory
> a. alternans
> a. gap
> a. percussion
> a. sign
> a. sound

Austin
> A. Flint murmur
> A. Flint phenomenon
> A. Flint respiration
> A. Flint rumble
> A. Medical Equipment

Australasian Society of Cardiology Perfusionists (ASCVP)

Australia antigen

Australian Q fever

australis
> *Rickettsia a.*

Austrian syndrome

autacoid, autocoid

Auth atherectomy

Autima II dual-chamber pacemaker

AutoAdjust CPAP device

autoanalyzer

autoantibody
> antiheart muscle a. (AHMA)
> antimyosin a.
> cardiac a.
> serum a.

autobiotic

autobullectomy
> inflammatory a.
> partial a.

autocapture
> ventricular a.

AutoCapture pacing system

AutoCAT intraaortic balloon pump

Autoclix

autocoid (*var. of* autacoid)

Autocorr
> A. Plus pulse oximeter
> A. portable pulse oximeter

autocorrelation
> serial a.

autocrine signaling

autodecremental
> a. mode
> a. pacing

autodigestion of connective tissue

autofluorescence bronchoscopy

autogamous

autogamy

autogenic
> a. drainage (AD)
> a. graft

autogenous
> a. saphenous vein (ASV)
> a. vein

autograft
> pulmonary a. (PA)

Autohaler

autohypnosis

autoimmune
> a. disorder
> a. pulmonary fibrosis
> a. thyroid disease (AITD)

autoimmunity
> cardiac a.

Auto-Injector

Autolet

autologous
> a. blood
> a. blood management system
> a. blood patch

a. blood selective aortic arch
  perfusion (AB-SAAP)
a. clot
a. fat graft
a. pericardial patch
a. saphenous vein (ASV)
a. transfusion
a. vein graft-coated stent (AVGCS)
automated
a. BNP assay
a. border detection (ABD)
a. boundary protection (ABP)
a. cardiac flow measurement
  (ACM)
a. cardiac output measurement
  (ACOM)
a. cervical cell screening system
a. edge detection
a. external defibrillator (AED)
automatic
a. atrial tachycardia (AAT)
a. beat
a. boundary detection (ABD)
a. capacitor formation interval
a. cell
a. device
a. dose rate control (ADRC)
a. ectopic tachycardia
a. electronic defibrillator
a. exposure system
a. external cardioverter-defibrillator
  (AECD)
a. external defibrillation
a. external defibrillator (AED)
a. implantable cardioverter-
  defibrillator (AICD, A-ICD)
a. implantable defibrillator (AID)
a. internal cardioverter-defibrillator
  (AICD, A-ICD)
a. internal defibrillator
a. mode conversion
a. mode conversion algorithm
a. mode switching (AMS)
a. mode-switching algorithm
a. oscillometric blood pressure
  monitor
a. pacemaker
a. positive airway pressure (APAP)
a. systolic blood pressure
  measurement (ABP)
a. titration system
a. ventricular contraction
automaticity
enhanced a.
pacemaker a.
sinus nodal a.
automatism
autonomic
a. dysreflexia

a. failure
a. hyperreflexia
a. modulation
a. nervous system (ANS)
a. perturbation
pulmonary branch of a.
a. response
a. seizure
a. sensory innervation
autonomici
rami pulmonales systematis a.
autoPEEP, intrinsic PEEP
unintended positive end-expiratory
  pressure
autoperfusion
a. balloon
a. balloon catheter
AutoPilot operational mode
Autoplex
A. Factor VIII inhibitor bypass
  product
A. T
autoprogramming
AutoPulse resuscitation system
autoradiography
quantitative a. (QAR)
autoregulate
autoregulation
cerebrovascular a.
heterometric a.
homeometric a.
orthostasis a.
autosensing
AutoSet
A. CS device
A. Portable II Plus device
A. T titration system
**autosomal-dominant familial aortic
  aneurysm disease**
autosome
Auto Suture Surgiclip
auto-threshold function
autotitrating CPAP
autotitration device
autotoxic cyanosis
Autotransfuser
Biosurge Synchronous A.
autotransfusion system (ATS)
autotransplantation
Autotrans system
Autovac LF autotransfusion system
autumnal catarrh
auxocardia
A-V, AV
arteriovenous
atrioventricular
A-V atrioventricular junctional
  rhythm
A-V branch block

A-V *(continued)*
- A-V bundle
- A-V canal
- A-V canal defect
- A-V conduction defect
- A-V delay
- A-V delay interval
- A-V dissociation
- A-V groove
- A-V groove block
- A-V interval
- A-V junction
- A-V junction ablation
- A-V junctional escape beat
- A-V junctional escape complex
- A-V junctional extrasystole
- A-V junctional tachycardia
- A-V nodal artery
- A-V nodal bigeminy
- A-V nodal conduction
- A-V nodal extrasystole
- A-V nodal modification
- A-V nodal reentry
- A-V nodal reentry tachycardia
- A-V nodal rhythm
- A-V nodal Wenckebach arrhythmia
- A-V node
- A-V node block
- A-V node reentrant tachycardia
- A-V node Wenckebach periodicity
- A-V reciprocating tachycardia
- A-V sequential pacemaker
- A-V sequential pacing
- A-V shunt
- A-V synchronous pacemaker
- A-V synchrony
- A-V universal (DDD)
- A-V Wenckebach block

AV
- aortic valve
- arteriovenous
- atrioventricular

A/V
- alanine/valine

AVA
- aortic valve anulus
- aortic valve area
- aortic valve atresia
- arteriovenous anastomosis
  - AVA 3Xi advanced venous access device

AVAD
- acute ventricular assist device

Avalide

Avanar
- A. intravascular ultrasound catheter
- A. IVUS catheter

Avanti introducer

Avapro HCT

avascularization

avascular necrosis

AVB
- atrioventricular block

AVC
- aberrant ventricular conduction
- aortic valve closure
- arteriovenous communication
- atrioventricular canal
- atrioventricular conduction

AVCO
- AVCO aortic balloon
- AVCO balloon pump

AVCS
- atrioventricular conduction system

AVCx
- atrioventricular circumflex branch

AVD
- aortic valvular disease
- atherosclerotic vascular disease
- atrioventricular delay
- atrioventricular dissociation

AVDO$_2$
- arteriovenous oxygen difference

AVDP
- average diastolic pressure

AVE
- aortic valve echocardiogram
- Arterial Vascular Engineering, Inc.
- atrioventricular extrasystole
  - AVE S540, S670 stent

Avelox
- A. IV
- A. tablet

avenaceus
- *Aspergillus a.*

average
- a. diastolic pressure (AVDP)
- a. mean pressure (AMP)
- a. peak velocity (APV)
- a. pulse magnitude
- spatial average pulse a. (I_{sapa})
- time-weighted a.

averaging
- acoustic quantification signal a.
- digital a.
- gated a.
- signal a.

AVF
- arteriovenous fistula

aVF
- unipolar limb lead on left leg in electrocardiography
  - aVF lead

AVG
- aortic valve gradient

AVGCS
- autologous vein graft-coated stent

AVHD
　　acquired valvular heart disease
AVHS
　　acquired valvular heart syndrome
avian
　　a. antigen
　　a. influenza A
　　a. influenza A (H5N1) virus
　　a. influenza pneumonia
　　a. influenza virus (AIV)
　　a. influenza virus strain H5N1
　　　(AIV H5N1, AIV H5N1, H5N1)
　　A. transport ventilator
　　a. tuberculosis
aviator
　　A. balloon
　　a.'s disease
AV-ICD
　　atrial and ventricular implantable
　　　cardioverter-defibrillator
avidin-biotin peroxidase
Avita PTCA dilation catheter
Avitene
avium
　　Mycobacterium a.
avium-intracellulare
　　Mycobacterium a.-i. (MAI)
AVJ
　　atrioventricular junction
AVJR
　　atrioventricular junctional rhythm
AVL
　　AVL Omni blood gas analyzer
　　AVL Opti Critical Care Analyzer
　　AVL Opti 1 portable blood gas
　　　analyzer
aVL
　　unipolar limb lead on left leg in
　　　electrocardiography
　　aVL lead
AVM
　　arteriovenous malformation
　　atrioventricular malformation
AVN
　　atrioventricular nodal conduction
　　atrioventricular node
AVND
　　atrioventricular node dysfunction
AVNFRP
　　atrioventricular node functional refractory
　　　period
AVNR
　　atrioventricular nodal reentry
AVNRT
　　atrioventricular nodal reentrant
　　　tachycardia
　　atrioventricular nodal reentry tachycardia
AVNT
　　atrioventricular nodal tachycardia

AVO
　　aortic valve opening
　　aortic valve orifice
　　atrioventricular opening
AvoSure PT monitor
**AVOXimeter 1000E whole blood
　oximeter**
AVP
　　abnormal vasopressin
　　ambulatory venous pressure
　　aqueous vasopressin
　　arginine vasopressin
　　arteriovenous passage time
AV-Paceport thermodilution catheter
AVR
　　accelerated ventricular rhythm
　　aortic valve replacement
aVR
　　unipolar limb lead on right arm in
　　　electrocardiography
　　late R in aVR
　　aVR lead
AVRP
　　atrioventricular refractory period
AVRT
　　atrial ventricular reciprocating
　　　tachycardia
　　atrioventricular reciprocating tachycardia
　　atrioventricular reentrant tachycardia
AVS
　　aortic valve stenosis
　　arteriovenous shunt
AVSD
　　acquired ventricular septal defect
　　atrioventricular septal defect
AVSV
　　aortic valve stroke volume
AVT
　　arginine vasotocin
avulsion
AVV
　　atrioventricular valve
Av3V
　　anteroventral third ventricle
AW
　　Anderson-Wilkins
　　anterior wall
　　AW acuteness score
AWAR
　　anterior wall of aortic root
A-wave spectral velocity waveform
AWESOME
　　Angina with Extremely Serious Operative
　　　Mortality Evaluation
AWI
　　anterior wall infarction
AWM
　　abnormal wall motion

AWMI
    anterior wall myocardial infarction
Axcis PMR system
axes (*pl. of* axis)
axial
    a. aneurysm
    a. computed tomography (ACT)
    a. control
    a. current
    a. flow pump
    a. interstitial disease
    a. interstitium
    a. plane
axillaris
    regio a.
axillary
    a. arch
    a. artery
    a. bifemoral bypass
    a. block
    a. lymph node
    a. nerve
    a. triangle
    a. vein
axilloaxillary bypass
axillofemoral bypass
axillofemoral-femoral bypass
axiom
    A. double sump pump
    A. thoracic trocar
Axios 04 pacemaker
axis, pl. **axes**
    celiac artery a.
    clockwise rotation of electrical a.
    a. deviation
    electrical a.
    frontal a.
    horizontal long a.
    hypophyseal-pituitary-adrenal a.
    hypothalamic-pituitary-adrenal a.
      (HPAA)
    instantaneous electrical a.
    J point electrical a.
    junctional a.
    long a. (LAX)
    mean electrical a.
    mean QRS a.
    normal electrical a.
    parasternal long a.
    parasternal short a.
    P-wave a.
    QRS a.
    R a.
    rightward a.
    a. shift
    short a. (SAX)
    Strong unbridling of celiac
      artery a.
    superior QRS a.

    T a.
    thoracic a.
    vertical long a.
    X, Y, Z a.
Axius Vacuum 2 stabilizer
axonal neuropathy
Axxion drug-eluting stent
Ayercillin
Ayers
    A. sphygmomanometer
    A. T piece
Ayerza
    A. disease
    A. syndrome
Aygestin
Ayr
    A. Saline mist
    A. saline nasal drops
    A. saline nasal gel
AZ
    acquisition zoom
      AZ technology
AZA
    azathioprine
Azactam
Azadirachta indica leaf extract
azalide class of antibiotics
Azan-Mallory stain
azapetine phosphate
azatadine maleate
azathioprine (AZA)
azidothymidine (AZT)
azimilide
    a. dihydrochloride
    a. supraventricular arrhythmia
      program
azithromycin
Azmacort Oral Inhaler
azole antifungal
azotemia
    extrarenal a.
    postrenal a.
    prerenal a.
    renal a.
AZT
    azidothymidine
AZTEC
    amplitude zone time epoch coding
      AZTEC algorithm
aztreonam
azurophil granule
azygography
azygos
    a. arch
    a. fissure
    a. lobe
    a. lobe of right lung
    a. node
    a. vein

Azzopardi effect

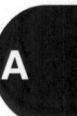

B

B bump
B bump on echocardiogram
B cell antibody
B cell lymphoma
B knuckle

b

branched

B₄

leukotriene B_4 (LTB_4)

B1 cell
B6 bronchus sign
B101 ET Tape II adhesive tape
BA

basilar artery
bilateral asymmetrical

Babcock operation
Babes-Ernst body
Babesia

B. bigemina
B. bovis
B. canis
B. divergens
B. major
B. microti
B. rodhaini

babesiosis

human b.

Babington-type nebulizer
Babinski

downgoing B.
B. reflex
B. syndrome
upgoing B.

baby

blue b.
b. lung concept

BABYbird respirator
babygram x-ray
Babyhaler spacer device
babyPac ventilator
BAC

bronchioloalveolar carcinoma

bacampicillin hydrochloride
Baccelli sign
Bachmann

anterior internodal tract of B.
B. bundle
internodal tract of B.
B. pathway

Baci-IM injection
bacillary

b. angiomatosis
b. embolism

b. phthisis
b. pneumonia

bacille Calmette-Guérin (BCG)
bacilli (*pl. of* bacillus)
bacilliformis

Bartonella b.

Bacillus

B. alvei
B. anthracis
B. cereus
B. circulans
B. laterosporus
B. licheniformis
B. megaterium
B. pneumoniae
B. polymyxa
B. pseudodiphtheriticum
B. pumilus
B. sphaericus
B. stearothermophilus
B. subtilis
B. subtilis enzyme

bacillus, pl. bacilli

acid-fast b. (AFB)
Battey b.
Bordet-Gengou b.
enteric gram-negative b.
Friedländer b.
gram-negative b. (GNB)
gram-positive b.
influenza b.
Klebs-Loeffler b.
Koch b.
Koch-Weeks b.
Loeffler b.
Much b.
Warthin-Starry-staining bacillus
Weeks b.

bacitracin
backflow
backflush
background subtraction technique
back pressure
backscatter

b. analysis
2-dimensional integrated b.
integrated b.
b. threshold

backup ventilation (BUV)
backward heart failure
baclofen
BACTEC

BACTEC MGIT 960 System
BACTEC radiometry

B

bacteremia, bacteriemia
    pneumococcal b.
    streptococcal b.
bacteremic
bacteria (*pl. of* bacterium)
bacteria-free
    b.-f. stage
    b.-f. stage of bacterial endocarditis
bacterial
    b. asthma
    b. colonization
    b. endocarditis (BE, BEC)
    b. endotoxin
    b. exacerbation
    b. myocarditis
    b. pericarditis
    b. pneumococcal pneumonia
    b. respiratory tract infection
    b. rhinosinusitis
    b. superinfection
    b. vegetation
bactericidal titer
bacteriemia (*var. of* bacteremia)
bacterioid
bacteriophage
bacteriostatic
    b. agent
    b. effect
bacterium, pl. **bacteria**
    facultative bacteria
Bacterium anitratum
Bacteroides
    B. corrodens
    B. fragilis
    B. furcosus
    B. melaninogenicus
    B. oralis
    B. pneumosintes
Bactrim DS
Bactroban Topical
BAE
    bovine aortic endothelium
    bronchial artery embolization
BAEC
    bovine aortic endothelial cell
BAEDP
    balloon aortic end-diastolic pressure
Baehr-Lohlein lesion
Baffes operation
baffle
    atrial b.
    fabric b.
    b. fenestration
    Gore-Tex b.
    intraatrial b.
    b. leak
    manual resuscitation b.
    Mustard atrial b.
    b. obstruction

    pericardial b.
    b. thrombosis
baffled jet nebulizer
bag
    Ambu b.
    disposable resuscitator b.
    Douglas b.
    Gamow b.
    Hope b.
    Lifesaver disposable resuscitator b.
    manual resuscitation b.
    rebreathing b.
    resuscitator b.
    SureGrip breathing b.
    Tedlar b.
    b. ventilation
    Voorhees b.
bagassosis
BagEasy disposable manual resuscitator
baggy heart
bag-mask
    b.-m. ventilation
    b.-m. ventilation device
bagpipe sign
bag-valve device
bag-valve-mask (BVM)
    b.-v.-m. ventilation
Bahnson aortic clamp
BAI
    breath-actuated inhaler
Bailey
    B. aortic clamp
    B. aortic valve rongeur
    B. catheter
    B. rib spreader
Bailey-Gibbon rib contractor
bailout
    emergency b.
    b. situation
    b. stenting
    b. valvoplasty
Baim pacing catheter
Bainbridge
    B. effect
    B. reflex
Bair
    B. Hugger
    B. Hugger blanket
Bairnsdale ulcer
baker's asthma
Bakes dilator
BAL
    bronchoalveolar lavage
    BAL brushing
Baladi Inverter device
balance
    acid-base b.
    B. Heavyweight guidewire
    micronutrient b.

B. Middle Weight guidewire
sympathovagal b.
B. Trek guidewire
Wilhelmy b.

balanced
b. coronary circulation
b. vasodilator

BALF
bronchoalveolar lavage fluid

Balke
B. exercise stress test
B. treadmill protocol

Balke-Ware
B.-W. test
B.-W. treadmill protocol

ball
carotid b.
Esmarch b.
fibrous b.
fungus b.
b. heart valve
b. mitral commissurotomy
NC Bandit b.
parietal b.
pleural fibrin b.
b. of Reil
sinuatrial b.
b. thrombus
b. valve prosthesis
b. variance

ball-and-cage, ball-in-cage
b.-a.-c. prosthesis
b.-a.-c. prosthetic valve

ballerina-foot pattern

ballet
cardiac b.

ball-in-cage (*var. of* ball-and-cage)

ballistocardiogram

ballistocardiograph (BCG)

ballistocardiography

ball-occluder valve

balloon
Accent-DG b.
ACS Alpha b.
b. angioplasty catheter
AngioSculpt scoring b.
b. aortic end-diastolic pressure (BAEDP)
b. aortic valvoplasty (BAV)
b. aortic valvotomy (BAV)
Arrow Berman angiographic b.
b. to artery ratio
b. atrial septoplasty
b. atrial septostomy (BAS)
b. atrioseptostomy
autoperfusion b.
AVCO aortic b.
Aviator b.
Bandit b.

Berman angiographic b.
Blue Max high-pressure b.
b. catheter angioplasty (BCA)
b. catheterization
b. catheter sealing device
b. coarctation angioplasty
compliant b.
Cook b.
Cordis Powerflex angioplasty b.
b. coronary angioplasty
b. coronary occlusion (BCO)
b. counterpulsation
counterpulsation b.
CrossSail b.
cutting b.
Datascope b.
b. dilation (BD)
b. dilation angioplasty (BDA)
Dispatch b.
b. dissector
b. distention test
Dynasty b.
Eliminator dilation b.
b. embolectomy catheter
Express b.
Extractor 3-lumen retrieval b.
Falcon Omniflex b.
fixed-wire b.
Force b.
Hartzler Micro II b.
Helix b.
Hunter-Sessions b.
b. inflation
b. inflation pressure
Inoue self-guiding b.
Integra II b.
intraaortic b. (IAB)
14K b.
Kay b.
Kontron b.
b. laser angioplasty
latex b.
liquid nitrous oxide-filled b.
Lo-Fold b.
low-profile semi-compliant b.
Mansfield b.
Maverick b.
Medtronic Evergreen b.
Micross SL b.
Microvasive Rigiflex TTS b.
b. mitral commissurotomy (BMC)
b. mitral valvoplasty (BMV)
Monorail Speedy b.
Multi-Link Tristar b.
NC b.
noncompliant b.
b. occlusion
b. occlusive intravascular lysis enhanced recanalization

balloon *(continued)*
    Olbert b.
    Owens b.
    Panther b.
    PE b.
    b. pericardiotomy
    Piccolino b.
    pillow-shaped b.
    polyethylene terephthalate b.
    polyolefin copolymer b.
    polyvinyl chloride b.
    Powerflex angioplasty b.
    PowerSail b.
    preperitoneal dilator b. (PDB)
    ProCross Rely b.
    b. pulmonary valvoplasty (BPV)
    b. pulmonary valvotomy
    b. pump
    QuickFurl SL b.
    radiofrequency hot b.
    Ranger b.
    Raptor PTCA b.
    right ventricular copulsation b.
      (RVCB)
    b. rupture
    b. septostomy
    b. septostomy catheter
    Shadow b.
    b. shunt
    Simpson PET b.
    Simpson positron emission
      tomography b.
    sizing b.
    Slalom b.
    Solo b.
    Spears laser b.
    Stack autoperfusion b.
    stealth angioplasty b.
    b. tamponade
    Target Therapeutics Stealth
      angioplasty b.
    b. test occlusion (BTO)
    trefoil Schneider b.
    b. tricuspid valvotomy
    Tyshak b.
    b. valvoplasty (BV)
    b. valvoplasty catheter
    b. valvoplasty registry (BVR)
    b. venography
    waisting of b.
    windowed b.
    workhorse b.
balloon-delivery system
balloon-expandable
    b.-e. flexible coil stent
    b.-e. intravascular stent
balloon-facilitated
    b.-f. PCT
    b.-f. percutaneous tracheostomy

balloon-flotation pacing catheter
balloon-imaging catheter
ballooning
    b. mitral cusp syndrome
    b. mitral valve syndrome
    b. posterior leaflet syndrome
balloon-occlusion pulmonary angiography
balloon-on-a-wire
    b.-o.-a-w. catheter
    b.-o.-a-w. dilation system
balloon-protected selective thrombin injection
balloon-shaped heart
balloon-tipped
    b.-t. angiographic catheter
    b.-t. flow-directed catheter
    b.-t. thermodilution catheter
ballpoint pen technique
ball-valve
    b.-v. effect
    b.-v. thrombus
Balme cough
Balminil-DM Children
Balminil Expectorant
BALT
    bronchus-associated lymphoid tissue
Baltaxe view
Baltherm catheter
Bamberger
    B. area
    B. bulbar pulse
    B. disease
    B. sign
Bamberger-Marie
    B.-M. disease
    B.-M. syndrome
Bamberger-Pins-Ewart sign
bambuterol
bamiphylline
Bamyl
banana-shaped left ventricle
Bancap HC
bancrofti
    Wuchereria b.
band
    A b.
    b. of adhesion
    annuloplasty b.
    atelectatic b.
    atrial anomalous b.
    contraction b.
    CPK-BB b.
    CPK-MB b.
    CPK-MM b.
    I b.
    Mach b.
    MB b.
    moderator b.
    myocardial b. (MB)

parietal b.
Pepper Medical tube neck b.
pulmonary artery b.
b. of Reil
b. saw effect
Vesseloops rubber b.
Z b.

bandage
Medicopaste b.
b. scissors

bandbox
b. resonance
b. sound

banding
Müller b.
PA b.
pulmonary artery b.
b. of pulmonary artery
Trusler rule for pulmonary
artery b.

bandit
B. balloon
B. PTCA catheter

bandlike
b. angina
b. intrapericardial echo

bandpass filter
bandwidth
bang artifact
bangungot syndrome
bank
tissue b.

Bannister disease
Bannwarth syndrome
Banophen Oral
BAO
basilar artery occlusion

Bapadin
BAPV
basal average peak velocity
baseline average peak velocity

BAR
beta-adrenergic receptor

Baratol
Barbeau radial guide catheter
barbed hook
Barbilixir
barbiturate
barbourin
bard
B. Clamshell septal occluder
B. Clamshell septal umbrella
B. Commander PTCA guidewire
B. percutaneous cardiopulmonary
support system
B. Safety Excalibur catheter
B. sign
B. Stinger S ablation catheter
B. XT coronary stent

Bardco catheter
Bard-Parker blade
bare metal stent (BMS)
baritosis
barium
b. enema
b. esophagram
b. swallow

BARK
beta-adrenergic receptor kinase

barking cough
Barlow syndrome
Barnard
B. mitral valve prosthesis
B. operation

baroceptor
barograph
barometer-maker's disease
barometric pressure
baroreceptor
cardiac b.
carotid b.
perturbed carotid b.
b. reflex
b. reflex sensitivity (BRS)
b. sensitivity
b. sensitization

baroreflex
arterial b. (ABR)
biochemical b.
carotid b.
b. sensitivity (BRS)
sinuatrial b.

baroscope
barosinusitis
barospirator
barotaxis
barotrauma
b. of ascent
dental b.
b. of descent
facial b.
pulmonary b.

Barraya forceps
barrel-hooping compression
barrel-shaped
b.-s. chest
b.-s. thorax

Barrett esophagus
barrier
blood-air b.
blood-brain b. (BBB)
blood-bronchoalveolar b.
blood-bronchus b.
blood-gas b.
blood-retina b.
placental b.

Barrow classification
Barsony-Polgar syndrome

B

Barthel
> B. ADL score
> B. index

Bartholin duct
Barth syndrome
Bartonella
> *B. bacilliformis*
> *B. elizabethae*
> *B. henselae*

Bartter syndrome
BAS
> balloon atrial septostomy
> beta-adrenergic stimulation

basal
> b. average peak velocity (BAPV)
> b. cell carcinoma
> b. collateral artery
> b. diastolic murmur
> b. fetal heart rate (BFHR)
> b. ganglion (BG)
> b. heart rate (BHR)
> b. interventricular septum
> b. metabolic rate (BMR)
> b. part of left and right inferior pulmonary
> b. pleural thickening
> b. segmental bronchus
> b. systolic
> b. tuberculosis

basalis communis
basaloid carcinoma
basal-septal hypertrophy
base
> b. of lung
> whole blood buffer b.

baseline
> b. arrhythmia
> b. artifact
> b. average peak velocity (BAPV)
> B. Dyspnea Index (BDI)
> b. ECG
> b. echocardiography
> b. rhythm
> b. shift
> b. ST-segment abnormality
> TP b.
> b. variability
> b. variability of fetal heart rate
> wandering b.

basement
> b. membrane
> reticular b.

baseplate
> winged b.

base-to-apex conduction
BASH
> body acceleration synchronous with heart rate

basic
> b. cardiac life support (BCLS)
> b. cycle length (BCL)
> b. drive cycle length
> b. fibroblast growth factor (bFGF)
> b. life support (BLS)
> b. life support ambulance
> b. life support-defibrillation (BLS-D)

Basidiomycetes
basilar
> b. artery (BA)
> b. artery fusiform aneurysm
> b. artery occlusion (BAO)
> b. bulla
> b. half ejection fraction
> b. rale
> b. sinus

basilaris ossis occipitalis
basilic vein
basiliximab
basipharyngeal canal
basis pulmonis
basket
> B. catheter
> Medi-Tech multipurpose b.
> pericardial b.

basophil
basophilic vascular streaking
Bassen-Kornzweig abetalipoproteinemia
bastadin-5
bat
> b. wing pattern
> b. wing shadow

bath
> film fixer b.
> film wash b.
> fixer b.
> Haake water b.
> Nauheim b.
> wash b.

bathycardia
bathypnea
batimastat-coated BiodivYsio vascular stent
Batista
> B. left ventricular reduction procedure
> B. left ventriculectomy procedure
> B. ventricular remodeling

batrachotoxin
Batson plexus
battery
> b. cell impedance
> b. cell voltage function
> Celsa b.
> b. elective replacement
> external pacemaker b.
> LiI b.

lithium iodine b.
nickel-cadmium b.
b. status
b. voltage
Battey
B. bacillus
B. disease
Bauer syndrome
baumannii
Acinetobacter b.
Baumanometer standard mercury sphygmomanometer
Baumès symptom
bauxite
b. pneumoconiosis
b. pneumonoconiosis
BAV
balloon aortic valvoplasty
balloon aortic valvotomy
bicommissural aortic valve
BAVFO
bradycardia after arteriovenous fistula occlusion
Bayer
B. Buffered Aspirin
B. Low Adult Strength
B. Select Chest Cold Caplets
B. Select Pain Relief Formula
Bayes theorem
Bayle granulation
Bayliss theory
Baylor
B. autologous transfusion system
B. rapid autologous transfusion (BRAT)
bayonet deformity
Bayou virus
Bazett
B. corrected QT interval
B. correction formula
Bazin disease
BB
blood buffer
bundle branch
BBB
blood-brain barrier
bundle branch block
BBBB
bilateral bundle branch block
BBM
brush border membrane
BBMV
brush border membrane vesicle
BBR
bundle branch reentry
BCA
balloon catheter angioplasty
bidirectional cavopulmonary anastomosis

BCC
Burkholderia cepacia complex
BCD Plus cardioplegic unit
BCG
bacille Calmette-Guérin
ballistocardiograph
bronchocentric granulomatosis
BCG vaccine
BCKD
branched chain alpha ketoacid dehydrogenase
BCL
basic cycle length
bcl-2 **expression**
BCLS
basic cardiac life support
BCM
blood-clotting mechanism
BCME
bischloromethyl ether
BCO
balloon coronary occlusion
biliary cholesterol output
B-complex
BCPR
bystander cardiopulmonary resuscitation
BCS
British Cardiac Society
BCT
blunt chest trauma
BD
balloon dilation
BD ProbeTec Direct TB System
B-D
Becton-Dickinson
B-D Potain thoracic trocar
B-D TwinPak dual cannula device
BDA
balloon dilation angioplasty
BDCS
Behavioral Dyscontrol Scale
BDG
bidirectional Glenn procedure
BDI
Baseline Dyspnea Index
BDT
bronchodilator
BDW
biphasic defibrillation waveform
BE
bacterial endocarditis
bead
Digoxin RIA B.
beading of arteries
Beall
B. circumflex artery scissors
B. disc valve prosthesis
B. mitral valve prosthesis
B. prosthetic valve

Beall-Surgitool ball-cage prosthetic valve
beam
> 4-b. laser Doppler probe
> b. splitter
> b. width artifact

bean
> castor b.
> green coffee b.

beanbag shotgun round ammunition
bean-spooning task
bear
> B. 1, 2 adult volume ventilator
> B. Cub infant ventilator
> B. 1000 ventilator

beat
> aberrant condition of
>   supraventricular b. (rSR)
> aberrantly conducted b.
> agonal b.
> apex b. (AB)
> Ashman b.
> atrial capture b.
> atrial ectopic b.
> atrial fusion b.
> atrial premature b. (APB)
> atrioventricular junctional escape b.
> auricular premature b.
> automatic b.
> A-V junctional escape b.
> capture b.
> combination b.
> coupled premature b.'s
> dependent b.
> Dressler b.
> dropped b.
> echo b.
> ectopic Ashman b.
> ectopic junctional b. (EJB)
> ectopic ventricular b.
> entrained b.
> escape b.
> extrasystolic b.
> fascicular b.
> forced b.
> frequency ectopic ventricular b.
>   (FEVB)
> fusion b.
> high-frequency b.
> b. inclusion index (BII)
> interference b.
> interpolated b.
> isolated ectopic b.
> junctional escape b.
> junctional premature b. (JPB)
> Lown class 4a, 4b ventricular
>   ectopic b.
> malignant b.
> missed b.
> mixed b.

> nodal premature b. (NPB)
> paced b.
> paired b.'s
> parasystolic b.
> b.'s per minute (BPM, bpm)
> b.'s per second (BPS)
> postextrasystolic b.
> premature b. (PB)
> premature atrial b. (PAB, PAC)
> premature junctional b.
> premature nodal b. (PNB)
> premature ventricular b. (PVB)
> pseudofusion b.
> reciprocal b.
> retrograde b.
> salvo of b.'s
> single premature atrial b.
> skipped b.
> summation b.
> supraventricular premature b.
>   (SVPB)
> total heart b.'s (THB)
> unifocal ventricular ectopic b.
>   (UVEB)
> ventricular capture b.
> ventricular ectopic b. (VEB)
> ventricular escape b.
> ventricular fusion b.
> ventricular premature b. (VPB)
> VP b.

beat-by-beat
> b.-b.-b. capture
> b.-b.-b. capture confirmation
> b.-b.-b. hemodynamic monitoring

beating
> b. action
> b. heart edge-to-edge technique
> b. heart surgery

beating-heart
> b.-h. bypass procedure
> b.-h. CABG
> b.-h. coronary artery bypass graft

beat-to-beat
> b.-t.-b. analysis
> b.-t.-b. finger arterial pressure
> b.-t.-b. variability (BTBV)
> b.-t.-b. variability of fetal heart
>   rate

Beatty-Bright friction sound
Beau
> B. asystole
> B. disease
> B. line
> B. syndrome

beaver
> B. blade
> B. knife

Beaver-DeBakey blade

BEB
blind esophageal brushing
BEC
bacterial endocarditis
Beck
B. cardiopericardiopexy
B. Depression Inventory
B. epicardial poudrage
B. I, II operation
B. miniature aortic clamp
B. triad
Becker disease
Becker-type tardive muscular dystrophy
Beckman
B. ICS Nephelometer system
B. O₂ analyzer
Beck-Potts aortic and pulmonic clamp
Béclard
B. anastomosis
B. hernia
Becloforte
beclomethasone
b. dipropionate
b. monopropionate (BMP)
Beclovent Oral Inhaler
Beconase AQ Nasal Inhaler
becquerel (Bq)
Becton-Dickinson (B-D)
B.-D. guidewire
B.-D. Teflon-sheathed needle
bed
adventitial b.
b. block
capillary b.
coronary b.
cyanosis of nail b.'s
distal b.
molecular sieve b.
myocardial b.
nail b.
perfusion b.
pulmonary vascular b.
rocking b.
Sanders b.
Stress Echo b.
time in b. (TIB)
vascular b.
venous capacitance b.
Bedbugg system
Bedfont carbon monoxide monitor
bedside
b. balloon atrial septoplasty
b. monitor
b. transthoracic echocardiography
beef
b. insulin
b. Lente Iletin II
beef-lung heparin

beer
b. and cobalt syndrome
b. heart
B. law
beer-drinker's cardiomyopathy
Beer-Lambert principle
bee venom
beginning-of-life rate
behavior
contractile b.
type A, B b.
behavioral
B. Dyscontrol Scale (BDCS)
b. factor
b. therapy
Behçet
B. disease
B. syndrome
Béhier-Hardy sign
beigelii
Trichosporon b.
Belhassen tachycardia
bell
b. sound
b. stethoscope
b. tympany
Bellavar medical support stockings
belli
Isospora b.
bellmetal resonance
bellows
chest b.
b. function
b. murmur
b. sound
Belos VR implantable cardioverter-defibrillator
BeLPT
beryllium lymphocyte proliferation test
Belsey
B. esophagoplasty
B. Mark IV fundoplication
belt
abdominal b.
stroke b.
Belzer solution
bemiparin
Bemis air purifier
Benadryl
B. injection
B. Oral
B. Topical
benazepril
amlodipine and b.
b. hydrochloride
b. and hydrochlorothiazide
bench surgery
bend
lytic b.

bendrofluazide
bendroflumethiazide
Benecol margarine
Benedict-Roth
    B.-R. apparatus
    B.-R. spirometer
benefit-risk ratio
Bengolea forceps
Benicar
benidipine
benign
    b. airway stenosis
    b. croupous angina
    b. early repolarization (BER)
    b. fibrous mesothelioma
    b. hypertension
    b. intracranial hypertension
    b. pleural disease
    b. teratoma
    b. transient hiccups
benigna
    endocarditis b.
benignum
    empyema b.
Benjamin
    B. binocular laryngoscope
    B. pediatric laryngoscope
Bennett
    B. Cascade II Servo Controlled Heated Humidifier
    B. MA-1, PR-2 ventilator
    Nellcor Puritan B. (NPB)
    B. twin
Bentall
    inclusion technique of B.
    B. inclusion technique
    B. operation
    B. procedure
bent bronchus sign
Bentley transducer
Benton Lines Test
Bentson
    B. exchange straight guidewire
    B. floppy-tip guidewire
    B. Plus cerebral wire guide
Bentson-Hanafee-Wilson catheter
Bentson-style guidewire
Benylin
    B. Expectorant
    B. Pediatric
benzalkonium chloride asthma
benzathine
    b. benzyl penicillin
    penicillin G b.
benzoate
    benzyl b.
    caffeine and sodium b.
    denatonium b.

benzocaine, butyl aminobenzoate, tetracaine, benzalkonium chloride
benzodiazepine
benzonatate
benzoporphyrin
benzothiadiazide
benzothiazepine
benzoylpas
    calcium b.
    b. calcium
benzthiazide
benzyl benzoate
benzylisoquinoline
benzylpenicillin
benzylpenicilloyl polylysine (PPL)
benzyl-thiourea
bepridil hydrochloride
BER
    benign early repolarization
beractant
beraprost sodium (BPS)
Berard aneurysm
Berenstein catheter
Berg Balance Scale
Berger operation
Bergmeister papilla
Bergstrom needle biopsy technique
beriberi
    cerebral b.
    dry b.
    b. heart
    infantile b.
    wet b.
Berkovits-Castellanos hexapolar electrode
Berlin
    B. nosology
    B. questionnaire
    B. TAH
    B. total artificial heart
Berman
    B. airway
    B. angiographic balloon
    B. angiographic catheter
Bernheim syndrome
Berning and Steensgaard-Hansen score
Bernoulli
    B. effect
    B. equation
    B. theorem
Bernstein
    B. procedure
    B. test
Berotec
berry aneurysm
berylliosis
beryllium
    b. lymphocyte proliferation test (BeLPT)
    b. sensitized (BeS)

beryllium-induced lung disease
beryllium-specific
  b.-s. CD4+ T_H1 cell
  b.-s. helper T cell
BeS
  beryllium sensitized
Besnier-Boeck-Schaumann
  B.-B.-S. disease
  B.-B.-S. syndrome
BeStent
  B. 2 coronary stent
  B. Rival coronary stent system
  B. Rival stent
  B. 2 with Discrete Technology
    Over-The-Wire and Rapid
    Exchange coronary stent delivery
    system
Bestneb nebulizer
besylate
  amlodipine b.
  cisatracurium b.
beta
  b. adrenoceptor
  b. adrenoceptor stimulation
  b. agonist
  b. antagonist
  b. ARK
  b. ARK-1
  b. AR kinase1 enzyme
  b. blockade
  b. blocker
  b. blocking agent
  b. carotene
  estrogen receptor b. (ER beta)
  b. lactamase
  b. lipoprotein
  b. ray
  b. receptor
  b. thromboglobulin
  b. variable (Vbeta, Vbeta3)
beta-1
  b.-1 adrenergic stimulation
  b.-1 antagonist
  b.-1 AR
  b.-1 blocker
  b.-1, -2 receptor
beta-1B adrenergic receptor (ADRA1B)
beta-2
  b.-2 adrenergic stimulation
  b.-2 adrenoreceptor stimulation
  b.-2 antagonist
  b.-2 AR
  b.-2 AR overexpression
  b.-2 integrin MAC-1
beta-adrenergic
  b.-a. agonist
  b.-a. blockade
  b.-a. blocker
  b.-a. blocking agent

  b.-a. receptor (BAR)
  b.-a. receptor kinase (BARK)
  b.-a. stimulation (BAS)
beta-adrenoceptor
  b.-a. agonist
  b.-a. antibody
  b.-a. blocker
  b.-a. blocking agent
beta-antagonist
  long-acting b.-a.
beta-Arr2
  beta-Arrestin-2
beta-Arrestin-2 (beta-Arr2)
beta-beta homodimer
beta-blocker therapy
Beta-Cath system
Betacel-Biotronik pacemaker
beta-D-glucan test
beta-endorphin
17-beta-estradiol
  transdermal 17-b.-e.
beta-galactosidase
beta-hydroxysteroid
  11--b.-h. dehydrogenase
betaine diet
beta-lactam
beta-lactamase
  CAZ b.-l.
  extended-spectrum b.-l.
  b.-l. inhibitor
Betaloc Durules
betamethasone
  systemic b.
betamethyliodophenyl pentadecanoic acid (BMIPP)
beta-MHC
  beta-myosin heavy chain
  beta-MHC gene
beta-myosin heavy chain (beta-MHC)
Betapace
  B. AF tablet
  B. Oral
Betapen-VK Oral
beta-radiation
  intracoronary b.-r.
Beta-Rail catheter
beta-receptor polymorphism
beta-sitosterol
beta-thalassemia
  homozygous b.-t.
beta-thromboglobulin
  b.-t. level
  plasma b.-t.
Beta-Tim
betaxolol hydrochloride
bethanechol chloride
bethanidine
Bethea sign
Bethune-Coryllos shears

B

Better Sleep Council
Bettman-Fovash thoracotome
Beuren syndrome
bevantolol
Bezalip
Bezold-Jarisch reflex
BF
 blood flow
 breathing frequency
  BF large core bronchoscope
BFE
 blood flow energy
bFGF
 basic fibroblast growth factor
BFHR
 basal fetal heart rate
BFR
 blood flow rate
BFV
 blood flow velocity
BG
 basal ganglion
BGO
 bismuth germanate
BH
 borderline hypertensive
 bundle of His
  BH interval
BH$_4$
 tetrahydrobiopterin
BHD
 bilateral hemisphere damage
BHF
 British Heart Foundation
BHI
 breathholding index
BHIA
 brain-heart infusion agar
BHIBA
 brain-heart infusion blood agar
B-H interval
BHIRS
 brain-heart infusion and rabbit serum
BHR
 basal heart rate
 bronchial hyperreactivity
 bronchial hyperresponsiveness
BHT
 borderline hypertension
 butylated hydroxytoluene
BI
 brain infarct
Bianchi
 B. nodule
 B. valve
bias
 b. flow
 b. flow system

biatrial
 b. anastomosis
 b. enlargement
 b. pacing
biatriatum
 cor pseudotriloculare b.
 cor triloculare b.
Biaxin Filmtabs
bibasally
bibasilar
 b. atelectasis
 b. coarse crackle
 b. rale
bible printer's lung
bicalutamide
BICAP
 bilateral circumactive probe
  BICAP unit
bicarbonate (HCO$_3$)
 sodium b.
bicarbonaturia
Bicarbon Sorin valve
bicardiogram
BiCAT
 bilateral carotid artery traction
bicaval
Bichat tunic
Bicillin
 B. C-R
 B. L-A injection
bicommissural aortic valve (BAV)
Bicor catheter
bicuspidalis
 cuspis anterior valvae b.
bicuspid aortic valve
bicuspidization
bicycle
 Aerodyne stationary b.
 Collins b.
 b. dynamometer
 b. echocardiography
 b. ergometer exercise stress test
 b. ergometry
 b. exercise
 stationary b.
 Tredex powered b.
BiDil
bidimensional echocardiography
bidirectional
 b. cavopulmonary anastomosis (BCA)
 b. cavopulmonary shunt
 b. conduction
 b. Glenn operation
 b. Glenn procedure (BDG)
 b. isthmus conduction block
 b. 4-pole Butterworth high-pass digital filter
 b. shunt calculation

b. superior cavopulmonary
  anastomosis (BSCA)
b. ventricular
b. ventricular tachycardia
Bier block anesthesia
Biermer sign
bifascicular heart block
biferious (*var. of* bisferious)
Bifidobacterium
bifid P wave
bifocal demand DVI pacemaker
bifoil balloon catheter
bifurcated
  b. aortofemoral prosthesis
  b. endograft
  b. graft
  b. stent
  b. vein graft for vascular
    reconstruction
bifurcating block
bifurcatio
  b. tracheae
  b. trunci
bifurcation
  b. of aorta
  aortic b.
  carotid b.
  coronary b.
  b. lesion (BL)
  b. lymph node
  moustache angiographic landmark
    of left anterior descending
    coronary artery b.
  pitchfork angiographic landmark of
    left anterior descending coronary
    artery b.
  b. prosthesis
  b. of pulmonary trunk
  b. of trachea
  tracheal b.
  whale's tail angiographic landmark
    of left anterior descending
    coronary artery b.
  Y-shaped b.
bifurcational coronary lesion
bigemina
  Babesia b.
bigeminal
  b. bisferious pulse
  b. pulse
  b. rhythm
bigemini
bigeminus
  pulsus b.
bigeminy
  atrial b.
  atrioventricular junctional b.
  atrioventricular nodal b.
  A-V nodal b.

escape-capture b.
junctional b.
nodal b.
reciprocal b.
rule of b.
ventricular b.
big endothelin
biglycan
biguanide
BII
  beat inclusion index
bilateral
  b. adrenal hyperplasia
  b. anterior flail chest
  b. aortoostial coronary artery
    disease
  b. asymmetrical (BA)
  b. bundle branch block (BBBB)
  b. carotid artery traction (BiCAT)
  b. circumactive probe (BICAP)
  b. hemisphere damage (BHD)
  b. internal mammary artery
    (BIMA)
  b. internal thoracic artery (BITA)
  b. lung transplant (BLT)
  b. sequential single lung transplant
  b. symmetrical (BS)
bile
  b. acid binding resin
  b. acid sequestrant
  b. solubility test
bileaflet
  b. mechanical prosthesis
  b. prolapse
  b. tilting disc prosthetic valve
bilevel
  b. positive airway pressure
    (BiPAP)
  b. positive pressure device
Bilharzia
bilharziasis
biliary
  b. cholesterol output (BCO)
  b. cirrhosis
  b. colic
  b. disease
BiliBlanket phototherapy system
Bili mask
bilious pneumonia
bilirubinemia
bilirubin oxidative metabolite
billiard ball effect
Billingham criteria
billowing
  cusp b.
  b. mitral leaflet syndrome (BMLS)
  mitral valve b.
  b. mitral valve syndrome
bilobate

B

bilobectomy
bilobed aneurysm
bilobular
biloculare
    cor b.
Biltricide
BIMA
    bilateral internal mammary artery
bimanual precordial palpation
Bimodality Lung Oncology Team (BLOT)
binary angiographic restenosis
binding
    albumin cobalt b. (ACB)
    antigen b.
    fragment antigen b. (Fab)
    guanine nucleotide modulatable b.
    ligand b.
    table b.
Bing stylet
Bing-Taussig heart procedure
Binswanger disease
binuclear
binucleate
bioabsorbable polymeric material (BPM)
bioassay
bioavailability
    nitric oxide b.
Biobrane adhesive
BioBypass gene-based drug delivery product
Biocef
Biocell RTV implant
biochanin A
biochemical
    b. assay procedure
    b. baroreflex
    b. enzyme assay
Bioclot protein S assay
biocompatibility
biocompatible stent
Biocontrol Technology/Coratomic lead
Biocor
    B. 200 high performance oxygenator
    B. porcine valve
biodegradable stent
Biodex System
BioDiamond
    B. F stent
    B. Micro stent
    B. S rapid exchange PTCA catheter
BiodivYsio
    B. added support stent
    B. AS PC-coated stent
    B. OC over-the-wire stent
    B. open cell stent
    B. PC stent

    B. phosphorylcholine-coated coronary stent
    B. small vessel stent
    B. SV PC-coated stent
    B. vascular stent
bioelectric
    b. current
    b. potential
bioelectricity
bioequivalence
bioerodible polymer stent coating
biofeedback
biofilm
biogenesis
    mitochondrial b.
BioGlue
    B. protein-based surgical adhesive
    B. surgical adhesive for aortic dissection
    B. surgical patch
biograft
    Dardik B.
    B. graft
biographer
    GlucoWatch G2 automatic glucose b.
bioimpedance
    b. electrocardiograph
    b. monitor
    thoracic electrical b. (TEB)
biologic
    GenStent b.
biological
    b. aortic valve
    b. effects of ionizing Radiation
    b. fibrous matrix
    b. fitness
    b. half-life
    b. prosthesis
biomarker
    intermediate endpoint b. (IEB)
    pharmacogenetic b.
    surrogate endpoint b. (SEB)
biomass fuel
biomaterial
    MycroMesh Plus b.
    Salubria b.
Biomatrix ocular implant
Bio-Medicus
    B.-M. arterial catheter
    B.-M. pump
Bio-Med MVP-10 pediatric ventilator
biomembrane
biondii
    Magnolia b.
bionic baroreflex system
BioPolyMeric vascular graft
Biopore membrane

bioprosthesis
> Carpentier-Edwards mitral Perimount pericardial b.
> Carpentier-Edwards Perimount RSR pericardial b.
> CryoLife-O'Brien stentless aortic porcine b.
> Edwards Prima Plus stentless porcine b.
> Freestyle aortic root b.
> Freestyle stentless b.
> Hancock II stented b.
> Hancock M.O. II porcine b.
> Medtronic Intact porcine b.
> Mosaic cardiac b.
> pericarbon b.
> Perimount RSR pericardial b.
> porcine b.
> Soprano b.
> stentless porcine b.
> Toronto SPV b.
> X-Cell cardiac b.

bioprosthetic
> b. endocarditis
> b. porcine heart valve
> b. valve (BPV)

biopsy, pl. **biopsies**
> aspiration b.
> bite b.
> blind needle b.
> bronchial brush b.
> bronchoscopic lung b. (BLB)
> bronchoscopic needle b.
> brush b.
> catheter-guided b.
> controlled lung b.
> cytological b.
> endomyocardial b. (EMB)
> endoscopic b.
> excisional b.
> fine-needle aspiration b.
> b. forceps
> lung b.
> mediastinal lymph node b.
> open lung b. (OLB)
> open pleural b.
> percutaneous needle aspiration b.
> percutaneous transthoracic needle b. (PTNB)
> pericardial b.
> pleural b.
> punch b.
> scalene fat pad b.
> scalene lymph node b.
> skeletal muscle b.
> supraclavicular lymph node b.
> surgical lung b. (SLB)
> thorascopic b.

> transbronchial b. (TBB, TBBX, TBBx)
> transbronchial lung b. (TBLB)
> transcatheter b. (TCB)
> transthoracic needle b. (TNB)
> transthoracic needle aspiration b.
> transvenous b.
> ultrasonically guided needle b. (UGNB)
> ventricular b.
> video-assisted thoracic surgical lung b.
> wedge b.

bioptic sampling

bioptome
> cardiac b.
> Caves-Schultz b.
> Cordis b.
> Kawai b.
> King b.
> Konno b.
> Mansfield b.
> Olympus b.
> Scholten endomyocardial b.
> Stanford b.

Bio-Pump

Biorate pacemaker

bioresorbable implant

Biosafe Hemo-Quant rapid anemia test

Biosense
> B. left ventricular mapping
> B. revascularization approach
> B. revascularization approach for viable endocardium (BRAVE)
> B. Webster NaviStar ablation deflectable tip catheter

Biosense-guided laser myocardial revascularization

Biosound
> B. Genesis II scanning system
> B. 2000 II ultrasound unit
> B. 3000 ultrasound unit

Biostent

Biosurge Synchronous Autotransfuser

biosynthesis
> collagen b.
> leukotriene b.

Biot
> B. breathing
> B. respiration
> B. sign

bioterrorism threat agent

biotin/streptavidin system

Biotrack coagulation monitor

biotransformation

biotrauma

Biotronik
> B. Home Monitoring System
> B. lead

Biotronik (*continued*)
    B. lead connector
    B. pacemaker
    B. Rithron-XR coronary stent
    B. Tenax stent
    B. Tensum stent
Bio-Vascular prosthetic valve
BI-OX III ear oximeter
BioZ
    B. hemodynamic monitoring system
    B. ICG Module
    B. ICG Monitor
    B. impedance cardiography
    technology
    B. noninvasive cardiac function
    monitoring system
BioZ.com cardiac output monitor
BioZ.pc system
BioZtect sensor
BIP
    bronchiolitic interstitial pneumonia
    bronchiolitis with interstitial pneumonitis
BiPAP
    bilevel positive airway pressure
    BiPAP duet system
    BiPAP S/T-D 30 system
    BiPAP S/T-D ventilatory support
    system
    BiPAP unit
    BiPAP Vision system
biperiden
biphasic
    b. defibrillation waveform (BDW)
    b. defibrillator
    b. mesothelioma
    b. response
    b. shock
    b. stridor
    b. waveform transthoracic
    defibrillation
biplanar tomography
biplane
    b. aortography
    b. area-length method
    b. fluoroscopy
    b. formula
    b. imaging
    b. orthogonal angiography
    b. pelvic arteriography
    b. quantitative coronary
    arteriography
    b. ventriculography
bipolar
    b. catheter
    b. circumactive probe
    b. coagulating forceps
    b. electrocardiogram
    b. electrocoagulation (BPEC)
    b. esophageal recording

    b. generator
    b. lead
    b. pacemaker
    b. radiofrequency surgical ablation
    instrument
BiPort hemostasis introducer sheath kit
bipyridine derivative
Biquin Durules
Birbeck granules
bird
    B. Ascension ventilator
    b. breeder's lung
    b. fancier's lung
    b. fever
    b. handler's lung
    b.'s eye catheter
    B. sign
    b.'s nest lesion
    b.'s nest vena cava filter
    B. VDR ventilator
birefringence
birminghamensis
    Legionella b.
Birmingham Vasculitis Activity Score
    (BVAS)
birth control pill
bischloroethylnitrosourea chemotherapy
bischloromethyl ether (BCME)
bisferiens
    pulsus b.
bisferient
bisferious, biferious
    b. pulse
bishop
    b.'s hat
    b.'s nod
    B. sphygmoscope
bishydroxycoumarin
bismesylate
bismuth
    b. germanate (BGO)
    b. subsalicylate
Bisolvon
bisoprolol
    b. fumarate
    b. and hydrochlorothiazide
Bisping electrode
bistoury
    Jackson b.
bisulfate
    clopidogrel b.
BITA
    bilateral internal thoracic artery
bitartrate
    hydrocodone b.
    metaraminol b.
    norepinephrine b.
bite biopsy
biteblock, bite block

B

bitolterol mesylate
Bitpad digitizer
Bitrex
BIVAD (*var. of* BVAD)
bivalirudin
bivalve
biventricular
    b. assist device (BVAD, BIVAD)
    b. direct cardiac compression
    b. dysfunction
    b. endomyocardial fibrosis
    b. hypertrophy (BVH)
    b. ICD
    b. pacing
    b. pacing and defibrillator device
      (BiV-ICD)
    b. pacing stimulation
    b. pacing wire
    b. resynchronization technology
    b. support (BVS)
biventriculare
    cor triloculare b.
BiV-ICD
    biventricular pacing and defibrillator
    device
Bivona
    B. Fome-Cuff tube
    B. TTS tracheostomy tube
bizarre QRS complex
Björk
    B. method
    B. method of Fontan procedure
Björk-Shiley (B-S)
    B.-S. aortic valve prosthesis
    B.-S. convexoconcave (BSCC)
    B.-S. convexoconcave 60-degree
      valve prosthesis
    B.-S. convexoconcave disc
      prosthetic valve
    B.-S. floating disc prosthesis
    B.-S. graft
    B.-S. heart valve holder
    B.-S. heart valve sizer
    B.-S. mitral valve
    B.-S. monostrut valve
BK
    human polyomavirus BK (BKV)
BKV
    human polyomavirus BK
BL
    bifurcation lesion
    buffered lidocaine
black
    b. blood angiography
    b. blood magnetic resonance
      imaging
    B. Creek Canal virus
    b. hole phenomenon
    b. lung

    b. lung disease
    b. phthisis
    b. pleura
    b. pleura sign
    b. tea
    b. widow spider venom
Blackfan-Diamond syndrome
blackfoot disease
Blackman window
blackout
    shallow water b.
    b. spell
black-white interface technique (BWIT)
    BWIT arterial blood filter
blade
    Acra-Cut Spiral craniotome b.
    Atherotome microsurgical b.
    b. atrial septostomy
    Bard-Parker b.
    Beaver b.
    Beaver-DeBakey b.
    CLM articulating laryngoscope b.
    b. control wire holder
    DeBakey b.
    electrosurgical b.
    knife b.
    Lite B.
    Macintosh b.
    microsurgical b.
    Miller b.
    RAD airway laryngeal b.
    rotating b.'s
    b. septostomy catheter
    straight b.
Blake exercise stress test
Blalock-Hanlon
    B.-H. atrial septectomy
    B.-H. operation
Blalock-Park procedure
Blalock pulmonary stenosis clamp
Blalock-Taussig (BT)
    B.-T. operation
    B.-T. procedure
    B.-T. shunt (BTS)
blanche
    tache b.
blanch test
bland
    b. diet
    b. edema
    b. embolism
    b. thrombus
Bland-Altman
    B.-A. method
    B.-A. technique
Bland-Garland-White syndrome
Bland-White-Garland syndrome
blanket
    Bair Hugger b.

blanket *(continued)*
   bronchial mucus b.
   circulating water b.
   cooling b.
   hypothermia b.
blanking
   b. period
   postventricular atrial b. (PVAB)
   total atrial b. (TAB)
blast
   b. chest
   b. lung
   b. wave
blastoma
   pleuropulmonary b.
   pulmonary b.
Blastomyces dermatitidis
blastomycosis
   North American b.
blazer
   B. II cardiac ablation catheter
   B. RPM navigation and ablation
      catheter
BLB
   bronchoscopic lung biopsy
   BLB oxygen mask
BLE
   buffered lidocaine with epinephrine
bleb
   apical pleural b.
   emphysematous b.
   pleural b.
   sarcolemmal b.
   b. stapling
bleed
   retroperitoneal b.
bleeding
   arterial b.
   b. blush
   cerebral b.
   b. diathesis
   extraparenchymal b.
   b. globe
   microvascular b. (MVB)
   b. time (BLT, BT)
blender
   Virtis b.
blending
   sensor b.
blennothorax
Blenoxane
bleomycin sulfate
BLES
   bovine lavage extract surfactant
blind
   b. coronary dimple
   b. cul-de-sac
   b. esophageal brushing (BEB)

   b. needle biopsy
   b. thoracentesis
bloater
   blue b.
Blocadren Oral
Bloch equation
block
   alveolar-capillary b.
   anatomic b.
   antegrade b.
   anterograde b.
   arborization b.
   atrial tachycardia with b. (ATB)
   atrioventricular b. (AVB)
   atrioventricular junctional heart b.
   atrioventricular node b.
   A-V branch b.
   A-V groove b.
   A-V node b.
   A-V Wenckebach b.
   axillary b.
   bed b.
   bidirectional isthmus conduction b.
   bifascicular heart b.
   bifurcating b.
   bilateral bundle branch b. (BBBB)
   bundle branch b. (BBB)
   1-b. claudication
   2-b. claudication
   3-b. claudication
   complete A-V b.
   complete heart b. (CHB)
   complete right bundle branch b.
      (CRBBB)
   conduction b.
   congenital complete heart b.
   congenital heart b. (CHB)
   congenital symptomatic A-V b.
   connector b.
   b. cycle length
   diffuse intraventricular b.
   divisional heart b.
   entrance b.
   exercise-induced left bundle
      branch b.
   exit b.
   familial atrioventricular b.
   fascicular heart b.
   first-degree A-V b.
   first-degree heart b.
   focal b.
   functional b.
   heart b. (HB)
   3:1 heart b.
   3:2 heart b.
   heart-lung b.
   heparin b.
   high-degree atrioventricular b.
   His bundle heart b.

incomplete atrioventricular b.
incomplete bilateral bundle
  branch b. (IBBBB)
incomplete left bundle branch b.
  (ILBBB)
incomplete right bundle branch b.
  (IRBBB)
infrahisian b.
interatrial b.
intercostal nerve b.
intraatrial b.
intrahisian b.
intraventricular b. (IVB)
left anterior bundle branch b.
  (LABBB)
left bundle branch b.
left bundle branch system b.
  (LBBsB)
Luciani-Wenckebach
  atrioventricular b.
Mobitz first-degree b.
Mobitz second-degree b.
Mobitz type I, II
  atrioventricular b.
Mobitz types of atrioventricular b.
nonspecific intraventricular b.
paraffin b.
partial heart b.
periinfarction b.
Perspex b.
protective b.
protoplasmic b.
pseudo-A-V b.
rate-dependent bundle branch b.
retrograde b.
right bundle branch b. (RBBB)
right bundle branch system b.
  (RBBsB)
second-degree A-V b.
second-degree heart b.
shock b.'s
sinoauricular b.
sinuatrial b. (SAB)
sinuatrial entrance b. (SAEB)
sinuatrial exit b.
sinus exit b.
subjunctional heart b.
suprahisian b.
third-degree atrioventricular b.
third-degree A-V b.
third-degree heart b.
total atrioventricular b. (TAVB)
transient heart b.
trifascicular b.
unidirectional b.
unifascicular b.
vagal b.
ventricular b.
voltage-dependent b.

Wenckebach atrioventricular b.
Wenckebach A-V b.
Wenckebach exit b.
Wenckebach periodicity b.
Wilson b.

blockade
aggressive platelet b.
alpha-1 adrenoceptor b.
angiotensin II receptor b.
beta b.
beta-adrenergic b.
left stellate ganglionic b. (LSGB)
neuromuscular b.
platelet glycoprotein IIb/IIIa b.
reuptake b.
sodium channel b.
stellate ganglion b.

blockage
arterial b.

blocked
b. APC
b. fascicle
b. heart artery
b. pleurisy

blocker
adrenoceptor b.
aldosterone-receptor b.
alpha-adrenergic b.
alpha-adrenoreceptor b.
angiotensin II receptor b. (ARB)
angiotensin receptor b.
beta b.
beta-1 b.
beta-adrenergic b.
beta-adrenoceptor b.
bronchial b.
calcium channel b. (CCB)
calcium entry b.
ganglionic b.
integrin b.
L-type calcium b.
nondihydropyridine calcium b.
platelet glycoprotein IIb/IIIa b.
receptor b.
renin-angiotensin b.
selectin b.
slow channel b.
sodium channel b.
vasopressin b.

blocking
b. vagal afferent fiber
b. vagal efferent fiber

Blom-Singer valve
blood
arterial b. (a)
arterialized capillary b. (ACB)
artificial b.
autologous b.
b. buffer (BB)

blood *(continued)*
    b. cardioplegia
    b. cast
    b. clot
    b. clot lysis time
    b. column
    b. count
    b. dyscrasia
    b. expander
    b. flow (BF)
    b. flow energy (BFE)
    b. flow enhancement device
    b. flow measurement
    b. flowmeter
    b. flow probe
    b. flow rate (BFR)
    b. flow reserve
    b. flow velocity (BFV)
    Fluosol artificial b.
    frank b.
    b. gas
    1620 b. gas analyzer
    840 b. gas analyzer
    b. gas sensor
    mixed venous b.
    b. monocyte stimulation
    b. murmur
    b. oxygen
    oxygenated b.
    b. oxygenation level-dependent
      (BOLD)
    b. oxygenation level-dependent
      technique
    b. oxygen level
    oxygen saturation of hemoglobin of
      arterial b.
    b. patch injection
    b. perfusion
    b. perfusion monitor (BPM)
    b. platelet thrombus
    b. pneumonitis
    b. pool
    b. pressure (BP, B/P)
    b. pressure assembly (BPA)
    b. pressure cuff (BPC)
    b. pressure decrease (BPD)
    b. pressure gauge (BPG)
    b. pressure increase (BPI)
    b. pressure index (BPI)
    b. pressure, left arm (BPLA)
    b. pressure and pulse (BP&P)
    b. pressure recorder (BPR)
    b. pressure return
    b. pressure, right arm (BPRA)
    b. pump
    b. replacement
    b. sampling
    b. sampling instrument

    shear rate of b.
    shunted b.
    sludged b.
    b. substitute
    b. sugar
    b. supply
    tonometered whole b.
    b. urea nitrogen (BUN)
    venous b. (VB)
    b. vessel (BV)
    b. vessel disease
    b. vessel invasion (BVI)
    b. vessel prosthesis (BVP)
    b. viscosity (BlV)
    b. volume (BLV, BlV)
    b. volume distribution
    b. volume expander (BVE)
    b. volume pulse (BVP)
    b. warmer
blood-air barrier
blood-borne
    b.-b. infectious agent
    b.-b. signal
blood-brain barrier (BBB)
blood-bronchoalveolar barrier
blood-bronchus barrier
blood-clotting mechanism (BCM)
blood-gas barrier
bloodless phlebotomy
bloodletting
blood-pool imaging
blood-retina barrier
bloodstream infection (BSI)
blood-surface interaction
blood-tinged sputum
blood-vascular system
Bloodwell forceps
bloody
    b. effusion
    b. sputum
    b. tap
bloom
    B. programmable stimulator
    B. syndrome
blooming
    b. artifact
    b. effect
BLOT
    Bimodality Lung Oncology Team
blot
    Northern b.
    slot b.
    Southern b.
    b. test
    Western b.
blow
    b. bottle
    diastolic b.

blow-by
>   b.-b. oxygen
>   b.-b. ventilator

blowing
>   b. murmur
>   b. wound

BLS
>   basic life support

BLS-D
>   basic life support-defibrillation

BLT
>   bilateral lung transplant
>   bleeding time

blubbery diastolic murmur

blue
>   b. asphyxia
>   b. baby
>   b. bloater
>   code b. (CB)
>   b. Cook sheath
>   b. digit syndrome
>   b. disease
>   Evans b.
>   b. finger syndrome
>   B. FlexTip catheter
>   B. Line cuffed endotracheal tube
>   B. Max high-pressure balloon
>   methylene b.
>   b. phlebitis
>   B. Rhino dilator
>   b. sclera
>   Sulphan B.
>   b. toe syndrome
>   b. velvet syndrome

Blumenau test

Blumenthal lesion

blunt
>   b. cardiac rupture
>   b. chest impact-induced cardiac arrest
>   b. chest injury
>   b. chest trauma (BCT)
>   b. dissection
>   b. eversion
>   b. eversion carotid endarterectomy
>   b. pulmonary injury
>   b. thoracic trauma
>   b. torso injury

blunted
>   b. costophrenic angle
>   b. ejection fraction
>   b. exercise response
>   b. heart rate
>   b. systolic pulmonary venous flow
>   b. systolic velocity
>   b. waveform

blunting
>   apical b.
>   nocturnal cardiovascular b.

blush
>   bleeding b.
>   capillary b.
>   myocardial b.
>   percutaneous coronary intervention myocardial b.
>   b. phenomenon
>   b. score
>   tumor b.
>   vascular b.

BLV
>   blood volume

Blv
>   blood viscosity
>   blood volume

BMC
>   balloon mitral commissurotomy
>   bone mineral content

BME
>   brief maximal effort

BMI
>   body mass index

BMIPP
>   betamethyliodophenyl pentadecanoic acid

BMLS
>   billowing mitral leaflet syndrome

B-mode
>   B-m. echocardiography
>   B-m. ultrasonography
>   B-m. ultrasound

BMP
>   beclomethasone monopropionate

BMP-2
>   bone morphogenetic protein type 2

BMPR
>   bone morphogenetic protein receptor

BMR
>   basal metabolic rate

BMS
>   bare metal stent

BMST
>   Bruce maximum stress test

BMV
>   balloon mitral valvoplasty

BNA
>   bronchoscopic needle aspiration

BNP
>   brain natriuretic peptide
>   B-type natriuretic peptide

BO
>   bronchiolitis obliterans

boat-shaped heart

Bobath
>   B. exercise
>   B. physiotherapy approach

bocavirus
>   parvovirus human b. (HBoV)

Bochdalek hernia

Bock ganglion

Bodai adapter
body, pl. **bodies**
   b. acceleration synchronous with heart rate (BASH)
   aortic b.
   Arantius b.
   b. of Arantius
   artificial b.
   asbestos bodies
   Aschoff b.
   aspiration of foreign b.
   asteroid b.
   Auer b.
   Babes-Ernst b.
   b. box method
   Bracht-Wächter bodies
   carotid b. (CB)
   central fibrous b.
   creola b.
   b. density analysis
   Döhle inclusion bodies
   b. fat
   ferruginous b.
   fibrin b.
   fibrous b.
   foreign b.
   Gamna-Gandy bodies
   gelatin compression b.
   Gordon elementary b.
   b. habitus
   Heinz b.
   LCL bodies
   b. mass index (BMI)
   Masson b.
   Medlar b.
   multilamellar b.
   Negri b.
   neuroepithelial b.
   b. packer
   paraaortic bodies
   b. of phalanx
   b. plethysmograph
   b. position
   psammoma bodies
   psittacosis inclusion bodies
   b. surface area (BSA)
   b. surface Laplacian mapping (BSLM)
   b. temperature, ambient pressure, saturated with water vapor (BTPS)
   thoracic vertebral b.
   tracheobronchial foreign b. (TFB)
   vagal b.
   Weibel-Palade bodies
   Zuckerkandl bodies
bodybuilder electromechanical criteria

Boeck
   B. disease
   B. sarcoid
Boehringer
   B. Mannheim standard
   B. suction regulator
Boerema hernia repair
Boerhaave
   B. syndrome
   B. tear
Boettcher forceps
Bogalusa criteria
boggy edema
Bogros space
Bohr
   B. effect
   B. equation
   B. formula
   B. isopleth method
bois
   bruit de b.
BOLD
   blood oxygenation level-dependent
   BOLD technique
Bolling procedure
bolometer
bolster
   Teflon felt b.
Boltzmann distribution
bolus
   b. cardiac output calculation
   b. glucocorticoid
   heparin b.
   b. intravenous injection
   b. of medication
   b. tracking
bombesin
bond
   soldered b.
bone
   b. cyst
   fibrous dysplasia of b.
   lingual b.
   b. loss
   b. marrow aplasia
   b. marrow-derived stem cell
   b. marrow embolism
   b. marrow injection
   b. marrow mononuclear cell
   b. marrow stromal cell
   b. marrow toxic therapy
   b. marrow transplant
   b. mineral content (BMC)
   b. morphogenetic protein receptor (BMPR)
   b. morphogenetic protein type 2 (BMP-2)
   Paget disease of b.
   b. sialoprotein

Bonferroni
    B. adjustment
    B. correction
    B. method
Bonhoeffer valve
boning
    dog b.
bony heart
Bonzel Monorail balloon catheter
bookeri
    Alcaligenes b.
book lung
Bookwalter retractor
Boomerang ClosureWire vascular closure system
booming rumble
BOOP
    bronchiolitis obliterans with organizing pneumonia
    steroid-resistant BOOP
booster heart
boot
    Bunny b.
    Circulator B.
    compression b.
    Cryo/Cuff pressure b.
    gelatin compression b.
    IPC b.'s
    PNS Unna b.
    sheepskin b.
Boothby-Lovelace-Bulbulian oxygen mask
boot-shaped heart
bootstrap
    b. dilation
    b. 2-vessel angioplasty
    b. 2-vessel technique
border
    anterior b.
    cardiac b.
    b. of cardiac dullness
    endocardial cardiac b.
    epicardial cardiac b.
    inferior b.
    b. rale
    sternal b.
    ventricular endocardial b.
    b. zone
    b. zone myocardium
    b. zone region
borderline
    b. cardiomegaly
    b. ECG
    b. hypertension (BHT)
    b. hypertensive (BH)
Bordetella pertussis
Bordet-Gengou
    B.-G. bacillus
    B.-G. test

Borg
    B. category-ratio
    B. dyspnea rating
    B. numerical scale (1-20)
    B. rating of perceived exertion
    B. rating of perceived exertion scale
    B. scale (1-20)
    B. treadmill exertion scale
Born aggregometry
Bornholm disease
Borrelia burgdorferi
borreliosis
    Lyme b.
Borst side-arm introducer set
BOS
    bronchiolitis obliterans syndrome
Bosch ERG 500 ergometer
bosentan
Bostock
    B. catarrh
    B. disease
Botallo duct
both ventricles inhibited (VDI)
botryomycosis
    pulmonary b.
Böttcher space
bottle
    blow b.
    Castaneda b.
    b. neck stenosis
    roller b.
    b. sound
    2-b. thoracic drainage system
botulinum
    Clostridium b.
    b. toxin type A
Bouchut respiration
bougie
    b. dilation
    EndoLumina illuminated b.
bougienage
    esophageal b.
Bouillaud
    B. disease
    B. sign
    B. tinkle
bound
    creatine kinase, myocardial b. (CK-MB)
bounding pulse
bouquet of vessels
Bourassa catheter
Bourdon gauge
Bourns-Bear ventilator
Bourns infant ventilator
bout
    hiccup b.
Bouveret disease

B

Bovie electrocautery
bovine
    b. aortic endothelial cell (BAEC)
    b. aortic endothelium (BAE)
    b. heart
    b. heart valve
    b. heterograft
    b. lavage extract surfactant (BLES)
    pegademase b.
    b. pericardial tissue
    b. pericardial valve
    b. pericardium strip
    b. serum antigen
bovinum
    cor b.
bovis
    Actinomyces b.
    Babesia b.
    Mycobacterium b.
Bowditch
    B. law
    B. phenomenon
    B. staircase effect
bowing
    leftward ventricular septal b.
    (LVSB)
    b. of mitral valve leaflet
box
    b. plot
    SunBox light b.
    b. of whistles
box-and-whisker plot
box-like heart
Boyce sign
Boyd
    B. perforating vein
    B. point
Boyden
    B. chamber
    B. classification
boydii
    Petriellidium b.
    Pseudallescheria b.
bozemanii
    Legionella b.
Bozzolo sign
BP
    blood pressure
    British Pharmacopeia
    bronchopulmonary
    bypass
    BP fistula
B/P
    blood pressure
BPA
    blood pressure assembly
BPC
    blood pressure cuff

BPD
    blood pressure decrease
    bronchopulmonary dysplasia
BPEC
    bipolar electrocoagulation
BPF
    bronchopleural fistula
BPG
    blood pressure gauge
    bypass graft
BPI
    blood pressure increase
    blood pressure index
BPLA
    blood pressure, left arm
BPM
    beats per minute
    bioabsorbable polymeric material
    blood perfusion monitor
bpm
    beats per minute
BP&P
    blood pressure and pulse
BPR
    blood pressure recorder
BPRA
    blood pressure, right arm
BPS
    beats per second
    beraprost sodium
    breaths per second
    systolic blood pressure
BPSA
    bronchopulmonary segmental artery
BPV
    balloon pulmonary valvoplasty
    bioprosthetic valve
BPXG body plethysmograph
Bq
    becquerel
BR
    breathing reserve
    bronchial responsiveness
brachial
    b. arteriogram
    b. arteriotomy
    b. artery
    b. artery approach
    b. artery cutdown
    b. artery pressure (BrAP)
    b. artery thrombosis
    b. bypass
    b. catheter
    b. dance
    b. nerve
    b. plexopathy
    b. plexus
    b. plexus injury
    b. plexus tension test

b. pulse
b., radial, femoral (BRAFE)
b. syndrome
b. vein
brachial-ankle index
brachioaxillary bridge graft fistula
brachiocephalic
b. arteritis
b. artery
b. ischemia
b. system
b. trunk
b. vein
b. vessel angioplasty
brachiocephalicus
truncus b.
brachiofemoral delay
brachiogram
brachiosubclavian bridge graft fistula
Bracht-Wächter
B.-W. bodies
B.-W. lesion
brachycardia
brachytherapy
endobronchial b.
intracoronary b.
intravascular b.
b. system
vascular b.
Bradbury-Eggleston syndrome
Bradshaw-O'Neill aorta clamp
bradyarrhythmia
sinus b.
bradyarrhythmic arrest
bradyasystolic arrest
bradycardia
b. after arteriovenous fistula
occlusion (BAVFO)
apnea and b. (A&B)
artifactual b.
atrial b.
Branham b.
cardiomuscular b.
central b.
clinostatic b.
essential b.
fetal b.
idiopathic b.
idioventricular b.
junctional b.
nodal b.
b. pacing support
postinfectious b.
postinfective b.
pulseless b.
sinuatrial b.
sinus b. (SB)
vagal b.
ventricular b.

bradycardiac
bradycardia-dependent aberrancy
bradycardia-tachycardia syndrome (BTS)
bradycardic
bradycrotic
bradydiastole
bradydysrhythmia (var. of
bradyrhythmia)
bradykinin perfusion
bradykinin-stimulated cells
bradypnea
bradyrhythmia, bradydysrhythmia
bradysphygmia
bradytachycardia syndrome
BRAFE
brachial, radial, femoral
BRAFE approach for elective
coronary stent implantation
Bragg-Paul respirator
braid-like lesion
brain
b. aneurysm
b. band enzyme of CPK
b. death
b. infarct (BI)
b. isoenzymes of creatine
phosphckinase (CPK-BB)
b. murmur
b. natriuretic peptide (BNP)
b. stem stroke
b. wave
brain-heart
b.-h. infusion
b.-h. infusion agar (BHIA)
b.-h. infusion blood agar (BHIBA)
b.-h. infusion and rabbit serum
(BHIRS)
branch, pl. **branches**
accessory meningeal b.
acetabular b.
anastomotic b.
atrioventricular circumflex b.
(AVCx)
bundle b. (BB)
conus b.
descending anterior b.
descending posterior b.
dorsal lingual b.
esophageal b.
external b.
faucial b.
internal b.
jailed side b.
left anterior descending b. (LADB)
left bundle b. (LBB)
left coronary circumflex b. (LCXB)
b. lesion
lingual b.
marginal b. #1

B

branch (*continued*)
    obtuse marginal b. (OMB)
    pharyngeal b.
    posterior descending b.
    posterolateral circumflex b. (PLCx)
    posterolateral descending b.
    b. pulmonary artery stenosis
    b. retinal artery occlusion (BRAO)
    b. retinal vein occlusion (BRVO)
    right bundle b. (RBB)
    branches of segmental bronchi
    septal perforator b.
    side b.
    tracheal b.
    b. vein occlusion
    ventricular extension b.
    b. vessel
    b. vessel occlusion (BVO)
    b. vessel pruning
branched (b)
    b. chain alpha ketoacid
        dehydrogenase (BCKD)
branching
    airway b.
    mirror-image brachiocephalic b.
branchiogenic
branchiomere
branchiomerism
branchiomotor
Branham
    B. bradycardia
    B. sign
Branhamella catarrhalis
BRAO
    branch retinal artery occlusion
BRAP
    burst of rapid atrial pacing
BrAP
    brachial artery pressure
Brasdor method
Brasfield chest radiograph score
brash
    water b.
brasiliensis
    Nocardia b.
    Paracoccidioides b.
brassy cough
BRAT
    Baylor rapid autologous transfusion
    BRAT system
Brauer cardiolysis
Braunwald
    B. classification I–IIIB
    B. sign
BRAVE
    Biosense revascularization approach for
    viable endocardium
brawny edema

braziliense
    Ancylostoma b.
bread-and-butter
    b.-a.-b. pericardium
    b.-a.-b. textbook sign
Breas
    B. PV10 CPAP device
    B. ventilator
breast
    b. artifact
    chicken b.
    b. pang
    thrush b.
breath
    b. analysis
    b. excretion test
    exercise-induced shortness of b.
    expiratory b.
    b. gas analyzer
    inspiratory b.
    b. marker
    b. pentane test
    b.'s per second (BPS)
    shortness of b. (SB, SOB)
    b. sounds
    b. sounds bilateral and equal
        (BSBE)
    b. stacking
    wide-open b.
breath-actuated inhaler (BAI)
breathe
    B. Right nasal strip
    B. with EEZ nasal dilator
breather
    The Sports B.
breathhold
    inspiratory b.
    b. maneuver
    b. turbo-flash tagged imaging
breathholding
    b. index (BHI)
    b. spell
    b. test
breathing
    agonal b.
    apneustic b.
    ataxic b.
    b. bag sign
    Biot b.
    bronchial b.
    b. capacity
    Cheyne-Stokes b. (CSB)
    controlled b.
    controlled diaphragmatic b. (CDBR)
    b. exercise
    exercise-induced periodic b.
    b. frequency (BF)
    frog b.
    glossopharyngeal b.

intermittent positive pressure b. (IPPB)
Kussmaul b.
Ondine b.
oxygen cost of b.
b. pacemaker
periodic b.
positive-negative pressure b. (PNPB)
pursed lip b. (PLB)
b. reserve (BR)
resting tidal b.
RfB System-I for controlled diaphragmatic b.
shallow b.
sign mechanism for ventilator b.
sleep-disordered b. (SDB)
b. technique
tidal b.
work of b. (WOB)
breath-methylated alkane contour
Brechenmacher fiber
Brecher and Cronkite technique
Breeze E150 ventilation system
bregmocardiac reflex
Brehmer treatment
Bremer AirFlo Vest
brequinar sodium
Brescia-Cimino A-V fistula
Breslow-Day
B.-D. test
B.-D. test for homogeneity
Brethaire Inhalation Aerosol
Brethine
B. injection
B. Oral
Bretonneau angina
Bretschneider-HTK cardioplegic solution
Brett syndrome
Bretylate
bretylium
b. infusion
b. loading
b. therapy
b. tosylate
Breuer-Hering
B.-H. deflation index
B.-H. inflation reflex
Brevibloc injection
Brevital
Bricanyl Turbuhaler
bridge
arteriolovenular b.
B. Assurant balloon-expandable stent
B. balloon-expandable stent
cytoplasmic b.
disulfide b.

B. extra support over-the-wire renal stent system
muscle b.
myocardial b.
Wheatstone b.
B. X3 renal stent system
bridging
b. anticoagulant
b. collateral
b. leaflets
muscular b.
myocardial b. (MB)
brief maximal effort (BME)
bright
B. disease
b. echo
B. murmur
brightness modulation
Brilliant lead
Brill-Zinsser disease
Brisbane method
brisk wall motion abnormality
Brite
B. Tip catheter
B. Tip sheath
British
B. Cardiac Society (BCS)
B. Heart Foundation (BHF)
B. Pharmacopeia (BP)
B. Thoracic Society (BTS)
brittle
b. asthma
b. asthmatic
BRK series transseptal needle
broadband ultrasound attenuation (BUA)
Broadbent inverted sign
broad QRS complex
Brock
B. infundibulectomy
B. operation
B. procedure
B. syndrome
Brockenbrough
B. atrial septoplasty
B. atrial stenting
B. curved needle
B. effect
B. sign
B. technique
B. transseptal commissurotomy
Brockenbrough-Braunwald-Morrow sign
Brockenbrough-Braunwald sign
brocresine
Broders index
Brodie abscess
Brodie-Trendelenburg tourniquet test
brodifacoum
Brodmann area 7, 9, 24, 40

broken heart syndrome
Bromanyl Cough Syrup
bromazepam
bromhexine hydrochloride
bromide
    ethidium b.
    hydrogen b.
    ipratropium b.
    methyl b.
    oxitropium b.
    pancuronium b.
    pipecuronium b.
    tiotropium b.
bromocriptine
bromodiphenhydramine and codeine
Bromotuss w/Codeine Cough Syrup
brompheniramine, phenylpropanolamine, codeine
Brompton
    B. cocktail
    B. solution
    B. technique
Brom repair
Bronalide
broncatar
bronchadenitis, bronchoadenitis
bronchi (*pl. of* bronchus)
bronchia (*pl. of* bronchium)
bronchial
    b. allergy
    b. anastomosis
    b. arteries
    b. arteriography
    b. artery
    b. artery embolization (BAE)
    b. asthma
    b. atresia
    b. blocker
    b. breathing
    b. breath sounds
    b. brush biopsy
    b. brushings
    b. bud
    b. calculus
    b. carcinoma
    b. cast
    b. challenge test
    b. collateral
    b. collateral artery murmur
    b. contusion
    b. crisis
    b. cyst
    b. dehiscence
    b. disruption
    b. epithelial cell
    b. fremitus
    b. gland
    b. hyperreactivity (BHR)
    b. hyperresponsiveness (BHR)

    b. inflammatory polyp
    b. lavage
    b. lumen
    b. marking
    b. meniscus sign
    b. microflora
    b. mucous gland adenoma
    b. mucous membrane
    b. mucus blanket
    b. mucus inhibitor
    b. pneumonia
    b. polyp
    b. provocation
    b. rale
    b. reactivity
    b. respiration
    b. responsiveness (BR)
    b. sarcoidosis
    b. sleeve resection
    b. smooth muscle
    b. smooth muscle tone
    b. spasm
    b. stenosis
    b. stump
    b. stump failure
    b. synechia
    b. toilet
    b. tree
    b. tube
    b. vein
    b. voice
    b. washing
    b. washings cytology
    b. wheezing
bronchiales
    rami b.
    venae b.
bronchiectasia sicca
bronchiectasis
    chemical b.
    cylindrical b.
    cystic b.
    dry b.
    fibronodular b.
    follicular b.
    fusiform b.
    pseudocylindrical b.
    saccular b.
    suppurative b.
    traction b.
    varicose b.
bronchiectatic
    b. cavity
    b. rale
bronchiloquy
bronchiocele
bronchiogenic
bronchiolar
    b. adenocarcinoma

b. carcinoma
b. exocrine cell
b. inflammatory infiltrate

bronchiole
alveolar b.
respiratory b.
terminal b.

bronchiolectasia
bronchiolectasis, bronchiolectasia
traction b.

bronchioli (*pl. of* bronchiolus)
bronchiolitic interstitial pneumonia (BIP)
bronchiolitis
acute obliterating b.
chronic obliterative b.
constrictive b.
b. exudativa
exudative b.
b. fibrosa obliterans
follicular b.
infectious b.
b. obliterans (BO)
b. obliterans syndrome (BOS)
b. obliterans with organizing pneumonia (BOOP)
obliterative b. (OB)
proliferative b.
respiratory b. (RB)
vesicular b.
viral b.
b. with interstitial pneumonitis (BIP)

bronchioloalveolar
b. adenocarcinoma
b. carcinoma (BAC)
b. communication

bronchiolocentric
bronchiologram
air b.

bronchiolopulmonary
bronchiolus, pl. **bronchioli**
bronchioli respiratorii
b. terminalis

bronchiomediastinalis
truncus lymphaticus b.

bronchiorum
tunica muscularis b.

bronchiostenosis
bronchitic asthma
bronchitis
acute bacterial exacerbation of chronic b. (ABECB)
acute exacerbation of chronic b. (AECB)
acute laryngotracheal b.
arachidic b.
asthmatic b.
capillary b.

Castellani b.
catarrhal b.
cheesy b.
chemical b.
chronic asthmatic b.
chronic obstructive b.
croupous b.
dry b.
eosinophilic b.
epidemic capillary b.
ether b.
exudative b.
fibrinous b.
hemorrhagic b.
industrial b.
infectious asthmatic b.
mechanic's b.
membranous b.
nonasthmatic eosinophilic b.
obliterative b.
phthinoid b.
plastic b.
polypoid b.
productive b.
protracted bacterial b.
pseudomembranous b.
putrid b.
radiation b.
secondary b.
b. sicca
simple chronic b.
smoker's b.
staphylococcal b.
streptococcal b.
suffocative b.
vegetal b.
verminous b.
vesicular b.
wheezy b.
winter b.

Bronchitrac L flexible suction catheter
bronchium, pl. **bronchia**
bronchoadenitis (*var. of* bronchadenitis)
bronchoalveolar
b. carcinoma
b. fluid
b. lavage (BAL)
b. lavage fluid (BALF)
b. washing

bronchoalveolitis
bronchoaspergillosis
bronchobiliary fistula
bronchoblastomycosis
bronchoblennorrhea
bronchocandidiasis
Broncho-Cath double-lumen endotracheal tube
bronchocavernous respiration
bronchocavitary fistula

B

bronchocele
bronchocentric granulomatosis (BCG)
bronchoconstriction
    hyperpnea-induced b. (HIB)
    reflex vagal b.
bronchoconstrictive effect
bronchoconstrictor
bronchodilatation
bronchodilating agent
bronchodilation, bronchodilatation
bronchodilator (BDT)
    b. administration
    aerosolized b.
    anticholinergic b.
    b. effect
    inhaled b.
    long-acting beta-2 agonist b.
      (LABA)
    Marax b.
    nebulized b.
    b. response
    b. therapy
bronchoedema
bronchoegophony
bronchoesophageal
    b. fistula
    b. muscle
bronchoesophageus
    musculus b.
bronchoesophagology
bronchoesophagoscopy
bronchofiberscope
bronchogenic
    b. adenocarcinoma
    b. carcinoma
    b. cyst
bronchogram
    air b.
    tantalum b.
bronchography
    Cope method b.
    inhalation b.
    percutaneous transtracheal b.
broncholith
broncholithiasis
bronchomalacia
bronchomediastinal lymphatic trunk
bronchomotor
bronchomycosis
bronchophony
    pectoriloquous b.
    sniffling b.
    whispered b.
bronchoplasty
bronchopleural-cutaneous fistula
bronchopleural fistula (BPF)
bronchopleuropneumonia
bronchopneumonia
    acute hemorrhagic b.

    confluent b.
    diffuse b.
    focal b.
    hemorrhagic b.
    hypostatic b.
    necrotizing b.
    sequestration b.
    subacute b.
    tuberculous b.
    virus b.
bronchopneumonic infiltrate
bronchopneumonitis
bronchoprovocant
bronchoprovocation test
bronchopulmonale
    segmentum b.
bronchopulmonales
    nodi lymphoidei b.
bronchopulmonary (BP)
    b. aspergillosis
    b. carcinoid tumor
    b. cyst
    b. dysplasia (BPD)
    b. lymph node
    b. segment
    b. segmental artery (BPSA)
    b. sequestration
    b. spasm
    b. spirochetosis
    b. tissue
    b. tract
    b. venous fistula
    b. washing
bronchorrhea
Broncho Saline
bronchoscope
    BF large core b.
    Dumon b.
    Dumon-Harrell b.
    fiberoptic b.
    flexible fiberoptic b.
    Fujinon flexible b.
    Kernan-Jackson b.
    Michelson b.
    Moersch b.
    Negus b.
    Olympus XBF-UC40P b.
    Pentax b.
    Pilling b.
    respiration b.
    Safar b.
    Storz b.
    ventilation b.
    Waterman b.
    Yankauer b.
bronchoscopic
    b. brush
    b. electrocautery
    b. lung biopsy (BLB)

b. needle aspiration (BNA)
b. needle biopsy
b. smear
b. ultrasound
bronchoscopist
bronchoscopy
autofluorescence b.
diagnostic b.
fiberoptic b. (FB, FOB)
flexible fiberoptic b. (FFB)
fluorescence b.
laser b.
b. quality improvement project
rigid b.
surveillance b.
therapeutic b.
ultrasound-guided b.
virtual b. (VB)
white light b. (WLB)
bronchospasm
allergic b.
allergically induced b.
cold-induced b.
exercise-induced b. (EIB)
paradoxical b.
reversible b.
bronchospasmolytic
bronchospastic
b. component
b. event
bronchospirography
bronchospirometer
bronchospirometry
differential b.
bronchostenosis
bronchostomy
bronchotracheal aspirate
bronchovascular bundle
bronchovenous fistula
bronchovesicular
b. breath sounds
b. marking
b. respiration
bronchovideoscope
novel high magnification b.
bronchus, pl. **bronchi**
anomalous b.
apical b.
basal segmental b.
branches of segmental bronchi
cardiac b.
ectopic b.
eparterial b.
hyparterial bronchi
intermediate b.
b. intermedius
left main b.
lingular b.
lobar b.

bronchi lobares
lower lobe b.
mainstem b.
middle lobe b.
mucosa of b.
muscular coat of b.
primary b.
b. principalis dexter
b. principalis sinister
right main b.
secondary b.
segmental b.
b. segmentalis
stem b.
subsegmental b.
b. suis
supernumerary b.
tertiary b.
tracheal b.
tunica mucosa bronchi
upper lobe b.
bronchus-associated lymphoid tissue (BALT)
bronchus-grasping forceps
Bronkodyl
Brontex Liquid
Brookfield viscometer
broth
heart infusion b. (HIB)
b. test
Todd-Hewitt b. (THB)
brown
b. atrophy
b. edema
b. induration
b. induration of lung
b. sputum
b. urine
Brown-Adson forceps
Brown-Dodge method
Brown-McHardy pneumatic dilator
Brozek formula
BRS
baroreceptor reflex sensitivity
baroreflex sensitivity
Bruce
B. bundle
B. exercise stress test
B. maximum stress test (BMST)
B. treadmill protocol
brucei
Trypanosoma b.
Brucella melitensis
brucellosis
Brugada syndrome
Brugia
B. *malayi*
B. *timori*
bruissement

bruit
    abdominal b.
    aneurysmal b.
    asymptomatic carotid b. (ACB)
    carotid b.
    b. de bois
    b. de canon
    b. de choc
    b. de clapotement
    b. de claquement
    b. de craquement
    b. de cuir neuf
    b. de diable
    b. de drapeau
    b. de frolement
    b. de frottement
    b. de galop
    b. de la roue de moulin
    b. de lime
    b. de parchemin
    b. de piaulement
    b. de rappel
    b. de Roger
    b. de scie
    b. de scie ou de rape
    b. de soufflet
    b. de tabourka
    b. de tambour
    b. de triolet
    epigastric b.
    false b.
    midepigastric b.
    musical b.
    Roger b.
    seagull b.
    systolic b.
    thyroid b.
    Traube b.
    Verstraeten b.
Bruker Avance spectrometer
Brunelli equation
brunetti
    Chlamydia b.
Brunnstrom-Fugl-Meyer Scale for motor test
brush
    Air-Lon tracheal tube b.
    b. biopsy
    b. border membrane (BBM)
    b. border membrane vesicle (BBMV)
    bronchoscopic b.
    b. cell
    Edwards-Carpentier aortic valve b.
    B. electrocardiographic score
    Mill-Rose protected specimen microbiology b.
    OTW thrombolytic b.
    protected specimen b. (PSB)

Brushfield spot
brushing
    BAL b.
    blind esophageal b. (BEB)
    bronchial b.'s
    double-sheath bronchial b.'s
    microbiologic b.
    protected catheter b. (PCB)
    protected specimen b. (PSB)
    washings and b.'s
brusque
    b. dilation
    b. dilation of esophagus
bruxism
    sleep b.
BRVO
    branch retinal vein occlusion
Bryant ampulla
BS
    bilateral symmetrical
B-S
    Björk-Shiley
    B-S valve
BSA
    body surface area
BSBE
    breath sounds bilateral and equal
BSCA
    bidirectional superior cavopulmonary anastomosis
B-scan frame
BSCC
    Björk-Shiley convexoconcave
    BSCC heart valve
BSI
    bloodstream infection
BSLM
    body surface Laplacian mapping
BT
    Blalock-Taussig
    bleeding time
    BT shunt
BTBV
    beat-to-beat variability
BTF-37 arterial blood filter
BTO
    balloon test occlusion
BTPS
    body temperature, ambient pressure, saturated with water vapor
BTS
    Blalock-Taussig shunt
    bradycardia-tachycardia syndrome
    British Thoracic Society
B-type natriuretic peptide (BNP)
BUA
    broadband ultrasound attenuation
bubble
    arterial gas b.

b. contrast echocardiography
b. cushion
gastric b.
b. humidifier
b. oxygenation
b. oxygenator
b. study
bubbling rale
bubbly lung syndrome
bubonic plague
bucardia
buccal
Nitrogard B.
buccalis
Leptotrichia b.
buccolingual apraxia
buccopharyngeal
Buchbinder Thruflex over-the-wire catheter
Buckberg cardioplegia
buckled aorta
buckling
b. of aorta
chordal b.
midsystolic b.
bud
bronchial b.
lung b.
Budd-Chiari syndrome
budesonide
formoterol and b.
b. inhalation powder
b. inhalation suspension
Buerger-Allen exercise
Buerger disease
buffalo chest
buffer
blood b. (BB)
Krebs-Henseleit b.
buffered
b. aspirin
b. lidocaine (BL)
b. lidocaine with epinephrine (BLE)
Bufferin
buffy coat smear
BUFUL
bumetanide and furosemide on lipid
BUFUL profile
Buhl desquamative pneumonia
buildup time (T$_b$)
bulb
b. of aorta
aortic b.
carotid b.
thrombosis of jugular b.
bulbar
b. feeder

b. pulse
b. stroke
bulboventricular
b. fold
b. foramen
b. groove
b. loop
b. sulcus
b. tube
bulbus cordis
bulge
precordial b.
spare tire b.
bulging
diastolic b.
infarct b.
systolic b.
bulk convection
bulla, pl. **bullae**
basilar b.
emphysematous b.
pulmonary b.
b. resorption
Bullard intubating laryngoscope
bulldog clamp
bullectomy
transaxillary apical b.
bullet-tip catheter
bullet wound
bullous
b. emphysema
b. lung disease
b. lung tissue
bull's-eye
b.-e. plot
b.-e. polar coordinate mapping
bumetanide and furosemide on lipid (BUFUL)
Bumex
bump
B b.
ductus b.
BUN
blood urea nitrogen
bunch-of-grapes appearance
bundle
AH b.
atrioventricular b.
atrium-His b.
A-V b.
Bachmann b.
b. branch (BB)
b. branch block (BBB)
b. branch fibrosis
b. branch reentrant tachycardia
b. branch reentry (BBR)
bronchovascular b.
Bruce b.
central bronchovascular b.

bundle *(continued)*
    commissural b.
    Gantzer accessory b.
    His b. (HB)
    b. of His (BH)
    image b.
    James b.
    Keith b.
    Kent b.
    Kent-His b.
    Killian b.
    left b. (LB)
    Mahaim b.
    main b.
    Marshall b.
    neurovascular b.
    right b. (RB)
    b. of Stanley Kent
    Thorel b.
    vascular b.
Bunnell Life Pulse high frequency jet ventilator
Bunny boot
Bunyaviridae
bupivacaine
bupropion SR
bur, burr
    diamond-coated b.
    b. hole
burden
    atheroma b.
    atherosclerotic plaque b.
    ischemic b.
    plaque b.
    radiation b.
    thrombus b.
Burdick
    B. ECG machine
    B. electrocardiogram
Burette multiple patient delivery system
Burford-Finochietto rib spreader
burgdorferi
    Borrelia b.
burger
    B. scalene triangle
    B. technique for scapulothoracic disarticulation
Bürger-Grütz
    B.-G. disease
    B.-G. syndrome
Burghart symptom
Burhenne steerable catheter
Burinex
Burkholderia
    B. cenocepacia
    B. cepacia
    B. cepacia complex (BCC)
    B. dolosa
    B. multivorans

    B. stabilis
    B. ubonensis
Burkitt lymphoma
burned out viral myocarditis
burnetii
    Coxiella b.
burning pain
Burns
    space of B.
Burow
    B. quantitative method
    B. solution
    B. vein
burr *(var. of* bur)
bursa, pl. **bursae**
    Calori b.
    Fleischmann b.
    laryngeal b.
    b. subcutanea
    subcutaneous b.
    sublingual b.
    b. sublingualis
burst
    b. of arrhythmia
    b. atrial pacing
    paroxysmal b.
    b. of rapid atrial pacing (BRAP)
    respiratory b.
    b. shock
    spider b.
    b. of ventricular pacing (BVP)
    b. of ventricular tachycardia
bur-to-artery ratio
Buschke
    B. disease
    scleredema of B.
Buselmeier shunt
buspirone transdermal patch
Busse-Buschke disease
buster
    clot b.
busulfan lung syndrome
butanedione monoxime
butorphanol
butterfly
    b. catheter
    b. heart valve
    b. needle
    b. pattern
    b. shadow
Butterworth bidirectional filter
buttock claudication
button
    b. of aorta
    cell b.
    coronary artery b.
    b. electrode
    Moore tracheostomy b.
    Panje voice b.

skin b.
b. technique
tracheal b.
tracheostomy b.
voice b.

buttoned device

buttonhole
b. deformity
mitral b.
b. mitral stenosis

buttress
Teflon pledget suture b.

butylated hydroxytoluene (BHT)

butyrophenone

BUV
backup ventilation

BV
balloon valvoplasty
blood vessel

BVA-100 blood volume analyzer

BVAD, BIVAD
biventricular assist device

BVAS
Birmingham Vasculitis Activity Score

BVE
blood volume expander

BvgAS regulon

BvgS protein

BVH
biventricular hypertrophy

BVI
blood vessel invasion

BVM
bag-valve-mask
BVM device
BVM ventilation

BVO
branch vessel occlusion

BVP
blood vessel prosthesis
blood volume pulse
burst of ventricular pacing

BVR
balloon valvoplasty registry

BVS
biventricular support
BVS 5000 biventricular support
system
BVS pump

BWIT
black-white interface technique

Bx
Bx Velocity coronary artery stent
Bx Velocity stent with Raptor
OTW delivery system
Bx Velocity with Hepacoat on
Raptor stent system

BxSonic coronary stent

ByCPR
bystander cardiopulmonary resuscitation

bypass (BP)
aortobiiliac b.
aortocarotid b.
aortocoronary b. (A-C, ACB)
aortocoronary saphenous vein b.
aortocoronary venous b. (ACVB)
aortofemoral b. (AFB)
aortoiliac b.
aortoiliofemoral b.
aortorenal b.
aortosubclavian b.
aortosubclavian-carotid-
axilloaxillary b.
atrial-femoral artery b.
axillary bifemoral b.
axilloaxillary b.
axillofemoral b.
axillofemoral-femoral b.
brachial b.
cardiopulmonary b. (CPB)
carotid-axillary b.
carotid-carotid b.
carotid-subclavian b.
b. circuit
coronary artery b. (CAB)
crossover femorofemoral b.
descending thoracic aortofemoral-
femoral b.
diagonal coronary b.
femoral-tibial-peroneal b.
femoroaxillary b.
femorofemoral b.
femorofemoral crossover b.
femoropopliteal b.
femorotibial b.
gastric b. (GBP)
b. graft (BPG)
b. graft catheterization
heart-lung b.
iliopopliteal b.
internal mammary artery b.
(IMAB)
left heart b.
Litwak left atrial-aortic b.
low-flow cardiopulmonary b. (LFB)
b. machine
midcoronary artery b.
minimally invasive combined mitral
valve repair and direct coronary
artery b.
minimally invasive coronary
artery b. (MICAB)
minimally invasive direct coronary
artery b. (MIDCAB)
off-pump coronary artery b.
(OPCAB)
partial ileal b. (PIB)

bypass *(continued)*
>percutaneous cardiopulmonary b. (PCPB)
>percutaneous in situ b.
>percutaneous left heart b. (PLHB)
>perfusion-assisted direct coronary artery b. (PADCAB)
>peripheral artery b.
>portacaval b. (PCB)
>ramus coronary b.
>renal artery-reverse saphenous vein b.
>reversed b.
>right heart b. (RHB)
>saphenous vein b. (SVB)
>B. Speedy stent
>subclavian-carotid b.
>subclavian-subclavian b.
>superior mesenteric artery b.

>b. surgery
>b. time
>total b. (TBP)
>total arterial off-pump coronary artery b.
>total cardiopulmonary b. (TCB)
>totally endoscopic coronary artery b. (TECAB)
>b. tract

bypassable
by-product
>eosinophil b.-p.
>nicotine b.-p.

byssinosis
bystander
>b. cardiopulmonary resuscitation (BCPR, ByCPR)
>b. effect

C
    cardiac
    cardiovascular disease
    chest lead in electrocardiography
    cholesterol
        calphostin C
        cystatin C
        C oxygen cylinder
        C point
        C point of cardiac apex pulse
        C valvular leaflet
        C wave
        C wave of jugular venous pulse
^{11}C, C-11
    carbon-11
^{13}C-triolein breath test
^{14}C-triolein breath test
C1qR gene
C1r deficiency
3C
    craniocerebellocardiac
C_4
    leukotriene C_4
c4b purified human complement
c7 E3 Fab
CA
    cardiac arrest
        CA monitor
        CA virus
CAA
    cardiac allograft atherosclerosis
    cerebral amyloid angiopathy
    circulating anodic antigen
Ca-activated C1 channel
CAA-related hemorrhage
CAAS
    Cardiovascular Angiography Analysis
    System
CAB
    coronary artery bypass
cabergoline
CABF
    coronary artery blood flow
CABG
    coronary artery bypass graft
    coronary artery bypass grafting
        beating-heart CABG
        off-pump CABG
        open heart CABG
CABGS
    coronary artery bypass graft surgery
cable
        OxyLead interconnect c.
        TempLink extension c.
Cabot-Locke murmur

CABRI
    coronary artery bypass revascularization
        investigation
CABS
    continuous ambulatory blood sampler
    coronary artery bypass surgery
CA-BSI
    catheter-associated bloodstream infection
CAC
    cardiac-accelerator center
    cardiac arrest code
    circulating anticoagulant
    cold air challenge
    coronary artery calcium
CACh
    cold air challenge
cachectic endocarditis
cachecticorum
    melanoderma c.
cachexia
    cancer c.
    cardiac c.
    pretransplant c.
    thyroid c.
cacoon seed asthma
CAD
    computer-assisted diagnostic
    coronary artery disease
    angiographically significant CAD
CADASIL
    cerebral autosomal dominant arteriopathy
        with subcortical infarct and
        leukoencephalopathy
CADD-Plus intravenous infusion pump
**Cadence tiered therapy defibrillator
    system**
cadet
        C. high voltage can implantable
            cardioverter-defibrillator
        C. V-115 implantable cardioverter-
            defibrillator
cadherin
    vascular c.
CADI
    coronary artery disease index
cadmiosis
cadmium (Cd)
    c. lung
    c. oxide
    c. oxide fumes
CADR
    coronary artery descriptors and restenosis
Caduet
CAE
    coronary artery embolism

C

CAESAR
  computer-assisted evaluation of stenosis
    and restenosis
    CAESAR analysis system
caesiellus
    Aspergillus c.
CAF
  continuous atrial fibrillation
  coronary artery fistula
Cafcit
    C. injection
    C. oral solution
café-au-lait spot
café coronary
Cafergot
caffeine
    aspirin, phenacetin, c. (APC)
    c. citrate
    citrated c.
    c. citrate oral solution
    phenacetin, aspirin, c. (PAC)
    c. and sodium benzoate
CAG
  coronary angiography
  coronary arteriography
CagA
  cytotoxin-associated gene product A
    CagA antigen
cage
    chest c.
    Faraday c.
    nitinol c.
    rib c.
    thoracic c.
    titanium c.
caged
    c. ball valve
    c. ball valve prosthesis
CAGEIN
  catheter-guided endoscopic intubation
CAH
  combined atrial hypertrophy
CAHD
  coronary arteriosclerotic heart disease
CAI
  cortical arousal index
c-a interval
caisson disease
CAL
  chronic airflow limitation
Calan SR
calcicardiogram
calcicosilicosis
calcicosis
calcific
    c. aortic stenosis (CAS)
    c. aortic valve disease
    c. debris
    c. embolus

c. mitral stenosis
c. nodular aortic stenosis
c. pericarditis
calcification
    anular c.
    arterial c.
    central c.
    conduit c.
    dystropic c.
    eccentric c.
    eggshell c.
    hilar c.
    metastatic c.
    mitral anular c. (MAC)
    Mönckeberg c.
    napkin-ring c.
    pericardial c.
    popcorn c.
    pulmonary c.
    senescent c.
    soft tissue c.
    stippled c.
    c. of tips of mitral valve
    valvular c.
calcified
    c. aortic valve
    c. lesion
    c. mitral leaflet
    c. nodule
    c. papillary muscle in right
      ventricle
    c. pericardium
    c. plaque
    c. thrombus
Calcilean
calcineurin inhibitor
calcinosis, Raynaud phenomenon, esophageal involvement, sclerodactyly, telangiectasia (CREST)
calciphylaxis
calcitonin gene-related peptide (CGRP)
calcium
    c. antagonist
    arc of c.
    atorvastatin c.
    c. benzoylpas
    benzoylpas c.
    c. channel agonist
    c. channel antagonist (CCA)
    c. channel blocker (CCB)
    c. channel blocking agent
    c. chloride
    coronary c.
    coronary artery c. (CAC)
    c. current (I_{Ca})
    c. deposit
    c. entry blocker
    fenoprofen c.
    c. gluceptate

c. gluconate
c. heparin (CH)
c. influx
c. ion
c. ionophore A23187
mitral anular c.
myoplasmic c.
nadroparin c.
c. oxalate
c. oxalate deposition
c. paradox
perivascular c.
c. product
c. rigor
c. score
c. sign
c. spark
spotty coronary c.
c. transient
calcium-sensitizing agent
Calciviridae virus
calcoaceticus
   Acinetobacter c.
calcofluor stain
Calculair spirometer
calculated minute volume
calculation
bidirectional shunt c.
bolus cardiac output c.
calculator
risk c.
calculosa
pericarditis c.
calculus, pl. calculi
bronchial c.
cardiac c.
pleural c.
caldesmon
calf, pl. calves
c. aortic microsome (CAM)
c. claudication
c. cramp
c. embryonic heart cell (CEHC)
c. lung surfactant extract (CLSE)
c. pain
calfactant intratracheal suspension
calf-vein thrombosis
Calgary Sleep Apnea Quality of Life Index
calibration chamber
calibrator
Flow-Volume c.
Califf score
California disease
calipers
AccuGage vessel c.
digital c.
electronic c.
Lange c.

callosa
pericarditis c.
callosomarginal artery
Calmette-Guérin
bacille C.-G. (BCG)
calmodulin
Calm-X Oral
Calmylin Expectorant
Calori bursa
calorie
ratio of ingested saturated fat and cholesterol to c.'s
calorie-restricted diet
calorimetry
myocardial indirect c.
Calot triangle
CALP
congenital absence of left pericardium
calpain inhibition
calphostin C
calsarcin
calsequestrin (CASQ)
Caltrac accelerometer
Caluso PEG tube
calves (*pl. of* calf)
Calypso Rely PTCA balloon angioplasty catheter
CAM
calf aortic microsome
cell adhesion molecule
child-adult mist
circulating adhesion molecule
Cam-Ap-Es
Cambridge
C. electrocardiograph
C. Heart CH2000 stress test system
camera
Anger scintillation c.
cine c.
DSX Sopha c.
gamma scintillation c.
multicrystal gamma c.
multiwire gamma c.
scintillation c.
Siemens Orbiter gamma c.
single-crystal gamma c.
Sopha Medical gamma c.
SPOT 3-shot Insight QE c.
video c.
cameral fistula
Cameron-Haight elevator
CAMP
cyclophosphamide, doxorubicin, methotrexate, procarbazine
CAMP test
cAMP
cyclic adenosine monophosphate
Campbell De Morgan spot

C

camptodactyly
    pericarditis, arthropathy, c. (PAC)
Camptosar
Campylobacter
camsylate
    trimethaphan c.
CAN
    cardiac autonomic neuropathy
    continuous albuterol nebulization
can
    high voltage c. (HVC)
    pacemaker c.
Canadian
    C. Cardiovascular Coalition (CCC)
    C. Cardiovascular Society (CCS)
    C. Cardiovascular Society angina
      score (CCSAS)
    C. Cardiovascular Society
      classification (CCSC)
    C. Cardiovascular Society functional
      classification
    C. class I–IV angina
    C. Heart Classification (CHC)
    C. Infectious Disease Society
    C. Registry of Atrial Fibrillation
      (CARAF)
    C. Thoracic Society
canal
    adductor c.
    c. of Arantius
    atrioventricular c. (AVC)
    A-V c.
    basipharyngeal c.
    carotid c.
    common atrioventricular c.
    complex atrioventricular c.
    c. of Cuvier
    facial c.
    femoral c.
    hiatus of facial c.
    His c.
    Holmgren-Golgi c.
    Hunter c.
    c. of Lambert
    palatovaginal c.
    partial atrioventricular c.
    perivascular c.
    persistent common
      atrioventricular c.
    pharyngeal c.
    pleuroperitoneal c.
    pulmoaortic c.
    Rivinus c.'s
    unbalanced A-V c.
    van Horne c.
    ventricular c.
    Verneuil c.
canalicular period
canalization

cANCA
    circulating antineutrophil cytoplasmic
    antibody
cancer
    American Joint Committee on C.
    (AJCC)
    c. cachexia
    c. embolus
    International Staging System for
    Lung C. (ISSLC)
    metachronous lung c.
    non-AIDS-defining c. (NADC)
    non-small-cell lung c. (NSCLC)
    roentgenographically occult lung c.
    (ROLC)
    scar c.
cancerization
    field c.
cancer-related retinopathy
Cancidas
Cancion cardiac recovery system
candesartan
    c. cilexetil
    c., cilexetil, hydrochlorothiazide
Candida
    C. albicans
    C. glabrata
    C. guilliermondii
    C. krusei
    C. lusitaniae
    C. parapsilosis
    C. pneumonia
candidemia
candidiasis
    invasive c.
    oral c.
    pulmonary c.
candidum
    Geotrichum c.
candidus
    Aspergillus c.
    Thermoactinomyces c.
candle flame pattern
candoxatril
candoxatrilat
candy-cane esophagus
candy wrapper edge effect
canine fossa
caninum
    Ancylostoma c.
canis
    Babesia c.
    Toxocara c.
cannabinoid
Cann-Ease
    C.-E. moisturizing nasal gel
    C.-E. nasal moisturizer
cannon
    C. formula

c. sound
C. theory
c. wave
cannonball
c. metastases
c. pulse
cannula, pl. **cannulae, cannulas**
Abelson c.
Aegis aortic c.
aortic arch c.
aortic perfusion c.
Argyle CPAP nasal c.
ascending balloon c. (ABC)
Cardeon ascending balloon c.
cardiovascular c.
Cimochowski cardiac c.
endovenous drainage c.
Entree thoracoscopy c.
femoral perfusion c.
Flexicath silicone subclavian c.
Fluoro Tip c.
Gregg c.
Grüntzig femoral stiffening c.
Heartport endovenous drainage c.
nasal c.
O_2 via nasal c.
oxygen-conserving nasal c.
PercuQuick tracheostomy c.
Polystan perfusion c.
QuickDraw venous c.
RAP c.
remote access perfusion c.
reservoir c.
Rockey ventricular c.
saphenous vein c.
Sarns aortic arch c.
Sarns soft-flow aortic c.
Sarns 2-stage c.
Softip oxygen nasal c.
2-stage c.
StraightShot arterial c.
Thora-Port c.
Tibbs arterial c.
triport c.
vein graft c.
vena cava c.
venous c.
Wallace Flexihub central venous pressure c.
washout c.
cannulate
cannulation
femoral arterial c. (FAC)
canola oil
canon
bruit de c.
canrenoate potassium
canrenone
cantering rhythm

canthomeatal slice
Cantlie line
Cantrell
C. pentalogy
C. syndrome
CAO
chronic airflow obstruction
coronary artery obstruction
CAO_2
arterial oxygen content
CAOD
coronary artery occlusive disease
CAP
central apical part
community-acquired pneumonia
coronary artery perforation
coupled atrial pacing
cyclic alternating pattern
cyclophosphamide, doxorubicin, cisplatin
CA4P
combretastatin A4 prodrug
cap
apical c.
atheromatous c.
collagenous c.
Drixoral Cough & Congestion Liquid C.'s
Drixoral Cough & Sore Throat Liquid C.'s
fibrous c.
c. inflammation
left apical c.
mesenchymal c.
pleural c.
c. repair
Sudafed Cold & Cough Liquid C.
c. thickness
capacitance
segmental venous c. (SVC)
venous c. (VC)
c. vessel
capacitor
c. deformation
c. forming time
c. reform
capacity
aerobic c. (VO_2max)
breathing c.
carbon monoxide diffusing c.
cerebrovascular reserve c. (CRC)
closing c. (CC)
diffusing c.
diffusion c.
exercise c.
forced expiratory c. (FEC)
forced inspiratory c. (FIC)
forced inspiratory vital c. (FIVC)
forced vital c. (FVC)
force-generating c.

C

123

capacity *(continued)*
    functional aerobic c.
    functional reserve c. (FRC)
    functional residual c. (FRC)
    inspiratory c. (IC)
    inspiratory reserve c. (IRC)
    inspiratory vital c. (IVC)
    lung transfer c.
    maximal breathing c.
    maximal sustainable ventilatory c. (MSVC)
    maximal vital c. (MVC)
    maximum aerobic c.
    maximum breathing c. (MBC)
    maximum expiratory flow at 50% vital c. (MEF_{50})
    membrane diffusing c. (Dm)
    metabolic vasodilatory c.
    myocardial vascular c. (MVC)
    normal vital c. (NVC)
    oxygen c.
    oxygen-binding c.
    oxygen-carrying c.
    oxygen-diffusing c.
    pulmonary diffusion c. (D_{CO})
    residual lung c.
    residual volume/total lung c. (RV/TLC)
    respiratory c.
    serum reserve cholesterol binding c. (SRCBC)
    slow vital c. (SVC)
    timed vital c.
    total lung c. (TLC)
    ventilatory c.
    vital c. (VC)
    work c.
Capastat Sulfate
capecitabine
Capetown prosthetic valve
capillaries (*pl. of* capillary)
capillaritis
    pulmonary c.
capillaropathy
capillary, pl. **capillaries**
    c. apoplexy
    c. bed
    c. blood flow (CBF)
    c. blood gas (CBG)
    c. blood sugar (CBS)
    c. blush
    c. bronchitis
    c. congestion
    c. embolism
    extraalveolar c.
    c. filling
    c. filtration coefficient
    c. hydrostatic pressure (CHP)
    c. leak syndrome (CLS)

    c. lumen
    peritubular c. (PTC)
    c. pressure (CP)
    c. pulse
    c. recruitment
    c. sclerosis
    c. thrombi
    c. wedge pressure
Capintec nuclear VEST monitor
Capiscint
Caplan
    C. nodule
    C. syndrome
Caplets
    Advil Cold & Sinus C.
    Bayer Select Chest Cold C.
    Dimacol C.
    Dristan Sinus C.
Capnocheck
    C. handheld capnometer
    C. II hand-held CO2/SpO2 monitor
    C. Plus capnograph monitor
    C. quantitative capnometer
Capnocytophaga canimorsus **sepsis**
capnogram
    volumetric c.
capnograph
    Clarity c.
    Microcap handheld c.
    Microstream c.
    Novametrix Tidal Wave handheld c.
    SC-300 portable c.
    SC-210 sidestream c.
    Tidal Wave handheld c.
capnography
    color c.
    c. ventilation monitoring
capnometer
    Capnocheck handheld c.
    Capnocheck quantitative c.
capnometry
    end-tidal c.
CapnoProbe
    C. model 2000 system
    C. SL system
    C. sublingual CO_2 system
Capnostat CO_2 sensor
Capoten
Capozide
capped lead
Capps reflex
capreomycin sulfate
CAPRI
    Cardiopulmonary Research Institute
capriloquism
caprisans
    pulsus c.
caprizant

caproate
    hydroxyprogesterone c.
capsaicin
capsid binding agent
CAPSO
    cautery-assisted palatal stiffening
    operation
capsula fibrosa glandula
capsulatum
    Histoplasma c.
capsule
    CellCept c.
    fibrous c.
    internal c.
    mycophenolate mofetil c.
    Neoral cyclosporine c.
    Ordrine AT Extended Release C.
    posterior limb of internal c.
      (PLIC)
    Rescaps-D C.
    Tiazac extended-release c.
    TriCor c.
CapSure
    C. cardiac pacing lead
    C. SP lead
    C. VDD lead
CapSureFix lead
captopril
    c. and hydrochlorothiazide
    c. renography
    c. scintigraphy
capture
    atrial c.
    c. beat
    beat-by-beat c.
    c. complex
    c. confirmation
    failure to c.
    functional failure to c.
    loss of c.
    pacemaker c.
    retrograde arterial c.
    c. threshold
    ventricular c.
caput medusae
CAQ
    Childhood Asthma Questionnaire
CAR
    cardiac ambulation routine
    carvedilol
Carabelli tube
Carabello sign
CARAF
    Canadian Registry of Atrial Fibrillation
caramiphen and phenylpropanolamine
CAR AMP
    carotid pulse amplitude
CARB
    coronary artery bypass graft

carbachol
    c. inhalation challenge (CIC)
    c. provocation test
carbamazepine
carbapenem
carbazochrome salicylate
carbenicillin
    indanyl c.
carbetapentane
    chlorpheniramine, ephedrine,
      phenylephrine, c.
carbide
    aluminum c.
    amorphous hydrogenated silicon c.
      (a-SiC:H)
    cobalt in tungsten c.
carbinoxamine
    c. and pseudoephedrine
    c., pseudoephedrine,
      dextromethorphan
Carbocaine
carbocholine
carbocysteine
Carbodec DM
Carbofilm
carbogen
carbohydrate
    c. intolerance
    c. utilization test
Carbomedics
    C. bileaflet prosthetic heart valve
    C. cardiac valve prosthesis
    C. top-hat supra-anular valve
    C. valve device
carbomethoxyisopropyl isonitrile
carbon
    c. dioxide (CO_2)
    c. dioxide dissociation curve
    c. dioxide elimination
    c. dioxide pressure
    c. dioxide production
    c. dioxide tension
    c. dioxide TMR laser
    c. disulfide
    hemocompatible turbostratic c.
    c. monoxide (CO)
    c. monoxide diffusing capacity
    c. monoxide oximetry (CO-
      oximetry)
    c. monoxide sleuth
    c. monoxide transfer factor (TLCO,
      TLco)
    pyrolytic c.
    thromboresistant turbostratic c.
carbon-11 (^{11}C, C-11)
    c.-11 acetate
    c.-11 hydroxyephedrine
    c.-11 palmitic acid radioactive
      tracer

C

carbon-11-labeled fatty acids
carbonate
    ammonium c.
    lithium c.
    magnesium c. ($MgCO_3$)
carbonica
    asphyxia c.
carbonic anhydrase inhibitor
carboplatin and etoposide (CE)
Carbo-Seal
    C.-S. ascending aortic prosthesis
    C.-S. graft material
Carbostent coronary stent
carboxyhemoglobin (COHb, $HbCO_2$)
carboxyhemoglobinemia
carbuterol hydrochloride
carcinoembryonic antigen (CEA)
carcinogen
carcinogenesis
    field c.
carcinogenicity
carcinoid
    c. heart disease
    c. murmur
    c. plaque
    c. syndrome
    c. tumor
    c. valve disease
carcinoma, pl. carcinomata
    adenoid cystic c.
    adenosquamous c.
    alveolar cell c.
    anaplastic c.
    basal cell c.
    basaloid c.
    bronchial c.
    bronchiolar c.
    bronchioloalveolar c. (BAC)
    bronchoalveolar c.
    bronchogenic c.
    clear cell c.
    ductal cell c.
    epidermoid c.
    giant cell c.
    hair-matrix c.
    infiltrating lobular c.
    large-cell neuroendocrine c.
      (LCNEC)
    large-cell undifferentiated c.
    lung c.
    lymphangitic c.
    lymphoepithelioma-like c.
    melanotic c.
    metastatic c.
    mucinous c.
    mucoepidermoid c.
    nasopharyngeal c.
    non-small-cell lung c. (NSCLC)
    oat cell c.

    occult bronchogenic c.
    papillary c.
    poorly differentiated c.
    prickle cell c.
    primary lung c.
    reserve cell c.
    scar c.
    scirrhous c.
    signet-ring cell c.
    c. simplex
    c. in situ
    small-cell c.
    small-cell lung c. (SCLC)
    spindle cell c.
    squamous cell bronchogenic c.
    thymic c.
    transitional cell c.
    undifferentiated small-cell c.
    verrucous c.
    well-differentiated c.
carcinomatosa
    lymphangitis c.
carcinomatosis
    lymphangitic c. (LC)
    pleural c.
carcinomatous
    c. neuromyopathy
    c. pericarditis
carcinosarcoma
CARD
    cardiac automatic resuscitative device
card
    C. Guard C.iac event recorder
    TruZone asthma action plan
      wallet c.
Cardarelli sign
Cardec DM
Cardec-S Syrup
Cardene SR
Cardeon ascending balloon cannula
cardia
    C. Horizon Legacy cannulated
     implant system
    c. mucosa (CM)
    C. Salt alternative
cardiac (C)
    C. Ablation Registry
    c. accident
    c. action potential
    c. adjustment scale (CAS)
    c. adrenergic activity
    c. allograft
    c. allograft atherosclerosis (CAA)
    c. allograft vascular disease
     (CAVD)
    c. allograft vasculopathy (CAV)
    c. alternation
    c. ambulation routine (CAR)
    c. amyloidosis

c. aneurysm
c. angiography
c. antimyosin antibody uptake
c. antrum
c. apex
c. apnea monitor
c. arrest (CA)
c. arrest code (CAC)
c. arrhythmia
c. assist system
c. asthma
c. atrophy
c. auscultation
c. autoantibody
c. autoimmunity
c. automatic resuscitative device (CARD)
c. autonomic neuropathy (CAN)
c. ballet
c. baroreceptor
c. bioluminescence imaging
c. bioptome
c. blood-pool imaging
c. border
c. border of dullness
c. bronchus
c. cachexia
c. calculus
c. care unit (CCU)
c. catheter
c. catheterization (CC)
c. catheter-microphone
c. center (CC)
c. chamber
c. cirrhosis
c. cocktail
c. coil
c. compensation
c. competence
c. compression
c. conduction
c. conduction system (CCS)
c. contour
C. Control Systems lead
c. contusion (CC)
c. cooling jacket
c. crisis
c. cushion
c. cycle (CC)
c. death
c. decompensation
c. decompression
c. decortication
c. defects, abnormal facies, thymic hypoplasia, cleft palate, hypocalcemia (CATCH-22)
c. defibrillation
c. depressant
c. depressor reflex

c. destabilization syndrome
c. diagnostic unit (CDU)
c. diastole
c. diet
c. dilation
c. disease (CD)
c. disturbance syndrome
c. diuretic
c. dropsy
c. dullness (CD)
c. dyspnea
c. dysrhythmia (CD)
c. echodensity
c. edema
c. effect
c. electrical defect
c. enlargement (CE)
c. enzyme
c. event
c. event recorder
c. examination
c. failure (CF)
c. fibrillation
c. fibrosis
FluoroPlus C.
c. function
c. gap junction protein
c. gating
c. gland
c. glands of esophagus
c. glycogenosis
c. glycoside
c. hemoptysis
c. hemosiderosis
c. herniation
c. heterotaxia
c. histiocyte
c. hybrid revascularization procedure
c. hypertrophy
c. impression
c. impression on lung
c. impulse
c. index (CI)
c. infarction
C. Infarction Injury Score
c. infiltration
c. insufficiency (CI)
c. insult
c. intensive care unit (CICU)
c. interstitium
c. ischemia
c. jelly
c. laboratory panel (CLP)
c. lithomyxoma
c. liver
c. lymphatic ring
c. malformation
c. mapping

cardiac *(continued)*
    c. marker
    c. mass
    c. massage
    c. memory
    c. metastasis
    c. minute output (CMO)
    c. monitoring (CM)
    c. monitor strip
    c. murmur (CM)
    c. muscle (CM)
    c. muscle wrap
    c. myocyte
    c. myocyte apoptosis
    c. myocyte hypertrophy
    c. myosin
    c. myxoma
    c. neural crest
    c. neurosis
    c. notch
    c. notch of left lung
    c. observation unit (COU)
    c. orifice
    c. output (CO, Q, QT, Q-T)
    c. output demand
    c. output index
    c. output measurement
    c. output recorder (COR)
    c. output shock
    c. output by thermodilution
      (COTD)
    c. pacemaker
    c. pacing (CP)
    c. patch
    c. perforation
    c. performance (CP)
    c. perfusion
    c. polyp
    c. power
    c. power output (CPO)
    c. preload
    c. probe
    C. Protect tomography
    c. pulmonary edema (CPE)
    c. recovery system (CRS)
    c. rehabilitation (CR)
    c. rehabilitation and prevention
      program
    c. rehabilitation protocol
    c. rehabilitation unit (CRU)
    c. remodeling
    c. reserve
    c. resuscitation (CR)
    c. resuscitation team (CRT)
    c. resynchronization
    c. resynchronization device
    c. resynchronization therapy (CRT)
    c. resynchronization therapy
      defibrillator (CRT-D)

c. resynchronization therapy
  implantable cardioverter-defibrillator
  (CRT-ICD)
c. rhabdomyoma
c. rhythm (CR)
c. risk
c. risk factor
c. risk index (CRI)
c. rotation
c. rupture
c. sarcoidosis myocarditis
c. sarcoma
c. sensory nerve
c. shadow
c. shock wave therapy (CSWT)
c. shunt
c. signal
c. silhouette
c. situs
c. skeleton
c. sling
C. Society of Great Britain and
  Ireland (CSGBI)
c. sodium channel gene
c. souffle
c. sound
c. standstill
c. status
C. STATus CK-MB/myoglobin
  panel test
C. STATus CK-MB test
C. STATus rapid assay
C. STATus rapid format troponin
  I panel test
c. stress test (CST)
c. stretch device
c. stump
c. surgery
c. surgery reporting system (CSRS)
c. surgical intensive care unit
  (CSICU)
c. sympathetic denervation
c. sympathetic nerve (CSN)
c. symphysis
c. synchronicity
c. syncope
c. syndrome X
c. systole
c. tamponade (CT)
c. telemetry
c. thrombosis
c. thrust
c. transplant
c. transplantation (CTx)
C. Transplant Research Database
  (CTRD)
C. T rapid assay
c. troponin I (CTI, cTnI, cTn-I)
c. troponin I assay

c. troponin T (cTnT)
c. tumor
c. tumor plop
c. ultrasound
c. ultrasound machine
c. unit (CU)
c. vagal tone
c. valve
c. valve prosthesis
c. valvular incompetence
c. variability
c. vasculitis
c. vein
c. ventricular contraction
c. vest
C. View Probe
c. volume (CV)
c. waist
c. wall hypokinesis
c. wall thickening
c. work (CW)
c. work index (CWI)
cardiaca
adiposis c.
steatosis c.
cardiac-accelerator center (CAC)
cardiac-specific overexpression
cardiacum
segmentum c.
cardialgia
cardiataxia
cardiatelia
cardiectasia
cardiectopia
Cardima surgical ablation system
cardinal
c. symptom
c. vein
cardioacceleration
cardioaccelerator center
cardioactive
cardioangiography
cardioaortic
cardioarterial interval
cardioauditory syndrome
Cardiobacterium hominis
cardioballistic
CardioBeeper CB 12L cardiac monitor
Cardioblate
C. BP, RF surgical ablation
system
C. BP2 surgical ablation system
C. RF generator
C. RF surgical ablation system
C. surgical ablation pen
C. XL pen
cardiocairograph
Cardiocap/5 monitor
cardiocele

cardiocentesis
cardiochalasia
CardioCoil coronary stent
Cardio-Cool myocardial protection pouch
Cardio-Cuff
cardiocyte
cardiodiaphragmatic angle
cardiodynamics
cardiodynia
cardioembolic stroke (CES)
cardioembolism
cardioesophageal (CE)
c. junction
c. reflex
c. reflux
c. sphincter
cardiofacial syndrome
cardiofaciocutaneous (CFC)
c. syndrome
CardioFix
C. pericardium patch
C. pericardium with PhotoFix
technology
Cardioflon suture
cardiogenesis
CardioGenesis TMR system
cardiogenic
c. mixing
c. pulmonary edema
c. sheath
c. shock (CGS, CS)
c. stroke
c. syncope
cardiogram
esophageal c.
impedance c. (IC, ICG)
cardiograph
Minnesota Impedance C.
cardiography (CG)
Doppler c.
echo-Doppler c.
impedance c. (ICG)
ultrasonic c. (UCG, USCG)
ultrasound c.
variance c. (VC)
vector c.
CardioGrip cardiovascular trainer
cardiohemothrombus
cardiohepatic triangle
cardiohepatomegaly
cardioinhibitory
c. carotid sinus hypersensitivity
c. center (CIC)
c. response
c. type
c. vasovagal syncope
cardiokinetic
cardiokymogram

cardiokymograph
cardiokymography (CKG)
CardioLab 2000 single monitor EP system
cardiolipin (CL)
    c. flocculation test (CFT)
    c. microflocculation test (CMFT)
    c. natural lecithin (CNL)
    c. synthetic lecithin (CSL)
Cardiolite
    C. scan
    C. stress test
cardiolith
cardiological workspace manager (CWM)
cardiologist
    Fellow of the American College of C.'s (FACC)
    interventional c.
cardiology
    American College of C. (ACC)
    digital interchange standards for c. (DISC)
    fetal c.
    C. II stethoscope
    International Society of C. (ISC)
    International Society and Federation of C. (ISFC)
    interventional c.
    pediatric c. (PDC, PdC)
    telecollaboration for signal analysis in c. (TECSAC)
cardiolysis
    Brauer c.
cardiomalacia
cardiomediastinal silhouette
cardiomegaly
    borderline c.
    false c.
    glycogen c.
    glycogenic c.
    idiopathic c.
Cardiomemo device
cardiometabolic risk factor
cardiometry
cardiomotility
cardiomuscular bradycardia
cardiomyocyte apoptosis
cardiomyoliposis
cardiomyopathy (CM, C-M, CMP)
    African c.
    alcoholic c.
    anthracycline-induced c.
    arrhythmogenic right ventricular c. (ARVC)
    arrhythmogenic ventricular c.
    atrophic c.
    beer-drinker's c.
    cobalt c.

    concentric hypertrophic c.
    congestive c. (CCM, COCM)
    diabetic c.
    dilated c. (DCM)
    doxorubicin c.
    doxorubicin-induced c.
    drug-induced c.
    dystrophinopathic c.
    false c.
    familial hypertrophic c. (FHC)
    familial hypertrophic obstructive c.
    fibroplastic c.
    genetic hypertrophic c.
    HIV c.
    hypertensive hypertrophic c.
    hypertrophic c. (HC, HCM, HCMP)
    hypertrophic obstructive c. (HOCM)
    idiopathic congestive c. (ICCM)
    idiopathic dilated c. (IDC)
    idiopathic restrictive c.
    infiltrative c.
    inflammatory c.
    ischemic c.
    Keshan c.
    latent c. (LCM)
    maternally inherited c.
    mildly dilated congestive c. (MDCM)
    mitochondrial c.
    nephropathic c.
    nonischemic dilated c. (NIDCM)
    obliterative c.
    obstructive hypertrophic c. (OHC)
    pacing in c. (PIC)
    parasitic c.
    pediatric c.
    peripartal c.
    peripartum c.
    postpartum c. (PPCM)
    primary restrictive c.
    rejection c.
    restrictive c.
    right ventricular c.
    secondary c.
    spiral hypertrophic c.
    storage c.
    tachycardia-induced c.
    takotsubo c. (TTC)
    valvular c.
    viral c.
    X-linked dilated c. (XLCM)
cardiomyoplasty
    dynamic c.
cardionector
cardioneural
cardioneurogenic syncope
cardioneuropathy
cardioneurosis

CardioNow telecardiology imaging
cardioomentopexy
cardiopaludism
CardioPass
    C. coronary artery bypass graft
    C. layered microporous small-bore vascular graft
cardiopath
cardiopathia nigra
Cardio-Path plaque excision device
cardiopathy
cardiopericardiopexy
    Beck c.
cardiopexy
    ligamentum teres c.
cardiophobia
cardiophone
cardiophony
cardiophrenia
cardiophrenic angle
cardioplegia
    adenosine-supplemented blood c.
    antegrade c.
    blood c.
    Buckberg c.
    cold blood c.
    cold crystalloid c.
    cold potassium c.
    c. cooling
    crystalloid potassium c.
    hyperkalemic c.
    ice c.
    c. infusion
    normothermic c.
    nutrient c.
    potassium chloride c.
    St. Thomas Hospital c.
    whole blood c.
cardioplegic
    c. arrest
    c. perfusion solution (CPS)
    c. solution
cardiopneumographic recording (CPG)
Cardiopoint needle
cardiopressor
cardioprotection
cardioprotective role
cardioptosia
cardiopulmonary (CP)
    c. arrest (CPA)
    c. blood volume (CPBV)
    c. bypass (CPB)
    c. bypass pump
    c. bypass surgery
    c. cerebral resuscitation (CPCR)
    c. coupling
    c. decompression sickness (the chokes)
    c. disease (CPD)

    c. exercise (CPX)
    c. exercise testing (CPET)
    c. gas exchange
    c. murmur
    C. Research Institute (CAPRI)
    c. reserve (CPR)
    c. resuscitation (CPR)
    c. risk index (CPRI)
    c. splanchnic nerves
    c. support (CPS)
CardioPump
    Ambu C.
cardioreparative drug agent intervention
cardiorespiratory (CR)
    c. arrest
    c. depression
    c. murmur
    c. sign
cardiorespirogram (CRG)
CardioRhythm generator
cardiorrhaphy
cardiorrhexis (CR)
cardioschisis
Cardioscint
    C. ambulatory vest detector
    C. nuclear detector
cardiosclerosis
    postinfarct c.
cardioscope
CardioSEAL
    C. septal occluder
    C. septal occlusion system
    C. septal occlusion system with QwikLoad
cardioselectivity
Cardioserv defibrillator
CardioShield
    MedNova C.
cardiosphygmograph
CardioSync cardiac synchronizer
cardiotachometer (CTM)
Cardiotec scan
CardioTek
    C. electrophysiologic tracer
    C. electrophysiologic tracer system
Cardiotest portable electrograph
cardiothoracic (CT)
    c. intensive care unit (CTICU)
    c. ratio (CTR)
    c. surgery (CTS)
    c. unit (CTU)
cardiothrombus
cardiothyrotoxicosis
cardiotocography (CTG)
cardiotomy reservoir
cardiotonic drug
cardiotoxicity
    Adriamycin c.
    doxorubicin c.

C

cardiotoxic myolysis
cardiotoxin
Cardiotrast
cardiotrophin-1
cardiovalvotomy
cardiovalvulitis
cardiovalvulotomy
CardioVascular
    Zynergy C. Inc. (ZCV)
cardiovascular (CV)
    c. accident (CVA)
    acute c. (ACV)
    C. Angiography Analysis System (CAAS)
    c. bifurcation disease
    c. cannula
    c. clamp
    c. clinic (CC)
    c. collapse
    c. complication
    c. computed tomography (CVCT)
    C. Credentialing International (CCI)
    c. death
    c. disability
    c. disease (C, CD, CVD)
    c. event
    c. excitatory center
    c. failure (CVF)
    c. fitness
    c. function
    c. function assessment
    c. imaging system (CVIS)
    c. incident (CVI)
    c. inhibitory center
    c. insufficiency (CVI)
    c. intensive care unit (CVICU)
    C. and Interventional Radiological Society of Europe (CIRSE)
    c. magnetic resonance (CMR, CVMR)
    c. measurement system (CMS)
    c. monitor (CVM)
    c. pressure
    c. recovery room (CVRR)
    c. reflex conditioning (CRC)
    c. reflex conditioning system (CRCS)
    c. risk factor
    c. self-assessment tool (CST)
    c. steady state
    c. surgery (CVS)
    c. syphilis
    c. system (CVS)
    c. technologist (CVT)

cardiovasculare
    systema c.
cardiovascular-renal (CVR)
    c.-r. disease (CVRD)
cardiovascular-respiratory (CVR)
cardioventricular pacing (CVP)
cardioversion
    chemical c.
    DC c.
    direct current c. (DCCV)
    elective c.
    electrical c.
    external c. (ECV)
    external electric c.
    internal c.
    low-energy intracardiac c.
    low-energy synchronized c.
    c. paddles
    pharmacological c.
    synchronized DC c.
    synchronized direct current c.
    c. threshold
    transthoracic direct current electrical c.
    transvenous c. (TVCV)
    transvenous internal c.
cardioverter
    Lyra 2020 implantable c.
cardioverter-defibrillator (*See also* defibrillator)
    Angstrom MD implantable single-lead c.-d.
    Atlas DR implantable c.-d.
    Atlas VR implantable c.-d.
    atrial implantable c.-d. (AICD, A-ICD)
    atrial and ventricular implantable c.-d. (AV-ICD)
    automatic external c.-d. (AECD)
    automatic implantable c.-d. (AICD, A-ICD)
    automatic internal c.-d. (AICD, A-ICD)
    Belos VR implantable c.-d.
    Cadet high voltage can implantable c.-d.
    Cadet V-115 implantable c.-d.
    cardiac resynchronization therapy implantable c.-d. (CRT-ICD)
    Contour LTV-135D implantable c.-d.
    Contour MD implantable single-lead c.-d.
    Contour V-145D implantable c.-d.
    DR-Atrial TX implantable c.-d.
    EnTrust implantable c.-d.
    external c.-d. (ECD)
    Gem II DR/VR implantable c.-d.
    Gem III AT implantable c.-d.

Gem III AT implantable c.-d.
Gem III DR dual-chamber c.-d.
Gem II VR implantable c.-d.
Guardian ATP 4210 implantable c.-d.
Guidant Ventak implantable c.-d.
implantable c.-d. (ICD)
implantable automatic c.-d. (IACD)
InSync c.-d.
Intermedics Res-Q implantable c.-d.
Jewel AF implantable c.-d.
Lifecor wearable c.-d.
Lyra 2020 implantable c.-d.
Medtronic external c.-d.
Medtronic GEM III AT
implantable c.-d.
Medtronic Jewel AF 7250 dual-chamber implantable c.-d.
Medtronic PCD implantable c.-d.
MycroPhylax implantable c.-d.
nonthoracotomy lead implantable c.-d.
Ovatio implantable c.-d.
Photon DR implantable c.-d.
Photon Micro DR/VR
implantable c.-d.
Phylax AV dual-chamber
implantable c.-d.
Phylax 06 implantable c.-d.
Powerheart automatic external c.-d.
programmable c.-d. (PCD)
PRx implantable c.-d.
Res-Q ACD implantable c.-d.
Res-Q Micron implantable c.-d.
Sentinel 2010 implantable c.-d.
subpectoral implantation of c.-d.
Telectronics ATP implantable c.-d.
tiered-therapy implantable c.-d.
tiered-therapy programmable c.-d.
transthoracic implantable c.-d.
Transvene nonthoracotomy
implantable c.-d.
Ventak A-V III DR automatic
implantable c.-d.
Ventak Mini II and III automatic
implantable c.-d.
Ventak Prizm 2 automatic
implantable c.-d.
Ventak PRx c.-d.
ventricular implantable c.-d. (VICD, V-ICD)
Ventritex Angstrom MD
implantable c.-d.
Ventritex Cadence implantable c.-d.
WCD 2000 system wearable c.-d.
wearable c.-d. (WCD)
cardiovirus

CardioWest
C. TAH
C. temporary total artificial heart
CardIQ software
carditis
coxsackievirus c.
rheumatic c.
streptococcal c.
verrucous c.
Cardizem
C. CD
C. Lyo-Ject
C. Monovial
C. Tablet
Cardura
care
American Association for
Respiratory C. (AARC)
continuity of c.
coronary c. (CC)
emergency cardiac c. (ECC)
end-of-life c.
intensive coronary c. (ICC)
kangaroo c.
long-term c. (LTC)
National Board for Respiratory C. (NBRC)
precoronary c. (PCC)
subacute c.
c. vigilance (CV)
Caregiver Strain Test
CareLink
C. monitor
C. network for patient monitoring
C. patient monitoring network
carer strain
Carey Coombs short mid-diastolic murmur
CARhd
high-dose carvedilol
carina, pl. **carinae**
c. not splayed
c. sharp and mobile
c. of trachea
c. tracheae
carinal lymph node
carinatum
pectus c.
carindacillin
Carinia domestica
carinii
Pneumocystis c.
cariporide
Carlen double-lumen endotracheal tube
Carmalt forceps
Carmeda BioActive Surface
C-arm fluoroscopy
Carmol topical
carmustine-impregnated water

carneae
  trabeculae c.
carneus
  Aspergillus c.
Carney
  C. complex
  C. triad
carnitine deficiency
Carnoy solution
Carolon life support antiembolism stockings
carotene
  beta c.
carotenoid
caroticotympanic artery
caroticovertebral stenosis
carotid
  c. angiography
  c. angioplasty and stenting (CAS)
  c. angioplasty and stent placement
  c. arch
  c. arteriography
  c. artery
  c. artery disease
  c. artery murmur
  c. artery shunt
  c. artery stenosis (CAS)
  c. artery stenting
  c. augmentation index
  c. ball
  c. baroreceptor
  c. baroreflex
  c. bifurcation
  c. B-mode sonography
  c. body (CB)
  c. body tumor
  c. bruit
  c. bulb
  c. canal
  c. Doppler
  c. duplex scan
  c. ejection time
  c. endarterectomy (CE, CEA)
  external c. (EC)
  c. impulse
  c. intima-media complex
  c. intima-medial thickness (CIMT)
  c. occlusive disease
  c. patch angioplasty
  c. phonoangiography
  c. plaque
  c. pulse
  c. pulse amplitude (CAR AMP)
  c. pulse tracing
  c. sheath
  c. shudder
  c. sinus
  c. sinus hypersensitivity
  c. sinus hypersensitivity syndrome
  c. sinus massage
  c. sinus nerve
  c. sinus reflex
  c. sinus stimulation
  c. sinus syncope
  c. sinus syndrome
  c. sinus test
  c. siphon
  c. steal syndrome
  c. stenosis
  c. stent
  c. stent-supported angioplasty (CSSA)
  c. triangle
  c. upstroke
  c. vascular disease
carotid-axillary bypass
carotid-carotid bypass
carotid-cavernous fistula (CCF)
carotid-subclavian bypass
carotodynia, carotidynia
carpal
  c. arch anterior
  c. arch dorsal
  c. arch palmar
Carpenter syndrome
Carpentier
  C. annuloplasty
  C. pericardial valve
  C. rigid ring
  C. technique
  C. tricuspid valvoplasty
Carpentier-Edwards
  C.-E. aortic valve prosthesis
  C.-E. glutaraldehyde-preserved porcine xenograft prosthesis
  C.-E. mitral annuloplasty valve
  C.-E. mitral Perimount pericardial bioprosthesis
  C.-E. pericardial valve
  C.-E. Perimount mitral valve
  C.-E. Perimount PSR pericardial prosthesis
  C.-E. Perimount RSR pericardial bioprosthesis
  C.-E. Physio annuloplasty ring
  C.-E. Physio annuloplasty ring with Duraflo
  C.-E. porcine prosthetic valve
  C.-E. porcine supraannular valve
carperitide
carpopedal spasm
Carrel method
Carrie coronary stent placement technique
Carrington
  C. disease
  C. pneumonia

CARS
  compensatory antiinflammatory response
  syndrome
cart
  crash c.
  MedGraphics CPX/D metabolic c.
  metabolic c.
  resuscitation c.
  SensorMedics 2900 metabolic c.
carteolol hydrochloride
Carter equation
Cartia XT
Cartilade
cartilage
  anular c.
  articular surface of arytenoid c.
  arytenoid c.
  cricoid c.
  epiglottic c.
  c. of larynx
  Luschka c.
  Meyer c.
  Seiler c.
  tracheal c.
  xiphoid c.
cartilagines tracheales
cartilago
  c. cricoidea
  c. sesamoidea laryngis
Carto
  C. electroanatomical mapping
  C. EP navigation system
  C. XP system
Cartomerge image integration module
Cartrol Oral
carumonam
caruncula, pl. **carunculae**
  c. salivaris
  sublingual c.
  c. sublingualis
Carvallo sign
carvedilol (CAR)
  high-dose c. (CARhd)
Cary 118C spectrophotometer
CAS
  calcific aortic stenosis
  cardiac adjustment scale
  carotid angioplasty and stenting
  carotid artery stenosis
  coronary artery scan
  coronary artery spasm
CAS-8000V general angiography
  positioner
Casale-Devereux criteria
cascade
  AA c.
  arachidonic acid c.
  coagulation c.
  downstream signaling c.

  immune c.
  ischemic c.
  leukocyte-endothelial cell
    adhesion c.
  neurohumeral c.
  pathological c.
  c. phenomenon
  renin-angiotensin-aldosterone c.
case
  M6/C cylinder carrying c.
caseated tissue
caseating granulomatous inflammation
caseation
  tuberculous c.
case-control study
CASE exercise testing system
casein asthma
caseous
  c. abscess
  c. osteitis
  c. pneumonia
  c. tonsillitis
CASHD
  coronary arteriosclerotic heart disease
casing
  Silastic electrode c.
Casodex
Casoni test
caspase inhibitor
CASPER
  computer-assisted pericardial puncture
  computer-assisted pericardial surgery
caspofungin acetate
CASQ
  calsequestrin
CASS
  continuous aspiration of subglottic
    secretions
Cassinari
  artery of Bernasconi and C.
cast
  blood c.
  bronchial c.
Castaneda
  C. bottle
  C. principle
Castellani
  C. bronchitis
  C. disease
  C. point
castellanii
  Acanthamoeba c.
Castellino sign
Castillo catheter
Castleman disease (CD)
castor
  c. bean
  c. bean asthma
Castroviejo needle holder

C

CAT
computerized axial tomography
cat
c. asthma
c. cry syndrome
catabolic illness
catabolism of rt-PA
catacrotic
c. pulse
c. wave
catacrotism
catacrotus
pulsus c.
catadicrotic
c. pulse
c. wave
catadicrotism
catadicrotus
pulsus c.
Cat-a-Kit analyzer
catalase
superoxide c.
catamenial
c. hemoptysis
c. hemothorax
c. pneumothorax
cataplectic
cataplexy
Catapres Oral
Catapres-TTS-1, -2, -3
Catapres-TTS Transdermal
catarrh
atrophic c.
autumnal c.
Bostock c.
hypertrophic c.
Laënnec c.
postnasal c.
sinus c.
suffocative c.
catarrhal
c. asthma
c. bronchitis
c. croup
c. fever
c. laryngitis
c. pharyngitis
c. pneumonia
catarrhalis
Branhamella c.
Moraxella c.
Neisseria c.
catastrophic hemorrhage
catatricrotic pulse
catatricrotism
Catatrol

CATCH-22
cardiac defects, abnormal facies, thymic hypoplasia, cleft palate, hypocalcemia CATCH-22 syndrome
catecholamine
c. action
plasma c.
c. release
catecholaminergic polymorphic ventricular tachycardia (CPVT)
category-ratio
Borg c.-r.
catenoid
Cath
Ash Split C.
Ash Split C. II
Cathcor LX hemodynamic recording system
cathepsin G
catheter
ablation c.
c. ablation
c. ablation of atrial fibrillation
Accent balloon angioplasty c.
Accu-Vu c.
ACE fixed-wire balloon c.
Achiever balloon dilation c.
ACS Endura coronary dilation c.
ACS Enhanced Torque 8/7.5-F Taper Tip c.
ACS Mini c.
ACS Monorail c.
ACS OTW Lifestream coronary dilation c.
ACS OTW Photon coronary dilation c.
ACS OTW Solaris coronary dilation c.
ACS Photon coronary dilation c.
ACS RX Comet angioplasty c.
ACS RX Comet VP coronary dilation c.
ACS RX Lifestream coronary dilation c.
ACS RX perfusion balloon c.
ACS RX Solaris coronary dilation c.
Active Response C. (ARC)
AcuNav ultrasound c.
c. adapter
AFocus steerable diagnostic c.
afterloading c.
Ag-AgCl$_2$ electrode bipolar c.
Agiltrac 0.018, 0.035 peripheral dilation c.
Ahn thrombectomy c.
Alert c.
alignment c.
AL I, II guiding c.

Amazr ablation c.
Amcath c.
Amplatz left I, II c.
Amplatz right coronary c.
Amplatz right I, II c.
A2 multipurpose c.
Angiocath c.
AngioDynamics SOS Omni
  selective c.
Angioflow high-flow c.
angiographic c.
AngioJet saline jet/vacuum
  device c.
AngioJet thrombectomy c.
Angio-Kit c.
Angiomedics c.
angioplasty guiding c.
angled balloon c.
angled pigtail c.
angle-tipped c.
angulated multipurpose c.
Anthron II c.
Anthron heparinized
  antithrombogenic c.
antiseptic-impregnated central
  venous c.
aortic c.
AR-1 c.
ARC-22 coronary balloon
  angioplasty c.
Argyle c.
Arrow balloon wedge c.
Arrow Flex intraaortic balloon c.
ARROWgard Blue antiseptic-
  coated c.
ARROWgard Blue Line c.
ARROWgard central venous c.
Arrow-Howes multilumen c.
Arrow Pullback atherectomy c.
Arrow QuadPolar electrode c.
Arrow QuadPolar pulmonary
  artery c.
arterial embolectomy c.
c. arteriography
Asahi Tornus specialty c.
Ascent guiding c.
aspiration c.
Aspirex PE c.
atherectomy c.
AtheroCath Bantam coronary
  atherectomy c.
AtheroCath GTO coronary
  atherectomy c.
Atlantis SR PRO coronary
  imaging c.
Atlas DG balloon angioplasty c.
Atlas ULP balloon dilation c.
ATRAC-II double-balloon c.
ATRAC multipurpose balloon c.

Attain Select 6238 TEL guide c.
Aurous centimeter sizing c.
Aurous graduate sizing c.
autoperfusion balloon c.
Avanar intravascular ultrasound c.
Avanar IVUS c.
Avita PTCA dilation c.
AV-Paceport thermodilution c.
Bailey c.
Baim pacing c.
balloon angioplasty c.
balloon embolectomy c.
balloon-flotation pacing c.
balloon-imaging c.
balloon-on-a-wire c.
balloon septostomy c.
balloon-tipped angiographic c.
balloon-tipped flow-directed c.
balloon-tipped thermodilution c.
balloon valvoplasty c.
c. balloon valvoplasty (CBV)
Balthern c.
Bandit PTCA c.
Barbeau radial guide c.
Bardco c.
Bard Safety Excalibur c.
Bard Stinger S ablation c.
Basket c.
Bentson-Hanafee-Wilson c.
Berenstein c.
Berman angiographic c.
Beta-Rail c.
Bicor c.
bifoil balloon c.
BioDiamond S rapid exchange
  PTCA c.
Bio-Medicus arterial c.
Biosense Webster NaviStar ablation
  deflectable tip c.
bipolar c.
bird's eye c.
blade septostomy c.
Blazer II cardiac ablation c.
Blazer RPM navigation and
  ablation c.
Blue FlexTip c.
Bonzel Monorail balloon c.
Bourassa c.
brachial c.
Brite Tip c.
Bronchitrac L flexible suction c.
Buchbinder Thruflex over-the-
  wire c.
bullet-tip c.
Burhenne steerable c.
butterfly c.
Calypso Rely PTCA balloon
  angioplasty c.
cardiac c.

C

catheter *(continued)*

Castillo c.
catheter introducing forceps c.
Cath-Finder c.
Cathlon IV c.
Cathmark suction c.
CCOmbo c.
central venous c. (CVC)
cerebral ablation c.
Chilli cooled-tip ablation c.
chronic indwelling venous c.
circular mapping c.
Clark rotating cutter c.
closed-end, noncentering c.
Closer-Closure c.
Cloverleaf c.
CoAxia NeuroFlo c.
cobra-shaped c.
coil-tipped c.
Comet c.
conductance c.
Constellation advanced mapping c.
c. contamination
Cook Cardiovascular infusion c.
Cook NIH Torcon blue c.
Cook Spectrum c.
Cook TPN c.
cool-tip c.
COPACtherm pulmonary artery c.
Cordis BriteTip guiding c.
Cordis Ducor I, II, III c.
Cordis Predator PTCA balloon c.
Cordis Titan balloon dilation c.
Cordis-Webster ablation c.
Cordis-Webster mapping c.
coronary angiographic c.
coronary angiography c.
coronary guiding c.
coronary sinus thermodilution c.
Cournand Tip Arrow QuadPolar electrode c.
CritiCath thermodilution c.
Critikon balloon temporary pacing c.
Critikon balloon-tipped end-hole c.
Critikon balloon wedge pressure c.
CrossPoint TransAccess c.
CrossSail coronary dilation c.
c. cryoablation
cutdown c.
Cynosar c.
Dacron c.
Daig decapolar c.
c. damping
Datascope CL-II percutaneous translucent balloon c.
Davies c.
decapolar electrode c.

deflectable circular-tipped self-expanding c.
deflectable quadripolar c.
c. delivery system
Desai VectorCath mapping c.
diagnostic ultrasound imaging c.
c. dilation
directional atherectomy c.
Dispatch infusion c.
Dispatch over-the-wire c.
disposable mapping c.
distal balloon c. (DBC)
dog-leg c.
Doppler coronary c.
Dotter caged-balloon c.
double-balloon c.
double-chip micromanometer c.
double-J c.
double-lumen Hickman c.
double-thermistor coronary sinus c.
drill-tip c.
D114S balloon c.
dual balloon perfusion c. (DBPC)
dual-sensor micromanometric high-fidelity c.
Ducor-Cordis pigtail c.
Duett c.
duodecapolar c.
EAC c.
EchoMark angiographic c.
EDM infusion c.
Edwards c.
EID c.
Elecath electrophysiologic stimulation c.
electrode c.
El Gamal coronary bypass c.
El Gamal guiding c.
c. embolectomy
embolectomy c.
c. embolism
c. embolus
Encapsulon epidural c.
Endeavor nondetachable silicone balloon c.
end-hole balloon-tipped c.
end-hole 7-French c.
endocoronary sinus c.
EndoCPB c.
endopulmonary vent c.
EndoSonics IVUS/balloon dilation c.
Endotak C lead transvenous c.
Enhanced Torque 8F guiding c.
EnSite multielectrode array transvenous c.
EN Snare endovascular c.
Eppendorf c.
e-TRAIN 110 AngioJet c.

c. exchange
expandable access c. (EAC)
expandable circular cryoablation c.
Explorer 360-degree rotational
  diagnostic EP c.
Expo diagnostic c.
Export c.
Express PTCA c.
Extra Back-up guiding c.
extra-strength 100-PSI c.
Extreme II peripheral excimer
  laser c.
Extreme laser disposable c. (sizes
  0.9 mm, 2.0 mm, 2.2 mm, 2.5
  mm)
8F c.
Falcon coronary c.
Falcon Omniflex balloon c.
Falcon Omniflex PTCA c.
Falcon single-operator exchange
  balloon c.
Fast-Cath hemostasis introducer c.
Feldman aortic stenosis c.
7F extended-curve thermistor c.
7F fused-tip c.
fiberoptic oximeter c.
fiberoptic pressure c.
Finesse guiding c.
Fino DVT c.
first generation cryoablation c.
fixed-wire coronary balloon c.
Flexguard Tip c.
flexible balloon-tipped c.
Flexxicon Blue dialysis c.
flotation c.
flow-assisted short-term balloon c.
flow-directed balloon
  cardiovascular c.
flow-directed end-hole c.
Flow Rider flow-directed c.
fluid-filled balloon cardiovascular c.
fluid-filled balloon-tipped flow-
  directed c.
fluid-filled pigtail c.
7F mapping c.
2F Millar Instrument c.
focal dilation c.
Fogarty adherent clot c.
Fogarty embolectomy c.
Fogarty graft thrombectomy c.
Foltz-Overton cardiac c.
Force balloon dilation c.
c. fragment
Franz monophasic action
  potential c.
Freeway PTCA c.
Freezor cardiac cryoablation c.
French double-lumen c.
French JR4 Schneider c.

6-French Judkins c.
6.2-French 12.5-MHz c.
7-French 20-pole deflectable
  mapping c
French shaft c.
French c. (size 3-34)
French sizing of c.
5-Fr MPC500 micromanometer-
  tipped c.
Frontrunner coronary c.
Frontrunner CTO c.
Frontrunner XP c.
fused-tip c.
FX miniRAIL RX PTCA c.
Ganz-Edwards coronary infusion c.
Gazelle balloon dilation c.
Gensini coronary arteriography c.
Gensini Teflon c.
Gentle-Flo suction c.
Glidecath hydrophilic coated c.
Goeltec c.
Goodale-Lubin c.
Gorlin c.
Gould PentaCath 5-lumen
  thermodilution c.
graft-seeking c.
Grollman pulmonary artery-
  seeking c.
Groshong double-lumen c.
Grüntzig balloon c.
Grüntzig Dilaca c.
Guardian c.
guide c.
c. guide
c. guidewire
guiding c.
Halo XP electrophysiology c.
Hancock embolectomy c.
Hancock fiberoptic c.
Hancock hydrogen detection c.
Hancock luminal electrophysiologic
  recording c.
Hancock wedge-pressure c.
Hands-Off thermal dilution c.
Hartzler LPS dilation c.
Hartzler Micro-600 c.
Hartzler Micro II c.
Hartzler Micro XT c.
Hartzler RX-014 balloon c.
headhunter angiography c.
Heartport endocoronary sinus c.
Heartport endopulmonary vent c.
Heartport endovascular c.
Helix PTCA dilation c.
HemoSplit hemodialysis c.
HemoSplit long-term dialysis c.
high-density sector basket c.
high-flow c.
HighSail coronary dilation c.

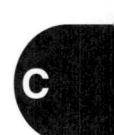

catheter *(continued)*

high-speed rotation dynamic angioplasty c.
Hilal modified headhunter c.
His bundle c.
hockey-stick c.
1-hole angiographic c.
1-hole angioplastic c.
HP SONOS 30-MHz imaging c.
c. hub
HydroCath c.
Hydrolyser hydrodynamic thrombectomy c.
Hydrolyser percutaneous thrombectomy c.
Hydromer-coated central venous c.
IAB c.
IBI Therapy Dual 8 ablation c.
ICE c.
Imager Torque selective c.
c. impact artifact
impedance c.
implantable cardioverter-defibrillator c. (ICDC)
Impulse diagnostic c.
indwelling central venous c.
Infiniti diagnostic c.
InfusaSleeve II c.
injection c.
Innervision ventricular c.
Inoue balloon c.
c. insertion
c. instability
Integra c.
Intellicath pulmonary artery c.
intercostal c.
internal mammary artery c.
c. interventional coronary sinus cerclage
intraaortic balloon c.
intraarterial c.
intracardiac c.
intrapleural c.
intravascular ultrasound c.
intraventricular c. (IVC)
Intrepid balloon c.
Intrepid PTCA c.
c. introduction method
irrigated coiled c.
irrigated-tip quadripolar ablation c.
irrigation ablation c.
ITC balloon c.
IVUS c.
Jackman coronary sinus electrode c.
Jackman orthogonal c.
JL4 c.
JL5 c.
Jocath Maestro coronary balloon c.

Jography angiographic c.
Joguide coronary guiding c.
Josephson quadripolar c.
Josephson Tip Arrow QuadPolar electrode c.
Jostra c.
JR4 c.
JR5 c.
Judkins coronary c.
Judkins curve LAD c.
Judkins curve LCX c.
Judkins curve STD c.
Judkins 4 diagnostic c.
Judkins guiding c.
Judkins pigtail left ventriculography c.
Judkins torque control c.
jugular venous c. (JVC)
Katzen long balloon dilation c.
Kawai flexible endomyocardial biopsy c.
Kerberos Rinspiration c.
Kimny guiding c.
Kimny radial guide c.
Kimny Wiseguide c.
King guiding c.
King multipurpose c.
Konigsberg c.
Kontron balloon c.
large-bore c.
laser delivery c.
Laserprobe c.
Laserprobe-PLR Flex c.
laser transluminal angioplasty c. (LASTAK)
Lasso c.
left coronary c.
left heart c.
left Judkins c.
left ventricular sump c.
Lehman ventriculography c.
Levin c.
Lifestream coronary dilation c.
LifeValve central venous c.
Livewire TC Compass ablation c.
Livewire TC steerable electrophysiology c.
long ACE fixed-wire balloon c.
Long Brite Tip guiding c.
Longdwel Teflon c.
long skinny over-the-wire balloon c.
Lo-Profile II c.
low-profile balloon-positioning c.
low-speed rotation angioplasty c.
Lumax Flex guiding c.
LuMend Frontrunner X39, XP c.
8-lumen manometry c.
Mallinckrodt angiographic c.

c. manipulation
manometer-tipped c.
Mansfield orthogonal electrode c.
Mansfield Scientific dilation
  balloon c.
Mansfield-Webster c.
mapping c.
c. mapping
mapping/ablation c.
mapping and ablation
  electrophysiology c.
Marathon guiding c.
marker c.
Maverick balloon dilation c.
Maverick OTW c.
MaxForce balloon dilation c.
Maxi LD PTA dilation c.
Medi-Tech balloon c.
Medi-Tech steerable c.
Medtronic Export aspiration c.
Medtronic Zuma guiding c.
MegaSonics PTCA c.
memory c.
Mercator atrial high-density
  array c.
Metras c.
Metricath 1000 console c.
Metricath measurement c.
Mewi-5 sidehole infusion c.
Mewissen infusion c.
MicroFerret-18 infusion c.
Micro Guide c.
micromanometer c.
MicroMewi multiple sidehole
  infusion c.
Micross dilation c.
Mikro-Tip micromanometer-tipped c.
Millar Doppler c.
Millar MPC-500 c.
Miller septostomy c.
Mini-Profile c.
Mirage over-the-wire balloon c.
Mogul 3-French steerable decapolar
  electrophysiology diagnostic c.
Molina needle c.
Monorail angioplasty c.
Monorail imaging c.
More-Flow long-term high-flow c.
Morph steerable and deflectable
  vascular c.
MS Classique balloon dilation c.
MTC c.
Mullins transseptal c.
multiaccess c. (MAC)
multielectrode basket c.
multielectrode impedance c.
multilimb c.
multipolar electrode c.
multisensor c.

multispine c.
MVP c.
Namic c.
NarrowFlex intraaortic balloon c.
National Institutes of Health left
  ventriculography c.
National Institutes of Health
  marking c.
NavAblator c.
Naviport deflectable tip guiding c.
Naviport hollow-lumen guiding c.
NaviStar Celsius DS
  diagnostic/ablation c.
NaviStar diagnostic/ablation
  deflectable tip c.
NaviStar DS diagnostic/ablation c.
NaviStar mapping/ablation c.
NC Bandit c.
NC Raptor over-the-wire coaxial
  PTCA dilation balloon c.
Neptune high-pressure PTCA
  balloon c.
NeuroVasx submicroinfusion c.
Newton c.
Nexus 2 linear ablation c.
NIH Cardiomarker c.
Ninja FX series over-the-wire
  coaxial PTCA dilation balloon c.
Norton flow-directed Swan-Ganz
  thermodilution c.
Novoste c.
Nycore pigtail c.
Nylex diagnostic c.
Nyman pigtail c.
octapolar c.
Olbert balloon c.
Olympix II PTCA dilation c.
Omega NV angioplasty c.
OmniCath atherectomy c.
Omni Flush c.
OpenSail balloon dilation c.
OpenSail coronary dilation c.
Opta 5 c.
Opta Pro PTA dilation c.
optical fiber c.
Opticath oximeter c.
Opti-Flow c.
Opti-Plast XT balloon c.
Oracle Focus imaging c.
Oracle Focus PTCA c.
Oracle Micro Plus PTCA c.
OTW HighSail coronary dilation c.
OTW perfusion c.
Outback re-entry c.
over-the-needle c.
over-the-wire balloon dilation c.
over-the-wire PTCA balloon c.
Owens balloon c.
Owens Lo-Profile dilation c.

C

catheter *(continued)*
oximetric c.
Pace bipolar pacing c.
pacemaker c.
Paceport c.
pacing c.
ParCA c.
Parodi balloon c.
c. patency
pediatric pigtail c.
Peel-Away banana c.
PE-MT balloon dilation c.
Pentalumen c.
Percor Stat-DL intraarotic
  balloon c.
PercuSurge Export aspiration c.
percutaneous endocoronary sinus c.
percutaneous intraaortic balloon
  counterpulsation c.
percutaneous radiofrequency c.
percutaneous rotational
  thrombectomy c.
Performa diagnostic c.
perfusion c.
perfusion balloon c. (PBC)
Periflow balloon dilation c.
peripherally inserted c. (PIC)
peripherally inserted central c.
  (PICC)
Per-Q-Cath percutaneously inserted
  central venous c.
pervenous c.
Phantom V Plus c.
PIBC c.
Piccolino Monorail c.
pigtail angiographic c.
pigtail rotation c.
Pinkerton .018 balloon c.
Pleurx pleural c.
plugged telescoping c.
POC Bandit c.
Polaris-DX steerable diagnostic c.
20-pole steerable mapping c.
Polystan venous return c.
Positrol II c.
Powerflex Extreme PTA balloon c.
Powerflex P3 high pressure
  balloon c.
PowerLine c.
PowerSail coronary dilation c.
Predator PTCA c.
preshaped c.
Pro-Bal Protected balloon-tipped c.
probe balloon c.
probing sheath exchange c.
Procath electrophysiology c.
ProCross Rely over-the-wire
  balloon c.
Profile Plus balloon dilation c.

Proflex 5 c.
Pronto thrombectomy c.
Proxis c.
PTCA dilation c.
pulmonary artery flotation c.
Pursuit balloon angioplasty c.
Quad-Lumen c.
quadripolar diagnostic c.
quadripolar pacing c.
quadripolar steerable electrode c.
quadripolar steerable
  mapping/ablation c.
quadripolar thermocouple-equipped
  ablation c.
QuickFlash arterial c.
Quinton PermCath c.
Radii-T c.
radiopaque ERCP c.
Ranger over-the-wire balloon c.
rapid-exchange c.
Raptorail c.
Rashkind septostomy balloon c.
recessed balloon septostomy c.
Redha-cut c.
reference c.
Ref-Star EP c.
Rentrop c.
reperfusion c.
Rescue aspiration c.
Response electrophysiology c.
Revelation Helix c.
Revelation T-Flex c.
Revelation Tx linear ablation c.
RF-generated thermal balloon c.
RF Marinr c.
rheolytic thrombectomy c.
Rhyder diagnostic c.
Rhythm c.
right coronary c.
right heart c.
right Judkins c.
Rigiflex TTS balloon c.
R2L rapid exchange balloon
  dilation c.
RMI antegrade cardioplegia c.
rotational dynamic angioplasty c.
Roubin infusion c.
Royal Flush Plus high-flow
  angiographic flush c.
RX CrossSail coronary dilation c.
RX Streak balloon c.
Sable PTCA balloon c.
Safe-Steer support c.
Sarns wire-reinforced c.
Savvy PTA dilation c.
Schmitz-Rode c.
Scimed angioplasty c.
Scoop 1, 2 c.
self-guiding c.

self-positioning balloon c.
semirigid c.
Sensation intraaortic balloon c.
Seroma-Cath c.
serrated c.
SET c.
Shadow over-the-wire balloon c.
sheath-based IVUS c.
Sherpa guiding c.
Shiley c.
SHJL4 c.
SHJR4 c.
SHJR4s c.
short monorail imaging c.
shredding embolectomy
    thrombectomy c.
sidewinder percutaneous intra-aortic
    balloon c.
Silastic c.
Simmons II, III c.
Simmons-type sidewinder c.
Simpson atherectomy c.
Simpson AtheroCath c.
Simpson-Robert c.
Slalom PTA dilation c.
sliding rail c.
Smec balloon c.
snare c.
Softip c.
Softouch diagnostic c.
Soft-Vu Omni flush c.
Solera thrombectomy c.
Solo c.
Sones coronary c.
Sones Hi-Flow c.
Sones woven Dacron c.
Spectranetics Extreme C laser c.
Spiroflex thrombectomy c.
Spring c.
Spyglass angiography c.
Stack perfusion c.
standard Lehman c.
steerable decapolar electrode c.
steerable diagnostic c.
steerable guidewire c.
steerable quadripolar c.
Steerocath-Dx Spec. Procedure
    Octa C.
Steerocath-T temperature ablation c.
Steri-Cath c.
Stertzer brachial c.
Stertzer guiding c.
stimulation c.
Stinger S ablation c.
Stormer OTW balloon dilation c.
straight flush percutaneous c.
straight tipped c.
Straub Aspirex pulmonary
    embolectomy c.

subselection c.
Sub-4 small vessel balloon
    dilation c.
Super Torque Plus c.
Supreme electrophysiology c.
Surpasse Superfusion perfusion c.
Swan-Ganz balloon flotation c.
Swan-Ganz bipolar pacing c.
Swan-Ganz flow-directed c.
Swan-Ganz Pacing TD c.
Syntel graft cleaning c.
Syntel latex-free embolectomy c.
systemic arterial c.
Talon balloon dilation c.
TEC extraction c.
TEC guide c.
Teflon c.
Tempo diagnostic c.
tennis racket peripheral
    angiographic c.
Terumo SP coaxial c.
tetrapolar esophageal c.
thermodilution balloon c.
thermodilution Swan-Ganz c.
thin-walled c.
c. thrombectomy
ThromCat thrombectomy c.
through-the-needle c.
Tidal balloon c.
Titan Mega XL PTCA dilation c.
Torcon NB Advantage coronary
    angiographic c.
Torcon NB selective
    angiographic c.
torque control balloon c.
torque tube c.
Tourguide guiding c.
TransAccess c.
transcutaneous extraction c.
transducer-tipped c.
transfemoral endoaortic occlusion c.
transjugular c.
transluminal angioplasty c.
transluminal endarterectomy c.
    (TEC)
transluminal extraction c. (TEC)
Transport dilation balloon c.
Transport drug delivery c.
transseptal c.
transtracheal oxygen c.
trefoil balloon c.
tripolar with Damato curve c.
True Sheathless intraaortic
    balloon c.
Twin-Pass dual access c.
Tyshak balloon valvoplasty c.
Uldall subclavian hemodialysis c.
ULP c.
Ultra 8 balloon c.

C

catheter *(continued)*
>UltraCross profile imaging c.
>UltraFuse infusion c.
>Ultra ICE c.
>ultra low profile fixed-wire balloon dilation c.
>ultrasound ablation c.
>ultrasound-tipped c.
>Ultra-Thin balloon c.
>UMI c.
>urinary c.
>URx intravascular Sonotherapy c.
>USCI c.
>valve mapper Steerocath-Dx mapping c.
>van Aman pulmonary pigtail c.
>van Andel c.
>Vantex central venous c.
>vascular access c.
>Vaxcel c.
>vector phased-array ultrasound tipped c.
>Vector-X coronary guiding c.
>Velocimed Proxis c.
>Venaport coronary sinus access c.
>Venaport coronary sinus guiding c.
>ventriculoatrial shunt c.
>ventriculography c.
>Veripath peripheral guiding c.
>vessel-sizing c.
>Viggo Spectramed c.
>Viking Bard c.
>Viking coronary guiding c.
>Visa II ST PTCA balloon c.
>Vision PTCA c.
>Vista Brite Tip large lumen guiding c.
>Vitek c.
>Vitesse E c.
>Vitesse 0.9-mm c.
>Viva Primo balloon c.
>Voda guiding c.
>vortex effect c.
>VTK c.
>Vueport balloon occlusion guiding c.
>VVDL c.
>waist of c.
>Webster halo c.
>Webster orthogonal electrode c.
>wedge pressure balloon c.
>Wexler arterial bypass c.
>c. whip
>c. whip artifact
>White vessel sizing c.
>Wilton Webster coronary sinus thermodilution c.
>Wilton Webster thermodilution flow and pacing c.
>Wiseguide c.
>WorkHorse II PTA balloon c.
>woven Dacron c.
>XMI thrombectomy c.
>Xpeedior t120 c.
>X-Sept transition c.
>Z cardiac c.
>Z-Med c.
>Zuma coronary guiding c.

catheter-associated bloodstream infection (CA-BSI)

catheter-based
>c.-b. revascularization
>c.-b. sensor
>c.-b. thrombolysis

catheter-directed thrombolysis and endovascular stent placement

catheter-guided
>c.-g. biopsy
>c.-g. endoscopic intubation (CAGEIN)

catheter-induced
>c.-i. ablation
>c.-i. coronary artery spasm
>c.-i. embolus
>c.-i. linear lesion
>c.-i. spasm (CIS)
>c.-i. thrombosis

catheterization
>balloon c.
>bypass graft c.
>cardiac c. (CC)
>combined heart c.
>coronary sinus c.
>diagnostic c.
>hepatic vein c.
>interventional cardiac c.
>left heart c. (LHC)
>Mullins modification of transseptal c.
>percutaneous transhepatic cardiac c.
>c. procedure
>pulmonary artery c. (PAC)
>retrograde c.
>right heart c. (RHC)
>selective cardiac c.
>selective venous c. (SVC)
>subclavian approach for cardiac c.
>subclavian vein c. (SVC)
>c. technique
>transradial cardiac c.
>transseptal left heart c.
>Y wave pressure on right atrial c.
>Z point pressure on left atrial c.
>Z point pressure on right atrial c.

catheterize

catheter-microphone
>cardiac c.-m.

catheter-related
    c.-r. bloodstream infection (CR-BSI)
    c.-r. infection (CRI)
    c.-r. peripheral vessel spasm
catheter-snare system
catheter-tip
    c.-t. micromanometer system
    c.-t. occluder
    c.-t. spasm
Cath-Finder
    C.-F. catheter
    C.-F. catheter tracking system
Cathflo Activase
Cath-Gard
    C.-G. catheter contamination shield
    TwistLock C.-G.
CathLink 20 implanted port
Cath-Lok catheter locking device
Cathlon IV catheter
Cathmark suction catheter
cathodal
    c. closing (KC)
    c. closing contraction (KCC)
    c. closure clonus (CCCl)
    c. closure contraction (CCC)
    c. closure tetanus (CCTe)
    c. duration tetanus (CDTe)
    c. opening clonus (COCl)
    c. opening contraction (COC, KOC)
    c. opening tetanus (COTe)
cat-scratch disease
cat's eye syndrome
cattaire
    frémissement c.
cauda equina syndrome
caudally angled balloon occlusion aortography
caudal plane angulation
caudate
    c. hemorrhage
    c. hemorrhagic stroke
    c. infarct
    c. ischemic stroke
    c. nucleus
caudocephalad
caudocranial hemiaxial view
causality assessment
cautery-assisted palatal stiffening operation (CAPSO)
CAV
    cardiac allograft vasculopathy
    cyclophosphamide, doxorubicin, vincristine
cava, pl. cavae
    foramen venae cavae
    inferior vena c. (IVC)
    interrupted inferior vena c.
    left inferior vena c. (LIVC)

    left superior vena c. (LSVC)
    membranous obstruction of inferior vena c. (MOIVC, MOVC)
    orifice of superior vena c.
    persistent left superior vena c. (PLSVC)
    right inferior vena c. (RIVC)
    right superior vena c. (RSVC)
    Spencer plication vena c.
    superior vena c. (SVC)
    thoracic inferior vena c. (TIVC)
    vena c. (VC)
cavae (*pl. of* cava) (*pl. of* cavum)
caval
    c. snare
    c. valve
Cavalieri method
CAVB
    complete atrioventricular block
CAVD
    cardiac allograft vascular disease
    complete atrioventricular dissociation
cave-in
    tracheal wall c.-i.
caveolae
    intracellular c.
Caverject injection
cavernoma
cavernous
    c. angioma
    c. hemangioma
    c. rale
    c. respiration
    c. sinus (CS)
    c. sinus thrombosis
    c. vein
    c. vein of penis
    c. voice
cave sickness
Caves-Schultz bioptome
CAVG
    coronary artery vein graft
CAVH
    continuous arteriovenous hemofiltration
CAVHD
    continuous arteriovenous hemodialysis
CAVHDF
    continuous arteriovenous hemodiafiltration
caviae
    Aeromonas c.
cavitary
    c. lesion
    c. lung disease
cavitas
    c. laryngis
    c. pharyngis
    c. pleuralis
cavitating lesion

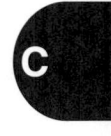
C

cavitation
    pulmonary c.
    c. sign
cavities (*pl. of* cavity)
cavitis
Cavitron ultrasonic surgical aspirator (CUSA)
cavity, pl. **cavities**
    bronchiectatic c.
    celomic c.
    inferior laryngeal c.
    intermediate laryngeal c.
    c. of larynx
    neoplastic c.
    pharyngonasal c.
    pleural c.
    pleuroperitoneal c.
    pulmonary c.
    superior laryngeal c.
    thrombus-filled c.
    ventricular c.
CAVO
    common atrioventricular orifice
cavoatrial anastomosis
cavocaval shunt
cavography
    radionuclide superior c. (RNSC)
cavopulmonary
    c. anastomosis
    c. channel
    c. connection
    c. shunt
cavotricuspid
    c. isthmus (CTI)
    c. isthmus-dependent flutter
    c. isthmus mapping
CAVR
    continuous arteriovenous rewarming
CAVU
    continuous arteriovenous ultrafiltration
cavum, pl. **cavae**
    c. pharyngis
    c. pleurae
CAZ beta-lactamase
CB
    carotid body
    code blue
        CB lead
C4B
    human gene C4B
CBA
    congenital bronchial atresia
    cutting balloon angioplasty
CBBEST
    cutting balloon before stent
CBC
    complete blood count
CBD
    chronic beryllium disease

CBF
    capillary blood flow
    cerebral blood flow
    coronary blood flow
CBFV
    cerebral blood flow velocity
    coronary blood flow velocity
CBG
    capillary blood gas
    coronary bypass graft
CBP
    cyclophosphamide, bleomycin, cisplatin
CBS
    capillary blood sugar
CBT
    code blue team
CBV
    catheter balloon valvoplasty
    central blood volume
    circulating blood volume
    corrected blood volume
C-C
    convexoconcave
        C-C heart valve
CC
    cardiac catheterization
    cardiac center
    cardiac contusion
    cardiac cycle
    cardiovascular clinic
    closing capacity
    coronary care
        CC chemokine I-309
        Touro CC
CCA
    calcium channel antagonist
    cephalin cholesterol antigen
    circumflex coronary artery
CCA-IMT
    common carotid artery intima-media thickness
CCAVF
    congenital coronary arteriovenous fistula
CCB
    calcium channel blocker
CCBV
    central circulating blood volume
CCC
    Canadian Cardiovascular Coalition
    cathodal closure contraction
    common carotid compression
    craniocerebellocardiac
CCCl
    cathodal closure clonus
CCCR
    closed chest cardiac resuscitation
CCCU
    comprehensive cardiac care unit

CCD
  clinical cardiovascular disease
  crossed cerebellar diaschisis
  cumulative cardiotoxic dose
CCE
  clubbing, cyanosis, edema
CCF
  carotid-cavernous fistula
  cephalin-cholesterol flocculation
CCI
  Cardiovascular Credentialing
    International
  cholesterol crystallization inhibitor
  chronic coronary insufficiency
  coherent contrast imaging
C-clamp
CCM
  congestive cardiomyopathy
CCN
  coronary care nursing
CCO
  continuous cardiac output
CCOmbo catheter
CCP
  Certified Cardiology Perfusionist
CCPD
  continuous cyclical peritoneal dialysis
CCPR
  closed chest cardiopulmonary
    resuscitation
CCS
  Canadian Cardiovascular Society
  cardiac conduction system
CCSAS
  Canadian Cardiovascular Society angina
    score
CCSC
  Canadian Cardiovascular Society
    classification
CCSP
  Clara cell secretory protein
CCT
  controlled clinical trial
CCT.2 CryoConsole system
CCTe
  cathodal closure tetanus
CC-TGA
  congenitally corrected transposition of
    great arteries
  congenitally corrected transposition of
    great vessels
CCTP
  coronary care training program
CCU
  cardiac care unit
  coronary care unit
CCVD
  chronic cerebrovascular disease

CCVM
  congenital cardiovascular malformation
CD
  cardiac disease
  cardiac dullness
  cardiac dysrhythmia
  cardiovascular disease
  Castleman disease
  conduction defect
    Cardizem CD
    Ceclor CD
Cd
  cadmium
CD18 antibody
CD4+
    CD4+ cell
    CD4+ measure
CD3 cell
CD4 cell
CD5 cell
CD8 cell
CD20 cell
CD68 cell
CD45 cell surface protein
CD63 platelet activation marker
**CD62p (p-selectin) platelet activation
  marker**
CD8+ T cell
CDBR
  computerized diaphragmatic breathing
    retraining
  controlled diaphragmatic breathing
    CDBR respiratory muscle training
CDC
  Centers for Disease Control and
    Prevention
CDE
  color Doppler energy
cDGS
  complete form of DiGeorge syndrome
CDH
  congenital diaphragmatic hernia
CD-HV
  hyaline-vascular type variant of
    Castleman disease
CDI 2000 blood gas monitoring system
CDM
  change description master
cDNA
  human cloned DNA
CDP
  certified distinct part
  coronary drug project
CD-PC
  plasma cell-type variant of Castleman
    disease
CDTe
  cathodal duration tetanus

C

CDU
cardiac diagnostic unit
CE
carboplatin and etoposide
cardiac enlargement
cardioesophageal
carotid endarterectomy
CEA
carcinoembryonic antigen
carotid endarterectomy
cholesterol-esterifying activity
CEAP
chronotropic exercise assessment protocol
clinical manifestation, etiologic factor,
anatomic involvement, pathophysiologic
feature
CEAP classification
CEAT
chronic ectopic atrial tachycardia
CECCC
confidential enquiry into cardiac
catheterization complications
Ceclor CD
cedar
Western red c.
Cedars-Sinai classification
Cedax
Cedocard-SR
CEE
conjugated equine estrogen
CEEA
curved end-to-end anastomosis
CEEA stapler
Ceelen disease
Ceelen-Gellerstedt
C.-G. disease
C.-G. syndrome
CeeNU Oral
cefaclor
cefadroxil monohydrate
cefazolin sodium
cefdinir
cefditoren pivoxil
cefepime HCl
cefixime
Cefizox
cefmetazole sodium
cefonicid sodium
cefoperazone sodium
ceforanide
cefotaxime sodium
cefotetan disodium
cefoxitin sodium
cefpiramide
cefpodoxime proxetil
cefprozil
ceftazidime
ceftibuten
Ceftin Oral

ceftizoxime sodium
ceftriaxone sodium
cefuroxime
Cefzil
Cegka sign
CEH
cholesterol ester hydrolase
CEHC
calf embryonic heart cell
ceiling
c. effect
c. effect in hypertension
Celacade
celecoxib
celer
pulsus c.
Celermajer method
celerrimus
pulsus c.
Celestin esophageal tube
Celestone
C. Oral
C. Phosphate Injection
C. Soluspan
celiac
c. artery
c. artery axis
c. disease
celiacus
truncus c.
celiprolol
cell
activated Jurkat T c.
c. adhesion molecule (CAM)
adventitial c.
air c.
alveolar c.
ameboid c.
Anitschkow c.
apoptotic c.
Aschoff c.
automatic c.
B1 c.
beryllium-specific CD4+ T_H1 c.
beryllium-specific helper T c.
bone marrow-derived stem c.
bone marrow mononuclear c.
bone marrow stromal c.
bovine aortic endothelial c.
(BAEC)
bradykinin-stimulated c.
bronchial epithelial c.
bronchiolar exocrine c.
brush c.
c. button
calf embryonic heart c. (CEHC)
CD3 c.
CD4+ c.
CD4 c.

CD5 c.
CD8 c.
CD8+ T c.
CD20 c.
CD68 c.
chicken-wire myocardial c.
ciliated epithelial c.
clear c.
c. cycle
dendritic c.
desquamated alveolar epithelial c.
effector c.
embryonal c.
endodermal c.
endothelial progenitor c. (EPC)
epithelial c.
equator of c.
foam c.
foamy myocardial c.
giant c.
goblet c.
c. granulation
great alveolar c.
heart failure c.
HeLa c.
hematopoietic stem c. (HSC)
human aortic endothelial c.
  (HAEC)
human aortic smooth muscle c.
  (HASMC)
hyperplastic mucus-secreting
  goblet c.
IgE-sensitized c.
interdigitating dendritic c.
Jurkat T c.
Kulchitsky c.
Kupffer c.
Langerhans giant c.
Langhans c.
Langhans-type giant c.
macrophage-derived foam c.
mast c.
c. membrane
c. membrane-bound adenylate
  cyclase
mesangial c.
mesenchymal intimal c.
mesenchymal stem c. (MSC)
mesothelial c.
metaplastic mucus-secreting c.
mononuclear c.
mucous c.
multinucleated giant c.
multipotent adult progenitor c.
  (MAPC)
myocardial c.
N c.
neoplastic c.
NPM c.'s

oat c.
open c. (OC)
P c.
pancreatic acinar c.
Pelger-Huet c.
peripheral blood mononuclear c.
  (PBMC)
perivascular epithelioid c.
perivascular foam c.
phagocytic natural killer c.
plasma c. (PC)
progenitor c.
prolactin-producing decidual c.
c. proliferation-to-apoptosis ratio
pup c.
Purkinje c.
RA c.
red blood c. (RBC)
renal juxtaglomerular c.
c. respiration
Sala c.
C. Saver
C. Saver autologous blood recovery
  system
C. Saver Haemonetics
  Autotransfusion system
c. seeding
sensitized c.
septal c.
smooth muscle c. (SMC)
somatic stem c.
c. sorter
squamous alveolar c.
stave c.
c. strain
T c.
c. therapy
transitional c.
c. type
typical small c.
unrestricted somatic stem c.
  (USSC)
vacuolated c.
vascular smooth muscle c. (VSMC)
vasofactive c.
c. wall defect (CWD)
whorling of myocardial c.
WI-38 c.
X-gal-positive c.
cell-based myocardial regenerative
  therapy
CellCept
  C. capsule
  C. Intravenous
  C. oral suspension
  C. tablet
cell-coated stent
Cellegesic ointment
cell-free extract

C

cell-mediated
>> c.-m. immune response
>> c.-m. immunity

cellophane rale
cell-seeded stent
Celltrifuge
cellular
>> c. apoptosis
>> c. cholesterol efflux
>> c. embolism
>> c. infiltrate
>> c. metaplasia
>> c. sheets

cellulase
cellulitis
cellulose
>> oxidized c.

celomic cavity
celophlebitis
CELP
>> code excited linear prediction
>> CELP ECG

Celsa battery
Celsior solution
Cel-U-Jec Injection
CEMRA, CE-MRA
>> contrast-enhanced magnetic resonance
>> angiography

Cenafed Plus Tablet
cenocepacia
>> *Burkholderia c.*

Cenolate
centenarian
center
>> cardiac c. (CC)
>> cardiac-accelerator c. (CAC)
>> cardioaccelerator c.
>> cardioinhibitory c. (CIC)
>> cardiovascular excitatory c.
>> cardiovascular inhibitory c.
>> central medullary cough c.
>> Chemetron HR-1 humidity c.
>> chest pain c. (CPC)
>> C.'s for Disease Control and
>> Prevention (CDC)
>> C.'s for Epidemiologic Studies
>> Depression scale (CES-D)
>> expiratory c.
>> inpatient exercise c. (IEC)
>> inspiratory c.
>> interventional cardiac c. (ICC)
>> Kronecker c.
>> C.'s for Medicare and Medicaid
>> Services (CMS)
>> musculoskeletal intervention c.
>> (MUSIC)
>> pneumotaxic c.
>> respiratory c.
>> vasoconstrictor c. (VCC)

>> vasodilator c. (VDC)
>> vasoinhibitory c.
>> vasomotor c. (VMC)
>> Veterans Affairs Medical C.

centerline
>> c. method
>> c. method of wall motion analysis

Centimist nebulizer
centimorgan (cM)
CentoRx
central
>> c. alveolar hypoventilation
>> c. apical part (CAP)
>> c. apnea
>> c. apnea-hypopnea index
>> c. approach
>> c. baroreflex failure
>> c. blood volume (CBV)
>> c. bradycardia
>> c. bridging strut
>> c. bronchovascular bundle
>> c. calcification
>> c. circulating blood volume
>> (CCBV)
>> c. cyanosis
>> c. fibrous body
>> c. hypopnea
>> c. medullary cough center
>> c. motor conduction time (CMCT)
>> c. nervous system (CNS)
>> c. pneumonia
>> c. respiration
>> c. respiratory drive
>> c. retinal artery occlusion (CRAO)
>> c. sleep apnea (CSA)
>> c. sleep apnea syndrome (CSAS)
>> c. splanchnic venous thrombosis
>> (CSVT)
>> c. tendon of diaphragm
>> c. terminal electrode
>> c. vein
>> c. vein occlusion (CVO)
>> c. venous (CV)
>> c. venous access device (CVAD)
>> c. venous catheter (CVC)
>> c. venous line
>> c. venous luminal diameter
>> c. venous oximetry
>> c. venous oxygen (CVO)
>> c. venous pressure (CVP)
>> c. venous temperature (CVT)

centriacinar emphysema
centrifugal
>> c. left and right ventricular assist
>> device
>> c. pump

centrilobular
>> c. axial interstitial disease
>> c. cyst

c. emphysema
c. nodule
centripetal
c. diffusion
c. rub (CPR)
c. venous pulse
centroid
centronuclear myopathy
centrum tendineum diaphragmatis
Century heart-lung machine
CEP
chronic eosinophilic pneumonia
cepacia
Burkholderia c.
Pseudomonas c.
Cepacia syndrome
C-E Perimount stented valve
cephalexin monohydrate
cephalic
c. approach
c. artery
c. vasomotor response (CVR)
c. vein
cephalin
c. cholesterol antigen (CCA)
c. flocculation
cephalin-cholesterol flocculation (CCF)
cephalization of pulmonary flow pattern
cephalocaudad
cephalometrics
cephalometry
lateral c.
radiographic c.
cephalopharyngeus
cephalosporin
first-generation c.
fourth-generation c.
second-generation c.
third-generation c.
cephalothin sodium
cephapirin sodium
cephradine
Ceporacin
Ceptaz
ceramide
cerclage
catheter interventional coronary
sinus c.
cerebra (*pl. of* cerebrum)
cerebral
c. ablation catheter
c. air embolism
c. amyloid angiopathy (CAA)
c. aneurysm
c. angiography
c. anoxia
c. anthrax
c. apoplexy
c. arteriosclerosis

c. autosomal dominant arteriopathy with subcortical infarct and leukoencephalopathy (CADASIL)
c. beriberi
c. bleeding
c. blood flow (CBF)
c. blood flow velocity (CBFV)
c. edema
c. embolization
c. embolus
c. event
c. HT
c. hyperthermia
c. hypoxia
c. infarct
c. infarction
c. ischemia
c. lupus
c. microangiopathy (CMA)
c. oximetry
c. palsy (CP)
c. perfusion
c. perfusion pressure (CPP)
c. pneumonia
c. protective therapy
c. rate
c. rate of glucose metabolism (CMR$_{gic}$)
c. rate of oxygen metabolism (CMRO$_2$)
c. red blood cell volume (CRCV)
c. respiration
c. thromboangiitis obliterans (CTAO)
c. thrombosis
c. transit time (cTT)
c. tuberculosis
c. vasculopathy
c. vasospasm (CVS)
c. venous thrombosis (CVT)
cerebritis
cerebroprotective
cerebrospinal fluid (CSF)
cerebrovascular (CV)
c. accident (CVA)
c. amyloid peptide (CVAP)
c. autoregulation
c. disease (CeVD)
c. event
c. ferrocalcinosis
c. incident (CVI)
c. infarction (CVI)
c. insufficiency (CVI)
c. reactivity (CVR)
c. reserve capacity (CRC)
c. resistance (CVR)
c. syncope
c. thrombosis

cerebrovasculopathy
    hypertensive c.
cerebrum, pl. **cerebrums, cerebra**
Ceredase injection
cereolysin
cereus
        bacillus c.
Cerezyme
Cerfolio
        Robert David C. (RDC)
cerivastatin
        c. sodium
        c. sodium tablet
Cerose-DM
Certec hyperbaric chamber
certified
        C. Cardiology Perfusionist (CCP)
        c. distinct part (CDP)
Certoparin
ceruleus
        locus c.
cervical
        c. aortic arch
        c. aortic knuckle
        c. disc
        c. heart
        c. part
        c. part of esophagus
        c. pleura
        c. plexus block for carotid
          endarterectomy surgery
        c. radiculitis
        c. rib syndrome
        c. spine deformity
        c. venous hum
        c. vertebra (CV)
cervicalis
        ansa c.
cervicothoracic sympathectomy
CES
        cardioembolic stroke
CESD
        cholesterol ester storage disease
CES-D
        Centers for Epidemiologic Studies
        Depression scale
cesium chloride
cESS
        circumferential end-systolic stress
cessation
        airflow c.
        smoking c.
cestodic tuberculosis
CET
        cholesterol ester transfer
Cetacaine
CE-TCCS
        contrast-enhanced transcranial color-
        coded real-time sonography

cethromycin
cetirizine
CETP
        cholesterol ester transfer protein
CEU
        contrast-enhanced ultrasound
CeVD
        cerebrovascular disease
CF
        cardiac failure
        chest and left leg lead in
          electrocardiography
        clotting factor
        complex fixation
        contractile force
        coronary flow
        cystic fibrosis
            CF lead
            CF lead in electrocardiography
            Synacol CF
            CF transmembrane ion regulator
CFA
        cryptogenic fibrosing alveolitis
CFC
        cardiofaciocutaneous
        chlorofluorocarbon
CFC-free
            CFC-f. delivery system
            CFC-f. metered-dose inhaler
            CFC-f. product
CFC syndrome
C-fiber
        unmyelinated C-f.
CFQ
        Cognitive Failures Questionnaire
CFR
        coronary flow reserve
CFS
        chronic fatigue syndrome
CFT
        cardiolipin flocculation test
CFTR
        cystic fibrosis transmembrane regulator
CFVR
        coronary flow velocity reserve
CFX
        circumflex coronary artery
CFZ
        clofazimine
CG
        cardiography
cGMP
        cyclic guanosine monophosphate
CGN
        compressor-generated nebulizer
CGR biplane angiographic system
CGRP
        calcitonin gene-related peptide

CGS
    cardiogenic shock
CGVD
    chronic graft vascular disease
CH
    calcium heparin
    cholesterol
    chronic hypertension
    chronic hypoxia
    continuous heparin
        CH 2000 cardiac diagnostic system
        CH infusion
Ch, ch
    chest
Chagas
    C. heart disease
    C. myocarditis
chagasic myocardiopathy
chagoma
chain
    alpha-myosin heavy c. (alpha-MHC)
    beta-myosin heavy c. (beta-MHC)
    heavy c.
    HLA-DP beta c.
    imaging c.
    light c.
    myosin heavy c.
    myosin light c.
    paratracheal c.
    c. smoker
    2-c. urokinase plasminogen activator
      (tcu-PA)
chain-compensated spirometer
chalcosis
challenge
    antiarrhythmic c.
    carbachol inhalation c. (CIC)
    cold air c. (CAC, CACh)
    cold dry air c.
    ergonovine c.
    fluid c.
    histamine c.
    hypercapnic c.
    methacholine bronchoprovocation c.
    osmotic c.
    pharmacological c.
chamber
    AeroChamber Plus valved
      holding c.
    anterior c. (AC)
    atrialized c.
    Boyden c.
    calibration c.
    cardiac c.
    Certec hyperbaric c.
    compression c.
    c. compression
    c. dilation
    dual c. (DC)

    EasiVent valved holding c.
    false aneurysmal c.
    c.'s of the heart
    hyperbaric c.
    lower c.
    monoplace c.
    MR 290 humidification c.
    multiplace c.
    OptiChamber valved holding c.
    plasma clot diffusion c. (PCDC)
    recompression c.
    rudimentary c.
    c. rupture
    c. stiffness
    upper c.
    valved holding c. (VHC)
    ventricular c.
    5-c. view
2-chamber
    apical 2-c.
    2-c. view
4-chamber
    apical 4-c.
    4-c. view
chambered
    3-c. heart
chamberlain
    C. mediastinoscopy
    C. procedure
Chandler V-pacing probe
change
    apoptotic c.
    arterial pulsatile volume c.
    arteriovenous crossing c.
    concordant c.'s
    cystic c.
    c. description master (CDM)
    environmental c.
    E-to-A c.
    fibrinoid c.
    fractional area c. (FAC)
    Gerhardt c.
    honeycomb cystic c.'s
    hyaline fatty c.
    ischemic ECG c.
    malignancy-associated c. (MAC)
    myxomatous c.
    nonspecific climatic c.
    obstructive sleep apnea-induced
      cardiovascular c.
    polyneuropathy, organomegaly,
      endocrinopathy, monoclonal
      gammopathy, skin c.'s (POEMS)
    pulse generator c.
    QRS c.
    rheologic c.
    serial c.
    skin c.
    ST-segment c.'s

C

change *(continued)*
  ST-T segment c.'s
  ST-T wave c.'s
  trophic c.'s
  T-wave c.
  vascular c. (VC)
  ventricular geometry c.
channel
  Ca-activated C1 c.
  cavopulmonary c.
  collateral c.
  common pulmonary venous c. (CPVC)
  fast c.
  HERG potassium c.
  ion c.
  K^+ c.
  c.'s of Lambert
  lymphatic c.
  marker c.
  membrane c.
  receptor-operated calcium c.
  sarcolemmal calcium c.
  slow c.
  sodium c. (I_{Na})
  transmural c.
  transmyocardial laser c.
  transnexus c.
  triphosphate-dependent potassium c.
  T-type calcium c.
  voltage-dependent calcium c.
  voltage-gated c.
  voltage-sensitive calcium c. (VSCC)
  water c.
3-channel
  3-c. electrocardiogram
  3-c. Holter monitor
channeling
  mechanical myocardial c. (MMC)
  myocardial c. (MC)
  percutaneous myocardial c. (PMC)
  transmyocardial mechanical c. (TMC)
Chantix
chaos theory
chaotic
  c. atrial tachycardia
  c. heart
  c. rhythm
Chapman index
charcoal
  c. heart
  c. hemoperfusion
Charcot
  C. sign
  C. syndrome
Charcot-Bouchard
  C.-B. aneurysm
  C.-B. microaneurysm

Charcot-Leyden crystal
Charcot-Marie-Tooth disease
Charcot-Neumann crystal
Charcot-Robin crystal
Charcot-Weiss-Baker syndrome
Chardack-Greatbatch
  C.-G. implantable cardiac pulse generator
  C.-G. pacemaker
Chardack Medtronic pacemaker
CHARGE
  colomba, heart anomaly, choanal atresia, retardation, genital and ear anomalies
  CHARGE association
  CHARGE syndrome
charge-coupled device transducer
charge time
Charles
  C. law
  C. procedure
Charlson comorbidity index
Char syndrome
CHART
  continuous hyperfractionated accelerated radiotherapy
charybdotoxin
chaser
  Scot-Tussin DM Cough C.'s
Chassaignac axillary muscle
Chaussier tube
CHB
  complete heart block
  congenital heart block
CHC
  Canadian Heart Classification
CHD
  congenital heart disease
  congestive heart disease
  coronary heart disease
  cyanotic heart disease
Chealamide
CHEC
  community hypertension evaluation clinic
check
  magnet c.
Check-Flo
  C.-F. introducer
  C.-F. performer introducer set for radial artery access
  C.-F. sheath obturator
checklist
  Hopkins Symptom C.
checkmate
  C. gamma brachytherapy system
  C. intravascular brachytherapy system
Chédiak-Higashi syndrome
Chedoke-McMaster Stroke Assessment

cheese
    c. handler's lung
    c. washer's disease
    c. washer's lung
    c. worker's lung
    c. worker's lung disease
cheesy
    c. bronchitis
    c. pneumonia
chelate
    gadolinium c.
chelator
    iron c.
chelonae
    Mycobacterium c.
Chemetron HR-1 humidity center
chemical
    c. ablation
    acaricidal c.
    c. bronchiectasis
    c. bronchitis
    c. cardioversion
    c. exposure
    c. inhalation injury
    c. pleurodesis
    c. pneumonia
    c. pneumonitis
    c. shift artifact
    c. shift imaging (CSI)
    c. stimulus
chemiluminescence
chemoattractant
chemoattracting
    c. agent
    c. molecule
    c. property
    c. stimuli
chemodectoma
chemokine
    CXC c.
    c. proteolysis
Chemo-Port perivena catheter system device
chemoprophylaxis
    secondary c.
chemoreceptor
    peripheral c.
    c. reflex
    c. syndrome
chemoreflex
chemosensitivity
chemosis
chemotactic
    c. anaphylatoxin
    c. cytokine
    c. response
chemotaxis
    eosinophilic c.

    leukocyte c.
    neutrophil c.
chemotherapeutic
    c. agent
    c. index
chemotherapy (CMT)
    antimycobacterial c.
    antituberculous c.
    bischloroethyl nitrosourea c.
    intraarterial c.
    molecular c.
    neoadjuvant c.
    tuberculous c.
ChemTrak AccuMeter theophylline test
Cheracol D
cherry angioma
cherry-picking procedure
chest (Ch, ch)
    alar c.
    anterior flail c.
    anterolateral flail c.
    barrel-shaped c.
    c. bellows
    bilateral anterior flail c.
    blast c.
    buffalo c.
    c. cage
    cobbler's c.
    c. compression
    c. cuirass
    dirty c.
    dropsy c.
    emphysematous c.
    empyema of c.
    flail c.
    foveated c.
    funnel c.
    c. index
    keeled c.
    lateral flail c.
    c. lead
    c. lead in electrocardiography (C)
    c. and left arm lead in electrocardiogram (CL)
    c. and left leg lead in electrocardiography (CF)
    musical c.
    noisy c.
    c. pain (CP)
    c. pain center (CPC)
    c. pain observation unit (CPOU)
    c. pain onset to hospital arrival (CPOTHA)
    c. pain order sheet (CPOS)
    c. pain policy (CPP)
    c. pain syndrome (CPS)
    c. pain of unknown etiology (CPUE)
    paralytic c.

C

chest *(continued)*
c. percussion
c. percussion and vibration
phthinoid c.
c. physical therapy (CPT)
c. physiotherapy (CPT)
pigeon c.
c. port
pressure-like sensation in c.
c. PT
pterygoid c.
quiet c.
c. radiograph (CXR, CxR)
c. and right arm lead in
  electrocardiogram (CR)
c. roentgenogram (CR)
c. roentgenography (CR)
c. shell
c. shield
tetrahedron c.
c. thump
c. tightness
c. tube (CT)
c. wall
c. wall adhesion
c. wall compliance
c. wall elastic recoil pressure (Pth)
c. wall injury
c. wall motion
c. wall movement
c. wall patch
c. wall stimulation (CWS)
c. x-ray (CX, CXR, CxR)
chewable
E.E.S. C.
Cheyne-Stokes
C.-S. asthma
C.-S. breathing (CSB)
C.-S. respiration
C.-S. sign
CHF
chronic heart failure
congestive heart failure
CHFDT
congestive heart failure data tool
Chiari
C. network
C. syndrome
Chiari-Budd syndrome
Chiba needle
chicken
c. breast
c. fat clot
chicken-wire myocardial cell
child-adult mist (CAM)
Child classification
childhood
C. Asthma Questionnaire (CAQ)

c. nitrosopnea
c. tuberculosis
childhood-type tuberculosis
children
Balminil-DM C.
Koffex DM C.
C.'s Motrin Suspension
chilli
C. cooled ablation system
C. cooled-tip ablation catheter
CHIME
coloboma, heart anomaly, ichthyosis,
  mental retardation, ear abnormality
chimeric-7E3
c.-7E3 antiplatelet therapy
c.-7E3 Fab
chimerism
hematopoietic c.
mixed hematopoietic c.
China clay pneumoconiosis
Chinese
C. licorice
C. restaurant asthma syndrome
chink
posterior diamond-shaped c.
chinking
Chito-Seal topical hemostasis pad
Chlamydia
C. *brunetti*
C. *pecorum*
C. *pneumonia*
C. *pneumoniae*
C. *psittaci*
C. *trachomatis*
Chlamydiaceae
chlamydial
chloral hydrate
chlorambucil
chloramine
chloramine-albumin conjugate
chloramine-T technique
chloramphenicol transferase
chlordiazepoxide
chlorella asthma
chlorhexidine gluconate mouthwash
chloride
Adrenalin C.
ammonium c.
Anectine C.
benzocaine, butyl aminobenzoate,
  tetracaine, benzalkonium c.
bethanechol c.
calcium c.
cesium c.
c. current (I_{Cl})
edrophonium c.
hydrogen c.
c. ion

lauryl dimethyl benzyl
ammonium c.
methacholine c.
polyvinyl c. (PVC)
potassium c. (KCl)
c. secretion
c. shift
sodium c.
succinylcholine c.
tetraethylammonium c.
thallous c. (^{201}Tl)
triphenyl tetrazolium c.
vinyl c.
xenon c.
zinc c.
chlorine
c. dioxide
c. induced paradoxical vocal cord
dysfunction
chlormethiazole (*var. of* clomethiazole)
chlorofluorocarbon (CFC)
chloroquine phosphate
chlorothiazide
c. and methyldopa
c. and reserpine
chlorotica
aorta c.
chlorotic phlebitis
chlorotrianisene
chloroxylenol
chlorpheniramine
c., ephedrine, phenylephrine,
carbetapentane
hydrocodone, phenylephrine,
pyrilamine, phenindamine, c.
c. maleate
c., phenylephrine, codeine
c., phenylephrine, dextromethorphan
c., phenylpropanolamine,
dextromethorphan
c. and pseudoephedrine
c., pseudoephedrine, codeine
Chlorprom
Chlorpromanyl
chlorpromazine hydrochloride
chlorpropamide
chlortetracycline sensitivity
chlorthalidone
atenolol and c.
clonidine and c.
Chlor-Trimeton
C.-T. injection
C.-T. Oral
choc
bruit de c.
chocolate sauce sputum
ChoICE
C. Floppy guidewire
C. PT guidewire

Choice PT plus wire
choir
vascular c.
chokes
cholangiogram
intravenous c. (IVC)
cholangiography
intravenous c. (IVC, IVCf)
cholangitis
sclerosing c.
cholecystitis
cholecystokinin
Choledyl SA
cholelithiasis
cholerae
Vibrio c.
choleraesuis
Salmonella c.
cholera vaccine reaction
cholestasis
cystic fibrosis induced c.
Cholestech LDX system
cholesterol (C, CH)
C. 1,2,3 test
c. cleft
c. crystallization inhibitor (CCI)
c. embolism
c. emboli syndrome
c. embolization
c. ester
c. ester hydrolase (CEH)
c. ester storage disease (CESD)
c. ester transfer (CET)
c. ester transfer protein (CETP)
free c. (FC)
low c.
low fat and c. (LFC)
c. monitoring system
nonesterified c. (NEC)
c. pericarditis
c. pleurisy
c. pneumoritis
remnant lipoprotein c.
c. saturation index (CSI)
serum c.
skin c.
c. stone (CS)
c. sulfate (CS)
c. thorax
total c. (TC)
total plasma c. (TPC)
unesterified c.
cholesterol-esterifying activity (CEA)
cholesterol-lecithin (CL)
c.-l. flocculation (CLF)
cholesterol-lowering lipid (CLL)
cholesterol-phospholipid (C/P, C/PL)
Cholesterol-Saturated Fat Index (CSFI)
cholesterol-triglyceride (C/TG)

C

Cholestin
Cholestron Pro II handheld device
cholestyramine resin
choline
    c. magnesium trisalicylate
    c. salicylate
    c. theophyllinate
cholinergic
    c. agent
    c. receptor
    c. response
    c. tone
    c. vasodilation
cholinesterase inhibitor
chondral disarticulation
chondralgia
chondrocostal disarticulation
chondroitin sulfate
chondroma
chondrosarcoma
chondrosternal
chondrosternoplasty
chondroxiphoid
chorda, pl. chordae
    flail c.
    chordae tendineae
    chordae tendineae cordis
    chordae tendineae rupture
    c. vocalis
chordal
    c. buckling
    c. length
    c. rupture
    c. structure
    c. transfer
chordalis
    endocarditis c.
chordoplasty
chorea
    amyotrophic c.
    c. cordis
    Huntington c.
    Sydenham c.
choriocarcinoma
chorionic villus sampling
choroidopathy
    Pneumocystis c.
CHP
    capillary hydrostatic pressure
Christmas
    C. disease
    C. factor
chromaffin cell tumor
chromate
chromatin
    coarse c.
chromatography
    affinity c.

    denaturing high performance
      liquid c. (DHPLC)
    gas c.
    high-performance liquid c. (HPLC)
    high-pressure liquid c. (HPLC)
    Sephadex G24 c.
chromic catgut suture
chromium
chromogenic method
chromogranin
chromosome
    c. 5q
    c. 11q
chronic
    c. airflow limitation (CAL)
    c. airflow obstruction (CAO)
    c. airway rejection
    c. aortic stenosis
    c. asthma
    c. asthmatic bronchitis
    c. atrial fibrillation
    c. beryllium disease (CBD)
    c. catarrhal laryngitis
    c. catarrhal tonsillitis
    c. cavitary histoplasmosis
    c. cerebrovascular disease (CCVD)
    c. constrictive pericarditis
    c. contractile dysfunction
    c. coronary insufficiency (CCI)
    c. coronary occlusions
    c. cor pulmonale
    c. ectopic atrial tachycardia
      (CEAT)
    c. endocarditis
    c. eosinophilic pneumonia (CEP)
    c. fatigue syndrome (CFS)
    c. fibrosing alveolitis
    c. fibrous pneumonia
    c. fusiform aneurysm
    c. graft vascular disease (CGVD)
    c. heart failure (CHF)
    c. hemolytic anemia
    c. hiccups
    c. hypercarbia
    c. hypertension (CH)
    c. hypertensive disease
    c. hypertrophic emphysema
    c. hyperventilation syndrome
    c. hypoxia (CH)
    c. idiopathic orthostatic hypotension
    c. indwelling venous catheter
    c. inflammatory airway disease
    c. innate immune response
    c. interstitial lung disease
    c. invasive pulmonary aspergillosis
    c. lunger
    c. lymphocytic thyroiditis
    c. mediastinal histoplasmosis
    c. metabolic acidosis

c. mucocutaneous moniliasis
c. myocarditis
c. necrotizing aspergillosis (CNA)
c. nonvalvular atrial fibrillation (CNAF)
c. obliterative bronchiolitis
c. obstruction outflow disease (COOD)
c. obstructive airways disease
c. obstructive bronchitis
c. obstructive lung disease (COLD)
c. obstructive pulmonary disease (COPD)
c. obstructive pulmonary emphysema (COPE)
c. obstructive respiratory disease (CORD)
c. occlusive in-stent restenosis (COISR)
c. passive congestion
c. peripheral arterial disease (CPAD)
c. pharyngitis
c. pleurisy
c. pulmonary cystic lymphangiectasis
c. pulmonary edema
c. pulmonary emphysema (CPE)
c. pulmonary insufficiency
c. pulmonary insufficiency of prematurity
c. recurrent chemical injury
c. renal failure
c. respiratory disease (CRD)
C. Respiratory Disease Questionnaire (CRQ)
c. respiratory failure (CRF)
C. Respiratory Questionnaire (CRQ)
c. restrictive pulmonary disease (CRPD)
c. sheath
c. shock
c. silicosis
c. sinus arrest
c. stable angina
c. stable asthmatic
c. suppurative lung disease (CSLD)
c. tamponade
c. thromboembolic pulmonary hypertension (CTEPH)
c. thrombotic pulmonary vascular obstruction (CTPVO)
c. total occlusion (CTO)
c. total occlusion recanalization
c. upper respiratory obstruction
c. valvular heart disease (CVHD)
c. valvulitis
c. vascular rejection
c. venous insufficiency (CVI)

c. ventilatory failure (CVF)
c. volume load
chronicity
Chronicle implantable hemodynamic monitor
Chrono-log
C.-l. lumi-aggregometer
C.-l. optical aggregometer
C.-l. platelet aggregometer
chronolog
nebulizer c.
Chrono-Lume reagent
Chrono-Par aggregation reagent
chronophysiology
chronotherapeutic
chronotherapeutics
chronotherapy
chronotropic
c. effect
c. exercise assessment protocol (CEAP)
c. incompetence
c. response
chronotropism
negative c.
positive c.
Chrysalin
chrysotile asbestos
CHUK
conserved helix-loop-helix ubiquitous kinase
Church cardiovascular scissors
Churchill-Cope reflex
Churg-Strauss
C.-S. angiitis
C.-S. syndrome (CSS)
C.-S. vasculitis
Chuter endovascular device
Chvostek sign
chyliform
c. pleural effusion
c. pleurisy
chylomicron
c. remnant (CMR)
c. remnant receptor
chylomicronemia syndrome
chylopericarditis
chylopericardium
idiopathic c.
primary idiopathic c.
primary isolated c.
chylopleura
chylopneumothorax
chyloptysis
chylothorax, pl. **chylothoraces**
traumatic c.
chylous
c. ascites
c. hydrothorax

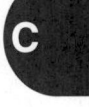

chylous *(continued)*
    c. pericardial effusion
    c. pleural effusion
    c. pleurisy
    c. spill
chymase gene locus
CI
    cardiac index
    cardiac insufficiency
    colloidal iron
    confidence interval
    constraint-induced
    coronary insufficiency
        CI therapy
Ciaglia
    C. Blue Dolphin tracheostomy
    C. Blue Rhino single-step dilator
        kit
    C. percutaneous tracheostomy
    C. percutaneous tracheostomy
        introducer
    C. sequential dilator kit
    C. serial dilation technique
Ciba-Corning 2500 CO-Oximeter
cibenzoline
cibum
    ante c. (a.c.)
CIC
    carbachol inhalation challenge
    cardioinhibitory center
cicaprost
cicatricial stenosis
cicatrization atelectasis
ciclesonide
cicletanine
CICU
    cardiac intensive care unit
cidal effect
Cidecin
cidofovir
Cidomycin
cifenline succinate
cigarette
    c. cough
    c. smoke (CS)
    c. smoking
CIIA
    common internal iliac artery
cilastatin
    imipenem and c.
cilazapril
cilexetil
    candesartan c.
cilia (*pl. of* cilium)
ciliary
    c. beat frequency
    c. dysfunction
    c. efficacy

    c. impairment
    c. movement
ciliastatic
ciliated
    c. epithelial cell
    c. epithelium
ciliocytophthoria
ciliogenesis
ciliotoxicity
cilium, pl. **cilia**
cilnidipine
cilomilast
cilostazol
cimetidine
Cimino arteriovenous shunt
Cimino-Brescia arteriovenous fistula
Cimochowski cardiac cannula
CIMT
    carotid intima-medial thickness
        CIMT regression
cinchonism
cincinnatiensis
    Legionella c.
cine
    c. camera
    c. computed tomography
    c. CT
    c. evaluation
    c. gradient-echo MRI
    c. loop
    c. scan
    c. sequence
    c. technique
    TruFisp c.
    c. view
cineangiocardiography
    radionuclide c.
cineangiogram
cineangiographic system
cineangiography
    conventional c.
cinearteriography
cinefilm
cinefluorography
cinefluoroscopy
cineless recording system
cine-loop
cine-pulse system
cineventriculogram
cineventriculography
CineView Plus Freeland system
cinnarizine
Cinobac Pulvules
cinoxacin
Cin-Quin
CIPF
    classic interstitial pneumonitis with
        fibrosis
CIP-Fenofibrate

Cipro
    C. injection
    C. Oral
ciprofibrate
ciprofloxacin hydrochloride
ciprostene
Circadia dual-chamber rate-adaptive pacemaker
circadian
    c. blood pressure pattern
    c. disruption
    c. event recorder
    c. pacemaker
    c. periodicity
    c. rhythm
    c. secretion
    c. variation
circannual cycle
circaseptan cycle
circle
    c. of death
    c. of Vieussens
    c. of Willis (CW)
circuit
    Adam c.
    aortoiliofemoral c.
    arrhythmia c.
    bypass c.
    FilterLine c.
    fluidic c.
    Intertech anesthesia breathing c.
    macroreentrant c.
    output c.
    reentrant c.
    sensing c.
    shunting c.
    timing c.
circuitry
    low-prime c.
Circulaire
    C. aerosol drug delivery device
    C. aerosol drug delivery system
    C. inhaled medication delivery device
circulans
    bacillus c.
circular
    c. mapping catheter
    c. plane
circulating
    c. adhesion molecule (CAM)
    c. anodic antigen (CAA)
    c. anticoagulant (CAC)
    c. antineutrophil cytoplasmic antibody (cANCA)
    c. bacterial endotoxin
    c. blood volume (CBV)
    c. endothelin
    c. interleukin-6
    c. water blanket
circulation
    airway, breathing, c. (ABC)
    allantoic c.
    anterior c. (AC)
    arterial c.
    assisted c.
    balanced coronary c.
    codominant coronary c.
    collateral c.
    compensatory c.
    coronary collateral c.
    derivative c.
    extracorporeal c. (ECC)
    fetal c.
    Fontan c.
    general c. (GC)
    left dominant coronary c.
    lesser c.
    native arterial c.
    peripheral c.
    persistent fetal c. (PFC)
    placental c.
    portal c.
    posterior c. (PC)
    pulmonary c. (PC)
    restoration of spontaneous c. (ROSC)
    return of spontaneous c. (ROSC)
    c., sensation, motion (CSM)
    splanchnic c.
    systemic c.
    thebesian c.
    c. time
    transient spontaneous c. (TSC)
    c. volume
Circulator
    C. Boot
    C. Boot therapy
circulatory
    c. arrest
    c. collapse
    c. compromise
    compromise systemic c.
    c. congestion
    c. depression
    c. embarrassment
    c. failure
    c. hypoxemia
    c. hypoxia
    c. instability
    c. overload
    c. shock
    c. stability
    c. support system
circumaortic
    c. venous collar
    c. venous ring

C

circumference
　　left ventricular end-diastolic c. (LVEDC)
circumferential
　　c. end-systolic stress (cESS)
　　c. ESS
　　c. fiber shortening
　　c. wall stress (CWS)
circumflex (CX)
　　anomalous c. (ACx)
　　c. aortic arch
　　c. artery (CX)
　　c. coronary artery (CCA, CFX)
　　left c. (LC, LCF, LCX)
　　left atrial c. (LAC)
　　c. occlusion
circumoral cyanosis
circumscribed
　　c. edema
　　c. pleurisy
circus
　　c. movement
　　c. movement tachycardia (CMT)
　　c. senilis
CIRF
　　cocaine-induced respiratory failure
CirKuit-Guard
　　C.-G. device
　　C.-G. pressure relief valve
cirrhosis
　　biliary c.
　　cardiac c.
　　congestive c.
　　Laënnec c.
　　c. of liver
　　stasis c.
cirrhotic
CIRSE
　　Cardiovascular and Interventional Radiological Society of Europe
cirsoid
　　c. aneurysm
　　c. varix
CIS
　　catheter-induced spasm
　　coronary implant system
cisapride
cisatracurium besylate
cisplatin (DDP)
　　cyclophosphamide, bleomycin, c. (CBP)
　　cyclophosphamide, doxorubicin, c. (CAP)
　　doxorubicin, 5-fluorouracil, c. (AFP)
　　c. and etoposide (PE)
　　mitomycin, ifosfamide, c. (MIC)
　　mitomycin, vinblastine, c. (MVP)

　　c., vincristine, doxorubicin, etoposide (CODE)
cisterna, pl. **cisternae**
　　cylindrical confronting c.
　　perinuclear c.
　　subsarcolemmal c.
　　terminal c.
CIT
　　cold ischemic time
citicoline
citrate
　　caffeine c.
　　diethylcarbamazine c.
　　esprolol plus sildenafil c.
　　c. exchange
　　nesiritide c.
　　piperazine c.
　　sildenafil c.
　　sufentanil c.
citrated caffeine
citric acid cycle
Citrobacter
　　C. amalonatica
　　C. freundii
Citrol Smoking alternative
citrovorum rescue
CIV
　　continuous intravenous infusion
c-Jun
　　c-Jun gene
　　c-Jun N-terminal kinase (JNK)
CK
　　color kinesis
　　creatine kinase
　　　CK image
CK19 level
CKG
　　cardiokymography
CK-MB
　　creatine kinase, myocardial bound
CK-MB elevation
CL
　　cardiolipin
　　chest and left arm lead in electrocardiogram
　　cholesterol-lecithin
　　cycle length
　　　CL lead
CLA
　　clarithromycin
　　closed-loop algorithm
　　　CLA for infusion of catecholamine in heart stress test
Clado anastomosis
Cladosporium
Claforan
Clagett
　　C. closure
　　C. procedure

clamp

Allis c.
anastomosis c.
aortic aneurysm c.
Atlee c.
Bahnson aortic c.
Bailey aortic c.
Beck miniature aortic c.
Beck-Potts aortic and pulmonic c.
Blalock pulmonary stenosis c.
Bradshaw-O'Neill aorta c.
bulldog c.
cardiovascular c.
Cooley anastomosis c.
Cooley aortic c.
Cooley-Beck vessel c.
Cooley bronchus c.
Cooley-Derra anastomosis c.
Cooley-Satinsky c.
Craafoord coarctation c.
Crile c.
Crutchfield c.
Davidson c.
DeBakey aortic aneurysm c.
DeBakey arterial c.
DeBakey-Bahnson c.
DeBakey-Bainbridge c.
DeBakey-Derra anastomosis c.
DeBakey-Harken auricle c.
DeBakey-Howard aortic
  aneurysmal c.
DeBakey-Kay aortic c.
DeBakey-McQuigg-Mixter
  bronchial c.
DeBakey pediatric c.
DeBakey peripheral vascular c.
DeBakey-Satinsky vena cava c.
DeBakey-Semb ligature-carrier c.
Demos tibial artery c.
Derra aortic c.
Derra vena caval c.
dreamer c.
Edwards c.
endoaortic c.
euglycemic glucose c.
Favaloro proximal anastomosis c.
Glassman c.
Grant abdominal aortic
  aneurysmal c.
Grover c.
Halsted c.
Hartmann c.
Heartport endoaortic c.
Hopkins aortic c.
Hufnagel ascending aortic c.
Jacobson microbulldog c.
Jacobson modified vessel c.
Jacobson-Potts c.
Javid carotid artery bypass c.

Kantrowitz thoracic c.
Kelly c.
Kindt carotid artery c.
Koala vascular c.
Lambert aortic c.
Lambert-Kay aortic c.
Liddle aorta c.
Mattox aorta c.
microvascular c.
mosquito c.
Müller vena caval c.
myocardial c.
noncrushing vascular c.
Noon A-V fistula c.
partial occlusion c.
pediatric vascular c.
Reich-Nechtow c.
resection c.
Rochester Kocher c.
Rochester Péan c.
Ruel aorta c.
Rumel c.
Sarot bronchus c.
Satinsky c.
Schumacher aorta c.
side-biting c.
Sideris c.
Subramanian c.
suprahepatic caval c.
VascuClamp vascular c.
vascular c.
vessel c.
Wylie carotid artery c.
Wylie vascular c.
Yasargil carotid c.

clamping

partial c.

clamshell

c. closure of atrial septal defect
C. II device
c. incision
c. septal occluder
C. septal umbrella

clandestine myocardial ischemia

clapotement

bruit de c.

claquement

bruit de c.

Clara cell secretory protein (CCSP)

clarithromycin (CLA)

Claritin

Claritin-D 24-Hour

clarity

C. capnograph
C. multiparameter monitoring
  system
C. software

Clark

C. classification

Clark *(continued)*
    C. classification of malignant
      melanoma
    C. oxygen electrode
    C. rotating cutter catheter
Clarke-Hadfield syndrome
classic
    c. angina
    c. expectorant
    C. II stethoscope
    c. interstitial pneumonitis with
      fibrosis (CIPF)
    c. mucolytic
    c. risk factor
classification, class
    Allen and Davis c.
    Ambrose c.
    American Heart Association c.
    American Heart Association Stroke
      Outcome C. (AHA.SOC)
    antiarrhythmic drug c. (Ia, Ib, Ic,
      II, III, IV)
    Astler-Coller c.
    Barrow c.
    Boyden c.
    Braunwald c. I–IIIB
    Canadian Cardiovascular Society c.
      (CCSC)
    Canadian Cardiovascular Society
      functional c.
    Canadian Heart C. (CHC)
    CEAP c.
    Cedars-Sinai c.
    Child c.
    Clark c.
    Cohen-Rentrop c.
    congestive heart failure c. I-IV
    Croften c.
    DeBakey c.
    Dexter-Grossman c.
    Diamond c.
    Dukes c.
    Efron jackknife c.
    Fontaine lower limb ischemia c.
    Forrester Therapeutic C. (grade
      I–IV)
    Fredrickson c.
    Fukunaga-Hayes unbiased
      jackknife c.
    functional capacity c.
    Gray-Weale plaque c.
    Hannover c.
    Heath-Edwards c.
    Hinkle-Thaler c.
    hip c.
    ILO c.
    International Labor Office C.
    Jackson-Huber c.
    Kiel lymphoma c.
    Killip heart disease c.
    Killip heart failure c.
    Killip-Kimball heart failure c.
    KWB hypertension c.
    Levine-Harvey c.
    Liebow c.
    Lipton c. (LI, LII-A, LII-B, LII-P,
      RII-A, RII-B)
    Loesche c.
    Lown c.
    Mallampati airway c. I-IV
    Mallampati-Samsoon airway c. I-IV
    Mayo c.
    Minnesota ECG c.
    New York Heart Association
      functional c. I–IV
    Novacode serial ECG c.
    NYHA functional c. I–IV
    RDC c.
    Reid c.
    Rentrop c.
    Robert David Cerfolio c.
    round-robin c.
    Rutherford claudication c.
    Sellers mitral regurgitation c.
    Shaher-Puddu c.
    Singh-Vaughan-Williams
      arrhythmia c.
    Stanford c.
    Stary histology c.
    TIMI c.
    TNM c.
    Vaughan-Williams antiarrhythmic
      drug c.
    Walter Reed c.
    WHO/Fredrickson c.
    Wood c.
    Yacoub and Radley-Smith c.
claudicant limb
claudication
    1-block c.
    2-block c.
    3-block c.
    buttock c.
    calf c.
    2-flights-of-stairs c.
    intermittent c.
claudicatory
Claudius fossa
Clauss
    C. assay
    C. method
clavicle
    acromial articular facies of c.
    acromial articular surface of c.
    sternal extremity of c.
clavicular facet
clavipectoral triangle
clavulanate

clavulanic acid
Clavulin
cleaner
　　VT Mercury Vac organic mercury vacuum c.
clear
　　C. Advantage Spirometry Filter
　　c. cell
　　c. cell carcinoma
　　c. cell tumor
　　Scot-Tussin Senior C.
clearance
　　airway c.
　　c. assistive device
　　creatinine c.
　　drug c.
　　gas c.
　　lung mucociliary c.
　　mucociliary c. (MCC)
　　peripheral zone radioaerosol c.
　　c. technique
　　tracheobronchial c.
Clearglide
　　C. endoscopic vessel harvesting system
　　C. precision bipolar device
CLeaRS cardiac lead removal system
ClearView
　　C. intracoronary shunt
　　C. intravascular arteriotomy shunt
Clearview Troponin I test
cleavage
　　abnormal c.
cleft
　　c. anterior leaflet
　　c. of aortic leaflet
　　c. A-V valve
　　cholesterol c.
　　laryngeal c.
　　c. limb-heart (CLH)
　　c. mitral valve
　　Schmidt-Lanterman c.
clemastine fumarate
clenched fist sign
clentiazem
Cleocin
　　C. HCl
　　C. HCl Oral
　　C. Pediatric
　　C. Pediatric Oral
　　C. Phosphate
　　C. Phosphate Injection
clevidipine
CLF
　　cholesterol-lecithin flocculation
CLH
　　cleft limb-heart
　　　CLH syndrome

click
　　ejection c. (EC)
　　Hamman c.
　　late systolic c. (LSC)
　　metallic c.
　　midsystolic c (MSC)
　　mitral c.
　　mitral valve prolapse-systolic c. (MVP-SC)
　　c. murmur
　　nonejection systolic c.
　　palmar c.
　　pulmonary ejection c. (PEC)
　　c. syndrome
　　systolic c. (SC)
Clickhaler
clicking
　　c. pneumothorax
　　c. rale
click-murmur syndrome
climbing
　　stair c.
clindamycin
clinic
　　cardiovascular c. (CC)
　　community hypertension evaluation c. (CHEC)
　　lipid research c. (LRC)
clinical
　　c. cardiovascular disease (CCD)
　　c. manifestation, etiologic factor, anatomic involvement, pathophysiologic feature (CEAP)
　　c. practice guidelines (CPG)
　　c. pulmonary infection score (CPIS)
　　c. research unit (CRU)
　　c. well-being
clinicoradiographic heart failure
CliniFLO breathing exerciser
Clinitron air-fluidized therapy
clinocephaly
Clinoril
clinostatic bradycardia
clip
　　Adams-DeWeese vena caval serrated c.
　　alligator c.
　　Astro-Trace Universal adapter c.
　　Atrauclip hemostatic c.
　　crankshaft c.
　　Elgiloy-Heifitz aneurysm c.
　　Fogarty spring c.
　　Horizon surgical ligating and marking c.
　　ligation c.
　　microbulldog c.
　　Miles vena cava c.
　　Moretz c.

C

clip *(continued)*
  nose c.
  C. On torquer
  partial occlusion inferior vena
    cava c.
  Smith c.
  Sugar c.
  Sugita c.
  vascular c.
  vena cava c.
ClipTip reusable sensor
Clivarine
CLL
  cholesterol-lowering lipid
CLM articulating laryngoscope blade
cloacae
  Enterobacter c.
clockwise
  c. flutter
  c. loop
  c. rotation
  c. rotation of electrical axis
  c. torque
clofazimine (CFZ)
  c. palmitate
clofibrate
clofilium
clomethiazole, chlormethiazole
clone
  antiadhesion c.
clonidine
  c. and chlorthalidone
  c. hydrochloride
cloning
  DNA c.
Cloninger Temperament and Character
  Inventory
clonogenic technique
Clonorchis sinensis
clonus
  anodal opening c.
  cathodal closure c. (CCCl)
  cathodal opening c. (COCl)
clopidogrel bisulfate
clorprenaline hydrochloride
closed
  c. chest cardiac massage
  c. chest cardiac resuscitation
    (CCCR)
  c. chest cardiopulmonary
    resuscitation (CCPR)
  c. chest commissurotomy
  c. chest pneumothorax
  c. chest thoracostomy
  c. chest water-seal drainage
  c. endarterectomy
  c. heart surgery
  c. transventricular mitral
    commissurotomy

closed-circuit
  c.-c. method
  c.-c. spirometer
closed-end, noncentering catheter
closed-loop
  c.-l. algorithm (CLA)
  c.-l. delivery
  c.-l. device
  c.-l. pacing
  c.-l. sedative administration
closed-tube thoracostomy
Closer-Closure catheter
closing
  c. capacity (CC)
  cathodal c. (KC)
  c. slope
  c. snap
  c. volume (CV)
clostridial myocarditis
Clostridium
  C. botulinum
  C. perfringens
  C. septicum
  C. tetani
Clo-Sur
  C.-S. P.A.D.
  C.-S. P.A.D. dressing
  C.-S. P.A.D. external vascular
    closure device
closure
  abrupt c.
  airway c.
  Angiolink staple-mediated c.
  aortic c. (AC)
  aortic valve c. (AVC)
  C. catheter/radiofrequency generator
  Clagett c.
  delayed primary c. (DPC)
  double umbrella c.
  early mitral valve c. (EMVC)
  King ASD umbrella c.
  mitral c. (Mc)
  nonoperative c.
  paradoxical inspiratory c.
  patch c.
  percutaneous patent ductus
    arteriosus c.
  premature mitral c. (PMC)
  premature valve c.
  primary c.
  PTFE c.
  pulmonic c. (PC)
  pulmonic valve c.
  saphenous vein patch c.
  semilunar valve c.
  threatened abrupt c.
  transcatheter c. (TCC)
  tricuspid c. (Tc)
  tricuspid valve c.

umbrella c.
vacuum-assisted c. (VAC)
wound c.

clot
agonal c.
agony c.
antemortem c.
autologous c.
blood c.
c. buster
C. Buster Amplatz thrombectomy
device
chicken fat c.
currant jelly c.
fibrin c.
laminated c.
c. lysis
c. lysis time (CLT)
passive c.
postmortem c.
c. retraction time
C. Stop drain
clot-bound thrombin
cloth
Dacron c.
clot-promoting factor (CPF)
clotrimazole
clotted hemothorax
clotting
c. abnormality
c. disorder
c. factor (CF)
c. time (CLT, CT)
cloud
signal-loss c.
clouded sensorium
clouding
hilar c.
mental c.
cloudy
Cloverleaf catheter
cloxacillin sodium
CLP
cardiac laboratory panel
CLS
capillary leak syndrome
CLSE
calf lung surfactant extract
CLT
clot lysis time
clotting time
clubbing
c., cyanosis, edema (CCE)
digital c.
c. of fingers
c. of toes
cluster
microcalcification c. (MCC)
cluster-of-grapes appearance

C-M
cardiomyopathy
CM
cardiac monitoring
cardiac murmur
cardiac muscle
cardia mucosa
cardiomyopathy
congestive myocardiopathy
continuous murmur
C/M
counts per minute
cM
centimorgan
CM3 cocktail
CMA
cerebral microangiopathy
CMAD
count median aerodynamic diameter
CMAP
compound motor action potential
CMC
corticomedullary contrast
CMCT
central motor conduction time
CMD
count median diameter
CMFT
cardiolipin microflocculation test
CMH
congenital malformation of heart
CMN
cystic medial necrosis
CMN-AA
cystic medial necrosis of ascending aorta
CMO
cardiac minute output
CMP
cardiomyopathy
CMR
cardiovascular magnetic resonance
chylomicron remnant
CMR$_{gic}$
cerebral rate of glucose metabolism
CMRO$_2$
cerebral rate of oxygen metabolism
CMS
cardiovascular measurement system
Centers for Medicare and Medicaid
Services
CMS AccuProbe 450 system
CMSD
congenital myocardial sympathetic
dysinnervation
CMT
chemotherapy
circus movement tachycardia
CMV
conventional mechanical ventilation

CMV *(continued)*
    cytomegalovirus
        CMV IE-2 gene expression
        CMV IE-2 riboprobe
        CMV pneumonitis
        CMV seronegative
        CMV seropositive
CMVIG
    cytomegalovirus immune globulin
CNA
    chronic necrotizing aspergillosis
CNAF
    chronic nonvalvular atrial fibrillation
CNL
    cardiolipin natural lecithin
cNOS
    constitutive nitric oxide synthase
CNP
    C-type natriuretic peptide
CNS
    central nervous system
CNT
    continuous nebulization therapy
CO
    carbon monoxide
    cardiac output
        CO oximeter
        CO oximetry
        CO Sleuth
        CO Sleuth carbon monoxide monitor
        CO Sleuth handheld carbon monoxide analyzer
CO2
    CO2 heart laser angina relief therapy
    CO2 TMR Heart Laser 2
CO$_2$
    carbon dioxide
    arterial partial pressure of CO$_2$ (PaCO$_2$)
    CO$_2$ oximetry
    partial pressure of end-tidal CO$_2$ (PETCO$_2$)
    pulse oximeter/end tidal CO$_2$ (POET)
    sublingual CO$_2$
    CO$_2$ waveform
CoA
    coarctation of aorta
    coenzyme A
Coach incentive spirometer
coaching whistle
Coag-A-Mate coagulometer
CoaguChek
    C. aPTT testing system
    C. Pro DM monitor
coagulation
    c. activity

argon plasma c. (APC)
c. cascade
c. defect
diffuse intravascular c. (DIC)
disseminated intravascular c. (DIC, DIVC)
disseminated intravascular blood c. (DIVBC)
c. factor
c. forceps
F2R blood c.
intravascular c. (IVC)
intravascular blood c. (IVBC)
local intravascular c. (LIC)
c. necrosis
c. protein
c. thrombosis
c. time (CT)
coagulative myocytolysis
coagulator
    argon beam c.
    argon plasma c. (APC)
    Concept bipolar c.
coagulometer
    Coag-A-Mate c.
coagulopathy
    consumption c.
    disseminated intravascular c. (DIC)
    hemorrhagic c.
    intravascular consumption c. (IVCC)
coagulum formation
coal
    c. miner's lung
    c. miner's pneumoconiosis
    c. tar
    c. worker's pneumoconiosis (CWP)
coalescence
coalition
    Canadian Cardiovascular C. (CCC)
Coanda effect
Coapsys
    C. device
    C. surgical treatment
coapt
coaptation height
coarctation
    angulated c.
    c. of aorta (CoA)
    aortic c.
    distorted c.
    juxtaductal c.
    low-plaque c.
    native c.
    c. of pulmonary artery
    reversed c.
coarctectomy
coarse
    c. breath sounds

c. chromatin
c. crackle
c. murmur
c. rale
c. thrill
CoA-set fibrin monomer assay
coat
muscular c.
Coat-a-Count radioimmunoassay
coating
bioerodible polymer stent c.
Dura-Trac hydrophilic c.
Hydrocoat hydrophilic c.
Hydro/Pel c.
hydrophilic c.
Pro/Pel c.
Teflon c.
coaxial
c. cannulae configuration
c. pressure
CoAxia NeuroFlo catheter
cobalt
c. alloy coronary stent
c. asthma
c. cardiomyopathy
c. chromium alloy
c. chromium stent (CoStar)
c. exposure
c. fumes
c. lung
c. pneumoconiosis
c. toxicity
c. in tungsten carbide
cobalt-induced airway disease
cobalt-related
c.-r. asthma
c.-r. lung disease
c.-r. pulmonary fibrosis
Cobas Fara centrifugal analyzer
Cobb
C. angle
C. measure
cobbler's chest
cobblestoning
Cobe-Stöckert heart-lung machine
Coblation technology
cobra-head anastomosis
cobra-shaped catheter
COC
cathodal opening contraction
cocaine
c. abuse
alkaloidal c.
cocaine-induced
c.-i. hypertension
c.-i. respiratory failure (CIRF)
cocaine-related sudden death
cocci (*pl. of* coccus)
coccidioidal meningitis

Coccidioides immitis
coccidioidin test
coccidioidoma
coccidioidomycosis
disseminated c.
meningeal c.
miliary c.
primary c.
pulmonary c.
coccobacillus
coccus, pl. cocci
cocci country
gram-negative cocci
gram-positive cocci
cocci granuloma
Cochrane Library
cocillana
Cockayne syndrome
Cockett procedure
cockroach asthma
Cockroft-Gault equation
cocktail
Brompton c.
cardiac c.
CM3 c.
scintillation c.
COCl
cathodal opening clonus
COCM
congestive cardiomyopathy
coctum
sputum c.
Codafed Expectorant
CODE
cisplatin, vincristine, doxorubicin,
etoposide
code
c. blue (CB)
c. blue team (CBT)
cardiac arrest c. (CAC)
c. excited linear prediction (CELP)
ICHD pacemaker c.
Minnesota Q-QS c.
pacing c.
c. response team (CRT)
codeine
bromodiphenhydramine and c.
brompheniramine,
phenylpropanolamine, c.
chlorpheniramine, phenylephrine, c.
chlorpheniramine,
pseudoephedrine, c.
Deproist Expectorant With C.
guaifenesin and c.
guaifenesin, pseudoephedrine, c.
Guiatussin with C.
Mallergan-VC with C.
Phenergan With C.
c. phosphate

C

codeine *(continued)*
    promethazine, phenylephrine, c.
    c. sulfate
    triprolidine, pseudoephedrine, c.
CodeMaster defibrillator
Codeprex
Codiclear DH
coding
    amplitude zone time epoch c.
    (AZTEC)
Co-Diovan
codominant
    c. coronary circulation
    c. system
    c. vessel
coefficient
    apparent diffusion c. (ADC)
    capillary filtration c.
    damping c.
    c. of diffusion
    distribution c. (Kd)
    fat-absorption c.
    Hill c.
    Spearman c.
coenzyme
    c. A (CoA)
    hydroxymethylglutaryl c. A (HMG-CoA)
    3-hydroxy-3-methylglutaryl coenzyme A (HMG-CoA)
    c. Q
    c. Q10
COER-24 delivery system
coeur
    c. en sabot
    c. en sabot configuration
Coe virus
coexistent
    c. cardiac alterations
    c. pathology
cofactor
    c. FVIIIa
    heparin c. (HCF)
coffee bean asthma
Cogan syndrome
Co-Gesic
cognitive
    c. deficit
    C. Failures Questionnaire (CFQ)
cogwheel
    c. phenomenon
    c. respiration
COHb
    carboxyhemoglobin
Cohen-Rentrop classification
coherent contrast imaging (CCI)
cohesiveness
Cohn cardiac stabilizer
cohort

coil
    cardiac c.
    Cook detachable PDA c.
    detachable embolization c.
    distal shocking c.
    c. electrode
    elliptical end-capped quadrature radiofrequency c.
    c. embolization
    Gianturco c.
    Guglielmi detachable c.
    Helmholtz head c.
    magnetic resonance c.
    c. obliteration
    phased array receiver c.
    platinum c.
    prolapse c.
    quadrature birdcage c.
    quadrature head c.
    spring c.
    c. stent
    c. thrombogenicity
    Tornado embolization c.
coil-tipped catheter
coin
    c. artifact
    c. lesion
    c. lesion of lungs
    c. percussion
    c. sound
    c. test
coincidence detection
coinfection
COISR
    chronic occlusive in-stent restenosis
coital hemoptysis
coitus-induced myocardial infarction
colander-like lesion
Colapinto compression device
colchicine
COLD
    chronic obstructive lung disease
cold
    c. abscess
    c. agglutinin
    c. agglutinin pneumonia
    c. air challenge (CAC, CACh)
    c. blood cardioplegia
    c. crystalloid cardioplegia
    c. dry air challenge
    c. dry air-induced asthma
    c. exposure
    c. gangrene
    c. hemagglutinin disease
    c. ischemic arrest
    c. ischemic time (CIT)
    c. nodule
    c. potassium cardioplegia
    c. pressor test

c. pressor testing maneuver
c. spot
Sudafed Severe C.

cold-induced
c.-i. angina
c.-i. bronchospasm

cold-mist humidifier
Cole-Cecil murmur
colesevelam HCl
Colestid
colestipol hydrochloride
colfosceril palmitate
colic
biliary c.
c. flexure

Colin VP-2000 automatic measuring device
colistimethate sodium
colistin
collaboration
Antiplatelet Trialists' C. (ATC)

collagen
c. biosynthesis
c. deposition
endomysial c.
c. fatigue
fibrillar c.
matrix c.
c. plug
c. replacement
c. sponge
c. type I–V
c. vascular graft
c. vascular lung disease
c. vascular sealing (CVS)
c. volume fraction (CVF)

collagenase
neutrophil c. (MMP 8)

collagenolysis
collagenous
c. cap
c. pneumoconiosis

collapse
absorption c.
cardiovascular c.
circulatory c.
dynamic c.
end-expiratory alveolar c.
hemodynamic c.
lobar c.
massive c.
c. rale
respiratory c.
right ventricular diastolic c. (RVDC)
systolic true lumen c.
c. therapy
tracheobronchial c.
vascular c.

collapsed lung
collapsibility
pharyngeal c.

collapsin
collapsing pulse
collar
circumaortic venous c.
c. incision
c. prosthesis
c. of Stokes

collateral
adequate c.
antegrade c.
aortopulmonary c.
arcade c.
bridging c.
bronchial c.
c. channel
c. circulation
c. filling
c. flow
c. flow index
c. hyperemia
perfusion via c.
reconstitution via c.
c. respiration
septal c.
systemic c.
venous c.
c. vessel

collateralization
compensatory c.
pial c.
ventilation c.

collateralizing vessel
collecting duct
collection
expired air c.

college
Tokyo Medical C. (TMC)

collier's
c.'s lung
c.'s phthisis

collimation
x-ray scatter c.

collimator
511-keV c.
LEAP c.
slant-hole c.
variable angle slant-hole c.

Collins
C. bicycle
C. chain compensated gasometer technique
C. respirometer
C. solution
C. Survey spirometer
C. SurveyTach with MicroTach assembly

C

Collis-Belsey fundoplication
Collis-Nissen fundoplication
colloid
 c. oncotic pressure (COP)
 c. osmotic pressure
colloidal
 c. iron (CI)
 c. osmotic pressure (COP)
Collostat hemostatic sponge
coloboma
 c., heart anomaly, choanal atresia,
  retardation, genital and ear
  anomalies (CHARGE)
 c., heart anomaly, ichthyosis,
  mental retardation, ear abnormality
  (CHIME)
Colombo inverted Y technique
colon
 angiodysplasia of c.
 marginal artery of c.
colonic ischemia
colonization
 airway bacterial c.
 atypical mycobacterial c.
 bacterial c.
 oropharyngeal c.
colonopathy
 fibrosing c.
colony-stimulating factor (CSF)
color
 c. capnography
 c. Doppler energy (CDE)
 c. Doppler flow convergence
 c. flow Doppler
 c. flow mapping
 c. kinesis (CK)
 c. kinesis echocardiographic display
 c. kinesis image
 c. kinesis imaging
 c. M-mode Doppler
  echocardiography
 c. power angiography
 c. tissue Doppler imaging
color-coded flow mapping
colorimetric detector
ColorZone
 C. Management system
 C. tape
Columbia SK virus
column
 blood c.
 plasma exchange c.
Coly-Mycin M Parenteral
coma
 apoplectic c.
 diabetic c.
Combicath

combination
 c. beat
 c. syndrome
combined
 c. atrial hypertrophy (CAH)
 c. heart catheterization
 c. M-mode echophonocardiography
 penicillin G benzathine and
  procaine c.
 c. ventricular hypertrophy (CVH)
Combitube airway
Combivent inhaler
Combivir
combo technique
combretastatin A4 prodrug (CA4P)
comet
 C. catheter
 c. tail sign
Comfeel Ulcus dressing
Comfit endotracheal tube holder
ComfortSeal mask
commissural
 c. bundle
 c. fusion
 c. mitral regurgitation
 c. splitting
commissurales
 cuspides c.
commissure
 aortic c.
 fused c.
 scalloped c.
 split fused c.
 valve c.
commissuroplasty
commissurotomy
 ball mitral c.
 balloon mitral c. (BMC)
 Brockenbrough transseptal c.
 closed chest c.
 closed transventricular mitral c.
 mitral c. (MC)
 mitral balloon c.
 mitral valve c.
 open mitral valve c. (OMVC)
 percutaneous balloon mitral c.
  (PBMC)
 percutaneous mechanical mitral c.
  (PMMC)
 percutaneous mitral c. (PMC)
 percutaneous mitral balloon c.
  (PMBC)
 percutaneous transatrial mitral c.
 percutaneous transvenous mitral c.
  (PTMC)
 transventricular mitral valve c.
 tricuspid c.
committed mode pacemaker

committee
American Heart Association
Nutrition C.

common
c. atrioventricular canal
c. atrioventricular orifice (CAVO)
c. atrium
c. carotid artery
c. carotid artery intima-media
thickness (CCA-IMT)
c. carotid compression (CCC)
c. femoral artery
c. femoral vein
c. hepatic artery
c. iliac artery
c. internal iliac artery (CIIA)
c. pulmonary venous channel
(CPVC)
c. variable immunodeficiency
(CVID)

commotio cordis

communication
arteriovenous c. (AVC)
bronchioloalveolar c.
interalveolar c.
interarterial c.
narrow c.

communis
basalis c.
truncus arteriosus c. (TAC)

community-acquired
c.-a. infection
c.-a. pneumonia (CAP)

**community hypertension evaluation
clinic (CHEC)**

compact
c. A-V node
C. II desktop spirometer
c. silent nebulizer

Compactin

COmpact Smokerlyzer

compages thoracis

CompAir
C. Elite compressor nebulizer
system
C. Elite nebulizer compressor

Companion 314 nasal CPAP

comparator

compartment
c. procedure
c. syndrome

Compazine
C. injection
C. Oral

compensated
c. congestive heart failure
c. edentulism
c. sheath
c. shock

compensating emphysema

compensation
cardiac c.
depth c.
electronic distance c.
time-gain c. (TGC)

compensatory
c. antiinflammatory response
syndrome (CARS)
c. circulation
c. collateralization
c. emphysema
c. hypertrophy
c. hypertrophy of heart
integral pulse frequency
modulation/Smith delay c.
(IPFM/SDC)
c. mechanism
c. pause
c. polycythemia
c. vessel enlargement

competence
cardiac c.

competing risks

complement
c. activation
c4b purified human c.
c. component C1r deficiency
c. inhibitor
c. system

complemental air

complementary
c. air
c. balloon angioplasty

complement-fixation test

complete
c. atrioventricular
c. atrioventricular block (CAVB)
c. atrioventricular dissociation
(CAVD)
c. A-V block
c. A-V dissociation
c. blood count (CBC)
c. form of DiGeorge syndrome
(cDGS)
c. heart block (CHB)
c. pacemaker patient testing system
(CPPTS)
c. right bundle branch block
(CRBBB)
C. stent delivery platform
c. transposition of great arteries
(CTGA)

completed myocardial infarction

completely positive deflection flutter

complex
aberrant QRS c.
*Acinetobacter calcoaceticus-
baumannii* c.

complex *(continued)*
  amphotericin B cholesteryl sulfate c.
  amphotericin B lipid c. (ABLC)
  anisoylated plasminogen streptokinase activator c. (APSAC)
  anomalous c.
  antiinhibitor coagulant c.
  AP-1 c.
  c. atheroma
  atrial c.
  atrial premature c.
  c. atrioventricular canal
  atrioventricular junctional escape c.
  auricular c.
  A-V junctional escape c.
  bizarre QRS c.
  broad QRS c.
  Burkholderia cepacia c. (BCC)
  capture c.
  Carney c.
  carotid intima-media c.
  diphasic c.
  Eisenmenger c.
  electrocardiographic c.
  electrocardiographic wave c.
  equiphasic c.
  extrinsic tenase c.
  factor IX c. (human)
  far-field QRS c.
  ferrous sulfate, ascorbic acid, vitamin B c.
  filtered QRS c.
  first positive deflection during the QRS c. (R)
  c. fixation (CF)
  frequent spontaneous premature c.
  fusion c.
  Ghon c.
  Golgi c.
  heterodimer c.
  high-density lipoprotein-cholesterol c. (HDL-C)
  HLA-DQ gene c.
  HLA-DR gene c.
  intermediate-density lipoprotein-cholesterol c. (IDL-C, IDL-c)
  interpolated premature c.
  intrinsic tenase c.
  iron dextran c.
  isodiphasic c.
  junctional c.
  c. lesion
  LIP/PLH c.
  low-density lipoprotein-cholesterol c. (LDL-C, LDL-c)
  Lutembacher c.
  MAI c.
  membrane attack c. (MAC)

  monophasic c.
  monophasic contour of QRS c.
  monophasic negative QRS c.
  multiform premature ventricular c.
  Mycobacterium avium c. (MAC)
  Mycobacterium avium-intracellulare c. (MAIC)
  Mycobacterium fortuitum-chelonae c.
  nadir of QRS c.
  c. plaque
  plasminogen-streptokinase c.
  pleomorphic premature ventricular c.
  c. pleural effusion
  polymorphic premature ventricular c.
  polysaccharide-iron c.
  premature atrial c.
  premature atrioventricular junctional c.
  premature ventricular c.
  primary c.
  prothrombin c. (PTC)
  prothrombinase c.
  QRS c.
  QRS-T c.
  c. of Q, R, S, waves corresponding to depolarization of ventricles (QRS)
  QS c.
  Ranke c.
  R-on-T premature ventricular c.
  RS c.
  second positive deflection during QRS c. (R′)
  Shone c.
  sling ring c.
  sodium ferric gluconate c.
  Steidele c.
  streptokinase-plasminogen c.
  supraventricular premature c. (SVPC)
  Taussig-Bing c.
  tenase c.
  thrombin-antithrombin III c.
  time between P wave and beginning of QRS c. (PR)
  transposition c.
  VATER c.
  ventricular c.
  ventricular premature c. (VPC)
  c. ventricular septal defect
  very low density lipoprotein-triglyceride c. (VLDL-TG)

compliance
  aortic c. (AC)
  chest wall c.
  dynamic c.
  c. of heart

left ventricular chamber c.
left ventricular muscle c.
lung c.
patient c.
pulmonary c. (PC)
c., rate, oxygenation, pressure
  (CROP)
c., rate, oxygenation, pressure
  index
specific c.
static lung c.
thoracic c.
total lung c.
ventilatory c.
compliant balloon
complicated myocardial infarction
complication
angioplasty c.
cardiovascular c.
confidential enquiry into cardiac
  catheterization c.'s (CECCC)
groin c.
late angioplasty c.
noninfectious c.
nonpulmonary c.
postoperative pulmonary c. (POPC)
pulmonary c.
c. rate
thromboembolic c. (TEC)
component
bronchospastic c.
elastic c.
harmonic c.
mitral c. (M1)
plasma thromboplastin c. (PTC,
  PTH)
pulmonary c.
thrombogenic c.
composite valve graft replacement
compound
antimony c.
artificial lung-expanding c. (ALEC)
c. cyst
glycyl c.
Hurler-Scheie c.
Hycomine C.
c. motor action potential (CMAP)
nitinol polymeric c.
selenium c.
volatile organic c. (VOC)
compPAC ventilator
**comprehensive cardiac care unit
  (CCCU)**
compressed-air sickness
compressed Ivalon patch graft
compressible volume
compression
anterior thoracic c.
anteroposterior thoracic c.

aortic root c.
c. atelectasis
barrel-hooping c.
biventricular direct cardiac c.
c. boot
cardiac c.
c. chamber
chamber c.
chest c.
common carotid c. (CCC)
c. cough
direct cardiac c. (DCC)
dynamic tracheal c.
external cardiac c. (ECC)
extrinsic c.
c. gloves
high-frequency chest wall c.
  (HFCC)
intermittent pneumatic c. (IPC)
interposed abdominal c.
intrathoracic gas c.
nonuniform direct cardiac c.
selective chamber c.
sternal c.
c. stockings
c. thrombosis
c. ultrasonography
compression-decompression
active c.-d. (ACD)
compressor
AM-50 portable air c.
CompAir Elite nebulizer c.
Deschamps c.
DeVilbiss Pulmo-Aide LT c.
Easy Air 15 c.
Easy Neb c.
external inflatable c.
Freeway Lite portable aerosol c.
Proneb Ultra nebulizer c.
Pulmo-Mist c.
Puritan all purpose c.
compressor-generated nebulizer (CGN)
compressor-nebulizer
Pulmo-Aide aerosol c.-n.
PulmoMate aerosol c.-n.
compromise
airway c.
circulatory c.
coronary c.
functional c.
hemodynamic c.
respiratory c.
side-branch c.
c. systemic circulatory
vascular c.
Compton
C. effect
C. scatter
Compu-Neb ultrasonic nebulizer

Compuscan Hittman computerized electrocardioscanner
computed
    c. radiography (CR)
    c. tomographic scan
    c. tomography (CT)
    c. tomography angiographic portography (CTAP)
    c. tomography angiography (CTA)
    c. tomography in arterial portography (CTAP)
    c. tomography scanner
computer
    digital c.
computer-assisted
    c.-a. diagnostic (CAD)
    c.-a. evaluation
    c.-a. evaluation of stenosis and restenosis (CAESAR)
    c.-a. pericardial puncture (CASPER)
    c.-a. pericardial surgery (CASPER)
computerized
    c. axial tomography (CAT)
    c. diaphragmatic breathing retraining (CDBR)
    c. sleep analysis system
    c. texture analysis
conal
    c. septal defect
    c. septum
Concato disease
concave pattern
concealed
    c. accessory conduction
    c. accessory pathway
    c. bypass tract
    c. entrainment
    c. retrograde conduction
    c. rhythm
concentration
    EBC keratin c.
    fractional inspired oxygen c. (FIO_2, FiO_2)
    gas c.
    hydrogen ion c. (pH)
    intracellular calcium c.
    lactic acid c.
    lymphocyte c.
    minimal alveolar c. (MAC)
    minimum bactericidal c.
    minimum inhibitory c. (MIC)
    plasma endothelin c.
    plasma homocysteine c.
    regional gas c.
    venous plasma norepinephrine c.
concentration-effect relation
concentrator
    NewLife Elite c.
    NewLife oxygen c.

    oxygen c.
    Puritan Bennett Aeris 590 oxygen c.
    SolAiris III, V oxygen c.
concentric
    c. hypertrophic cardiomyopathy
    c. left ventricular hypertrophy
    c. narrowing
    c. remodeling
    C. retriever system
concept
    baby lung c.
    C. bipolar coagulator
    leading circle c.
    solid angle c.
Concerto CRT-D device
Conchapak
concordance
    atrioventricular situs c.
    ventriculoarterial c.
concordant
    c. alternans
    c. alternation
    c. atrioventricular connection
    c. changes
    c. changes electrocardiogram
    c. ventriculoarterial connection
concretio
    c. cordis
    c. pericardii
concussion
    myocardial c.
condensate
    exhaled breath c. (EBC)
condition
    isocapnic c.
    mucus-producing respiratory c.
    preexisting c.
conditioning
    cardiovascular reflex c. (CRC)
    c. program
conduct
    Health On the Net code of c. (HONcode)
conductance
    c. catheter
    c. catheter method
    epicardial flow c.
    S-segment airway c.
    c. stroke volume
    upstream airway c.
    c. vessel
conducting airway
conduction
    2:1 c.
    aberrant ventricular c. (AVC)
    accelerated A-V node c.
    anisotropic c.
    anomalous c.

antegrade c.
anterograde c.
antidromic c.
atrioventricular c. (AVC)
atrioventricular nodal c. (AVN)
A-V nodal c.
base-to-apex c.
bidirectional c.
c. block
cardiac c.
concealed accessory c.
concealed retrograde c.
decremental c.
c. defect (CD)
c. delay
delayed c.
c. disorder
c. disturbance
EAVN c.
electrotonic c.
enhanced atrioventricular c. (EAVC)
forward c.
His-Purkinje c.
c. impairment
impulse c.
internodal c.
c. interval
intraatrial c.
intraventricular c.
nondecremental retrograde
  ventriculoatrial c.
orthodromic c.
orthograde c.
c. pathway
Purkinje c.
c. ratio
retrograde atrioventricular c.
  (RAVC)
retrograde VA c.
sinoventricular c.
c. slowing
supernormal c.
c. system
c. time
transseptal c.
VA c.
c. velocity
ventricular c.
ventriculoatrial c. (VAC)

conductive
  c. ability
  c. coupling
  c. system

conduit
  c. augmentation
  c. calcification
  Contegra pulmonary valved c.
  extracardiac c. (ECC)
  extracardiac ventriculopulmonary c.

c. lumen
c. placement
RA-RV c.
respiratory syncytial virus c.
c. stenting
c. surgery

cone
  arterial c.
  elastic c.
  pulmonary c.

coned-down view
Conexus wireless telemetry
Confianza guidewire
confidence interval (CI)
**confidential enquiry into cardiac
  catheterization complications (CECCC)**
configuration
  anteroposterior paddle c.
  atrial sensing c.
  coaxial cannulae c.
  coeur en sabot c.
  dome-and-dart c.
  doughnut c.
  horseshoe c.
  QRS complex c.
  snowman c.
  spade-like c.
  spike-and-dome c.
  ventricular sensing c.
  wringer wrap c.
confirmation
  beat-by-beat capture c.
  capture c.
confirmatory evaluation
confluence
  pulmonary venous c. (PVC)
confluent bronchopneumonia
confocal microscopy
conformability
  optimized c. (OC)
congenita
  arthrogryposis multiplex c.
  myotonia c.
congenital
  c. absence
  c. absence of left pericardium
    (CALP)
  c. adenomatoid malformation
  c. adrenal hyperplasia
  c. anomaly of mitral valve
  c. aortic aneurysm
  c. aortic stenosis
  c. aspiration pneumonia
  c. atelectasis
  c. bronchial atresia (CBA)
  c. cardiovascular malformation
    (CCVM)
  c. central alveolar hypoventilation
  c. central hypoventilation syndrome

congenital *(continued)*
- c. complete heart block
- c. conotruncal anomaly
- c. coronary arteriovenous fistula (CCAVF)
- c. coronary ostia web
- c. cystic adenomatoid malformation
- c. diaphragmatic hernia (CDH)
- c. heart block (CHB)
- c. heart disease (CHD)
- c. interrupted aortic arch
- c. laryngeal stridor
- c. lobar emphysema
- c. lobar overinflation
- c. long QT interval syndrome
- c. malformation of heart (CMH)
- c. mitral stenosis
- c. murmur
- c. myocardial sympathetic dysinnervation (CMSD)
- c. peribronchial myofibroblastic tumor
- c. polyvalvular disease (CPVD)
- c. pseudocholinesterase deficiency
- c. pulmonary arteriovenous
- c. pulmonary arteriovenous fistula
- c. pulmonary stenosis
- c. single atrium
- c. symptomatic A-V block

congenitale
- P c.

congenitally
- c. absent pericardium
- c. corrected transposition of great arteries (CC-TGA)
- c. corrected transposition of great vessels (CC-TGA)

Congestac
congested
congestion
- active c.
- capillary c.
- chronic passive c.
- circulatory c.
- functional c.
- hypostatic c.
- passive c.
- physiologic c.
- pulmonary c.
- pulmonary venous c. (PVC)
- venous c.
- Vicks 44D Cough & Head C.

congestive
- c. cardiomyopathy (CCM, COCM)
- c. cirrhosis
- c. edema
- c. heart disease (CHD)
- c. heart failure (CHF)
- c. heart failure classification I-IV
- c. heart failure data tool (CHFDT)
- c. myocardiopathy (CM)
- c. pulmonary disease
- c. right ventricular failure (CRVF)

congophilic angiopathy
Coniel
coniofibrosis
conivaptan
conjoined cusp
conjugate
- chloramine-albumin c.
- polyribosylribitol phosphate-diphtheria toxoid c.

conjugated equine estrogen (CEE)
conjunctival hyperemia
connection
- accessory arteriovenous c.
- anomalous pulmonary venous c. (APVC)
- cavopulmonary c.
- concordant atrioventricular c.
- concordant ventriculoarterial c.
- Damus-Kaye-Stansel c.
- discordant atrioventricular c.
- discordant ventriculoarterial c.
- double inlet atrioventricular c.'s
- endotracheal tube c.
- Fontan c.
- hemianomalous pulmonary venous c. (HAPVC)
- partial anomalous pulmonary venous c. (PAPVC)
- pulmonary venous c.
- RA-RV c.
- systemic to pulmonary c.
- total anomalous pulmonary venous c. (TAPVC)
- total cavopulmonary c. (TCPC)
- univentricular atrioventricular c.

connective
- c. tissue
- c. tissue growth factor (CTGF)
- c. tissue lesion

connector
- Biotronik lead c.
- c. block
- Cordis c.
- Luer-Lok c.
- Medtronic c.
- Symmetry bypass system aortic c.
- unipolar c.
- Y c.

Connell airway
connexin
- c. 43
- C. 40 gene GJA5

connori
- *Nosema c.*

Conn syndrome

Conor stent
conotruncal
 c. abnormality
 c. anomaly
 c. heart malformation (CTHM)
 c. septation
conoventricular fold and groove
Conradi-Hünermann syndrome
Conradi line
Conray contrast medium
consanguineous
consanguinity
consciousness
 loss of c.
conscious sedation
consecutive vasculitis
conservative surgery (CS)
conserved helix-loop-helix ubiquitous
 kinase (CHUK)
conserver
 EX-2000 DeVilbiss c.
 Hideaway oxygen c.
 high-flow oxygen c. (HFOC)
 Oxymatic 411 electronic c.
 Oxymatic 401 electronic oxygen c.
 PulseDose EX2000D oxygen c.
 Walkabout oxygen c.
console
consolidated lung volume
consolidation
 airspace c.
 lobular c.
 c. of lung
 patchy c.
 peribronchiolar airspace c.
 pulmonary c.
consolidative process
consonating rale
constant
 atrial volume c. (Vak)
 c. coupling
 empiric c.
 gas c. (R)
 Gorlin c.
 Hodgkin-Huxley c.
 c. tilt wave
 ventricular volume c. (vvk)
constant-flow method
constant-workload cycle exercise
Constellation advanced mapping
 catheter
constellatus
 Peptococcus c.
constitutive
 c. nitric oxide synthase (cNOS)
 c. secretion

constraint
 pericardial c.
constraint-induced (CI)
 c.-i. movement therapy
constriction
 anular c.
 arterial c.
 esophageal c.
 neurohormonal arterial c.
 occult pericardial c.
 pericardial c.
 supraanular c.
constrictive
 c. bronchiolitis
 c. endocarditis
 c. heart disease
 c. pericarditis (CP)
 c. physiology
constrictor
 c. muscle
 c. muscle of pharynx
consumption
 c. coagulopathy
 maximum oxygen c.
 myocardial oxygen c. (MVO_2)
 oxygen c. (VO_2max)
 peak exercise oxygen c. (VO_2max)
 platelet c.
 volume oxygen c. (VO_2max)
consumptive
contact metastasis
contagiosum
 molluscum c.
contained rupture
Contak
 C. CD 2 cardiac resynchronization
  therapy defibrillator
 C. CD CRT-D
 C. CD pulse generator
 C. CD ventricular resynchronization
  pacemaker
 C. Renewal 3 cardiac
  resynchronization therapy
  defibrillator
 C. Renewal 3 system cardiac
  resynchronization therapy
contamination
 catheter c.
Contegra pulmonary valved conduit
content
 arterial oxygen c. (CAO_2)
 bone mineral c. (BMC)
 harmonic c.
 oxygen c.
contiguous ventricular septal defect
continuity
 c. of care
 c. equation

continuous
- c. air leak
- c. albuterol nebulization (CAN)
- c. ambulatory blood sampler (CABS)
- c. arrhythmia
- c. arteriovenous hemodiafiltration (CAVHDF)
- c. arteriovenous hemodialysis (CAVHD)
- c. arteriovenous hemofiltration (CAVH)
- c. arteriovenous rewarming (CAVR)
- c. arteriovenous ultrafiltration (CAVU)
- c. aspiration
- c. aspiration of subglottic secretions (CASS)
- c. atrial fibrillation (CAF)
- c. cardiac output (CCO)
- c. cardiac output with SvO$_2$
- c. cyclical peritoneal dialysis (CCPD)
- c. cyclic peritoneal
- c. electrogram storage
- c. full-thickness linear lesion
- c. heart murmur
- c. heparin (CH)
- c. hyperfractionated accelerated radiotherapy (CHART)
- c. intravenous infusion (CIV)
- c. loop exercise echocardiogram
- c. mandatory ventilation
- c. murmur (CM)
- c. nebulization therapy (CNT)
- c. noninvasive measurement
- c. noninvasive monitoring of ventilated infants
- c. pericardial lavage
- c. positive airway pressure (CPAP)
- c. positive pressure ventilation
- c. progesterone
- c. pulse oximetry
- c. ramp protocol
- c. venovenous hemofiltration (CVVH)
- c. wave Doppler echocardiogram

continuous-flow ventilation

continuous-wave
- c.-w. Doppler (CWD)
- c.-w. Doppler echocardiography
- c.-w. Doppler imaging
- c.-w. Doppler ultrasound
- c.-w. laser ablation

continuum
- Evolve Cardiac C.

contour
- aortic c.
- breath-methylated alkane c.

cardiac c.
- c. of heart
- C. high voltage can ICD
- C. II ICD
- left heart c.
- C. LT V-135D ICD
- C. LTV-135D implantable cardioverter-defibrillator
- C. MD implantable single-lead cardioverter-defibrillator
- Murgo pressure c.
- QRS c.
- C. V-145D ICD
- C. V-145D implantable cardioverter-defibrillator
- ventricular c.
- Ventritex C.

contracta
- vena c.

contracted heart

contractile
- c. amplitude
- c. behavior
- c. element
- c. force (CF)
- c. function
- c. protein
- c. reserve
- c. ring dysphagia
- c. work index

contractility
- increased c.
- isovolumetric c.
- left ventricular c.
- myocardial c.
- ventricular wall c.

contraction
- anodal closure c. (ACC, AnCC)
- anodal duration c. (ADC)
- anodal opening c. (AnOC, AOC)
- atrial c. (AC)
- atrial premature c. (APC)
- automatic ventricular c.
- c. band
- c. band necrosis
- cardiac ventricular c.
- cathodal closing c. (KCC)
- cathodal closure c. (CCC)
- cathodal opening c. (COC, KOC)
- endovascular c.
- escape ventricular c.
- Gowers c.
- high-amplitude peristaltic c. (HAPC)
- isometric c.
- isotonic c.
- isovolumic c.
- junctional premature c. (JPC)
- LAA c.

left atrial c. (LAC)
low-amplitude c. (LAC)
maximum voluntary c. (MVC)
muscular c.
nodal premature c. (NPC)
c. pattern
premature c.
premature atrial c. (PAC)
premature junctional c. (PJC)
premature ventricular c. (PVC)
pulse synchronized c. (PSC)
rested state c. (RSC)
R on T ventricular premature c.
supraventricular premature c.
synchronous atrial c.
tertiary c.
ventricular c. (VC)
ventricular premature c. (VPC)
volume c.
contractor
Bailey-Gibbon rib c.
contracture
ischemic c.
nodal c.
premature nodal c. (PNC)
contraindication
contrast
c. agent
angiographic c.
c. angiography
corticomedullary c. (CMC)
Definity c.
c. echocardiography
half-diluted c.
Iohexol c.
left atrial spontaneous echo c.
 (LASEC)
c. left ventriculography
Levovist c.
c. material
c. medium
c. medium delivery
negative c.
c. nephropathy
Optiray c.
Optison c.
c. ratio
sonicated albumin-dextrose c.
spontaneous echo c. (SEC)
c. stagnation
time-to-peak c.
Ultravist c.
c. venography
c. ventriculography (CV)
contrast-enhanced
c.-e. CT
dynamic susceptibility c.-e. (DSC)
c.-e. echocardiogram

c.-e. magnetic resonance
 angiography (CEMRA, CE-MRA)
c.-e. transcranial color-coded real-
 time sonography (CE-TCCS)
c.-e. ultrasound (CEU)
contrast-guided venipuncture
contrecoup injury
control
automatic dose rate c. (ADRC)
axial c.
CVC 123 calibration verification c.
damping c.
gain c.
C. III Elite disinfectant
intravenous accurate c. (IVAC)
pressure c. (PC)
pressure-regulated volume c.
 (PRVC)
QC 253 CO-oximetry c.
quality c.
RA 523 blood gas/CO-oximetry c.
rate c.
reject c.
Take C.
time-gain c. (TGC)
time-gain compensationtime-varied
 gain c.
time-varied gain c. (TGC, TVGC)
torque c.
volume c. (VC)
c. wire
controlled
c. breathing
c. clinical trial (CCT)
c. coughing
c. diaphragmatic breathing (CDBR)
c. diaphragmatic respiration
c. lung biopsy
c. mechanical ventilation
c. release (C-R)
c. ventricular response
controller
EPT-1000 XP cardiac ablation c.
flow c.
pressure c.
vacuum c.
venous flow c. (VFC)
volume c.
control-mode ventilation
ControlWire guidewire
contusion
bronchial c.
cardiac c. (CC)
lung c.
myocardial c.
c. pneumonia
pulmonary c.
conundrum

C

conus
- c. arteriosus
- c. branch
- c. cordis
- c. elasticus
- pulmonary c.
- tendon of c.

convalescent phase

convection
- bulk c.

convective
- c. cooling
- c. gas mixing

conventional
- amphotericin B (c.)
- c. cineangiography
- c. mechanical ventilation (CMV)
- c. ventilation (CV)

convergence
- color Doppler flow c.

conversion
- analog-to-digital c.
- automatic mode c.
- Fontan c.
- pressure c.

converter
- scan c.

converting enzyme inhibitor

convex linear array

convexoconcave (C-C)
- Björk-Shiley c.-c. (BSCC)

convulsion

ConXn

COOD
- chronic obstruction outflow disease

cooing
- c. murmur
- c. sign

cook
- C. balloon
- C. Cardiovascular infusion catheter
- C. County aspirator
- C. detachable PDA coil
- C. flexible biopsy forceps
- C. FlexStent
- C. intracoronary stent
- C. locking stylet
- C. multiple-assessment scale
- C. NIH Torcon blue catheter
- C. pacemaker
- C. Shuttle Flexor introducer
- C. Spectrum catheter
- C. TPN catheter

cookie
- Gelfoam c.

Cook-Medley hostility scale

Cook-Swartz Doppler flow monitoring system

cool
- c. head-warm body perfusion
- c. mist

Cooley
- C. anastomosis clamp
- C. anemia
- C. aortic clamp
- C. atrial retractor
- C. bronchus clamp
- C. dilator
- C. forceps
- C. intrapericardial anastomosis
- C. modification
- C. modification of Waterston anastomosis
- C. neonatal instrument
- C. sump tube

Cooley-Beck vessel clamp

Cooley-Bloodwell-Cutter valve

Cooley-Bloodwell mitral valve prosthesis

Cooley-Cutter disc prosthetic valve

Cooley-Derra anastomosis clamp

Cooley-Satinsky clamp

cooling
- c. blanket
- cardioplegia c.
- convective c.
- core c.
- topical c.
- c. vest

cool-tip
- c.-t. catheter
- c.-t. laser

Coomassie blue stain

Coombs
- C. murmur
- C. test

Coons Super Stiff long tip guidewire

Cooper ligament

Cooperman event probability

Cooper-Rand intraoral artificial larynx

coordinate
- c. reduction time encoding system (CORTES)
- c. system

CO-Oximeter
- Ciba-Corning 2500 C.-O.
- C.-O. module
- pHOx C.-O.

CO-oximetry
- carbon monoxide oximetry

COP
- colloidal osmotic pressure
- colloid oncotic pressure
- cryptogenic organizing pneumonia
- cryptogenic organizing pneumonitis

COPACtherm pulmonary artery catheter

COPD
chronic obstructive pulmonary disease
COPE
chronic obstructive pulmonary
emphysema
cope
C. method bronchography
C. Nitinol mandril wire guide
C. pleural biopsy needle
Copeland technique
Coping Strategies questionnaire
copious sputum
copolymer
Elast-Eon silicone urethane c.
polyolefin c. (POC)
copper (CU)
c. wiring
copper-62 (^{62}CU)
copper-wire
c.-w. artery
c.-w. effect
COR
cardiac output recorder
cor
c. adiposum
c. arteriosum
c. biloculare
c. bovinum
c. hirsutum
c. juvenum
c. mobile
c. pendulum
c. pseudotriloculare biatriatum
c. pulmonale (CP)
c. taurinum
c. triatriatum
c. triatriatum dexter
c. triatriatum dextrum
c. triatriatum sinistrum
c. triloculare
c. triloculare biatriatum
c. triloculare biventriculare
Coradur
coral thrombus
Coratomic R wave inhibited pacemaker
Corazonix Predictor
CorCap
Acorn C.
C. cardiac support device
CORD
chronic obstructive respiratory disease
cord
epidural spinal c. (ESC)
false vocal c.
Ferrein c.'s
paradoxical inspiratory closure of
vocal c.'s
true vocal c.
vocal c.

Cordarone
cordis
accretio c.
adipositas c.
C. Ancar pacing lead
angina c.
anulus fibrosus dexter/sinister c.
apex c.
ataxia c.
atrium c.
C. bioptome
C. Bioptome sheath
C. BriteTip guiding catheter
bulbus c.
C. Bx Velocity stent
C. Checkmate system
chordae tendineae c.
chorea c.
commotio c.
concretio c.
C. connector
conus c.
crena c.
C. CrossFlex coronary stent
delirium c.
diastasis c.
C. Ducor I, II, III catheter
ectasia c.
ectopia c
facies anterior c.
facies diaphragmatica c.
facies inferior c.
facies pulmonalis dextra/sinistra c.
facies sternocostalis c.
C. Hydrolyser
hypodynamia c.
ictus c.
incisura apicis c.
C. LC Multipurpose stent system
malum c.
C. Mini stent system
myasthenia c.
myofibrosis c.
myomalacia c.
myopathia c.
palpitatio cordis
C. Powerflex angioplasty balloon
C. Predator PTCA balloon catheter
pulsus c.
steatosis c.
C. Stockert generator
systema conducens c.
C. tantalum coil stent
theca c.
C. Titan balloon dilation catheter
C. TrapEase permanent vena cava
filter
trepidatio c.
tumultus c.

C

cordis *(continued)*
    venae c.
    vortex c.
Cordis-Webster
    C.-W. ablation catheter
    C.-W. mapping catheter
Cordox
cordy pulse
core
    c. of atheroma
    atheromatous c.
    c. cooling
    C. Exercise Testing Laboratory
    ischemic c.
    lipid c.
    c. pneumonia
    c. temperature
Coreg
Core-Vent implant
Corgard
Cori
    C. cycle
    C. disease
Corinthian stent
corkscrew artery
Corlopam
Cormed ambulatory infusion pump
corneal arcus
cornealis
    arcus c.
Cornelia de Lange syndrome
Cornell
    C. exercise protocol
    C. modification of the Bruce
      protocol
    C. voltage
    C. voltage-duration product criteria
corner vessel
corniculate tubercle
corniculum
Corometrics
    C. Doppler scanner
    C. material fetal monitor
Corometrics-Aloka echocardiograph
  machine
coronal
    c. cut
    c. plane
    c. slice
corona radiata
coronarism
coronaritis
coronarius
    sinus c.
coronary
    c. air embolism
    c. anastomotic shunt
    c. anatomy
    c. aneurysm

    c. angiographic catheter
    c. angiography (CAG)
    c. angiography catheter
    c. angioscopy
    c. arterial reserve
    c. arteriography (CAG)
    c. arteriosclerosis
    c. arteriosclerotic heart disease
      (CAHD, CASHD)
    c. arteritis
    c. artery
    c. artery angioplasty
    c. artery anomaly
    c. artery atherosclerosis
    c. artery blood flow (CABF)
    c. artery button
    c. artery bypass (CAB)
    c. artery bypass graft (CABG,
      CARB)
    c. artery bypass grafting (CABG)
    c. artery bypass grafting surgery
    c. artery bypass graft surgery
      (CABGS)
    c. artery bypass revascularization
      investigation (CABRI)
    c. artery bypass surgery (CABS)
    c. artery calcium (CAC)
    c. artery descriptors and restenosis
      (CADR)
    c. artery disease (CAD)
    c. artery disease index (CADI)
    c. artery dissection
    c. artery distensibility
    c. artery dominance
    c. artery ectasia
    c. artery embolism (CAE)
    c. artery fistula (CAF)
    c. artery lesion
    c. artery obstruction (CAO)
    c. artery occlusion
    c. artery occlusive disease (CAOD)
    c. artery perforation (CAP)
    c. artery probe
    c. artery-right ventricular fistula
    c. artery risk assessment and
      treatment
    c. artery scan (CAS)
    c. artery spasm (CAS)
    c. artery stenosis
    c. artery stent
    c. artery thrombosis
    c. artery vein graft (CAVG)
    c. atherectomy
    c. atheroma
    c. bed
    c. bifurcation
    c. blood flow (CBF)
    c. blood flow measurement
    c. blood flow velocity (CBFV)

c. branch occlusion
c. bypass graft (CBG)
c. bypass graft patency
café c.
c. calcium
c. calcium scanning
c. calcium score
c. care (CC)
c. care nursing (CCN)
c. care training program (CCTP)
c. care unit (CCU)
c. collateral circulation
c. compromise
c. conduit vessel
c. cushion
c. cusp
c. drug project (CDP)
c. endarterectomy
c. event
c. failure
c. flow (CF)
c. flow reserve (CFR)
c. flow reserve technique
c. flow velocity
c. flow velocity reserve (CFVR, CVR)
c. guiding catheter
c. heart disease (CHD)
c. implant system (CIS)
c. insufficiency (CI)
c. intravascular ultrasound
c. IVUS
left circumflex c. (LCC)
left interventricular c. (LIC)
left main c. (LMC)
c. luminal stenosis
c. luminology
c. macroangiopathy
c. magnetic resonance angiography
c. microangiopathy
c. microcirculatory vasoconstriction
c. microvascular disease
c. microvessel endothelium
c. nodal rhythm
c. occlusive disease
c. ostial dimple
c. ostial stenosis
c. ostium
percutaneous transluminal c.
c. perfusate solution (CPS)
c. perfusion gradient
c. perfusion pressure (CPP)
c. plaque
c. plaque regression
c. plaque rupture
c. prognostic index (CPI)
c. radiation therapy
c. recanalization
c. reflex

c. rehabilitation program (CRP)
c. remodeling
c. resistance vessel
c. restenosis
c. revascularization
right interventricular c. (RIC)
c. ring
c. risk factor
c. risk profile
c. roadmapping
c. rotational ablation
c. rotational atherectomy (CRA)
c. sclerosis (CS)
c. sinus (CS)
c. sinus blood flow (CSBF)
c. sinus catheterization
c. sinus electrogram
c. sinus flow
c. sinus guiding (CSG)
c. sinus intervention (CSI)
c. sinus lead
c. sinus occlusion pressure (CSOP)
c. sinus retroperfusion
c. sinus rhythm
c. sinus thermodilution
c. sinus thermodilution catheter
c. slow flow syndrome (CSFS)
c. spasm
c. spastic angina
c. steal
c. steal mechanism
c. steal phenomenon
c. stenting
c. sulcus
c. tendon
c. thrombolysis
c. thrombosis (CT)
c. tree
c. vascular reserve
c. vascular resistance
c. vascular turgor
c. vasculature
c. vasodilation
c. vasodilator reserve
c. vasomotion
c. vasospasm
c. vein
c. venous graft (CVG)
c. venous pressure
c. wire
coronary-pulmonary fistula (C-PF)
coronary-subclavian steal syndrome (CSSS)
Coronaviridae virus
coronavirus
　　human c.
　　human c. HKU1 (CoV-HKU1)
　　human c. NL63 (HCoV-NL63)
　　c. infection

185

coronavirus *(continued)*
    severe acute respiratory syndrome-associated c. (SARS-CoV)
corpectomy
corporeal
corpus, pl. **corpora**
    c. linguae
    c. phalangis
corpuscle
    Donné c.
    Drysdale c.
    Hassall c.
corrected
    c. blood volume (CBV)
    c. dextrocardia
    c. diffusing capacity for carbon monoxide ($DLCO_c$)
    c. ejection time (ETc)
    c. preejection period (PEPc)
    c. QT
    c. sinus node recovery time (CSNRT)
    c. time of sinuatrial node function recovery (CTSNFR)
    c. TIMI frame count (CTFC)
    c. transposition (CT)
    c. transposition of great vessels
correction
    Bonferroni c.
    metabolite c.
    Teichholz c.
    Yates c.
corrective therapy (CT)
Correra line
CorRestore
    C. implantable patch
    C. system
corridor procedure
Corrigan
    C. disease
    C. pneumonia
    C. pulse
    C. respiration
    C. sign
    C. wave
corrodens
    Bacteroides c.
    Eikenella c.
corrosive esophagitis
Cortef Oral
CORTES
    coordinate reduction time encoding system
    CORTES ECG
cortex, pl. **cortices**
    adrenal c.
    premotor c. (PMC)
    primary sensorimotor c. (SM1)
    sensorimotor c. (SMC)

cortical
    c. arousal index (CAI)
    c. neuronal apoptosis
    c. plasticity
    c. stroke
    c. vein thrombosis
    c. volume loss
corticale
    Cryptostroma c.
cortices (*pl. of* cortex)
corticobulbar tract
corticomedullary contrast (CMC)
corticosteroid
    inhaled c. (ICS)
    QVAR inhaled c.
    systemic c.
    c. therapy
corticosteroid-dependent asthmatic
corticosteroid-treated heart
corticotropin
corticotropin-releasing factor (CRF)
cortisol
    24-hour c.
cortisone acetate
Cortone Acetate
Cortrosyn injection
Corvert injection
Corvisart
    C. disease
    C. facies
Corvita
    C. endoluminal graft
    C. endoprosthesis stent graft
Coryllos-Bethune rib shears
Coryllos-Shoemaker rib shears
corymbifera
    Absidia c.
Corynebacterium
    C. diphtheriae
    C. jeikeium
coryza
coryzavirus
Corzide
CoSeal
    C. resorbable synthetic sealant
    C. surgical sealant
Cosgrove-Edwards
    C.-E. annuloplasty system
    C.-E. annuloplasty system with Duraflo treatment
    C.-E. ring
Cosgrove retractor
Cosmegen
CO₂SMO
    C. capnograph/pulse oximeter
    C. Plus
    C. Plus! respiratory profile monitor
Cosmos
    C. 283 DDD pacemaker

C. II DDD pacemaker
C. II pulse generator

cost

oxygen c.
Prescription Analyses and C. (PACT)

costal

c. margin
c. part of diaphragm
c. pit of transverse process
c. pleura
c. pleurisy
c. respiration
c. surface
c. surface of lung

costalis

pleura c.

CoStar

cobalt chromium stent
CoStar cobalt chromium paclitaxel-eluting coronary stent system
CoStar stent

costarum

arcus c.

costocervicalis

truncus c.

costochondral

c. junction
c. syndrome

costochondrectomy
costochondritis
costoclavicular

c. ligament
c. maneuver
c. rib syndrome

costodiaphragmatic

c. recess
c. recess of pleura

costomediastinal

c. recess
c. recess of pleura

costophrenic

c. angle
c. gutter
c. septal line
c. sinus
c. sulcus

costosternal syndrome
costotome
costoversion thoracoplasty
costovertebral angle (CVA)
cosyntropin
COTD

cardiac output by thermodilution

COTe

cathodal opening tetanus

cotransporter

monocarboxylate proton c.

co-trimoxazole

cottage-loaf appearance
cotton-dust asthma
cotton-mill fever
cottonoid patty
cotton-wool

c.-w. exudate
c.-w. spot

Cotunnius space
COU

cardiac observation unit

couch incrementation
cough

aneurysmal c.
Balme c.
barking c.
brassy c.
cigarette c.
compression c.
c. CPR
c. CPR technique
croupy c.
decubitus c.
Diphen C.
directed c.
dog c.
dry c.
c. efficiency
exercise-associated c.
extrapulmonary c.
c. fracture
habit c.
habitual c.
hacking c.
mechanical c.
minute-gun c.
Morton c.
multifactorial c.
musical c.
paroxysmal c.
privet c.
productive c.
psychogenic c.
c. receptor
reflex c.
c. reflex
c. resonance
seal-bark c.
Silphen C.
smoker's c.
stomach c.
c. suppressant
Sydenham c.
c. syncope
tea taster's c.
c. threshold
c. transportability
trigeminal c.
c. variant asthma
wet c.

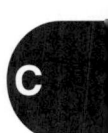

cough *(continued)*
    whooping c.
    winter c.
    workplace-related c.
coughing
    controlled c.
    expulsive c.
    Huff c.
    paroxysm of c.
    quad c.
cough-specific quality of life questionnaire
cough-thrill
cough-variant asthma
Coulter
    C. counter
    C. RapidVUE particle shape and size analyzer
CoumaCare
    C. Coumadin management system
    C. patient management system
Coumadin
coumadinization
coumaric anhydride
coumarin pulsed dye laser
Coumel tachycardia
coumestan
coumetarol
council
    Better Sleep C.
    National Advisory Heart C. (NAHC)
    National Health and Medical Research C.
count
    blood c.
    complete blood c. (CBC)
    corrected TIMI frame c. (CTFC)
    differential blood c.
    double c.
    end-diastolic c. (EDC)
    end-systolic c. (ESC)
    first shock c.
    kick c.
    c. median aerodynamic diameter (CMAD)
    c. median diameter (CMD)
    myocardial infarction frame c.
    c.'s per minute (C/M)
    c. rate
    relative lymphocyte c.
    second through fifth shock c.
    shock c.
    thrombolysis in myocardial infarction frame c.
    TIMI frame c.
    total patient shock c.
    touch shock c.
    white blood cell c.

counter
    Coulter c.
    event/episode c.
    mechanical lap c.
    pacing c.
    time-based c.
counterclockwise
    c. flutter
    c. rotation
counterimmunoelectrophoresis
counteroccluder
counterpressor
    Acland-Buncke c.
counterpulsation
    aortic c.
    c. balloon
    balloon c.
    enhanced external c. (EECP)
    intraaortic c. (IACP)
    intraaortic balloon c. (IABC, IABCP)
    intraarterial c.
    percutaneous intraaortic balloon c. (PIBC)
    pulmonary artery c. (PACP)
countershock
    electrical c.
counting
    double c.
count-rate linearity
country
    cocci c.
coupled
    c. atrial pacing (CAP)
    c. premature beats
    c. pulse
    c. rhythm
    c. suturing
coupler
    Y c.
couplet
    ventricular c.
coupling
    arterial c.
    cardiopulmonary c.
    conductive c.
    constant c.
    electromechanical c.
    excitation-contraction c.
    fixed c.
    intercellular c.
    c. interval
    neuromuscular c.
    variable c.
    vasoneuronal c.
    ventriculoarterial c.
Cournand
    C. dip
    C. needle

C. Tip Arrow QuadPolar electrode
catheter
Cournand-Grino angiography needle
Cournand-Potts needle
coved ST-segment elevation
cove plane
cover
Gore-Tex c.
OxiLink oximeter probe c.
Covera-HS
Cover-Strip wound closure strip
Coversyl
CoV-HKU1
human coronavirus HKU1
coving
ST-segment c.
COX
cyclooxygenase
cytochrome c oxidase
Cox
C. maze operation
C. organism
COX-1, -2 enzyme
Coxiella burnetii
coxsackie A, B, B3, B4 virus
coxsackievirus
c. carditis
c. myocarditis
Cozaar
CP
capillary pressure
cardiac pacing
cardiac performance
cardiopulmonary
cerebral palsy
chest pain
constrictive pericarditis
cor pulmonale
Vancocin CP
C/P
cholesterol-phospholipid
C/P ratio
CPA
cardiopulmonary arrest
CPAD
chronic peripheral arterial disease
CPAP
continuous positive airway pressure
AirSep CPAP
autotitrating CPAP
Companion 314 nasal CPAP
fixed-pressure CPAP
intelligent CPAP
nasal CPAP
Phantom nasal mask CPAP
REMstar auto CPAP
Sullivan III CPAP
CPB
cardiopulmonary bypass

CPBV
cardiopulmonary blood volume
CPC
chest pain center
CP-Cardiosol
CPCR
cardiopulmonary cerebral resuscitation
CPD
cardiopulmonary disease
CPE
cardiac pulmonary edema
chronic pulmonary emphysema
CPET
cardiopulmonary exercise testing
C-PF
coronary-pulmonary fistula
CPF
clot-promoting factor
CPG
cardiopneumographic recording
clinical practice guidelines
CPHV OptiForm mitral valve
CPI
coronary prognostic index
CPI endocardial defibrillation/rate-
sensing/pacing lead
CPI Endotak transvenous electrode
CPI Mini device
CPI/Guidant
CPI/G lead
CPI/G pacemaker
CPI-PRx pulse generator
CPIS
clinical pulmonary infection score
CPK
creatine phosphokinase
brain band enzyme of CPK
CPK isoenzyme
MB enzymes of CPK
muscle fraction enzyme of CPK
(CPK-MM, CPK-3)
myocardial band enzymes of CPK
(CPK-MB, CPK-2)
CPK-3 (*var. of* CPK-MM)
CPK-BB
brain isoenzymes of creatine
phosphokinase
CPK-BB band
CPK-MB, CPK-2
myocardial band enzymes of CPK
CPK-MB band
CPK-MB fraction
CPK-MM, CPK-3
muscle fraction enzyme of CPK
CPK-MM band
C/PL
cholesterol-phospholipid
C/PL ratio

C

CPO
cardiac power output
CPOS
chest pain order sheet
CPOTHA
chest pain onset to hospital arrival
CPOU
chest pain observation unit
CPP
cerebral perfusion pressure
chest pain policy
coronary perfusion pressure
CPPTS
complete pacemaker patient testing
system
CPR
cardiopulmonary reserve
cardiopulmonary resuscitation
centripetal rub
cough CPR
4-phase Lifestick CPR
simultaneous compression-ventilation
CPR (SCV-CPR)
CPRI
cardiopulmonary risk index
CPS
cardioplegic perfusion solution
cardiopulmonary support
chest pain syndrome
coronary perfusate solution
CPS system
CPT
chest physical therapy
chest physiotherapy
CPUE
chest pain of unknown etiology
CPVC
common pulmonary venous channel
CPVD
congenital polyvalvular disease
CPVT
catecholaminergic polymorphic
ventricular tachycardia
CPX
cardiopulmonary exercise
CPX test
C-R
controlled release
Bicillin C-R
CR
cardiac rehabilitation
cardiac resuscitation
cardiac rhythm
cardiorespiratory
cardiorrhexis
chest and right arm lead in
electrocardiogram
chest roentgenogram
chest roentgenography

computed radiography
CR lead
metoprolol CR
Norpace CR
CRA
coronary rotational atherectomy
cracked-pot
c.-p. resonance
c.-p. sound
cracking
environmental stress c.
crackle
bibasilar coarse c.
coarse c.
end-inspiratory Velcro c.
inspiratory c.
pleural c.
Velcro c.
crackling rale
crack lung
cradle
foot c.
Crafoord
C. coarctation clamp
C. lobectomy scissors
Crafoord-Sellor hemostatic forceps
cramp
calf c.
Crampton test
cranial
c. angulation
c. arteritis
c. nerves I–XII
craniocardiac reflex
craniocaudal view
craniocerebellocardiac (3C, CCC)
c. dysplasia
c. syndrome
craniopharyngeal
c. duct
c. duct tumor
cranking
arm c.
crankshaft clip
CRAO
central retinal artery occlusion
craquement
bruit de c.
crash
c. cart
c. technique
crassamentum
Crawford graft inclusion technique
crazy paving pattern
CRBBB
complete right bundle branch block
CR-BSI
catheter-related bloodstream infection

CRC
    cardiovascular reflex conditioning
    cerebrovascular reserve capacity
CRCS
    cardiovascular reflex conditioning system
CRCV
    cerebral red blood cell volume
CRD
    chronic respiratory disease
C-reactive protein (CRP)
cream
    EMLA c.
    Gormel c.
crease
    ear lobe c. (ELC)
creatine
    c. kinase (CK)
    c. kinase, myocardial bound (CK-
    MB)
    c. phosphokinase (CPK)
creatinine clearance
Creech
    manner of C.
    C. manner
    C. technique
creep
    stent c.
creeping thrombosis
Crego traction
crena cordis
crenulated tantalum wire
creola body
Creo-Terpin
crepitant rale
crepitation
crepitus
crescendo
    c. angina
    c. murmur
    c. sleep
    c. snoring
    c. TIA
**crescendo-decrescendo diamond-shaped
  systolic ejection murmur**
crescent
    c. sign
    sublingual c.
crescentic glomerulonephritis
CREST
    calcinosis, Raynaud phenomenon,
      esophageal involvement, sclerodactyly,
      telangiectasia
        CREST syndrome
crest
    cardiac neural c.
    supraventricular c.
    vagal neural c.
Crestor

CRF
    chronic respiratory failure
    corticotropin-releasing factor
CRG
    cardiorespirogram
CRI
    cardiac risk index
    catheter-related infection
Cribier
    C. method
    C. valve
Cribier-Edwards percutaneous valve
Cricket pulse oximeter
cricoarytenoid arthritis
cricoesophageal tendon
cricoesophageus
    tendo c.
cricoid
    c. cartilage
    c. pressure
cricoidea
    cartilago c.
cricoideae
    arytenoidea c.
cricopharyngeal
    c. achalasia syndrome
    c. obstruction
cricothyroid
    c. artery
    c. membrane
cricothyroidotomy
cricotracheotomy
cri du chat syndrome
Crile
    C. clamp
    C. tip occluder
crimper
crimping
Crinone
crinophagy
crisis, pl. crises
    anaphylactic c.
    bronchial c.
    cardiac c.
    hypertensive c.
    laryngeal c.
    myasthenic c.
    pharyngeal c.
    sickle cell c.
    thoracic c.
Crisp aneurysm
crisscross
    c. atrioventricular valve
    c. fashion
    c. heart
    c. heart malposition
crista
    c. supraventricularis

crista *(continued)*
    c. terminalis
    c. ventricularis
criteria, sing. **criterion**
    Airlie House c.
    Akaike information c.
    Allen-Brown c.
    Billingham c.
    bodybuilder electromechanical c.
    Bogalusa c.
    Casale-Devereux c.
    Cornell voltage-duration product c.
    Dallas c.
    Duke infective endocarditis c.
    Eagle c.
    Estes ECG c.
    exclusion c.
    Framingham heart failure c.
    Ghent c.
    Gubner-Ungerleider voltage c.
    Heath-Edwards c.
    Heffner c.
    Jones c.
    12-lead voltage-duration product c.
    light c.
    MADIT II c.
    Minnesota c.
    pathologic c.
    Penn Convention c.
    process-based c.
    pseudodisappearance c.'s
    Rand appropriateness selection c.
    Rautaharju ECG c.
    Romhilt-Estes point score c.
    Saccomanno morphologic c.
    scintigraphic c.
    Sellers c.
    Sgarbossa c.
    Sokolow-Lyon voltage c.
    TIMI c.
    voltage c.
    von Reyn c.
    Weitzman c.
    Wilks lambda c.'s
critical
    c. aortic stenosis
    c. care unit
    C. Care Ventilator
    c. closing pressure of collapsible segment (Ptm')
    c. coronary stenosis
    c. coupling interval
    c. flicker frequency
    c. flicker fusion
    c. limb ischemia
    c. malperfusion syndrome
    c. rate
    c. valvular stenosis
Criticare pulse oximeter

CritiCath thermodilution catheter
Critikon
    C. automated blood pressure cuff
    C. balloon temporary pacing catheter
    C. balloon-tipped end-hole catheter
    C. balloon wedge pressure catheter
    C. guidewire
CritScan hematocrit sensor
Crixivan
crochetage EKG pattern
crocidolite
Crocq disease
Croften classification
cromafiban
cromakalim
cromoglycate
    disodium c. (DSCG)
    PMS-Sodium C.
    sodium c.
cromolyn
    c. sodium
    c. sodium inhalation solution
CROP
    compliance, rate, oxygenation, pressure
cross
    yellow c.
crossbridge
    actin-myosin c.
cross-checking
    sensory c.-c.
cross-clamp
    aortic c.-c.
    c.-c. time
cross-clamping of aorta
crossed
    c. cerebellar diaschisis (CCD)
    c. embolism
cross-femoral graft
CrossFlex
    C. coil stent
    C. LC-stainless steel, laser-cut coronary stent
Cross-IT guidewire
Cross-Jones
    C.-J. disc prosthetic valve
    C.-J. mitral valve
crosslinkage
    DNA c.
    c. theory
crosslinked D fragment
crossover
    femorofemoral c.
    c. femorofemoral bypass
CrossPoint TransAccess catheter
cross-reactive antibody
CrossSail
    C. balloon
    C. coronary dilation catheter

cross-sectional
>c.-s. area (CSA)
>c.-s. 2-dimensional echocardiogram
>c.-s. echocardiography (CSE)

crosstalk pacemaker

Crosswire
>C. nitinol hydrophilic guidewire
>C. NT guidewire

Crotalus

croup
>catarrhal c.
>diphtheritic c.
>false c.
>membranous c.
>pseudomembranous c.
>spasmodic c.
>c. tent

croup-associated virus

Croupette child tent

crouposa
>angina c.

croupous
>c. bronchitis
>c. laryngitis
>c. pharyngitis
>c. pneumonia

croupy cough

crowded oropharynx

Crow-Fukase syndrome

crowing
>c. breath sounds
>c. inspiration

Crown-Crisp index

Crown stent

CRP
>coronary rehabilitation program
>C-reactive protein
>>high-sensitivity CRP

CRPD
>chronic restrictive pulmonary disease

CRQ
>Chronic Respiratory Disease
>>Questionnaire
>Chronic Respiratory Questionnaire

CRS
>cardiac recovery system

CRT
>cardiac resuscitation team
>cardiac resynchronization therapy
>code response team

CRT-D
>cardiac resynchronization therapy
>>defibrillator
>>Contak CD CRT-D

CRT-ICD
>cardiac resynchronization therapy
>>implantable cardioverter-defibrillator
>>InSync II Marquis remote
>>>monitoring CRT-ICD

CRU
>cardiac rehabilitation unit
>clinical research unit

cruces (*pl. of* crux)

cruciate anastomosis

crude stroke

crudum
>sputum c.

cruentum
>sputum c.

crunch
>Hamman c.
>mediastinal c.

crunching sound

crural
>c. artery
>c. diaphragm

crus, pl. **crura**
>angina c.
>c. dextrum diaphragmatis
>c. dextrum fasciculi
>>atrioventricularis
>c. sinistrum diaphragmatis
>c. sinistrum fasciculi
>>atrioventricularis

crush
>c. artifact
>c. stent technique

crushing chest pain

Crutchfield clamp

Cruveilhier
>C. nodes
>C. sign

Cruveilhier-Baumgarten
>C.-B. murmur
>C.-B. sign

crux, pl. **cruces**
>c. dextrum fasciculi
>>atrioventricularis
>c. of heart
>c. sinistrum fasciculi
>>atrioventricularis

cruzi
>*Trypanosoma c.*

CRVF
>congestive right ventricular failure

CryCor cardiac cryoablation system

cryoablation
>arrhythmia circuit c.
>catheter c.
>encircling c.
>c. lesion

cryocardioplegia

Cryocare cardiac surgical system

cryocatheter
>Freezor c.

CryoCor cryoablation system

cryocrit

Cryo/Cuff pressure boot

Cryo-Cut microtome
cryoenergy
cryoglobulinemia
CryoHit system
cryolesion
CryoLife-O'Brien
    C.-O. stentless aortic porcine
      bioprosthesis
    C.-O. stentless aortic porcine valve
cryomapping
    efficacy c.
cryomicroscope
cryomicroscopy
CryoPlasty therapy
cryoprecipitate
cryopreservation
cryopreserved
    c. heart valve allograft
    c. homograft valve
    c. human aortic allograft
    c. valved allograft
    c. vein
cryoprobe
    Erbe c.
    Spembly c.
cryoprotectant
cryosurgical technique
cryotherapy
    endobronchial c.
    c. probe
cryptococcal
    c. capsular antigen
    c. myocarditis
    c. pulmonary disease
cryptococcoma
cryptococcosis
    disseminated c.
    pulmonary c.
Cryptococcus
    C. albidus
    C. histolyticus
    C. laurentii
    C. neoformans
cryptogenic
    c. fibrosing alveolitis (CFA)
    c. hemoptysis
    c. organizing pneumonia (COP)
    c. organizing pneumonitis (COP)
    c. stroke
cryptophthalmos syndrome
cryptosporidiosis
Cryptosporidium
Cryptostroma corticale
crystal
    asthma c.
    Charcot-Leyden c.
    Charcot-Neumann c.
    Charcot-Robin c.
    Doppler c.

    Leyden c.
    piezoelectric c.
    silica tetrahedral c.
    sonomicrometer piezoelectric c.
crystalline nicotine
crystalloid
    airway, breathing, circulation,
      intravenous c. (ABCIC)
    c. cardioplegic solution
    c. fluid
    c. potassium cardioplegia
    c. prime
    c. resuscitation
CS
    cardiogenic shock
    cavernous sinus
    cholesterol stone
    cholesterol sulfate
    cigarette smoke
    conservative surgery
    coronary sclerosis
    coronary sinus
    cycloserine
CSA
    central sleep apnea
    cross-sectional area
CsA
    cyclosporin A
CSAS
    central sleep apnea syndrome
CSB
    Cheyne-Stokes breathing
CSBF
    coronary sinus blood flow
CSE
    cross-sectional echocardiography
CSF
    cerebrospinal fluid
    colony-stimulating factor
CSFI
    Cholesterol-Saturated Fat Index
CSFS
    coronary slow flow syndrome
CSG
    coronary sinus guiding
CSGBI
    Cardiac Society of Great Britain and
      Ireland
CSI
    chemical shift imaging
    cholesterol saturation index
    coronary sinus intervention
CSICU
    cardiac surgical intensive care unit
CSL
    cardiolipin synthetic lecithin
CSLD
    chronic suppurative lung disease

CSM
circulation, sensation, motion
CSN
cardiac sympathetic nerve
CSNRT
corrected sinus node recovery time
CSO
ostium of coronary sinus
CSOP
coronary sinus occlusion pressure
CSRS
cardiac surgery reporting system
CSS
Churg-Strauss syndrome
CSSA
carotid stent-supported angioplasty
CSSS
coronary-subclavian steal syndrome
CST
cardiac stress test
cardiovascular self-assessment tool
CSVT
central splanchnic venous thrombosis
CSWT
cardiac shock wave therapy
^{13}C-triolein breath test
^{14}C-triolein breath test
CT
cardiac tamponade
cardiothoracic
chest tube
clotting time
coagulation time
computed tomography
coronary thrombosis
corrected transposition
corrective therapy
   CT angiography
   cine CT
   contrast-enhanced CT
   HeartView CT
   helical CT
   high-resolution CT (HRCT)
   multidetector-row chest CT
   reference phantom CT
   CT scan
   Siemens Evolution electron beam
    CT
   Technicare Omega 500 CT
   thin-section CT
CTA
computed tomography angiography
CTAO
cerebral thromboangiitis obliterans
   isolated CTAO
CTAP
computed tomography angiographic
  portography

computed tomography in arterial
  portography
CTB
cytotrophoblast
CTEPH
chronic thromboembolic pulmonary
  hypertension
C-terminal peptide
CTFC
corrected TIMI frame count
CTG
cardiotocography
C/TG
cholesterol-triglyceride
   C/TG ratio
CTGA
complete transposition of great arteries
CTGF
connective tissue growth factor
CT-guided stereotaxic technique
CTHM
conotruncal heart malformation
CTI
cardiac troponin I
cavotricuspid isthmus
CTICU
cardiothoracic intensive care unit
CTI-dependent flutter
CTLA4Ig protein
CTM
cardiotachometer
cTnI, cTn-I
cardiac troponin I
   cTnI assay
cTnT
cardiac troponin T
CTO
chronic total occlusion
   CTO guidewire
C-to-E amplitude
CTPVO
chronic thrombotic pulmonary vascular
  obstruction
CTR
cardiothoracic ratio
CTRD
Cardiac Transplant Research Database
CTS
cardiothoracic surgery
CTSNFR
corrected time of sinuatrial node function
  recovery
cTT
cerebral transit time
CTU
cardiothoracic unit
CTx
cardiac transplantation
C-type natriuretic peptide (CNP)

C

CU
    cardiac unit
    copper
⁶²CU
    copper-62
cubitus valgus
cuff
        antimicrobial catheter c.
        aortic c.
        Astropulse c.
        atrial c.
        blood pressure c. (BPC)
        Critikon automated blood pressure c.
        Dinamap blood pressure c.
        endotracheal tube c.
        Finapres finger c.
        finger c.
        c. plethysmography
        pneumatic c.
        c. sign
        c. suctioning
        c. test
        tracheostomy c.
cuffed
        c. endotracheal tube
        c. hypertension
        c. tracheostomy tube
cuffing
        peribronchial c.
cuff-leak test
cuirass
        chest c.
        c. respirator
        tabetic c.
        c. ventilation
        c. ventilator
culbertsoni
        Acanthamoeba c.
cul-de-sac
        blind c.-d.-s.
culotte
        c. coronary stenting technique
        c. fashion
        c. stent technique
culprit
        c. lesion
        c. lesion angioplasty
        c. stenosis
        c. vessel angioplasty
culture
        endoscopic tissue c. (ETC)
        pericardial fluid c. (PFC)
culture-negative endocarditis
cumetharol
cumethoxaethane
cumulative cardiotoxic dose (CCD)
cuneiform tubercle
Cunninghamella

cupping artifact
cuprophane membrane
cupula, pl. **cupulae**
        c. of pleura
        c. pleurae
        pleural c.
curare
curative irradiation
curd
        soap c.
curettage, curettement
curette, curet
Curosurf intratracheal suspension
currant
        c. jelly clot
        c. jelly sputum
        c. jelly thrombus
current
        alternating c. (AC)
        axial c.
        bioelectric c.
        calcium c. (I_{Ca})
        chloride c. (I_{Cl})
        diastolic c.
        direct c. (DC)
        eddy c.
        fast sodium c.
        injury c.
        K c.
        low energy direct c. (LEDC)
        membrane c.
        pacemaker c. (I_F)
        pseudoalternating c.
        pump c.
        radiofrequency c. (RFC)
        range-alternating c.
        sodium c. (I_{Na})
        systolic c.
        toxin-insensitive c.
        transient inward c.
        transsarcolemmal calcium c.
Curry needle
Curschmann spiral
curse
        Ondine c.
curve
        actuarial survival c.
        AH c.
        ascorbate dilution c.
        carbon dioxide dissociation c.
        deflation c.
        dissociation c.
        dose-effect curve dose-response c.
        dye-dilution c.
        flow volume c.
        Frank-Starling c.
        function c.
        green dye c.
        hemoglobin-oxygen dissociation c.

indocyanine dilution c.
intracardiac pressure c.
isovolume pressure flow c. (IVPF)
J c.
left ventricular pressure-volume c.
length-active tension c.
length-tension c. (LT)
mitral E velocity c.
nitrogen c.
oxygen dissociation c.
oxyhemoglobin disassociation c.
 (OHDC)
oxyhemoglobin dissociation c.
pressure-natriuresis c.
pressure-volume c.
pulse c.
PV c.
single-breath nitrogen c.
Starling c.
thermal dilution c.
thermodilution c.
time-activity c.
Traube c.
venous return c.
venovenous dye dilution c.
ventricular function c. (VFC)
volume-time c.
ZEEP PV c.

curved
    c. end-to-end anastomosis (CEEA)
    c. M mode
    c. tapered Tefcor movable core
      wire guide

Curvularia lunata
CUSA
    Cavitron ultrasonic surgical aspirator
Cushing
    C. forceps
    C. pressure response
    C. reflex
    C. syndrome
    C. triad

cushingoid facies
cushion
    atrioventricular canal c.
    bubble c.
    cardiac c.
    coronary c.
    endocardial c.
    pharyngoesophageal c.'s
    Sullivan bubble c.

Cushman assay
cusp
    accessory c.
    anterior c.
    aortic c.
    aortic sinus c.
    c. billowing
    conjoined c.

coronary c.
c. degeneration
c. eversion
c. excursion
c. fenestration
fish-mouth c.
left coronary c. (LCC)
c. motion
noncoronary c. (NCC)
c. prolapse
c. retraction
right coronary c. (RCC)

cuspis, pl. **cuspides**
    c. anterior valvae bicuspidalis
    c. anterior valvae tricuspidalis
    c. commissurales

cut
    coronal c.
    DCA c.
    c. point
    sagittal c.

cutaneous
    c. anthrax
    c. asthma
    c. emphysema
    c. hyperesthesia
    c. malignancy
    c. necrotizing venulitis
    c. vasculopathy
    c. xanthoma

cutaneum
    Trichosporum c.
cutdown
    arterial c.
    brachial artery c.
    c. catheter
    saphenous vein c. (SVC)
    c. technique
    venous c.

cut-film arteriography
Cutinova Hydro dressing
cutis
    c. laxa
    c. laxa syndrome
    c. marmorata

Cutler-Ederer method
cutpoint
cutter
    C. aortic valve prosthesis
    EZ45 thoracic linear c.
    rib c.

Cutter-Smeloff
    C.-S. aortic valve prosthesis
    C.-S. disc valve
    C.-S. mitral valve

cutting
    c. balloon
    c. balloon angioplasty (CBA)

C

cutting (*continued*)
    c. balloon before stent (CBBEST)
    c. balloon Ultra^2 Monorail device
cuvette
    dye c.
Cuvier
    canal of C.
    duct of C.
Cu/Zn superoxide dismutase
CV
    cardiac volume
    cardiovascular
    care vigilance
    central venous
    cerebrovascular
    cervical vertebra
    closing volume
    contrast ventriculography
    conventional ventilation
        CV wave
        CV wave of jugular venous pulse
CVA
    cardiovascular accident
    cerebrovascular accident
    costovertebral angle
CVAD
    central venous access device
CVAP
    cerebrovascular amyloid peptide
CVC
    central venous catheter
        CVC 123 calibration verification
        control
CVCT
    cardiovascular computed tomography
CVD
    cardiovascular disease
C-Vest
    C-V. ambulatory radionuclide
        detector
    C-V. radiation detector system
CVF
    cardiovascular failure
    chronic ventilatory failure
    collagen volume fraction
CVG
    coronary venous graft
CVH
    combined ventricular hypertrophy
CVHD
    chronic valvular heart disease
CVI
    cardiovascular incident
    cardiovascular insufficiency
    cerebrovascular incident
    cerebrovascular infarction
    cerebrovascular insufficiency
    chronic venous insufficiency
        multiple CVIs

CVICU
    cardiovascular intensive care unit
CVID
    common variable immunodeficiency
        partial CVID
CVIS
    cardiovascular imaging system
        CVIS imaging device
CVM
    cardiovascular monitor
CVMR
    cardiovascular magnetic resonance
CVO
    central vein occlusion
    central venous oxygen
CVP
    cardioventricular pacing
    central venous pressure
        CVP line
CVProfilor
    C. DO-2020 cardiovascular profiling
        device
    C. DO-2020 system
CVR
    cardiovascular-renal
    cardiovascular-respiratory
    cephalic vasomotor response
    cerebrovascular reactivity
    cerebrovascular resistance
    coronary flow velocity reserve
CVRD
    cardiovascular-renal disease
CVRR
    cardiovascular recovery room
CVS
    cardiovascular surgery
    cardiovascular system
    cerebral vasospasm
    collagen vascular sealing
CVT
    cardiovascular technologist
    central venous temperature
    cerebral venous thrombosis
CVVH
    continuous venovenous hemofiltration
CVX-300 excimer laser system
CW
    cardiac work
    circle of Willis
CWD
    cell wall defect
    continuous-wave Doppler
CWI
    cardiac work index
CWM
    cardiological workspace manager
CWP
    coal worker's pneumoconiosis

CWS
    chest wall stimulation
    circumferential wall stress
CX
    chest x-ray
    circumflex
    circumflex artery
CXC chemokine
CxCor
CXR, CxR
    chest radiograph
    chest x-ray
cyanide
    c. antidote kit
    hydrogen c. (HCN)
cyanmethemoglobin method
cyanoacrylate
    n-butyl c. (n-BCA)
2-cyanoacrylate
    isobutyl 2-c.
cyanochroic, cyanochrous
cyanogen bromide method
cyanosed
cyanose tardive
cyanosis
    autotoxic c.
    central c.
    circumoral c.
    edema, clubbing, c. (ECC)
    false c.
    hereditary methemoglobinemic c.
    late c.
    c. of nail beds
    peripheral c.
    pulmonary c.
    c. retinae
    reverse differential c.
    shunt c.
    tardive c.
cyanotic
    c. asphyxia
    c. atrophy
    c. atrophy of liver
    c. congenital heart disease
    c. congenital heart disease
      arrhythmia
    c. heart defect
    c. heart disease (CHD)
cyanotica
    asphyxia c.
Cyberlith pacemaker
Cybertach
    C. automatic-burst atrial pacemaker
    C. 60 bipolar pacemaker
Cybex isokinetic dynamometer
cyclandelate
cyclase
    adenylate c.
    adenylyl c. (AC)

    cell membrane-bound adenylate c.
    guanylate c.
    guanylyl c.
cycle
    cardiac c. (CC)
    cell c.
    circannual c.
    circaseptan c.
    citric acid c.
    Cori c.
    c. ergometer
    c. ergometry
    forced c.
    isometric period of cardiac c.
    Krebs c.
    c. length (CL)
    c. length alternans
    c. length alternation
    c. length window
    moiety-conserved c.
    ratio of expiration time and total
      time of breathing c. (tE/tTOT)
    ratio of inspiration time and total
      time of breathing c. (tI/tTOT)
    respiratory c.
    restored c.
    returning c.
    RR c.
    short-long-short c.
    sound wave c.
    Wenckebach c.
cyclic
    c. adenosine monophosphate
      (cAMP)
    c. alternating pattern (CAP)
    c. guanosine monophosphate
      (cGMP)
    c. nucleotide adenosine
      monophosphate
    c. progesterone
    c. respiration
cyclin A gene
cyclocumarol
cycloergometer
cycloheximide
cyclohexylamine
Cyclomen
cyclooxygenase (COX)
    c. inhibitor
cyclooxygenase-2
cyclooxygenase-1 inhibitor
cyclopentamine hydrochloride
cyclopenthiazide
cyclopentylpropionate
    hydrocortisone c.
cyclophosphamide
    c., bleomycin, cisplatin (CBP)
    c., doxorubicin, cisplatin (CAP)

C

cyclophosphamide *(continued)*
    c., doxorubicin, methotrexate,
      procarbazine (CAMP)
    c., doxorubicin, vincristine (CAV)
    vindesine, cisplatin, lomustine, c.
      (VCPC)
cyclopropane
cycloserine (CS)
cyclosporin A, cyclosporine (CsA)
cyclothiazide
cyclotron-produced F-18
  fluorodeoxyglucose
CYFRA
    cytokeratin 19 fragment
      CYFRA 21-1 tumor marker
Cyklokapron
    C. injection
    C. Oral
Cylexin
cylinder
    C oxygen c.
    M6 oxygen c.
    oxygen c.
    portable oxygen c.
cylindrical
    c. bronchiectasis
    c. confronting cisterna
cylindroadenoma
cylindroid aneurysm
cylindroma
cylindruria
Cylos pacemaker
Cynosar catheter
CYP1A2 isoform
CYP2C9 isoform
CYP2C19 isoform
CYP2D6 isoform
CYP3A isoform
CYP3A4 isoform
Cypher sirolimus-eluting coronary stent
cypionate
    hydrocortisone c.
cyproheptadine hydrochloride
cyproterone
Cyriax syndrome
cys-LT
    cysteinyl leukotriene
cyst
    aneurysmal bone c.
    apoplectic c.
    bone c.
    bronchial c.
    bronchogenic c.
    bronchopulmonary c.
    centrilobular c.
    compound c.
    echinococcal c.
    enterogenous c.
    esophageal duplication c.

    hemorrhagic c.
    hepatic hydatid c.
    honeycomb c.
    hydatid c.
    locular c.
    loculated c.
    mucoretention c.
    mucous retention c.
    multilocular c.
    multiseptate c.
    necrotic c.
    neurenteric c.
    neuroenteric c.
    pericardial c.
    pleuropericardial c.
    renal c.
    retention c.
    springwater c.
    thymic c.
    Tornwaldt c.
    true c.
    unilocular c.
cystathionine synthase deficiency
cystatin
    c. C
    c. C test
    c. C test for predicting heart
     death
cysteine
cysteinyl leukotriene (cys-LT)
cystic
    c. adenomatoid malformation
    c. bronchiectasis
    c. change
    c. disease of lung
    c. emphysema
    c. fibrosis (CF)
    c. fibrosis induced cholestasis
    c. fibrosis transmembrane
     conductance regulator
    c. fibrosis transmembrane regulator
     (CFTR)
    c. lesion
    c. lung disease
    c. medial necrosis (CMN)
    c. medial necrosis of ascending
     aorta (CMN-AA)
    c. periventricular leukomalacia
    c. space
cystica
    medionecrosis aortae idiopathica c.
    osteitis tuberculosa multiplex c.
cysticercosis
Cytadren
cytarabine hydrochloride
cytobrush
cytocentrifugation
cytochalasin B

cytochrome
- c. c oxidase (COX)
- c. P450-3A4 isoform
- c. P450 system

CytoGam

cytokeratin 19 fragment (CYFRA)

cytokine
- chemotactic c.
- c. expression
- inflammatory c.
- pleiotropic c.
- proinflammatory c.
- c. release syndrome
- c. snowstorm

cytokine-induced endothelial synthesis

cytological biopsy

cytology
- aspiration biopsy c. (ABC)
- bronchial washings c.
- sputum c.

cytomegalic inclusion disease

cytomegalovirus (CMV)
- c. encephalitis
- human c. (HCMV)
- c. immune globulin (CMVIG)
- c. immune globulin intravenous, human
- c. pneumonitis

Cytomel Oral

cytometer

cytometric indirect immunofluorescence

cytometry
- flow c.

cytomitome

cytomorphology

cytomorphosis

cytoplasmic bridge

cytoprotective
- c. agent
- c. effect

Cytosar-U

cytosine-thymine-guanine trinucleotide

cytoskeletal protein

cytoskeleton
- actin c.

cytosolic protein

cytosome

cytotoxic
- c. edema
- c. gene therapy
- c. singlet oxygen

cytotoxicity

cytotoxin-associated gene product A (CagA)

cytotrophoblast (CTB)

Cytovene

Cytoxan
- C. injection
- C. Oral

Czaja-McCaffrey rigid stent introducer/endoscope

C

D
  diastole
  dipyridamole
  disease
  donor
    Cheracol D
    D, F, H, M gate
    D, I allele
    D loop
    D point
    D sleep
    D wave
D2
  prostaglandin D2
2D
  2-dimensional
    2D echocardiogram
    2D echocardiography
    2D gradient-echo sequence
    2D TEE system Ultra-Neb 99
3D
  3-dimensional
    3D IVUS
    3D motion evaluation
    3D segmented-FLASH imaging
      sequence
    3D SPGR image
    3D tagged magnetic resonance
      imaging
    3D TF magnetic resonance
      angiography
    3D time-of-flight magnetic
      resonance angiographic sequence
    3D TOF MRA
    3D transesophageal echocardiogram
D_4
Do_2
  oxygen delivery
D_{CO}
  pulmonary diffusion capacity
D114S balloon catheter
D1790G mutant gene
D2L OTW balloon dilation catheter
  with extended pressure range
DA
  daytime asthma
  descending aorta
  digital angiography
  ductus arteriosus
D-A
  donor-acceptor
Da
  dalton
d(A)
  primary donor

Daae disease
dabigatran etexilate
DAC
  Guiatuss DAC
  Guiatussin DAC
  Halotussin DAC
  Mytussin DAC
dacarbazine
daclizumab
DaCosta syndrome
Dacron
  D. catheter
  D. cloth
  D. fiber
  D. intracardiac patch
  D. onlay patch-graft
  D. tube
  D. tube graft
dactinomycin
DAD
  delayed afterdepolarization
  diffuse alveolar damage
Dae-Jo-Hwan
dagger-shaped aortic envelope
Daggett procedure
DAH
  diffuse alveolar hemorrhage
  disordered action of heart
daidzein
Daig
  D. decapolar catheter
  D. sheath
Dakin solution
Dalalone
Dale-Schwartz tube
Dale tracheostomy tube holder
dalfopristin
Dallas
  D. Classification System
  D. criteria
dalteparin
  d. sodium
  d. sodium injection
dalton (Da)
Dalton-Henry law
Dalton law
DALY
  disability-adjusted life year
damage
  bilateral hemisphere d. (BHD)
  diffuse alveolar d. (DAD)
  enzyme-induced d.
  left brain d. (LBD)
  left hemisphere d. (LHD)
  myocardial d. (MD)

D

damage *(continued)*
  parietal pleural d.
  regional alveolar d. (RAD)
  right brain d. (RBD)
  right hemisphere d. (RHD)
  silent ischemic brain d. (SIBD)
D'Amato sign
DAMIA
  direct acute myocardial infarction
  angioplasty
Damian graft procedure
dampened waveform
damping
  Accudynamic adjustable d.
  catheter d.
  d. coefficient
  d. control
Damus-Kaye-Stansel (DKS)
  D.-K.-S. connection
  D.-K.-S. operation
  D.-K.-S. procedure
  D.-K.-S. procedure for single
  ventricle physiology
DAN
  diabetic autonomic neuropathy
danaparoid sodium
danazol
dance
  brachial d.
  hilar d.
  St. Vitus d.
dancer's foot malformation
dander
  animal d.
Dane particle
Danielson method
Danocrine
Danon disease
danshen
Dantrium
dantrolene sodium
DAo
  descending aorta
DAP
  depolarizing afterpotential
  diastolic aortic pressure
dapsone (DDS)
daptomycin for injection
Daranide
Daraprim
DAR breathing system
Dardik Biograft
darkfield microscopy
Darling disease
Darox cutaneous thoracic patch
  electrode
darusentan

DASE
  dobutamine atropine stress
  echocardiography
DASH
  dietary approaches to stop hypertension
Dash single-chamber rate-adaptic
  pacemaker
DASI
  Duke Activity Status Index
DAT
  direct amplification test
data
  measured d.
  nonparametric d.
  pressure-volume d.
database
  Cardiac Transplant Research D.
  (CTRD)
  Duke Carcinoid D.
  GenBank genome sequence d.
  low-density lipoprotein receptor
  mutation d. (LDLR, LDL-R)
Datascope
  D. Accutorr bedside monitor
  D. balloon
  D. CL-II percutaneous translucent
  balloon catheter
  D. pulse oximeter
  D. System 90 intraaortic balloon
  pump
Datex-Ohmeda
  D.-O. S/5 telemetry system
  D.-O. ventilator
DATI
  diastolic amplitude time index
daughter radionuclide
DaunoXome
DAVF
  dural arteriovenous fistula
DAVID
  dual-chamber and VVI implantable
  defibrillator
David reimplantation operation
Davidson
  D. clamp
  D. protocol exercise test
  D. scapular retractor
  D. thoracic trocar
Davies
  D. catheter
  D. disease
  D. endomyocardial fibrosis
  D. myocardial fibrosis
  D. technique
da Vinci robotic surgical system
Davis
  D. double-end soft tissue retractor
  D. sign

DAVM
　　dural arteriovenous malformation
Daxas
day
　　milligram per kilogram per d.
　　4-d. syndrome
　　total ventilator d.'s
daytime asthma (DA)
Dazamide
dazoxiben
DBC
　　distal balloon catheter
DBCL
　　dilute blood clot lysis
　　　　DBCL method
DBP
　　diastolic blood pressure
DBPC
　　dual balloon perfusion catheter
DC
　　direct current
　　dual chamber
　　　　DC cardioversion
　　　　DC discharge
　　　　DC electric shock
DCA
　　dichloroacetate
　　directional color angiography
　　directional coronary angioplasty
　　　　DCA cut
　　　　DCA debulking technique
DCABG
　　double coronary artery bypass graft
DCAF
　　dilated cardiomyopathy and atrial
　　　fibrillation
DCAPI
　　Duke Coronary Angiographic Prognostic
　　　Index
DCBF
　　dynamic cardiac blood flow
DCC
　　direct cardiac compression
DCCV
　　direct current cardioversion
DCFM
　　Doppler color flow mapping
DCG
　　dynamic electrocardiography
DCHS
　　dysarthria-clumsy hand syndrome
DCI
　　delayed cerebral ischemia
　　digital cardiac imaging
**DCI-S automated coronary analysis
　system**
DCLHb
　　diaspirin cross-linked hemoglobin

DCM
　　dilated cardiomyopathy
DCMAG-1 gene
DCOP
　　distal coronary occlusion pressure
DCOR
　　dopachrome oxidoreductase
DCP
　　dual-chamber pacemaker
DCS
　　decompression sickness
　　distal coronary sinus
　　　　neurologic DCS
　　　　pulmonary DCS
DCV
　　delayed cerebral vasoconstriction
D2CV
　　Doppler 2-chamber view
D4CV
　　Doppler 4-chamber view
D-cycloserine
DDAVP, dDAVP
　　deamino-8-D-arginine vasopressin
　　desmopressin acetate
　　　　DDAVP injection
　　　　DDAVP Nasal
ddC
　　dideoxycytidine
DDD
　　A-V universal
　　dual-mode, dual-pacing, dual-sensing
　　　　DDD pacemaker
　　　　DDD pacing
DDDR
　　　　DDDR mode
　　　　DDDR pacing
DDFP
　　dodecafluoropentane
DD genotype
DDI
　　　　DDI mode pacemaker
　　　　DDI pacing
ddI
　　didanosine
D-dimer
　　　　D-d. enzyme-linked immunosorbent
　　　　　assay
　　　　fibrin D-d.
　　　　Simplify D-d.
　　　　D-d. test
DDIR pacing
DDP
　　cisplatin
DDR
　　diastolic descent rate
DD2R
　　dopamine D2 receptor
DDS
　　dapsone

D

DDx
　differential diagnosis
DE
　dobutamine echocardiography
　dural ectasia
2DE
　2-dimensional echocardiography
3DE
　3-dimensional echocardiography
de
　　de Lange syndrome
　　De Martel scissors
　　De Morgan spots
　　de Musset sign (aortic aneurysm)
　　de Mussy point
　　de Mussy sign (pleurisy)
　　de novo
　　de novo atherosclerosis
　　de novo disease
　　de novo malignancy
　　de novo narrowing
　　de novo native coronary artery
　　　lesion
　　de Quervain thyroiditis
deacetylase
　　histone d. 2 (HDAC2)
dead
　　d. space
　　d. space gas volume to tidal gas
　　　volume ratio (V_{DS}/V_T)
　　d. space/tidal volume ratio
　　d. space ventilation
　　d. time
deadly quartet syndrome
deafness
　　lentigines, electrocardiographic
　　abnormalities, ocular hypertelorism,
　　pulmonary stenosis, abnormalities
　　of genitalia, retardation of
　　growth, d. (LEOPARD)
deaired
deairing procedure
deaminase
　　adenosine d. (ADA)
**deamino-8-D-arginine vasopressin
(DDAVP, dDAVP)**
deamino-4-valine-D-arginine
　　1--d.-v.-D.-a. vasopressin (dVDAVP)
dearterialization
　　hepatic d.
death
　　aborted sudden d.
　　apoptotic cell d.
　　arrhythmic d.
　　brain d.
　　cardiac d.
　　cardiovascular d.
　　circle of d.
　　cocaine-related sudden d.

cystatin C test for predicting
　heart d.
heart d.
ischemic sudden d.
late sudden d.
out-of-hospital sudden cardiac d.
　(OOH-SCD)
postresuscitative d.
pump failure d.
sudden cardiac d. (SCD)
sudden coronary d. (SCD)
sudden heart d. (SHD)
sudden unexplained d.
sudden unexplained nocturnal d.
　(SUND)
vascular d.
voodoo d.
DeBakey
　　D. aortic aneurysm clamp
　　D. aortic dissection (type I, II, III,
　　　IIIa, IIIb)
　　D. arterial clamp
　　D. arterial forceps
　　D. Atraugrip forceps
　　D. ball valve prosthesis
　　D. blade
　　D. chest retractor
　　D. classification
　　manner of D.
　　D. pediatric clamp
　　D. peripheral vascular clamp
　　D. rib spreader
　　D. tissue forceps
　　D. VAD
　　D. VAD child device
　　D. VAD continuous-axial-flow
　　　pump
　　D. Vasculour-II vascular prosthesis
DeBakey-Bahnson clamp
DeBakey-Bainbridge clamp
**DeBakey-Colovira-Rumel thoracic
forceps**
DeBakey-Creech
　　D.-C. aneurysm repair
　　D.-C. manner
DeBakey-Derra
　　D.-D. anastomosis clamp
　　D.-D. anastomosis forceps
**DeBakey-Diethrich coronary artery
forceps**
DeBakey-Harken auricle clamp
**DeBakey-Howard aortic aneurysmal
clamp**
DeBakey-Kay aortic clamp
**DeBakey-McQuigg-Mixter bronchial
clamp**
DeBakey-Mixter thoracic forceps
**DeBakey-NASA axial-flow ventricular-
assist device**

DeBakey-Péan cardiovascular forceps
DeBakey-Satinsky vena cava clamp
DeBakey-Semb ligature-carrier clamp
DeBakey-Surgitool prosthetic valve
debilis
    pulsus d.
debility
Debove
    D. membrane
    D. treatment
debris
    atheromatous d.
    atherosclerotic d.
    calcific d.
    grumous d.
    pultaceous d.
    valve d.
debrisoquine sulfate
debt
    oxygen d.
debubbling procedure
debulking
    d. device
    mechanical d.
    d. procedure
Decabid
Decadron
    D. Injection
    D. Oral
Decadron-LA
Deca-Durabolin
Decaject
Decaject-LA
decamethonium
decannulation
decanoate
    Hybolin D.
    nandrolone d.
decapolar electrode catheter
decarboxylase
    histidine d.
decay
    isovolumic pressure d.
    pressure d.
deceleration
    early d.
    horizontal anteroposterior d.
    late d.
    d. time (DT)
    variable d.
    vertical d.
deceleration-dependent aberrancy
decerebrate posturing
declamping
    d. shock
    d. shock syndrome
decline
    neurocognitive d.
Declomycin

DE-CMR
    delayed contrast-enhanced cardiovascular
    magnetic resonance
Decofed Syrup
Decohistine
    D. DH
    D. Expectorant
decompensate
decompensated
    d. heart failure
    d. shock
decompensation
    cardiac d.
decompression
    cardiac d.
    d. disorder
    d. illness
    microvascular d. (MVD)
    d. sickness (DCS)
    d. table
decompressive chest tube
Deconamine
    D. SR
    D. Syrup
    D. Tablet
deconditioning
Deconsal II
decontamination
decortication
    arterial d.
    cardiac d.
    d. of heart
    d. of lung
decrease
    blood pressure d. (BPD)
decreased
    d. breath sounds
    d. respiration
    d. valve excursion
decrement
decremental
    d. atrial pacing
    d. conduction
decrescendo murmur
decrudescence
decrudescent arteriosclerosis
decubitus
    angina d.
    d. angina
    angina pectoris d.
    d. cough
    d. ulcer
dedicated bipolar lead
Dedo-Pilling laryngoscope
deductive echocardiography
deendothelialization
deenergization
    myocyte d.

D

207

deep

d. chest therapy
d. driveline infection
d. hypothermia circulatory arrest (DHCA)
d. lingual artery
d. lingual vein
d. pathologic Q wave
d. sleep
d. sulcus sign
d. vein thrombosis (DVT)
d. venous insufficiency (DVI)
d. venous pressure (DVP)
d. venous thrombosis (DVT)
d. venous thrombosis/pulmonary embolism (DVT/PE)
d. white matter hyperintensity (DWMHI)
d. white matter lesion (DWML)

de-epicardialization
deer-antler vascular pattern
Defares rebreathing method
defecation

salivation, lacrimation, urination, d. (SLUD)
d. syncope

defect

acquired ventricular septal d. (AVSD)
aortic septal d.
aortopulmonary septal d. (APSD)
atrial ostium primum d.
atrial septal d. (ASD)
atrial ventricular canal d.
atrioventricular canal d.
atrioventricular conduction d.
atrioventricular septal d. (AVSD)
A-V canal d.
A-V conduction d.
cardiac electrical d.
cell wall d. (CWD)
clamshell closure of atrial septal d.
coagulation d.
complex ventricular septal d.
conal septal d.
conduction d. (CD)
contiguous ventricular septal d.
cyanotic heart d.
Eisenmenger reaction with septal d.
endocardial cushion d. (ECD)
extrafusion d.
factor V Leiden coagulation d.
filling d.
fixed perfusion d.
fixed-rate perfusion d.
Gerbode d.
humoral immune d.
hydrogen-detected ventricular septal d. (HVSD)

iatrogenic atrial septal d.
infundibular septal d.
interatrial septal d. (IASD)
interauricular septal d.
interventricular septal d. (ISD, IVSD)
intimal d.
intraarterial conduction d.
intraventricular conduction d. (IVCD)
isolated conduction d. (ICD)
lucent d.
match d.
muscular ventricular septal d. (MVSD)
myocardial long-chain fatty acid uptake d.
napkin-ring d.
nonsegmental perfusion d.
nonuniform rotational d. (NURD)
obstructive ventilatory d. (OVD)
ostium primum d.
ostium secundum d.
panconduction d.
partial A-V canal d.
perfusion d.
periinfarction conduction d. (PICD)
perimembranous ventricular septal d.
postinfarction ventricular septal d.
primum atrial septal d.
pterygia, heart defects, autosomal recessive inheritance, vertebral defects, ear anomalies, radial d.'s (PHAVER)
pulmonary artery filling d. (PAFD)
pulmonary atresia with ventricular septal d. (PAVSD)
restrictive airways d.
restrictive ventilatory d.
reversible ischemic neurologic d. (RIND)
scintigraphic perfusion d.
secundum atrial septal d. (ASD2)
secundum-type atrial septal d.
septal d. (SD)
sinus venosus atrial septal d.
supracristal ventricular septal d.
Swiss cheese d.
T cell d.
thallium uptake d.
transcatheter closure of atrial d.
transcatheter occlusion of atrial septal d.
ventilation/perfusion d.
ventricular septal d. (VSD)
ventricular septal heart d. (VSHD)
V̇/Q̇ d.

defects syndrome

defense
    antiproteolytic d.
defensin
    human beta d. 2 (HBD2)
defensiveness
    emotional d. (ED)
deferoxamine mesylate
defervesce
defervescence
defibrillate
    airway, breathing, circulation, d.
    (ABCD)
defibrillation (DF)
    automatic external d.
    biphasic waveform transthoracic d.
    cardiac d.
    d. device
    external d.
    life-saving d.
    Moe multiple wavelet hypothesis
    of atrial d.
    d. paddles
    d. patch
    public access to d. (PAD, P.A.D.)
    public access d. (PAD, P.A.D.)
    d. response interval (DRI)
    d. shock
    1-shock d.
    3-shock d.
    d. threshold (DFT, DT)
    d. waveform
defibrillator
    Alert Companion II biphasic d.
    Atrioverter implantable atrial d.
    automated external d. (AED)
    automatic electronic d.
    automatic external d. (AED)
    automatic implantable d. (AID)
    automatic internal d.
    biphasic d.
    cardiac resynchronization therapy d.
    (CRT-D)
    Cardioserv d.
    CodeMaster d.
    Contak CD 2 cardiac
    resynchronization therapy d.
    Contak Renewal 3 cardiac
    resynchronization therapy d.
    dual-chamber and VVI
    implantable d. (DAVID)
    electric d.
    Endotak lead d.
    external d.
    ForeRunner automatic external d.
    Gem II DR dual-chamber d.
    Gem DR implantable d.
    Guidant d.
    Guidant Triad d.
    Heart Aid 80 d.

    HeartStart MRx d.
    Hewlett-Packard d.
    d. implant
    implantable d.
    implantable atrial d. (IAD)
    InSync implantable cardioverter d.
    Intec implantable d.
    Jewel AF implantable d.
    Lifepak d.
    LifeVest wearable d.
    manual d.
    Marquette Responder 1500
    multifunctional d.
    Medtronic GEM automatic
    implantable d.
    Medtronic InSync Sentry cardiac
    resynchronization therapy d.
    Medtronic Micro Jewel II
    implantable d.
    Metrix implantable atrial d.
    d. paddles
    PD 2000 d.
    Philips Electronics' HeartStart
    Home D.
    Philips HeartStart Home OTC d.
    Porta Pulse 3 d.
    Powerheart automated external d.
    Prizm d.
    public access d. (PAD, P.A.D.)
    semiautomatic external d. (SAED)
    smart d.
    transvenous implantable d.
    d. unit
    Ventak Prizm dual-chamber
    implantable d.
    wearable d.
    Zoll PD 1200 external d.
defibrillator-monitor
    Powerheart d.-m.
deficiency, pl. **deficiencies**
    acetylcholinesterase d.
    acid maltase d.
    ADA d.
    adenosine deaminase d.
    alpha-1 antitrypsin d.
    antithrombin III d.
    antitrypsin d.
    apolipoprotein A1 d.
    carnitine d.
    complement component C1r d.
    congenital pseudocholinesterase d.
    C1r d.
    cystathionine synthase d.
    dopamine beta-hydroxylase d.
    enzymatic d.
    factor III d.
    familial apoA-I d.
    familial HDL d.
    familial high-density-lipoprotein d.

D

deficiency *(continued)*
    galactosidase d.
    glucosidase d.
    hemostatic d.
    heparin cofactor II d.
    hexosaminidase d.
    homogentisic acid oxidase d.
    HRF d.
    hydroxylase d.
    17-hydroxylase d.
    magnesium d.
    maltase d.
    Owren factor V d.
    protein-calorie d.
    protein C, S d.
    pseudocholinesterase d.
    selenium d.
    surfactant d.
    thiamine d.
    tissue plasminogen activator
      release d.
    vasopressor d.

deficit
    cognitive d.
    neurologic d.
    postoperative cognitive d. (POCD)
    pulse d.
    spectacular shrinking d.

definition
    endocardial d.

Definity
    D. contrast
    D. perflutren

deflated profile

deflation curve

deflazacort

deflectable
    d. circular-tipped self-expanding
      catheter
    d. quadripolar catheter

deflection
    atrial d.
    delta d.
    His bundle d.
    d. in His bundle in electrogram
    intrinsic d.
    intrinsicoid d.
    negative d.
    QS d.
    RS d.
    undulating d.

deflector

deformans
    arteritis d.
    endarteritis d.
    osteitis d.

deformation
    capacitor d.
    myocardial d.

deformity, pl. **deformities**
    bayonet d.
    buttonhole d.
    cervical spine d.
    gooseneck outflow tract d.
    hockey-stick d.
    joint d.
    parachute d.
    pectus d.
    pigeon breast d.
    shepherd's crook d.

degeneration
    angiolithic d.
    atheromatous d.
    cusp d.
    endothelial cell d.
    fatty d.
    fibrinoid d.
    glassy d.
    Mönckeberg d.
    mucoid medial d.
    myxomatous d.
    olivopontocerebellar d.
    Quain fatty d.
    spinocerebellar d.
    Wallerian d. (WD)

degenerative aortic stenosis

deglutition
    d. apnea
    d. mechanism
    d. murmur
    d. pneumonia
    d. syncope

Degos disease

degradation
    aortic d.

degranulation
    adenosine-induced mast cell d.
    goblet cell d.

degrees of freedom

Dehio test

dehiscence
    anular d.
    bronchial d.
    sternal d.

dehydrocholesterol (DHC)

dehydroemetine

dehydrogenase
    d. activity
    alpha-hydroxybutyrate d.
    11-beta-hydroxysteroid d.
    branched chain alpha ketoacid d.
      (BCKD)
    glucose-6-phosphate d. (G6PD)
    hydroxybutyrate d. (HBDH)
    lactate d.

lactic d. (LDH)
lactic acid d.
placental 11 b-hydroxysteroid d.
  type 2
pyruvate d. (PDH)
dehydromonocrotaline
Deklene II cardiovascular suture
Del
  D. Mar Avionics Scanner
  D. Mar Avionics three-channel
    recorder
Delaborde tracheal dilator
Delatestryl Injection
delavirdine
delay
  atrioventricular d. (AVD)
  A-V d.
  brachiofemoral d.
  conduction d.
  electromechanical d.
  intramyocardial conduction d.
  intraventricular conduction d.
  ischemia-induced intramyocardial
    conduction d.
  nonspecific intraventricular
    conduction d. (NSIVCD)
  radiofemoral d.
delayed
  d. afterdepolarization (DAD)
  d. cerebral ischemia (DCI)
  d. cerebral vasoconstriction (DCV)
  d. conduction
  d. contrast-enhanced cardiovascular
    magnetic resonance (DE-CMR)
  d. depolarization
  d. primary closure (DPC)
  d. pulmonary toxicity syndrome
    (DPTS)
  d. xenograft rejection (DXR)
delayed-type hypersensitivity (DTH)
Delbet sign
deletion
  allelic d.
  22q11 d.
delimitation
delineation
  endocardial border d.
delirium
  d. cordis
  D. Rating Scale
  toxic d.
delivery, pl. deliveries
  adaptive aerosol d. (AAD)
  closed-loop d.
  contrast medium d.
  energy d.
  oxygen d. (Do_2)
  pulmonary drug d.

radiofrequency energy d.
  d. wire
Delmege sign
Delorme thoracoplasty
Delphian node
Delrin
  D. frame of valve prosthesis
  D. heart valve
Delsym
delta
  d. deflection
  d. pressure (delta P)
  d. wave
Delta-Cortef Oral
delta P
  delta pressure
Deltasone Oral
Deltatrac
  D. II metabolic monitor
  D. II metabolic rate meter
Deltavasc
deltopectoral groove
Deltran disposable transducer
Demadex
  D. injection
  D. Oral
demand
  cardiac output d.
  d. delivery device
  d. hypoxia
  d. mode
  myocardial oxygen d.
  d. oxygen delivery system (DODS)
  d. pacemaker
  d. pacing
  d. pulse generator
demand-triggered
  ventricular d.-t. (VVD)
Demarquay sign
demeclocycline hydrochloride
dementia
  multiinfarct d.
  thalamic d.
  vascular d.
Demerol
demethylating agent
demineralization technology
Demos tibial artery clamp
Demser
denatonium benzoate
denatured homograft
**denaturing high performance liquid
  chromatography (DHPLC)**
dendritic
  d. cell
  d. lesion
Dendroaspis **natriuretic peptide (DNP)**
denervated

denervation
  cardiac sympathetic d.
  sinoaortic d. (SAD)
  d. supersensitivity
dengue fever
Denhardt solution
denileukin diftitox
Dennis dissecting scissors
densa
  lamina d.
dense
  d. hemiplegia
  d. thrill
densities (*pl. of* density)
densitogram
  ear d.
densitometry
  acoustic d.
  video d.
density, pl. densities
  dependent d.
  echo d.
  echogenic d.
  echo tissue d.
  full caloric d.
  hydrogen d.
  lipid core d.
  nontissue d.
  power spectral d. (PSD)
  proton d.
  spin d.
density-exposure relationship of film
dental
  d. antisnoring device
  d. barotrauma
dentis
  anterior d.
dentocariosa
  Rothia d.
dentrificans
  Alcaligenes d.
denudation
  endothelial d.
Denver pleural effusion shunt
deoxycorticosterone
deoxygenated hemoglobin
2-deoxyglucose
deoxyhemoglobin
deoxyribonuclease (DNAse, DNase)
  human recombinant d.
deoxyribonucleic acid (DNA)
15-deoxyspergualin
dependence
  nicotine d.
  oxygen d.
  use d.
dependency
  ventilator d.

dependent
  d. beat
  d. density
  d. edema
  exquisitely d.
  d. lobe
  non-CTI d.
  d. rubor
dephosphorylation
deplasmolysis
depletion
  glycogen d.
  volume d.
deployment
  high-pressure stent d.
  stent d.
depolarization
  alternating failure of response,
    mechanical, to electrical d.
    (AFORMED)
  atrial premature d. (APD)
  delayed d.
  diastolic d.
  His bundle d.
  intrinsic d.
  myocardial d.
  premature ventricular d. (PVD)
  rapid d.
  transient d.
  ventricular ectopic d. (VED)
  ventricular premature d. (VPD)
  d. wave
depolarization-repolarization
depolarizing
  d. afterpotential (DAP)
  d. drug
depolymerization
depolymerized porcine mucosal heparin
Depo-Medrol injection
Depopred injection
Depo-Provera injection
deposit
  calcium d.
  exogenous antigen d.
  intraalveolar d.
deposition
  aerosol d.
  amyloid d.
  calcium oxalate d.
  collagen d.
  immune-complex d.
  mitochondrial calcium d.
depot
  Androcur D.
  Lupron D.
Depot-Ped
  Lupron D.-P.
depreotide
  technetium d.

depressant
    cardiac d.
depressed
    d. cough response
    d. ejection fraction
    d. ST segment
    d. ventricular function
depression
    aldosterone d.
    cardiorespiratory d.
    circulatory d.
    downhill ST-segment d.
    downsloping ST segment d.
    horizontal ST-segment d.
    Hospital Anxiety and D. (HAD)
    junctional d.
    myocardial d.
    postanesthesia respiratory d.
    postdrive d.
    P-Q segment d.
    precordial ST d.
    reciprocal ST d.
    rectilinear ST-segment d.
    respiratory d.
    spreading d. (SD)
    ST-segment d. (STD)
    upsloping ST-segment d.
    vascular d.
    X, Y d.
depression-induced altered autonomic tone
depressor reflex
depressurization
deprivation
    sleep d.
Deproist Expectorant With Codeine
depth
    d. compensation
    echocardiographic coaptation d.
    d. of paralysis
    volumetric lung d. (Vp)
DEQ
    digital echo quantification
deranged fibrotic septa
derecruit
derecruitment
derivative
    bipyridine d.
    d. circulation
    ergotamine d.'s
    hematoporphyrin d. (HPD)
    JTV519 1,4-benzothiazepine d.
    methanesulfonanilide d.
    purified protein d. (PPD)
    quaternary ammonium atropine d.
    thiazolidinedione d.
derived 12-lead electrocardiogram
DermaFlex Gel
Dermalon suture

dermatan sulfate
dermatitidis
    Ajellomyces d.
    Blastomyces d.
    Wangiella d.
dermatitis, pl. **dermatitides**
    exfoliative d.
    livedoid d.
    stasis d.
    weeping d.
dermatomyositis (DM)
    anti-Jo-1-negative amyopathic d.
Dermatophagoides
    D. farinae
    D. pteronyssinus
dermonecrotic
Derra
    D. aortic clamp
    D. valve dilator
    D. vena caval clamp
DES
    diethylstilbestrol
    diffuse esophageal spasm
    drug-eluting stent
Desai
    D. VectorCath
    D. VectorCath mapping catheter
    D. VectorCath mapping system
desaturation
    arterial d.
    arterial oxygen d. (AOD)
    nocturnal d.
descendens
    aorta d.
    ramus anterior d.
    ramus posterior d.
descending
    d. anterior branch
    d. aorta (DA, DAo)
    left anterior d. (LAD)
    d. necrotizing mediastinitis (DNM)
    d. phlebitis
    d. posterior branch
    Stanford type B anterior d.
    d. thoracic aneurysm
    d. thoracic aorta (DTA)
    d. thoracic aorta-to-femoral artery (DTAFA)
    d. thoracic aorta-to-femoral artery bypass graft
    d. thoracic aortic-femoral-femoral (DTAF-F)
    d. thoracic aortofemoral-femoral bypass
descent
    barotrauma of d.
    rapid Y d.
    X, Y d.
Deschamps compressor

D

deserpidine
    methyclothiazide and d.
desert
    d. fever
    d. rheumatism
    D. Storm syndrome
desethylamiodarone
Desferal Mesylate
desferrioxamine
desflurane
desglycinamide-9-arginine-8-vasopressin
  (DGAVP)
desiccation
    mucous d.
designed after natural anatomy
Desilets-Hoffman
    D.-H. catheter introducer
    D.-H. sheath
desipramine hydrochloride
desirudin
deslanoside
desloratadine
desmethyldiazepam
desmin gene
desmoplastic
    d. mesothelioma
    d. small round cell tumor
desmopressin acetate (DDAVP, dDAVP)
desmosine
desmosome
desmoteplase
desoxycholate
    amphotericin B d.
desoxycorticosterone
desoxyephedrine
    phenacetin, aspirin, d. (PAD,
      P.A.D.)
Desoxyn
d'Espine sign
desquamated alveolar epithelial cell
desquamation
    peribronchial d.
desquamative
    d. alveolitis
    d. interstitial pneumonia (DIP)
    d. interstitial pneumonitis (DIP)
destabilization
    plaque d.
destruction
    alveolar d.
    apoptotic d.
    lung tissue d.
    plasmatic vascular d.
desulfatohirudin
    recombinant d.
desynchronized sleep
DET
    dipyridamole echocardiography test
detachable embolization coil

detachment velocity
detection
    d. algorithm
    atrial fibrillation d.
    automated border d. (ABD)
    automated edge d.
    automatic boundary d. (ABD)
    coincidence d.
    echocardiographic automated
      border d.
    edge d.
    d. enhancement
    manual edge d.
    microarousal d.
    molecular coincidence d. (MCD)
    noninvasive d.
    shunt d.
    single-photon d.
detective quantum efficiency
detector
    ambulatory nuclear d.
    Cardioscint ambulatory vest d.
    Cardioscint nuclear d.
    colorimetric d.
    C-Vest ambulatory radionuclide d.
    Doppler blood flow d.
    multihead d.
    TubeChek esophageal intubation d.
detect time
Detensol
detergent worker's lung
deterioration
    d. following improvement (DFI)
    structural valve d. (SVD)
Determann syndrome
determination
    acid-base d.
    metabolic parameter d.
    serial enzyme d.
detrusor-sphincter dyssynergia
Detsky
    D. modified risk index
    D. score
detumescence
deuterosome
devascularization
DeVega tricuspid valve annuloplasty
Devereux formula
Devereux-Reichek method
deviation
    abnormal left axis d. (ALAD)
    abnormal right axis d. (ARAD)
    axis d.
    left axis d. (LAD)
    right axis d. (RAD)
    ST d.
    standard d.
    ST-T d.
    tracheal d.

device

abdominal aortic counterpulsation d. (AACD)
abdominal left ventricular assist d. (ALVAD)
Abiomed implantable heart-replacement d.
ablative d.
acapella chest physical therapy d.
access d.
Accutorr oscillometric d.
Accutracker blood pressure d.
ACIST CVi d.
Acorn CorCap cardiac support d.
ACS anchor exchange d.
acute ventricular assist d. (AVAD)
Adams-DeWeese d.
advanced venous access d.
AeroChamber spacing d.
Aerosomes drug delivery d.
AERx drug delivery d.
A-MED percutaneous ventricular assist d.
AME tongue retaining d.
A-mode echo-tracking d.
Amplatzer d.
Amplatz thrombectomy d. (ATD)
Amplatz ventricular septal defect d.
Anaconda d.
AngioGuard catheter d.
AngioGuard embolic protection d.
AngioGuard filter d.
AngioGuard XP emboli protection d.
AngioJet Xpeedior d.
Angio-Seal hemostatic puncture closure d.
Angio-Seal vascular closure d.
Aquatherm radiant heat d.
arachnophlebectomy surgical d.
arrhythmia control d. (ACD)
Arrow-Clarke thoracentesis d.
Arrow LionHeart heart assist d.
Arrow LionHeart left ventricular assist d.
ASD closure d.
assist d.
Atrioverter implantable defibrillator d.
AutoAdjust CPAP d.
automatic d.
AutoSet CS d.
AutoSet Portable II Plus d.
autotitration d.
AVA 3Xi advanced venous access d.
Babyhaler spacer d.
bag-mask ventilation d.
bag-valve d.

Baladi Inverter d.
balloon catheter sealing d.
B-D TwinPak dual cannula d.
bilevel positive pressure d.
biventricular assist d. (BVAD, BIVAD)
biventricular pacing and defibrillator d. (BiV-ICD)
blood flow enhancement d.
Breas PV10 CPAP d.
buttoned d.
BVM d.
Carbomedics valve d.
cardiac automatic resuscitative d. (CARD)
cardiac resynchronization d.
cardiac stretch d.
Cardiomemo d.
Cardio-Path plaque excision d.
Cath-Lok catheter locking d.
central venous access d. (CVAD)
centrifugal left and right ventricular assist d.
Chemo-Port perivena catheter system d.
Cholestron Pro II handheld d.
Chuter endovascular d.
Circulaire aerosol drug delivery d.
Circulaire inhaled medication delivery d.
CirKuit-Guard d.
Clamshell II d.
clearance assistive d.
Clearglide precision bipolar d.
closed-loop d.
Clo-Sur P.A.D. external vascular closure d.
Clot Buster Amplatz thrombectomy d.
Coapsys d.
Colapinto compression d.
Colin VP-2000 automatic measuring d.
Concerto CRT-D d.
CorCap cardiac support d.
CPI Mini d.
cutting balloon Ultra^2 Monorail d.
CVIS imaging d.
CVProfilor DO-2020 cardiovascular profiling d.
DeBakey-NASA axial-flow ventricular-assist d.
DeBakey VAD child d.
debulking d.
defibrillation d.
demand delivery d.
dental antisnoring d.
Digiflator digital inflation d.

D

device (*continued*)

Dinamap automated blood pressure d.
directional atherectomy d.
displacement sensing d.
Doppler d.
double-disc ASD closure d.
double-umbrella d.
DPAP Stealth d.
Duett arterial closure d.
Duett vascular sealing d.
Durathane cardiac d.
El Gamal cardiac d.
emergency infusion d. (EID)
Enclose anastomosis assist d.
Enclose proximal anastomotic assist d.
Encore inflation d.
Endo Grasp d.
EpiClose d.
Epicor cardiac ablation d.
EPI FilterWire EX emboli protection d.
Equinox EEG acquisition d.
esophageal detection d. (EDD)
Everest disposable inflation d.
excluder d.
extended collection d.
external negative pressure d.
extraction atherectomy d.
ExtreSafe phlebotomy d.
EZ Hold manual compression d.
FemoStop inflatable pneumatic compression d.
fiberoptic delivery d.
Finesse cardiac d.
finger photoplethysmographic d.
FloSeal FAST sealing d.
Flutter hands-free chest percussion therapy d.
Flutter mucus clearance d.
ForeRunner automatic external defibrillator d.
Frontier 3 x 2 multi-chamber stimulation d.
Gianturco-Grifka vascular occlusion d.
Goetz cardiac d.
Goodale-Lubin cardiac d.
GoodKnight bilevel CPAP d.
grip torque d.
heart assist d.
HeartMate implantable ventricular assist d.
Helix clot buster thrombectomy d.
HemoBand hemostasis d.
HemoNIR portable cooximetry d.
hemostatic occlusive leverage d. (HOLD)

hemostatic puncture closure d. (HPCD)
Horizon CPAP d.
HSRA d.
ICD-ATP d.
Imed infusion d.
impedance threshold d. (ITD)
implantable circulatory support d.
implantable ventricular assist d. (IVAD)
implanted pacing d.
ImPulse elite oxygen conserving d.
In-Exsufflator respiratory d.
InfaMyst aerosol spray d.
Infiltrator local drug delivery d.
infusion d.
Innervasc percutaneous vascular access d.
InspirEase d.
Inspiron d.
Insuflon d.
InSync III CRT-P d.
InSync II Marquis CRT-D d.
InSync Maximo CRT-D d.
InSync Sentry CRT-D d.
Intellitemp EP energy management d.
Interceptor emboli protection d.
Interceptor wire distal protection d.
interrogation d.
intraaortic balloon d.
intracaval d.
intracorporeal ventricular assist d.
inverted buttoned d.
IVAC d.
Jewel AF implantable arrhythmia management d.
Jewel atrial fibrillation dual chamber d.
Kangaroo Web d.
Kendall sequential compression d.
King cardiac d.
King interlocking d.
lead locking D. (LLD)
left ventricular assist d. (LVAD)
Lehman cardiac d.
light Talker d.
Linx guidewire extension cardiac d.
Lock Clamshell d.
locking d.
D.'s, Ltd. pacemaker
mandibular advancement d. (MAD)
Matrix VSG sealing d.
MDILog therapy monitoring d.
mechanical circulatory support d. (MCSD)
mechanical ventricular assist d. (MVAD)

Medtronic Activa tremor control
therapy d.
Medtronic defibrillator implant
support d.
Medtronic external tachyarrhythmia
control D.
Medtronic-Hall d.
Medtronic-Hancock d.
Medtronic Hemopump cardiac
assist d.
Medtronic Inspire implantable d.
Medtronic InSync Maximo CRT-
D d.
Medtronic InSync Sentry CRT-D d.
Medtronic Jewel AF implantable
arrhythmia management d.
Medtronic Jewel 7219D and C d.
Medtronic Octopus tissue
stabilizing d.
microarousal scoring d.
MicroDigitrapper-S apnea
screening d.
MicroMed DeBakey ventricular
assist d.
Miltner constraint compliance d.
21 Mini d.
26 Mini II d.
Monarch 25 inflation d.
motorized transducer pullback d.
mucus clearance d.
Mullins cardiac d.
multi-chamber stimulation d.
Myosplint d.
Needle-Pro needle protection d.
NeoMend arterial closure d.
NeuroShield cerebral protection d.
NeuroShield emboli protection d.
Nit-Occlud d.
nonthoracotomy system
antitachycardia d. (NTS-AICD)
Novacor Diasys cardiac d.
Novacor left ventricular assist d.
Novel d.
O$_2$ Advantage oxygen
conserving d.
occlusion d.
Octopus tissue stabilizing d.
Olcott torque d.
OxiMax pulse oximetry d.
OxyALERT d.
pacing d.
Pavcnik Monodisk d.
PediPump ventricular assist d.
Perclose vascular closure d.
percutaneous thrombolytic d. (PTD)
percutaneous ventricular assist d.
(pVAD)
PerDUCER percutaneous pericardial
access d.

permanent occlusion d.
personal heart d. (PHD)
PET balloon atherectomy d.
phased array ultrasonographic d.
Philips Integris 3000 biplane digital
subtraction angiography d.
PhotoDerm VL d.
Pierce-Donachy Thoratec ventricular
assist d.
plaque-trapping d.
Pleur-evac d.
PlexiPulse compression d.
pneumatic peripheral circulation
improvement d.
POCT d.
point-of-care testing d.
portable aerosol delivery d.
portable monitoring d.
portable oxygen d.
Port-A-Cath d.
power infusion d.
PPCID sequential foot
compression d.
Prima total occlusion d.
Pro/Pel coating cardiac d.
Prostar Plus percutaneous vascular
surgical d.
Prostar XL hemostatic puncture
closure d.
pullback atherectomy d.
pulsatile assist d. (PAD, P.A.D.)
pulsatile ventricular assist d.
pulse delivery d.
pulse oximetry d.
QuicKlamp hemostasis d.
QuickSeal arterial closure d.
QuickSeal sealing d.
radiant heat d. (RHD)
Rashkind double umbrella d.
rate-adaptive d.
ReadMyHeart handheld ECG d.
RESPeRATE interactive
breathing d.
Respiradyne pulmonary function d.
Res-Q arrhythmia control d.
right ventricular assist d. (RVAD)
RotaLink rotational atherectomy d.
rotary atherectomy d.
rotary ventricular assist d.
rotational atherectomy d.
Rubicon filter d.
Sarns ventricular assist d.
Selute Picotip steroid-eluting d.
Sentinel ICD d.
sequential compression d. (SCD)
Servo Screen 390 ventilator
monitoring d.
Sideris adjustable buttoned d.

D

device *(continued)*
 Silent Night diagnostic and
  screening d.
 SilverHawk System plaque
  excision d.
 Smart CapnoLine O2 monitoring d.
 SmartFlow multiple lesion d.
 Smart MAC-Line O2 sedation
  monitoring d.
 snare d.
 Softclix lancet d.
 SomaSensor d.
 SphygmoCor Px Aortic BP Profile
  cardiovascular data collection d.
 Spider embolic protection d.
 SpideRX embolic protection d.
 STARFlex d.
 StatLock Arterial Plus
  securement d.
 stent-anchoring d.
 St. Jude cardiac d.
 subcutaneous tunneling d.
 Sub-Q-Set subcutaneous continuous
  infusion d.
 Sunshine Heart C-Pulse implantable
  mechanical heart assist d.
 SuperStitch suture-mediated d.
 surgical closure d.
 Surveyor recording d.
 Symbion cardiac d.
 Tandem cardiac d.
 TandemHeart centrifugal
  pump/ventricular assist d.
 TEC atherectomy d.
 Techstar d.
 Telectronics Guardian ATP 4210 d.
 d. therapy
 Thermedics cardiac d.
 Thermocardiosystems left ventricular
  assist d.
 Thoratec biventricular assist d.
 Thoratec cardiac d.
 Thoratec right ventricular assist d.
 Threshold PEP d.
 tiered-therapy antiarrhythmic d.
 tongue-retaining d. (TRD)
 TQa d.
 Trak Back pullback d.
 Tranquility Bilevel airway patency
  maintenance d.
 Tranquility Bilevel positive airway
  pressure therapy d.
 Tranquility Quest CPAP d.
 transcatheter d.
 transvenous d.
 Trapper catheter exchange d.
 Turboaire Challenger cold-air
  bronchial provocation d.
 Unilink anastomotic d.

 Valleylab Force 2 electrosurgical d.
 Vanguard d.
 Vascugel d.
 vascular hemostatic d. (VHD)
 vascular sealing d.
 VasoSeal vascular hemostasis d.
 VasoView balloon dissection d.
 venous access d. (VAD)
 VentrAssist d.
 ventricular assist d. (VAD)
 ventricular containment d.
 Venture demand oxygen delivery d.
 Veriflex cardiac d.
 Vingmed System Five d.
 Viringe vascular access flush d.
 wearable cardioverter-defibrillator d.
 Wizard disposable inflation d.
 X-Press suture-mediated d.
 Zipper antidisconnect d.
DeVilbiss
 D. nebulizer
 D. Pulmo-Aide LT compressor
devil's grip
Dew sign
dexamethasone
 oral inhalation d.
 d. sodium phosphate (DSP)
 d. suppression test
 d. systemic
Dexasone L.A.
dexchlorpheniramine maleate
DExE
 dipyridamole-exercise stress
  echocardiography
dexfenfluramine (dFEN)
dexiocardia (*var. of* dextrocardia)
dexmedetomidine HCl
Dexone LA
Dexon Plus suture
dexrazoxane
dexter
 bronchus principalis d.
 cor triatriatum d.
 lobus d.
 pulmo d.
Dexter-Grossman classification
dextra, gen. and pl. **dextrae**
 arteria pulmonalis d.
 ramus lobi medii arteriae
  pulmonalis dextrae
 valvula semilunaris d.
 vena pulmonalis inferior d.
 vena pulmonalis superior d.
dextran
 d. 1, 70
 high molecular weight d.
 low molecular weight d. (LMD)
 d. solution
 d. sulfate

dextri
　　fissura horizontalis pulmonis d.
　　foramen venarum minimarum
　　　atria d.
　　lobus azygos pulmonis d.
　　lobus medius pulmonis d.
　　pars intralobaris intersegmentalis
　　　venae posterioris lobi superioris
　　　pulmonis d.
dextroamphetamine
　　d. sulfate
　　d. toxicity
dextrocardia, dexiocardia
　　corrected d.
　　false d.
　　isolated d.
　　mirror-image d.
　　pulmonary hypoplasia, hypoplasia
　　　of pulmonary artery, agonadism,
　　　omphalocele/diaphragmatic
　　　defect, d. (PAGOD)
　　secondary d.
　　type 1-4 d.
　　d. with situs inversus
dextrocardiogram
dextrogastria
dextrogram
dextro isomer
dextromethorphan (DM)
　　acetaminophen and d.
　　carbinoxamine, pseudoephedrine, d.
　　chlorpheniramine, phenylephrine, d.
　　chlorpheniramine,
　　　phenylpropanolamine, d.
　　guaifenesin and d.
　　guaifenesin, phenylpropanolamine, d.
　　guaifenesin, pseudoephedrine, d.
　　promethazine and d.
　　pseudoephedrine and d.
**dextroposed transposition of great
　arteries**
dextropositioned aorta
dextroposition of heart
dextropropoxyphene
dextrorotation
dextrorphan
**dextrose 5% in water (D5W, D-5-W,
　D_5W)**
Dextrostat
Dextrostix
dextrothyroxine sodium
dextrotransposition
dextroversion of heart
dextrum
　　atrium d.
　　cor triatriatum d.
Dey-Lute Isoetharine
DF
　　defibrillation

DFA
　　direct fluorescent antibody
dFEN
　　dexfenfluramine
DFI
　　deterioration following improvement
D/Flex filter
DFP
　　diastolic filling period
　　diastolic filling pressure
DFT
　　defibrillation threshold
3DFT
　　3-dimensional Fourier transform
DG
　　diastolic gallop
　　DiGeorge
　　diglyceride
DGA
　　DiGeorge anomaly
DGAVP
　　desglycinamide-9-arginine-8-vasopressin
DGCR
　　DiGeorge chromosome region
　　DiGeorge critical region
DGS
　　DiGeorge sequence
　　DiGeorge syndrome
DGSCR
　　DiGeorge syndrome critical region
DG/VCF
　　DiGeorge/velocardiofacial
　　　DG/VCF syndrome
DH
　　dynamic hyperinflation
　　　Codiclear DH
　　　Decohistine DH
　　　Dihistine DH
DHBP
　　direct His bundle pacing
DHC
　　dehydrocholesterol
DHCA
　　deep hypothermia circulatory arrest
D.H.E. 45 injection
DHF
　　diastolic heart failure
DHPLC
　　denaturing high performance liquid
　　　chromatography
DiaBeta
diabetes
　　hypertension in d. (HID)
　　d. mellitus (DM)
diabetic
　　d. autonomic neuropathy (DAN)
　　d. cardiomyopathy
　　d. coma
　　d. diet

D

219

diabetic *(continued)*
    d. gangrene
    d. HDL
    d. nephropathy
    d. neuropathy
    d. phthisis
    d. retinopathy
    D. Tussin DM
    D. Tussin EX
    d. ulcer
diabeticorum
    necrobiosis lipoidica d.
Diabinese
diable
    bruit de d.
diacetate
    triamcinolone d.
diacylglycerate pathway
diacylglycerol lipase
diagnosis, pl. **diagnoses (Dx)**
    airway, breathing, circulation,
      differential d.
    differential d. (DDx)
    d. of exclusion
    obligatory differential d.
    preimplantation d. (PID)
    Prospective Investigation of
      Pulmonary Embolism D.
      (PIOPED)
diagnostic
    d. algorithm
    d. aspiration
    d. bronchoscopy
    d. catheterization
    computer-assisted d. (CAD)
    d. electrophysiology
    d. electrophysiology procedure
    d. evaluation
    d. HRCT
    d. imaging agent
    d. peritoneal lavage (DPL)
    sleep d.
    d. ultrasound imaging catheter
diagnostic-related group (DRG)
diagonal
    d. coronary artery
    d. coronary bypass
    left anterior descending d. (LADD)
diagram
    Dieuaide d.
    ladder d.
    pressure-volume d.
Dialog pacemaker
dialysis
    continuous cyclical peritoneal d.
      (CCPD)
    peritoneal d.
    renal d.
dialyzer

diameter
    aerodynamic mass d.
    anteroposterior thoracic d.
    central venous luminal d.
    count median d. (CMD)
    count median aerodynamic d.
      (CMAD)
    end-diastolic d. (EDD)
    external d. (ED)
    geometric mean d. (GMD)
    D. Index Safety System (DISS)
    injury d.
    inlet d.
    internal d.
    internal orifice d. (IOD)
    left atrial d.
    left ventricular end-diastolic d.
      (LVEDD)
    left ventricular internal diastolic d.
      (LVIDD)
    luminal d.
    LV end-diastolic d.
    mass median aerodynamic d.
      (MMAD)
    mean luminal d. (MLD)
    mean reference d. (MRD)
    media-to-media d.
    minimal luminal d. (MLD)
    minimum lumen d. (MLD)
    outer d. (OD)
    particulate matter less than 10
      micrometers in d. (PM10)
    reference vessel d. (RVD)
    relative vessel d. (RVD)
    right atrium d. (RAD)
    right ventricular end-diastolic d.
      (RVEDD)
    d. stenosis (DS)
    stretched d.
    total end-diastolic d. (TEDD)
    total end-systolic d. (TESD)
    transverse cardiac d. (TCD)
    transverse heart d. (THD)
diamine oxidase (DO)
diaminobenzidine tetrahydrochloride
diamond
    D. classification
    d. ejection murmur
diamond-coated bur
Diamond-Forrester table
Diamond-Lite titanium instrument
diamond-shaped
    d.-s. ejection murmur
    d.-s. tracing
Diamox
diaphanoscopy
diaphoresis
diaphragm
    central tendon of d.

costal part of d.
crural d.
dome of d.
eventrated d.
eventration of d.
left crus of d.
lumbar part of d.
d. phenomenon
right crus of d.
d. of stent
sternal part of d.
d. transducer
vertebral part of d.
diaphragma
musculus d.
diaphragmalgia
diaphragmatic
d. artery
d. dysfunction
d. excursion
d. fatigue resistance
d. flutter
d. hernia
d. myocardial infarction (DMI)
d. pacing
d. paralysis
d. pericardium
d. phenomenon
d. pleura
d. pleurisy
d. respiration
d. rupture
d. surface
d. surface of heart
diaphragmatica
facies d.
pleura d.
diaphragmatis
centrum tendineum d.
crus dextrum d.
crus sinistrum d.
pars costalis d.
pars lumbalis d.
Diaqua
diary
event d.
Holter d.
sleep d.
DiaryCard
diarylquinoline
diaschisis
crossed cerebellar d. (CCD)
Diasonics transducer
diaspirin cross-linked hemoglobin (DCLHb)
diastasis cordis
diastatic
Diastat vascular access graft
diastema

diaster
diastole (D)
atrial d.
cardiac d.
electrical d.
late d.
ventricular d.
diastolic
d. afterpotential
d. amplitude time index (DATI)
d. aortic pressure (DAP)
d. blood pressure (DBP)
d. blow
d. bulging
d. closing velocity
d. current
d. current of injury
d. decrescendo murmur
d. depolarization
d. descent rate (DDR)
d. filling
d. filling pattern
d. filling period (DFP)
d. filling pressure (DFP)
d. fluttering
d. fluttering aortic valve
d. function
d. gallop (DG)
d. grunt
d. heart disease
d. heart failure (DHF)
d. hump
d. hypertension
d. lumen
d. motion
d. murmur (DM)
d. overload
d. potential
d. pressure (DP, Pd)
d. pressure-flow relationship (DPFR)
d. pressure gradient
d. pressure-time index (DPTI)
d. pressure-volume relation
pulmonary artery d. (PAD, P.A.D.)
d. pulmonary artery pressure
d. pulmonic regurgitation velocity
pulsed d. (PD)
d. relaxation
d. reserve
d. rumble
d. shock
d. slope
d. stiffness
d. suction
d. thrill
d. upstroke
d. velocity integral (DVI)

D

diastolic (*continued*)
    d. ventricular dysfunction
    d. wave
diastology
diathermy
diathesis, pl. **diatheses**
    allergic d.
    bleeding d.
diatrizoate
    sodium meglumine d.
diazepam
diazine
diazoxide
Dibenzyline
DIC
    diffuse intravascular coagulation
    disseminated intravascular coagulation
    disseminated intravascular coagulopathy
dichloramine
dichloroacetate (DCA)
    sodium d.
dichloroisoprenaline
dichloroisoproterenol
dichlorphenamide
dichotomization
dichotomy
diclofenac
dicloxacillin sodium
DICOM
    digital imaging and communications in
      medicine
      DICOM acquisition station
dicrotic
    d. notch (DN)
    d. pulse
    d. wave
dicrotism
dicumarol
dicumyl peroxide
didanosine (ddI)
didehydrodideoxythymidine
dideoxycytidine (ddC)
dideoxyinosine
dideoxynucleoside
dielectrography
diesel exhaust
diet
    AHA type I d.
    American Heart Association No-
      Fad D.
    American Heart Association type
      I d.
    arthrogenic d.
    Atkins d.
    betaine d.
    bland d.
    calorie-restricted d.
    cardiac d.
    diabetic d.

    Healthy Heart d.
    high-fiber d.
    Karell d.
    Kempner d.
    LFC d.
    low-fat d.
    low-methionine d.
    low-salt d.
    low sodium d.
    Mediterranean d.
    NCEP Step-One d.
    Ornish d.
    Portagen d.
    prudent d.
    renal d.
    salt-free d.
    Sauerbruch-Herrmannsdorfer-
      Gerson d.
    South Beach d.
    Step-One D.
    Step-Two D.
    d. and stress management in
      angina (DSMA)
    vegetarian d.
    very low calorie d. (VLCD)
dietary
    d. approach
    d. approaches to stop hypertension
      (DASH)
    d. fat
    d. fiber
    d. salt
    d. sodium
Dieterle stain
diethylcarbamazine citrate
diethylenetriamine
diethylenetriaminepentaacetate (DTPA)
    d. aerosol inhalation lung
      scintigraphy
**diethylenetriaminepentaacetic acid
  (DPTA, DTPA)**
diethylstilbestrol (DES)
Dieuaide
    D. diagram
    D. sign
difference
    alveolar-arterial PO_2 d. $(AaPO_2)$
    arterial-venous oxygen content d.
    arteriovenous oxygen d. $(AVDO_2)$
    nasal potential d.
    pulmonary A-V O_2 d.
differens
    pulsus d.
differential
    d. blood count
    d. blood pressure
    d. bronchospirometry
    d. diagnosis (DDx)

d. pressure transducer
d. stethoscope
differentiated ECG
differentiation
echocardiographic d.
pressure pulse d.
difficult airway
difficulty, pl. **difficulties**
rating of perceived breathing d.
(RPBD)
Diff-Quik stain
diffuse
d. airways disease
d. alveolar damage (DAD)
d. alveolar hemorrhage (DAH)
d. arterial ectasia
d. bronchopneumonia
d. cutaneous scleroderma
d. esophageal spasm (DES)
d. infiltrative lung disease (DILD)
d. in-stent restenosis
d. interstitial infiltrate
d. interstitial lung disease (DILD)
d. interstitial pulmonary fibrosis
d. intimal thickening
d. intravascular coagulation (DIC)
d. intraventricular block
d. lung injury
d. malignant mesothelioma (DMM)
d. malignant pleural mesothelioma
(DMPM)
d. obstructive emphysema
d. obstructive pulmonary syndrome
(DOPS)
d. panbronchiolitis (DPB)
d. parenchymal disease
d. paroxysmal slowing
d. pleurisy
d. pulmonary lymphangiomatosis
d. pulmonary ossification
d. sclerosing alveolitis
d. vasospasm
diffusing
d. capacity
d. capacity of lung (DL)
d. capacity of lung for carbon
monoxide (DLCO)
diffusion
d. anoxia
d. capacity
centripetal d.
coefficient of d.
d. hypoxia
lung d.
molecular d.
d. MRI
d. respiration
single-breath d.
d. tensor imaging (DTI)

diffusion-weighted
d.-w. imaging (DWI)
d.-w. MRI
diffusometry
NMR d.
diffusum
angiokeratoma corporis d.
Diflucan
D. injection
D. Oral
diflunisal
diftitox
denileukin d.
DIG
Digitalis Investigation Group
Digoxin Investigators Group
DiGeorge
D. anomaly (DG, DGA)
D. chromosome region (DGCR)
D. critical region (DGCR)
D. sequence (DGS)
D. syndrome (DGS)
D. syndrome critical region
(DGSCR)
DiGeorge/velocardiofacial (DG/VCF)
digestive system vascular disease
Digibind
D. digoxin immune Fab fragments
D. pneumatonometer
Digidote digoxin immune Fab fragments
Digiflator digital inflation device
digital
d. angiography (DA)
d. averaging
d. calipers
d. cardiac imaging (DCI)
D. Cardiac Imaging system
d. clubbing
d. color Doppler velocity
integration method
d. color Doppler velocity profile
integration
d. computer
d. echo quantification (DEQ)
d. endarteropathy
d. fluoroscopic unit
d. imaging and communications in
medicine (DICOM)
d. interchange standards for
cardiology (DISC)
d. necrosis
d. phase mapping (DPM)
d. pulse plethysmography (DPP)
d. radiography
d. runoff
d. smoothing
d. subtraction
d. subtraction angiography (DSA)

D

digital *(continued)*
  d. subtraction angiography mask image
  d. subtraction arteriography
  d. subtraction echocardiography (DSE)
  d. subtraction imaging
  d. subtraction supravalvular aortogram
  d. subtraction supravalvular aortography
  d. subtraction technique
  d. vascular imaging (DVI)
  d. vascular imaging system (DVIS)
  d. vascular reactivity (DVR)
  d. videoangiography
digitalate pulse
Digitaline
Digitalis
  D. *lanata*
  D. *purpurea*
digitalis
  d. effect
  d. glycoside
  d. intoxication
  D. Investigation Group (DIG)
  d. sensitivity
  d. toxicity
digitalis-specific antibody
digitalization
digitalize
Digitek
digitization
digitized caliper method
digitizer
  Bitpad d.
digitizing pad
digitoxicity
digitoxin
Digitrapper
  D. pH 400 ambulatory 24-hour pH recorder
  D. pH 400 monitor
digit span memory test
diglyceride (DG)
digoxigenin
digoxigenin-labeled DNA probe
digoxin (DO)
  d. effect
  d. immune Fab
  d. intoxication
  D. Investigators Group (DIG)
  d. level
  d. reduction product (DRP)
  D. RIA Bead
  d. toxicity
digoxin-induced hyperkalemia (DIH)
digoxin-like immunoreactive substance (DLIS)

digoxin-specific Fab
DIH
  digoxin-induced hyperkalemia
Dihistine
  D. DH
  D. Expectorant
dihydralazine
dihydrochloride
  azimilide d.
dihydrocodeine
dihydroergotamine mesylate
dihydropyridine calcium antagonist
dihydroxyphenylalanine
dihydroxypropyltheophylline
diisocyanate
  d. asthma
  diphenylmethane d.
  hexamethylene d.
  methylene diphenyl d. (MDI)
  toluene d. (TDI)
Dilacor XR
Dilantin
dilatable lesion
dilatancy
dilatation *(var. of* dilation*)*
dilated
  d. cardiomyopathy (DCM)
  d. cardiomyopathy and atrial fibrillation (DCAF)
dilating forceps
dilation, dilatation
  aneurysmal d.
  anular d.
  aortic d.
  ascending aorta d.
  balloon d. (BD)
  bootstrap d.
  bougie d.
  brusque d.
  cardiac d.
  catheter d.
  chamber d.
  endothelial-dependent arterial d.
  esophageal d.
  finger d.
  flow-mediated d. (FMD)
  d. of heart
  idiopathic right atrial d.
  interventional d.
  intrapulmonary vascular d.
  left ventricular cavity d.
  lymphatic d.
  nitroglycerin-induced d.
  onion bulb d.
  oscillating d.
  percutaneous transluminal d. (PTD)
  percutaneous transluminal balloon d. (PTBD)
  portal vein d. (PVD)

poststenotic d. (PSD)
d. pressure
reactive d.
sequential d.
serial d.
2-step d.
d. thrombosis
transient ischemic d. (TID)
venous d.
ventricular d.

dilator
Achiever balloon d.
AirMax external nasal d.
Amplatz d.
Bakes d.
Blue Rhino d.
Breathe with EEZ nasal d.
Brown-McHardy pneumatic d.
Cooley d.
Delaborde tracheal d.
Derra valve d.
Einhorn esophageal d.
14-French punch d.
Garrett d.
graded d.
Maloney mercury-filled
    esophageal d.
mitral valve d.
Mullins d.
Nozovent nasal valve d.
Quantum TTC balloon d.
Savary-Gilliard esophageal d.
d. and sheath technique
Silent Nite external nasal d.
Tubbs d.
ventricular d. (VD)
vessel d.
dilator-sheath system
Dilatrate-SR
DILD
diffuse infiltrative lung disease
diffuse interstitial lung disease
DILE
drug-induced lupus erythematosus
dilevalol
Dilor
Diltia XT
diltiazem
enalapril and d.
d. HCl extended-release tablet
d. hydrochloride
dilute blood clot lysis (DBCL)
dilution
gas d.
helium d.
thermal-dye d. (TDD)
transpulmonary thermal-dye d.
DILV
double-inlet left ventricle

Dimacol Caplets
dimenhydrinate
dimension
anteroposterior d.
aortic root d.
effective airspace d. (EAD)
end-diastolic d. (EDD)
end-systolic d. (ESD)
left atrial d.
left ventricular d. (LVDI)
left ventricular end-diastolic d.
    (LVEDD)
left ventricular end-systolic d.
    (LVESD)
left ventricular internal d. (LVID)
left ventricular internal diastolic d.
    (LVIDD)
left ventricular systolic d. (LVSD)
maximum transverse thoracic d.
right ventricular d. (RVD)
right ventricular internal d. (RVID)
superoinferior d.
2-dimensional (2D)
2-d. echocardiography (2DE)
2-d. integrated backscatter
2-d. tag
2-d. transcranial color-coded
    sonography (2D-TCCS)
3-dimensional (3D)
3-d. echocardiography (3DE)
3-d. Fourier transform (3DFT)
3-d. helical computed tomography
3-d. intravascular ultrasound
3-d. MSPECT software
3-d. reconstruction
3-d. spoiled gradient-recalled
    acquisition image
3-d. tagged magnetic resonance
    imaging
3-d. time-of-flight (3DTF)
3-d. time-of-flight magnetic
    resonance angiography
3-d. transesophageal echocardiogram
    (3D TEE)
dimensionality in imaging
dimer
excited d.'s
dimethyl
d. hydrazine
d. sulfate
d. sulfoxide
dimethylarginine
asymmetric d. (ADMA)
symmetric d.
1,1-dimethylbiguanide
dimethyl-L-arginine
dimorphic fungus
dimorphism

D

dimple
 blind coronary d.
 coronary ostial d.
Dinamap
 D. Accutorr A1, A3 blood
  pressure monitor
 D. automated blood pressure device
 D. blood pressure cuff
 D. pulse oximeter
 D. system
 D. ultrasound blood pressure
  manometer
dinitrate
 isosorbide d. (ISDN)
dinitrile
 pyridazinone d.
dinucleotide
 nicotinamide adenine d. (NAD)
diode
 light-emitting d. (LED)
 Zener d.
Diomycin
Diovan HCT
dioxide
 carbon d. (CO_2)
 chlorine d.
 end-tidal carbon d. ($ETCO_2$)
 fraction of expired carbon d.
  ($FECO_2$)
 fraction of inspired carbon d.
  ($FICO_2$)
 nitrogen d. (NO_2)
 partial pressure of carbon d.
  (pCO_2)
 selenium d.
 sulfur d. (SO_2)
DIP
 desquamative interstitial pneumonia
 desquamative interstitial pneumonitis
dip
 a d.
 Cournand d.
 midsystolic d.
 d. phenomenon
 septal d.
 type I, II d.
dipalmitoyl
 d. phosphatidylcholine (DPPC)
 d. phosphatidylcholine test
dip-and-plateau pattern
dipeptidyl peptidase
diphasic
 d. complex
 d. P, T wave
Diphen Cough
Diphenhist
diphenhydramine (DPHM)
 d. hydrochloride

diphenylhydantoin
diphenylmethane diisocyanate
diphosphate
 adenosine d. (ADP)
 histamine d.
5′-diphosphate
2,3-diphosphoglycerate (2,3-DPG)
diphosphonate
 methylene d. (MDP)
 technetium-99m methylene d.
diphtheria
 d. antitoxin
 d. and tetanus toxoid
 d., tetanus toxoids, acellular
  pertussis vaccine
 d., tetanus toxoids, whole-cell
  pertussis vaccine
 d., tetanus toxoids, whole-cell
  pertussis vaccine, *Haemophilus*
  type b conjugate vaccine
diphtheriae
 Corynebacterium d.
diphtherial tonsillitis
diphtheric
 d. paralysis
 d. pharyngitis
diphtherin
diphtheritic
 d. croup
 d. laryngitis
 d. myocarditis
 d. paralysis
 d. pharyngitis
diphtheroid
diplegia
 facial d.
diplocardia
diplococci
Diplococcus pneumoniae
dipole theory
dipper pattern
Diprivan injection
dipropionate
 beclomethasone d.
dipyridamole (D)
 d. and aspirin
 aspirin/extended-release d.
 d. echocardiography test (DET)
 d. handgrip test
 d. stress
 d. stress echocardiography
 d. thallium-201 scan
 d. thallium-201 scintigraphy
 d. thallium stress test
**dipyridamole-exercise stress
 echocardiography (DExE)**
dipyridamole-thallium imaging (DTI)
dipyrine

direct
> d. acute myocardial infarction angioplasty (DAMIA)
> d. amplification test (DAT)
> d. cardiac compression (DCC)
> d. cardiac massage
> d. cardiac puncture
> d. coronary angioplasty
> d. current (DC)
> d. current cardioversion (DCCV)
> d. current electric shock
> d. diaphragmatic irritation
> d. embolism
> d. excitation
> d. fluorescent antibody (DFA)
> d. Fourier transformation imaging
> d. His bundle pacing (DHBP)
> d. immunofluorescent stain
> d. insertion technique
> d. laryngoscopy
> d. lead
> d. mapping sequence
> d. mechanical ventricular actuation (DMVA)
> d. murmur
> Mycobacterium Tuberculosis D. (MTD)
> d. myocardial revascularization (DMR)
> d. percutaneous coronary intervention (d-PCI)
> d. respiration
> d. sinuatrial conduction time (DSACT, D-SACT)
> d. stenting
> d. stenting of coronary artery
> d. stimulation
> d. thrombin inhibitor

direct-current shock ablation
directed cough
directional
> d. atherectomy
> d. atherectomy catheter
> d. atherectomy debulking technique
> d. atherectomy device
> d. color angiography (DCA)
> d. coronary angioplasty (DCA)

directly
> d. observed therapy (DOT)
> d. observed treatment (DOT)

dirithromycin
Dirofilaria immitis
dirofilariasis
DIRP
> dose at the interventional reference point

dirty
> d. chest
> d. film
> d. lung

> d. lung appearance
> d. necrosis

Dirythmin
disability, pl. **disabilities**
> cardiovascular d.

disability-adjusted life year (DALY)
disappearance slope
disarray
> myocardial d.
> myofibrillar d.

disarticulation
> Burger technique for scapulothoracic d.
> chondral d.
> chondrocostal d.

DISA S-Flex coronary stent
DISA-SPECT
> dual-isotope simultaneous acquisition single-photon emission computed tomography

DISC
> digital interchange standards for cardiology

disc, disk
> atrial d.
> cervical d.
> intervertebral d.
> Molnar d.
> open atrial d.
> optic d.
> d. oxygenation
> d. oxygenator
> d. spring

disc-cage valve
discharge
> DC d.
> electric defibrillator using DC d.
> systolic d. (SD)

discission of pleura
discoid
disconnect
> airway pressure d. (APD)

discontinuity
> atrial-axis d.

discontinuous incremental threshold loading
discordance
> atrioventricular d.
> ventriculoarterial d.

discordant
> d. alternans
> d. alternation
> d. atrioventricular connection
> d. changes electrocardiogram
> d. ventriculoarterial connection

discovery, pl. **discoveries**
> D. DDDR pacemaker
> D. handheld spirometer
> D. portable spirometer

discrete
>   d. coronary lesion
>   d. subaortic stenosis (DSAS, DSS)
>   d. subvalvular aortic stenosis
>   (DSAS)
>   D. Technology coronary stent
>   system

discrimination
>   rhythm d.

disease (D)
>   Acosta d.
>   acquired valvular heart d. (AVHD)
>   acromegalic heart d.
>   acute cardiovascular d. (ACVD)
>   acute exacerbation of chronic
>   obstructive pulmonary d.
>   acute heart d. (AHD)
>   acute respiratory d. (ARD)
>   ACV d.
>   acyanotic heart d.
>   Adams d.
>   Adams-Stokes d.
>   Addison d.
>   adult congenital heart d. (ACHD)
>   airspace d.
>   alcoholic heart muscle d.
>   amyloid heart d.
>   Anderson-Fabry d.
>   antiglomerular basement
>   membrane d.
>   aortic aneurysmal d.
>   aortic thromboembolic d.
>   aortic valve d.
>   aortic valvular d. (AVD)
>   aortoiliac obstructive d. (AIOD)
>   aortoiliac occlusive d.
>   apple picker's d.
>   arrhythmogenic right ventricular d.
>   arterial occlusive d. (AOD)
>   arteriosclerotic cardiovascular d.
>   (ASCVD)
>   arteriosclerotic heart d. (AHD,
>   ASHD)
>   arteriosclerotic occlusive d. (AOD)
>   arteriosclerotic peripheral
>   vascular d. (ASPVD)
>   arteriosclerotic vascular d. (ASVD)
>   AS d.
>   aspiration-induced respiratory d.
>   asymptomatic coronary artery d.
>   (ACAD)
>   atherosclerotic aortic d.
>   atherosclerotic cardiovascular d.
>   (ACVD, ASCVD)
>   atherosclerotic carotid artery d.
>   atherosclerotic coronary artery d.
>   (ACAD, ASCAD)
>   atherosclerotic heart d. (AHD)
>   atherosclerotic hypertensive
>   cardiovascular d. (ASHCVD)
>   atherosclerotic occlusive d.
>   atherosclerotic peripheral vascular d.
>   (ASPVD)
>   atherosclerotic vascular d. (AVD)
>   atherothrombotic cardiovascular d.
>   atrioseptal heart d. (ASHD)
>   autoimmune thyroid d. (AITD)
>   autosomal-dominant familial aortic
>   aneurysm d.
>   aviator's d.
>   axial interstitial d.
>   Ayerza d.
>   Bamberger d.
>   Bamberger-Marie d.
>   Bannister d.
>   barometer-maker's d.
>   Battey d.
>   Bazin d.
>   Beau d.
>   Becker d.
>   Behçet d.
>   benign pleural d.
>   beryllium-induced lung d.
>   Besnier-Boeck-Schaumann d.
>   bilateral aortoostial coronary
>   artery d.
>   biliary d.
>   Binswanger d.
>   blackfoot d.
>   black lung d.
>   blood vessel d.
>   blue d.
>   Boeck d.
>   Bornholm d.
>   Bostock d.
>   Bouillaud d.
>   Bouveret d.
>   Bright d.
>   Brill-Zinsser d.
>   Buerger d.
>   bullous lung d.
>   Bürger-Grütz d.
>   Buschke d.
>   Busse-Buschke d.
>   caisson d.
>   calcific aortic valve d.
>   California d.
>   carcinoid heart d.
>   carcinoid valve d.
>   cardiac d. (CD)
>   cardiac allograft vascular d.
>   (CAVD)
>   cardiopulmonary d. (CPD)
>   cardiovascular d. (C, CD, CVD)
>   cardiovascular bifurcation d.
>   cardiovascular-renal d. (CVRD)
>   carotid artery d.

carotid occlusive d.
carotid vascular d.
Carrington d.
Castellani d.
Castleman d. (CD)
cat-scratch d.
cavitary lung d.
Ceelen d.
Ceelen-Gellerstedt d.
celiac d.
centrilobular axial interstitial d.
cerebrovascular d. (CeVD)
Chagas heart d.
Charcot-Marie-Tooth d.
cheese washer's d.
cheese worker's lung d.
cholesterol ester storage d. (CESD)
Christmas d.
chronic beryllium d. (CBD)
chronic cerebrovascular d. (CCVD)
chronic graft vascular d. (CGVD)
chronic hypertensive d.
chronic inflammatory airway d.
chronic interstitial lung d.
chronic obstruction outflow d.
  (COOD)
chronic obstructive airways d.
chronic obstructive lung d. (COLD)
chronic obstructive pulmonary d.
  (COPD)
chronic obstructive respiratory d.
  (CORD)
chronic peripheral arterial d.
  (CPAD)
chronic respiratory d. (CRD)
chronic restrictive pulmonary d.
  (CRPD)
chronic suppurative lung d.
  (CSLD)
chronic valvular heart d. (CVHD)
clinical cardiovascular d. (CCD)
cobalt-induced airway d.
cobalt-related lung d.
cold hemagglutinin d.
collagen vascular lung d.
Concato d.
congenital heart d. (CHD)
congenital polyvalvular d. (CPVD)
congestive heart d. (CHD)
congestive pulmonary d.
constrictive heart d.
Cori d.
coronary arteriosclerotic heart d.
  (CAHD, CASHD)
coronary artery d. (CAD)
coronary artery occlusive d.
  (CAOD)
coronary heart d. (CHD)
coronary microvascular d.

coronary occlusive d.
Corrigan d.
Corvisart d.
Crocq d.
cryptococcal pulmonary d.
cyanotic congenital heart d.
cyanotic heart d. (CHD)
cystic lung d.
cytomegalic inclusion d.
Daae d.
Danon d.
Darling d.
Davies d.
Degos d.
de novo d.
diastolic heart d.
diffuse airways d.
diffuse infiltrative lung d. (DILD)
diffuse interstitial lung d. (DILD)
diffuse parenchymal d.
digestive system vascular d.
Döhle d.
DRFS risk factors in coronary
  heart d.
drug-induced lung d.
Duke Databank for
  Cardiovascular D.
Duroziez d.
dust d.
Ebstein d.
effusive-constrictive d.
Eisenmenger d.
electrical d.
elevator d.
Emery-Dreifuss d.
endomyocardial d.
end-stage liver d. (ESLD)
end-stage renal d. (ESRD)
environmental lung d.
eosinophilic endomyocardial d.
epicardial coronary artery d.
Epstein d.
Erb-Goldflam d.
Erdheim d.
extracranial carotid d. (ECD)
extracranial carotid arterial d.
  (ECAD)
extracranial internal carotid d.
Fabry d.
Fahr d.
familial premature coronary
  heart d.
family history of heart d.
fibrocystic d.
fibroplastic d.
fibroproliferative d.
fish-meal worker's lung d.
flax-dresser's d.
flint d.

D

disease *(continued)*
 flow-limiting d.
 Fothergill d.
 Friedländer d.
 Friedreich d.
 fulminant peptic ulcer d.
 functional cardiovascular d.
 furrier's lung d.
 Gairdner d.
 gallbladder d.
 gannister d.
 gastroesophageal reflux d. (GERD)
 Gaucher d.
 giant bullous d.
 Gilchrist d.
 global cardiac d.
 global initiative of obstructive
  lung d. (GOLD)
 glycogen storage d. (type I-VIII)
 Goldflam d.
 Goldflam-Erb d.
 gold-induced lung d.
 gonadal d.
 graft coronary d. (GCD)
 graft-versus-host d. (GVHD)
 grain handler's d.
 granulomatous d.
 Graves d.
 grown-up congenital heart d.
  (GUCH)
 Hamman d.
 hand-foot-and-mouth d.
 Hand-Schüller-Christian d.
 hard metal d.
 heart d. (HD)
 Heller-Döhle d.
 hematologic d.
 hepatic d.
 heterogeneous d.
 Hodgkin d.
 Hodgson d.
 Horton d.
 Huchard d.
 humeroperoneal neuromuscular d.
 Hutinel d.
 hyaline membrane d. (HMD)
 hyaline-vascular type variant of
  Castleman d. (CD-HV)
 hypereosinophilic heart d.
 hypertension secondary to renal d.
  (HSRD)
 hypertensive arteriosclerotic
  cardiovascular d. (HASCVD)
 hypertensive arteriosclerotic heart d.
  (HASHD)
 hypertensive cardiovascular d.
  (HCVD, HTCVD)
 hypertensive heart d. (HHD,
  HTHD)

 hypertensive pulmonary vascular d.
  (HPVD)
 hypertensive vascular d. (HTVD,
  HVD)
 iatrogenic d.
 idiopathic venoocclusive d.
 immune-mediated d.
 immune restoration d. (IRD)
 inflammatory airway d.
 inorganic dust d.
 International Society for Adult
  Congenital Cardiac D. (ISACCD)
 Inter-Society Commission for
  Heart d.'s (ICHD)
 interstitial lung d. (ILD)
 intracranial atherosclerotic d. (IAD)
 intrastent recurrent d.
 intraventricular conduction d.
  (IVCD)
 intrinsic pulmonary vascular d.
 iron storage d.
 Isambert d.
 ischemic coronary d. (ICD)
 ischemic heart d. (IHD)
 isolated cerebral thromboangiitis
  obliterans d.
 Kawasaki d.
 Kennedy d.
 Keshan d.
 Kienböck d.
 Kikuchi d.
 kinky-hair d.
 Krishaber d.
 Kugelberg-Welander d.
 Kussmaul d.
 Kussmaul-Maier d.
 Leeuwenhoek d.
 left main d. (LMD)
 left main coronary d.
 left main coronary artery d.
  (LMCAD)
 left main stem coronary artery d.
  (LMS-CAD)
 Legionnaire d.
 Lemierre d.
 Lenègre d.
 Letterer-Siwe d.
 leukoencephalopathy d.
 Lev d.
 Lewis upper limb cardiovascular d.
 Libman-Sacks d.
 lipid coronary artery d. (LCAD)
 Little d.
 LMC d.
 Löffler d.
 lower extremity arterial d. (LEAD)
 Lucas-Championnière d.
 luetic d.
 lung parenchymal d.

lupus-associated valve d.
Lutz-Splendore-Almeida d.
Lyme d.
macrovascular artery d.
maple bark d.
Marek d.
McArdle d.
metastatic d.
microvascular artery d.
Mikity-Wilson d.
mineral-induced lung d.
mitral d. (MD)
mitral valve d. (MVD)
mixed aortic valve d. (MAVD)
mixed connective tissue d.
 (MCTD)
mixed mitral valve d. (MMVD)
Mondor d.
Monge d.
Morgagni d.
Morquio-Brailsford d.
Moschcowitz d.
moyamoya d.
multilobar d.
multisystem d.
multivalve d.
multivalvular d.
multivessel d. (MVD)
multivessel coronary artery d.
mushroom worker's d.
mycobacterial d.
myocardial d. (MD)
myxomatous valve d.
nail-patella d.
native coronary artery d.
Naxos d.
necrotizing arterial d.
neoplastic d.
neurodegenerative d.
neuromuscular d.
Niemann-Pick d.
nonculprit coronary artery d.
nonsegmental d.
nosocomial d.
obliterative vascular d.
obstructive airway d. (OAD)
obstructive lung d. (OLD)
occlusive d.
occupational-environmental lung d.
 (OELD)
occupational lung d.
oculocraniosomatic d.
organic heart d. (OHD)
Osler-Weber-Rendu d.
Owren d.
parenchymal d.
peribronchovascular d.
pericardial d.
peripartal heart d.

peripheral arterial d. (PAD, P.A.D.)
peripheral arterial occlusive d.
 (PAOD)
peripheral arteriosclerotic
 occlusive d. (PAOD)
peripheral atherosclerotic d.
peripheral conduction d.
peripheral interstitial d.
peripheral vascular d. (PVD)
pigeon breeder's d.
plasma cell-type variant of
 Castleman d. (CD-PC)
pleural d.
Plummer d.
pneumatic hammer d.
polycystic kidney d.
polysaccharide storage d.
Pompe d.
Posadas-Wernicke d.
primary electrical d.
primary myocardial d. (PMD)
primary pleuropulmonary d.
primary pulmonary parenchymal d.
prion d.
progression of coronary artery d.
 (PCAD)
proinflammatory d.
pseudo-heart d.
pulmonary parenchymal d.
pulmonary thromboembolic d.
 (PTED)
pulmonary valve d.
pulmonary vascular d. (PVD)
pulmonary vascular obstructive d.
 (PVOD)
pulmonary venooclusive d.
 (PVOD)
pulseless d.
Purkinje d.
Quincke d.
radiation-induced heart d. (RIHD)
radiation lung d.
ragpicker's d.
ragsorter's d.
Raynaud d.
reactive airways d. (RAD)
recalcitrant obstructive airways d.
Refsum d.
Reiter d.
renal artery d.
renal parenchymal d.
Rendu-Osler-Weber d.
Research Group on Instability in
 Coronary Artery D. (RISC)
respiratory bronchiolitis-interstitial
 lung d. (RB-ILD)
restrictive airways d.
restrictive heart d.
restrictive lung d.

D

disease *(continued)*
    reversible obstructive airways d. (ROAD)
    rheumatic heart d. (RHD)
    rheumatic valvular heart d. (RVHD)
    Roger d.
    Rokitansky d.
    Rosai-Dorfman d.
    Rougnon-Heberden d.
    Roussy-Lévy d.
    Sandhoff d.
    San Joaquin Valley d.
    saphenous vein graft d.
    Schaumann d.
    Shaver d.
    Shoshin d.
    shuttlemaker's d.
    sickle cell d.
    silo filler's d.
    single-vessel d. (SVD)
    sinus node d.
    Sjögren syndrome-associated interstitial lung d.
    skeletal myopathic d.
    slim d.
    Sly d.
    small airways d.
    Spatz-Lindenberg d. (SLD)
    spirochetal d.
    spontaneous coronary artery d. (SCAD, sCAD)
    Steinert d.
    stenotic valvular heart d.
    Still d.
    Stokes-Adams d.
    stress-related mucosal d. (SRMD)
    structural heart d. (SHD)
    subacute coronary d. (SCD)
    subclinical atherosclerotic d.
    sudden death heart d. (SDHD)
    sudden death ischemic heart d. (SDIHD)
    suspected coronary artery d.
    Sylvest d.
    symptomatic ischemic heart d.
    symptomatic peripheral arterial d.
    synchronous endobronchial d.
    Takayasu d.
    Takayasu-Onishi d.
    Tangier d.
    target organ disease/clinical cardiovascular d. (TOD/CCD)
    Taussig-Bing d.
    Tay-Sachs d.
    The Global Initiative for Chronic Obstructive Pulmonary D. (GOLD)
    Thomsen d.

    thromboembolic d. (TED)
    thyrocardiac d.
    thyroid d.
    thyrotoxic heart d.
    transplant coronary artery d. (TCAD, TxCAD)
    traumatic heart d.
    tricuspid valve d.
    TWAR d.
    Uhl d.
    unilocular hydatid d.
    unstable coronary artery d. (UCAD)
    valvular heart d. (VHD)
    van den Bergh d.
    Vaquez d.
    vascular d. (VD)
    vascular Parkinson d.
    vasospastic d.
    venoocclusive d. (VOD)
    vertebrobasilar occlusive d.
    3-vessel coronary d.
    vibration d.
    von Recklinghausen d.
    von Willebrand d.
    warfarin-aspirin symptomatic intracranial d. (WASID)
    Weber-Christian d.
    Weil d.
    Wenckebach d.
    Werlhof d.
    wheat weevil d.
    Whipple d.
    Wilkie d.
    Wilson d.
    Wilson-Kimmelsteil d.
    Winiwarter-Buerger d.
    winter vomiting d.
    Woillez d.
    Wolman d.
    wood pulp worker's lung d.
    woolsorter's d.
    woven coronary artery d.
    Yamaguchi d.
    Zamboni d.

diseased
    d. graft
    d. heart valve

disinfectant
    Control III Elite d.

disintegration rate

disk *(var. of* disc)

Diskhaler inhaler

Diskus
    Advair D.
    Flovent D.
    D. inhaler
    Serevent D.

dislodgment, dislodgement
    lead d.
dismutase
    Cu/Zn superoxide d.
    manganese superoxide d. (Mn-SOD)
    superoxide d.
disodium
    adenosine triphosphate d.
    cefotetan d.
    d. cromoglycate (DSCG)
    edetate d.
    ticarcillin d.
disopyramide phosphate
disorder
    acid-base d.
    arrhythmogenic d.
    autoimmune d.
    clotting d.
    conduction d.
    decompression d.
    dysbaric d.
    endocrine d.
    Fredrickson classification of
      lipid d.'s
    genetic d.
    glycosphingolipid d.
    iatrogenic d.
    International Classification of
      Sleep D.'s (ICSD)
    lipid d.
    lupus anticoagulant d.
    lymphocytic infiltrative d.
    mendelian d.
    mixed connective tissue d.
    movement d.
    multisystemic inflammatory d.
    neurological d.
    neuromuscular d.
    neuromyopathic d.
    panic d.
    periodic limb movement d.
      (PLMD)
    posttransplantation
      lymphoproliferative d. (PTLPD,
      PTLD)
    posttransplant lymphoproliferative d.
    sarcoid-like pulmonary d.
    Sheffield Screening Test for
      Acquired Language D.'s (STALD)
    single-gene d.
    skeletal myopathic d.
    sleep d.
    somatization d.
disordered action of heart (DAH)
disorganization
    segmental arterial d.
Disotate
dispar
    Entamoeba d.

dispatch
    D. balloon
    D. infusion catheter
    D. over-the-wire catheter
dispenser
dispersing electrode
dispersion
    aerosol bolus d. (AD)
    interlead QT d.
    intravoxel phase d.
    QT d. (QTd)
    QT interval d.
    QT/QTc d.
    d. of refractoriness
    Taylor d.
    temporal d.
dispersive electrode
displacement
    d. sensing device
    ST-segment d.
    d. waveform
display
    color kinesis echocardiographic d.
    liquid crystal d. (LCD)
    PerfTrak d.
    PerfTrak perfusion waveform d.
disposable
    d. electrode
    d. mapping catheter
    d. percutaneous entry thinwall
      needle
    d. pneumotachometer
    d. resuscitator bag
Disprin
disrupted plaque
disruption
    bronchial d.
    circadian d.
    great vessel d.
    plaque d.
    traumatic aortic d.
DISS
    Diameter Index Safety System
dissecans
    pneumonia d.
dissected tissue
dissecting
    d. aorta
    d. aortic aneurysm
    d. hematoma
    d. lamella
dissection
    acute aortic d. (AAD)
    acute type B aortic d. (ABAD)
    d. of aorta
    aortic d. (type A, B)
    arterial d.
    BioGlue surgical adhesive for
      aortic d.

D

dissection *(continued)*
blunt d.
coronary artery d.
DeBakey aortic d. (type I, II, III, IIIa, IIIb)
epiphenomena of d.
International Registry of Acute Aortic D. (IRAD)
intraluminal d.
long d.
spiral d.
spontaneous cervical artery d. (sCAD)
spontaneous coronary artery d. (SCAD, sCAD)
Stanford type A, B aortic d.
therapeutic d.
thoracic aortic d.

dissector
balloon d.
Holinger d.
SAPHfinder surgical balloon d.
SAPHtrak balloon d.
Spacemaker balloon d.

disseminated
d. aspergillosis
d. coccidioidomycosis
d. cryptococcosis
d. histoplasmosis
d. intravascular blood coagulation (DIVBC)
d. intravascular coagulation (DIC, DIVC)
d. intravascular coagulopathy (DIC)
d. lupus erythematosus
d. polyarteritis
d. tuberculosis

dissemination
hematogenous bacterial d.
micronodular d.

dissociation
atrial d.
atrioventricular d. (AVD)
A-V d.
complete atrioventricular d. (CAVD)
complete A-V d.
d. curve
electromechanical d. (EMD)
electromyocardial d.
incomplete atrioventricular d.
incomplete A-V d.
d. by interference
interference d.
intracavitary pressure-electrogram d.
isorhythmic d.
longitudinal d.

dissolution

distal
d. acinar emphysema
d. akinesia
d. anastomosis
d. balloon catheter (DBC)
d. bed
d. convoluted tubule
d. coronary occlusion pressure (DCOP)
d. coronary perfusion pressure
d. coronary sinus (DCS)
d. ectasia
d. intestinal obstruction syndrome
d. intestinal obstructive syndrome
d. lateral wall
d. perfusion system (DPS)
d. pyogenic abscess
d. reentry tear
d. runoff
d. shocking coil
d. splenorenal shunt
d. stenosis
d. vascular insufficiency
d. vessel embolization

distance
half-power d.
interelectrode d.
Mahalanobis d.
6-minute walk d. (6MWD)
walk d.

distant
d. breath sounds
d. heart sounds

distensibility
aortic d.
arterial d.
coronary artery d.
ventricular d.

distention, distension
jugular venous d. (JVD)
premature diastolic d.
d. waveform

disto-occlusal (DO)

distorted coarctation

distortion
peribronchovascular d.
pincushion d.

distress
respiratory d.

distribution
blood volume d.
Boltzmann d.
d. coefficient (Kd)
interstitial d.
microvascular flow d.
nonhomogeneous pulmonary time-constant d.
perilymphatic d.
perimetric d.

segmented extracardiac
   radioactive d.
smooth pseudo-Wigner-Ville d.
   (SPWVD)
stocking-glove d.
tracer d.
volume of d.
distributive shock
disturbance
conduction d.
electrolytic d.
d. of function occlusion syndrome
   (DOFOS)
rhythm d.
sleep d.
disturbed
d. circadian blood pressure pattern
d. flow
disulfide
d. bridge
carbon d.
glutathione d.
Dittrich
D. plug
D. stenosis
Diuchlor
Diulo
diurese
diuresis
loop d.
diuretic
d. agent
cardiac d.
high-ceiling d.
indirect d.
loop d.
osmotic d.
potassium-sparing d.
potassium-wasting d.
d. therapy
thiazide d.
Diurexan
Diuril
diurnal
d. peak flow variability
d. rhythm
d. sleep
d. variation
Diutensin-R
divarication
DIVBC
disseminated intravascular blood
   coagulation
DIVC
disseminated intravascular coagulation
divergens
Babesia d.
diversity
antigen binding d.

diver's syncope
diverticula (*pl. of* diverticulum)
diverticulectomy
Harrington esophageal d.
diverticuli
tracheal d.
diverticulum, pl. **diverticula**
apical d.
Heister d.
Kommerell d.
d. of Kommerell
laryngotracheal d.
tracheobronchial d.
Zenker d.
divided respiration
diving
d. air embolism
d. goiter
d. reflex
division
vascular ring d.
divisional heart block
Dixarit
dizziness
DKS
Damus-Kaye-Stansel
DKS operation
DL
diffusing capacity of lung
double lumen
DLCO
diffusing capacity of lung for carbon
   monoxide
DLCO$_c$
corrected diffusing capacity for carbon
   monoxide
DLIS
digoxin-like immunoreactive substance
D-looping
DLP cardioplegic needle
d,l-**sotalol**
DLT
double lung transplant
DM
dermatomyositis
dextromethorphan
diabetes mellitus
diastolic murmur
Anatuss DM
Carbodec DM
Cardec DM
Diabetic Tussin DM
Fenesin DM
Genatuss DM
Hold DM
Humibid DM
Iobid DM
Mytussin DM
Pseudo-Car DM

DM (*continued*)
    Respa DM
    Robafen DM
    Silphen DM
    Siltussin DM
    Tolu-Sed DM
    Touro DM
    Triaminic DM

Dm
    membrane diffusing capacity

DM-400 Holter ECG cassette recorder

DMI
    diaphragmatic myocardial infarction
    Doppler myocardial imaging
        DMI analyzer

DMM
    diffuse malignant mesothelioma

DMPM
    diffuse malignant pleural mesothelioma

DMR
    direct myocardial revascularization

DMVA
    direct mechanical ventricular actuation

DN
    dicrotic notch

DNA
    deoxyribonucleic acid
        DNA cloning
        DNA crosslinkage
        DNA histogram
        human cloned DNA (cDNA)
        DNA probe
        DNA sequencing
        DNA switch

DNA-coated stent

DNAR
    do not attempt resuscitation

DNAse, DNase
    deoxyribonuclease
        inhaled recombinant DNAse

DNI
    do not intubate

DNM
    descending necrotizing mediastinitis

DNP
    Dendroaspis natriuretic peptide

DNR
    do not resuscitate

DO
    diamine oxidase
    digoxin
    disto-occlusal

do
    do not attempt resuscitation
      (DNAR)
    do not intubate (DNI)
    do not resuscitate (DNR)

Doan
    Extra Strength D.'s
    D.'s Original

dobutamine
    d. atropine stress echocardiography
      (DASE)
    d. echocardiography (DE)
    d. holiday
    d. hydrochloride
    d. perfusion scintigraphy
    d. stress echocardiography (DSE)
    d. stress test

dobutamine-induced ischemia

docetaxel

Docke murmur

docking wire

dock wire

docosahexaenoic acid

documentation

Dodd perforating vein

dodecafluoropentane (DDFP)

dodecapeptide

Dodge area-length method

DODS
    demand oxygen delivery system

DOE
    dyspnea on exertion

dofetilide

DOFOS
    disturbance of function occlusion
     syndrome

dog
    d. boning
    d. cough

dog-leg catheter

Döhle
    D. disease
    D. inclusion bodies

Döhle-Heller aortitis

Dolacet

dolastatin

dolens
    phlegmasia alba d.
    phlegmasia cerulea d.

dolichoectatic aneurysm

dolichol

dolichostenomelia

Dolobid

dolore
    angina pectoris sine d.
    angina sine d.

dolosa
    Burkholderia d.

DOLV
    double-outlet left ventricle

domain
    time d.

dome
    d. of diaphragm
    d. excursion
dome-and-dart configuration
dome-shaped
domestica
    Carinia d.
dominance
    coronary artery d.
    T $_H$2-cell d.
dominant positive deflection flutter
doming
    d. of leaflet
    systolic d.
    tricuspid valve d.
domino procedure
domperidone
donation
    predeposit autologous d.
Donders pressure
Donné corpuscle
donor (D)
    d. heart
    d. organ ischemic time
    primary d. (d(A))
    unrelated d. (URD)
donor-acceptor (D-A)
donor-specific transfusion
door-to-balloon time
door-to-needle time
L-dopa
dopachrome oxidoreductase (DCOR)
Dopamet
dopamine
    d. antagonist
    d. beta-hydroxylase deficiency
    d. D2 receptor (DD2R)
    d. hydrochloride
dopaminergic
    d. agent
    d. function
Dopastat
dopexamine
Doppler
    Aloka color D.
    D. auto-correlation technique
    D. blood flow detector
    D. cardiography
    carotid D.
    D. 2-chamber view (D2CV)
    D. 4-chamber view (D4CV)
    D. color flow
    color flow D.
    D. color flow mapping (DCFM)
    D. color jet
    D. continuity equation
    continuous-wave D. (CWD)
    D. coronary catheter

    D. crystal
    D. deceleration time
    D. device
    D. echocardiography
    D. effect
    D. fetal heart monitor
    D. fetal stethoscope
    D. flow analysis
    D. flow probe
    FreeDop cordless D.
    D. index
    D. interrogation
    intravascular D.
    D. measurement
    D. myocardial imaging (DMI)
    D. peak flow velocity (Vmax)
    power M-mode transcranial D.
    D. pressure
    D. pressure gradient
    D. PR jet width
    pulsed myocardial D. (PMD)
    pulsed spectral D.
    pulsed-wave D. (PWD)
    pulsed-wave tissue D. (PWTD)
    quantitative D.
    D. recording
    D. shift
    D. signal
    D. sonography (DS)
    D. speckle
    spectral D.
    D. spectral analysis
    steady D.
    D. tissue imaging (DTI)
    D. transducer
    D. transesophageal color flow imaging
    D. ultrasonic flowmeter
    D. ultrasonography
    D. ultrasound
    D. velocimetry
    D. velocity probe
    D. velocity wire
    D. waveform analysis
Doppler-Cavin monitor
Doppler-derived index
Doppler-guided hemorrhoidal artery ligation
Doppler-tipped angioplasty guidewire
Dopram injection
DOPS
    diffuse obstructive pulmonary syndrome
Doptone monitoring
d'orange
    peau d'o.
Dorendorf sign
Dorian rib stripper
Dormin Oral

D

dornase
    d. alfa
    pancreatic d.
Dor procedure
dorsal
    carpal arch d.
    d. lingual branch
    d. lingual branches of lingual
        artery
    d. mesocardium
dorsalis pedis pulse
dorsi
    latissimus d.
dorsum linguae
DORV
    double-outlet right ventricle
Doryx Oral
dosage regimen
dose
    d. at the interventional reference
        point (DIRP)
    cumulative cardiotoxic d. (CCD)
    extra-fine particle d. (EFPD)
    fine particle d. (FPD)
    high heparin d. (HHD)
    maximum tolerated d.
    MIH d.
    minimum cumulative cardiotoxic d.
        (MCCD)
    nonpressor d.
    priming d.
    radiation absorbed d. (rad)
    subantihypertensive d.
    threshold d.
dose-effect curve dose-response curve
Dosepak
    Medrol D.
dose-volume histogram
dosimetry
dosing
    trough d.
Dos Santos needle
Dostinex
DOT
    directly observed therapy
    directly observed treatment
Dotter
    D. caged-balloon catheter
    D. effect
    D. intravascular retrieval set
    D. procedure
    D. technique
dottering
    d. effect
    d. of lesion
Dotter-Judkins
    D.-J. percutaneous transluminal
        angioplasty
    D.-J. technique

dotuse margin
double
    d. aortic arch
    d. aortic stenosis
    d. coronary artery bypass graft
        (DCABG)
    d. count
    d. counting
    d. ectopic tachyarrhythmia
    d. external direct current shock
    d. flexible tipped wire guide
    d. inlet atrioventricular connections
    d. lumen (DL)
    d. lung transplant (DLT)
    D. Play large-bore double Y
        hemostasis valve
    d. pleurisy
    d. pneumonia
    d. product
    d. simultaneous stimulation test
    d. strength (DS)
    d. switch procedure
    d. tachycardia (DT)
    d. umbrella
    d. umbrella closure
    d. valve replacement (DVR)
    d. ventricular extrastimulus
    d. ventricular response (DVR)
    d. voice
double-balloon
    d.-b. catheter
    d.-b. (9-11) technique
    d.-b. valvoplasty
    d.-b. valvotomy
double-barreled aorta
double-chain rt-PA
double-chip micromanometer catheter
double-disc
    d.-d. ASD closure device
    d.-d. occluder
double-dummy technique
double-flanged valve sewing ring
double-headed stethoscope
double-inlet left ventricle (DILV)
double-J
    d.-J catheter
    d.-J stent
double-lumen
    d.-l. endobronchial tube
    d.-l. Hickman catheter
    d.-l. sign
    venovenous d.-l. (VVDL)
double-oblique imaging
double-outlet
    d.-o. left ventricle (DOLV)
    d.-o. left ventricle malposition
    d.-o. right ventricle (DORV)
    d.-o. right ventricle malposition
double-rib fracture

double-sandwich IgM ELISA
double-sheath bronchial brushings
double-shock sound
double-syringe technique
doublet
double-thermistor coronary sinus
  catheter
double-umbrella device
double-wire technique
doubling time
doubly committed VSD
doughnut
    d. configuration
    d. sign
Douglas
    D. bag
    D. bag collection method
    D. bag technique
dove coo musical murmur
Dow
    D. Corning tube
    D. method
down
    D. flow generator
    D. syndrome (DS)
downgoing Babinski
downhill
    d. esophageal varix
    d. ST-segment depression
down-regulation
downsloping
    d. ST segment
    d. ST segment depression
downstream
    d. sampling method
    d. segment
    d. signaling cascade
    d. venous pressure (DSVP)
doxacurium
doxapram hydrochloride
doxazosin mesylate
doxepin hydrochloride
doxofylline
doxorubicin
    d. cardiomyopathy
    d. cardiotoxicity
    d., 5-fluorouracil, cisplatin (AFP)
    d. hydrochloride
doxorubicin-induced
    d.-i. cardiac toxicity
    d.-i. cardiomyopathy
Doxychel Oral
doxycycline pleurodesis
Doyen elevator
DP
  diastolic pressure
DPAP Stealth device
DPB
  diffuse panbronchiolitis

DPC
  delayed primary closure
d-PCI
  direct percutaneous coronary intervention
dP/dt_{MAX} end-diastolic volume
D-penicillamine
DPFR
  diastolic pressure-flow relationship
2,3-DPG
  2,3-diphosphoglycerate
D-Phe-L-Pro-L-Arg-chloromethyl ketone
  (PPACK)
DPHM
  diphenhydramine
DPI
  dry powder inhaler
DPL
  diagnostic peritoneal lavage
DPM
  digital phase mapping
DPP
  digital pulse plethysmography
DPPC
  dipalmitoyl phosphatidylcholine
    DPPC test
DPS
  distal perfusion system
    QuickFlow DPS
DPTA
  diethylenetriaminepentaacetic acid
DPTI
  diastolic pressure-time index
DPTS
  delayed pulmonary toxicity syndrome
DR-70 tumor marker test
drag
    d. force
    viscous d.
Dräger
    D. respirometer
    D. ventilator
drain
    Clot Stop d.
drainage
    anomalous pulmonary venous d.
     (APVD)
    autogenic d. (AD)
    closed chest water-seal d.
    external ventricular d. (EVD)
    hemianomalous pulmonary
     venous d. (HAPVD)
    partial anomalous pulmonary
     venous d. (PAPVD)
    percussion and postural d. (P&PD)
    postural d. (PD)
    pulmonary venous d.
    thoracic duct d. (TDD)
    total anomalous pulmonary
     venous d. (TAPVD)

D

drainage *(continued)*
    underwater seal d.
    water-seal suction d.
Dramamine Oral
Drapanas mesocaval shunt
drapeau
    bruit de d.
DR-Atrial TX implantable cardioverter-defibrillator
drawback stent deployment technique
dreamer clamp
dreaming sleep
dream pain
Drechslera hawaiiensis
dressing
    Clo-Sur P.A.D. d.
    Comfeel Ulcus d.
    Cutinova Hydro d.
    Kaltostat wound packing d.
    pressure applied d. (PAD, P.A.D.)
    stent d.
    Vigilon d.
    wet-to-dry d.
Dressler
    D. beat
    D. syndrome
DRFS
    Dundee rank factor score
    DRFS risk factors in coronary heart disease
DRG
    diagnostic-related group
DRI
    defibrillation response interval
drift
    antigenic d.
drill-tip catheter
drink
    HeartBar Orange D.
Drinker respirator
drip
    heparin d.
    postnasal d. (PND)
    silent postnasal d.
Dripps-American Surgical Association score
Dristan Sinus Caplets
drive
    central respiratory d.
    d. cycle length
    neuroendocrine d.
    respiratory d.
    d. train
    ventricular d.
driveline infection
driver
    D. coronary stent
    TLC-II portable VAD d.

Drixoral
    D. Cough & Congestion Liquid Caps
    D. Cough & Sore Throat Liquid Caps
    D. Nasal
Dromos pacemaker
dromotropic effect
dronabinol
droop
    facial d.
drop
    d. attack
    Ayr saline nasal d.'s
    falling d.
    d. heart
    Rondamine-DM d.'s
    Rondec D.'s
    Tussafed d.'s
droperidol
dropout
    septal d.
dropped
    d. beat
    d. lung sign
dropsy
    cardiac d.
    d. chest
    d. of pericardium
drowned
    d. lung
    d. newborn syndrome
drowning
    dry d.
drowsiness
    Tylenol Cold No D.
Droxia
DRP
    digoxin reduction product
drug
    d. abuse
    antiarrhythmic d. (AAD)
    antilipemic d.
    antituberculous d.
    cardiotonic d.
    d. clearance
    depolarizing d.
    hydrophobic d.
    hypnotic d.
    investigational new d. (IND)
    lipophilic d.
    neuroprotective d.
    nondepolarizing d.
    nonsteroidal antiinflammatory d. (NSAID)
    pressor d.
    sedative-hypnotic d.
    sympathomimetic d.

d. therapy
vasoactive d.
drug-associated pericarditis
drug-based regimen
drug-delivery stenting
drug-eluting stent (DES)
drug-induced
d.-i. cardiomyopathy
d.-i. lung disease
d.-i. lupus erythematosus (DILE)
d.-i. lupus syndrome
d.-i. pericarditis
d.-i. thrombocytopenia
drug-loaded biodegradable polymer stent
drug-refractory tachycardia
Drummond
marginal artery of D.
D. marginal artery
D. sign
dry
d. beriberi
d. bronchiectasis
d. bronchitis
d. cough
d. drowning
d. gangrene
d. pericarditis
d. pleurisy
d. powder inhaler (DPI)
d. rale
standard temperature and
pressure, d.
Drysdale corpuscle
DS
diameter stenosis
Doppler sonography
double strength
Down syndrome
duration of systole
Bactrim DS
Septra DS
Sulfatrim DS
%DS
percent diameter stenosis
DSA
digital subtraction angiography
DSACT, D-SACT
direct sinuatrial conduction time
DSAS
discrete subaortic stenosis
discrete subvalvular aortic stenosis
DSC
dynamic susceptibility contrast-enhanced
DSCG
disodium cromoglycate
DSC MRI
dynamic susceptibility contrast-enhanced
MRI

DSE
digital subtraction echocardiography
dobutamine stress echocardiography
DSI-III screw-in lead pacemaker
DSMA
diet and stress management in angina
D-sotalol block of HERG
DSP
dexamethasone sodium phosphate
DSPA
vampire bat salivary plasminogen
activator
DSS
discrete subaortic stenosis
DSVP
downstream venous pressure
DSX Sopha camera
DT
deceleration time
defibrillation threshold
double tachycardia
DTA
descending thoracic aorta
DTAFA
descending thoracic aorta-to-femoral
artery
DTAFA bypass graft
DTAF-F
descending thoracic aortic-femoral-
femoral
2D-TCCS
2-dimensional transcranial color-coded
sonography
3D TEE
3-dimensional transesophageal
echocardiogram
3DTF
3-dimensional time-of-flight
3DTF magnetic resonance
angiography
D-TGA, dTGA
D-transposition of great arteries
DTH
delayed-type hypersensitivity
DTI
diffusion tensor imaging
dipyridamole-thallium imaging
Doppler tissue imaging
DTIC-Dome
D-to-E
D-t.-E amplitude
D-t.-E slope
DTPA
diethylenetriaminepentaacetate
diethylenetriaminepentaacetic acid
DTPA aerosol inhalation lung
scintigraphy
D-transposition of great arteries (D-TGA, dTGA)

D

dual
    d. atrioventricular node
    d. balloon perfusion catheter (DBPC)
    d. chamber (DC)
    d. echophonocardiography
    d. marker
dual-chamber
    d.-c. defibrillation system
    d.-c. Maximo remote monitoring ICD
    d.-c. Medtronic Kappa 400 pacemaker
    d.-c. pacemaker (DCP)
    d.-c. pacing
    d.-c. rate-responsive
    d.-c. and VVI implantable defibrillator (DAVID)
dual-coil transvenous lead
dual-demand pacemaker
dual-energy digital radiography
dual-helical slice mode
dual-isotope simultaneous acquisition single-photon emission computed tomography (DISA-SPECT)
duality
dual-lead electrocardiogram
dual-loop intraatrial reentry
dual-lumen endotracheal tube
dual-mode, dual-pacing, dual-sensing (DDD)
dual-sensor micromanometric high-fidelity catheter
dual-site right atrial pacing
dual-slice mode
Dubois index
Du Bois-Reymond law
Duchenne
    D. muscular dystrophy
    D. sign
duckbill voice prosthesis
Duckworth phenomenon
Ducor-Cordis pigtail catheter
duct
    alveolar d.
    Bartholin d.
    Botallo d.
    collecting d.
    craniopharyngeal d.
    d. of Cuvier
    medullary collecting d.
    pharyngobranchial d.
    thoracic d.
    thyrolingual d.
ductal cell carcinoma
Duct-Occlud system
ductus
    d. arantii
    d. arteriosus (DA)

    d. bump
    patent d. (PD)
    percutaneous occlusion of d.
    d. sublinguales minores
    d. sublingualis major
    d. thoracicus
    d. venosus
Duet coronary stent
Duett
    D. arterial closure device
    D. catheter
    D. vascular sealing device
Duffield cardiovascular scissors
Duke
    D. Activity Status Index (DASI)
    D. bleeding time
    D. Carcinoid Database
    D. Coronary Angiographic Prognostic Index (DCAPI)
    D. Databank for Cardiovascular disease
    D. infective endocarditis criteria
    D. myocardial jeopardy score
    D. treadmill exercise score
    D. treadmill prognostic score
Dukes classification
dullness
    absolute d. (M3)
    absolute cardiac d. (ACD)
    area of cardiac d. (ACD)
    border of cardiac d.
    cardiac d. (CD)
    cardiac border of d.
    left border of d. (LBD)
    left border of cardiac d. (LBCD)
    marked d. (M2)
    percussion d.
    relative cardiac d. (RCD)
    right border of d. (RBD)
    right border cardiac d. (RBCD)
dull pain
dumoffii
    Legionella d.
Dumon
    D. bronchoscope
    D. endobronchial silicone stent
    D. tracheobronchial stent
    D. Y stent
Dumon-Harrell bronchoscope
Duncan syndrome
Dundee rank factor score (DRFS)
Dunham fan
duodecapolar catheter
duodenale
    Ancylostoma d.
duodenal string test
DuoNeb
Duostat rotating hemostatic valve
Duotan PD

Duo-Trach Injection
Dupel drug delivery system
duplex
    d. Doppler scan
    d. imaging
    d. pulsed-Doppler ultrasonography
    pulsus d.
    d. scanning
    d. ultrasound
DURAC
    duration of anticoagulation
Duracep biopsy forceps
Duraflo
    Carpentier-Edwards Physio
      annuloplasty ring with D.
Duragesic Transdermal
dural
    d. arteriovenous fistula (DAVF)
    d. arteriovenous malformation
      (DAVM)
    d. ectasia (DE)
Duralyn balloon material
Duramist Plus
Duran annuloplasty ring
Durapulse pacemaker
Durathane cardiac device
duration
    action potential d. (APD)
    anodal d. (AD)
    d. of anticoagulation (DURAC)
    d. of ECG wave
    d. of exercise
    d. of expiration (T_E)
    half amplitude pulse d.
    d. of inspiration (T_I)
    monophasic action potential d.
      (MAPD)
    D. Nasal Solution
    P d.
    pacing d.
    PR duration to diastolic d. (PRi)
    pulse d. (PD)
    pulse wave d.
    d. of P wave
    P-wave d.
    QRS complex d.
    QT interval d.
    signal-averaged P-wave d. (SAPD)
    sustained rate d.
    d. of systole (DS)
Dura-Trac hydrophilic coating
Duratuss
Duratuss-G
Durham tube
Duricef
Duromedics
    D. mitral valve
    D. valve prosthesis
duropleural fistula

Duroziez
    D. disease
    D. murmur
    D. sign
    D. symptom
Durules
    Betaloc D.
    Biquin D.
durus
    pulsus d.
duskiness
dusky
dust
    d. asthma
    d. disease
    grain d.
    inorganic d.
    d. mite
    d. mite powder
    mushroom d.
    organic d.
duteplase
duty factor
Duval-Coryllos rib shears
Duval lung-grasping forceps
dVDAVP
    1-deamino-4-valine-D-arginine
    vasopressin
DVI
    deep venous insufficiency
    diastolic velocity integral
    digital vascular imaging
      DVI pacemaker
      DVI pacing
DVIS
    digital vascular imaging system
DVP
    deep venous pressure
DVR
    digital vascular reactivity
    double valve replacement
    double ventricular response
DVT
    deep vein thrombosis
    deep venous thrombosis
      residual DVT
DVT/PE
    deep venous thrombosis/pulmonary
    embolism
dwarfism
    aortic d.
DWI
    diffusion-weighted imaging
DWMHI
    deep white matter hyperintensity
DWML
    deep white matter lesion
Dx
    diagnosis

D

DX-Portable spirometry
DXR
    delayed xenograft rejection
Dyazide
dyclonine
dye
    d. cuvette
    flashlamp excited pulsed d.
    Fox green d.
    indocyanine green d.
    d. injection
    d. laser
    radiocontrast d.
    Unisperse blue d.
dye-dilution
    d.-d. curve
    d.-d. method
    d.-d. technique
Dymedix sleep sensor
Dymer excimer delivery system
Dynabac
Dynacin Oral
DynaCirc
Dynalink biliary self-expanding stent
    system
dynamic
    d. aorta
    d. cardiac blood flow (DCBF)
    d. cardiomyoplasty
    d. collapse
    d. compliance
    d. compliance of lung
    d. CT scan
    d. electrocardiography (DCG)
    d. exercise
    d. frequency response
    d. hyperinflation (DH)
    d. intracavitary obstruction
    d. method
    d. MR perfusion imaging
    d. murmur
    d. pressure
    d. range
    d. relaxation
    d. stenosis
    d. stiffness
    d. susceptibility contrast-enhanced
    (DSC)
    d. susceptibility contrast-enhanced
    MRI (DSC MRI, DSC MRI)
    d. tracheal compression
    D. Y stent
dynamics
    fluid d.
    funnel d.
    left ventricular-left atrial
    crossover d.
    RR interval d.
dynamite heart

dynamometer
    bicycle d.
    Cybex isokinetic d.
    Jamar hand d.
    Jamar model 0030J4 d.
DynaPulse 5000A blood pressure
    monitor
Dynasty
    D. balloon
    D. delivery system
dynein
Dynepo
dyne seconds
dynorphin
dyphylline
Dyrenium
dysanapsis
    airway-parenchymal d.
dysanaptic growth
dysarteriotony
dysarthria
    isolated d.
    pure d. (PD)
dysarthria-clumsy hand syndrome
    (DCHS)
dysautonomia
    familial d.
dysbaric
    d. disorder
    d. osteonecrosis
dysbarism
dysbetalipoproteinemia
    familial d.
dyscontrol
dyscrasia
    blood d.
dysfibrinogenemia
dysfunction
    acute endothelial d.
    age-related endothelial d.
    asymptomatic left ventricular d.
    atrioventricular node d. (AVND)
    biventricular d.
    chlorine induced paradoxical vocal
     cord d.
    chronic contractile d.
    ciliary d.
    diaphragmatic d.
    diastolic ventricular d.
    endothelial d.
    erectile d.
    extrathoracic airway d.
    focal ventricular d.
    global ventricular d.
    intellectual d.
    irritant-associated vocal cord d.
    ischemic d.
    left ventricular d. (LVD)
    left ventricular systolic d.

lung d.
microvascular d.
M2 receptor d.
multiple-organ d.
myocardial d.
obstructive ventilatory d.
papillary muscle d.
postischemic d.
restrictive ventilatory d.
reversible left ventricular d.
sinuatrial node d.
sinus node d. (SND)
systolic d.
valvular d.
vascular endothelial d.
ventricular d.
vocal cord d. (VCD)

dysfunctional
d. airway immune response
d. myocardium

dysgenesis
gonadal d.

dysgeusia

dysinnervation
congenital myocardial
sympathetic d. (CMSD)

dyskinesia
d. intermittens
primary ciliary d. (PCD)
d. syndrome
tracheobronchial d.

dyskinesis
anterior wall d.
anteroapical d.
left ventricular d.
posteroinferior d.

dyskinetic segment

dyslipidemia
atherogenic d.
Fredrickson d. (type I, IIa, IIb,
III, IV, V)

dyslipidemic hypertension syndrome

dyslipoproteinemia

dysmetria

dysmodulation

dysmotility
esophageal d.

dysnystaxis

dyspeptica
angina d.

dysphagia, dysphagy
contractile ring d.
d. inflammatoria
d. lusoria
d. nervosa
d. paralytica
sideropenic d.
d. spastica

vallecular d.
d. valsalviana

dysphasia

dysphasic

dysphonia
abductor spasmodic d.

dysplasia
alveolar capillary d. (ACD)
angiogenic squamous d.
arrhythmogenic right ventricular d.
(ARVD)
atriodigital d.
bronchopulmonary d. (BPD)
craniocerebellocardiac d.
ectodermal d.
fibromuscular d. (FMD)
fibrous d.
mucoepithelial d.
polyostotic fibrous d.
right ventricular d.
triangle of d.
tricuspid valve d.
ventricular radial d. (VRD)
ventriculoradial d.
vertebral defects, imperforate anus,
transesophageal fistula, radial and
renal d. (VATER)

dysplasminogenemia

dysplastic
d. mitral valvar leaflet
d. valve

dyspnea
American Thoracic Society
classification of d.
d. at isotime
cardiac d.
effort d.
episodic d.
exercise-induced d. (EID)
exertional d. (ED)
expiratory d.
1-flight exertional d.
2-flight exertional d.
functional d.
D. Index
inspiratory d.
Monday d.
nocturnal d.
nonexpansional d.
d. on exertion (DOE)
orthostatic d.
paroxysmal nocturnal d. (PND)
d. of pregnancy
progressive d.
psychogenic d.
pulmonary d.
renal d.
rest d.
resting d.

D

245

dyspnea *(continued)*
    d. scale
    D. Scale questionnaire
    sighing d.
    d. target
    tracheal wall injury with intermittent stoppage of tracheostomy and episodes of d. (TWISTED)
    Traube d.
    workplace-related d.
dyspneic
dysreflexia
    autonomic d.
dysregulation
    thermal d.
dysrhythmia
    cardiac d. (CD)
dysrhythmic cardiac arrest
dysrhythmogenic
dyssynchronization
dyssynchronous thoracoabdominal excursion
dyssynchrony
    left ventricular d.
    mechanical d.
    thoracoabdominal d.
    ventricular d.
dyssynergia
    detrusor-sphincter d.

dyssynergic
    d. myocardial segment
    d. myocardium
dyssynergy
    regional d.
    ventricular d.
dystrophin
dystrophinopathic cardiomyopathy
dystrophinopathy
dystrophy
    asphyxiating thoracic d. (ATD)
    Becker-type tardive muscular d.
    Duchenne muscular d.
    Emery-Dreifuss muscular d.
    facioscapulohumeral d.
    familial asphyxiant thoracic d.
    Landouzy-Dejerine d.
    limb-girdle muscular d.
    muscular d.
    myotonic muscular d.
    reflex sympathetic d.
    Steinert myotonic d.
    tardive muscular d.
    thoracic asphyxiant d.
    thoracic-pelvic-phalangeal d.
dystropic calcification
dysvascular

E

E greater than A
E point
E point on echocardiogram
E point to septal separation (EPSS)
E sign
E wave
E wave to A wave (E:A)

7E3

7E3 glycoprotein IIb/IIIa platelet antibody
7E3 monoclonal Fab antibody

44E

Vicks Pediatric Formula 44E

E₄

leukotriene C_4, D_4, E, E_4

E-150 Breeze ventilator

EA

endocardiographic amplifier
endotracheal aspirate

E:A

early to late diastolic filling ratio
E wave to A wave
E:A wave ratio

EABV

effective arterial blood volume

EAC

expandable access catheter
EAC catheter

EAD

early afterdepolarization
effective airspace dimension

EAE

effective arterial elastance

EAG

endovascular aortic graft

eagle

E. criteria
E. equation
E. medium
E. portable ventilation system
E. risk score index
E. spirometer

EAM

experimental autoimmune myocarditis

EAMI

exercise training in anterior myocardial infarction

EAR

early asthmatic response

ear

e. densitogram
e. lobe crease (ELC)
e. oximeter

earclip

early

e. afterdepolarization (EAD)
e. asthmatic response (EAR)
e. deceleration
e. diastolic murmur (EDM)
e. diastolic relaxation (EDR)
e. graft failure (EGF)
e. ischemic recurrence (EIR)
e. to late diastolic filling ratio (E:A)
e. lung injury
e. mitral valve closure (EMVC)
e. opening valve
e. progressing stroke (EPS)
e. pulmonary injury
e. rapid repolarization
e. recurrence of atrial fibrillation (ERAF)
e. repolarization (ER)
e. repolarization syndrome
e. return to normal activities (ERNA)
e. secretory antigenic target-6 (ESAT-6)
e. systolic paradox (ESP)
e. systolic wave
e. tracheostomy
e. ventricular repolarization syndrome (EVRS)
e. wheezing

early-peaking systolic murmur

EARR

extended aortic root replacement

EARSS

European Antimicrobial Resistance Surveillance System

EasiVent

E. valved holding chamber
E. valved holding chamber mask

Easprin

easy

E. Air 15 compressor
E. Dial Reg oxygen regulator
E. Neb compressor

Easy-Breathe

Easyhaler

EasyOne spirometry system

Easytrak coronary venous steroid-eluting single-electrode pace/sense lead

EAT

ectopic atrial tachycardia

Eaton

E. agent
E. agent pneumonia

E

247

Eaton-Lambert syndrome
EAVC
    enhanced atrioventricular conduction
EAVN
    enhanced atrioventricular nodal
        EAVN conduction
EBA
    electronic beam angiography
EBC
    exhaled breath condensate
        EBC keratin concentration
EBCT
    electron beam computed tomography
EBDA
    effective balloon-dilated area
Eberth perithelium
EBM
    evidence-based medicine
EBNA
    Epstein-Barr nuclear antigen
Ebola
    Reston subtype of E.
    E. virus
EBR
    embolus-to-blood ratio
ebrantil
Ebstein
    E. angle
    E. anomaly
    E. disease
    E. malformation
    E. malformed valve
    E. sign
EBT
    electronic beam tomography
        HeartCam EBT
EBUS
    endobronchial ultrasonography
    endobronchial ultrasound
EBUS-NA
    endobronchial ultrasound-guided needle
    aspiration
EBUS-TBNA
    endobronchial ultrasound-guided
    transbronchial needle aspiration
        EBUS-TBNA scope
EBV
    effective blood volume
    Epstein-Barr virus
    estimated blood volume
EC
    ejection click
    external carotid
    extracorporeal
        EC artery
EC50 ToxCO breath carbon monoxide
monitor
ECA
    external carotid artery

E-CABG
    endarterectomy and coronary artery
    bypass grafting
    endoscopic coronary artery bypass graft
ECAD
    extracranial carotid arterial disease
ecadotril
ecallantide
ECAT III positron tomograph
ECBV
    effective circulating blood volume
ECC
    edema, clubbing, cyanosis
    emergency cardiac care
    external cardiac compression
    extracardiac conduit
    extracorporeal circulation
eccentric
    e. atrial activation
    e. calcification
    e. hypertrophy
    e. ledge
    e. lesion
    e. narrowing
    e. stenosis
    e. stenotic jet
eccentricity index
ecchymosis, pl. **ecchymoses**
ecchymotic
    e. facies
    e. mask
ECCO$_2$R
    extracorporeal carbon dioxide removal
Eccovision acoustic pharyngometer
ECD
    endocardial cushion defect
    external cardioverter-defibrillator
    extracranial carotid disease
    extracranial Doppler sonography
        Ventak ECD
ECF
    effective capillary flow
ECF-A
    eosinophil chemotactic factors of
    anaphylaxis
ECG, EKG
    electrocardiogram
    electrocardiograph
    electrocardiography
        abnormal rhythm on ECG (rSR)
        baseline ECG
        borderline ECG
        CELP ECG
        CORTES ECG
        differentiated ECG
        esophageal ECG
        intracardiac ECG
        ECG leads I, II, III; V1 through
        V6; aVF, aVL, aVR

LifeSync wireless ECG
Micro-Tracer portable ECG
Miniscope MS-3 pocket ECG
Minnesota classification of ECG
ECG monitor strip
PocketView ECG
ECG repolarization
ECG signal-averaging technique
ECG silence
straight-line ECG
EKG trigger
ECG triggering unit
ECG wave
Welch Allyn/Schiller AT-1 3-
  channel ECG
Welch Allyn/Schiller AT-2 full-size
  ECG
Welch Allyn/Schiller AT-10
  hospital grade ECG
Welch Allyn/Schiller AT-2*plus* full-
  size ECG
Welch Allyn/Schiller MS-3 pocket-
  size ECG

ecg@home heart monitor
ECG-synchronized digital subtraction
  angiogram
Echinacea
echinocandin
echinococcal cyst
echinococcosis
  pericardial e.
Echinococcus
  E. granulosus
  E. multilocularis
ECHO
  enteric cytopathogenic human orphan
  enterocytopathogenic human orphan
    ECHO virus
    ECHO virus myocarditis
echo, pl. **echoes**
  amphoric e.
  atrial e.
  bandlike intrapericardial e.
  e. beat
  bright e.
  e. delay time (TE)
  e. density
  gradient e.
  gradient recall e. (GRE)
  e. guidance
  high-density e.
  e. intensity
  intrapericardial e.
  linear e.
  metallic e.
  mitral valve e. (MVE)
  motion display e.
  nodus sinuatrialis e.
  NS e.

pericardial e.
e. planar imaging (EPI)
e. ranging
e. record access (ERA)
e. reverberation
RT3D e.
scattered e.
e. score
smokelike echoes
specular e.
e. tissue density
transcutaneous e.
transesophageal e.
turbo field e. (TFE)
ventricular e.
e. zone
echoaortography
echo-bright endocardium
echocardiogram (*See also*
  echocardiography)
  aortic valve e. (AVE)
  apical 2-chamber view e.
  apical 4-chamber view e.
  apical 5-chamber view e.
  B bump on e.
  continuous loop exercise e.
  continuous wave Doppler e.
  contrast-enhanced e.
  cross-sectional 2-dimensional e.
  2D e.
  3-dimensional transesophageal e.
    (3D TEE)
  3D transesophageal e.
  E point on e.
  exercise e. (EE)
  Feigenbaum e.
  long-axis parasternal view e.
  meridian e.
  mitral valve e.
  M-mode e.
  Ochsner-Mahorner e.
  parasternal long-axis view e.
  parasternal short-axis view e.
  postcontrast e.
  posterior left ventricular wall
    motion on e.
  postexercise e.
  signal-averaged e.
  transthoracic e. (TTE)
  e. with saline agitation
  W wave on e.
echocardiograph
  Acuson e.
  e. machine
  Ultramark 9 e.
echocardiographic
  e. assessment
  e. automated border detection

E

echocardiographic *(continued)*
- e. automated boundary detection system
- e. coaptation depth
- e. differentiation
- e. scoring system
- e. smoke
- e. strain rate imaging
- e. transducer

echocardiography *(See also* echocardiogram)
- adenosine e.
- American Society of E.
- A-mode e.
- any-plane e.
- AT-atropine stress e.
- baseline e.
- bedside transthoracic e.
- bicycle e.
- bidimensional e.
- B-mode e.
- bubble contrast e.
- color M-mode Doppler e.
- continuous-wave Doppler e.
- contrast e.
- cross-sectional e. (CSE)
- 2D e.
- deductive e.
- digital subtraction e. (DSE)
- 2-dimensional e. (2DE)
- 3-dimensional e. (3DE)
- dipyridamole-exercise stress e. (DExE)
- dipyridamole stress e.
- dobutamine e. (DE)
- dobutamine atropine stress e. (DASE)
- dobutamine stress e. (DSE)
- Doppler e.
- epiaortic e.
- ergonovine e.
- esophageal e.
- exercise stress e. (ESE, Ex-Echo)
- high-frequency epicardial e. (HFEE)
- interventional e.
- intracardiac e. (ICE)
- intraoperative e. (IOE)
- intraoperative transesophageal e. (IOTEE)
- intravenous myocardial contrast e. (IMCE)
- meridian e.
- M-mode e. (MME)
- multiplane transesophageal e.
- myocardial contrast e. (MCE)
- negative contrast e.
- paraplane e.
- pharmacologic stress e.
- pulmonary valve e.

- pulsed Doppler e. (PDE)
- pulsed Doppler e. (PDE)
- pulsed Doppler cross-sectional e. (PD-CSE)
- quantitative 2-dimensional e.
- real-time 3-dimensional dobutamine stress e.
- sector scan e.
- signal-averaged e.
- SonoHeart hand-carried e.
- stress e.
- stress-injected sestamibi-gated SPECT with e.
- supine bicycle stress e. (SBSE)
- TDI M-mode e.
- transesophageal e. (TEE)
- transesophageal atrial pacing stress e. (TAPSE)
- transesophageal contrast e.
- transesophageal dobutamine stress e.
- transesophageal echocardiography-dobutamine stress e. (TEE-DSE)
- transthoracic e. (TTE)
- transthoracic color Doppler e.
- transthoracic contrast e.
- transthoracic Doppler harmonic e.
- treadmill e.
- VIDA stress e.

echo-contrast variability imaging
echodense
- e. mass
- e. structure
- e. valve

echodensity
- cardiac e.
- intracavitary e.
- linear e.
- superimposed e.

echo-Doppler cardiography
echoendoscope
- Olympus e.

echoes *(pl. of* echo)
EchoFlow blood velocity meter system
echo-free space
echogenic
- e. density
- e. mass
- e. plaque

echogenicity
- end-diastolic wall e.

EchoGen injectable emulsion
echogram
echograph
- Siemens Sonoline CD e.

echography
- A-scan e.

echo-guided
- e.-g. pericardiocentesis
- e.-g. ultrasound

echolucent plaque
EchoMark angiographic catheter
echophonocardiography
    combined M-mode e.
    dual e.
echophony
echoreflective
echoreflectivity
echoscanner
echoscope
echo-signal shape
echo-spared area
Echovar Doppler system
echovirus myocarditis
Echovist
EC/IC
    extracranial/intracranial
Eck fistula
ECL
    euglobin clot lysis
ECLA
    excimer laser coronary angioplasty
eclampsia
eclipse
    E. holmium laser
    E. PTMR system
    E. TMR laser
ECLS
    extracorporeal life support
ECM
    external cardiac massage
    extracellular matrix
ECMO
    extracorporeal membrane oxygenation
    ECMO pump
    ECMO therapy
ecNOS
    endothelial constitutive nitric oxide
    synthase
    ecNOS gene
    ecNOS gene expression
    promotor region of eNOS
EcoCheck oxygen monitor
ECOM
    endotracheal cardiac output monitor
    endotracheal cardiac output monitoring
economy class syndrome
Ecotrin
ECP
    effective conduction period
    endocardial potential
    eosinophil cationic protein
    exercise cardiac power
    external cardiac pressure
ECPR
    external cardiopulmonary resuscitation
ECR
    electrocardiographic response

ECS
    endocannabinoid system
    extracellular-like, calcium-free solution
        ECS cardioplegic solution
Ecstasy
ECT
    esophageal combination tube
    euglobulin clot test
    Extracorporeal Circulation Technology
ectasia, ectasis
    alveolar e.
    anuloaortic e. (AAE)
    aortoannular e.
    artery e.
    e. cordis
    coronary artery e.
    diffuse arterial e.
    distal e.
    dural e. (DE)
    familial aortic e.
    vascular e.
ectatic
    e. aneurysm
    e. emphysema
ecto-ADPase
ectocardia
ectocardiac, ectocardial
Ectocor pacemaker
ectodermal dysplasia
ectopia
    e. cordis
    e. cordis abdominalis
    e. cordis pectoral
    e. lentis
ectopic
    e. Ashman beat
    atrial e. (AE)
    e. atrial tachycardia (EAT)
    e. bronchus
    e. focus
    e. impulse
    e. junctional beat (EJB)
    e. junctional tachycardia
    e. pacemaker
    e. rhythm
    e. ventricular beat
ectopy
    asymptomatic complex e.
    atrial e.
    supraventricular e.
    ventricular e.
ECV
    endocardial ventriculotomy
    external cardioversion
    extracorporeal volume
ED
    emotional defensiveness
    end-diastole

E

ED *(continued)*
　exertional dyspnea
　external diameter
EDA
　end-diastolic area
EDBP
　erect diastolic blood pressure
EDC
　end-diastolic count
EDCI
　energetic dynamic cardiac insufficiency
EDCS
　end-diastolic chamber stiffness
　end-diastolic circumferential stress
EDD
　end-diastolic diameter
　end-diastolic dimension
　esophageal detection device
eddy
　　e. current
　　e. sound
Edecrin
　　E. Oral
　　E. Sodium injection
edema
　　acute cardiogenic pulmonary e.
　　　(ACPE)
　　acute noncardiogenic pulmonary e.
　　acute pulmonary e. (APE)
　　airway e.
　　alveolar e.
　　angioneurotic e.
　　ankle e.
　　bland e.
　　boggy e.
　　brawny e.
　　brown e.
　　cardiac e.
　　cardiac pulmonary e. (CPE)
　　cardiogenic pulmonary e.
　　cerebral e.
　　chronic pulmonary e.
　　circumscribed e.
　　e., clubbing, cyanosis (ECC)
　　clubbing, cyanosis, e. (CCE)
　　congestive e.
　　cytotoxic e.
　　dependent e.
　　fingerprint e.
　　flash pulmonary e.
　　florid pulmonary e.
　　focal e.
　　hereditary angioneurotic e. (HANE)
　　high-altitude cerebral e. (HACE)
　　high-altitude pulmonary e. (HAPE)
　　high-pressure cardiogenic
　　　pulmonary e.
　　hydrostatic e.
　　idiopathic cyclic e.

　　increased permeability pulmonary e.
　　infective e.
　　interarytenoid e.
　　interstitial pulmonary e.
　　laryngeal e.
　　lung e.
　　e. of lung
　　lymphatic e.
　　Milton e.
　　mucosal e.
　　myocardial e.
　　negative pressure pulmonary e.
　　　(NPPE)
　　neurogenic pulmonary e.
　　noncardiac pulmonary e. (NCPE)
　　noncardiogenic pulmonary e.
　　nonpitting e.
　　obstructive e.
　　paroxysmal pulmonary e.
　　passive e.
　　pedal e.
　　periodic e.
　　periorbital e.
　　peripheral e.
　　perivascular e.
　　pitting e.
　　postanesthesia pulmonary e.
　　postcardioversion pulmonary e.
　　presacral e.
　　pretibial e.
　　e., proteinuria, hypertension (EPH)
　　pulmonary e. (PE)
　　pulmonary interstitial e.
　　pyemic e.
　　Quincke e.
　　reexpansion pulmonary e.
　　reperfusion pulmonary e.
　　sacral e.
　　septic e.
　　septic pulmonary e. (SPE)
　　stasis e.
　　subpleural e.
　　tense e.
　　terminal e.
　　tocolytic pulmonary e.
　　upper lobe pulmonary e. (ULPE)
　　vasogenic e.
　　vernal e.
　　woody e.
edematous
EdenTrace
　　E. II multichannel
　　　polysomnographic system
　　E. II Plus recorder
edentulism
　　compensated e.
Eder-Puestow wire
edetate disodium

edge
    e. detection
    leading e.
    shelving e.
    trailing e.
edge-detection
    e.-d. method
    e.-d. system
edge-to-edge technique mitral valve repair
EDHF
  endothelium-derived hyperpolarizing factor
Edinburgh Handedness Inventory (EHI)
EDL
  end-diastolic length
  end-diastolic load
EDM
  early diastolic murmur
    EDM infusion catheter
Edmark
    E. mitral valve
    E. monophasic waveform
EDNF
  endogenous digitalis-like natriuretic factor
EDNO
  endothelium-derived nitric oxide
EDP
  end-diastolic pressure
EDPS
  esophageal-directed pressure support
EDR
  early diastolic relaxation
EDRF
  endothelium-derived relaxing factor
edrophonium chloride
EDS
  Ehlers-Danlos syndrome
  excessive daytime sleepiness
EDT
  end-diastolic thickness
EDTA
  ethylenediaminetetraacetic acid
EDV
  end-diastolic volume
EDVI
  end-diastolic volume index
Edwards
    E. catheter
    E. clamp
    E. heart valve
    E. IMR ETlogix annuloplasty ring
    E. Lifesciences Perimount Magna stented prosthesis
    E. Prima Plus porcine tissue valve
    E. Prima Plus Stentless Bioprosthesis Model 2500P

    E. Prima Plus stentless porcine bioprosthesis
    E. Prima Plus valve
    E. septectomy
Edwards-Carpentier aortic valve brush
Edwards-Duromedics bileaflet heart valve
Edwards-Tapp arterial graft
EDWTH
  end-diastolic wall thickness
EE
  exercise echocardiogram
EECP
  enhanced external counterpulsation
    EECP therapy
EEE
  experimental enterococcal endocarditis
EEG
  electroencephalogram
  electroencephalograph
  electroencephalography
    Equinox digital EEG
EEL
  external elastic lamina
    EEL area
EELV
  end-expiratory lung volume
EEM
  external elastic membrane
E.E.S.
  erythromycin ethylsuccinate
    E.E.S. Chewable
    E.E.S. Granules
    E.E.S. Oral
EET acid
EEV
  elastic equilibrium volume
EF
  ejection fraction
efaroxan
efavirenz
EFE
  endocardial fibroelastosis
Efedron
efegatran
effect
    adverse cardiac e.'s
    Anrep e.
    antiapoptotic e.
    antiatherogenic e.
    antineoplastic e.
    Azzopardi e.
    bacteriostatic e.
    Bainbridge e.
    ball-valve e.
    band saw e.
    Bernoulli e.
    billiard ball e.
    blooming e.

E

effect *(continued)*
    Bohr e.
    Bowditch staircase e.
    Brockenbrough e.
    bronchoconstrictive e.
    bronchodilator e.
    bystander e.
    candy wrapper edge e.
    cardiac e.
    ceiling e.
    chronotropic e.
    cidal e.
    Coanda e.
    Compton e.
    copper-wire e.
    cytoprotective e.
    digitalis e.
    digoxin e.
    Doppler e.
    Dotter e.
    dottering e.
    dromotropic e.
    erectile e.
    extrapyramidal side e.
    Fahraeus e.
    Fenn e.
    first-night e.
    fish-scaling e.
    founder e.
    Haldane e.
    hamburger e.
    Hawthorne e.
    healthy worker e.
    horse-race e.
    implosion e.
    inertial e.
    inotropic e.
    jet e.
    Joule-Thompson e.
    late proarrhythmic e.
    lusitropic e.
    Mach e.
    mass e.
    mille feuilles e.
    neurotoxic e.
    neurotrophic e.
    nonhemodynamic e.
    partial volume e.
    passive girdle e.
    peripheral vasodilator e.
    postantibiotic e. (PAE)
    pressor e.
    Prinzmetal e.
    proarrhythmic e.
    proinflammatory e.
    protooncogenic e.
    Rivero-Carvallo e.
    second gas e.
    silver-wire e.
    snare-drum e.
    snowplow e.
    space-occupying e.
    spalling e.
    squeeze e.
    steal e.
    stochastic e.
    time-of-flight e.
    tongue-rolling e.
    training e.
    vasodilator e.
    Vaughan-Williams class e.
    Venturi e.
    volume of distribution e.
    Vroman e.
    waterfall e.
    watermelon seeding e.
    Wedensky e.
    white-coat e.
    windkessel e.
    work e.
    wrecking ball e.

effective
    e. airspace dimension (EAD)
    e. arterial blood volume (EABV)
    e. arterial elastance (EAE)
    e. balloon-dilated area (EBDA)
    e. blood volume (EBV)
    e. capillary flow (ECF)
    e. circulating blood volume (ECBV)
    e. conduction period (ECP)
    e. half-life
    e. orifice area (EOA)
    e. refractory period (ERP)
    e. refractory period of left ventricle (ERPLV)
    e. regurgitant orifice (ERO)
    e. renal blood flow (ERBF)
    e. stroke
    e. systolic pressure (ESP)

effector cell

efferent
    e. arteriole
    e. artery

efficacious

efficacy
    ciliary e.
    e. cryomapping
    e. of drug therapy
    therapeutic e.
    e. of treatment

efficiency
    cough e.
    detective quantum e.
    e. of gas exchange
    mucociliary e.

Effler hiatal hernia repair

efflux
    cellular cholesterol e.
effort
    e. angina
    angina of e.
    brief maximal e. (BME)
    e. dyspnea
    expiratory e.
    first e.
    inspiratory e.
    poor expiratory e.
    relative inspiratory e. (RIE)
    respiratory e.
    e. syndrome
    ventilatory e.
effort-independent lung volume
effort-induced thrombosis
effusion
    asbestos pleural e.
    bloody e.
    chyliform pleural e.
    chylous pericardial e.
    chylous pleural e.
    complex pleural e.
    eosinophilic e.
    exudative pleural e.
    hemorrhagic e.
    interlobar e.
    loculated pericardial e.
    malignant pleural e. (MPE)
    neoplastic pericardial e.
    parapneumonic e.
    partially coagulated e.
    pericardial e. (PE)
    pericarditis with e.
    pleurisy with e.
    pulmonary e.
    purulent e.
    serosanguineous e.
    serous e.
    silent pericardial e.
    stranding e.
    subpulmonic e.
    sympathetic e.
    transudative pleural e.
effusion-associated lymphocyte
effusive-constrictive
    e.-c. disease
    e.-c. pericarditis
Efidac/24
eflornithine
efonidipine
EFPD
    extra-fine particle dose
EFR
    extended field radiation
Efron jackknife classification
Efudex Topical

EG
    eosinophilic granuloma
EGF
    early graft failure
eGFP
    enhanced green fluorescent protein
eggcrate mattress
Eggleston method
egg-on-a-string silhouette
egg-on-its-side heart
egg-shaped heart
eggshell
    e. aorta
    e. calcification
    e. friability
    e. pattern
egg-yellow reaction
egg-yolk sputum
EGM
    electrogram
egobronchophony
egophony
EGT
    exuberant granulation tissue
EGTA
    esophagogastric tube airway
EH
    enlarged heart
    essential hypertension
EHC
    essential hypercholesterolemia
EHI
    Edinburgh Handedness Inventory
Ehlers-Danlos syndrome (EDS)
EHPH
    extrahepatic portal hypertension
Ehrenritter ganglion
Ehret phenomenon
ehrlichiosis
EHT
    essential hypertension
EHV
    electric heart vector
EI
    endovascular irradiation
E:I
    expiratory to inspiratory
      E:I ratio
EIA
    enzyme immunoassay
    exercise-induced asthma
EIB
    exercise-induced bronchospasm
Eichner index
Eicken method
eicosanoid excretion
eicosapentaenoic acid (EPA)
EID
    emergency infusion device

EID (*continued*)
  exercise-induced dyspnea
    EID catheter
Eikenella corrodens
EILV
  end-inspiratory lung volume
Einhorn esophageal dilator
Einthoven
    E. equation
    E. law
    E. lead
    E. string galvanometer
    E. triangle
EIR
  early ischemic recurrence
Eisenmenger
    E. complex
    E. disease
    E. physiology
    E. reaction
    E. reaction with septal defect
    E. syndrome
    E. tetralogy
    E. VSD
EIT
  electrical impedance tomography
EJ
  external jugular
EJB
  ectopic junctional beat
ejected volume (EV)
ejection
    area-length method for e.
    e. click (EC)
    e. fraction (EF)
    e. fraction at rest (REF)
    e. fraction during exercise (ExEF)
    e. fraction image
    left ventricular e. (LVE)
    e. murmur (EM)
    e. period
    e. phase
    e. phase index
    e. rate (ER)
    e. shell image
    e. sound (ES)
    e. systolic murmur (ESM)
    e. time (ET)
    e. velocity
Ejrup maneuver
EKG (*var. of* ECG)
  electrocardiogram
  electrocardiograph
EKY
  electrokymogram
El
    El Gamal cardiac device
    El Gamal coronary bypass catheter
    El Gamal guiding catheter

ELA
  excimer laser-assisted angioplasty
E-LAM
  endothelium-leukocyte adhesion molecule
Elantan
Elastalloy Ultraflex Strecker nitinol stent
elastance
    effective arterial e. (EAE)
    end-systolic e.
    maximum ventricular e. (Emax)
    pleural space e.
elastase
    human neutrophil e.
    leukocyte e.
    neutrophil e.
    Pseudomonas e.
    sputum e.
Elast-Eon silicone urethane copolymer
elastic
    e. component
    e. cone
    e. equilibrium volume (EEV)
    e. fibers
    e. fibers in sputum
    e. lamella
    e. lamina
    e. load
    e. mandibular advancement (EMA)
    e. pressure-volume (Pel-V)
    e. pulse
    e. recoil
    e. recoil pressure
    e. resistance
    e. stiffness
    e. stockings
    e. tissue hyperplasia
elasticity
    lung e.
    sputum viscosity and e.
    ventricular e. (VE)
elasticum
    pseudoxanthoma e.
elasticus
    conus e.
elastin
elastinolytic
elastogram
    intravascular e.
elastography
elastomeric half-face respirator
Elastorc catheter guidewire
elbow flexion
ELC
    ear lobe crease
ELCA
    excimer laser coronary angioplasty
elderly
    innocent murmur of e.

Elecath electrophysiologic stimulation catheter

Elecsys
  E. proBNP immunoassay
  E. troponin T immunoassay system

elective
  e. angiography
  e. cardioversion
  e. percutaneous coronary intervention
  e. replacement indicator (ERI)

electric
  e. cardiac pacemaker
  e. defibrillator
  e. defibrillator using DC discharge
  General E. (GE)
  e. heart vector (EHV)
  e. replacement indicator (ERI)
  e. storm

electrical
  e. activation abnormality
  e. activity
  e. alternans
  e. alternation
  e. alternation of heart
  e. axis
  e. cardioversion
  e. catheter ablation
  e. countershock
  e. diastole
  e. disease
  e. failure
  e. fulguration
  e. heart position
  e. impedance tomography (EIT)
  e. impulse
  e. injury
  e. isolation
  e. isolation of vein
  e. pathway
  e. potential
  e. signal
  e. systole

electrically unexcitable scar mapping

electroanatomical
  e. map
  e. mapping
  e. mapping system

electrocardiac shock

electrocardioanalyzer

electrocardiogram (ECG, EKG) (*See also* electrocardiography)
  ambulatory e. (AECG)
  bipolar e.
  Burdick e.
  3-channel e.
  chest and left arm lead in e. (CL)

chest and right arm lead in e. (CR)
concordant changes e.
derived 12-lead e.
discordant changes e.
dual-lead e.
exercise e.
fetal e. (FECG, FEKG)
FIESTA e.
Fourier analysis of e.
His bundle e.
12-lead e.
16-lead e.
left arm electrode for e. (VL)
left leg electrode for e. (VF)
orthogonal e.
right arm electrode for e. (VR)
scalar e.
signal-averaged e. (SAECG)
stored e.
stress MUGA e.
thallium e.
time domain signal-averaged e.
treadmill e.
unipolar e.
vector e. (VECG)
Wedensky modulated signal-averaged e.

electrocardiograph (ECG, EKG)
  bioimpedance e.
  Cambridge e.
  MAC-VU e.
  Marquette e.
  Micro-Induction 1000 e.
  Mingograf 62 6-channel e.

electrocardiographic
  e. complex
  e. fibrillatory wave
  e. gated SPECT myocardial perfusion imaging
  e. gating
  e. lead
  e. modeling
  e. response (ECR)
  e. strain pattern
  e. transtelephonic monitor
  e. wave complex
  e. wave corresponding to repolarization of ventricles (T)
  e. wave corresponding to wave of depolarization crossing atria (P)

electrocardiography (ECG, EKG) (*See also* electrocardiogram)
  ambulatory e.
  American Society of E. (ASE)
  CF lead in e.
  chest lead in e. (C)
  chest and left leg lead in e. (CF)
  dynamic e. (DCG)

E

electrocardiography *(continued)*
  esophageal e.
  exercise e.
  exercise stress e. (Ex-ECG)
  fetal e.
  high-resolution e. (HRE)
  intracavitary e.
  12-lead e.
  long-term e. (LT-ECG)
  myocardial e.
  precordial e.
  signal-averaged e. (SAECG)
  stress e. (SECG)
  time domain signal-averaged e.
  unipolar limb lead on left leg
    in e. (aVF, aVL)
  unipolar limb lead on right arm
    in e. (aVR)
electrocardiophonogram
electrocardiophonography
electrocardioscanner
  Compuscan Hittman
    computerized e.
electrocardioversion
electrocautery
  Bovie e.
  bronchoscopic e.
  needlepoint e.
electrochemical
  e. gradient
  e. polarization
electrochemiluminescence immunoassay
electrocoagulation
  bipolar e. (BPEC)
electroconvulsive therapy
electrode
  AE-60-I-2 implantable pronged
    unipolar e.
  AE-85-I-2 implantable pronged
    unipolar e.
  AE-60-KB implantable unipolar
    endocardial e.
  AE-85-KB implantable unipolar
    endocardial e.
  AE-60-K-10 implantable unipolar
    endocardial e.
  AE-85-K-10 implantable unipolar
    endocardial e.
  AE-60-KS-10 implantable unipolar
    endocardial e.
  AE-85-KS-10 implantable unipolar
    endocardial e.
  Arzbaecher pill e.
  Arzco Tapsul pill e.
  Berkovits-Castellanos hexapolar e.
  Bisping e.
  button e.
  e. catheter
  e. catheter ablation operation

central terminal e.
Clark oxygen e.
coil e.
CPI Endotak transvenous e.
Darox cutaneous thoracic patch e.
dispersing e.
dispersive e.
disposable e.
epicardial sock e.
esophageal pill e.
exploring e.
Fast-Patch disposable
  defibrillation/electrocardiographic e.
e. gel
Goetz bipolar e.
Hi-Res electrocardiogram e.
hydrogen e.'s
implantable cardioverter e.
indifferent e.
intravascular catheter e.
ion-selective e. (ISE)
e. jelly
J-shaped pacemaker e.
large-tip e.
Laserdish e.
Mansfield Polaris e.
monopolar temporary e.
multiple point e.
multipolar catheter e.
myocardial e.
pacemaker e.
e. pad
e. paddles
e. paste
PE-60-I-2 implantable pronged
  unipolar e.
PE-85-I-2 implantable pronged
  unipolar e.
PE-60-K-10 implantable unipolar
  endocardial e.
PE-85-K-10 implantable unipolar
  endocardial e.
PE-60-KB implantable unipolar
  endocardial e.
PE-85-KB implantable unipolar
  endocardial e.
PE-85-KS-10 implantable unipolar
  endocardial e.
platinum-iridium e.
QuadPolar e.
quadripolar Quad e.
Quik-Prep e.
reference e.
e. replacement interval
ring e.
scalp e.
screw-in epicardial e.
screw-in sutureless myocardial e.
Severinghaus e.

sew-on e.
silent e.
silver bead e.
silver-silver chloride e.
stab e.
stab-in epicardial e.
steroid-eluting e.
subcutaneous patch e.
sutured plaque e.
e. system
temporary atrial pacemaker e.
 (TAPE)
tined ventricular e.
Transvene tripolar e.
transvenous e.
tripolar defibrillation coil e.
unipolar defibrillation coil e.
USCI Goetz bipolar e.
USCI NBIH bipolar e.
VF e.
Vitatron catheter e.
VL e.
VR e.
electrodesiccation
electrode-skin interface
electrodispersive skin patch
Electrodyne pacemaker
electrodynogram
electroencephalogram (EEG)
electroencephalograph (EEG)
electroencephalography (EEG)
electrofluoroscopy
electrogenic
electrogram (EGM)
atrial e. (AEG)
coronary sinus e.
deflection in His bundle in e.
evoked endocardial e.
evoked ventricular e.
far-field e.
e. fractionation
Furman type II e.
high right atrium e. (HRAE)
His bundle e. (HBE)
intracardiac e.
sinus node e. (SNE)
e. storage
electrograph
Cardiotest portable e.
electrokymogram (EKY)
electrokymograph
electrokymography
electrolyte
e. abnormality
e. imbalance
e. and steroid cardiopathy with
 necrosis (ESCN)
electrolytic disturbance

electromagnetic
e. interference/radiofrequency
 interference (EMI/RFI)
e. mapping
e. navigation system
electromanometer
electromechanical
e. artificial heart
e. coupling
e. delay
e. dissociation (EMD)
e. interval
e. left ventricular mapping
e. systole
electromyocardial dissociation
electromyogram (EMG)
kinesiological e.
electromyograph (EMG)
electromyography (EMG)
e. unit
electron
e. beam angiography
e. beam computed tomography
 (EBCT)
e. beam fence
e. microprobe analysis
e. microscope
e. paramagnetic resonance
 spectroscopy
e. volt (eV)
electronic
e. beam angiography (EBA)
e. beam tomography (EBT)
e. calipers
e. distance compensation
e. fetal monitor
E. HouseCall system
e. pacemaker
e. pacemaker load
e. scanning
electrooculogram (EOG)
electrooculograph (EOG)
electrooculography (EOG)
electropharmacology
electrophoresis
agarose gel e.
gradient gel e.
hemoglobin e.
lipoprotein e. (LEP, LPE)
polyacrylamide gel e.
protein e.
sodium dodecylsulfate
 polyacrylamide gel e. (SDS-
 PAGE)
electrophrenic respiration
electrophysiologic
e. mapping
e. study
e. test

E

electrophysiologist
electrophysiology (EP)
    diagnostic e.
    e. evaluation
    intracardiac e.
    North American Society for Pacing
      and E. (NAPSE)
electrostethograph
electrosurgery
electrosurgical blade
electrotonic
    e. conduction
    e. transmission
electroversion
elegant study
Elema
    E. lead
    E. pacemaker
Elema-Schonander pacemaker
element
    contractile e.
    length contraction compensation e.
      (LCCE)
    peroxisome proliferator response e.
      (PPRE)
    series elastic e.
elephant
    e. trunk procedure
    e. trunk prosthesis
    e. trunk technique
elephantiasis
elephant-on-the-chest sensation
elevated gradient
elevation
    CK-MB e.
    coved ST-segment e.
    e. of enzyme
    e. MI
    1-natural-log-unit e.
    notched ST-segment e.
    e. pallor
    e. pallor of extremity
    ST-segment e.
    tombstoning ST-segment e.
    transient ST-segment e.
    upsloping ST e.
elevator
    Aufricht e.
    Cameron-Haight e.
    e. disease
    Doyen e.
    Lemmon sternal e.
    Matson rib e.
    e. muscle
    Phemister e.
    rib e.
ELF
  epithelial lining fluid
    ELF levels

elfin
    e. facies
    e. facies syndrome
Elgiloy-Heifitz aneurysm clip
Elgiloy stent
elimination
    carbon dioxide e.
    e. half-life
    single-breath nitrogen e.
Eliminator dilation balloon
eliprodil
ELISA
  enzyme-linked immunosorbent assay
    double-sandwich IgM ELISA
ELISPOT
  enzyme-linked immunospot
    ELISPOT test
Elite dual-chamber rate-responsive
  pacemaker
Elixicon
Elixophyllin
elizabethae
    Bartonella e.
Ellence
Ellestad
    E. exercise stress test
    E. protocol
Ellipse compact spacer
ellipsoid arteriole
elliptical
    e. end-capped quadrature
      radiofrequency coil
    e. loop
Elliptosphere cardiac catheter set
Ellis sign
Ellis-van Creveld syndrome
Eloesser flap
Elsner asthma
ELSO
  Extracorporeal Life Support Organization
Elspar
ELT
  endless loop tachycardia
eltrombopag
Eltroxin
eluting stent
elution
    abluminal e.
    isocratic e.
    steroid e.
ELVT
  endolaser venous therapy
EM
  ejection murmur
EMA
  elastic mandibular advancement
    EMA appliance
Emax
  maximum ventricular elastance

EMB
    endomyocardial biopsy
embarrassment
    circulatory e.
    hemodynamic e.
    respiratory e.
EmboGold microsphere
embolectomy
    catheter e.
    e. catheter
    femoral e.
    pulmonary e.
    surgical e.
emboli (*pl. of* embolus)
embolic
    e. abscess
    e. aneurysm
    e. event
    e. gangrene
    e. infarct
    e. necrosis
    e. obstruction
    e. phenomenon
    e. pneumonia
    e. shower
    e. stroke
    e. thrombosis
    e. volume
embolism (*See also* embolus)
    acute pulmonary e.
    air e. (AE)
    air pulmonary e.
    amnionic fluid e. (AFE)
    amniotic fluid e. (AFE)
    aortic e.
    arterial e.
    arterial gas e. (AGE)
    atheromatous e.
    bacillary e.
    bland e.
    bone marrow e.
    capillary e.
    catheter e.
    cellular e.
    cerebral air e.
    cholesterol e.
    coronary air e.
    coronary artery e. (CAE)
    crossed e.
    deep venous
      thrombosis/pulmonary e. (DVT/PE)
    direct e.
    diving air e.
    fat e.
    fatal pulmonary e. (FPE)
    gas e.
    hematogenous e.
    infective e.
    miliary e.

    multiple e.'s
    myxomatous pulmonary e.
    obturating e.
    oil e.
    pantaloon e.
    paradoxic e.
    paradoxical cerebral e.
    Plasmodium e.
    pulmonary e. (PE)
    pulmonary air e.
    pyemic e.
    retrograde e.
    riding e.
    saddle e.
    silent e.
    spinal e.
    straddling e.
    submassive pulmonary e.
    systemic arterial air e.
    trichinous e.
    tumor e.
    venous e.
    venous air e. (VAE)
embolization
    air e.
    bronchial artery e. (BAE)
    cerebral e.
    cholesterol e.
    coil e.
    distal vessel e.
    paradoxical e.
    e. particle
    plaque e.
    pulmonary e.
    septal artery e.
    septic e.
    stent e.
    subsegmental transcatheter
      arterial e. (STAE)
    e. therapy
    transcatheter e.
    transcatheter arterial e. (TAE)
embolized foreign material
embolomycotic aneurysm
embolotherapy
    percutaneous e.
    transcatheter e.
embolus, pl. **emboli** (*See also* embolism)
    air e.
    calcific e.
    cancer e.
    catheter e.
    catheter-induced e.
    cerebral e.
    emboli containment system
    femoral e.
    missile emboli
    paradoxical e.
    polyurethane foam e.

E

embolus *(continued)*
  pulmonary e.
  riding e.
  saddle e.
  threw an e.
  throw an e.
embolus-to-blood ratio (EBR)
Embol-X arterial cannula and filter system
Emboshield bare wire filter
embryocardia
  jugular e.
  e. rhythm
embryologic
embryology
embryoma
embryonal cell
embryonic
  e. phenotype pattern
  e. residua
embryopathy
EMC
  encephalomyocarditis
  EMC virus
Emcyt
EMD
  electromechanical dissociation
Emerald diagnostic guidewire
emergency
  e. bailout
  e. bailout stent
  e. cardiac care (ECC)
  hypertensive e.
  e. infusion device (EID)
  e. medical tag (EMT)
  e. medical treatment (EMT)
  e. medical treatment and active labor act (EMTALA)
  e. portocaval shunt (EPCS)
  e. reperfusion
emergent
  e. angioplasty
  e. thoracotomy
Emerson
  E. cuirass respirator
  E. postoperative ventilator
  E. pump
Emery-Dreifuss
  E.-D. disease
  E.-D. muscular dystrophy
emesis
  posttussive e.
emetine toxicity
EMF
  endomyocardial fibrosis
EMG
  electromyogram
  electromyograph
  electromyography

Eminase
EMI/RFI
  electromagnetic interference/radiofrequency interference
emission
  e. flame photometry
  single-photon e.
  stimulated acoustic e.
  vascular acoustic e.
emitter
  high-energy, low-penetration beta e.
  low-energy, high-penetration gamma e.
  positron e.
EMLA
  eutectic mixture of local anesthetics
  EMLA cream
emotional
  e. defensiveness (ED)
  e. laryngeal wheezing
  e. stress
Emphasys endobronchial valve
emphysema
  alveolar duct e.
  atrophic e.
  bullous e.
  centriacinar e.
  centrilobular e.
  chronic hypertrophic e.
  chronic obstructive pulmonary e. (COPE)
  chronic pulmonary e. (CPE)
  compensating e.
  compensatory e.
  congenital lobar e.
  cutaneous e.
  cystic e.
  diffuse obstructive e.
  distal acinar e.
  ectatic e.
  false e.
  familial e.
  focal e.
  gangrenous e.
  generalized e.
  glass blower's e.
  hereditary e.
  heterogenous e.
  hypertrophic e.
  hypoplastic e.
  idiopathic unilobar e.
  increased markings e.
  infantile lobar e.
  interlobular e.
  interstitial e.
  intestinal e.
  irregular e.
  Jenner e.
  lobar e.

localized obstructive e.
loculated e.
mediastinal e.
obstructive e.
panacinar e.
panlobular e.
paracicatricial e.
paraseptal e.
peripheral paracicatricial e.
predominant e.
protease-antiprotease theory of e.
proximal acinar e.
pulmonary e. (PE)
pulmonary interstitial e. (PIE)
scar e.
senile e.
subcutaneous e.
subgaleal e.
surgical e.
traumatic e.
unilateral lobar e.
vesicular e.
emphysematous
e. asthma
e. bleb
e. bulla
e. chest
e. gangrene
empiric
e. constant
e. therapy
Empirin
empyema
anaerobic e.
Aspergillus e.
e. benignum
e. of chest
exudative e.
fibrinopurulent e.
free-flowing e.
interlobar e.
latent e.
loculated e.
metapneumonic e.
e. necessitatis
organizing e.
e. of pericardium
pleural e.
pneumococcal e.
postinjury e.
postpneumonectomy tuberculous e.
pulsating e.
putrid e.
sacculated e.
streptococcal e.
synpneumonic e.
thoracic e.
e. thoracis
tuberculous e.

empyesis
tuberculous e.
EMS
eosinophilia-myalgia syndrome
EMT
emergency medical tag
emergency medical treatment
endocardial mapping technique
EMTA
endomethylene tetrahydrophthalic acid
EMTALA
emergency medical treatment and active
labor act
emulation
pectoral e.
emulsion
EchoGen injectable e.
fat e.
intravascular perfluorochemical e.
perflenapent injectable e.
emu oil
EMVC
early mitral valve closure
E-Mycin Oral
EN
EN Snare endovascular catheter
EN Snare endovascular snare
en
en bloc
en bloc bilateral lung transplant
en bloc face
en bloc face view
en bloc no-touch technique
ENA
extractable nuclear antigen
Enable aortic hear valve
enalapril
e. and diltiazem
e. and felodipine
e. and hydrochlorothiazide
e. maleate
enalaprilat
enalaprilic acid
enantiomer
Enbrel
encainide hydrochloride
Encap
Novo-Rythro E.
encapsulated organism
Encapsulon epidural catheter
encarditis
encased heart
encephalitis
cytomegalovirus e.
Encephalitozoon
encephalomyelitis
encephalomyocarditis (EMC)
e. virus

E

encephalopathy
> hypertensive e. (HE)
> hypoxic-ischemic e.
> metabolic e.
> subcortical vascular e. (SVE)

encircling
> e. cryoablation
> e. endocardial ventriculotomy
> e. endocardial ventriculotomy operation

enclose
> E. anastomosis assist device
> E. proximal anastomotic assist device

encode

encoding
> respiratory ordered phase e. (ROPE)
> velocity e.

Encompass cardiac network

Encor
> E. lead
> E. pacemaker

Encore inflation device

encroachment
> luminal e.

encrustation theory of atherosclerosis

encysted pleurisy

Endal

endangiitis

Endantadine

endaortitis

endarterectomy
> abdominal aortic e.
> aortoiliofemoral e.
> blunt eversion carotid e.
> carotid e. (CE, CEA)
> closed e.
> coronary e.
> e. and coronary artery bypass grafting (E-CABG)
> femoral e.
> gas e.
> pull-out e.
> traction e.
> transient ischemic attack plus carotid e.
> transluminal e.
> vertebral e.

endarterial

endarteritis
> e. deformans
> Heubner specific e.
> e. obliterans
> e. proliferans
> syphilitic e.

endarteropathy
> digital e.

end artery

end-diastole (ED)
> left ventricular e.-d. (LVED)
> left ventricular dimension in e.-d. (LVDd)

end-diastolic
> e.-d. area (EDA)
> e.-d. chamber stiffness (EDCS)
> e.-d. circumferential stress (EDCS)
> e.-d. count (EDC)
> e.-d. diameter (EDD)
> e.-d. dimension (EDD)
> e.-d. left ventricular pressure
> e.-d. length (EDL)
> e.-d. load (EDL)
> e.-d. murmur
> e.-d. pressure (EDP)
> e.-d. pulmonic regurgitation velocity
> right ventricular e.-d. (RVED)
> e.-d. thickness (EDT)
> e.-d. volume (EDV)
> e.-d. volume index (EDVI)
> e.-d. wall echogenicity
> e.-d. wall enlargement
> e.-d. wall thickness (EDWTH)

Endeavor nondetachable silicone balloon catheter

endemic
> e. fungal infection
> e. influenza

end-expiratory
> e.-e. alveolar collapse
> e.-e. apnea
> e.-e. esophageal pressure
> e.-e. film
> e.-e. lung volume (EELV)

end-flow
> right ventricular e.-f. (RVEF)

end-hole
> e.-h. balloon-tipped catheter
> e.-h. 7-French catheter
> e.-h. Tracker microcatheter

end-inspiratory
> e.-i. film
> e.-i. lung volume (EILV)
> e.-i. overdistention
> e.-i. Velcro crackle

endless loop tachycardia (ELT)

Endo
> E. GIA stapler
> E. Grasp device

endoaneurysmorrhaphy
> ventricular e.

endoaortic clamp

endoaortitis

endoauscultation

endobronchial
> e. brachytherapy
> e. cryotherapy

e. infection
e. laser therapy
e. obstruction
e. sarcoid
e. tamponade
e. tree
e. tube
e. tuberculosis
e. ultrasonography (EBUS)
e. ultrasound (EBUS)
e. ultrasound-guided needle
  aspiration (EBUS-NA)
e. ultrasound-guided transbronchial
  needle aspiration (EBUS-TBNA)
e. Watanbe spigot (EWS)
endobronchially
endocannabinoid system (ECS)
endocardiac
endocardial
e. bipolar lead
e. border delineation
e. cardiac border
e. catheter ablation
e. cushion
e. cushion defect (ECD)
e. definition
e. to epicardial resection operation
e. excursion
e. fibroelastosis (EFE)
e. fibrosis
e. flow
e. mapping
e. mapping technique (EMT)
e. mapping of ventricular
  tachycardia
e. motion
e. murmur
e. pacing
e. potential (ECP)
e. pressure
e. resection
e. sclerosis
e. shortening
e. stain
e. surface area (ESA)
e. thickening
e. triangle
e. tube
e. vegetation
e. ventriculotomy (ECV)
e. wire
endocardial-to-endocardial resection
endocardiographic amplifier (EA)
endocardiography
endocarditic
endocarditis
abacterial thrombotic e.
acute bacterial e. (ABE)
acute infective e. (AIE)

aortic e.
atypical verrucous e.
bacteria-free stage of bacterial e.
bacterial e. (BE, BEC)
e. benigna
bioprosthetic e.
cachectic e.
e. chordalis
chronic e.
constrictive e.
culture-negative e.
enterococcal e.
experimental enterococcal e. (EEE)
fungal e.
gonococcal e.
gram-negative e.
green strep e.
Haemophilus e.
infectious e.
infective e. (IE)
isolated parietal e.
e. lenta
Libman-Sacks e.
Löffler parietal fibroplastic e.
malignant e.
marantic e.
methicillin-sensitive right-sided e.
mitral valve e.
multivalve e.
mural e.
mycotic e.
native valve e. (NVE)
native valve fibroplastic e.
nonbacterial thrombotic e. (NBTE)
nonbacterial verrucous e.
noninfective valve e.
nosocomial e.
pacemaker e.
parietal e.
e. parietalis fibroplastica (EPF)
plastic e.
polypous e.
postoperative e.
prosthetic infectious e. (PIE)
prosthetic valve e. (PVE)
pulmonic e.
rheumatic e.
rickettsial e.
right-sided e.
septic e.
staphylococcal e.
streptococcal e.
subacute bacterial e. (SBE)
subacute infective e.
syphilitic e.
terminal e.
thrombotic e.
tricuspid valve e.
tuberculous e.

E

endocarditis *(continued)*
  ulcerative e.
  valvular e.
  vegetative e.
  verrucous e.
  viridans e.
endocardium
  Biosense revascularization approach
    for viable e. (BRAVE)
  echo-bright e.
  mural e.
  viable e.
endocoronary sinus catheter
EndoCPB catheter
endocrine
  e. disorder
  e. system
endocytosis
endoderm
endodermal
  e. cell
  e. sinus tumor
endoepicardial mapping
endofibrosis
Endoflator insufflator
Endoflex endotracheal tube
end-of-life (EOL)
  e.-o.-l. care
  e.-o.-l. pacemaker
  e.-o.-l. rate
endogenous
  e. digitalis-like natriuretic factor
    (EDNF)
  e. fibrinolysis
  e. kinin
  e. lipid
  e. thrombin potential (ETP)
endoglin gene
endograft
  aortic e.
  bifurcated e.
  Talent bifurcated e.
  Vanguard e.
Endoknot suture
endolaryngeal
endolaser venous therapy (ELVT)
endoleak type I–IV
Endologix PowerLink system
endolumen enlargement
EndoLumina illuminated bougie
endoluminal
  e. reconstruction
  e. reconstruction of basilar artery
    fusiform aneurysm
  e. stent graft
  e. stenting
endolymphatic hypertension
endolymphaticus
  saccus e.

endolysosome
**endomethylene tetrahydrophthalic acid
  (EMTA)**
endomyocardial
  African e.
  e. biopsy (EMB)
  e. disease
  e. fibroelastosis
  e. fibrosis (EMF)
endomyocarditis
endomysial
  e. collagen
  e. fibrosis
endomysium
end-on aortogram
endonuclease
  restriction e.
Endopath EZ45 thoracic linear stapler
endopeptidase
  e. inhibitor
  neutral e. (NEP)
endopericarditis
endoperimyocarditis
endoperoxide steal
endophthalmitis
endoplasmic reticulum
endopolyploidy
endoprosthesis
  Gore TAG thoracic e.
  Gore Viabahn e.
  Gore Viatorr Tips e.
  Wallgraft tracheobronchial e.
  Wallstent venous e.
endopulmonary vent catheter
end-organ ischemia
endorphin
Endosaph vein harvest system
endoscope
  lung imaging fluorescence e.
    (LIFE)
  Messerklinger e.
  velopharyngeal e.
endoscopic
  e. beating heart surgery
  e. biopsy
  e. coronary artery bypass graft (E-
    CABG)
  e. saphenous vein harvesting
    (ESVH)
  e. tissue culture (ETC)
  e. ultrasound-guided fine-needle
    aspiration (EUS-FNA)
  e. variceal sclerotherapy (EVS)
  e. vascular surgery (ESVS)
  e. vessel harvesting (EVH)
endoscopy
  videostroboscopic e.
**EndoSonics IVUS/balloon dilation
  catheter**

Endotak
    E. C lead transvenous catheter
    E. C tripolar transvenous lead
    E. DSP lead
    E. lead defibrillator
    E. lead system
    E. pacemaker
    E. Picotip defibrillation lead
    E. Reliance endocardial lead
endotension
endothelial
    e. cell activation
    e. cell adhesion molecule
    e. cell apoptosis
    e. cell degeneration
    e. constitutive nitric oxide synthase
    (ecNOS, eNOS)
    e. denudation
    e. dysfunction
    e. function
    e. nitric oxide synthase (eNOS)
    e. oxide synthase (eNOS)
    e. permeability
    e. progenitor cell (EPC)
    e. purinoceptor
endothelial-dependent arterial dilation
endothelial-derived relaxation factor
endothelialization
endothelin (ET)
    e. A, B receptor
    e. antagonist
    big e.
    circulating e.
    myocardial e.
endothelin-1 (ET-1)
    e.-1 immunoreactivity
endothelin-2 (ET-2)
    plasma e.-2
endothelin-3 (ET-3)
endothelin-converting enzyme
endothelioma
endothelium
    bovine aortic e. (BAE)
    coronary microvessel e.
    nonfenestrated e.
endothelium-dependent
    e.-d. dilator response to substance
    P
    e.-d. vascular relaxation
    e.-d. vasodilation
endothelium-derived
    e.-d. hyperpolarizing factor (EDHF)
    e.-d. nitric oxide (EDNO)
    e.-d. relaxing factor (EDRF)
endothelium-independent vascular
  relaxation
endothelium-leukocyte adhesion molecule
  (E-LAM)
endothelium-mediated relaxation

endotoxemia
endotoxic sepsis
endotoxin
    bacterial e.
    circulating bacterial e.
    e. shock
endotracheal (ET)
    e. aspirate (EA)
    e. cardiac output monitor (ECOM)
    e. cardiac output monitoring
    (ECOM)
    e. intubation
    e. tube (ETT)
    e. tube connection
    e. tube cuff
    e. tube placement
Endotrol
    E. endotracheal tube
    E. tracheal tube
endovascular
    e. aneurysm repair (EVAR)
    e. aortic graft (EAG)
    e. contraction
    e. edge-to-edge technique
    e. irradiation (EI)
    e. radiation therapy
    e. radiofrequency catheter ablation
    e. repair (EVR)
    e. snare
    e. stent grafting
    e. treatment
endovenous drainage cannula
endoventricular circular patch plasty
EndoWrist instrument
endpoint
    e. attachment
    hemodynamic e.
    therapeutic e.
end-pressure artifact
endralazine
Endrate
end-stage
    e.-s. heart failure (ESHF)
    e.-s. liver disease (ESLD)
    e.-s. lung
    e.-s. renal disease (ESRD)
end-systole (ES)
end-systolic
    e.-s. circumferential wall stress
    e.-s. count (ESC)
    e.-s. dimension (ESD)
    e.-s. elastance
    e.-s. force-length relationship
    (ESFL)
    e.-s. force-velocity index
    e.-s. left ventricular pressure
    e.-s. left ventricular stress
    e.-s. length (ESL)
    e.-s. murmur

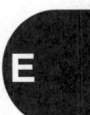

E

end-systolic *(continued)*
    e.-s. pressure (ESP)
    e.-s. pressure-volume relation
    e.-s. pressure-volume relationship
      (ESPVR)
    e.-s. stress (ESS)
    e.-s. stress-dimension relation
    e.-s. volume (ESV)
    e.-s. volume index (ESVI)
    e.-s. volume ratio
    e.-s. wall stress (ESWS)
end-tidal
    e.-t. capnometry
    e.-t. carbon dioxide ($ETCO_2$)
    e.-t. sample
end-to-end anastomosis
end-to-side suture
endurance
    expiratory muscle e.
    inspiratory muscle e.
Enduron
Enduronyl Forte
enema
    barium e.
    Kayexalate e.
    sodium polystyrene sulfonate e.
Enemol
energetic dynamic cardiac insufficiency
  (EDCI)
energometer
energy
    blood flow e. (BFE)
    color Doppler e. (CDE)
    e. delivery
    epicardial, off-pump, beating heart
      ablation with acoustic e.
    e. expenditure
    internal e.
    minimum defibrillation e. (MDE)
    myocardial e.
    noninvasive electrical e.
    perimetric distribution of
      radiofrequency e.
    e. production
    radiofrequency e.
    e. resolution
    e. supply
Enertrax 7100 pacemaker
e-Net headpiece
enflurane
Enforcer SDS coronary stent
enfuvirtide
engineering
    Arterial Vascular E., Inc. (AVE)
    tissue e.
Englert forceps
engorgement
    venous e.
engraftment syndrome (ES)

enhanced
    e. atrioventricular conduction
      (EAVC)
    e. atrioventricular nodal (EAVN)
    e. automaticity
    e. external counterpulsation (EECP)
    e. external counterpulsation unit
    e. green fluorescent protein (eGFP)
    e. oxygenation
    E. Torque 8F guiding catheter
enhancement
    detection e.
    leading edge e.
    mean contrast e.
    personalized aerobics for
      cardiovascular e.
enhancer
    aerosol cloud e. (ACE)
    universal aerosol cloud e.
enhancing lesion
enlarged heart (EH)
enlargement
    biatrial e.
    cardiac e. (CE)
    compensatory vessel e.
    end-diastolic wall e.
    endolumen e.
    left atrial e. (LAE)
    left ventricular e. (LVE)
    panchamber e.
    right atrial e. (RAE)
    right ventricular e. (RVE)
Enlon injection
eNO, ENO
    exhaled nitric oxide
    expired nitric oxide
enolase
    neuron-specific e. (NSE)
eNOS
    endothelial constitutive nitric oxide
     synthase
    endothelial nitric oxide synthase
    endothelial oxide synthase
      eNOS activation
      eNOS activity
      eNOS uncoupling
enoxacin
enoxaparin
    e. bridge therapy
    e. sodium
enoximone
EnRhythm pacemaker
EnSite
    E. 3000 electrophysiology
     workstation
    E. multielectrode array transvenous
     catheter

E. NavX intracardiac nonfluoroscopic navigation system

E. 3000 system

Entamoeba

   E. dispar

   E. histolytica

entangling technique

enteral

   e. nutrition

   e. tube feeding

enteric

   e. cytopathogenic human orphan (ECHO)

   e. cytopathogenic human orphan virus

   e. fistula

   e. gram-negative bacillus

enteric-coated aspirin

enteroadherent

enteroaggregative

Enterobacter

   E. cloacae

   E. pneumonia

Enterobacteriaceae

enterococcal endocarditis

Enterococcus

   E. faecalis

   E. faecium

enterococcus, pl. **enterococci**

   vancomycin-resistant e.

enterocolitica

   Yersinia e.

enterocolitis

enterocytopathogenic human orphan (ECHO)

enterogenous cyst

enterohemorrhagic

enteroinvasive

enteropathy

   protein-losing e. (PLE)

enterothorax

enterotoxin

   Escherichia coli e.

enteroviral

enterovirus

Entity pacemaker

entocyte

entoplasm

entoptic pulse

entrained beat

entrainment

   concealed e.

   epicardial e.

   high air flow with oxygen e. (HAFOE)

   e. mapping

   oxygen e.

   e. port

   e. of tachycardia

   transient e.

   e. with concealed fusion

entrance

   e. block

   e. wound

entrapment

   lung e.

Entrata aortic valve system

Entree

   E. thoracoscopy cannula

   E. thoracoscopy trocar

Entrophen

entropy

   approximate e. (ApEn)

EnTrust implantable cardioverter-defibrillator

entry

   air e.

   e. site

   transsarcolemmal calcium e.

ENT wash

enucleation of subaortic stenosis

envelope

   aortic e.

   dagger-shaped aortic e.

   flow e.

   maximal flow-volume e.

   spectral e.

env gene

environment

   normobaric e.

   pharmacologic e.

environmental

   e. allergen

   e. change

   e. irritant

   e. lung disease

   e. stress cracking

   e. survey

   e. tobacco smoke (ETS)

Enzygnost

   E. F1+2 ELISA kit

   E. TAT complex kit

   E. TAT ELISA assay

enzymatic

   e. deficiency

   e. infarct size

   e. reserve

enzyme

   allosteric modification of e.

   angiotensin-converting e. (ACE)

   angiotensin-converting e. DD (ACE-DD)

   angiotensin-converting e. ID (ACE-ID)

   angiotensin-converting e. II (ACE-II)

   angiotensin I-converting e.

   Bacillus subtilis e.

E

enzyme *(continued)*
>beta AR kinase1 e.
>cardiac e.
>COX-1, -2 e.
>elevation of e.
>endothelin-converting e.
>fibrinolytic e.
>glycolytic e.
>e. immunoassay (EIA)
>lysosomal e.
>mitochondrial e.
>pancreatic e.
>phosphodiesterase e.
>proteolytic e.
>pulmonary angiotensin I
> converting e.
>sarcoplasmic reticulum-associated
> glycolytic e.'s
>e. substrate

enzyme-induced damage
enzyme-linked
>e.-l. immunosorbent assay (ELISA)
>e.-l. immunospot (ELISPOT)

enzymology
EOA
>effective orifice area
>esophageal obturator airway

EOG
>electrooculogram
>electrooculograph
>electrooculography

EOL
>end-of-life

eosin
>hematoxylin and e. (H&E)

eosinophil
>e. by-product
>e. cationic protein (ECP)
>e. chemotactic factors of
> anaphylaxis (ECF-A)
>e. recruitment

eosinophilia
>angiolymphoid hyperplasia with e.
>nonallergic rhinitis with e.
> (NARES)
>peripheral blood e.
>prolonged pulmonary e.
>pulmonary infiltrate with e. (PIE)
>pulmonary infiltration with e. (PIE)
>sputum e.
>tropical pulmonary e. (TPE)

eosinophilia-myalgia syndrome (EMS)
eosinophilic
>e. bronchitis
>e. chemotaxis
>e. effusion
>e. endomyocardial disease
>e. granuloma (EG)
>e. granulomatosis

>e. lung
>e. lung syndrome
>e. pneumonia
>e. pneumonitis
>e. pneumonopathy
>e. pulmonary syndrome

eotaxin
EP
>electrophysiology
>extreme pressure
>>EP evaluation
>>EP mapping

EP-2104R injectable MRI agent
EPA
>eicosapentaenoic acid

Epanutin
EPAP
>expiratory positive airway pressure

eparterial bronchus
EPC
>endothelial progenitor cell

EPCA
>external pressure circulatory assistance

EPCS
>emergency portocaval shunt

E-peak velocity
EPF
>endocarditis parietalis fibroplastica

EPH
>edema, proteinuria, hypertension

ephedrine
>aminophylline, amobarbital, e.
>e. sulfate

ephelis, pl. **ephelides**
>nevi, atrial myxoma, myxoid
> neurofibromas, ephelides (NAME)

ephemeral pneumonia
EPI
>echo planar imaging
>>EPI FilterWire EX emboli
>> protection device

epiaortic echocardiography
**epibronchial right pulmonary artery
syndrome**
epicardial
>e. arterial spasm
>e. artery patency
>e. cardiac border
>e. coronary artery
>e. coronary artery disease
>e. defibrillator patch
>e. entrainment
>e. fat
>e. fat pad sign
>e. fat tag
>e. flow
>e. flow conductance
>e. lead

e., off-pump, beating heart ablation
with acoustic energy
e. pacing
e. poudrage
e. radiofrequency atrial lesion
e. radiofrequency catheter ablation
e. sock electrode
e. stenosis
e. vessel patency
epicardial-mesenchymal transformation
epicardiectomy
epicardin gene
epicardium
left ventricular e.
Epic HF ICD
EpiClose device
Epicoccum nigrum
Epicor cardiac ablation device
epidemic capillary bronchitis
epidermal
e. growth factor
e. hyperplasia
epidermidis
Staphylococcus e.
epidermoid carcinoma
epidural
e. analgesia
e. spinal cord (ESC)
epigastric bruit
epiglottic cartilage
epiglottidis
epiglottis
epiglottitis
thermal e.
epiglottoplasty
epi-illuminated microscope
epilepsy
epilepticus
status e.
epimysium
epinephrine
aortic arch e.
aqueous e.
buffered lidocaine with e. (BLE)
high-dose e.
lidocaine, atropine, naloxone, e.
[drugs that may be administered
via endotracheal tube] (LANE)
racemic e.
EpiPen
epiphenomena of dissection
epipodophyllotoxin
epirubicin
episcleritis
episode
presyncopal e.
transient ischemic e. (TIE)
vasovagal e.
ventilation e.

episodic
e. dyspnea
e. hypertension
epistaxis
epistenocardiac pericarditis
epistenocardica
pericarditis e.
epithelia (*pl. of* epithelium)
epithelial
e. cell
e. lining fluid (ELF)
e. mucin
e. 5'-nucleotide receptor
epithelial-mucus attachment
epithelioid
e. hemangioendothelioma
e. mesothelioma
epithelium, pl. **epithelia**
ciliated e.
human airway e.
pulmonary e.
sloughed bronchial e.
epithelized tracheostomy
epitope
epituberculous infiltration
Epivir
eplerenone
Epogen
epoprostenol
e. sodium
e. sodium for injection
epoxyeicosatrienoic acid
epoxy resin
EPP
equal pressure point
extrapleural pneumonectomy
Eppendorf catheter
eprosartan
EPS
early progressing stroke
epsilon wave
EPSS
E point to septal separation
Epstein-Barr
E.-B. nuclear antigen (EBNA)
E.-B. virus (EBV)
Epstein disease
EPT-1000
EPT-1000 XP cardiac ablation
controller
EPT-1000 XP cardiac ablation
system
eptacog alfa activated
ePTFE
expanded polytetrafluoroethylene
ePTFE graft
ePTFE polymer membrane
ePTFE vascular suture

E

eptifibatide
Epworth Sleepiness Scale (ESS)
equal
> breath sounds bilateral and e.
> (BSBE)
> e. pressure point (EPP)

equation
> ACSM regression e.
> alveolar-air e.
> American College of Sports
>   Medicine regression e.
> Bernoulli e.
> Bloch e.
> Bohr e.
> Brunelli e.
> Carter e.
> Cockroft-Gault e.
> continuity e.
> Doppler continuity e.
> Eagle e.
> Einthoven e.
> Fick e.
> Ford e.
> Framingham e.
> Friedewald e.
> Gorlin and Gorlin e.
> Hagenbach extension of
>   Poiseuille e.
> Harris-Benedict e.
> Henderson-Hasselbalch e.
> Kubicek e.
> Navier-Stokes e.
> Nernst e.
> Poiseuille e.
> regression e.
> Riley-Cournand e.
> Rodrigo e.
> Röhrer e.
> Siri e.
> Starling e.
> Teichholz e.
> Torricelli orifice e.

equator of cell
equi
> *Rhodococcus e.*

equilibrate
equilibration
equilibrium
> Hardy-Weinberg e.
> e. image
> e. multigated radionuclide
>   ventriculography
> e. radionuclide angiocardiography
>   (ERNA)
> e. radionuclide angiography
>   (ERNA)
> voltage e.

equine rabies immunoglobulin (ERIG)

equinovarus
equinox
> E. digital EEG
> E. digital EEG system
> E. EEG acquisition device
> E. occlusion balloon system

equiphasic complex
equipment
> Angiostar Plus vascular imaging e.
> Austin Medical E.

equipotency
equipotent
equivalency
> left main e.

equivalent
> Abell-Kendall e.
> anginal e.
> metabolic e. (MET)
> right anterior oblique e.
> ventilation e.
> ventilatory e.

equol
equuli
> *Actinobacillus e.*

ER
> early repolarization
> ejection rate
>   VoSpire ER

ERA
> echo record access
>   ERA 300 dual-chamber pacing
>   system analyzer

ERAF
> early recurrence of atrial fibrillation

ER alpha
> estrogen receptor alpha

Erb
> E. area
> E. atrophy
> limb-girdle dystrophy of E.
> E. point

Erbe cryoprobe
Erben reflex
ERBE surgical instrument
ER beta
> estrogen receptor beta

ERBF
> effective renal blood flow

Erb-Goldflam disease
erbium:YAG laser
erbumine
> perindopril e.

Erdheim
> E. cystic medial necrosis
> E. cystic medial necrosis of aorta
> E. disease
> medionecrosis aortae idiopathica E.

erect diastolic blood pressure (EDBP)

erectile
  e. dysfunction
  e. effect
Ergoline bicycle ergometer
ergometer
  Bosch ERG 500 e.
  cycle e.
  Ergoline bicycle e.
  Ergometrics ER 900 e.
  Gould-Godart type 18070 e.
  Lode BV Excalibur braked
    cycle e.
  Monark bicycle e.
  pedal-mode e.
  Siemens-Elema AG bicycle e.
  treadmill e.
  Tunturi EL400 bicycle e.
Ergometrics ER 900 ergometer
ergometry
  arm cycle e.
  bicycle e.
  cycle e.
  supine bicycle e.
ergonomic vascular access needle
  (EVAN)
ergonovine
  e. challenge
  e. echocardiography
  e. infusion
  e. injection
  e. maleate
  e. maleate provocation angina
  e. provocation test
ergonovine-induced
  e.-i. coronary vasospasm
  e.-i. spasm
ergoreceptor
  muscle e.
ergoreflex
ergot alkaloid
ergotamine derivative
ERI
  elective replacement indicator
  electric replacement indicator
Erie System
ERIG
  equine rabies immunoglobulin
    ERIG serum
ERK
  extracellularly responsive kinase
  extracellular-regulated kinase
Erlanger sphygmomanometer
ERNA
  early return to normal activities
  equilibrium radionuclide
    angiocardiography
  equilibrium radionuclide angiography
    ERNA after acute myocardial
    infarction

Erni sign
ERO
  effective regurgitant orifice
erosion
  intimal e.
  spark e.
erosive
  e. esophagitis
  e. reflux
ERP
  effective refractory period
ERPLV
  effective refractory period of left
    ventricle
ERS
  European Respiratory Society
ERT
  estrogen replacement therapy
ertapenem sodium
eruptive xanthoma
ERV
  expiratory reserve volume
Erwinia
Erybid
Eryc Oral
EryPed Oral
Erysipelothrix
Ery-Tab Oral
erythema
  e. marginatum
  e. migrans
  e. multiforme
  e. nodosum
  palmar e.
erythematosus
  disseminated lupus e.
  drug-induced lupus e. (DILE)
  lupus e. (LE)
  systemic lupus e. (SLE)
erythematous maculopapular rash
erythrityl tetranitrate
erythroblastosis fetalis
Erythrocin Oral
erythrocyte
  e. protoporphyrin
  e. sedimentation rate (ESR)
erythrocytosis
erythroderma
erythrogenin
erythromelalgia
erythromycin
  e. ethylsuccinate (E.E.S.)
  e. and sulfisoxazole
  systemic e.
erythropheresis
erythropoiesis
erythropoietin
  gene-activated e.
  plasma e.

E

273

Eryzole Oral

ES
ejection sound
end-systole
engraftment syndrome
extrasystole
ES 300-Cardiac T ELISA troponin T immunoassay system

ESA
endocardial surface area

ESAT-6
early secretory antigenic target-6
ESAT-6 protein *mycobacterium tuberculosis*

ESC
end-systolic count
epidural spinal cord

escalator
mucociliary e.

escape
e. beat
e. impulse
e. interval
junctional e.
nodal e.
e. pacemaker
e. rhythm
vagal e.
ventricular e.
e. ventricular contraction

escape-capture bigeminy

Escherichia coli **enterotoxin**

Escherich test

ESCN
electrolyte and steroid cardiopathy with necrosis

E-Scope II electronic stethoscope

ESD
end-systolic dimension

ESE
exercise stress echocardiography

E-selectin cell adhesion molecule

ESFL
end-systolic force-length relationship

ESHF
end-stage heart failure

Esimil

ESL
end-systolic length

ESLD
end-stage liver disease

ESM
ejection systolic murmur

Esmarch
E. ball
E. tourniquet

esmolol hydrochloride

esophagagram

esophagalgia

esophageae
glandulae e.

esophageal
e. achalasia
e. adventitious breath sounds
e. angina
e. atresia
e. bougienage
e. branch
e. branch of left gastric artery
e. branch of thoracic aorta
e. branch of vagus nerve
e. cardiogram
e. combination tube (ECT)
e. constriction
e. contraction ring
e. detection device (EDD)
e. dilation
e. duplication cyst
e. dysmotility
e. ECG
e. echocardiography
e. electrocardiography
e. gland
e. hiatus
e. lead
e. lumen
e. lung
e. manometry
e. motility
e. mucosa
e. nervous plexus
e. obturator airway (EOA)
e. opening
e. perforation
e. pill electrode
e. prosthesis
e. reflux
e. rupture
e. sling procedure
e. spasm
e. speech
e. sphincter
e. stricture
e. tamponade
e. temperature
e. transit time
e. varices
e. vein
e. web

esophageal-directed pressure support (EDPS)

esophageales
rami e.
venae e.

esophagectomy

esophageus, pl. **esophagei**
hiatus e.

plexus nervosus e.
rami esophagei
esophagi (*pl. of* esophagus)
esophagism
hiatal e.
esophagismus
esophagitis
corrosive e.
e. dissecans superficialis
erosive e.
infectious e.
monilial e.
peptic e.
reflux e.
esophagogastric
e. junction
e. orifice
e. tamponade
e. tube airway (EGTA)
e. vestibule
esophagomyotomy
Heller e.
esophagoplasty
Belsey e.
Grondahl e.
esophagoplication
esophagorespiratory fistula
esophagosalivary reflex
esophagoscope
Foregger rigid e.
Jesberg e.
Mikulicz-type e.
Schindler e.
esophagoscopy
fiberoptic e.
esophagospasm
esophagotracheal
esophagram
barium e.
esophagus, pl. **esophagi**
abdominal part of e.
Barrett e.
brusque dilation of e.
candy-cane e.
cardiac glands of e.
cervical part of e.
muscular coat of e.
nutcracker e.
pars abdominalis esophagi
pars cervicalis esophagi
pars thoracica esophagi
suspensory ligament of e.
thoracic part of e.
tunica mucosa esophagi
tunica muscularis esophagi
ESP
early systolic paradox
effective systolic pressure
end-systolic pressure

ESP radiation reduction examination
gloves
Esprit ventilator
esprolol
e. hydrochloride
e. plus sildenafil citrate
ESPVR
end-systolic pressure-volume relationship
ESR
erythrocyte sedimentation rate
ESRD
end-stage renal disease
ESS
end-systolic stress
Epworth Sleepiness Scale
European Stroke Scale
circumferential ESS
essential
e. asthma
e. bradycardia
e. brown induration
e. brown induration of lung
e. hemoptysis
e. hypercholesterolemia (EHC)
e. hypertension (EH, EHT)
e. pulmonary hemosiderosis
e. tachycardia
e. thrombocytopenia
EST
exercise stress test
expression sequence tagged
estazolam
ester
cholesterol e.
N^G-nitro-L-arginine methyl e. (L-NAME)
phorbol e.
Estes
E. ECG criteria
E. point system
E. score
Estes-Romhilt ECG point-score system
estimated
e. blood volume (EBV)
e. Fick method
e. MET
Estlander operation
estradiol
estramustine
estrogen
conjugated equine e. (CEE)
e. and medroxyprogesterone
e. receptor alpha (ER alpha)
e. receptor beta (ER beta)
e. replacement therapy (ERT)
estrone
ESV
end-systolic volume

E

ESVH
  endoscopic saphenous vein harvesting
ESVI
  end-systolic volume index
ESVS
  endoscopic vascular surgery
ESWS
  end-systolic wall stress
eszopiclone
ET
  ejection time
  endothelin
  endotracheal
  exercise test
  exercise treadmill
ET-1
  endothelin-1
ET-2
  endothelin-2
ET-3
  endothelin-3
ETA
  ethionamide
etanercept
ETC
  endoscopic tissue culture
ETc
  corrected ejection time
ETCO₂
  end-tidal carbon dioxide
    $ETCO_2$ multigas analyzer
    sidestream $ETCO_2$
etexilate
  dabigatran e.
ETFE
  ethylene tetrafluoroethylene
ETFVL
  exercise tidal flow-volume loop
ethacrynic acid
Ethalloy needle
ethambutol hydrochloride
ethamivan
Ethamolin injection
ethane
  exhaled e.
ethanol (EtOH)
  selective septal branch injection
    of e.
ethanolamide
ethanolamine oleate
ethaverine hydrochloride
Ethavex-100
ether
  bischloromethyl e. (BCME)
  e. bronchitis
  e. pneumonia
  e. test
Ethibond suture
Ethicon Endopath EZ45 stapler

ethidium bromide
ethionamide (ETA)
Ethmozine
ethoxysclerol
ethyl alcohol
ethylenediamine
  theophylline e.
ethylenediaminetetraacetic
  e. acid (EDTA)
  e. acid disodium salt
ethylene oxide (ETO)
ethylene tetrafluoroethylene (ETFE)
ethylnorepinephrine hydrochloride
ethylsuccinate
  erythromycin e. (E.E.S.)
Etibi
etilefrine
etiology
  chest pain of unknown e. (CPUE)
etiopathogenesis
ETO
  ethylene oxide
    ETO Sleuth
E-to-A change
E-to-F slope
EtOH
  ethanol
etomidate
Etopophos
etoposide
  Adriamycin, cyclophosphamide, e.
    (ACE)
  carboplatin and e. (CE)
  cisplatin and e. (PE)
  cisplatin, vincristine, doxorubicin, e.
    (CODE)
  e. phosphate
etoricoxib
ETP
  endogenous thrombin potential
e-TRAIN 110 AngioJet catheter
ETS
  environmental tobacco smoke
ETT
  endotracheal tube
  exercise tolerance test
  exercise treadmill test
ETView endotracheal tube
eucapnic voluntary hyperventilation
Eudal-SR
Euflex
euglobin
  e. clot lysis (ECL)
  e. clot test
euglobulin
  e. clot lysis time
  e. clot test (ECT)
euglycemia

euglycemic
  e. glucose clamp
  e. hyperinsulinemic glucose clamp
    test
eugonic
eukaryon
eukaryosis
eukaryote
Eulerian strain
Eulexin
eunuchoid voice
eupaverin
eupnea
Euro-Collins
  E.-C. multiorgan perfusion kit
  E.-C. solution
Euroglyphus maynei
Europe
  Cardiovascular and Interventional
    Radiological Society of E.
    (CIRSE)
European
  E. Antimicrobial Resistance
    Surveillance System (EARSS)
  E. Heart Survey
  E. Respiratory Society (ERS)
  E. Stroke Scale (ESS)
EUS-FNA
  endoscopic ultrasound-guided fine-needle
    aspiration
Eustace Smith murmur
eustachian
  e. ridge
  e. valve
eusystole
eusystolic
**eutectic mixture of local anesthetics
  (EMLA)**
euthyroid sick syndrome
euvolemic
EV
  ejected volume
eV
  electron volt
evacuation
  pleural space e.
evagination
evaluation
  Acute Physiology, Age, Chronic
    Health E. (APACHE)
  Angina with Extremely Serious
    Operative Mortality E.
    (AWESOME)
  anthropometric e.
  cine e.
  computer-assisted e.
  confirmatory e.
  diagnostic e.
  3D motion e.

electrophysiology e.
EP e.
medication use e. (MUE)
noninvasive e.
Physical Activity Scale for the
  Elderly E. (PASE)
quality-of-care e.
Randomized Outpatient
  Milrinone E. (ROME)
spirometric e.
EVAN
  ergonomic vascular access needle
Evans blue
EVAR
  endovascular aneurysm repair
EVD
  external ventricular drainage
Eve method
even-echo rephasing
event
  acute coronary e. (ACE)
  e. adjudication
  adverse e.
  apparent life-threatening e. (ALTE)
  bronchospastic e.
  cardiac e.
  cardiovascular e.
  cerebral e.
  cerebrovascular e.
  coronary e.
  e. diary
  embolic e.
  hard cardiac e.
  intracardiac e.
  ischemic e.
  life-threatening cardiac e.
  main adverse coronary e. (MACE)
  major adverse cardiac e. (MACE)
  nonfatal cardiac e.
  e. recorder
  e. recorder monitor
  reducing e.
  respiratory e.
  serious cardiac e. (SCE)
  sleep-disordered breathing e.
  soft e.
  transient ischemic e. (TIE)
  ventricular tachycardia e. (VTE)
  wave coronary e.
event/episode counter
eVent Inspiration ventilator system
event-link data system
eventrated diaphragm
eventration of diaphragm
Everest disposable inflation device
EverGrip clamp insert
eversion
  blunt e.
  cusp e.

E

everting mattress suture
EVH
    endoscopic vessel harvesting
evidence-based medicine (EBM)
EVLW
    extravascular lung water
evoked
    e. endocardial electrogram
    e. ventricular electrogram
evolution
    R-Test E.
    E. scanner
evolutus
    Peptostreptococcus e.
Evolve Cardiac Continuum
evolving
    e. myocardial infarction
    e. rupture
EVR
    endovascular repair
EVRS
    early ventricular repolarization syndrome
EVS
    endoscopic variceal sclerotherapy
    EVS vascular closure system
Ewald tube
Ewart sign
E-wave
    E-w. spectral velocity waveform
    E-w. velocity
Ewing sign
EWS
    endobronchial Watanbe spigot
EX
    expectorant
        Diabetic Tussin EX
        Naldecon Senior EX
ex
    ex vivo
    ex vivo aggregation
    ex vivo gene transfer
EX-2000 DeVilbiss conserver
exacerbation
    acute bacterial e.
    bacterial e.
    infective e.
    recurrent infective e.
ExacTech blood glucose meter
examination
    cardiac e.
    funduscopic e.
    limited Doppler e.
    neurologic e.
    parasternal e.
    supraclavicular e.
    suprasternal e.
excavatum
    pectus e.

excellence
    National Institute for Clinical E.
      (NICE)
Excelsior 1018 microcatheter
excessive daytime sleepiness (EDS)
exchange
    air e.
    alanine e.
    cardiopulmonary gas e.
    catheter e.
    citrate e.
    efficiency of gas e.
    FFA e.
    gas e.
    glucose e.
    glutamate e.
    e. guidewire
    oxygen e.
    perfluorocarbon-associated gas e.
      (PAGE)
    pulmonary gas e.
    rapid e. (RX)
    respiratory e.
    sodium-potassium e.
    e. technique
    e. tip deflecting wire guide handle
    e. transfusion
exchanger
    heat/moisture e. (HME)
    Na^+/H^+ e. (NHE)
    ThermoVent heat and moisture e.
excimer
    e. cool laser
    e. gas laser
    e. laser-assisted angioplasty (ELA)
    e. laser coronary angioplasty
      (ECLA, ELCA)
    e. laser coronary atherectomy
    e. sheath
    e. vascular recanalization
excision
    wedge e.
excisional
    e. atherectomy
    e. biopsy
    e. cardiac surgery
excitability
    supranormal e.
excitable gap
excitation
    anodal e.
    anomalous atrioventricular e.
    direct e.
    premature e.
    reentrant e.
    supranormal e.
    e. wave
excitation-contraction coupling
excited dimers

excitotoxic
excluder device
exclusion
 e. criteria
 diagnosis of e.
Excor temporary total artificial heart
excrescence
 Lambl e.
excretion
 absorption, distribution,
  metabolism, e. (ADME)
 eicosanoid e.
 sodium e.
 urinary equol e.
excursion
 cusp e.
 decreased valve e.
 diaphragmatic e.
 dome e.
 dyssynchronous thoracoabdominal e.
 endocardial e.
 mitral valve e. (MVE)
 phasic e.
 posterior wall e. (PWE)
 respiratory e.
 thoracoabdominal e.
 valve e.
Ex-ECG
 exercise stress electrocardiography
Ex-Echo
 exercise stress echocardiography
ExEF
 ejection fraction during exercise
exemption
 human device e. (HDE)
exenatide
exercise
 aerobic e. (AEX, AEx)
 ankle e.
 bicycle e.
 Bobath e.
 breathing e.
 Buerger-Allen e.
 e. capacity
 e. cardiac power (ECP)
 cardiopulmonary e. (CPX)
 constant-workload cycle e.
 duration of e.
 dynamic e.
 e. echocardiogram (EE)
 ejection fraction during e. (ExEF)
 e. electrocardiogram
 e. electrocardiography
 e. factor
 e. hyperemia
 e. hyperpnea
 e. hypertension
 e. imaging
 e. index

 e. intolerance
 isometric e.
 isotonic e.
 e. load
 low-intensity treadmill e. (LITE)
 e. LV function
 maximal resistive e. (MRE)
 mild-intensity e.
 passive vascular e. (pavex)
 peak e.
 e. prescription
 e. pressor reflex
 e. regimen
 rehabilitation e.
 So Much Improvement with a
  Little E. (SMILE)
 strenuous e.
 e. stress echocardiography (ESE,
  Ex-Echo)
 e. stress electrocardiography (Ex-
  ECG)
 e. stress test (EST)
 e. stress testing
 supine e.
 sustained physical e. (SPE)
 e. termination
 e. test (ET)
 e. thallium scintigraphy
 e. thallium-201 scintigraphy
 therapeutic e.
 e. tidal flow-volume loop (ETFVL)
 e. tolerance
 e. tolerance test (ETT)
 e. tomographic TI-201 imaging
 e. training in anterior myocardial
  infarction (EAMI)
 e. treadmill (ET)
 treadmill e. (TE)
 e. treadmill test (ETT)
 unsupported arm e. (UAE)
 upright e.
exercise-associated
 e.-a. cough
 e.-a. wheezing
exercise-induced
 e.-i. angina
 e.-i. arrhythmia
 e.-i. asthma (EIA)
 e.-i. bronchospasm (EIB)
 e.-i. dyspnea (EID)
 e.-i. fatigue
 e.-i. left bundle branch block
 e.-i. periodic breathing
 e.-i. shortness of breath
 e.-i. silent myocardial ischemia
 e.-i. ventricular tachycardia
exerciser
 CliniFLO breathing e.

E

exerciser *(continued)*
    low-flow breathing e.
    Voldyne 5000 volumetric e.

exertion
    Borg rating of perceived e.
    dyspnea on e. (DOE)
    paroxysmal dyspnea on e. (PDE)
    perceived e.
    rating of perceived e. (RPE)
    shortness of breath on e. (SBE, SOBOE)

exertional
    e. angina
    e. dyspnea (ED)
    e. hypotension
    e. syncope

exfoliative dermatitis
exhalation
exhaled
    e. breath condensate (EBC)
    e. ethane
    e. nitric oxide (eNO, ENO)

exhaust
    diesel e.

exhaustion
    vital e.

exit
    e. block
    e. block murmur
    e. point
    e. site
    e. surgical osteosynthesis
    e. wound

exocardia
exocardial murmur
exogenous
    e. antigen deposit
    e. lipid
    e. lipid pneumonia
    e. nitric oxide
    e. obesity
    e. substrate

exon
exophthalmica
    tachycardia e.

exophthalmos
exophytic
exopneumopexy
exopolysaccharide
    mucoid e.

Exorcist technique
Exosurf Neonatal
exotoxin
    Pseudomonas e.

expandable
    e. access catheter (EAC)
    e. circular cryoablation catheter

expanded
    e. polytetrafluoroethylene (ePTFE)
    e. polytetrafluoroethylene vascular graft

expander
    blood e.
    blood volume e. (BVE)
    Hespan plasma volume e.
    hetastarch plasma e.
    plasma volume e.
    PMT AccuSpan tissue e.
    E. stent

expansion
    infarct e.
    paradoxical systolic e. (PSE)
    stent e.
    T-cell e.
    volume e.

expectorant (EX)
    Balminil E.
    Benylin E.
    Calmylin E.
    classic e.
    Codafed E.
    Decohistine E.
    Dihistine E.
    liquifying e.
    Nucofed Pediatric E.
    Phenhist E.
    Ru-Tuss E.

expectorated sputum volume
expectoration
    prune juice e.
    sputum e.

expedited recovery program
expenditure
    energy e.
    resting energy e. (REE)

experiment
    Müller e.
    Weber e.

experimental
    e. autoimmune myocarditis (EAM)
    e. enterococcal endocarditis (EEE)

expiration
    duration of e. (T_E)
    prolongation of e.

expiratory
    e. airflow
    e. breath
    e. center
    e. dyspnea
    e. effort
    e. flow limitation
    e. flow rate
    e. grunt
    inspiratory to e. (I:E)
    e. to inspiratory (E:I)
    e. limb
    e. murmur
    e. muscle endurance

e. muscle training
e. positive airway pressure (EPAP)
e. reserve volume (ERV)
e. resistance
e. retard
e. rhonchus
e. tidal flow
e. time (T_E)
e. trapping of air
e. view
e. wheezing

expired
e. air collection
e. gas
e. nitric oxide (eNO, ENO)

expirograph
Godart e.

explant
explanted heart
Explorer 360-degree rotational diagnostic EP catheter
exploring electrode
Expo diagnostic catheter
Export catheter
exposure
air kerma e.
airway, breathing, circulation, disability, e. (ABCDE)
allergen e.
alternobaric e.
chemical e.
cobalt e.
cold e.
heptanal occupational e.
hyperbaric e.
hypobaric e.
toxin e.
workplace e.

exposure-response relationship
express
E. balloon
E. balloon-expandable stent
E. PTCA catheter

Express2 coronary stent system
expression
adenovirus-based phospholamban-antisense e.
bcl-2 e.
CMV IE-2 gene e.
cytokine e.
ecNOS gene e.
fibroblast growth factor e.
gene e.
P-selectin e.
e. sequence tagged (EST)

expressive aphasia
expulsive coughing
exquisitely dependent
exsanguinate

exsanguination protocol
exsanguinotransfusion
exsorption
extended
e. aortic root replacement (EARR)
e. collection device
e. field radiation (EFR)
e. pressure range
e. release (XL, XR, XT)

extended-release niacin/lovastatin
extended-spectrum beta-lactamase
extender
Taq e.

extension
anterior mitral leaflet e.
infarct e.
knee e.
Linx guidewire e.
PSG LOC guidewire e.
venous e. (VE)

Extentabs
Quinidex E.

external
e. branch
e. branch of superior laryngeal nerve
e. cardiac compression (ECC)
e. cardiac massage (ECM)
e. cardiac pressure (ECP)
e. cardiopulmonary resuscitation (ECPR)
e. cardioversion (ECV)
e. cardioverter-defibrillator (ECD)
e. carotid (EC)
e. carotid artery (ECA)
e. chest wall oscillation
e. defibrillation
e. defibrillator
e. diameter (ED)
e. elastic lamina (EEL)
e. elastic lamina area
e. elastic membrane (EEM)
e. electric cardioversion
e. grid
e. high-output ramp pacing
e. inflatable compressor
e. intercostal
e. jugular (EJ)
e. jugular approach
e. jugular vein
e. mammary artery
e. negative pressure device
e. pacemaker
e. pacemaker battery
e. pressure circulatory assistance (EPCA)
e. pudendal vein
e. respiration
e. ventricular drainage (EVD)

E

externum
> pericardium e.

extra
> E. Back-up guiding catheter
> E. Sport coronary guidewire
> E. Strength Bayer Enteric 500 Aspirin
> E. Strength Doan's

extraalveolar capillary

extracardiac
> e. cavopulmonary anastomosis
> e. conduit (ECC)
> e. Fontan operation
> e. Fontan procedure
> e. murmur
> e. shunt
> e. ventriculopulmonary conduit

extracellular
> e. F-actin
> e. lipid
> e. matrix (ECM)
> e. matrix metabolism
> e. N-terminus
> e. signal-regulated kinase

extracellular-like, calcium-free solution (ECS)

extracellularly responsive kinase (ERK)

extracellular-regulated kinase (ERK)

extracoronary

extracorporeal (EC)
> e. carbon dioxide removal (ECCO₂R)
> e. cardiac shock wave therapy
> e. circulation (ECC)
> E. Circulation Technology (ECT)
> e. exchange hypothermia
> e. heart
> e. life support (ECLS)
> E. Life Support Organization (ELSO)
> e. membrane differential filtration
> e. membrane oxygenation (ECMO)
> e. membrane oxygenation therapy
> e. membrane oxygenator
> e. photochemotherapy
> e. pump oxygenator
> e. volume (ECV)

extracranial
> e. carotid arterial disease (ECAD)
> e. carotid disease (ECD)
> e. carotid obstruction
> e. Doppler sonography (ECD)
> e. internal carotid disease

extracranial/intracranial (EC/IC)
> e./i. bypass surgery

extract
> Apocynum venetum leaf e.
> Azadirachta indica leaf e.
> calf lung surfactant e. (CLSE)
> cell-free e.
> pancreatic e.
> *Rauwolfia* e.
> shiitake mushroom e.
> thyroid e.

extractable nuclear antigen (ENA)

extraction
> e. atherectomy
> e. atherectomy device
> lactate e.
> myocardial lactate e.
> oxygen e.
> e. reserve
> transvenous catheter e.

Extractor 3-lumen retrieval balloon

extraesophageal reflux

extra-fine particle dose (EFPD)

extra-flexible wire

extrafusion defect

extrahepatic portal hypertension (EHPH)

extralobar

extramedullary plasmacytoma

extranuclear

extraparenchymal bleeding

extrapericardial patch

extrapleural
> e. air
> e. apicolysis
> e. catheter analgesia
> e. pneumonectomy (EPP)
> e. pneumothorax
> e. space

extrapontine myelinolysis

extrapulmonary
> e. cough
> e. site
> e. tuberculosis

extrapyramidal side effect

extrarenal azotemia

extrastimulation
> single premature e.

extrastimulus, pl. extrastimuli
> double ventricular e.
> premature atrial e.
> single e.
> e. test
> triple e.

extra-strength 100-PSI catheter

extra-support guidewire

extrasystole (ES)
> atrial e.
> atrioventricular e. (AVE)
> atrioventricular junctional escape e.
> atrioventricular nodal e.
> auricular e.
> auriculoventricular e.
> A-V junctional e.
> A-V nodal e.

infranodal e.
interpolated e.
junctional e.
lower nodal e.
midnodal e.
nodal e.
premature ventricular e. (PVE)
return e.
spontaneous e.
supraventricular e. (SVE)
tip e.
upper nodal e.
ventricular e. (VE)
extrasystolic beat
extrathoracic
    e. airway dysfunction
    e. airway obstruction
    e. neoplasm
    e. rale
    e. soft tissue
    e. tumor
extratracheal
extravasation
    plasma e.
extravascular
    e. granulomatous feature
    e. lung water (EVLW)
    e. space
extreme
    E. II peripheral excimer laser
      catheter
    E. laser disposable catheter (sizes
      0.9 mm, 2.0 m m, 2.2 mm, 2.5
      mm)
    e. pressure (EP)
extremis
    in e.
    respiratory e.
extremitas anterior lienis
extremity, pl. **extremities**

elevation pallor of e.
e. ischemia
mottling of extremities
extremity-artery aneurysm
ExtreSafe phlebotomy device
extrinsic
    e. allergic alveolitis
    e. asthma
    e. compression
    e. factor
    e. force
    e. tenase complex
extrusion
    Kensey rotation atherectomy e.
extubation time
exuberant granulation tissue (EGT)
exudate
    cotton-wool e.
    fibrinous e.
    fluffy cotton-wool e.
exudation
    plasma protein e.
exudativa
    bronchiolitis e.
exudative
    e. bronchiolitis
    e. bronchitis
    e. empyema
    e. pleural effusion
    e. pleurisy
    e. tuberculosis
eyeball compression reflex
eyeball-heart reflex
eyeless needle
EZ45 thoracic linear cutter
ezetimibe
EZ Hold manual compression device
Ezide

E

F, Fr
  French
    F point
    F point of cardiac apex pulse
    F wave
7F
    7F extended-curve thermistor
      catheter
    7F fused-tip catheter
    7F mapping catheter
f
  respiratory frequency
    f wave
    f wave of jugular venous pulse
F2-alpha prostaglandin analog
FA
  femoral artery
FAA plasty
Fab
  fragment antigen binding
    c7 E3 Fab
    chimeric-7E3 Fab
    digoxin immune Fab
    digoxin-specific Fab
    Fab fragment
    m7E3 Fab
FABF
  femoral artery blood flow
FABP
  fatty acid-binding protein
fabric baffle
Fabry disease
FAC
  femoral arterial cannulation
  fractional area change
FACC
  Fellow of the American College of
    Cardiologists
face
    en bloc f.
    moon f.
    f. shield
    f. squeeze
    transverse artery of f.
    f. validity
facet
    clavicular f.
    inferior costal f.
    superior costal f.
    transverse costal f.
facial
    f. barotrauma
    f. canal
    f. diplegia
    f. droop

    f. nerve
    f. vein
facies
    f. anterior cordis
    aortic f.
    f. articularis
    Corvisart f.
    f. costalis pulmonis
    cushingoid f.
    f. diaphragmatica
    f. diaphragmatica cordis
    ecchymotic f.
    elfin f.
    f. inferior cordis
    f. interlobares pulmonis
    f. medialis pulmonis
    f. mediastinalis pulmonis
    mitral f.
    f. mitralis
    mitrotricuspid f.
    f. pulmonalis dextra/sinistra cordis
    f. sternocostalis cordis
facilitated
    f. angioplasty
    f. reperfusion
facility, pl. facilities
    long-term care f.
    LTC f.
    skilled nursing f. (SNF)
facioscapulohumeral
    f. dystrophy
    f. dystrophy of Landouzy-Dejerine
FACS
  fluorescence-activated cell sorter
FACT
  Focus Angioplasty Catheter Technology
FACT-22
  Focus Angioplasty Catheter Technology
F-actin
  filamentous actin
    extracellular F-actin
factitious
    f. asthma
    f. syncope
Factive
factor
    f. I (fibrinogen)
    f. II (prothrombin)
    f. III (thromboplastin)
    f. IV (calcium ions)
    f. V (proaccelerin)
    f. VI (cannot be identified)
    f. VII antigen (FVIIag)
    f. VII (proconvertin)
    f. VIII (antihemophilic f.)

F

factor *(continued)*

porcine f. VIII
f. VIII:C (von Willebrand f.)
f. Xa
f. X (Stuart f. or Stuart-Prower f.)
f. XI (plasma thromboplastin
  antecedent f.)
f. XII (Hageman f.)
f. XIII (fibrin stabilizing f.)
accelerator globin blood
  coagulation f.
AcG blood coagulation f.
acidic fibroblast growth f. (aFGF)
activated f. VII (FVIIa)
activating transcription f. (ATF)
active-site inhibited f. VIIa
angiogenesis f.
antiarteriosclerosis polysaccharide f.
  (AAPF)
antihemophilic f. (recombinant)
antithrombotic f.
atrial natriuretic f. (ANF)
f. B
basic fibroblast growth f. (bFGF)
behavioral f.
carbon monoxide transfer f.
  (TLCO, TLco)
cardiac risk f.
cardiometabolic risk f.
cardiovascular risk f.
Christmas f.
classic risk f.
clot-promoting f. (CPF)
clotting f. (CF)
coagulation f.
colony-stimulating f. (CSF)
connective tissue growth f. (CTGF)
coronary risk f.
corticotropin-releasing f. (CRF)
f. D
duty f.
endogenous digitalis-like
  natriuretic f. (EDNF)
endothelial-derived relaxation f.
endothelium-derived
  hyperpolarizing f. (EDHF)
endothelium-derived relaxing f.
  (EDRF)
epidermal growth f.
exercise f.
extrinsic f.
fibrin-stabilizing blood
  coagulation f.
fibroblast growth f. (FGF)
Fletcher f.
Framingham risk f.
genetic f.
granulocyte/macrophage colony-
  stimulating f. (GM-CSF)

gravitation f.
growth f.
f. H
Hageman f.
heparin-binding epidermal growth f.
histamine release inhibitory f.
  (HRIF)
histamine-releasing f. (HRF)
human atrial natriuretic f. (hANF)
hypoxia-inducible f. (HIF)
f. III deficiency
f. II receptor (F2R)
insulin-like growth f. (IGF)
intravascular procoagulant f.
f. IX complex (human)
keratinocyte growth f. (KGF)
lipid risk f.
lymphocyte chemoattractant f.
  (LCF)
modifying f. (MF)
monocyte chemotactic and
  activating f. (MCAF)
Moody friction f.
myeloid progenitor inhibitory f.
  (MPIF)
myocardial depressant f. (MDF)
necrosis f.
neurohumoral f.'s
N-terminal proatrial natriuretic f.
f. P
paracrine f.
plasma thromboplastin f. (PTF)
platelet f. 4
platelet activating f. (PAF)
platelet-aggregating f.
platelet-derived growth f. (PDGF)
platelet-derived histamine-
  releasing f. (PDHRF)
proatherosclerotic f.
proatrial natriuretic f. (proANF)
proconvertin blood coagulation f.
profibrotic f.
proinflammatory f.
psychological f.
psychosocial f.
recombinant activated f. VII
  (rFVIIa)
recombinant human vascular
  endothelial growth f. (rhVEGF)
Rh f.
rheumatoid f.
risk f.
stem cell f. (SCF)
Stuart-Prower f.
thrombogenic f.
tissue f. (TF)
transcription f.
transforming growth f. (TGF)
transfusion f.

tumor necrosis f. (TNF)
up-regulated tissue f.
vascular endothelial growth f.
  (VEGF)
vascular permeability f. (VPF)
f. VII antigen (FVIIag)
f. V Leiden coagulation defect
f. V Leiden mutation
von Willebrand f. (vWF)
f. XII-kallikrein-kinin system
factor-2
tumor necrosis f.-2 (TNF2)
factor-AB
platelet-derived growth f.-AB
  (PDGF-AB)
factor-alpha
tumor necrosis f.-a. (TNF-alpha)
factor-beta
transforming growth f.-b.
factor-kappa B
nuclear f.-k. B (NF-kappa-B)
facultative bacteria
fading
nicotine f.
faecalis
Alcaligenes f.
Enterococcus f.
Streptococcus f.
faecium
Enterococcus f.
faeni
Micropolyspora f.
Fagerstrom
F. Tolerance Questionnaire (FTQ)
F. Tolerance Scale
Faget sign
Fahraeus effect
Fahr disease
FAI
functional aerobic impairment
failed rescue angioplasty
failing lung sign
failure
ACC/AHA heart f. (stage A-D)
acute congestive heart f.
acute decompensated heart f.
  (ADHF)
acute hypercapnic respiratory f.
acute hypoxemic respiratory f.
acute hypoxic respiratory f.
acute left ventricular f. (ALVF)
acutely decompensated congestive
  heart f. (ADCHF, AD-CHF)
acute-on-chronic hypercapnic
  respiratory f.
acute renal f.
acute respiratory f. (ARF)
advanced heart f.
autonomic f.

backward heart f.
bronchial stump f.
f. to capture
cardiac f. (CF)
cardiovascular f. (CVF)
central baroreflex f.
chronic heart f. (CHF)
chronic renal f.
chronic respiratory f. (CRF)
chronic ventilatory f. (CVF)
circulatory f.
clinicoradiographic heart f.
cocaine-induced respiratory f.
  (CIRF)
compensated congestive heart f.
congestive heart f. (CHF)
congestive right ventricular f.
  (CRVF)
coronary f.
decompensated heart f.
diastolic heart f. (DHF)
early graft f. (EGF)
electrical f.
end-stage heart f. (ESHF)
florid congestive heart f.
forward heart f.
heart f. (HF)
heart surgery-induced cognitive f.
hepatic f.
high-output heart f.
hypercapnic respiratory f.
hypoxemic respiratory f.
impending respiratory f.
insulation f.
left heart f. (LHF)
left-sided heart f.
left ventricular f. (LVF)
living with heart f. (LIFE)
low-output heart f.
multiple-organ f.
multisystem organ f. (MSOF)
myocardial f.
nonhypercapnic respiratory f.
NYHA classification of congestive
  heart f.
organ system f.
pacemaker f.
pacing-induced heart f.
peripartal heart f.
peripartum cardiac f. (PPCF)
power f.
primary graft f. (PGF)
progressive pump f.
pulmonary f.
pump f.
refractory congestive heart f.
renal f.
respiratory f.
right congestive heart f. (RCHF)

F

failure *(continued)*
    right heart f. (RHF)
    right-sided heart f.
    right ventricular f. (RVF)
    systolic heart f. (SHF)
    tachycardia-induced heart f.
    target vessel f.
    ventilatory f.
    ventricular f.
faint
    f. flow
    f. opacification
    f. pulmonary regurgitation
fainting
    hysterical f.
faintness
FAK
    focal adhesion kinase
falciparum
    Plasmodium f.
falcon
    F. coronary catheter
    F. Omniflex balloon
    F. Omniflex balloon catheter
    F. Omniflex PTCA catheter
    F. single-operator exchange balloon
       catheter
fallen lung sign
falling drop
falloff
    upstroke and f.
Fallot
    pentalogy of F.
    F. pentalogy
    pink tetralogy of F.
    F. tetrad
    tetralogy of F. (Tet, tet, TF, TOF)
    F. tetralogy (FT)
    total repair of tetralogy of F.
    F. triad
    trilogy of F.
    F. trilogy
false
    f. aneurysmal chamber
    f. angina
    f. aortic aneurysm
    f. apex
    f. bruit
    f. cardiomegaly
    f. cardiomyopathy
    f. combined hyperlipidemia
    f. croup
    f. cyanosis
    f. dextrocardia
    f. emphysema
    f. hypercholesterolemia
    f. lumen
    f. mass
    f. negative

    f. positive
    f. tendon
    f. vocal cord
false-positive result
FAMA, FAMAT
    fluorescence antimembrane antibody
    fluorescent antimembrane antibody
famciclovir
familial
    f. abetalipoproteinemia
    f. amyloidosis
    f. amyloid polyneuropathy (FAP)
    f. aortic ectasia
    f. aortic ectasia syndrome
    f. apoA-I deficiency
    f. asphyxiant thoracic dystrophy
    f. atrial myxoma
    f. atrial myxoma syndrome
    f. atrioventricular block
    f. cholestasis syndrome
    f. chylomicronemia syndrome
    f. combined hyperlipidemia (FCHL)
    f. congenital cardiac abnormality
       (FCCA)
    f. defective apolipoprotein B (FDB)
    f. dysautonomia
    f. dysbetalipoproteinemia
    f. dyslipidemic hypertension
    f. emphysema
    f. HDL deficiency
    f. high-density-lipoprotein deficiency
    f. hypercholesterolemia (FH, FHC)
    f. hyperchylomicronemia
    f. hypertension (FH)
    f. hypertriglyceridemia (FHTG)
    f. hypertrophic cardiomyopathy
       (FHC)
    f. hypertrophic obstructive
       cardiomyopathy
    f. hypobetalipoproteinemia (FHBL)
    f. hypocalciuric hypercalcemia
    f. intracranial aneurysm
    f. Mediterranean fever
    f. multifocal fibrosclerosis
    f. nephritis
    f. paroxysmal polyserositis
    f. polymorphic ventricular
       tachycardia (FPVT)
    f. premature coronary heart disease
    f. primary pulmonary hypertension
       (FPPH)
    f. pulmonary fibrosis
    f. recurrence
    f. tachycardia
family, pl. **families**
    f. history
    f. history of heart disease
    f. history of myocardial infarction

signal transducer and activator of transcription protein f.

STAT protein f.

family-witnessed resuscitation

Famvir

fan

Dunham f.

Fansidar

Fansimef

Fantoni

F. translaryngeal tracheostomy

F. translaryngeal tracheostomy technique

FAP

familial amyloid polyneuropathy

Faraday cage

Fareston

far-field

f.-f. electrogram

f.-f. QRS complex

f.-f. R-wave sensing

f.-f. visualization

FARI

filtered atrial rate interval

farinae

Dermatophagoides f.

farmer's lung

farnesyl

f. pyrophosphate

f. transferase inhibitor

Farr test

FAS

fetal alcohol syndrome

Fas

F. ligand (FasL)

F. receptor

Fasarium vasinfectum

fascia, gen. **fasciae**, pl. **fasciae, fascias**

pectoral f.

f. pectoralis

Scarpa f.

fascial layer

fascicle

blocked f.

fascicular

f. beat

f. heart block

f. tachycardia

fasciculation

fasciculoventricular Mahaim fiber

fascioperitoneal

f. flap

f. graft

f. infection

f. layer

f. patch repair

fasciotomy

Fas-Fas ligand pathway

fashion

crisscross f.

culotte f.

stoichiometric f.

FasL

Fas ligand

FasL pathway

FAST

flow-assisted short-term

Fourier-acquired steady-state technique

Frenchay Aphasia Screening Test

fast

f. channel

f. cine magnetic resonance imaging

f. Fourier

f. Fourier spectral analysis

f. Fourier transform (FFT)

f. imaging employing steady-state acquisition (FIESTA)

f. induction steady state potential

f. low-angle shot (FLASH)

f. pathway

f. sodium current

f. tissue

f. wave sleep

Fast-Cath

F.-C. Duo introducer

F.-C. hemostasis introducer catheter

F.-C. sheath

Fast-Fit vascular stockings

fasting

f. blood sugar

f. plasma lipid (FPL)

f. plasma norepinephrine

Fast-Patch disposable defibrillation/electrocardiographic electrode

fast-pathway radiofrequency catheter ablation

FastPlaqueTB assay

Fastrach

LMA F.

fasudil

fat

body f.

dietary f.

f. embolism

f. embolism syndrome (FES)

f. emulsion

epicardial f.

high f. (HF)

monosaturated f.

polyunsaturated f.

preperitoneal f.

f. substitute

trans f.

truncal distribution of body f.

fat-absorption coefficient

F

fatal
- f. cardiac arrest
- f. pulmonary embolism (FPE)

fat-free mass (FFM)

Fathom guidewire

fatigue
- collagen f.
- exercise-induced f.
- inspiratory muscle f.
- respiratory muscle f.
- f. testing method

fat-laden microphages

fatty
- f. acid
- f. acid-binding protein (FABP)
- f. degeneration
- f. degeneration of heart
- f. streak

faucial
- f. branch
- f. branches of lingual nerve

faucium
- *Mycoplasma f.*

Faught sphygmomanometer

Fauvel granules

FAV
- floppy aortic valve

Favaloro
- F. proximal anastomosis clamp
- F. saphenous vein bypass graft

Favaloro-Morse rib spreader

FB
- fiberoptic bronchoscopy

FBAO
- foreign body airway obstruction

FBN1 gene

FBP
- femoral blood pressure

FBPM
- forward-backward Prony method
  - FBPM spectral analysis of heart sounds

FC
- free cholesterol

FCCA
- familial congenital cardiac abnormality

FCF
- fetal cardiac frequency

FCHL
- familial combined hyperlipidemia

FCP
- functional conduction period

Fc receptor

FDB
- familial defective apolipoprotein B

FDG
- fluorodeoxyglucose

FDG-PET
- fluorodeoxyglucose-positron emission tomography

FDP
- fibrin degradation product

Fe
- iron
  - Slow Fe

fear of food syndrome

feature
- alexithymic personality f.'s
- clinical manifestation, etiologic factor, anatomic involvement, pathophysiologic f. (CEAP)
- extravascular granulomatous f.

febrile
- agglutinin f.
- f. neutropenia

FEC
- forced expiratory capacity

FECG, FEKG
- fetal electrocardiogram

Fechtner syndrome

$FECO_2$
- fraction of expired carbon dioxide

Federici sign

feedback
- mechanoelectrical f.
- respiratory f. (RFb)

feeder
- bulbar f.
- f. vessel

feeding
- enteral tube f.
- nasogastric tube f. (NTF)

feeleii
- *Legionella f.*

feeling
- suction f.

FEES
- fiberoptic endoscopic evaluation of swallowing

feet (*pl. of* foot)

FEF
- forced expiratory flow

$FEF_{25-75\%}$
- mean midexpiratory flow rate

FEFmax
- maximal forced expiratory flow

Feiba VH Immuno

Feigenbaum echocardiogram

FEKG (*var. of* FECG)

Feldman aortic stenosis catheter

Fell-O'Dwyer apparatus

Fellow of the American College of Cardiologists (FACC)

felodipine
- enalapril and f.

Felson
　　silhouette sign of F.
felt strip
female
　　f. hormone
　　f. pattern obesity
Femara
Femiron
femoral
　　f. approach
　　f. arterial cannulation (FAC)
　　f. arteriography
　　f. artery (FA)
　　f. artery blood flow (FABF)
　　f. artery occlusion
　　f. artery pressure
　　f. artery puncture site
　　f. artery thrombosis
　　f. blood pressure (FBP)
　　brachial, radial, f. (BRAFE)
　　f. canal
　　f. embolectomy
　　f. embolus
　　f. endarterectomy
　　percutaneous f.
　　f. perfusion cannula
　　f. pseudoaneurysm
　　f. vascular injury
　　f. vein
　　f. vein occlusion
　　f. venous sheath
　　f. venous thrombosis
　　f. vessel
femoral-popliteal (*var. of* femoropopliteal)
femoral-tibial (*var. of* femorotibial)
femoral-tibial-peroneal bypass
femoris
femoroaxillary bypass
femorofemoral
　　f. bypass
　　f. crossover
　　f. crossover bypass
femoropopliteal, femoral-popliteal
　　f. bypass
　　f. stenting
femorotibial, femoral-tibial
　　f. bypass
FemoStop
　　F. femoral compression system
　　F. inflatable pneumatic compression device
femtoliter (fL)
fenbufen
fence
　　electron beam f.
　　Kirklin f.
Fenesin DM

fenestrated
　　f. Fontan operation
　　f. Fontan procedure
　　f. tracheostomy tube
fenestration
　　aortopulmonary f.
　　baffle f.
　　cusp f.
fenfluramine
　　f. hydrochloride
　　f. and phentermine (fen-phen)
Fenn effect
FENO
　　total exhaled nitric oxide
fenofibrate
fenoldopam mesylate
fenoprofen calcium
fenoterol
fen-phen
　　fenfluramine and phentermine
fentanyl
Feosol
Feostat
FEP-ringed Gore-Tex vascular graft
Feratab
Fergie needle
Fergon
Ferguson needle
Fergus percutaneous introducer kit
Fer-In-Sol
Fer-Iron
Fernandez reaction
Fero-Grad 500
Ferrans
　　F. and Powers Quality of Life Index
　　F. and Powers Quality of Life Index, Cardiac Version
Ferrein cords
ferricytochrome assay
ferritin
Ferrlecit
ferrocalcinosis
　　cerebrovascular f.
Ferro-Sequels
ferrous
　　f. fumarate
　　f. gluconate
　　f. salt and ascorbic acid
　　f. sulfate
　　f. sulfate, ascorbic acid, vitamin B complex
　　f. sulfate, ascorbic acid, vitamin B complex, folic acid
ferrugination
ferruginous body
FES
　　fat embolism syndrome

F

FES *(continued)*
flame emission spectroscopy
forced expiratory spirogram
FET
forced expiratory time
fetal
f. alcohol syndrome (FAS)
f. aspiration syndrome
f. atrial wall motion
f. bradycardia
f. cardiac frequency (FCF)
f. cardiology
f. circulation
f. electrocardiogram (FECG, FEKG)
f. electrocardiography
f. heart (FH)
f. heart frequency (FHF)
f. heart heard (FHH)
f. heart monitor tracing
f. heart not heard (FHNH)
f. heart rate (FHR)
f. heart rate nonstress test
  (FHRNST)
f. heart rhythm
f. heart sound (FHS)
f. heart tone (FHT)
f. intervention
f. magnetocardiography (FMCG)
f. origins hypothesis
f. oxygenation
f. PR interval
f. souffle
f. tachycardia
f. ventricular myocyte proliferative
  response
f. ventricular wall motion
fetalis
erythroblastosis f.
hydrops f.
fetal-type
f.-t. PCA
f.-t. posterior cerebral artery
fetid sputum
fetuin-A gene
FEV
forced expiratory volume
FEV$_1$
forced expiratory volume in 1 second
FEVB
frequency ectopic ventricular beat
fever
acute rheumatic f. (ARF)
Australian Q f.
bird f.
catarrhal f.
cotton-mill f.
dengue f.
desert f.
familial Mediterranean f.

hay f.
hemorrhagic f.
Jaccoud dissociated f.
Katayama f.
Korean hemorrhagic f.
Lassa f.
lung f.
Mediterranean f.
metal fume f. (MFF)
Monday f.
Omsk hemorrhagic f.
parrot f.
pharyngoconjunctival f.
pneumonic f.
polymer fume f. (PFF)
Pontiac f.
pulmonary f.
Q f.
Queensland f.
query f.
rabbit f.
relapsing f.
rheumatic f. (RF)
Rocky Mountain spotted f.
San Joaquin Valley f.
scarlet f.
septic f.
shoddy f.
sthenic f.
thermic f.
threshing f.
typhoid f.
valley f.
yellow f.
zinc fume f.
FEV/FVC
forced expiratory volume timed to forced
vital capacity ratio
FEV$_1$/FVC
forced expiratory volume in 1 second to
forced vital capacity ratio
fexofenadine hydrochloride
FF
fibrillation-flutter
FFA
free fatty acid
FFA exchange
FFB
flexible fiberoptic bronchoscopy
F-18 FDG
fluorine-18 fluorodeoxyglucose
f-f interval
F-fluorodeoxyglucose imaging
FFM
fat-free mass
FFP
fresh frozen plasma
FFR
fractional flow reserve

FFR_{myo}
 myocardial fractional flow reserve
FFT
 fast Fourier transform
 free-floating thrombus
ff waves
FGF
 fibroblast growth factor
FH
 familial hypercholesterolemia
 familial hypertension
 fetal heart
FHBL
 familial hypobetalipoproteinemia
FHC
 familial hypercholesterolemia
 familial hypertrophic cardiomyopathy
FHF
 fetal heart frequency
FHH
 fetal heart heard
FHNH
 fetal heart not heard
FHR
 fetal heart rate
FHRNST
 fetal heart rate nonstress test
FHS
 fetal heart sound
FHT
 fetal heart tone
FHTG
 familial hypertriglyceridemia
FI
 fundamental imaging
fiber
 accelerator f.
 actin f.
 afferent nerve f.'s
 atrio-His f.
 blocking vagal afferent f.'s
 blocking vagal efferent f.'s
 Brechenmacher f.
 Dacron f.
 dietary f.
 elastic f.'s
 fasciculoventricular Mahaim f.
 His-Purkinje f.'s
 James f.'s
 Kent f.'s
 laser f.
 Mahaim f.'s
 manmade vitreous f. (MMVF)
 nerve f.
 nodoventricular f.
 nylon f.
 parasympathetic nerve f.'s
 pseudo-Mahaim f.
 Purkinje f.'s

 f. shortening
 f. shortening velocity (V_{cf})
 sinospiral f.
 spindle f.
 sympathetic f.
 terminal Purkinje f.'s
 vitreous f.
 wavy f.
fiberoptic
 f. bronchoscope
 f. bronchoscopy (FB, FOB)
 f. catheter delivery system
 f. delivery device
 f. endoscopic evaluation of swallowing (FEES)
 f. esophagoscopy
 f. oximeter catheter
 f. pressure catheter
 f. rhinoscopy
fibrate
fibremia
fibric acid
fibrillar
 f. collagen
 f. collagen network
 f. mass of Fleming
fibrillary wave
fibrillate
fibrillation
 atrial f. (AF)
 auricular f.
 Canadian Registry of Atrial F. (CARAF)
 cardiac f.
 catheter ablation of atrial f.
 chronic atrial f.
 chronic nonvalvular atrial f. (CNAF)
 continuous atrial f. (CAF)
 dilated cardiomyopathy and atrial f. (DCAF)
 early recurrence of atrial f. (ERAF)
 focal atrial f.
 idiopathic ventricular f.
 inducible polymorphic ventricular f.
 lone atrial f.
 medically refractory atrial f.
 nonatrial f.
 nonprimary ventricular f.
 nonvalvular atrial f. (NVAF)
 paroxysmal atrial f. (PAF, PAFIB)
 pharmacological intervention in atrial f. (PIAF)
 postoperative atrial f.
 f. potential
 preexcited atrial f.
 primary ventricular f. (PVF)
 prognosis in atrial f. (PIAF)

F

fibrillation *(continued)*
    f. rhythm
    spontaneous f. (SF)
    spontaneous paroxysmal atrial f.
      (SPAF)
    f. threshold
    vagal atrial f.
    ventricular f. (VF)
    ventricular tachycardia/ventricular f.
      (VT/VF)
fibrillation-flutter, fibrilloflutter (FF)
    atrial f.-f. (AFF)
fibrillatory wave
fibrillin-1
fibrilloflutter *(var. of* fibrillation-flutter)
Fibrimage diagnostic imaging agent
fibrin
    f. bodies of pleura
    f. body
    f. clot
    f. D-dimer
    f. degradation product (FDP)
    f. formation
    f. gel
    f. glue
    f. monomer (FM)
    f. split product
    f. thrombus
fibrinogen
    f. degradation product
    plasma f.
    radiolabeled f. (RLF)
fibrinogen-fibrin
    f.-f. conversion syndrome
    f.-f. degradation product
fibrinogenolysis
fibrinohematic material
fibrinoid
    f. arteritis
    f. change
    f. degeneration
    f. necrosis
fibrinolysis
    endogenous f.
fibrinolytic
    f. abnormality
    f. agent
    f. enzyme
    f. medium
    f. reaction
    f. system
    f. therapy
fibrinopeptide A, B
fibrinopurulent
    f. empyema
    f. phase
fibrinous
    f. acute lobar pneumonia
    f. acute pleuritis

    f. adhesion
    f. bronchitis
    f. exudate
    f. pericarditis
    f. pleurisy
fibrin-specific antibody
**fibrin-stabilizing blood coagulation
factor**
fibroatheroma
fibroblast
    adventitial f.
    f. growth factor (FGF)
    f. growth factor expression
    human fetal lung f. (HFL)
fibrobronchoscope
fibrobullous
fibrocalcification
fibrocalcific lesion
fibrocystic
    f. disease
    f. disease of pancreas
    f. lung
    f. sarcoidosis
fibroelastoma
    papillary f. (PFE)
fibroelastosis
    endocardial f. (EFE)
    endomyocardial f.
    primary endocardial f.
fibrofatty plaque
fibrogenesis
fibroid
    f. heart
    f. lung
    f. phthisis
fibroma
fibromuscular dysplasia (FMD)
fibromusculoelastic lesion
fibromyxoid
    f. connective tissue
    f. lesion
fibronectin
fibronodular bronchiectasis
fibroplastic
    f. cardiomyopathy
    f. disease
fibroplastica
    endocarditis parietalis f. (EPF)
fibroproliferative
    f. disease
    f. phase
fibrosa
    intervalvular f.
fibrosarcoma
    neurogenic f.
fibrosclerosis
    familial multifocal f.
fibrosing
    f. alveolitis

f. colonopathy
f. mediastinitis
fibrosis
adeno-associated virus for cystic f.
African endomyocardial f.
aluminum oxide f.
amiodarone pulmonary f.
autoimmune pulmonary f.
biventricular endomyocardial f.
bundle branch f.
cardiac f.
classic interstitial pneumonitis
 with f. (CIPF)
cobalt-related pulmonary f.
cystic f. (CF)
Davies endomyocardial f.
Davies myocardial f.
diffuse interstitial pulmonary f.
endocardial f.
endomyocardial f. (EMF)
endomysial f.
familial pulmonary f.
focal f.
hard metal-related lung f.
idiopathic alveolar f. (IAF)
idiopathic interstitial f.
idiopathic pulmonary f. (IPF)
interstitial pulmonary f. (IPF)
intraalveolar f.
Löffler endocardial f.
lung f.
mediastinal f.
myocardial f. (MF)
nonspecific idiopathic pulmonary f.
nonspecific lung f.
nontransmural f.
occult cystic f.
parahilar f.
parenchymal f.
partial intermixed f.
patchwork f.
periarteriolar f.
peribronchial f.
perielectrode f.
perimyocytic f.
perivascular f.
progressive interstitial pulmonary f.
progressive massive f. (PMF)
pulmonary f.
radiation f.
rejection-associated pulmonary f.
subendocardial f.
subepithelial f.
tropical endomyocardial f.
fibrosum
pericardium f.
fibrosus
anulus a.

fibrothorax
fibrotic
f. mass
f. scar
fibrous
f. ball
f. body
f. cap
f. cap lesion
f. capsule
f. capsule of thyroid gland
f. dysplasia
f. dysplasia of bone
f. infiltrate
f. mediastinitis
f. pericarditis
f. pericardium
f. plaque
f. pneumonia
f. ring
f. skeleton
f. subaortic stenosis
f. tumor
FIC
forced inspiratory capacity
Fick
F. cardiac output
F. equation
F. oxygen method
F. principle
F. relationship
F. technique
FICO$_2$
fraction of inspired carbon dioxide
Fiedler myocarditis
field
f. cancerization
f. carcinogenesis
f. flow velocity
lung f.
near f.
stippling of lung f.
f. of view (FOV)
FIESTA
fast imaging employing steady-state
acquisition
FIESTA electrocardiogram
FIF
forced inspiratory flow
fifth Korotkoff sound (K5)
fight-or-flight
f.-o.-f. reaction
f.-o.-f. response
figure-of-8
f.-o.-8 abnormality
f.-o.-8 heart
f.-o.-8 intraatrial reentry
f.-o.-8 suture

F

filament
- actin f.
- myosin f.

filamentous actin (F-actin)

filarial infection

filariasis

Filcard vena cava filter

filiform
- f. pulse
- f. stenosis

filiformis
- pulsus f.

filling
- capillary f.
- collateral f.
- f. defect
- diastolic f.
- f. fraction
- f. gallop
- LAA f.
- parameterized diastolic f. (PDF)
- period of ventricular f.
- f. pressure (FP)
- rapid f.
- retrograde f.
- f. rumble
- superior mesenteric artery f.
- ventricular f.

film
- absorbable gelatin f.
- density-exposure relationship of f.
- dirty f.
- end-expiratory f.
- end-inspiratory f.
- f. fixer bath
- f. oxygenation
- f. processing
- Repel-CV bioresorbable adhesion-barrier f.
- scout f.
- serial cut f.'s
- f. wash bath

Filmtabs
- Biaxin F.
- Rondec F.

Filoviridae virus

filter
- Accunet f.
- AngioGuard f.
- arterial f.
- bandpass f.
- bidirectional 4-pole Butterworth high-pass digital f.
- bird's nest vena cava f.
- BTF-37 arterial blood f.
- Butterworth bidirectional f.
- Clear Advantage Spirometry F.
- Cordis TrapEase permanent vena cava f.
- D/Flex f.
- Emboshield bare wire f.
- Filcard vena cava f.
- Gianturco-Roehm bird's nest vena cava f.
- Greenfield IVC f.
- Greenfield vena cava f.
- Günther Tulip vena cava MReye f.
- HEPA f.
- heparin arterial f.
- 2H Technology Breathing Circuit F. (2HBCF)
- Interface arterial blood f.
- Jostra arterial blood f.
- Kim-Ray Greenfield caval f.
- KoKo Moe pulmonary function f.
- LeukoNet F.
- low-pass f.
- mediastinal sump f.
- MedNova f.
- MicroGard f.
- Millipore f.
- Mobin-Uddin vena cava f.
- MultiSPIRO Clear Advantage pulmonary function f.
- nitinol f.
- Re/Flex f.
- Rubicon Embolic F.
- Simon nitinol inferior vena cava f.
- Simon nitinol IVC f.
- Spider f.
- temporary f.
- third-order Butterworth f.
- titanium Greenfield IVC f.
- TrapEase permanent vena cava f.
- triple-bandpass f.
- umbrella f.
- vena cava f.
- Vena Tech IVC f.
- Vena Tech LGM f.
- Vitalograph Bacterial/Viral F.
- Wiener f.
- William Harvey arterial blood f.

filtered
- f. atrial rate interval (FARI)
- f. QRS complex

filtering
- 4-pole Butterworth f.

FilterLine
- F. circuit
- F. sampling technology

FilterWatch sensor

FilterWire EX embolic protection system

filtragometry

filtration
- extracorporeal membrane differential f.
- gel f.

tangential flow f. (TFF)
x-ray beam f.

FIM
functional independence measure

final
f. common pathway
f. rapid repolarization

Finapres
F. blood pressure monitor
F. finger cuff
F. technique

finder
lumen f.

finding
sonographic f.

fine-needle
f.-n. aspiration (FNA)
f.-n. aspiration biopsy

fine particle dose (FPD)

finesse
F. cardiac device
F. guiding catheter

finger
clubbing of f.'s
f. cuff
f. dilation
f. oximetry
F. Phantom pulse oximeter testing system
f. photoplethysmographic device
f. systolic blood pressure (FSBP)

finger-in-glove appearance
fingerprint edema
FingerPrint handheld pulse oximeter
finned pacemaker lead
Finochietto
F. forceps
F. retractor
F. rib spreader

Finochietto-Geissendorfer rib retractor
Fino DVT catheter
FIO$_2$, FiO$_2$
fractional inspired oxygen concentration
fraction of inspired oxygen

firing
laser f.
repetitive atrial f. (RAF)

first
f. effort
f. generation cryoablation catheter
f. heart sound (S$_1$)
f. obtuse marginal (OM1)
f. obtuse marginal artery
f. positive deflection during the QRS complex (R)
F. Response manual resuscitator
f. shock count

first-degree
f.-d. A-V block
f.-d. heart block

first-effort angina
first-generation cephalosporin
first-line therapy
first-night effect
first-order kinetics
first-pass
f.-p. radionuclide angiocardiography
f.-p. radionuclide angiography
f.-p. technique
f.-p. view

first-phase tilt
first-third filling fraction
Fischer
F. pneumothoracic needle
F. sign
F. symptom

Fischl index
FISH
fluorescent in situ hybridization

fish
f. meal lung
f. oil

Fisher murmur
fishhook lead
fish-meal worker's lung disease
fish-mouth
f.-m. cusp
f.-m. incision
f.-m. mitral stenosis

fishnet pattern
fish-scaling effect
F$_2$-isoprostane
fissura
f. horizontalis pulmonis dextri
f. obliqua pulmonis

fissure
azygos f.
horizontal f.
inferior accessory f.
f. of lung
major f.
minor f.
oblique f.
plaque f.
f. sign
sphenoidal f.
Sylvian f.
tissue f.
transverse f.

fissuring
plaque f.

fist percussion
fistula, pl. **fistulae, fistulas**
alveolar-pleural f.
aortobronchopulmonary f.
aortocaval f.

F

fistula *(continued)*
    aortoenteric f. (AEF)
    arteriovenous f. (AVF)
    atrial f.
    atrioesophageal f.
    BP f.
    brachioaxillary bridge graft f.
    brachiosubclavian bridge graft f.
    Brescia-Cimino A-V f.
    bronchobiliary f.
    bronchocavitary f.
    bronchoesophageal f.
    bronchopleural f. (BPF)
    bronchopleural-cutaneous f.
    bronchopulmonary venous f.
    bronchovenous f.
    cameral f.
    carotid-cavernous f. (CCF)
    Cimino-Brescia arteriovenous f.
    congenital coronary arteriovenous f. (CCAVF)
    congenital pulmonary arteriovenous f.
    coronary artery f. (CAF)
    coronary artery-right ventricular f.
    coronary-pulmonary f. (C-PF)
    dural arteriovenous f. (DAVF)
    duropleural f.
    Eck f.
    enteric f.
    esophagorespiratory f.
    Gore-Tex AF f.
    gross tracheoesophageal f.
    H-type tracheoesophageal f.
    pancreaticopleural f.
    pancreatopleural f.
    pleuroesophageal f.
    pulmonary arteriovenous f. (PAF, PAVF)
    renal f.
    silent coronary artery f.
    solitary pulmonary arteriovenous f.
    spontaneous closure of f.
    subclavian arteriovenous f.
    systemic pulmonary f. (SPF)
    TE f.
    tracheoesophageal f. (TEF)
    traumatic f.
fistulectomy
fistulous opening
FITC
    fluorescein isothiocyanate
Fitch obturator
fitness
    biological f.
    cardiovascular f.
Fitzgerald forceps
FIVC
    forced inspiratory vital capacity

fixation
    complex f. (CF)
    f. mechanism
    screw-in f.
    tumor f.
fixative
    Saccomanno f.
fixed
    f. airflow obstruction
    f. coupling
    f. lead
    f. lymphadenopathy
    f. orifice resistor
    f. perfusion defect
    f. upper airway obstruction
fixed-pressure CPAP
fixed-rate
    f.-r. mode
    f.-r. pacemaker
    f.-r. perfusion defect
    f.-r. pulse generator
fixed-wire
    f.-w. balloon
    f.-w. balloon dilation system
    f.-w. coronary balloon catheter
fixer bath
FL
    flow limitation
fL
    femtoliter
flabby airways
flaccid areflexia
Flack node
flagellar
flagellum, pl. **flagella**
Flagyl Oral
flail
    f. chest
    f. chorda
    f. leaflet
    f. mitral leaflet (FML)
    f. mitral valve
    f. segment
FLAIR
    fluid-attenuated inversion recovery
    FLAIR image
flame emission spectroscopy (FES)
flame-shaped hemorrhage
flap
    Abbe f.
    Eloesser f.
    fascioperitoneal f.
    intimal f.
    intraluminal f.
    Linton f.
    liver f.
    microvascular free f.
    pericardial f.

subclavian f.
f. tracheostomy
flapping
f. sound
f. tremor
f. valve syndrome
flare
wheal and f.
flaring
alar f.
nasal f.
FLASH
fast low-angle shot
FLASH MRI
FLASH sequence
flash
F. portable spirometer
f. pulmonary edema
flashing checkerboard test
flashlamp excited pulsed dye
flashlamp-pulsed Nd:YAG laser
flask-shaped heart
flat
f. diastolic slope
f. tube pressure sensor
f. wire coil stent
flattened T wave
flattening
inspiratory limb f.
T-wave f.
flavonoid
flavus
Aspergillus f.
flax-dresser's disease
flaxseed oil
flea-bitten kidney
flecainide
fleeting
f. infiltrate
f. palpitations
Fleet Phospho-Soda
Fleischmann bursa
Fleischner
F. line
F. syndrome
Fleisch pneumotachograph
Fleming
fibrillar mass of F.
Fletcher factor
flex
F. DIC tracheostomy tube
F. stent
F. Tip guidewire
Flex-4 procedure
Flexguard Tip catheter
Flexguide intubation guide
flexibility
flexible
f. balloon-tipped catheter

f. coil stent
f. fiberoptic bronchoscope
f. fiberoptic bronchoscope (FFB)
f. guidewire
f. myocardial biopsy forceps
flexible-tip nitinol guidewire
Flexicath silicone subclavian cannula
flexion
elbow f.
hip f.
shoulder horizontal f.
trunk forward f.
Flexipath surgical thoracic trocar
flexor
F. Check-Flo introducer set
F. introducer
FlexStent
Cook F.
Flextend
F. pacing lead
F. steroid-eluting, transvenous
pace/sense lead
flexure
colic f.
Flexxicon Blue dialysis catheter
flicker fusion threshold
flight
1-f. exertional dyspnea
2-f. exertional dyspnea
time of f. (TOF)
flights-of-stairs
2-f.-o.-s. claudication
flint
f. disease
F. murmur
flip
f. angle
LDH f.
flipped T wave
flitter
floating lead
flocculation
cephalin f.
cephalin-cholesterol f. (CCF)
cholesterol-lecithin f. (CLF)
flock worker's lung
Flolan injection
FloMap
F. guidewire
F. velocimeter
Flonase
flooding
alveolar f.
floppy
f. aortic valve (FAV)
f. guidewire
f. mitral valve (FMV)
f. valve syndrome
floppy-tipped guidewire

F

flora
> mixed f.
> oral f.
> respiratory f.
> tracheobronchial f.

Flo-Rester vascular occluder

Florex medical compression stockings

florid
> f. congestive heart failure
> f. pulmonary edema

Florinef Acetate

FloSeal
> F. FAST sealing device
> F. Matrix hemostatic sealant

flosequinan

flotation
> f. catheter
> f. catheter technique

Flo-Thru intraluminal shunt

Flovent
> F. aerosol
> F. Diskus
> F. HFA metered-dose inhaler
> F. Rotadisk

flow
> f. acceleration
> accessory pulmonary blood f. (APBF)
> f. across orifice
> adequate blood f.
> air f.
> aliasing f.
> antegrade diastolic f.
> anterograde f.
> anular f.
> aortic f. (AF)
> aortic blood f. (ABF)
> aortic ductal f.
> arterial blood f.
> f. artifact
> f. augmentation
> bias f.
> blood f. (BF)
> blunted systolic pulmonary venous f.
> capillary blood f. (CBF)
> cerebral blood f. (CBF)
> collateral f.
> f. controller
> f. convergence method
> coronary f. (CF)
> coronary artery blood f. (CABF)
> coronary blood f. (CBF)
> coronary sinus f.
> coronary sinus blood f. (CSBF)
> f. cytometry
> disturbed f.
> Doppler color f.
> dynamic cardiac blood f. (DCBF)

> effective capillary f. (ECF)
> effective renal blood f. (ERBF)
> endocardial f.
> f. envelope
> epicardial f.
> expiratory tidal f.
> faint f.
> femoral artery blood f. (FABF)
> forced expiratory f. (FEF)
> forced inspiratory f. (FIF)
> forced midexpiratory f. (FMF)
> forearm blood f.
> global f.
> graft f.
> great cardiac vein f. (GCVF)
> hepatofugal f.
> hepatopetal f.
> high f. (HF)
> holodiastolic f.
> infradiaphragmatic venous f.
> f. injector
> isovolume f.
> laminar blood f.
> left ventricular minute f. (LVMF)
> limb blood f.
> f. limitation (FL)
> f. mapping
> f. mapping technique
> maximal forced expiratory f. (FEFmax)
> maximal midexpiratory f. (MMEF, MMF)
> mean forced midexpiratory f.
> mean inspiratory f. (MIF)
> midinspiratory f.
> mitral regurgitant f. (MRF)
> mitral valve f. (MVF)
> f. murmur
> myocardial blood f. (MBF)
> pansystolic f.
> f. parameter
> peak f. (PF)
> peak cough f. (PCF)
> peak expiratory f. (PEF)
> peak inspiratory f. (PIF)
> peak tidal expiratory f. (PTEF)
> peak tidal inspiratory f. (PTIF)
> percent predicted peak expiratory f. (%PEF)
> perigraft f.
> peripheral blood f. (PBF)
> petal-fugal f.
> portal venous f. (PVF)
> pressure f. (P-Q, PQ)
> pressure-compensated f.
> f. profile
> pulmonary blood f. (PBF, Qp)
> pulmonary capillary blood f. (Qc, Qpc)

pulmonary venous f. (PVF)
pulsatile f.
f. rate
f. ratio
ratio of tidal expiratory flow at
  25% of tidal volume and peak
  tidal expiratory f. (TEF$_{25}$/PTEF)
regional cerebral blood f. (rCBF)
regional myocardial blood f.
  (RMBF)
renal cortical blood f. (RCBF)
renal plasma f. (RPF)
f. reserve
F. Rider flow-directed catheter
shunt f. (SF)
shunted blood to total blood f.
  (Qs/Qt)
splanchnic blood f.
systemic blood f. (Qs, SBF)
systodiastolic f.
thrombolysis in myocardial
  infarction f.
tidal f.
time to peak expiratory f. (tPTEF)
time to peak inspiratory f. (tPTIF)
TIMI f.
total coronary f. (TCF)
total pulmonary blood f. (TPBF)
transcutaneous access f. (TQa)
transvalvular f.
tricuspid valve f.
f. velocity
f. volume curve
f. volume loop (FVL)
vortex f.
f. wire
Wright peak f.

flow-assisted
f.-a. short-term (FAST)
f.-a. short-term balloon catheter

flow-delivery waveform

flow-directed
f.-d. balloon cardiovascular catheter
f.-d. end-hole catheter

FloWire Doppler guidewire

flow-limiting
f.-l. disease
f.-l. stenosis

FlowMaker
Pediatric Jarvik 2000 F.

flow-mediated
f.-m. dilation (FMD)
f.-m. vasodilation

flowmeter (*See also* meter)
AirZone peak f.
asmaPLAN+ peak f.
Assess peak f.
Astech peak f.
Asthma Check peak f.

AsthmaMentor peak f.
blood f.
Doppler ultrasonic f.
FM color-coded f.
Gould electromagnetic f.
laser Doppler f.
Narcomatic f.
Parks 800 bidirectional Doppler f.
peak f. (PFM)
Periflux PF 1 D blood-f.
Personal Best peak f.
Pocketpeak peak f.
SensorMedics mass flow sensor
  heated wire f.
SpiroFlow children's peak f.
Thorpe f.
Transonic f.
TruZone peak f.
Youlten nasal inspiratory peak f.

flowmetry
laser-Doppler f.
magnetic resonance f. (MRF)
pulsed Doppler f.

flow-responsive remodeling

flow-sensing
f.-s. pneumotachograph
f.-s. spirometer

flow-time registration

Flowtron
F. DVT pump
F. DVT pump system

flow-volume
F.-v. calibrator
f.-v. loop studies
f.-v. syringe

Floxin
F. injection
F. Oral

floxuridine

FLU
flunisolide

flucloxacillin

fluconazole

fluctuation
heart rate f. (HRF)

flucytosine

Fludara

fludrocortisone acetate

fluens
pulsus f.

fluffy
f. alveolar infiltrate
f. cotton-wool exudate

fluffy-cuffed tube

fluid
arterial f.
arterial pressure of arterial f. (P$_A$)
f. aspiration
bronchoalveolar f.

301

fluid *(continued)*
    bronchoalveolar lavage f. (BALF)
    cerebrospinal f. (CSF)
    f. challenge
    crystalloid f.
    f. dynamics
    epithelial lining f. (ELF)
    interstitial f.
    intravascular f. (IVF)
    intravenous f. (IVF)
    isotonic f.
    f. mechanics
    nasal lavage f.
    partial pressure of arterial f. (PA)
    pericardial f. (PF)
    periciliary f.
    pleural f.
    proteinaceous edema f.
    pulmonary edema f. (PEF)
    respiratory tract lining f. (RTLF)
    retained lung f. (RLF)
    f. shift
    standard perfusion f. (SPF)
    f. therapy
    ventricular f. (VF)
    vesicular f.
    viscoelastic f.
fluid-attenuated
    f.-a. inversion recovery (FLAIR)
    f.-a. inversion recovery image
fluid-filled
    f.-f. balloon cardiovascular catheter
    f.-f. balloon-tipped flow-directed catheter
    f.-f. pigtail catheter
    f.-f. pressure monitoring guidewire
fluidic circuit
fluindione
fluke
    lung f.
Flumadine Oral
flumazenil
FluMist
flunarizine
flunisolide (FLU)
    f. HFA
flunitrazepam
Fluogen
fluorescein
    f. angiography
    f. isothiocyanate (FITC)
fluorescence
    f. antimembrane antibody (FAMA, FAMAT)
    f. bronchoscopy
    laser-induced arterial f. (LIAF)
    f. polarization
    f. spectroscopy
fluorescence-activated cell sorter (FACS)

fluorescence-guided smart laser
fluorescent
    f. antimembrane antibody (FAMA, FAMAT)
    f. in situ hybridization (FISH)
    f. treponemal antibody absorption (FTA-ABS)
    f. treponemal antibody absorption test
fluoride
    hydrogen f.
    f. toxicity
fluorine-18 fluorodeoxyglucose (F-18 FDG)
fluorocarbon poisoning
5-fluorocytosine
fluorodeoxyglucose (FDG)
    cyclotron-produced F-18 f.
    fluorine-18 f. (F-18 FDG)
2-fluoro-2-deoxyglucose
fluorodeoxyglucose-positron emission tomography (FDG-PET)
fluorodeoxyuridine (FUDR)
fluorodopamine positron emission tomographic scanning
fluorogenic
    f. substrate
    f. thrombin substrate Z-Gly-Gly-Arg-AMC
fluorography
    spot-film f.
fluorohydrocortisone
fluorometry
Fluoropassiv thin-wall carotid patch
Fluoroplex Topical
FluoroPlus
    F. angiography
    F. Cardiac
fluoropolymer molecule
fluoroquinolone
fluoroscopic
    f. guidance
    f. isthmus ablation
    f. visualization
fluoroscopy
    biplane f.
    C-arm f.
    kV f.
Fluoro Tip cannula
5-fluorouracil (5-FU)
Fluosol artificial blood
Fluotec vaporizer
fluoxetine hydrochloride
fluoxymesterone
flurazepam
flush
    aortic arch f. (AAF)
    f. aortogram
    f. aortography

f. and bathe technique
heparin f.
mahogany f.
malar f.
warm heparinized saline f.
flushed
aspirated and f.
flushing
f. time
vasomotor f. (VMF)
flutamide
fluticasone
f. propionate (FP)
f. propionate and salmeterol
inhalation powder
flutter
atrial f. (AF, AFL)
atrial noncavotricuspid isthmus-
dependent f.
atypical f.
auricular f.
cavotricuspid isthmus-dependent f.
clockwise f.
completely positive deflection f.
counterclockwise f.
CTI-dependent f.
f. cycle length
diaphragmatic f.
dominant positive deflection f.
F. hands-free chest percussion
therapy device
impure f.
inferior axis f.
isthmus-dependent atrial f.
left septal f.
mediastinal f.
mitral anulus f.
F. mucus clearance device
pure f.
f. R interval
scar and pulmonary vein-related f.
ventricular f. (VF)
f. wave
f. wave morphology
flutter-fibrillation wave
fluttering
diastolic f.
fluvastatin
Fluviral
flux
soldering f.
transmembrane calcium f.
fluxionary hyperemia
Fluzone
fly ash
flying W sign
FM
fibrin monomer
FM color-coded flowmeter

FMCG
fetal magnetocardiography
FMD
fibromuscular dysplasia
flow-mediated dilation
FMF
forced midexpiratory flow
FMIV
forced mandatory intermittent ventilation
FML
flail mitral leaflet
FMLP
formyl methionyl leucyl phenylalanine
FMLP receptor
fMRI
functional magnetic resonance imaging
FMV
floppy mitral valve
FNA
fine-needle aspiration
FO
foramen ovale
forced oscillation
foam
f. cell
polyurethane f.
f. stability test
foamy
f. macrophage
f. myocardial cell
FOB
fiberoptic bronchoscopy
focal
f. activation
f. adhesion kinase (FAK)
f. atrial fibrillation
f. block
f. bronchopneumonia
f. dilation catheter
f. eccentric stenosis
f. edema
f. emphysema
f. fibrosis
f. media aplasia
f. motion abnormality
f. myocytosis
f. myositis of heart
f. pulmonary vein stenosis
f. vasospasm
f. ventricular dysfunction
FocalSeal-L surgical sealant
focus, pl. **foci**
F. Angioplasty Catheter Technology
(FACT, FACT-22)
arrhythmia f.
Assmann f.
ectopic f.
Ghon f.
Kampmeier foci

F

focus *(continued)*
    Simon foci
    subpleural caseous f.
    F. technology
Foerster forceps
Fogarty
    F. adherent clot catheter
    F. embolectomy catheter
    F. forceps
    F. graft thrombectomy catheter
    F. spring clip
Foix-Cavany-Marie syndrome
fold
    adipose f.
    bulboventricular f.
    Marshall f.
    pleuroperitoneal f.
    Rindfleisch f.
    vestibular f.
    vestigial f.
folded lung syndrome
Folgard RX
folic acid
follicular
    f. bronchiectasis
    f. bronchiolitis
    f. pharyngitis
followup
    postinterventional f.
Foltz-Overton cardiac catheter
Fome-Cuf tracheostomy tube
fomite-mediated spread
fomivirsen
fondaparinux sodium
Fontaine lower limb ischemia classification
Fontan
    F. atriopulmonary anastomosis
    F. circulation
    F. connection
    F. conversion
    F. modification
    F. modification of Norwood procedure
    F. operation
    F. palliation
    F. pathway
    F. repair
    F. right atrium
Fontan-Baudet procedure
Fontan-Kreutzer procedure
food
    f. angina
    f. asthma
    F. Guide Pyramid
    sodium content of f.
    whole-grain f.
foot, pl. **feet**
    f. cradle

feet of sea water (fsw)
superficial medial artery of f.
trash f.
f. ulcer
footprint of transducer
Foradil Aerolizer
foramen, pl. **foramina**
    bulboventricular f.
    f. diaphragmatis sellae
    Galen f.
    interventricular f. (IVF)
    jugular f. (JF)
    Lannelongue f.
    f. of Luschka
    f. of Monro
    f. of Morgagni
    oval f.
    f. ovale (FO)
    f. quadratum
    f. rotundum
    round f.
    f. secundum
    thebesian foramina
    f. of veins of heart
    vena caval f.
    f. venae cavae
    f. venarum minimarum atria dextri
force
    atrial ejection f.
    F. balloon
    F. balloon dilation catheter
    contractile f. (CF)
    drag f.
    extrinsic f.
    left ventricular f.
    life f.
    myocardial contraction f. (MCF)
    negative inspiratory f.
    peak twitch f.
    potentiated twitch f.
    P terminal f.
    f. and rhythm (F and R)
    shear f.
    Starling f.
    twitch f.
    unpotentiated twitch f.
    Venturi f.
forced
    f. beat
    f. cycle
    f. expiratory capacity (FEC)
    f. expiratory flow (FEF)
    f. expiratory maneuver
    f. expiratory spirogram (FES)
    f. expiratory technique
    f. expiratory time (FET)
    f. expiratory volume (FEV)
    f. expiratory volume in 1 second (FEV_1)

f. expiratory volume in 1 second
to forced vital capacity ratio
(FEV₁/FVC)

f. expiratory volume timed to
forced vital capacity ratio
(FEV/FVC)

f. inspiratory capacity (FIC)
f. inspiratory flow (FIF)
f. inspiratory vital capacity (FIVC)
f. ischemia-reperfusion transition
f. mandatory intermittent ventilation
(FMIV)
f. midexpiratory flow (FMF)
f. oscillation (FO)
f. oscillation technique (FOT)
f. respiration
f. spirometry
f. vital capacity (FVC)
f. vital capacity analysis (FVCA)

force-frequency relation
force-generating capacity
force-length relation
forceps

Barraya f.
Bengolea f.
biopsy f.
bipolar coagulating f.
Bloodwell f.
Boettcher f.
bronchus-grasping f.
Brown-Adson f.
Carmalt f.
coagulation f.
Cook flexible biopsy f.
Cooley f.
Crafoord-Sellor hemostatic f.
Cushing f.
DeBakey arterial f.
DeBakey Atraugrip f.
DeBakey-Colovira-Rumel thoracic f.
DeBakey-Derra anastomosis f.
DeBakey-Diethrich coronary
artery f.
DeBakey-Mixter thoracic f.
DeBakey-Péan cardiovascular f.
DeBakey tissue f.
dilating f.
Duracep biopsy f.
Duval lung-grasping f.
Englert f.
Finochietto f.
Fitzgerald f.
flexible myocardial biopsy f.
Foerster f.
Fogarty f.
Fraenkel f.
Gerald f.
Gerbode f.
guidewire dilating f.

Harken f.
Hopkins f.
Howard-Kelly f.
Jawz disposable biopsy f.
Julian thoracic f.
Kahler bronchial biopsy f.
Magill f.
McGill f.
Mount-Mayfield f.
National Institutes of Health mitral
valve-grasping f.
NIH mitral valve-grasping f.
Pilling Weck Y-stent f.
Potts bronchial f.
renal artery f.
Samuels f.
Scholten biopsy f.
Tuttle thoracic f.
Varco thoracic f.

force-velocity-length relation
force-velocity relation
force-velocity-volume relation
Ford equation
forearm blood flow
Foregger

F. laryngoscope
F. rigid esophagoscope

foregut
foreign

f. body
f. body airway obstruction (FBAO)
f. body aspiration

ForeRunner (FR2)

F. automatic external defibrillator
F. automatic external defibrillator
device

foreshortening
fork

f. stent
f. stenting technique

Forlanini treatment
form

myocardial infarction in
dumbbell f.
pentamidine in aerosol f.

formaldehyde
format

quad screen f.
scanning f.

formation

aspergilloma f.
coagulum f.
fibrin f.
hyaline membrane f.
impulse f.
rouleau f.
sinus node f. (SNF)
spinnaker f.
syncytium f.

F

305

forme
  f. fruste
  f. fruste of TS
  f. fruste of tuberous sclerosis
formicans
  pulsus f.
formicant pulse
formononetin
formoterol
  f. and budesonide
  f. fumarate
  f. fumarate powder
  f. fumarate powder for inhalation
formula, pl. **formulas, formulae**
  Bayer Select Pain Relief F.
  Bazett correction f.
  biplane f.
  Bohr f.
  Brozek f.
  Cannon f.
  Devereux f.
  Framingham f.
  Fridericia f.
  Friedewald f.
  Ganz f.
  geometric cube f.
  Gorlin hydraulic f.
  Hakki f.
  Hamilton-Stewart f.
  heart rate correction f.
  Janz f.
  f. of Mirsky
  Penn f.
  Poiseuille resistance f.
  Sramek f.
  Teichholz f.
  Triaminic AM Decongestant F.
  Vicks F. 44
  Vicks Formula 44 Pediatric F.
  Yeager f.
formulation
  Sicilian Gambit f.
formyl methionyl leucyl phenylalanine (FMLP)
Forney syndrome
Forrester
  F. syndrome
  F. Therapeutic Classification (grade I–IV)
forskolin
  adenylate cyclase stimulator f.
Forssmann technique
Fortaz
forte
  Aristocort F.
  Enduronyl F.
  Robinul F.
fortis
  pulsus f.

Fortovase
fortuitum
  Mycobacterium f.
forward
  f. conduction
  f. flow of velocity
  f. heart failure
  f. pressure waveform
  f. stroke volume (FSV)
  f. triangle method
  f. triangle technique
forward-backward Prony method (FBPM)
foscarnet
Foscavir injection
fos **gene**
fosinoprilat
fosinoprilic acid
fosinopril sodium
FOSQ
  Functional Outcomes of Sleep Questionnaire
fossa, pl. **fossae**
  antecubital f.
  canine f.
  Claudius f.
  Gerdy hyoid f.
  f. glandulae lacrimalis
  Malgaigne f.
  f. ovalis
  supraclavicular f.
FOT
  forced oscillation technique
Fothergill disease
foundation
  British Heart f. (BHF)
  Heart Disease Research f. (HDRF)
  HON F.
  National Heart f. (NHF)
founder effect
Fourier
  F. analysis of electrocardiogram
  F. 2-dimensional imaging
  F. series analysis
  F. transform
  F. transform analysis
Fourier-acquired steady-state technique (FAST)
Fourmentin thoracic index
Fournier gangrene
fourth
  f. heart sound (S_4)
  f. Korotkoff sound (K4)
fourth-generation cephalosporin
FOV
  field of view
fovea
  f. articularis inferior atlantis
  f. articularis superior atlantis

f. costalis inferior
f. costalis processus transversi
f. costalis superior
f. dentis atlantis

foveated chest

Fowler

F. single-breath test
F. solution
F. thoracoplasty

Fox green dye

FP

filling pressure
fluticasone propionate

FPD

fine particle dose

FPE

fatal pulmonary embolism

FPL

fasting plasma lipid

FPPH

familial primary pulmonary hypertension

FPVT

familial polymorphic ventricular
tachycardia

F and R

force and rhythm

FR2

ForeRunner

F2R

factor II receptor
F2R blood coagulation

Fr (*var. of* F)

fractal

Fractalkine

fraction

atrial filling f. (AFF)
basilar half ejection f.
blunted ejection f.
collagen volume f. (CVF)
CPK-MB f.
depressed ejection f.
ejection f. (EF)
f. of expired carbon dioxide
  (FECO$_2$)
filling f.
first-third filling f.
global left ventricular ejection f.
heparin-precipitable f. (HPF)
f. of inspired carbon dioxide
  (FICO$_2$)
f. of inspired oxygen (FIO$_2$, FiO$_2$)
intrapulmonary shunt f. (Q$_s$/Q$_t$)
left atrial active emptying f.
left ventricular ejection f. (LVEF)
light pen-determined ejection f.
lipoprotein-deficient f. (LPDF)
MB f.
oxygen extraction f. (OEF)
physiologic dead space f.

physiologic shunt f.
regurgitant f.
residual volume f. (RVF)
rest ejection f.
right ventricular ejection f. (REF,
  RVEF)
shortening f.
Teichholz ejection f.
ventricular ejection f. (VEF)
ventriculogram-derived ejection f.
ventriculographic ejection f.

fractional

f. area change (FAC)
f. flow reserve (FFR)
f. inspired oxygen concentration
  (FIO$_2$, FiO$_2$)
f. myocardial shortening
f. velocity reserve (FVR)

fractionation

electrogram f.

fracture

anterior rib f.
cough f.
double-rib f.
gross stent f.
J retention wire f.
lead f.
outlet strut f. (OSF)
pacemaker lead f.
plaque f.
posterior rib f.
rib f.
sternal f.
suprastomal ring f.

Fraenkel

F. forceps
F. node
F. pneumococcus

**fragile X-mental retardation (FRAX-
  MR)**

fragilis

Bacteroides f.

fragilitas sanguinis

fragility

hereditary capillary f. (HCF)
RBC osmotic f.
red blood cell osmotic f.

fragment

f. antigen binding (Fab)
antimyosin Fab f.
antimyosin monoclonal antibody
  with Fab f. (AMA-Fab)
catheter f.
crosslinked D f.
cytokeratin 19 f. (CYFRA)
Digibind digoxin immune Fab f.'s
Digidote digoxin immune Fab f.'s
Fab f.

F

fragmentation
maximum atrial f. (MAF)
f. myocarditis
f. of myocardium
sleep f.
ventricular diastolic f. (VDF)
Fragmin injection
frame
B-scan f.
Framingham
F. equation
F. formula
F. heart failure criteria
F. risk factor
F. risk index
F. risk score
Francisco
Francisella tularensis
frank
f. blood
F. ECG lead placement system
F. XYZ orthogonal lead
F. XYZ orthogonal lead system
Frankel treatment
Frank-Starling
F.-S. curve
F.-S. law
F.-S. mechanism
F.-S. reserve
Frank-Straub-Wiggers-Starling principle
Fräntzel murmur
Franzen needle guide
Franz monophasic action potential
catheter
frappage
Fraser Harlake respirometer
Fraunhofer zone
Fraxiparine
FRAX-MR
fragile X-mental retardation
FRAX-MR syndrome
FRC
functional reserve capacity
functional residual capacity
Fredrickson
F. classification
F. classification of lipid disorders
F. dyslipidemia (type I, IIa, IIb, III, IV, V)
free
f. cholesterol (FC)
f. fatty acid (FFA)
f. liquid
f. liquid migration
f. liquid silicone
f. protoporphyrin
f. radical
f. RIMA
f. RIMA graft

f. root
f. thyrotoxin index
f. wall
free-beam laser
free-breathing coronary magnetic resonance angiography
freedom
Accu-Chek II F.
degrees of f.
Pericarbon F.
FreeDop
F. cordless Doppler
F. portable Doppler unit
free-floating
f.-f. thrombus (FFT)
f.-f. vena caval thrombus
free-flowing empyema
freeing up of adhesion
free-radical scavenger
freestyle
F. aortic root bioprosthesis
F. bioprosthetic heart valve
F. stentless aortic heart valve
F. stentless bioprosthesis
free-wall accessory pathway
freeway
F. Lite portable aerosol compressor
F. PTCA catheter
Freezor
F. cardiac cryoablation catheter
F. CryoAblation system
F. cryocatheter
Freitag stent
frémissement cattaire
fremitus
auditory f.
bronchial f.
friction f.
hydatid f.
pectoral f.
pericardial f.
pleural f.
rhonchal f.
subjective f.
tactile f.
tussive f.
vocal f.
French (F, Fr)
F. catheter (size 3-34)
F. double-lumen catheter
F. JR4 Schneider catheter
6.2-F. 12.5-MHz catheter
3.2-F. Monorail system
F. paradox
7-F. 20-pole deflectable mapping catheter
14-F. punch dilator
F. scale
F. shaft catheter

F. sheath
F. sizing of catheter
6-French
6-F. Angio-Seal
6-F. Judkins catheter
Frenchay
F. Activities Index
F. Aphasia Screening Test (FAST)
frequency, pl. **frequencies**
breathing f. (BF)
ciliary beat f.
critical flicker f.
f. domain imaging
f. ectopic ventricular beat (FEVB)
fetal cardiac f. (FCF)
fetal heart f. (FHF)
fundamental f.
heart f.
high pulse repetition f. (HiPRF)
Larmor f.
natural f.
pulse repetition f. (PRF)
resonant f.
respiratory f. (f)
f. response
f. shifter
f. to tidal volume (f/VT)
f. tracer
frequency-domain analysis
frequens
pulsus f.
frequent spontaneous premature complex
fresh
f. frozen plasma (FFP)
f. gas
Fresnel zone
Freund
F. anomaly
F. operation
freundii
Citrobacter f.
Frey-Sauerbruch rib shears
friability
eggshell f.
friable wall
friction
f. fremitus
f. murmur
f. rub
f. sound
Fridericia formula
Friedewald
F. approximation
F. equation
F. formula
Friedländer
F. bacillus
F. bacillus pneumonia

F. disease
F. pneumobacillus
Friedreich
F. ataxia
F. disease
F. phenomenon
F. sign
frog breathing
frolement
bruit de f.
frond
papillary f.
sea f.
wispish intraluminal f.
frontal axis
Frontier 3 x 2 multi-chamber stimulation device
Frontrunner
F. coronary catheter
F. CTO catheter
F. XP catheter
frosted heart
frosting heart
Frostline linear cryoablation system
frothy sputum
frottement
bruit de f.
frozen
f. elephant trunk technique
f. thorax
FRP
functional refractory period
fructosamine
Frumil
frusemide
fruste
forme f.
frustrate systole
FS-069 contrast agent
FSBP
finger systolic blood pressure
FSV
forward stroke volume
fsw
feet of sea water
FT
Fallot tetralogy
FTA-ABS
fluorescent treponemal antibody absorption
FTA-ABS test
fTCD
functional transcranial Doppler sonography
FTQ
Fagerstrom Tolerance Questionnaire
5-FU
5-fluorouracil
fucose residue

F

fucosidosis
FUDR
    fluorodeoxyuridine
fuel
    biomass f.
fugax
    amaurosis partialis f.
Fugl-Meyer
    F.-M. motor test scale
    F.-M. motor test score
Fujinon flexible bronchoscope
Fukunaga-Hayes unbiased jackknife
  classification
Fulcrum balloon material
fulguration
    electrical f.
full
    f. caloric density
    f. compensatory pause
    f. PSG
fuller's earth pneumoconiosis
full-night attended polysomnography
full-thickness linear lesion
fully automatic pacemaker
fulminans
    purpura f.
fulminant
    f. myocarditis
    f. peptic ulcer disease
fumagillin
fumarate
    bisoprolol f.
    clemastine f.
    ferrous f.
    formoterol f.
    ibutilide f.
fume
    cadmium oxide f.'s
    cobalt f.'s
    metallic oxide f.'s
    soldering f.'s
    toxic f.'s
fumigatus
    Aspergillus f.
function
    atrial transport f.
    auto-threshold f.
    battery cell voltage f.
    bellows f.
    cardiac f.
    cardiovascular f.
    contractile f.
    f. curve
    depressed ventricular f.
    diastolic f.
    dopaminergic f.
    endothelial f.
    exercise LV f.
    global left ventricular f.

    hepatic f.
    intramyocardial f.
    left atrial appendage f.
    left ventricular f. (LVF)
    left ventricular systolic/diastolic f.
    lung f.
    mechanical contractile f.
    mitochondrial f.
    myocardial f.
    neurohormonal f.
    neuromuscular f.
    parasympathetic f.
    perturbed autonomic nervous
     system f.
    phagocytic f.
    platelet f.
    preserved left ventricular systolic f.
    probability density f. (PDF)
    pulmonary f. (PF)
    pump f.
    renal f.
    respiratory f.
    resting systolic f.
    right ventricular f.
    sigh f.
    sinus node f.
    stress perfusion and rest f.
    systolic f.
    valvular f.
    ventilatory f.
    ventricular f. (VF)
functional
    f. aerobic capacity
    f. aerobic impairment (FAI)
    f. assessment
    f. block
    f. capacity classification
    f. cardiovascular disease
    f. compromise
    f. conduction period (FCP)
    f. congestion
    f. dyspnea
    f. failure to capture
    f. image
    f. imaging
    f. independence measure (FIM)
    f. magnetic resonance imaging
     (fMRI)
    f. magnetic stimulation
    f. mitral regurgitation
    f. MRI
    f. murmur
    F. Outcomes of Sleep
     Questionnaire (FOSQ)
    f. pacing abnormality
    f. pain
    f. pulmonary atresia
    f. recovery
    f. refractory period (FRP)

f. reserve capacity (FRC)
f. residual air
f. residual capacity (FRC)
f. status
f. subtraction
f. transcranial Doppler sonography (fTCD)
f. undersensing
functionalism
fundamental
f. frequency
f. imaging (FI)
fundoplication
Belsey Mark IV f.
Collis-Belsey f.
Collis-Nissen f.
laparoscopic Nissen f.
Nissen f. (NF)
Nissen 360-degree wrap f.
Rossetti modification of Nissen f.
fundus, pl. **fundi**
funduscopic examination
fungal
f. endocarditis
f. infection
fungating mass
fungi (*pl. of* fungus)
Fungizone Intravenous
fungoides
mycosis f.
fungus, pl. **fungi**
f. ball
dimorphic f.
invasive filamentous f.
funic
f. pulse
f. souffle
funnel
f. chest
f. dynamics
mitral f.
vascular f.
Furadantin
furcosus
Bacteroides f.
furifosmin
Furman type II electrogram
furoate
mometasone f.

furosemide
Furoside
furrier's
f. lung
f. lung disease
furrow
atrioventricular f.
Schmorl f.
Fusarium solani
fused commissure
fused-tip catheter
fusidic acid
fusiform
f. aortic aneurysm
f. bronchiectasis
fusion
atrial f. (AF)
f. beat
commissural f.
f. complex
critical flicker f.
entrainment with concealed f.
f. QRS
Fusobacterium
F. necrophorum
F. nucleatum
f/V_t
FVC
forced vital capacity
FVCA
forced vital capacity analysis
FVIIa
activated factor VII
FVIIag
factor VII antigen
FVIIIa
cofactor FVIIIa
FVL
flow volume loop
FVR
fractional velocity reserve
f/VT
frequency to tidal volume
respiratory rate to tidal volume ratio
F-wave pattern
Fxa
phospholipid-bound activated factor X
FX miniRAIL RX PTCA catheter

G
>gallop
>>cathepsin G
>>G protein

G5
>G5 massage and percussion machine
>G5 Neocussor percussor

G₂

GA
>general angiography

Ga
>gallium

⁶⁸Ga
>gallium-68

GABA
>gamma-aminobutyric acid

gabapentin

Gabbay-Frater valve suture

Gad hypothesis

gadodiamide

gadolinium chelate

gadolinium-diethylenetriamine pentaacetic acid (Gd-DTPA)

gadoteridol injection

Gaertner (*var. of* Gärtner)

Gaffky scale

GAG
>glycosaminoglycan

gag
>g. gene
>g. reflex

gain
>g. control
>time-compensated g.
>time compensation g. (TCG)
>time-varied g. (TVG)

Gairdner disease

Gaisböck syndrome

gait
>ataxic g.

gaiter perforator

galactomannan
>g. antigen test
>g. enzyme immunoassay

galactophlebitis

galactose

galactosidase deficiency

Galanti-Giusti colorimetric method

Galaxy IVUS imaging system

Galen foramen

Galileo
>G. intravascular radiotherapy system
>G. ventilator

gallamine triethiodide

Gallavardin
>G. murmur
>G. phenomenon

gallbladder disease

gallinatum
>pectus g.

gallium (Ga)
>g. imaging
>radiolabeled g.
>g. scan

gallium-67
>g.-67 imaging
>g.-67 scan
>g.-67 scintigraphy

gallium-68 (⁶⁸Ga)

gallop (G)
>atrial g. (AG)
>atrial diastolic g. (ADG)
>diastolic g. (DG)
>filling g.
>g., murmur, rub (GMR)
>presystolic g. (PSG)
>protodiastolic g.
>g. rhythm
>S₃ g.
>S₄ g.
>S₇ g.
>g. sound
>summation g. (S₇)
>systolic g.
>ventricular g. (VG)

gallopamil

galop
>bruit de g.

GALT
>gut-associated lymphoid tissue

galvanometer
>Einthoven string g.

gambiense
>*Trypanosoma* g.

Gambro
>G. Lundia Minor hemodialyzer
>G. oxygenator

Gamimune N

gamma
>g. globulin
>g. hydroxybutyrate (GHB)
>interferon g.
>g. knife
>g. radiation
>g. radiation therapy system
>g. ray
>g. scintillation camera

gamma-aminobutyric acid (GABA)

gamma-1b
    interferon g-1b
Gammagard S/D
gamma-linolenic acid
Gammar-P IV
gammopathy
    monoclonal immunoglobulin M g.
    polyclonal g.
Gamna-Gandy bodies
Gamow bag
ganciclovir (GCV)
ganglion, pl. **ganglia**
    basal g. (BG)
    Bock g.
    Ehrenritter g.
    inferior g.
    g. inferius nervi
    g. inferius nervi vagi
    left stellate g.
    petrosal g.
    pharyngeal branch of
      pterygopalatine g.
    pterygopalatine g.
    stellate g.
    g. superius nervi
    Wrisberg g.
ganglionectomy
ganglioneuroblastoma
ganglioneuroma
ganglionic blocker
ganglioside
gangliosidosis
gangrene
    angiosclerotic g.
    arteriosclerotic g.
    cold g.
    diabetic g.
    dry g.
    embolic g.
    emphysematous g.
    Fournier g.
    gas g.
    hot g.
    intracardiac gas g.
    Raynaud g.
gangrenosa
    angina g.
gangrenosum
    pyoderma g.
gangrenous
    g. emphysema
    g. pharyngitis
    g. pneumonia
gannister disease
gantry
Gantzer accessory bundle
Ganz-Edwards coronary infusion
  catheter
Ganz formula

gap
    anion g.
    auscultatory g.
    g. conduction phenomenon
    excitable g.
    g. junction
    silent g.
Garatec
Garfield-Holinger laryngoscope
gargoylism
garlic
    Kwai G.
garment
    antishock g.
    Jobst pressure g.
    pneumatic antishock g. (PASG)
    pressure g.
garnet
    yttrium-aluminum-g. (YAG)
Garrett dilator
Gärtner, Gaertner
    G. method
    G. tonometer
    G. vein phenomenon
GAS
    generalized arteriosclerosis
    group A *Streptococcus*
gas, pl. **gases**
    alveolar g.
    ambient g.
    arterial blood g. (ABG)
    blood g.
    capillary blood g. (CBG)
    g. chromatography
    g. chromatography-mass
      spectrometry (GC-MS)
    g. clearance
    g. clearance measurement
    g. clearance method
    g. concentration
    g. constant (R)
    g. dilution
    g. embolism
    g. endarterectomy
    g. exchange
    g. exchange analysis
    expired g.
    fresh g.
    g. gangrene
    ideal alveolar g.
    inspired g.
    intrathoracic g.
    mixed expired g.
    g. mixing
    serial blood g.
    subphysiological volumes of g.
    suffocating g.
    g. supply
    thoracic g.

trapped g.
g. trapping
VX nerve g.

gaseous
g. microembolus (GME)
g. pulse
gas-exchanging region
Gas-Lyte ABG syringe
gasometer
gasometric
gasometry
gasp reflex
gastri
   Mycobacterium g.
gastric
g. acid suppressor
g. aspiration
g. bubble
g. bypass (GBP)
g. inhibitory polypeptide (GIP)
g. insufflation
g. lung
gastric-intrapleural pressure (Pg-Ppl)
gastrocardiac syndrome
Gastrocrom
gastroepiploic artery (GEA)
gastroesophageal
g. reflux (GER)
g. reflux disease (GERD)
g. scintigraphy
g. sphincter
g. vestibule
Gastrolyzer breath hydrogen monitor
gastropneumonic
gastropulmonary
gate
acquisition g.
D, F, H, M g.
gated
g. averaging
g. blood-pool angiography
g. blood-pool imaging
g. blood-pool scanning
g. blood-pool scintigraphy
g. cardiac scan
g. computed tomography
g. equilibrium ventriculography, frame-mode acquisition
g. equilibrium ventriculography, list-mode acquisition
g. list mode
g. nuclear angiogram
g. radionuclide angiography
g. SPECT
g. sweep magnetic resonance imaging
g. system
g. technique

g. view
g. wall motion
gatifloxacin
gating
cardiac g.
electrocardiographic g.
in-memory g.
g. mechanism
prospective g.
respiratory g.
R-wave g.
g. signal
Gaucher disease
gauge
blood pressure g. (BPG)
Bourdon g.
mercury-in-Silastic strain g.
pounds per square inch g. (psig)
Silastic strain g.
gaussian
gauze
Surgicel g.
Xeroform g.
Gazelle balloon dilation catheter
GBM
glioblastoma multiforme
GBP
gastric bypass
   GBP scintigraphy
GC
general circulation
GCD
graft coronary disease
GCI
global cerebral ischemia
GC-MS
gas chromatography-mass spectrometry
G-couple surface receptor
Gc protein
GCS
Glasgow Coma Scale
graduated compression stockings
GCV
ganciclovir
great cardiac vein
GCVF
great cardiac vein flow
Gd-DTPA
gadolinium-diethylenetriamine pentaacetic acid
Gd-DTPA-enhanced MRI
GDP
guanosine 5'-diphosphate
GE
General Electric
   GE Advantx system
   GE CT Advantage high-speed CT system
   GE 9800 CT scanner

G

GE *(continued)*
 GE Lightspeed CT scanner
 GE Signa Horizon SR 120 whole-body scanner
 GE Signa 1.5-T MRI
 GE Signa 1.5-T MRI system
GEA
 gastroepiploic artery
 GEA graft
gefitinib
Ge Gen
gel
 agarose g.
 aluminum hydroxide g.
 Ayr saline nasal g.
 Cann-Ease moisturizing nasal g.
 DermaFlex G.
 electrode g.
 fibrin g.
 g. filtration
 H.P. Acthar G.
 mucous g.
 Nasal Moist G.
 SDS-polyacrylamide g.
gelatin
 absorbable g.
 g. compression body
 g. compression boot
 g. sponge
 g. sponge slurry
 zinc g.
 g. zymography
gelatinase
 92-kDa g.
gelatinous
 g. acute pneumonia
 g. infiltration
 g. sputum
gel-filtered platelet (GFP)
Gelfoam
 G. cookie
 G. sponge
 thrombin-soaked G.
 G. Topical
Gelpi retractor
Gelsoft vascular graft
gelsolin
Gelweave
 G. Ante-Flo
 G. 3-branch Plexus
 G. Valsalva
 G. Valsalva graft
 G. vascular graft
gem
 G. DR implantable defibrillator
 G. II DR dual-chamber defibrillator
 G. II DR/VR implantable cardioverter-defibrillator
 G. III AT implantable cardioverter-defibrillator
 G. III DR dual-chamber cardioverter-defibrillator
 G. II VR implantable cardioverter-defibrillator
 G. Premier Plus blood gas/electrolyte analyzer
 G. SensiCath blood gas monitoring system
gemcitabine
Gemcor
gemfibrozil
gemifloxacin mesylate
Gemini sensor
Gemzar
Gen
 Ge G.
Genac Tablet
Genahist Oral
Genatuss DM
genavense
 Mycobacterium g.
GenBank
 G. genome sequence database
 G. information system
gene
 actin g.
 angiotensinogen g.
 beta-MHC g.
 cardiac sodium channel g.
 c-Jun g.
 C1qR g.
 cyclin A g.
 DCMAG-1 g.
 desmin g.
 D1790G mutant g.
 ecNOS g.
 endoglin g.
 env g.
 epicardin g.
 g. expression
 FBN1 g.
 fetuin-A g.
 fos g.
 gag g.
 glycoprotein Ia g.
 HER2/neu g.
 human ether-a-go-go-related g. (HERG)
 human preproendothelin-1 g.
 IL-4 g.
 Jumonji g.
 Jun g.
 kallikrein g.
 mef(A) g.
 methylase *erm*(B) g.
 methylenetetrahydrofolate reductase g.

MTHFR g.
MTP g.
MyBP-C g.
myosin-binding protein C g.
Panton-Valentine leucocidin g.
g. polymorphism
PVL g.
g. secretor
sodium channel g.
superoxide dismutase g.
g. therapy
g. therapy product
g. transcription
g. transfection
g. transfer injection site
TSC2 g.
TT form of MTP g.
TUPLE-1 g.
zinc finger g.
gene-activated erythropoietin
general
g. angiography (GA)
g. circulation (GC)
G. Electric (GE)
G. Electric Vivid 3, 4, and 7 echocardiology system
g. ward
G. Well-Being Index
generalized
g. arteriosclerosis (GAS)
g. emphysema
g. tuberculosis
generation
neointimal g.
peak of thrombin g. (PTG)
thrombin g. (TG)
generator
Angeion 2000 ICD g.
asynchronous pulse g.
atrial synchronous pulse g.
atrial triggered pulse g.
bipolar g.
Cardioblate RF g.
CardioRhythm g.
Chardack-Greatbatch implantable cardiac pulse g.
Closure catheter/radiofrequency g.
Contak CD pulse g.
Cordis Stockert g.
Cosmos II pulse g.
CPI-PRx pulse g.
demand pulse g.
Down flow g.
fixed-rate pulse g.
IBI 1500T6 g.
implantable pulse g.
Intec AID cardioverter-defibrillator g.
magnet application over pulse g.

Maxilith pacemaker pulse g.
Medtronic pulse g.
Microny II SR+ pulse g.
Minilith pacemaker pulse g.
multiprogrammable pulse g.
PCD ICD g.
g. pocket
pulse g.
quadripolar Itrel 2 pulse g.
Radionics radiofrequency g.
radionuclide g.
rate-responsive pulse g.
Regency SR, SR+ pulse g.
SensorMedics g.
single-chamber pulse g.
small-particle aerosol g. (SPAG)
standby pulse g.
Stockert 70 RF g.
subpectoral implantation of pulse g.
Synchrony II, III DDDR pulse g.
tantalum-178 g.
Trilogy DC, DR, SR pulse g.
ventricular inhibited pulse g.
ventricular synchronous pulse g.
ventricular triggered pulse g.
VNUS Closure catheter/radiofrequency g.
VPAP II ST-A bilevel flow g.
x-ray g.
generator/defibrillator
Ventak Prizm AVT pulse g./d.
Generx gene therapy
GenESA
G. closed-loop delivery system
G. system for radionuclide imaging stress test
Genesis
G. balloon-expandable stent
G. system
genetic
g. disorder
g. factor
g. heterogeneity
g. hypertension (GH)
g. hypertrophic cardiomyopathy
g. locus
g. modeling
g. testing
g. transmission
Genic coronary stent delivery system
geniculate
genioglossal
g. advancement
g. advancement procedure
genioglossus
genistein
Gen-Minoxidil
Gen-Nifedipine
genomic

genotype
ACE-II g.
ACE-DD g.
ACE-ID g.
angiotensin-converting enzyme DD, ID, II g.
DD g.
glutathione-S-transferase g.
methylenetetrahydrofolate reductase g.
mitochondrial g.
MTHFR g.
QQ, QR, TT g.
GenoType MTBDR assay
Gen-Pindolol
Genpril
Gensini
G. coronary arteriography catheter
G. index
G. score
G. Teflon catheter
GenStent biologic
gentamicin sulfate
Gen-Timolol
Gentle-Flo suction catheter
Gentran
Genus stent
Geocillin
geometric
g. cube formula
g. mean diameter (GMD)
g. orifice area (GOA)
geometry
left ventricular g.
normal g.
g. of stenosis
ventricular g.
George-Lewis technique
George Washington strut
geotrichosis
Geotrichum candidum
GER
gastroesophageal reflux
Gerald forceps
geranyl pyrophosphate
Gerbode
G. annuloplasty
G. defect
G. forceps
GERD
gastroesophageal reflux disease
Gerdy
G. hyoid fossa
G. intraauricular loop
Gerhardt
G. change
G. syndrome
G. triangle
Geriatric Depression Scale

geriatrician
Gerlach tonsil
germanate
bismuth g. (BGO)
germanium-68 external source
germanium sesquioxide
germ cell tumor
gerontology
gestational
g. asthma
g. hypertension
GEWS
Gianturco expandable wire stent
Gey fixative solution
GFP
gel-filtered platelet
GFR
glomerular filtration rate
GFT
gradient field transform
GFX
grepafloxacin
GFX 2 coronary stent system
GFX Micro stent III
GFX over-the-wire coronary stent
GGA
ground-glass attenuation
GG/DM
Kolephrin GG/DM
GH
genetic hypertension
GHB
gamma hydroxybutyrate
Ghent criteria
Ghon
G. complex
G. focus
G. primary lesion
G. tubercle
ghosting artifact
ghost vessel
ghrelin
GIA
Global Initiative for Asthma
Global Institute for Asthma
giant
g. aneurysm
g. a wave
g. bullous disease
g. cell
g. cell aortitis
g. cell arteritis
g. cell carcinoma
g. cell interstitial pneumonitis (GIP)
g. cell myocarditis
g. cell pneumonia
g. lymph node hyperplasia

g. TU fusion wave
g. T, V wave

Gianturco
G. coil
G. expandable wire stent (GEWS)
G. Z stent

Gianturco-Grifka vascular occlusion device

Gianturco-Roehm bird's nest vena cava filter

Gianturco-Roubin
G.-R. Flex II stent
G.-R. Flex-Stent coronary stent

Gibbon-Landis test

Gibson
G. circularity index
G. murmur
G. rule

Giemsa stain

Giertz-Shoemaker rib shears

GIK
glucose, insulin, potassium

Gilchrist disease

Gill-Jonas modification of Norwood procedure

GINA
Global Initiative for Asthma

gingivalis
Porphyromonas g.

GIP
gastric inhibitory polypeptide
giant cell interstitial pneumonitis
glucose, insulin, potassium

G$_i$ protein

girdle-like action

gitalin

giving-in/giving-up response

GJA5
Connexin 40 gene GJA5

GKI
glucose, potassium, insulin

glabrata
Candida g.
Torulopsis g.

Glagov
G. remodeling
G. remodeling response

gland
adrenal g.
arytenoid g.
bronchial g.
cardiac g.
esophageal g.
fibrous capsule of thyroid g.
Knoll g.
laryngeal g.
levator muscle of thyroid g.
Nuhn g.
pharyngeal g.

Philip g.
Rivinus g.
sublingual g.
submucosal g.
thyroid g.
tracheal g.

glandula, pl. glandulae
capsula fibrosa g.
glandulae esophageae
glandulae laryngeae
g. lingualis anterior
glandulae pharyngeales
g. sublingualis
glandulae tracheales

glandular pharyngitis

Glanzmann thrombasthenia

glare
veiling g.

Glasgow
G. Coma Scale (GCS)
G. sign

glass blower's emphysema

Glassman clamp

glassy degeneration

Glattelast compression pantyhose

glebae
Acanthamoeba g.

Glenn
G. anastomosis
G. anastomosis procedure
G. operation
G. shunt

glibenclamide

Glidecath hydrophilic coated catheter

Glidewire
G. Gold surgical guidewire
long taper/stiff shaft G.
Microvasive G.
Radifocus G.
Terumo Radifocus G.

glioblastoma multiforme (GBM)

gliosarcoma

glipizide

glissonitis

glistening yellow coronary plaque

global
g. amnesia
g. aphasia
g. asynchrony
g. cardiac disease
g. cerebral ischemia (GCI)
g. flow
g. hypokinesis
G. Initiative for Asthma (GIA, GINA)
G. Initiative for Chronic Obstructive Lung Disease guidelines

G

global *(continued)*
    g. initiative of obstructive lung disease (GOLD)
    G. Institute for Asthma (GIA)
    g. left ventricular ejection fraction
    g. left ventricular function
    G. Therapeutics V-Flex stent
    g. tissue hypoxia
    g. ventricular dysfunction

globe
    bleeding g.

globin
    accelerator g. (AcG)

globoid heart

globular
    g. heart
    g. sputum
    g. thrombus

globulin
    antilymphocyte g. (ALG)
    antithymocyte g.
    cytomegalovirus immune g. (CMVIG)
    gamma g.
    intravenous gamma g. (IVGG)
    intravenous immune g.
    lymphocyte immune g.
    Minnesota antilymphocyte g. (MAG)
    rabbit antithymocyte g.
    respiratory syncytial virus IV immune g.
    Rho(D) immune g.

globus
    g. hystericus
    g. pharyngis

glomangiosis
    pulmonary g.

glomeriform

glomerular
    g. filtration rate (GFR)
    g. hyperfiltration

glomerulonephritis
    acute g. (AGN)
    crescentic g.
    idiopathic g.
    mesangial proliferative g.
    pauciimmune g.
    poststreptococcal g.

glomerulosa

glomerulosclerosis

glomus
    g. pulmonale
    g. tumor

glossectomy

glossopharyngeal
    g. breathing
    g. nerve
    g. neuralgia

glossopharyngeo
    ramus communicans cum nervo g.

glossopharyngeus, pl. **glossopharyngei**

glottic
    g. atresia
    g. constrictor muscles

glottidis
    atrium g.

glottis
    inspiratory narrowing of g.
    g. respiratoria

glove
    compression g.'s
    ESP radiation reduction examination g.'s

gloved
    g. finger sign
    g. fist technique

glucagon

glucarate
    technetium g.

gluceptate
    calcium g.

Gluck rib shears

glucocorticoid
    bolus g.
    inhaled g.
    g. resistance

glucocorticoid-induced hypertension

glucocorticosteroid

glucometer

gluconate
    calcium g.
    ferrous g.
    potassium g.
    quinidine g.

Glucophage

glucoregulatory

glucoronate
    trimetrexate g.

glucose
    g. exchange
    g., insulin, potassium (GIK, GIP)
    g. intolerance
    g. metabolism
    g., potassium, insulin (GKI)
    regional metabolic rate of g. (rMRGlu)
    sarcolemmal g.
    g. transporter 4
    g. uptake

glucose-6-phosphate dehydrogenase (G6PD)

glucose-6-phosphatase

glucosidase deficiency

glucotoxicity

Glucotrol

GlucoWatch G2 automatic glucose biographer

glucuronate
glucuronidation
glue
    fibrin g.
Glu-plasminogen
glutamate exchange
glutamer-250
    hemoglobin g.-250
glutamic-oxaloacetic transaminase (GOT)
glutaraldehyde
glutaraldehyde-tanned
    g.-t. bovine collagen tube
    g.-t. bovine heart valve
    g.-t. porcine heart valve
glutathione (GSH)
    g. disulfide
glutathione-S-transferase genotype
gluteal
    left ventrolateral g. (LVLG)
glutethimide
Glutose
glyburide
glyceraldehyde 3-phosphate
glycerin
glyceroltrinitrate (GTN)
glyceryl
    g. guaiacolate
    g. trinitrate
glycinate
    theophylline sodium g.
glycine site
glycocalicin
    g. index
    plasma g.
glycocalix, glycocalyx
glycoconjugate
    respiratory g. (RGC)
glycogen
    g. cardiomegaly
    g. depletion
    g. loading
    g. phosphorylase
    g. storage disease (type I-VIII)
    g. synthase
glycogenic cardiomegaly
glycogenosis
    cardiac g.
    g. type III
glycol
    polyethylene g. (PEG)
    recombinant polyethylene g. (r-
    PEG)
glycolated
glycolipid antibody
glycolysis
glycolytic enzyme
glycometabolic state
glycopeptide teicoplanin
glycoprotein (GP)

histidine-rich g.
    g. Ia gene
    g. IIb/IIIa antagonist
    g. IIb/IIIa inhibitor
    g. IIb/IIIa receptor
    multikringle g.
    platelet membrane g.
    platelet receptor g.
glycopyrrolate
glycosaminoglycan (GAG)
    g. molecule
glycoside
    cardiac g.
    digitalis g.
glycosphingolipid disorder
glycosylated hemoglobin
glycosylation of intracellular proteins
glycoxidation
glycyl compound
glycyrrhizinic acid
Glydeine
Glynase PresTab
Glyrol
Glytuss
GM-CSF
    granulocyte/macrophage colony-
    stimulating factor
GMD
    geometric mean diameter
GME
    gaseous microembolus
GMP
    guanosine monophosphate
GMR
    gallop, murmur, rub
GMS stain
GNB
    gram-negative bacillus
GOA
    geometric orifice area
goblet
    g. cell
    g. cell degranulation
    g. cell hypertrophy
    g. cell metaplasia
Godart expirograph
Godwin tumor
Goeltec catheter
Goethlin test
Goetz
    G. bipolar electrode
    G. cardiac device
goiter
    diving g.
    mediastinal g.
    plunging g.
    suffocative g.
    wandering g.
Golaski knitted Dacron graft

G

Golaski-UMI vascular prosthesis
GOLD
> global initiative of obstructive lung
> disease
> The Global Initiative for Chronic
> Obstructive Pulmonary Disease
> GOLD staging system

gold (Au)
> g. marker
> g. salt

gold-195m radionuclide
Goldberg-MPC mediastinoscope
Goldblatt
> G. hypertension
> G. kidney
> 2-kidney G.
> G. phenomenon

gold-coated
> g.-c. Inflow coronary stent
> g.-c. NIR stent

golden
> g. hour
> G. sign of S
> G. S sign

Goldenhar syndrome
Goldflam disease
Goldflam-Erb disease
gold-induced lung disease
Goldman
> G. cardiac risk index score
> G. index of risk
> G. risk-factor index

Goldner trichrome stain
Goldscheider percussion
GoldSeal nasal mask
Goldsmith operation
gold-standard method
Goldstein hemoptysis
Golgi
> G. complex
> G. tendon organ

Gomco thoracic drainage pump
gomenol
Gomori methenamine silver stain
gonadal
> g. disease
> g. dysgenesis

gondii
> *Toxoplasma* g.

gonion to pogonion (GO-POG)
gonococcal endocarditis
gonorrhoeae
> *Neisseria* g.

Goodale-Lubin
> G.-L. cardiac device
> G.-L. catheter

GoodKnight
> G. 418A, 418G, 418P CPAP
> system

> G. bilevel CPAP device
> G. home care system

good lung down position
goodness-of-fit test
Goodpasture syndrome
Goodwin protocol
goose-honk murmur
gooseneck, goose neck
> g. outflow tract deformity
> g. snare

Goosen vascular punch
GO-POG
> gonion to pogonion

gordonae
> *Mycobacterium* g.

Gordon elementary body
gore
> G. Eze-Sit valvulotome kit
> G. TAG thoracic endoprosthesis
> G. Viabahn endoprosthesis
> G. Viatorr Tips endoprosthesis

Gore-Tex
> G.-T. Acuseal cardiovascular patch
> G.-T. AF fistula
> G.-T. baffle
> G.-T. bifurcated vascular graft
> G.-T. cover
> G.-T. jump graft
> G.-T. shunt
> G.-T. soft tissue patch
> G.-T. surgical membrane
> G.-T. tube

Goris background subtraction technique
Gorlin
> G. catheter
> G. constant
> G. and Gorlin equation
> G. hydraulic formula
> G. syndrome

gormanii
> *Legionella* g.

Gormel Cream
goserelin
GOT
> glutamic-oxaloacetic transaminase

Gott
> G. butterfly heart valve
> G. shunt

Gott-Daggett heart valve prosthesis
Gottron
> G. papule
> G. rash

Gould
> G. electromagnetic flowmeter
> G. Instrument Systems spirometer
> G. PentaCath 5-lumen
> thermodilution catheter
> G. Statham pressure transducer

Gould-Godart type 18070 ergometer

gout
gouty phlebitis
Gowers
    G. contraction
    G. sign
    G. syndrome
GP
    glycoprotein
gp91^{phox} protein
G6PD
    glucose-6-phosphate dehydrogenase
gp100 protein
grabbing technique
gracile habitus
gradational step exercise stress test
grade
    g. 1-6 murmur
    myocardial blush g. (MBG)
    Sellers g.
    thrombus g.
    TIMI flow g. 0–3
    TIMI myocardial perfusion g.
graded
    g. dilator
    g. exercise test (GXT)
gradient
    A-a g.
    alveolar-arterial g. (AAG)
    alveolar-arterial oxygen g. ((A-a)O$_2$)
    alveolocapillary partial pressure g.
    aortic pressure g.
    aortic valve g. (AVG)
    apicobasal g.
    arm-leg g.
    atrial-to-pulmonary venous g.
    atrioventricular g.
    coronary perfusion g.
    diastolic pressure g.
    Doppler pressure g.
    g. echo
    g. echo-cine MRI
    electrochemical g.
    elevated g.
    g. field transform (GFT)
    g. gel electrophoresis
    hemodynamic g.
    interatrial pressure g. (IAPG)
    intracavitary pressure g.
    intraventricular pressure g. (IVPG)
    mean diastolic g. (MDG)
    mitral valve g. (MVG)
    myocardial velocity g. (MVG)
    peak instantaneous Doppler g.
    peak systolic g. (PSG)
    peak-to-peak g.
    peak transaortic valve g.
    portal pressure g. (PPG)
    pressure g.
    pulmonary bed g.

    pulmonary valve g. (PVG)
    g. recall echo (GRE)
    g. recalled acquisition in a steady
     state (GRASS)
    g. reduction
    residual g.
    g. reversal image
    systolic g.
    transaortic valve g.
    transcardiac g.
    transmitral g.
    transprosthetic g.
    transpulmonary g. (TPG)
    transstenotic pressure g.
    transvalvular aortic g.
    transvalvular pressure g. (TPG)
    ventricular g.
gradient-echo imaging
grading
    Stary histology g.
graduated compression stockings (GCS)
Graduate measuring wire guide
graft
    activated g.
    albumin-coated vascular g.
    aldehyde-tanned bovine carotid
     artery g.
    AneuRx stent g.
    aortic tube g.
    aortocoronary g. (ACG)
    aortocoronary bypass g. (ACBG)
    aortocoronary saphenous vein
     bypass g. (ACSVBG)
    aortocoronary snake g.
    aortofemoral bypass g. (AFBG)
    aortoiliac bypass g.
    aortomonoiliac g.
    Aria coronary artery bypass g.
    Artegraft natural collagen
     vascular g.
    autogenic g.
    autologous fat g.
    beating-heart coronary artery
     bypass g.
    bifurcated g.
    Biograft g.
    BioPolyMeric vascular g.
    Björk-Shiley g.
    bypass g. (BPG)
    CardioPass coronary artery
     bypass g.
    CardioPass layered microporous
     small-bore vascular g.
    collagen vascular g.
    compressed Ivalon patch g.
    coronary artery bypass g. (CABG,
     CARB)
    coronary artery vein g. (CAVG)
    coronary bypass g. (CBG)

G

graft (continued)
g. coronary disease (GCD)
coronary venous g. (CVG)
Corvita endoluminal g.
Corvita endoprosthesis stent g.
cross-femoral g.
Dacron tube g.
descending thoracic aorta-to-femoral
   artery bypass g.
Diastat vascular access g.
diseased g.
double coronary artery bypass g.
   (DCABG)
DTAFA bypass g.
Edwards-Tapp arterial g.
endoluminal stent g.
endoscopic coronary artery
   bypass g. (E-CABG)
endovascular aortic g. (EAG)
ePTFE g.
expanded polytetrafluoroethylene
   vascular g.
fascioperitoneal g.
Favaloro saphenous vein bypass g.
FEP-ringed Gore-Tex vascular g.
g. flow
free RIMA g.
GEA g.
Gelsoft vascular g.
Gelweave Valsalva g.
Gelweave vascular g.
Golaski knitted Dacron g.
Gore-Tex bifurcated vascular g.
Gore-Tex jump g.
Hancock pericardial valve g.
Hancock vascular g.
Hemashield Gold 1, 4 branch
   AAA g.
Hemashield Gold Microvel knitted
   double velour g.
Hemashield Vantage vascular g.
HUV bypass g.
IEA g.
IMA g.
Impra Carboflo ePTFE vascular g.
Impra Distaflo bypass g.
inferior epigastric artery g.
infrainguinal bypass g.
Inoue triple-branched stent g.
InterGard heparin vascular g.
internal mammary artery g.
internal thoracic artery g.
Ionescu-Shiley vascular g.
ITA g.
Jomed Jostent coronary stent g.
Jostent coronary stent g.
jump g.
Kimura cartilage g.
knitted polyester crimped g.

left internal mammary artery g.
left internal thoracic artery g.
LIMA g.
LITA g.
lower extremity bypass g.
mammary artery g.
mandrel g.
Meadox g.
Medtronic AneuRx stent g.
mesenteric bypass g.
Microknit arterial g.
Microknit patch g.
Microvel double velour g.
minimally invasive direct coronary
   artery bypass g. (MIDCABG)
modified human graft umbilical
   vein g.
nonvalved g.
g. occlusion
off-pump coronary artery bypass g.
   (OPCABG)
Passager stent-g.
g. patency
pedicle g.
Perma-Flow coronary bypass g.
2-piece bifurcated intraluminal g.
polytetrafluoroethylene-covered
   coronary stent g.
polytetrafluoroethylene stent g.
portacaval H g.
post g. (PG)
Powerlink endovascular g.
predilated polytetrafluoroethylene g.
PTFE stent g.
radial artery g.
g. rejection
renal artery bypass g.
reversed saphenous vein g.
right internal mammary artery g.
right internal thoracic artery g.
RIMA g.
RITA g.
saphenous vein g. (SVG)
g. seeding
single coronary artery bypass g.
   (SCABG)
g. sizer
skip g.
snake g.
stent g. (SG)
straight tube g.
subclavian artery bypass g.
T g.
Talent g.
T-composite arterial g.
Teflon g.
thoracic stent g.
transluminally placed endovascular
   branched stent g.

triple coronary artery g. (TCAG)
triple coronary artery bypass g.
  (TCABG)
Ultramax woven velour vascular g.
Vanguard III endovascular aortic g.
vascular access g. (VAG)
VascuLink vascular access g.
g. vasculopathy
Vascutek Gelseal vascular g.
Vascutek knitted vascular g.
Vascutek woven vascular g.
Vectra vascular access g.
vein g.
velour collar g.
venous bypass g. (VBG)
vertebral artery bypass g.
Vitagraft vascular g.
Weavenit patch g.
woven Dacron fabric g.
woven Dacron tube g.
Y g.
Y-composite arterial g.
Y-shaped g.
GraftAssist vein-graft holder
grafted vessel
grafting
arrested heart totally endoscopic
  coronary artery bypass g.
  (AHTECAB)
coronary artery bypass g. (CABG)
endarterectomy and coronary artery
  bypass g. (E-CABG)
endovascular stent g.
minimally invasive coronary
  bypass g. (MICABG)
Port-Access coronary artery
  bypass g.
saphenous vein bypass g. (SVBG)
sequential g.
GraftMaster
Jostent G.
graft-seeking catheter
graft-versus-host disease (GVHD)
Graham
G. law
G. Steell murmur
grain
g. dust
g. handler's disease
g. handler's lung
refined g.
gram-negative
g.-n. bacillus (GNB)
g.-n. cocci
g.-n. endocarditis
g.-n. organism
g.-n. pericarditis
gram-positive
g.-p. bacillus

g.-p. cocci
g.-p. organism
Gram stain
granarius
  Sitophilus g.
Grancher
G. sign
G. triad
granoplasm
Grant abdominal aortic aneurysmal
  clamp
granular
g. cell tumor
g. pharyngitis
g. respiration
granulation
Bayle g.
cell g.
g. stenosis
g. tissue
granule
aleuronoid g.
azurophil g.
Birbeck g.'s
E.E.S. G.'s
Fauvel g.'s
Much g.'s
sho-seiryu-to g.
Granulex
granulocyte activation
granulocyte/macrophage colony-
  stimulating factor (GM-CSF)
granulocytopenia
granulocytopenic host
granuloma
cocci g.
eosinophilic g. (EG)
hyalinizing g.
interstitial g.
necrotizing g.
noncaseating g.
pulmonary hyalinizing g.
sarcoid g.
swimming pool g.
granulomatosis
allergic angiitis and g.
bronchocentric g. (BCG)
eosinophilic g.
Langerhans cell g.
lymphomatoid g. (LYG)
necrotizing sarcoid g.
talc g.
Wegener g. (WG)
granulomatous
g. arteritis
g. disease
g. hepatitis
g. inflammation

G

granulomatous *(continued)*
    g. mediastinitis
    g. pneumonitis
granulosus
    Echinococcus g.
graphite
    g. furnace atomic absorption
      spectroscopy
    g. pneumoconiosis
GRASS
    gradient recalled acquisition in a steady
      state
    GRASS MRI
Grass S88 muscle stimulator
gratus
    Strophanthus g.
Gräupner method
Graves disease
gravis
    myalgia g.
    myasthenia g.
gravitation factor
gray (Gy)
    g. hepatization
    g. induration
    g. infiltration
    g. scale
grayout spell
gray-scale ultrasound
Gray-Weale plaque classification
GRE
    gradient recall echo
great
    g. alveolar cell
    g. artery
    g. cardiac vein (GCV)
    g. cardiac vein flow (GCVF)
    G. Ormond Street tracheostomy
    g. vessel
    g. vessel disruption
    g. vessel tear
green
    g. coffee bean
    g. dye curve
    g. sputum
    g. strep endocarditis
Greene sign
Greenfield
    G. IVC filter
    G. vena cava filter
Gregg
    G. cannula
    G. phenomenon
grepafloxacin (GFX)
grid
    external g.
Griesinger sign
Griess test
Griggs tracheostomy

grinder's
    g. asthma
    g. phthisis
grip
    devil's g.
    NEO-fit endotracheal tube g.
    G. Technology stent crimping
      process
    g. torque device
gripping heart
griseofulvin
groaning murmur
Grocco sign
Grocott
    G. methenamine silver
    G. stain
groin
    g. approach
    g. complication
Grollman pulmonary artery-seeking
    catheter
Grönblad-Strandberg syndrome
Grondahl esophagoplasty
Grondahl-Finney operation
Groningen voice prosthesis
groove
    arterial g.
    atrioventricular g.
    auriculoventricular g.
    A-V g.
    bulboventricular g.
    conoventricular fold and g.
    deltopectoral g.
    Harrison g.
    laryngotracheal g.
    nasopharyngeal g.
    pharyngotympanic g.
    terminal g.
    vascular g.
    venous g.
    Waterston g.
Groshong double-lumen catheter
gross
    g. stent fracture
    g. tracheoesophageal atresia
    g. tracheoesophageal fistula
Grossman
    G. scale
    G. sign
ground-glass
    g.-g. appearance
    g.-g. attenuation (GGA)
    g.-g. infiltrate
    g.-g. opacification
    g.-g. opacity
    g.-g. pattern
group
    g. A streptococcal pneumonia
    g. A *Streptococcus* (GAS)

diagnostic-related g. (DRG)
Digitalis Investigation G. (DIG)
Digoxin Investigators G. (DIG)
NICE g.
protein sulfuryl g.
VACTERL Association Support G.
Grover clamp
grown-up congenital heart disease (GUCH)
growth
    dysanaptic g.
    g. factor
    g. factor-beta-1 staining
    g. hormone
    lepidic g.
gruberi
    Naegleria g.
gruel
    atheromatous g.
grumous debris
grunt
    diastolic g.
    expiratory g.
Grüntzig
    G. balloon catheter
    G. balloon catheter angioplasty
    G. Dilaca catheter
    G. femoral stiffening cannula
    G. technique
GSH
    glutathione
GS Modular pulmonary testing system
GSNO
    S-nitrosoglutathione
G-strophanthin
G-suit
GTN
    glyceroltrinitrate
GTP
    guanosine triphosphate
    guanosine 5'-triphosphate
GTPase
    Rho G.
guaiacolate
    glyceryl g.
Guaifed
guaifenesin
    g. and codeine
    g. and dextromethorphan
    hydrocodone, pseudoephedrine, g.
    g. and phenylpropanolamine
    g., phenylpropanolamine, dextromethorphan
    g., phenylpropanolamine, phenylephrine
    g. and pseudoephedrine
    g., pseudoephedrine, codeine

    g., pseudoephedrine, dextromethorphan
    theophylline and g.
Guaifenex
    G. LA
    G. PSE
Guaimax-D
Guai-Vent/PSE
guanabenz acetate
guanadrel sulfate
guanethidine
    g. monosulfate
    g. sulfate
guanfacine
    g. acetate
    g. hydrochloride
Guangzhou GD-1 prosthetic valve
guanine
    g. nucleotide exchange factor protein
    g. nucleotide modulatable binding
guanosine
    g. 5'-diphosphate (GDP)
    g. monophosphate (GMP)
    g. triphosphate (GTP)
    g. 5'-triphosphate (GTP)
guanylate cyclase
guanylyl cyclase
GUARD
    saphenous vein graft intervention using AngioGuard
GuardDOG Embolic Protection System
guardian
    G. AICD
    G. ATP 4210 implantable cardioverter-defibrillator
    G. catheter
    G. ICD
    G. pacemaker
GuardWire
    PercuSurge G.
    G. Plus system
guar gum
Gubner-Ungerleider
    G.-U. voltage
    G.-U. voltage criteria
GUCH
    grown-up congenital heart disease
Guéneau de Mussy point
guggulipid
Guglielmi detachable coil
Guiatex
Guiatuss DAC
Guiatuss-DM
Guiatussin
    G. DAC
    G. with Codeine
guidance
    echo g.

G

guidance *(continued)*
    fluoroscopic g.
    video-assisted endoscopic g.
Guidant
    G. cardiac resynchronization therapy defibrillator system
    G. CRM pacemaker
    G. defibrillator
    G. Heart Rhythm Technologies Linear Ablation system
    G. Hi-Torque Wiggle guidewire
    G. Multi-Link Tetra coronary stent system
    G. Triad defibrillator
    G. Ventak implantable cardioverter-defibrillator
    G. Vision Multi-Link Stent
guide
    ACS LIMA g.
    Amplatz tapered extra stiff wire g.
    Amplatz tube g.
    Amplatz ultra stiff wire g.
    Bentson Plus cerebral wire g.
    g. catheter
    catheter g.
    Cope Nitinol mandril wire g.
    curved tapered Tefcor movable core wire g.
    double flexible tipped wire g.
    Flexguide intubation g.
    Franzen needle g.
    Graduate measuring wire g.
    intubation g.
    Lunderquist extra-stiff wire g.
    McNamara renal exchange wire g.
    movable core straight safety wire g.
    Müller catheter g.
    needle g.
    New York catheter exchange wire g.
    Reuter tip deflecting wire g.
    Roadrunner extra-support wire g.
    tapered movable core curved wire g.
    Tefcor movable core straight wire g.
    Torq-Flex wire g.
    variable stiffness wire g.
    Vista Brite Tip IG introducer g.
    wire g.
guided imagery
guideline
    ACC/AHA pacemaker implantation g.'s
    American College of Cardiology/American Heart Association Task Force on Practice g.'s

American Heart Association g.'s
clinical practice g.'s (CPG)
Global Initiative for Chronic Obstructive Lung Disease g.'s
implantation g.'s
McGoon g.'s
National Cholesterol Education Panel g.'s
NCEP g.'s
NCEP-II g.'s
guider
GuideRight guidewire
guidewire, guide wire (gw)
    ACS Amplatz g.
    ACS exchange g.
    ACS extra-support g.
    ACS Hi-Torque Balance middleweight g.
    ACS LIMA g.
    Amplatz Super Stiff g.
    AngioGuard XP emboli capture g.
    Asahi Prowater g.
    Asahi Soft g.
    atherolytic reperfusion g.
    Athlete g.
    ATW steerable g.
    Balance Heavyweight g.
    Balance Middle Weight g.
    Balance Trek g.
    Bard Commander PTCA g.
    Becton-Dickinson g.
    Bentson exchange straight g.
    Bentson floppy-tip g.
    Bentson-style g.
    catheter g.
    ChoICE Floppy g.
    ChoICE PT g.
    Confianza g.
    ControlWire g.
    Coons Super Stiff long tip g.
    Critikon g.
    Cross-IT g.
    Crosswire nitinol hydrophilic g.
    Crosswire NT g.
    CTO g.
    g. dilating forceps
    Doppler-tipped angioplasty g.
    Elastorc catheter g.
    Emerald diagnostic g.
    exchange g.
    Extra Sport coronary g.
    extra-support g.
    Fathom g.
    flexible g.
    flexible-tip nitinol g.
    Flex Tip g.
    FloMap g.
    floppy g.
    floppy-tipped g.

FloWire Doppler g.
fluid-filled pressure monitoring g.
Glidewire Gold surgical g.
Guidant Hi-Torque Wiggle g.
GuideRight g.
Hi-Torque Floppy exchange g.
Hi-Torque Floppy II g.
Hi-Torque Floppy intermediate g.
Hi-Torque Standard g.
hydrophilic coated g.
HydroSteer hydrophilic g.
intermediate-stiffness steerable g.
intravascular Doppler-tipped g.
Ironman g.
J g.
J-tip g.
Kayak hydrophilic g.
Linx exchange g.
Linx extension g.
g. loop
Magic Torque g.
Magnum g.
Mailman coronary g.
Micropuncture g.
Microvasive stiff piano wire g.
Microvena nitinol g.
Mirage hydrophilic g.
Monorail g.
Newton g.
Patriot moderate support g.
g. perforation
Phantom g.
Pilot g.
Platinum Plus g.
PressureWire g.
Prima laser g.
PT^2 g.
PT Graphix g.
Radifocus catheter g.
g. reflection
Reflex steerable g.
RotaWire Floppy Gold g.
Safe-Cross g.
Safe-Cross-RF g.
Safe-Steer g.
safety g.
Schwarten LP g.
Seeker g.
Shinobi steerable g.
silk g.
Silver Speed hydrophilic g.
Sniper hydrophilic Nitinol g.
SOS g.
Spectranetics Prima laser g.
Stabilizer balanced performance g.
Stabilizer marker wire steerable g.
Stabilizer Plus steerable g.
Stabilizer XS steerable g.
stainless steel g.

steerable angioplastic g.
g. technique
Teflon-coated g.
Terumo Crosswire g.
Terumo Crosswire NT g.
Tomcat PTCA g.
g. traversal test
Trooper extra support g.
Ultra-Select nitinol PTCA g.
Whisper g.
Wholey Hi-Torque Floppy g.
Wholey Hi-Torque modified J g.
Wholey Hi-Torque standard g.
Wiggle coronary g.
Wizdom PTCA steerable g.
Wizdom ST steerable g.

guiding
g. catheter
coronary sinus g. (CSG)

Guillain-Barré syndrome

guilliermondii
Candida g.

guillotine
rib g.

Guiraudon corridor operation

gulae
plexus g.

Gulf War syndrome

gum
g. acacia
g. elastic bougie introducer
guar g.
Nicorette G.
nicotine g.
polacrilex chewing g.

Gunn crossing sign

gunshot wound

Günther
G. Tulip vena cava MReye filter
G. Tulip Vena Cava MReye filter
and retrieval system

gurgling rale

Gurvich biphasic waveform

gut-associated lymphoid tissue (GALT)

gutter
costophrenic g.

guttural
g. pulse
g. rale

Guyatt questionnaire

GVHD
graft-versus-host disease

gw
guidewire

GXT
graded exercise test

Gy
gray

gynoid obesity

G

gyri (*pl. of* gyrus)
Gyrocaps
Gyroscan HP Philips 15S whole-body
  system
gyrus, pl. gyri

angular g. (AG)
inferior frontal g. (IFG)
middle frontal g. (MFG)
superior temporal g. (STG)
supramarginal g. (SMG)

H
- heart
- heparin
    - H space
    - H spike
    - H wave
    - H zone

h
- h peak
- h plateau

H1 receptor

H$_2$
- prostaglandin D2, E, Eq, G$_2$, H$_2$

HA
- Hispanic American
- Horton arteritis

Haake water bath

HAART
- highly active antiretroviral therapy

Haber-Weiss reaction

habit
- alimentary h.'s
- h. cough

Habitrol Patch

habitual cough

habitus
- body h.
- gracile h.

HACE
- high-altitude cerebral edema

HACEK
- *Haemophilus aphrophilus, Actinobacillus actinomycetemcomitans, Cardiobacterium hominis, Eikenella corrodens, Kingella kingae*

hacking cough

HAD
- Hospital Anxiety and Depression

HADS
- Hospital Anxiety and Depression Scale

HAEC
- human aortic endothelial cell

H-Ae interval

haemagglutinin

haematobium
- *Schistosoma h.*

Haemolite autologous blood recovery system

haemolyticus
- *Haemophilus h.*

Haemonetics
- H. Cell Saver
- H. Cell Saver system

haemophilum
- *Mycobacterium h.*

Haemophilus
- *H. aphrophilus*
- *H. aphrophilus, Actinobacillus actinomycetemcomitans, Cardiobacterium hominis, Eikenella corrodens, Kingella kingae* (HACEK)
- *H.* endocarditis
- *H. haemolyticus*
- *H. influenzae*
- *H. parahaemolyticus*
- *H. parainfluenzae* (HPI)
- *H. pertussis*
- *H.* type b conjugate vaccine

haemostasis (*var. of* hemostasis)

Hafnia

HAFOE
- high air flow with oxygen entrainment

Hageman factor

Hagenbach extension of Poiseuille equation

hair-matrix carcinoma

hairspray thesaurosis

hairy heart

Hakki formula

Halbrecht syndrome

Haldane
- H. effect
- H. transformation

Haldane-Priestley
- H.-P. sample
- H.-P. tube

Hales piesimeter

half amplitude pulse duration

half-diluted contrast

half-life
- biological h.-l.
- effective h.-l.
- elimination h.-l.

half-normal saline

half-power distance

Halfprin

half-time
- h.-t. method
- pressure h.-t. (PHT)

half-value layer

hall
- H. prosthetic heart valve
- H. sign
- H. valvulotome

Haller plexus

Hallion test

Hall-Kaster prosthetic valve

H

hallucination
> hypnagogic h.
> hypnopompic h.

halo
> h. sheathing
> h. sign
> H. XP electrophysiology catheter

haloether

halofantrine

halogenated
> h. anesthetic
> h. hydrocarbon
> h. hydrocarbon propellant

HaloLite AAD system

haloperidol

Haloscale respirometer

Halotestin

halothane

Halotussin DAC

Halsted clamp

Haltran

hamartoma
> myocardial h.
> pulmonary h.

hamburger
> h. effect
> H. test

Hamilton-Stewart formula

Hamilton ventilator

Hamman
> H. click
> H. crunch
> H. disease
> H. murmur
> H. sign
> H. syndrome

Hamman-Rich syndrome (HRS)

Hammersmith mitral prosthesis

hammocking of posterior mitral leaflet

Hampton hump

Ham test

Hancock
> H. bipolar balloon pacemaker
> H. embolectomy catheter
> H. fiberoptic catheter
> H. hydrogen detection catheter
> H. II stented bioprosthesis
> H. II tissue valve
> H. luminal electrophysiologic recording catheter
> H. mitral valve prosthesis
> H. modified orifice valve
> H. M.O. II bioprosthesis porcine valve
> H. M.O. II porcine bioprosthesis
> H. pericardial valve graft
> H. porcine heterograft
> H. temporary cardiac pacing wire

> H. vascular graft
> H. wedge-pressure catheter

hand
> h. agitated solution
> h. injection

hand-foot-and-mouth disease

handgrip
> h. apexcardiographic test (HAT)
> isometric h.
> h. stress

handheld
> h. nebulizer
> 8500 h. pulse oximeter

Handi oxygen analyzer

handle
> exchange tip deflecting wire guide h.

Hand-Schüller-Christian disease

hands-off
> H.-o. infusion port heparin-coated thermodilution catheter with TwistLock
> H.-o. thermal dilution catheter

HANE
> hereditary angioneurotic edema

hANF
> human atrial natriuretic factor

hanging heart

hangout interval

Hank's balanced salt solution

Hanley-McNeil method

Hanning window

Hannover classification

hANP
> human atrial natriuretic peptide

Hans Rudolph nonbreathing valve

Hantaan virus

Hantavirus pulmonary syndrome

HAP
> high-amplitude peristalsis
> hospital-acquired pneumonia

HAPC
> high-amplitude peristaltic contraction

HAPE
> high-altitude pulmonary edema

HAPE-r
> high-altitude pulmonary edema resistant

HAPE-s
> high-altitude pulmonary edema susceptible

haploinsufficiency

haplotype
> HLA-DQA1 gene h.
> HLA-DQB1 gene h.

happy tachypnea

HAPVC
> hemianomalous pulmonary venous connection

HAPVD
    hemianomalous pulmonary venous
      drainage
HAPVR
    hemianomalous pulmonary venous return
hard
    h. cardiac event
    h. metal disease
    h. metal pneumoconiosis
    h. metal-related lung fibrosis
    h. pulse
hardening
    x-ray beam h.
Hardy-Weinberg equilibrium
HAREM
    heparin assay rapid easy method
Hare syndrome
Harken
    H. ball valve
    H. forceps
    H. rib spreader
HARM
    heparin assay rapid method
harmonic
    h. component
    h. content
    h. gray-scale imaging
    h. imaging (HI)
    h. imaging mode
    h. imaging ultrasound technique
    h. phase (HARP)
    h. phase image
    h. power Doppler imaging
harness
    Heart Hugger sternum support h.
HARP
    harmonic phase
    Hospital Admission Risk Profile
    HARP image
Harpoon suture anchor
Harrington esophageal diverticulectomy
Harris adapter
Harris-Benedict equation
Harrison groove
harsh
    h. murmur
    h. respiration
Hartmann
    H. clamp
    H. solution
HARTS
    heat-activated recoverable temporary
      stent
Hartzler
    H. LPS dilation catheter
    H. Micro-600 catheter
    H. Micro II balloon
    H. Micro II catheter

    H. Micro XT catheter
    H. RX-014 balloon catheter
Harvard pump
harvester's lung
harvesting
    endoscopic saphenous vein h.
      (ESVH)
    endoscopic vessel h. (EVH)
    saphenous vein h. (SVH)
Harvey Elite stethoscope
HASCVD
    hypertensive arteriosclerotic
      cardiovascular disease
HASHD
    hypertensive arteriosclerotic heart disease
Hashimoto thyroiditis
HASMC
    human aortic smooth muscle
    human aortic smooth muscle cell
Hassall corpuscle
HAST
    high-altitude simulation test
HAT
    handgrip apexcardiographic test
    heparin-associated thrombocytopenia
hat
    bishop's h.
Hatafuku fundus onlay patch
esophageal repair
hatchetti
    Acanthamoeba h.
Hatle method
HATT
    heparin-associated thrombocytopenia and
      thrombosis
hawaiiensis
    Drechsiera h.
Hawksley random zero mercury
sphygmomanometer
hawthorn
Hawthorne effect
Hayek oscillator
Hayfebrol Liquid
hay fever
Haynes 25 material
haze
    hilar h.
    perihilar h.
hazy
    h. appearance
    h. infiltrate
    h. lesion
HB
    heart block
    His bundle
Hb
    hemoglobin
    Hb oximetry

2HBCF
2H Technology Breathing Circuit Filter
HbCO$_2$
carboxyhemoglobin
HBD2
human beta defensin 2
HBDH
hydroxybutyrate dehydrogenase
HBE
His bundle electrogram
HBHA
heparin-binding hemagglutinin
hBMSC transplantation
HBO
hyperbaric oxygen
HBO therapy
HbO$_2$
oxyhemoglobin
HbO$_2$ oximetry
HbOC vaccine
HBOT
hyperbaric oxygen therapy
HBoV
parvovirus human bocavirus
HBP
heartbeat period
high blood pressure
HBT Sleuth portable hydrogen monitor
HC
hypercholesterolemia
hypertrophic cardiomyopathy
Bancap HC
HCAP
healthcare-associated pneumonia
HCF
heparin cofactor
hereditary capillary fragility
HCl
hydrochloride
anagrelide HCl
cefepime HCl
colesevelam HCl
dexmedetomidine HCl
isoetharine HCl
isoproteronol HCl
levalbuterol HCl
moxifloxacin HCl
sotalol HCl
verapamil HCl
HCM, HCMP
hypertrophic cardiomyopathy
HCMV
human cytomegalovirus
HCN
hydrogen cyanide
HCO$_3$
bicarbonate
HCoV-NL63
human coronavirus NL63

HCT, HCTZ
hydrochlorothiazide
Atacand HCT
Avapro HCT
Diovan HCT
Lotensin HCT
HCTS
high cholesterol and tocopherol
supplement
HCVD
hypertensive cardiovascular disease
HD
heart disease
HDAC2
histone deacetylase 2
HDE
human device exemption
HDH
heart disease history
HDL
high-density lipoprotein
diabetic HDL
isolated low HDL
nascent HDL
pre-beta 1 HDL
HDLBP
high-density lipoprotein binding protein
HDL-C
high-density lipoprotein-cholesterol
complex
HDL-c
high-density lipoprotein-cell surface
HDLP
high-density lipoprotein
HDM
house dust mite
HDM allergen
HDRF
Heart Disease Research Foundation
HDU
high-dependency unit
HE
hypertensive encephalopathy
H&E
hematoxylin and eosin
H&E stain
He
heart
head
H. area
H. paradoxical reflex
H. zone
headache
migraine h.
syncopal migraine h.
head-down tilt test
headhunter angiography catheter
head-out water immersion

headpiece
    e-Net h.
head-tilt
    h.-t., chin-lift maneuver
    h.-t. method
head-up
    h.-u. tilt (HUT)
    h.-u., tilt-induced syncope
    h.-u. tilt-table test (HUTTT)
    h.-u. tilt test
Heaf test
healed
    h. myocardial infarct (HMI)
    h. tuberculosis
healing
    per primam h.
    per secundum h.
health
    H. behavior model
    H. Insurance Portability and
      Accountability Act of 1996
      (HIPAA)
    H. level 7 (HL7)
    H. Locus of Control Scale
    National Institute of Occupational
      Safety and H. (NIOSH)
    National Institutes of H. (NIH)
    H. On the Net (HON)
    H. On the Net code of conduct
      (HONcode)
healthcare
healthcare-associated pneumonia (HCAP)
Healthdyne Quantum PSV ventilator
health-related quality of life (HRQL,
  HRQOL)
healthy
    H. Early Alarm Recognition and
      Telemonitoring System (HEARTS)
    H. Heart diet
    h. worker effect
heard
    fetal heart h. (FHH)
    fetal heart not h. (FHNH)
heart (H, He, HT, ht)
    abdominal h.
    AbioCor implantable replacement h.
    AbioCor mechanical h.
    acute margin of h.
    H. Aid 80 defibrillator
    H. Aide Etd recorder
    air-driven artificial h.
    Akutsu III total artificial h.
    anterior surface of h.
    armor h.
    armored h.
    h. arrest
    artificial h. (AH)
    h. assist device
    athlete's h.

athletic h.
atrium of h.
h. attack
baggy h.
balloon-shaped h.
beer h.
beriberi h.
Berlin total artificial h.
h. block (HB)
3:1 h. block
3:2 h. block
boat-shaped h.
bony h.
booster h.
boot-shaped h.
bovine h.
box-like h.
CardioWest temporary total
  artificial h.
cervical h.
3-chambered h.
h. chamber remodeling
chambers of the h.
chaotic h.
charcoal h.
compensatory hypertrophy of h.
compliance of h.
congenital malformation of h.
  (CMH)
contour of h.
contracted h.
corticosteroid-treated h.
crisscross h.
crux of h.
h. death
decortication of h.
dextroposition of h.
dextroversion of h.
diaphragmatic surface of h.
dilation of h.
h. disease (HD)
h. disease history (HDH)
H. Disease Research Foundation
  (HDRF)
disordered action of h. (DAH)
donor h.
drop h.
dynamite h.
egg-on-its-side h.
egg-shaped h.
electrical alternation of h.
electromechanical artificial h.
encased h.
enlarged h. (EH)
Excor temporary total artificial h.
explanted h.
extracorporeal h.
h. failure (HF)
h. failure cell

H

heart *(continued)*
    H. Failure Knowledge Test
    H. Failure Society of America
      (HFSA)
    fatty degeneration of h.
    fetal h. (FH)
    fibroid h.
    figure-of-8 h.
    flask-shaped h.
    focal myositis of h.
    foramen of veins of h.
    h. frequency
    frosted h.
    frosting h.
    globoid h.
    globular h.
    gripping h.
    hairy h.
    hanging h.
    height of h. (Ht)
    h. helper
    holiday h.
    Holmes h.
    horizontal h.
    H. Hugger sternum support harness
    hyperthyroid h.
    hypertrophied h.
    hypoplastic h.
    hypoplastic left h. (HPLH)
    icing h.
    implantable artificial h. (IAH)
    h. infusion (HI)
    h. infusion broth (HIB)
    intermediate h.
    intracorporeal h.
    irritable h.
    h. jacket
    Jarvik-7 artificial h.
    Jarvik 7-70 artificial h.
    Jarvik 2000 artificial h.
    H. Laser
    h. laser revascularization
    H. Laser system
    H. Laser for TMR
    law of the h.
    left h. (LH)
    left auricle of h.
    left margin of h.
    Liotta total artificial h.
    h., liver, kidneys (H-L-K)
    h. loop
    h. and lung (H&L)
    h. massage
    mechanical h.
    mechanical alternation of h.
    h. minute output (HMO)
    movable h.
    moyamoya of h.
    h. murmur (HM)

    myocytolysis of h.
    myxedema h.
    natural failing h.
    H. nebulizer
    Norwood operation for hypoplastic
      left-sided h.
    obtuse margin of h.
    orthotopic univentricular artificial h.
    ox h.
    h. palpitations
    paracorporeal h.
    parchment h.
    partial artificial h.
    pear-shaped h.
    pectoral h.
    pendulous h.
    h. position
    postischemic h.
    pulmonary h.
    h. pump
    Quain fatty h.
    h. rate (HR, HRT)
    h. rate audiometry (HRA)
    h. rate correction formula
    h. rate fluctuation (HRF)
    h. rate-pressure product
    h. rate range (HRR)
    h. rate recovery (HRR)
    h. rate reserve (HRR)
    h. rate retardation index (HRRI)
    h. rate-systolic blood pressure
      product (RPP)
    h. rate turbulence
    h. rate variability (HRV)
    h. rate variability test
    recipient h.
    h. reflex
    reinnervation in transplanted h.
    rheumatism of the h.
    h. rhythm
    right h. (RH)
    right auricle of h.
    right margin of h.
    round h.
    sabot h.
    semihorizontal h.
    semivertical h.
    senescent h.
    septation of h.
    h. shock protein antigen
    skeleton of h.
    skin h.
    snowman h.
    soldier's h.
    h. sound (HS)
    h. sounds S_1, S_2, S_3, S_4
    stiff h.
    stone h.
    h. stroke

superoinferior h.
h. surgery-induced cognitive failure
suspended h.
swinging h.
Symbion total artificial h.
h. synchronized evoked potential (HSEP)
systemic h.
tabby cat h.
takotsubo h.
h. tamponade
Taussig-Bing h.
teardrop h.
temporary total artificial h. (TAH-t)
tendinous zones of h.
thrush breast h.
tiger lily h.
tobacco h.
h. tone (HT, Ht, ht)
total artificial h. (TAH)
total implantation of artificial h. (TIAH)
h. transplant (HT)
h. transplantation (HT)
transplanted h.
transverse section of h.
Traube h.
triatrial h.
trilocular h.
univentricular h.
upstairs-downstairs h.
Utah total artificial h.
h. valve
h. valve prosthesis
h. valve replacement surgery
valvular disease of h. (VDH)
venous h.
1-ventricle h.
vertical h.
Vienna total artificial h.
h. volume (HV)
waist of h.
h. wall
wandering h.
water-bottle h.
h. weight (HW)
wooden-shoe h.
HeartBar Orange Drink
heartbeat
AE h.
h. period (HBP)
HeartCam
H. EBT
H. electronic beam tomography
HeartCard
H. monitor
H. 3X cardiac event recorder
heart-hand syndrome

heart-lung
h.-l. block
h.-l. bypass
h.-l. machine
h.-l. resuscitation (HLR)
h.-l. transplant (HLT, HLTx)
h.-l. transplantation (HLT)
HeartMate
H. implantable pneumatic left ventricular assist system
H. implantable ventricular assist device
H. LVAD
H. LVAS
H. pump
H. SNAP-VE LVAS
H. vented electric left ventricular assist system
Heartport
H. endoaortic clamp
H. endocoronary sinus catheter
H. endopulmonary vent catheter
H. endovascular catheter
H. endovenous drainage cannula
H. Port-Access system
H. technique
HEARTS
Healthy Early Alarm Recognition and Telemonitoring System
HeartSaver VAD
Heartscan heart attack prediction test
HeartStart MRx defibrillator
Heartstream
H. FR2 AED
H. FR2 AED with attenuated defibrillation pad
Heartstring Proximal Seal System
heart-type fatty acid binding protein (H-FABP)
HeartView CT
HearTwave system
heat
h. load
h. shock protein (HSP, hsp)
h. shock protein 47 (HSP47)
h. shock protein 70 (HSP70)
h. stroke
heat-activated recoverable temporary stent (HARTS)
Heath-Edwards
H.-E. classification
H.-E. criteria
heating
ohmic h.
resistive h.
volume h.
heat/moisture exchanger (HME)
heat-treated
Profilnine H.-T.

H

heave
    parasternal h.
    precordial h.
    right ventricular h.
heavy
    h. chain
    h. chain cardiac myosin (MYHC)
    h. chain cardiac myosin alpha
      (MYHCA)
    h. metal
Heberden
    H. angina
    H. asthma
    H. node
Hecht pneumonia
HED
    hydroxyephedrine
heel strike
Heffner criteria
Hegglin syndrome
HEHR
    highest equivalent heart rate
height
    AR jet h.
    coaptation h.
    h. of heart (Ht)
    left ventricle outflow h. (LVOH)
    right hemidiaphragm h.
    Z score weight-Z score h.
heightened immunity
Heim-Kreysig sign
Heimlich
    H. chest drainage valve
    H. heart valve
    H. maneuver
    H. sign
Heinecke method
Heiner syndrome
Heinz body
Heister diverticulum
HeLa cell
Helex septal occluder
helical
    h. coil stent
    h. CT
    h. CT scanning
    h. CT venography
helices (*pl. of* helix)
Helicobacter pylori
HELiOS oxygen delivery system
heliox
    helium-oxygen mixture
      heliox nebulizer
Helistat
Helistent
helium
    h. dilution

    h. dilution method
    h. washout
helium-oxygen mixture (heliox)
helix, pl. **helices**
    amphipathic h.
    H. balloon
    H. clot buster thrombectomy device
    H. PTCA dilation catheter
Helixate
Heller-Belsey operation
Heller-Döhle disease
Heller esophagomyotomy
Heller-Nissen operation
HELLP
    hemolysis, elevated liver enzymes, low
    platelets
      HELLP syndrome
Helmholtz head coil
helminth
helminthic myocarditis
Helminthosporium
HELP
    heparin-induced extracorporeal low-
    density lipoprotein precipitation
HELP-apheresis treatment
helper
    heart h.
HEM780 blood pressure monitor
hemadostenosis
Hemaflex
    H. PTCA sheath
    H. PTCA sheath with obturator
hemagglutinin
    heparin-binding h. (HBHA)
hemangioendothelioma
    epithelioid h.
    pulmonary h.
hemangioma
    cavernous h.
    lobular capillary h.
    sclerosing h.
hemangioma-thrombocytopenia syndrome
hemangiomatosis
    pulmonary capillary h.
hemangiopericytoma
hemangiosarcoma
Hemaquet
    H. introducer
    H. introducer sheath
    H. PTCA sheath
    H. PTCA sheath with obturator
hemarthrosis
Hemashield
    H. Gold 1, 4 branch AAA graft
    H. Gold Microvel knitted double
    velour graft
    H. Vantage vascular graft
hemathorax (*var. of* hemothorax)
hematin

hematocrit
hematogenous
  h. bacterial dissemination
  h. embolism
  h. metastasis
  h. nodule
  h. pneumonia
  h. tuberculosis
hematologic disease
hematoma
  aneurysmal h.
  aortic intramural h. (AIH)
  apical h.
  dissecting h.
  intramural h. (IH, IMH)
  intramyocardial h.
  intraparenchymal h.
  irregular h.
  lobular h.
  loculated pericardial h.
  parenchymal h. (PH)
  periaortic h.
  pouch h.
  pulmonary h.
  retroperitoneal h.
  round h.
  subdural h. (SDH)
hematopoiesis
hematopoietic
  h. chimerism
  h. stem cell (HSC)
  h. system
hematoporphyrin derivative (HPD)
hematosis
hematoxylin
  h. and eosin (H&E)
  h. and eosin stain
hematuria
hemianomalous
  h. pulmonary venous connection
    (HAPVC)
  h. pulmonary venous drainage
    (HAPVD)
  h. pulmonary venous return
    (HAPVR)
hemianopia
hemiaxial view
hemiazygos vein
hemiblock
  left anterior h. (LAH)
  left anterior superior h. (LASH)
  left middle h.
  left posterior h.
  left posterior inferior h. (LPIH)
  left septal h.
hemic
  h. hypoxia
  h. murmur
  h. systole

hemicardia
hemidesmosome
hemidiaphragm
  h. paralysis
  tenting of h.
hemi-Fontan
  h.-F. operation
  h.-F. procedure (HFP)
hemifundoplication
  Toupet h.
hemin
hemineglect
  motor-exploratory h.
hemiosteoporosis
hemiparesis
  atactic h.
  ataxic h. (AH)
  pure motor h. (PMH)
hemiplegia
  dense h.
hemisphere
  left h. (LH)
hemisystole
hemithorax
hemitruncus
hemizygosity
hemizygous
Hemobahn
  H. endovascular prosthesis
  H. stent-graft
HemoBand hemostasis device
hemochromatosis
Hemochron
  H. high-dose thrombin time assay
  H. monitor
hemoclastic reaction
hemoclip
  Samuels h.
hemocompatible turbostratic carbon
hemoconcentrator
HemoCue photometer
hemocyanin
  keyhole-limpet h.
Hemocyte
hemocytometer
hemodiafiltration
  continuous arteriovenous h.
    (CAVHDF)
hemodialysis
  continuous arteriovenous h.
    (CAVHD)
hemodialyzer
  Gambro Lundia Minor h.
hemodilution
  isovolemic h.
  normovolemic h.
hemodilutional anemia
hemodynamic
  h. abnormality

H

hemodynamic *(continued)*
  h. analysis
  h. assessment
  h. collapse
  h. compromise
  h. embarrassment
  h. endpoint
  h. gradient
  h. instability
  h. maneuver
  h. measurement
  h. mental stress response
  h. monitoring (HM)
  h. parameter
  h. principle
  h. profile
  h. shock
  h. stability
  h. tolerance
  h. vise
hemodynamically
  h. significant stenosis
  h. weighted MRI (HW)
hemodynamics
  intraoperative h.
  pulmonary h.
  systemic h.
  transvalvular h.
Hemofil M
hemofiltration
  continuous arteriovenous h.
    (CAVH)
  continuous venovenous h. (CVVH)
hemoglobin (Hb)
  deoxygenated h.
  diaspirin cross-linked h. (DCLHb)
  h. electrophoresis
  h. glutamer-250
  glycosylated h.
  oxygenated h.
  h. P50
  h. product substitute
  pyridoxalated stroma-free h. (SFHb)
  reduced h.
  total h.
hemoglobin-based therapeutic system
hemoglobinemia
hemoglobinopathy
  sickle cell h.
hemoglobin-oxygen dissociation curve
hemoglobinuria
  paroxysmal nocturnal h. (PNH)
hemograft
Hemolink investigational hemoglobin product or blood substitute
hemolysis
  h., elevated liver enzymes, low
    platelets (HELLP)

  h., elevated liver function tests,
    low platelets syndrome
hemolytic anemia
hemomediastinum
HemoNIR portable cooximetry device
hemoperfusion
  charcoal h.
  pump-assisted coronary h.
hemopericardium
  traumatic h.
hemophagocytic histiocyte
hemopneumopericardium
hemopneumothorax
hemopoietic
hemoptysis
  cardiac h.
  catamenial h.
  coital h.
  cryptogenic h.
  essential h.
  Goldstein h.
  life-threatening h.
  massive h.
  nonmassive h.
  oriental h.
Hemopump
  H. cardiac assist system
  Johnson & Johnson H.
  Medtronic H.
  Nimbus H.
hemorheology
hemorrhage
  alveolar h.
  anticoagulant-related h.
  aortic intramural h. (AIH)
  CAA-related h.
  catastrophic h.
  caudate h.
  diffuse alveolar h. (DAH)
  flame-shaped h.'s
  hypertensive intracerebral h. (HIH)
  intracavitary h.
  intracerebral h. (ICH)
  intracranial h. (ICH)
  intramural h. (IMH)
  intraparenchymal h.
  intrapericardial h.
  intraventricular h. (IVH)
  juxtaluminal h.
  multiple lobar h. (MLH)
  parenchymal h. (PH)
  peribronchovascular h.
  petechial h.
  postoperative h. (POH)
  primary intracerebral h. (PICH)
  pulmonary alveolar h.
  h. pulmonary nodule
  recurrent lobar h. (RLH)
  reperfusion-induced h.

splinter h.
spontaneous intracerebral h. (SICH)
subarachnoid h. (SAH)
supratentorial intracerebral h.
symptomatic h.
thrombolysis-related intracranial h.
(TICH)
traumatic h.
hemorrhagic
h. bronchitis
h. bronchopneumonia
h. coagulopathy
h. cyst
h. effusion
h. fever
h. hereditary telangiectasia
h. hypotension
h. infarction (HI)
h. mediastinitis
h. pericarditis
h. pleurisy
h. sputum
h. stroke
h. transformation (HT)
hemosiderin-laden macrophage
hemosiderosis
cardiac h.
essential pulmonary h.
idiopathic pulmonary h. (IPH)
pulmonary h.
transfusional h.
HemoSplit
H. hemodialysis catheter
H. long-term dialysis catheter
hemostasis, haemostasis
International Society on Thrombosis
and H. (ISTH)
h. valve
hemostat
Kelly h.
Mayo h.
microfibrillar collagen h.
mosquito h.
straight h.
hemostatic
h. deficiency
h. occlusive leverage device
(HOLD)
h. puncture closure device (HPCD)
h. sheath
h. splittable valved sheath system
hemoSTATUS assay
**HemoTec activated clotting time
monitor**
Hemotene
hemothorax, hemathorax,
pl. **hemothoraces (HTX)**
catamenial h.
clotted h.

Hemovac
hen-cluck stertor
Henderson-Hasselbalch equation
Henipavirus
Henke space
Henle
ascending loop of H.
H. elastic membrane
H. fenestrated membrane
H. loop
Henle-Coenen test
Henoch-Schönlein
H.-S. purpura
H.-S. syndrome
H.-S. vasculitis
Henry-Gauer response
Henry law
henselae
Bartonella h.
Rochalimaea h.
HEPA
high-efficiency particulate air
HEPA filter
HepaCoat coronary stent
Hepamed-coated stent
heparin (H, HP)
h. arterial filter
h. assay rapid easy method
(HAREM)
h. assay rapid method (HARM)
beef-lung h.
h. block
h. bolus
calcium h. (CH)
h. cofactor (HCF)
h. cofactor II deficiency
continuous h. (CH)
depolymerized porcine mucosal h.
h. drip
h. and early patency
h. flush
immobilized h.
h. infusion
h. injection
h. lock (HL)
low-dose h. (LDH)
low-dose unfractionated h. (LDUH)
low molecular weight h. (LMWH)
minimal intermittent h. (MIH)
h. neutralizing activity (HNA)
standard h. (SH)
unfractionated h. (UFH)
heparin-associated
h.-a. thrombocytopenia (HAT)
h.-a. thrombocytopenia and
thrombosis (HATT)
heparin-binding
h.-b. epidermal growth factor
h.-b. hemagglutinin (HBHA)

H

341

heparin-dihydroergotamine
heparin-induced
    h.-i. extracorporeal low-density lipoprotein precipitation (HELP)
    h.-i. platelet activation (HIPA)
    h.-i. thrombocytopenia (HIT)
    h.-i. thrombocytopenia and thrombosis (HITT)
    h.-i. thrombosis-thrombocytopenia syndrome (HITTS)
heparinization
    intermittent h. (IH)
heparinized saline
heparinoid
heparin-precipitable fraction (HPF)
HEPAtech air purification system
hepatic
    h. artery
    h. dearterialization
    h. disease
    h. failure
    h. function
    h. hydatid cyst
    h. hydrothorax
    h. lipoprotein lipase
    h. sphincter
    h. steatosis
    h. vein
    h. vein catheterization
hepaticopulmonary
hepatis
    porta h.
hepatitis
    h. A, B, C, D, E
    granulomatous h.
    viral h.
hepatization
    gray h.
    red h.
    yellow h.
hepatocyte
hepatoesophageum
    ligamentum h.
hepatofugal flow
hepatojugular
    h. reflux (HJR)
    h. reflux test
hepatoma
hepatomegaly
hepatopetal flow
hepatopneumonic
hepatopulmonary syndrome (HPS)
hepatosplenic mansonic schistosomiasis
hepatosplenomegaly
hepatotoxicity
HEPES
    hydroxyethyl piperazine-ethanesulfonic acid
hep-lock injection

heptachlorodibenzodioxin
heptachlorodibenzofuran
heptahelical protein G
heptahydrate
    magnesium sulfate h.
heptanal occupational exposure
heptapeptide
Heptest clotting assay
HER2/neu gene
Herceptin
Herculink balloon-expandable stent
hereditary
    h. angioneurotic edema (HANE)
    h. ataxia
    h. capillary fragility (HCF)
    h. emphysema
    h. hemorrhagic telangiectasia (HHT)
    h. methemoglobinemic cyanosis
heredopathia atactica polyneuritiformis
HERG
    human ether-a-go-go-related gene
    HERG potassium channel
Hering
    nerve of H.
    H. phenomenon
Hering-Breuer reflex
heritability
Hermansky-Pudlak syndrome
Herner syndrome
hernia
    Béclard h.
    Bochdalek h.
    congenital diaphragmatic h. (CDH)
    diaphragmatic h.
    hiatal h.
    Larrey h.
    Morgagni h.
    paraesophageal h.
    rolling h.
    Serafini h.
    sliding hiatal h.
    Velpeau h.
herniation
    cardiac h.
heroics
heroic snoring
heroin
herpangina pharyngitis
herpes
    h. simplex
    h. simplex pneumonia
    h. simplex pneumonitis
    h. simplex virus (HSV)
    h. zoster
Herpesviridae
herpesvirus
    human h. 8 (HHV-8)
herpetic
herzstoss

HES
HydroCoil embolization system
Hespan plasma volume expander
Hess capillary test
hetastarch plasma expander
20-HETE
20-hydroxyeicosatetraenoic acid
heterochronicus
pulsus h.
heterodimer complex
heterogeneity
genetic h.
myocardial h.
heterogeneous
h. disease
h. parenchymal attenuation
h. plaque
heterogenous emphysema
heterograft
bovine h.
Hancock porcine h.
porcine h.
heterologous
h. cardiac transplant
h. surfactant
heterometric autoregulation
heterophony
phase h.
heterophyiasis
heteroscedastic
heterotaxia
cardiac h.
heterotaxy
h. syndrome
visceral h.
heterotopic
h. cardiac transplant
h. heart transplant (HHT)
h. heart transplantation (HHT)
h. stimulus
heterotrimeric protein G
heterotypic adhesion
heterozygosity
heterozygote
heterozygous familial
hypercholesterolemia (hFH)
Heubner
H. recurrent artery
H. specific endarteritis
Hewlett-Packard (HP)
H.-P. 77020 A phased-array sector
scanner
H.-P. biplane 5-MHz probe
H.-P. defibrillator
H.-P. ear oximeter
H.-P. 500, 1000 Echo-Doppler
machine
H.-P. Omniplane 5-MHz probe

H.-P. 2500 Sonos ultrasound
H.-P. Sonos 1000, 1500 2500
ultrasound system
HEWS
histamine equivalent wheal size
Hexabrix contrast material
hexachlorophene
Hexadrol Phosphate
hexafluoride
sulfur h. (SF_6)
hexahydrophthalic anhydride (HHPA)
Hexalen
hexamethonium
hexamethylene diisocyanate
hexamethylmelamine
hexarelin
hexaxial reference system
hexokinase reaction
Hexonate
hexosaminidase deficiency
HF
heart failure
high fat
high flow
HF infrared laser
HFA
hydrofluoroalkane
flunisolide HFA
Proventil HFA
Ventolin HFA
H-FABP
heart-type fatty acid binding protein
HFCC
high-frequency chest wall compression
HFCWO
high-frequency chest wall oscillation
HFCWO ventricular resynchronizer
HFEE
high-frequency epicardial
echocardiography
HFH
homozygous familial
hypercholesterolemia
hFH
heterozygous familial
hypercholesterolemia
HFJV
high-frequency jet ventilation
HFL
human fetal lung fibroblast
HFO
high-frequency oscillation
HFOC
high-flow oxygen conserver
H-form myocardial infarction
HFOV
HFP
hemi-Fontan procedure

H

HFPPV
   high-frequency positive pressure
      ventilation
HFPV
   high-frequency percussive ventilation
HFSA
   Heart Failure Society of America
HFV
   high-frequency ventilation
Hg
   mercury
195mHg
   mercury-195m
HHCS
   high-altitude hypertrophic
      cardiomyopathy syndrome
HHD
   high heparin dose
   hypertensive heart disease
H₁-H₂ interval
HHPA
   hexahydrophthalic anhydride
HHS
   hyperkinetic heart syndrome
HHT
   hereditary hemorrhagic telangiectasia
   heterotopic heart transplant
   heterotopic heart transplantation
   hypertensive hypervolemic therapy
HHV-8
   human herpesvirus 8
HI
   harmonic imaging
   heart infusion
   hemorrhagic infarction
HIA
   hyperventilation-induced asthma
hiatal
   h. esophagism
   h. hernia
hiatus
   aortic h.
   h. aorticus
   esophageal h.
   h. esophageus
   h. of facial canal
HIB
   heart infusion broth
   hyperpnea-induced bronchoconstriction
hibernating myocardium
hibernation
   myocardial h.
HibTITER
Hib-VAX
**Hi-Care closed suction and pulmonary
   hygiene system**
HIC-CPR
   high-impulse compression
      cardiopulmonary resuscitation

hiccup, hiccough
   benign transient h.'s
   h. bout
   chronic h.'s
   intractable h.'s
   persistent h.'s
   h. reflex arc
   transient h.'s
HICOR system
HI-CPR
   high-impulse cardiopulmonary
      resuscitation
HID
   hypertension in diabetes
Hideaway oxygen conserver
HIF
   hypoxia-inducible factor
Hi-Flex lead
high
   h. air flow with oxygen
      entrainment (HAFOE)
   h. arched palate
   h. blood pressure (HBP)
   h. cholesterol and tocopherol
      supplement (HCTS)
   h. fat (HF)
   h. flow (HF)
   h. heparin dose (HHD)
   h. lung volume
   h. molecular weight dextran
   h. pressure connecting tube
   h. pulse repetition frequency
      (HiPRF)
   h. regional wall motion velocity
      (Vhigh)
   h. right atrium
   h. right atrium electrogram
      (HRAE)
   h. R wave
   h. setting
   h. spatial resolution
   h. vacuum (HV)
   h. voltage can (HVC)
high-altitude
   h.-a. cerebral edema (HACE)
   h.-a. hypertrophic cardiomyopathy
      syndrome (HHCS)
   h.-a. peristalsis
   h.-a. pulmonary edema (HAPE)
   h.-a. pulmonary edema resistant
      (HAPE-r)
   h.-a. pulmonary edema susceptible
      (HAPE-s)
   h.-a. simulation test (HAST)
   h.-a. syncope
high-amplitude
   h.-a. peristalsis (HAP)
   h.-a. peristaltic contraction (HAPC)
high-ceiling diuretic

high-concentration oxygen mask
high-degree atrioventricular block
high-density
    h.-d. echo
    h.-d. electroanatomical and
        entrainment mapping
    h.-d. lipoprotein (HDL, HDLP)
    h.-d. lipoprotein binding protein
        (HDLBP)
    h.-d. lipoprotein-cell surface (HDL-
        c)
    h.-d. lipoprotein-cholesterol complex
        (HDL-C)
    h.-d. sector basket catheter
high-dependency unit (HDU)
high-dose
    h.-d. carvedilol (CARhd)
    h.-d. epinephrine
    h.-d. steroid
high-efficiency particulate air (HEPA)
high-energy
    h.-e. defibrillation shock
    h.-e. laser
    h.-e., low-penetration beta emitter
    h.-e. transthoracic shock
high-esophageal pH probe
highest equivalent heart rate (HEHR)
high-fat meal
high-fiber diet
high-fidelity microtransducer
high-flow
    h.-f. catheter
    h.-f. oxygen conserver (HFOC)
high-frequency
    h.-f. beat
    3100B h.-f. oscillatory ventilator
    h.-f. breath volume
    h.-f. burst pacing
    h.-f. chest wall compression
        (HFCC)
    h.-f. chest wall oscillation
        (HFCWO)
    h.-f. chest wall oscillation
        ventricular resynchronizer
    h.-f. chest wall ventilator
    h.-f. epicardial echocardiography
        (HFEE)
    h.-f. jet ventilation (HFJV)
    h.-f. jet ventilator
    h.-f. murmur
    h.-f. oscillation (HFO)
    h.-f. oscillation ventilator
    h.-f. percussion
    h.-f. percussive ventilation (HFPV)
    h.-f. positive pressure ventilation
        (HFPPV)
    h.-f. ventilation (HFV)
high-grade stenosis

high-impulse
    h.-i. cardiopulmonary resuscitation
        (HI-CPR)
    h.-i. compression cardiopulmonary
        resuscitation (HIC-CPR)
high-intensity transient signal (HITS)
**highly active antiretroviral therapy
    (HAART)**
high-output
    h.-o. extended aerosol respiratory
        therapy
    h.-o. heart failure
**high-performance liquid chromatography
    (HPLC)**
high-pitched murmur
high-powered (HP)
    h.-p. laser
high-pressure
    h.-p. adjunctive percutaneous
        transluminal coronary angioplasty
    h.-p. balloon stenting
    h.-p. cardiogenic pulmonary edema
    h.-p. gas supply
    h.-p. inflation technique
    h.-p. liquid chromatography (HPLC)
    h.-p. neurologic syndrome (HPNS)
    h.-p. stent deployment
high-ramp protocol
**high-renin essential hypertension
    (HREH)**
high-resolution
    h.-r. B-mode ultrasonography
    h.-r. computed tomography (HRCT)
    h.-r. CT (HRCT)
    h.-r. deep penetration 2D
        intracardiac ultrasound
    h.-r. electrocardiography (HRE)
    h.-r. thin section computed
        tomographic
high-risk
    h.-r. angioplasty
    h.-r. phenotype
    h.-r. repolarization abnormality
    h.-r. staged procedure
HighSail coronary dilation catheter
high-sensitivity
    h.-s. C-reactive protein (hs-CRP,
        hsCRP)
    h.-s. CRP
high-speed
    h.-s. directional coronary
        atherectomy
    h.-s. rotational atherectomy (HSRA)
    h.-s. rotation dynamic angioplasty
        catheter
    h.-s. volumetric imaging
high-volume cuffed endotracheal tube
HIH
    hypertensive intracerebral hemorrhage

H

Hilal
  H. embolization microcoil
  H. modified headhunter catheter
hilar
  h. adenopathy
  h. calcification
  h. clouding
  h. dance
  h. haze
  h. lymphadenopathy
  h. lymph node
hill
  H. coefficient
  H. phenomenon
  H. sign
Hillis-Müller maneuver
hills-and-valley morphology
Hi-Lo
  H.-L. Evac endotracheal tube
  H.-L. Jet tracheal tube
Hilton sac
hilum
  h. convergence sign
  h. of lung
  h. of lymph node
  h. nodi lymphatici
  h. overlay sign
  pulmonary h.
  h. pulmonis
  h. tuberculosis
Hines-Brown test
hinge point
Hinkle-Thaler classification
hip
  h. classification
  h. flexion
HIPA
  heparin-induced platelet activation
HIPAA
  Health Insurance Portability and
    Accountability Act of 1996
hippocampal neuronal apoptosis
hippocratic
  h. angina
  h. nails
  h. sound
  h. succussion
  h. succussion sound
HiPRF
  high pulse repetition frequency
Hi-Res electrocardiogram electrode
hirsutum
  cor h.
hirudin
  recombinant h. (r-hirudin)
Hirudo medicinalis
his
  bundle of H. (BH)
  H. bundle (HB)

  H. bundle ablation
  H. bundle catheter
  H. bundle deflection
  H. bundle depolarization
  H. bundle electrocardiogram
  H. bundle electrogram (HBE)
  H. bundle heart block
  H. bundle potential
  H. canal
  H. perivascular space
  H. spindle
His-Hass procedure
Hispanic American (HA)
His-Purkinje
  H.-P. conduction
  H.-P. fiber
  H.-P. system
  H.-P. tissue
Histalet Syrup
histaminase
histamine
  h. acid phosphate
  h. challenge
  h. challenge testing
  h. diphosphate
  h. equivalent wheal size (HEWS)
  h. provocation
  h. release inhibitory factor (HRIF)
histamine-releasing factor (HRF)
His-Tawara node
histidine decarboxylase
histidine-rich glycoprotein
histidyl-tRNA synthetase
histiocyte
  cardiac h.
  hemophagocytic h.
  palisading h.
histiocytoma
  malignant fibrous h. (MFH)
histiocytosis
  Langerhans cell h.
  primary pulmonary Langerhans
    cell h.
  primary pulmonary h. X
  pulmonary Langerhans cell h.
Histoacryl Blue tissue adhesive
histocompatability
histocompatibility agent B27
histogram
  DNA h.
  dose-volume h.
  h. mode
histologic staining
histolytica
  Entamoeba h.
  Torula h.
histolyticus
  Cryptococcus h.

histomorphometry
histone deacetylase 2 (HDAC2)
histopathology
Histoplasma
    H. capsulatum
    H. myocarditis
    H. polysaccharide antigen
histoplasmic pericarditis
histoplasmoma
histoplasmosis
    acute pulmonary h.
    African h.
    chronic cavitary h.
    chronic mediastinal h.
    disseminated h.
    progressive disseminated h. (PDH)
history, pl. histories
    family h.
    heart disease h. (HDH)
    natural h.
    pack-year smoking h.
    smoking h.
histotoxic hypoxia
Histussin D Liquid
His-ventricle (HV)
    H.-v. conduction time
    H.-v. interval
HIT
    heparin-induced thrombocytopenia
Hitachi
    H. PCT-3600W PET system
    H. U-2000 spectrophotometer
Hi-Torque
    H.-T. balance middleweight
        universal guide wire
    H.-T. Floppy exchange guidewire
    H.-T. Floppy II guidewire
    H.-T. Floppy intermediate guidewire
    H.-T. Standard guidewire
HITS
    high-intensity transient signal
HITT
    heparin-induced thrombocytopenia and
        thrombosis
HITTS
    heparin-induced thrombosis-
        thrombocytopenia syndrome
Hitzenberg test
HIV
    human immunodeficiency virus
    HIV cardiomyopathy
    HIV fusion inhibitor
    HIV seropositive
HIV-1 riboprobe
HIVAGEN test
HIV-associated pulmonary hypertension
Hivid

HIV-PH
    human immunodeficiency virus-
        associated pulmonary hypertension
HJR
    hepatojugular reflux
HL
    heparin lock
    hyperlipidemia
HL7
    Health level 7
H&L
    heart and lung
HLA
    human leukocyte antigen
    HLA-6
    HLA-129
    HLA-A11
    HLA-DPGlu69
HLA-DP beta chain
HLA-DQA1 gene haplotype
HLA-DQB1 gene haplotype
HLA-DQ gene complex
HLA-DR gene complex
HLHS
    hypoplastic left heart syndrome
H-L-K
    heart, liver, kidneys
HLR
    heart-lung resuscitation
HLT
    heart-lung transplant
    heart-lung transplantation
    human lipotropin
HLTx
    heart-lung transplant
HLV
    hypoplastic left ventricle
HLVS
    hypoplastic left ventricle syndrome
HM
    heart murmur
    hemodynamic monitoring
    Holter monitoring
HMB45 antibody
HMCAS
    hyperdense middle cerebral artery sign
HMD
    hyaline membrane disease
HME
    heat/moisture exchanger
        Tracheolife HME
HMG-CoA
    hydroxymethylglutaryl coenzyme A
    3-hydroxy-3-methylglutaryl coenzyme A
HMG-CoA-reductase inhibitor
HMI
    healed myocardial infaret
HMO
    heart minute output

H

347

hMPV
human metapneumonovirus
HMSAS
hypertrophic muscular subaortic stenosis
H5N1
avian influenza virus strain H5N1
AIV H5N1
avian influenza virus strain H5N1
HNA
heparin neutralizing activity
HO
Holt-Oram
HO syndrome
hoarseness
hockey-stick
h.-s. catheter
h.-s. deformity
h.-s. tricuspid valve
HOCM
hypertrophic obstructive cardiomyopathy
Hodgkin
H. disease
H. lymphoma
Hodgkin-Huxley
H.-H. constant
H.-H. model
Hodgkin-Key murmur
Hodgson disease
Hoffman reflex
hoist
HOLD
hemostatic occlusive leverage device
Hold DM
holder
Björk-Shiley heart valve h.
blade control wire h.
Castroviejo needle h.
Comfit endotracheal tube h.
Dale tracheostomy tube h.
GraftAssist vein-graft h.
Lewy chest h.
LifePort endotracheal tube h.
Marsupial Pouch postsurgical
drain h.
needle h.
NEO-fit neonatal endotracheal
tube h.
Thomas LT endotracheal tube h.
Thomas Quick Block endotracheal
tube h.
Vital-Ryder microvascular needle h.
Watson heart valve h.
wire h.
holding
hole
bur h.
silicone suture h.
suture h.

1-hole
1-h. angiographic catheter
1-h. angioplastic catheter
holiday
dobutamine h.
h. heart
h. heart syndrome
Holinger
H. anterior commissure
laryngoscope
H. dissector
holism
Hollenberg treadmill exercise score
Hollenhorst plaque
hollow-core needle
hollow viscus
Holmes heart
Holmes-Rahe scale
Holmgren-Golgi canal
holmium laser
holmium:yttrium-aluminum-garnet
(Ho:YAG)
holodiastolic
h. decrescendo murmur
h. flow
h. flow reversal
holography
ultrasound h.
holosystolic murmur (HSM)
Holter
H. diary
Marquette 3-channel laser H.
H. monitor
H. monitoring (HM)
H. tube
Holter-guided antiarrhythmic drug
therapy
Holt-Oram (HO)
H.-O. syndrome (HOS)
Holzknecht space
Homans sign
homatropine
hydrocodone and h.
home
h. monitor
h. unattended polysomnography
home-based cardiac rehabilitation
homeometric autoregulation
homeostasis
homeostatic lag
homeothermic
hominis
Actinobacillus h.
Cardiobacterium h.
Mycoplasma h.
Pentatrichomonas h.
HomMed
H. monitor
H. monitoring system

homocysteine
    plasma h.
    total h. (tHcy)
homocystine
homocystinuria syndrome
homodimer
    alpha-alpha h.
    beta-beta h.
homogeneity
    Breslow-Day test for h.
    tracer h.
homogeneous plaque
homogentisic acid oxidase deficiency
homograft
    antibiotic sterilized aortic valve h.
      (ASAH)
    aortic h.
    denatured h.
    homovital h.
    h. insertion
    h. insertion for pulmonary
      regurgitation
    mitral valve h.
    pulmonary artery h.
homolateral lymph node
homologous cardiac transplant
homoscedastic
homotypic adhesion
homovital homograft
homozygosity
homozygote
homozygous
    h. beta-thalassemia
    h. familial hypercholesterolemia
      (HFH)
HON
    Health On the Net
    HON Foundation
HONcode
    Health On the Net code of conduct
honeycomb
    h. cyst
    h. cystic changes
    h. lesion
    h. lung
    h. pattern
honeycombing
    h. of lung
    subpleural h.
Hong Kong influenza
honk
    precordial h.
    systolic h.
honking murmur
Hood stoma stent
hook
    Adson h.
    barbed h.

hook-and-loop fastener strap
Hooke law
Hoover sign
hope
    H. bag
    H. continuous & Heliox nebulizer
    H. resuscitator
    h. sign
Hopkins
    H. aortic clamp
    H. forceps
    H. Symptom Checklist
Horder spots
horehound lozenge
horizon
    H. AutoAdjust CPAP system
    H. CPAP device
    H. LT CPAP system
    H. nasal CPAP system
    H. PFT spirometer
    H. surgical ligating and marking
      clip
horizontal
    h. anteroposterior deceleration
    h. fissure
    h. heart
    h. long axis
    h. long-axis tomogram
    h. long-axis view
    h. ST segment
    h. ST-segment depression
    h. VAS
hormone
    adrenocorticotropic h. (ACTH)
    antidiuretic h. (ADH)
    female h.
    growth h.
    mineralocorticoid h.
    natriuretic h.
    parathyroid h. (PTH)
    h. replacement therapy (HRT)
    syndrome of inappropriate
      antidiuretic h. (SIADH)
    thyroid-stimulating h. (TSH)
Horner
    H. sign
    H. syndrome
horripilation
horse asthma
horse-race effect
horseshoe
    h. configuration
    h. lung
Horton
    H. arteritis (HA)
    H. disease
HOS
    Holt-Oram syndrome

H

hose
Juzo h.
TED h.
Hosmer-Lemeshow Goodness-of-Fit test
hospital
H. Admission Risk Profile (HARP)
H. Anxiety and Depression (HAD)
H. Anxiety and Depression Scale (HADS)
Veterans Affairs Non-Q-Wave Infarction Strategies in H.
hospital-acquired
h.-a. infection
h.-a. pneumonia (HAP)
host
granulocytopenic h.
humoral h.
immunocompetent h.
immunocompromised h. (ICH)
nonimmunocompromised h.
host-generated neutrophils recruitment
hot
h. gangrene
h. nose sign
h. potato voice
h. spot
Hotelling T2 test
hot-tip laser probe
hot-wire
h.-w. anemometer
h.-w. pneumotachometer
Hounsfield unit (HU)
hour
12-h. antiplatelet therapy
golden h.
4-h. scan
24-hour
24-h. ambulatory electrocardiographic recorder
Claritin-D 24-H.
24-h. cortisol
hourglass
h. murmur
h. pattern
h. stenosis
house
h. dust mite (HDM)
h. dust mite allergen
Housecall transtelephonic monitoring system
Howard-Kelly forceps
Howard method
Howel-Evans syndrome
Howell test
Ho:YAG
holmium:yttrium-aluminum-garnet
Ho:YAG laser
Ho:YAG laser angioplasty
Hoyer anastomosis

HP
heparin
Hewlett-Packard
high-powered
hypersensitivity pneumonitis
HP SONOS 30-MHz imaging catheter
HP SONOS 2500 transducer
HP Sonos 2000 ultrasound system
HPA
hypothalamic-pituitary-adrenal
HPAA
hypothalamic-pituitary-adrenal axis
H.P. Acthar Gel
HPB-Artery Klenz
HPCD
hemostatic puncture closure device
HPD
hematoporphyrin derivative
HPETE
5-HPETE acid
HPF
heparin-precipitable fraction
HPI
Haemophilus parainfluenzae
H′P interval
HPLC
high-performance liquid chromatography
high-pressure liquid chromatography
HPLH
hypoplastic left heart
HPN
hypertension
HPNS
high-pressure neurologic syndrome
H-proline
HPS
hepatopulmonary syndrome
HPV
human papillomavirus
hypoxic pulmonary vasoconstriction
HPVD
hypertensive pulmonary vascular disease
H-Q interval
H-QRS interval
HR
heart rate
HR conduction time
HRA
heart rate audiometry
HRAE
high right atrium electrogram
HRCT
high-resolution computed tomography
high-resolution CT
diagnostic HRCT
HRCT scan
HRE
high-resolution electrocardiography

HREH
high-renin essential hypertension
HRF
heart rate fluctuation
histamine-releasing factor
HRF deficiency
HRIF
histamine release inhibitory factor
Hrmax
maximal heart rate
HRQL, HRQOL
health-related quality of life
HRR
heart rate range
heart rate recovery
heart rate reserve
HRRI
heart rate retardation index
HRS
Hamman-Rich syndrome
HRT
heart rate
hormone replacement therapy
hyperfractionated radiation
HRV
heart rate variability
power spectrum of HRV
HRV test
HS
heart sound
HSAS
hypertrophic subaortic stenosis
HSC
hematopoietic stem cell
hs-CRP, hsCRP
high-sensitivity C-reactive protein
HSEP
heart synchronized evoked potential
HSM
holosystolic murmur
HSP, hsp
heat shock protein
HSP antigen
HSP47
heat shock protein 47
HSP70
heat shock protein 70
hsp (*var. of* HSP)
HSRA
high-speed rotational atherectomy
HSRA device
HSRD
hypertension secondary to renal disease
HSS
hypertrophic subaortic stenosis
HSV
herpes simplex virus
HSV meningitis
HSV pneumonia

HT
heart
heart tone
heart transplant
heart transplantation
hemorrhagic transformation
hypertension
hypertensive
cerebral HT
5-HT receptor mechanism
5HT
5-hydroxytryptamine
Ht
heart tone
height of heart
ht
heart
heart tone
HTCVD
hypertensive cardiovascular disease
HTG
hypertriglyceridemia
HTHD
hypertensive heart disease
HTLV
human T-cell lymphotropic virus
HTLV-I, II
HTN
hypertension
hypertensive nephropathy
HTVD
hypertensive vascular disease
HTX
hemothorax
hypertension
H-type tracheoesophageal fistula
HU
Hounsfield unit
hub
catheter h.
h. and spoke referral system
Huchard
H. disease
H. sign
Hudson
H. Lifesaver resuscitator
H. Multi-Vent
Huff coughing
Hufnagel
H. ascending aortic clamp
H. prosthetic valve
Hugger
Bair H.
Hughes-Stovin syndrome
Hull triad
hum
cervical venous h.
venous h.

human
    h. airway epithelium
    h. amylin analog
    h. analog amylin AC137
    antihemophilic factor (h.)
    h. aortic endothelial cell (HAEC)
    h. aortic smooth muscle (HASMC)
    h. aortic smooth muscle cell
    (HASMC)
    h. atrial natriuretic factor (hANF)
    h. atrial natriuretic peptide (hANP)
    h. babesiosis
    h. beta defensin 2 (HBD2)
    h. cloned DNA (cDNA)
    h. coronavirus
    h. coronavirus HKU1 (CoV-HKU1)
    h. coronavirus NL63 (HCoV-NL63)
    h. cosmid library
    h. cytomegalovirus (HCMV)
    cytomegalovirus immune globulin
    intravenous, h.
    h. device exemption (HDE)
    h. ether-a-go-go-related gene
    (HERG)
    h. fetal lung fibroblast (HFL)
    h. gene C4B
    h. herpesvirus 8 (HHV-8)
    h. herpesvirus 8 infection
    h. immunodeficiency virus (HIV)
    h. immunodeficiency virus-
    associated pulmonary hypertension
    (HIV-PH)
    h. leukocyte antigen (HLA)
    h. lipotropin (HLT)
    h. lymphocyte antigen typing
    h. menopausal gonadotropin
    coenzyme A reductase inhibitor
    h. metapneumonovirus (hMPV)
    h. neuropeptide
    h. neutrophil elastase
    h. papillomavirus (HPV)
    h. polyomavirus BK (BKV)
    h. pooled AAT
    h. preproendothelin-1 gene
    h. recombinant deoxyribonuclease
    h. T-cell lymphotropic virus
    (HTLV)
    h. umbilical vein (HUV)
    Velosulin H.
Humate-P
Humatin
humeral
    anterior circumflex h.
humeroperoneal neuromuscular disease
Humibid DM
humid asthma
humidification
humidified oxygen

humidifier
    Bennett Cascade II Servo
    Controlled Heated H.
    bubble h.
    cold-mist h.
    jet h.
    h. lung
    Mistogen passover h.
    passover h.
    Respironics Oasis h.
    Sullivan HumidAire heated h.
    Whisper Mist h.
humidity
    absolute h.
    relative h. (RH)
humming murmur
humming-top murmur
humoral
    h. host
    h. immune defect
hump
    diastolic h.
    Hampton h.
Humulin L, N, R, U insulin
huN901-DM1 antibody
hunger
    air h.
hunt
    H. angiographic trocar
    H. and Hess grades I through V
    aneurysm grading system
hunter
    H. canal
    H. detachable balloon occluder
    H. operation
    H. syndrome
Hunter-Hurler syndrome
Hunter-Sessions balloon
hunting reaction
Huntington chorea
Hurler-Scheie compound
Hurler syndrome
Hurricaine spray
Hürthle
    H. cell tumor
    H. manometer
Hustead needle
HUT
    head-up tilt
Hutinel disease
HUTTT
    head-up tilt-table test
HUV
    human umbilical vein
    HUV bypass graft
Huygens principle
HV
    heart volume
    high vacuum

His-ventricle
hyaline-vascular
hypervolemic
    HV conduction time
    HV interval

HVC
    high voltage can

HVD
    hypertensive vascular disease

HVR
    hypoxic ventilatory response

HVS
    hyperventilation syndrome

HVSD
    hydrogen-detected ventricular septal
    defect

HW
    heart weight
    hemodynamically weighted MRI

hwaotang

hyaline
    h. arterionecrosis
    h. arteriosclerosis
    h. fatty change
    h. membrane disease (HMD)
    h. membrane disease of the
      newborn
    h. membrane formation
    h. membrane syndrome
    h. thrombus

hyaline-vascular (HV)
    h.-v. type variant of Castleman
      disease (CD-HV)

hyalinizing granuloma

hyalinosis
    arteriolar h.

hyaloserositis
    progressive multiple h.

hyaluronan

hyaluronic
    h. acid
    h. acid polymer

hyaluronidase

Hyate:C

Hybolin Decanoate

Hybond ECL nitrocellulose membrane

hybrid
    h. revascularization
    h. stent
    h. unit

hybridization
    fluorescent in situ h. (FISH)
    in situ h.

Hybritech immunoradiometric assay

Hycamtin

Hycodan

Hycomine Compound

Hycotuss Expectorant Liquid

HYD
    hydrocortisone

hydantoin

hydatid
    h. cyst
    h. fremitus
    h. sand

hydralazine
    h. hydrochloride
    h. and hydrochlorothiazide
    h., hydrochlorothiazide, reserpine

Hydrap-ES

hydrate
    chloral h.

hydration
    systemic h.

hydraulic
    h. resistance
    h. vein stripper

hydrazine
    dimethyl h.

Hydrea

hydride
    lithium h.

hydrobromic acid

hydrobromide
    hydroxyamphetamine h.

hydrocarbon
    h. aspiration
    halogenated h.
    polycyclic aromatic h. (PAH)
    h. toxicity

HydroCath catheter

Hydrocet

hydrochloric acid

hydrochloride (HCl)
    acebutolol h.
    acecainide h.
    alfentanil h.
    alprenolol h.
    amantadine h.
    amiloride h.
    amiodarone h.
    amprolium h.
    bacampicillin h.
    benazepril h.
    bepridil h.
    betaxolol h.
    bromhexine h.
    carbuterol h.
    carteolol h.
    chlorpromazine h.
    ciprofloxacin h.
    clonidine h.
    clorprenaline h.
    colestipol h.
    cyclopentamine h.
    cyproheptadine h.
    cytarabine h.

H

hydrochloride *(continued)*
   demeclocycline h.
   desipramine h.
   diltiazem h.
   diphenhydramine h.
   dobutamine h.
   dopamine h.
   doxapram h.
   doxepin h.
   doxorubicin h.
   encainide h.
   esmolol h.
   esprolol h.
   ethambutol h.
   ethaverine h.
   ethylnorepinephrine h.
   fenfluramine h.
   fexofenadine h.
   fluoxetine h.
   guanfacine h.
   hydralazine h.
   idarubicin h.
   isoprenaline h.
   isoprophenamine h.
   isopropylarterenol h.
   isoproterenol h.
   isosorbide dinitrate/hydralazine h.
   isoxsuprine h.
   labetalol h.
   levamisole h.
   levobupivacaine h.
   lidocaine h.
   lincomycin h.
   lomefloxacin h.
   mecamylamine h.
   mechlorethamine h.
   mefloquine h.
   meperidine h.
   mepivacaine h.
   methamphetamine h.
   methoxamine h.
   methoxyphenamine h.
   metoclopramide h.
   mexiletine h.
   minocycline h.
   mitoxantrone h.
   moexipril h.
   Mustargen H.
   nalmefene h.
   naloxone h.
   nicardipine h.
   nortriptyline h.
   odansetron h.
   oxytetracycline h.
   papaverine h.
   phenoxybenzamine h.
   phentolamine h.
   phenylephrine h.
   phenylpropanolamine h.

   prazosin h.
   prenalterol h.
   procainamide h.
   procaine h.
   promethazine h.
   propafenone h.
   propranolol h.
   protokylol h.
   protriptyline h.
   pyridoxine h.
   quinapril h.
   rimantadine h.
   sematilide h.
   sertraline h.
   sotalol h.
   spirapril h.
   terazosin h.
   tetracaine h.
   thioridazine h.
   ticlopidine h.
   tiprenolol h.
   tizanidine h.
   tocainide h.
   tolazoline h.
   trazodone h.
   vancomycin h.
   verapamil h.
   yohimbine h.
hydrochlorothiazide (HCT, HCTZ)
   amiloride and h.
   benazepril and h.
   bisoprolol and h.
   candesartan, cilexetil, h.
   captopril and h.
   enalapril and h.
   hydralazine and h.
   irbesartan and h.
   lisinopril and h.
   h. and lisinopril
   losartan and h.
   methyldopa and h.
   moexipril and h.
   propranolol and h.
   quinapril and h.
   h. and reserpine
   h. and spironolactone
   h. and triamterene
   valsartan and h.
Hydrocoat hydrophilic coating
hydrocodone
   h. and acetaminophen
   h. bitartrate
   h. and homatropine
   h., phenylephrine, pyrilamine,
      phenindamine, chlorpheniramine
   h. and phenylpropanolamine
   h. and pseudoephedrine
   h., pseudoephedrine, guaifenesin
HydroCoil embolization system (HES)

Hydrocort
hydrocortisone (HYD)
    h. cyclopentylpropionate
    h. cypionate
    h. hydrogen succinate
    h. sodium phosphate
    h. sodium succinate
    systemic h.
hydrocyanic acid
HydroDot neuromonitoring system
hydroflumethiazide and reserpine
hydrofluoric acid
hydrofluoroalkane (HFA)
hydrogen
    h. appearance time
    h. bromide
    h. chloride
    h. cyanide (HCN)
    h. density
    h. electrodes
    h. fluoride
    h. inhalation technique
    h. ion concentration (pH)
    h. peroxide
    h. sulfide
hydrogen-3 mazindol
hydrogen-detected ventricular septal defect (HVSD)
hydrolase
    cholesterol ester h. (CEH)
    lysosomal h.
Hydrolyser
    Cordis H.
    H. hydrodynamic thrombectomy catheter
    H. percutaneous thrombectomy catheter
hydrolyser
hydrolysis
    ATP h.
    sphingomyelin h.
    h. of surfactant
hydromediastinum
Hydromer-coated central venous catheter
Hydromet
hydromorphone
hydronephrosis
Hydropane
Hydro/Pel coating
hydropericarditis
hydropericardium
Hydrophen
hydrophilic
    h. agent
    h. coated guidewire
    h. coating
hydrophobic drug
hydropneumatosis

hydropneumopericardium
hydropneumothorax
hydrops
    h. fetalis
    h. pericardii
hydroquinidine
Hydro-Serp
Hydroserpine
hydrosoluble asthmogen
hydrosphere
hydrosphygmograph
hydrostatic
    h. edema
    h. suction
HydroSteer hydrophilic guidewire
Hydro-T
hydrothorax
    chylous h.
    hepatic h.
hydroxide
    potassium h. (KOH)
hydroxocobalamin
hydroxyamphetamine hydrobromide
hydroxyapatite
hydroxybutyrate
    h. dehydrogenase (HBDH)
    gamma h. (GHB)
hydroxychloroquine sulfate
18-hydroxycorticosterone
20-hydroxyeicosatetraenoic acid (20-HETE)
hydroxyephedrine (HED)
    carbon-11 h.
hydroxyethyl
    h. piperazine-ethanesulfonic acid (HEPES)
    h. starch
hydroxylase
    h. deficiency
    17-h. deficiency
    tyrosine h.
hydroxyl radical
hydroxymethylglutaryl
    h. coenzyme A (HMG-CoA)
    h. coenzyme A reductase inhibitor
3-hydroxy-3-methylglutaryl
    3-h.-3-m. coenzyme A (HMG-CoA)
    3-h.-3-m. coenzyme A reductase
    3-h.-3-m. coenzyme A reductase inhibitor
hydroxyprogesterone caproate
hydroxyproline
    h. analysis
    lavage h.
5-hydroxypropafenone
hydroxytoluene
    butylated h. (BHT)
5-hydroxytryptamine (5HT)
hydroxyurea

H

hydroxyzine
theophylline, ephedrine, h. (TEH)
Hylutin injection
Hynes pharyngoplasty
hyoid
mandibular plane to h. (MP-H)
h. myotomy
h. suspension
hyopharyngeus
Hypaque
hyparterial bronchi
hyperabduction syndrome
hyperacute
h. rejection
h. T wave
hyperadrenergic activity
hyperaldosteronism
hyperalgesia
hyperalimentation
intravenous h. (IVH)
hyperalphalipoproteinemia
hyperammonemia
hyperapobetalipoproteinemia
hyperapolipoprotein B syndrome
hyperbaric
h. chamber
h. exposure
h. oxygen (HBO)
h. oxygenation
h. oxygen therapy (HBOT)
h. pressure
hyperbradykinism
hypercalcemia
familial hypocalciuric h.
h. syndrome
hypercalciuria
hypercapnia
oxygen-induced h.
permissive h. (PHC)
hypercapnic
h. acidosis
h. challenge
h. respiratory failure
h. stimulus
h. ventilatory response
hypercarbia
chronic h.
oxygen-induced h.
hypercardia
hyperchloremic acidosis
hypercholesterolemia (HC)
essential h. (EHC)
false h.
familial h. (FH, FHC)
heterozygous familial h. (hFH)
homozygous familial h. (HFH)
polygenic h.
h. (types IIa, IIb)
hypercholesterolemic

hyperchylomicronemia
familial h.
hypercirculation
hypercoagulability
hypercoagulable state
hypercontractile
hypercontractility
hypercortisolemia
hypercortisolism
hypercyanotic
h. angina
h. spell
hyperdense middle cerebral artery sign (HMCAS)
hyperdiastole
hyperdicrotic
hyperdicrotism
hyperdynamic
h. septic shock
h. state
hyperemia
active h.
adenosine-induced h.
arterial h.
collateral h.
conjunctival h.
exercise h.
fluxionary h.
passive h.
peripheral h.
peristatic h.
postocclusion h.
reactive h.
venous h.
hyperemic
h. stimulus
h. velocity
hyperenhancement
hypereosinophilia syndrome
hypereosinophilic
h. heart disease
h. syndrome
hyperesthesia
cutaneous h.
hyperestrogenemia
hyperfibrinogenemia
hyperfiltration
glomerular h.
Hyperflex tracheostomy tube
hyperfractionated radiation (HRT)
hypergammaglobulinemia
hyperglobulinemia
hyperglycemia
hyperhomocysteinemia
hyperimmunoglobulin E syndrome
hyperinfection
hyperinflated
hyperinflation
dynamic h. (DH)

hyperinsulinemia
hyperinsulinemic euglycemic clamp
  metabolic state
hyperinsulinism
hyperintense heterogeneous signal
hyperintensity
      deep white matter h. (DWMHI)
      patchy h.
      periventricular h. (PVH, PVHI)
      pontine h. (PHI)
      punctate h.
      white matter h. (WMHI)
hyperirritability
hyperkalemia
      digoxin-induced h. (DIH)
hyperkalemic cardioplegia
hyperkinemia
hyperkinesia
hyperkinesis
hyperkinetic
      h. heart syndrome (HHS)
      h. pulse
      h. state
hyperlactatemia
hyperleukocytosis
hyperlipidemia (HL)
      false combined h.
      familial combined h. (FCHL)
      multiple lipoprotein-type h.
      polygenic h.
      primary h.
      WHO/Fredrickson classification of
        primary h.
hyperlipoproteinemia type I, IIa, IIb,
  III, IV, V
hyperlucency
      unilateral h.
hyperlucent
      h. lung
      h. lung syndrome
hypermagnesemia
hypermetabolism
hypernatremia
hyperoxaluria
hyperoxia
hyperparathyroidism
hyperperfusion
      septal h.
      h. syndrome
hyperphosphatemia
hyperpiesis, hyperpiesia
hyperpietic
hyperpigmentation
hyperplasia
      adrenal h.
      angiofollicular lymph node h.
      atypical alveolar h.
      bilateral adrenal h.
      congenital adrenal h.

      elastic tissue h.
      epidermal h.
      giant lymph node h.
      intimal h. (IH)
      intravascular papillary endothelial h.
       (IPEH)
      localized mediastinal lymph
       node h.
      lymph node h.
      lymphoid h.
      lymphoid interstitial
       pneumonia/pulmonary lymphoid h.
       (LIP/PLH)
      mucous gland h.
      multifocal micronodular
       pneumocyte h.
      neointimal h.
      nodular lymphoid h.
      reactive mesothelial h.
      thymic h.
      type II cell h.
hyperplastic
      h. mucus-secreting goblet cell
      h. osteoarthritis
      h. response
hyperplastica
      arteritis h.
hyperpnea
      exercise h.
      isocapnic h.
      normocapnic h.
hyperpnea-induced bronchoconstriction
  (HIB)
hyperpolarization
      afterspike h. (AHP)
HyperQ system
hyperreactivity
      airway h. (AHR)
      bronchial h. (BHR)
      nonspecific bronchial h.
      work-related bronchial h.
hyperreflexia
      autonomic h.
hyperreninemia
hyperresonance
hyperresonant
hyperresponsive airways
hyperresponsiveness
      airway h. (AHR)
      bronchial h. (BHR)
hypersecretion
      airway h.
      mucus h.
hypersecretory
hypersensitive
      h. carotid sinus syndrome
      h. xiphoid syndrome
hypersensitivity
      aminosalicylic acid h.

H

hypersensitivity *(continued)*
    h. angiitis
    cardioinhibitory carotid sinus h.
    carotid sinus h.
    delayed-type h. (DTH)
    h. myocarditis
    h. pneumonia
    h. pneumonitis (HP)
    sirolimus-induced pulmonary h.
    h. vasculitis
hyperserotonemia
    vasculocardiac syndrome of h.
hypersialorrhea
hypersignal
hypersomnia
    idiopathic h.
hypersomnolence
hypersphyxia
Hyperstat IV
hypersystole
hypersystolic
hypertelorism
hypertension (HPN, HT, HTN, HTX)
    accelerated h.
    acquired pulmonary h.
    adrenal h.
    alveolar h.
    arterial h. (AH)
    benign h.
    benign intracranial h.
    borderline h. (BHT)
    ceiling effect in h.
    chronic h. (CH)
    chronic thromboembolic
      pulmonary h. (CTEPH)
    cocaine-induced h.
    cuffed h.
    h. in diabetes (HID)
    diastolic h.
    dietary approaches to stop h.
      (DASH)
    edema, proteinuria, h. (EPH)
    endolymphatic h.
    episodic h.
    essential h. (EH, EHT)
    exercise h.
    extrahepatic portal h. (EHPH)
    familial h. (FH)
    familial dyslipidemic h.
    familial primary pulmonary h.
      (FPPH)
    genetic h. (GH)
    h. genetic epidemiology network
    gestational h.
    glucocorticoid-induced h.
    Goldblatt h.
    high-renin essential h. (HREH)
    HIV-associated pulmonary h.

    human immunodeficiency virus-
      associated pulmonary h. (HIV-PH)
    hypoxic pulmonary h.
    idiopathic portal h. (IPH)
    idiopathic pulmonary h. (IPH)
    idiopathic pulmonary arterial h.
      (IPAH)
    induced h.
    International Society of H. (ISH)
    intracranial h. (ICH)
    intrathoracic h.
    isolated systolic h.
    labile h.
    left atrial h.
    low-renin essential h. (LREH)
    malignant h. (MH)
    masked h.
    mineralocorticoid-induced h.
    neuromuscular h.
    nonprimary pulmonary h.
    obesity h.
    obliterative pulmonary h. (OPH)
    office h.
    oral contraceptive-induced h.
    orthostatic h.
    Page episodic h.
    pale h.
    paroxysmal h.
    pediatric h.
    portal h. (PHT)
    portal systemic h.
    portopulmonary h.
    postcapillary h.
    postoperative h.
    postpartum h.
    precapillary pulmonary h.
    pregnancy-induced h. (PIH)
    primary h.
    primary pulmonary h. (PPH)
    progressive pulmonary h.
    pulmonary h. (PH, PHT)
    pulmonary arterial h.
    pulmonary artery h. (PAH)
    pulmonary venous h. (PVH)
    recalcitrant h.
    red h.
    renal h.
    renoprival h.
    renovascular h. (RVH)
    resistant h.
    resting h.
    retrograde h.
    salt and water dependent h.
    sarcoidosis-induced pulmonary h.
    secondary pulmonary h.
    h. secondary to renal disease
      (HSRD)
    splenoportal h.
    h. standard

stress-related h.
superimposed pregnancy-induced h.
  (SPIH)
systemic vascular h.
systemic venous h.
systolic h.
thromboembolic pulmonary h.
venous h.
white coat h.
hypertensive (HT)
  h. agent
  h. arteriopathy
  h. arteriosclerosis
  h. arteriosclerotic cardiovascular
    disease (HASCVD)
  h. arteriosclerotic heart disease
    (HASHD)
  borderline h. (BH)
  h. cardiovascular disease (HCVD,
    HTCVD)
  h. cerebrovasculopathy
  h. crisis
  h. emergency
  h. encephalopathy (HE)
  h. heart disease (HHD, HTHD)
  h. hypertrophic cardiomyopathy
  h. hypervolemic therapy (HHT)
  h. intracerebral hemorrhage (HIH)
  h. nephropathy (HTN)
  h. pulmonary polyarteritis
  h. pulmonary vascular disease
    (HPVD)
  h. retinopathy
  spontaneously h. (SH)
  h. urgency
  h. vascular disease (HTVD, HVD)
  h. vasculopathy
hyperthermia
  cerebral h.
  whole-body h.
hyperthyroid heart
hyperthyroidism
  amiodarone-induced h.
  apathetic h.
hypertonic
  h. saline
  h. saline inhalation
  h. saline solution
hypertonica
  polycythemia h.
hypertriglyceridemia (HTG)
  familial h. (FHTG)
hypertriglyceridemic waist
hypertrophic
  h. adenoid
  h. cardiomyopathy (HC, HCM,
    HCMP)
  h. catarrh
  h. emphysema

h. muscular subaortic stenosis
  (HMSAS)
h. obstructive cardiomyopathy
  (HOCM)
h. pulmonary osteoarthropathy
h. smooth muscle layer
h. subaortic stenosis (HSAS, HSS)
hypertrophied
  h. apex
  h. heart
  h. myocardium
hypertrophy
  adenotonsillar h.
  apical h.
  asymmetric septal h. (ASH)
  basal-septal h.
  biventricular h. (BVH)
  cardiac h.
  cardiac myocyte h.
  combined atrial h. (CAH)
  combined ventricular h. (CVH)
  compensatory h.
  concentric left ventricular h.
  eccentric h.
  goblet cell h.
  idiopathic myocardial h. (IMH)
  isolated septal h. (ISH)
  left atrial h. (LAH)
  left ventricular h. (LVH)
  lipomatous h.
  load-induced cardiac h.
  mucous gland h.
  myocardial cell h.
  myocyte h.
  pressure-overload h.
  right atrial h. (RAH)
  right ventricular h. (RVH)
  secondary septal h.
  septal h.
  stretch-induced cardiomyocyte h.
  submucosal gland h.
  trabecular h.
  transcoronary ablation of septal h.
    (TASH)
  ventricular h. (VH)
  volume load h.
hyperuricemia
hyperuricemic nephropathy
hyperventilation
  alveolar h.
  h. challenge test
  eucapnic voluntary h.
  hypocapnic h.
  isocapnic h.
  h. maneuver
  h. syndrome (HVS)
hyperventilation-induced
  h.-i. asthma (HIA)
  h.-i. hypotension

H

hyperviscosity syndrome
hypervitaminosis
hypervolemia
hypervolemic (HV)
hypha, pl. hyphae
hyphemia
hypnagogic hallucination
hypnagogue
hypnalgia
hypnic
hypnology
Hypnomidate
hypnopompic hallucination
hypnosis
hypnotic drug
hypoadrenalism
hypoaeration
hypoalbuminemia
hypoaldosteronism
    hyporeninemic h.
hypoalphalipoproteinemia
hypobaric
    h. exposure
    h. hypoxia
hypobetalipoproteinemia
    familial h. (FHBL)
hypocalcemia
    cardiac defects, abnormal facies, thymic hypoplasia, cleft palate, h. (CATCH-22)
hypocapnia
hypocapnic hyperventilation
hypocarbia
hypochloremia
hypochloremic metabolic alkalosis
hypochlorite
hypocholesterolemia
hypochondrial reflex
hypochondriasis
hypocomplementemia
hypodynamia cordis
hypoechoic plaque
hypofunction
hypogammaglobulinemia
hypoglossal nerve
hypoglycemia
hypoglycemic
    h. agent
    h. syncope
hypokalemia
hypokalemia-induced arrhythmia
hypokalemic periodic paralysis
hypokinemia
hypokinesis, hypokinesia
    anteromesial h.
    cardiac wall h.
    global h.
hypokinetic pulse
hypomagnesemia

hyponatremia
hyponatremic-hypertensive syndrome
hypoparathyroidism
hypoperfused myocardium
hypoperfusion
    apical h.
    h. index
    myocardial h.
    septal h.
    tissue h.
hypopharyngeal obstruction
hypophosphatemia
hypophyseal-pituitary-adrenal axis
hypophyseos
    pars pharyngea h.
hypopiesis
    orthostatic h.
hypoplasia
    isthmic h.
    mitral valve h.
    h. of right ventricle
    right ventricular h.
hypoplasminogenemia
hypoplastic
    h. emphysema
    h. heart
    h. left heart (HPLH)
    h. left heart syndrome (HLHS)
    h. left ventricle (HLV)
    h. left ventricle syndrome (HLVS)
hypopnea
    central h.
    obstructive h.
hypopneic
hyporeninemia
hyporeninemic hypoaldosteronism
hyposphygmia
hypostasis
    pulmonary h.
hypostatic
    h. bronchopneumonia
    h. congestion
    h. pneumonia
hyposystole
hypotension
    acute severe h.
    arterial h.
    chronic idiopathic orthostatic h.
    exertional h.
    hemorrhagic h.
    hyperventilation-induced h.
    idiopathic orthostatic h. (IOH)
    intractable h.
    orthostatic h.
    paradoxical h.
    postprandial h.
    postural h.
    pulmonary artery h. (PAH)
    sympathetic orthostatic h. (SOH)

vasodilatory h.
vasovagal h.
hypotensive agent
hypothalamic-pituitary-adrenal (HPA)
h.-p.-a. axis (HPAA)
hypothermia
h. blanket
extracorporeal exchange h.
h. mattress
moderate h.
therapeutic h.
topical h.
hypothermic fibrillating arrest
hypothesis, pl. **hypotheses**
fetal origins h.
Gad h.
leading circle h.
lipid h.
Lyon h.
Moe multiple wavelet h.
monoclonal h.
multiple wavelet h.
null h.
premature ventricular complex-
trigger h.
response-to-injury h.
sulfhydryl depletion h.
Wu-Hoak h.
hypothrombogenic
hypothyroidism
subclinical h.
hypotonia
hypotonicity
hypotonus, hypotony
hypotube
nitinol h.
Hypovase
hypoventilation
alveolar h.
central alveolar h.
congenital central alveolar h.
nocturnal h.
primary alveolar h.
pulmonary alveolar h. (PAH)
hypovolemia
hypovolemic shock
hypoxanthine
hypoxemia
arterial h.
circulatory h.
intraoperative h.
reflecting chronic h.
refractory h.
REM sleep-related h.

rest h.
h. test
hypoxemic respiratory failure
hypoxia
altitude h.
alveolar h.
anemic h.
cerebral h.
chronic h. (CH)
circulatory h.
demand h.
diffusion h.
global tissue h.
hemic h.
histotoxic h.
hypobaric h.
hypoxic h.
ischemic h.
myocyte h.
sleep h.
stagnant h.
tissue h.
h. warning system
hypoxia-inducible factor (HIF)
hypoxic
h. hypoxia
h. lap swimming
h. pulmonary hypertension
h. pulmonary vasoconstriction
(HPV)
h. spell
h. syncope
h. vasoconstriction
h. ventilatory response (HVR)
hypoxic-ischemic encephalopathy
hypoxidosis
hysteresis
airway h.
pacemaker h.
pacing h.
rate h.
hysterical
h. fainting
h. syncope
hysteric angina
hystericus
globus h.
hysterosystole
Hy-Tape waterproof adhesive tape
Hytinic
Hytrin
Hytuss
Hytuss-2X
Hyzaar

H

IASD
    interatrial septal defect
iatrogenic
    i. atrial septal defect
    i. disease
    i. disorder
    i. pneumothorax
    i. trauma
IAV
    intraarterial vasopressin
IAVP
    immunoreactive arginine vasopressin
IBBBB
    incomplete bilateral bundle branch block
Iberet-Folic-500
iberiotoxin
IBI
    internal borderzone infarct
        IBI 1500T6 generator
        IBI Therapy cardiac ablation
        system
        IBI Therapy Dual 8 ablation
        catheter
ibopamine
IBP
    intraaortic balloon pump
IBPMS
    indirect blood pressure measuring system
ibuprofen
        pseudoephedrine and i.
Ibuprohm
Ibu-Tab
ibutilide fumarate
IC
    impedance cardiogram
    inspiratory capacity
    intracardiac
ICA
    internal carotid artery
ICAM
    intercellular adhesion molecule
ICAM-1
    intercellular adhesion molecule-1
ICAO standard atmosphere
ICAT
    intracoronary aspiration thrombectomy
icatibant pretreatment
ICC
    immunocytochemistry
    intensive coronary care
    interventional cardiac center
ICCM
    idiopathic congestive cardiomyopathy
ICCU
    intensive coronary care unit
ICD
    implantable cardioverter-defibrillator
    ischemic coronary disease
    isolated conduction defect

        Angstrom II ICD
        Angstrom MD ICD
        Atlas ICD
        Atlas DR ICD
        Atlas VR ICD
        biventricular ICD
        Contour high voltage can ICD
        Contour II ICD
        Contour LT V-135D ICD
        Contour V-145D ICD
        dual-chamber Maximo remote
          monitoring ICD
        Epic HF ICD
        Guardian ICD
        internet monitoring of ICD
        ICD lead
        Medtronic InSync ICD
        ICD parameters
        Photon DR dual-chamber ICD
        Phylax AV implantable ICD
        remotely monitored ICD
        Res-Q Micron ICD
        single-chamber Maximo remote
          monitoring ICD
        Telectronics Guardian ATP II ICD
        transthoracically implanted ICD
        Ventritex Cadence ICD
        Vitatron Diamond ICD
ICD-9
    International Classification of Diseases,
      Ninth Revision
ICD-ATP
    implantable cardioverter-
      defibrillator/atrial tachycardia pacing
        ICD-ATP device
ICDC
    implantable cardioverter-defibrillator
      catheter
ICE
    intracardiac echocardiography
        ICE catheter
ice
        i. cardioplegia
        i. mapping
iceberg tumor
iced
        i. saline
        i. saline lavage
        i. saline perfusion
        i. saline solution
ice-pick view
ICER
    incremental cost-effectiveness ratio
ICEUS
    intracaval endovascular ultrasonography
ICG
    impedance cardiogram
    impedance cardiography

ICG-PDR
indocyanine green plasma disappearance rate
ICH
immunocompromised host
intracerebral hemorrhage
intracranial hemorrhage
intracranial hypertension
infratentorial ICH
supratentorial ICH
ICHD
Inter-Society Commission for Heart Diseases
ICHD pacemaker code
ichorous pleurisy
ICI
intracardiac infection
icing heart
ICM
intelligent cardiovascular monitor
isolated cardiovascular malformation
ICO
impedance cardiac output
intracellular organism
ICOPER
International Cooperative Pulmonary Embolism Registry
ICP
intracranial pressure
ICR
intracardiac catheter recording
ICRT
intracoronary radiation therapy
ICS
inhaled corticosteroid
intercostal space
intracellular-like, calcium-bearing crystalloid solution
ICS cardioplegic solution
ICSD
International Classification of Sleep Disorders
ICSI
intracoronary stent implantation
ICSK
intracoronary streptokinase
ICSO
intermittent coronary sinus occlusion
ICT
intracardiac thrombus
icteric sputum
ictometer
ICTP
type I collagen telopeptide
ictus
i. cordis
i. sanguinis
ICUS
intracoronary ultrasound

ICV
internal cerebral vein
ICXA
intermediate circumflex artery
ID
immunodiffusion
Idamycin PFS
idarubicin hydrochloride
IDC
idiopathic dilated cardiomyopathy
IDDM
insulin-dependent diabetes mellitus
ideal alveolar gas
ideational apraxia
IDEC-Y2B8 antibody
identity
I. DR model 5370 pacemaker
I. SR model 5172 pacemaker
I. XL DR model 5376 pacemaker
ideomotor apraxia
idiojunctional rhythm
idionodal rhythm
idiopathic
i. acute eosinophilic pneumonia
i. alveolar fibrosis (IAF)
i. arterial calcification of infancy (IACI)
i. arteritis of Takayasu
i. bradycardia
i. brown induration
i. cardiomegaly
i. central sleep apnea
i. chylopericardium
i. congestive cardiomyopathy (ICCM)
i. cyclic edema
i. dilated cardiomyopathy (IDC)
i. disease of myocardium (IDM)
i. glomerulonephritis
i. hypereosinophilic syndrome (IHES, IHS)
i. hyperkinetic heart syndrome (IHHS)
i. hypersomnia
i. hypertrophic subaortic stenosis (IHSS)
i. interstitial fibrosis
i. interstitial pneumonia (IIP)
i. left bundle branch block-shaped ventricular tachycardia
i. long QT interval syndrome
i. mitral valve prolapse (IMVP)
i. myocardial hypertrophy (IMH)
i. myocarditis
i. orthostatic hypotension (IOH)
i. pericarditis
i. pneumonia syndrome (IPS)
i. polyneuropathy
i. portal hypertension (IPH)

idiopathic *(continued)*
    i. pulmonary arterial hypertension (IPAH)
    i. pulmonary fibrosis (IPF)
    i. pulmonary hemosiderosis (IPH)
    i. pulmonary hypertension (IPH)
    i. restrictive cardiomyopathy
    i. right atrial dilation
    i. thrombocytopenia
    i. thrombocytopenic purpura (ITP)
    i. unilobar emphysema
    i. venoocclusive disease
    i. ventricular fibrillation
    i. ventricular tachycardia (IVT)
idiosyncratic asthma
idioventricular
    i. bradycardia
    i. kick
    i. rhythm (IVR)
    i. tachycardia
IDIS
    intraoperative digital subtraction
IDISA
    intraoperative digital subtraction angiography
IDL
    intermediate-density lipoprotein
IDL-C, IDL-c
    intermediate-density lipoprotein-cholesterol complex
IDM
    idiopathic disease of myocardium
idoxuridine
idraparinux
IDV
    intermittent demand ventilation
IE
    infective endocarditis
I:E
    inspiratory to expiratory
        I:E ratio
IE-2 riboprobe
IEA
    inferior epigastric artery
        IEA graft
IEB
    intermediate endpoint biomarker
IEC
    inpatient exercise center
IEL
    internal elastic lamina
I-ELCAP
    International Early Lung Cancer Action Program
IEM
    internal elastic membrane
        IEM rupture
IETT
    immediate exercise treadmill testing

Ifex
IFG
    inferior frontal gyrus
IFL
    inferior frontal lobe
IFN
    interferon
IFN-gamma
    interferon-gamma
ifosfamide
IFP
    intimal fibrous proliferation
Ig
    immunoglobulin
Igaki-Tamai stent
IgAN
    immunoglobulin A neuropathy
IgA neuropathy
IgE
    immunoglobulin E
        serum IgE
IgE-independent occupational asthma
IgE-mediated
    IgE-m. asthma
    IgE-m. food allergy
IgE-sensitized cell
IGF
    insulin-like growth factor
IGF-1 overexpression
IgG
    immunoglobulin G
        ACLA IgG
        IgG avidity test
IgG1–4
IgM
    immunoglobulin M
        ACLA IgM
IGT
    impaired glucose tolerance
IH
    intermittent heparinization
    intimal hyperplasia
    intramural hematoma
IHD
    ischemic heart disease
IHDI
    ischemic heart disease index
IHD QUERI
    ischemic heart disease quality enhancement research initiative
IHES
    idiopathic hypereosinophilic syndrome
IHHS
    idiopathic hyperkinetic heart syndrome
IHR
    intrinsic heart rate
IHS
    idiopathic hypereosinophilic syndrome

IHSS
    idiopathic hypertrophic subaortic stenosis
IIFT
    intraoperative intraarterial fibrinolytic
        therapy
IIP
    idiopathic interstitial pneumonia
IJ
    internal jugular
Ikorel
IL
    interleukin
        IL Synthesis analyzer
IL-4 gene
IL-10
        IL-10 production
        recombinant human IL-10 (rhuIL-
            10)
Ilbawi
        I. operation
        I. procedure
ILBBB
    incomplete left bundle branch block
ILCOR
    International Liaison Committee on
        Resuscitation
ILD
    interleukin D
    interstitial lung disease
        SS-associated ILD
ileal artery
ileocolic artery
Iletin
        beef Lente I. II
        pork NPH I. II
        pork Regular I. II
ileus
        meconium i.
ILHDL
    isolated low high-density lipoprotein
iliac
        i. artery
        i. artery occlusion
        i. steal
        i. vein
        i. vein thrombosis
iliofemoral
        i. artery
        i. venous system
iliopopliteal bypass
Illinois Test of Psycholinguistic Abilities
illness
        catabolic i.
        decompression i.
illusion
ILMA
    intubating laryngeal airway mask

ILO
    International Labor Office
        ILO classification
Iloprost
Ilosone
Ilotycin
ILR
    insertable loop recorder
IL-4R
    interleukin 4 receptor
ILUS
    intraluminal ultrasound
IM
    innocent murmur
    internal mammary
    intramuscular
        IM artery
        Rocephin IM
IMA
    inferior mesenteric artery
    internal mammary artery
        IMA graft
        IMA retractor
IMAB
    internal mammary artery bypass
image
        i. aliasing
        amplitude i.
        i. analysis
        i. bundle
        CK i.
        color kinesis i.
        digital subtraction angiography
            mask i.
        3-dimensional spoiled gradient-
            recalled acquisition i.
        3D SPGR i.
        ejection fraction i.
        ejection shell i.
        equilibrium i.
        FLAIR i.
        fluid-attenuated inversion
            recovery i.
        functional i.
        gradient reversal i.
        harmonic phase i.
        HARP i.
        i. intensifier
        paradox i.
        parametric i.
        phase i.
        phase-encoded velocity i.
        postpump i.
        prepump i.
        regional ejection fraction i. (REFI)
        respiratory-gated 2D segmented-
            FLASH MRCA i.
        SE i.
        short-axis i.

image *(continued)*
    stress washout myocardial
      perfusion i.
    supine rest gated equilibrium i.
    T1-weighted i.
Image-Measure morphometry software
Imagent contrast agent
imager
    Sonos 2000, 5500 ultrasound i.
    I. Torque selective catheter
imagery
    guided i.
ImageView system
ImageVue software
imaging
    acoustic i.
    ADC i.
    adenosine nuclear perfusion i.
    adenosine radionuclide perfusion i.
    i. agent
    antifibrin antibody i.
    antimyosin antibody i.
    apparent diffusion coefficient i.
    arrhythmia-insensitive flow-sensitive
      alternating inversion recovery i.
    biplane i.
    black blood magnetic resonance i.
    blood-pool i.
    breathhold turbo-flash tagged i.
    cardiac bioluminescence i.
    cardiac blood-pool i.
    CardioNow telecardiology i.
    i. chain
    chemical shift i. (CSI)
    coherent contrast i. (CCI)
    color kinesis i.
    color tissue Doppler i.
    continuous-wave Doppler i.
    diffusion tensor i. (DTI)
    diffusion-weighted i. (DWI)
    digital cardiac i. (DCI)
    digital subtraction i.
    digital vascular i. (DVI)
    dimensionality in i.
    3-dimensional tagged magnetic
      resonance i.
    dipyridamole-thallium i. (DTI)
    direct Fourier transformation i.
    Doppler myocardial i. (DMI)
    Doppler tissue i. (DTI)
    Doppler transesophageal color
      flow i.
    double-oblique i.
    3D tagged magnetic resonance i.
    duplex i.
    dynamic MR perfusion i.
    echocardiographic strain rate i.
    echo-contrast variability i.
    echo planar i. (EPI)

    electrocardiographic gated SPECT
      myocardial perfusion i.
    exercise i.
    exercise tomographic TI-201 i.
    fast cine magnetic resonance i.
    F-fluorodeoxyglucose i.
    Fourier 2-dimensional i.
    frequency domain i.
    functional i.
    functional magnetic resonance i.
     (fMRI)
    fundamental i. (FI)
    gallium i.
    gallium-67 i.
    gated blood-pool i.
    gated sweep magnetic resonance i.
    gradient-echo i.
    harmonic i. (HI)
    harmonic gray-scale i.
    harmonic power Doppler i.
    high-speed volumetric i.
    ^{123}I BMIPP i.
    indium-111-labeled lymphocyte i.
    infarct-avid i.
    Integris cardiovascular i.
    krypton-81m ventilation i.
    long-echo-train-length fast-spin-
      echo i.
    long-ETL FSE i.
    magnetic resonance i. (MRI)
    magnetic source i. (MSI)
    mask-mode cardiac i.
    MCD i.
    molecular i.
    MR cine i.
    myocardial perfusion i. (MPI)
    native tissue harmonic i.
    nuclear magnetic resonance i.
     (NMRI)
    nuclear perfusion i.
    parametric i.
    perfusion-weighted i.
    perfusion-weighted magnetic
      resonance i. (PWI)
    pharmacologic stress perfusion i.
    phase i.
    planar myocardial i.
    planar thallium i.
    platelet i.
    power motion i.
    pulsed Doppler tissue i.
    pulse inversion harmonic i.
    PYP i.
    pyrophosphate i.
    radionuclide i.
    radiopharmaceutical i.
    real-time perfusion i.
    reconstructed pulsed-wave Doppler
      myocardial i.

redistribution i.
rest-redistribution thallium-201 i.
rubidium-82 i.
second harmonic i. (SHI)
sestamibi perfusion i.
single-photon emission computed
 tomographic i.
single-photon emission
 tomography i.
SPECT i.
SPET i.
spin-echo i.
stress-redistribution-reinjection
 thallium-201 i.
stress SPECT perfusion i.
stress thallium-201 myocardial
 perfusion i.
i. surveillance
tagged magnetic resonance i.
^{99m}Tc sestamibi i.
^{99m}Tc tetrofosmin i.
teboroxime i.
technetium-99m MIBI i.
technetium-99m sestamibi
 tomographic i.
technetium-99m tetrofosmin i.
thallium perfusion i.
thallium SPECT i.
tissue Doppler i. (TDI)
tomographic radionuclide i.
transient response i. (TRI)
transmission i.
triggered harmonic power
 Doppler i.
ultrasonic integrated backscatter i.
velocity-encoded cine-magnetic
 resonance i. (VE-cMRI)
ventilation/perfusion i.
video i.
VScore with AutoGate cardiac i.
i. window
xenon lung ventilation i.
IMAI
internal mammary artery implant
Imatron C-150XP electron beam CT scanner
IMAX
internal maxillary artery
imazodan
imbalance
acid-base i.
electrolyte i.
protease-antiprotease i.
sympathovagal i.
ventricular i.
IMCE
intravenous myocardial contrast
 echocardiography
imciromab pentetate

Imdur
Imed
I. infusion device
I. infusion pump
I-Methasone
IMGU
insulin-mediated glucose uptake
IMH
idiopathic myocardial hypertrophy
intramural hematoma
intramural hemorrhage
IMI
impending myocardial infarction
inferior myocardial infarction
^{125}I MIBG
^{123}-I MIBG
imidazoline
i. receptor (I-receptor)
i. receptor agonist
imiglucerase
imipenem and cilastatin
imipramine
Immedia PT system
immediate
i. exercise treadmill testing (IETT)
i. silhouette
immersion
head-out water i.
immitis
Coccidioides i.
Dirofilaria i.
immobilized heparin
immotile cilia syndrome
ImmuCyst
immune
i. adherence immunosorbent assay
 (IAIA)
i. cascade
i. reconstitution inflammatory
 reaction (IRIS)
i. reconstitution syndrome
i. restoration disease (IRD)
i. thrombocytopenia
immune-complex deposition
immune-mediated
i.-m. disease
i.-m. injury
i.-m. membranous nephritis
i.-m. vasculitis
immunity
cell-mediated i.
heightened i.
Immuno
Feiba VH I.
immunoadsorption
immunoassay
AfeCTA i.
Elecsys proBNP i.
electrochemiluminescence i.

immunoassay *(continued)*
> enzyme i. (EIA)
> galactomannan enzyme i.
> nifedipine enzyme i.
> NT-proBNP ELISA enzyme i.
> Thrombus Precursor Protein i.

immunoblot
> antiphosphotyrosine i.

immunoblotting
immunochemical abnormality
immunocompetent host
immunocompromised host (ICH)
immunocytochemistry (ICC)
immunodeficiency
> common variable i. (CVID)

immunodetected
immunodiffusion (ID)
immunofluorescence
> i. assay
> cytometric indirect i.
> i. microscopy

immunofluorescent technique
immunogenicity
immunoglobulin (Ig)
> i. A neuropathy (IgAN)
> i. E (IgE)
> equine rabies i. (ERIG)
> i. G (IgG)
> intravenous polyspecific i. G (IVIG)
> i. M (IgM)
> respiratory syncytial virus i. (RSV-IG)
> varicella-zoster i. (VZIG)

immunohistochemical staining
immunohistochemistry
immunological theory
immunology
> American College of Allergy, Asthma and I.

immunometric sandwich method
immunomodulator
immunonephelometry
> rate i.

immunoperoxidase stain
immunophenotype
immunophenotyping
immunophilin
immunoprecipitation
immunoprecipitin analysis
immunoprophylaxis
immunoradiometric assay (IRMA)
immunoreactive
> i. arginine vasopressin (IAVP, irAVP)
> i. atrial natriuretic peptide (iANP, irANP)

immunoreactivity
> endothelin-1 i.

immunoregulator
> IMREG-1 i.

immunoseparation
immunosorbent
immunospot
> enzyme-linked i. (ELISPOT)

immunostaining technique
immunostimulatory sequence (ISS)
immunosuppressant
immunosuppression
> postinjury i.
> i. therapy

immunosuppressive
immunotherapy
immunoturbidimetric assay
Imovax vaccine
impact
> I. portable aspirator model 326
> I. Uni-Vent ventilator

impaction
> mucoid i.

impaired
> i. glucose tolerance (IGT)
> i. relaxation mitral flow pattern

impairment
> i. of activities of daily living (IADL)
> ciliary i.
> conduction i.
> functional aerobic i. (FAI)
> memory i.
> restrictive functional i.
> ventricular systolic i.

impedance
> acoustic i.
> i. aggregometry
> aortic i.
> arterial i.
> atrial lead i.
> battery cell i.
> i. cardiac output (ICO)
> i. cardiogram (IC, ICG)
> i. cardiography (ICG)
> i. catheter
> lead i.
> i. modulus
> pacemaker i.
> pacing lead i.
> i. plethysmography (IPG)
> i. rise
> thoracic i.
> i. threshold device (ITD)
> i. threshold valve (ITV)
> transthoracic i.
> i. variables
> vascular i.
> ventricular i.

impeller pump

impending
> i. myocardial infarction (IMI)
> i. respiratory failure

imperfecta
> osteogenesis i.

implant
> adrenal medullary i.
> Biocell RTV i.
> Biomatrix ocular i.
> bioresorbable i.
> Core-Vent i.
> defibrillator i.
> internal mammary artery i. (IMAI)
> laser-sculpted i.
> polytef i.
> supraanular i.
> SynerGraft i.
> Thoratec HeartMate i.
> Zoladex i.

implantable
> i. artificial heart (IAH)
> i. atrial defibrillator (IAD)
> i. automatic cardioverter-defibrillator (IACD)
> i. cardioverter-defibrillator (ICD)
> i. cardioverter-defibrillator/atrial tachycardia pacing (ICD-ATP)
> i. cardioverter-defibrillator catheter (ICDC)
> i. cardioverter-defibrillator lead
> i. cardioverter electrode
> i. circulatory support device
> i. defibrillator
> i. left ventricular assist system (IPLVAS)
> i. loop recorder
> i. pulse generator
> i. ventricular assist device (IVAD)

implantation
> BRAFE approach for elective coronary stent i.
> i. guidelines
> intracoronary stent i. (ICSI)
> i. metastasis
> prophylactic implantable cardioverter-defibrillator i.
> rescue stent i.
> i. response
> stent i.
> subcoronary aortic valve i.
> i. test (IT)
> total i.
> transcatheter valve i.

implanted pacing device
implosion effect
Import vascular access port
impotence
> vasculogenic i.

Impra
> I. Carboflo ePTFE vascular graft
> I. Distaflo bypass graft

impressio cardiaca pulmonis
impression
> cardiac i.

ImPressure sensor
improvement
> deterioration following i. (DFI)

impulse
> afferent i.
> apex i.
> apical i. (AI)
> cardiac i.
> carotid i.
> i. conduction
> I. diagnostic catheter
> ectopic i.
> electrical i.
> escape i.
> i. formation
> overlapping biphasic i. (OLBI)
> pacing i. (PI)
> paradoxic rocking i.
> point of maximal i. (PMI)
> point of maximum i. (PMI)
> i. propagation
> right parasternal i.
> right parasternal i.'s
> i. summation
> systolic apical i.

ImPulse elite oxygen conserving device
impure flutter
IMREG-1 immunoregulator
IMT
> inspiratory muscle training
> intimal-medial thickness

Imulyse tPA ELISA kit
IMV
> intermittent mandatory ventilation
> intermittent mechanical ventilation

IMVP
> idiopathic mitral valve prolapse

^{111}In
> indium-111

in
> in extremis
> in situ
> in situ hybridization
> in situ thrombosis
> in situ zymography
> in vitro
> in vitro allergy test
> in vitro effective orifice area
> in vitro pharmacology
> in vivo
> in vivo effective orifice area
> in vivo gene transfer

inactivated poliovirus vaccine

371

inactivation
  recovery from i.
  tumor suppressor gene i.
inactive tuberculosis
inactivity
  physical i.
inaequalis
  pulsus i.
inamrinone
inappropriate sinus tachycardia (IST)
INCA
  infant nasal cannula assembly
  INCA system
incannulated
Incardia valve system
incentive
  i. spirometer
  i. spirometry
incessant
  i. atrial tachycardia
  i. ventricular tachycardia
inch
  pounds per square i. (psi)
incidence
  peak i.
incident
  cardiovascular i. (CVI)
  cerebrovascular i. (CVI)
  i. pressure waveform
  vascular i.
incidental murmur
incision
  clamshell i.
  collar i.
  fish-mouth i.
  ladder i.
  longitudinal midline i.
  median sternotomy i.
  pleuropericardial i.
  racquet i.
  stab i.
  sternal-splitting i.
  stocking-seam i.
  thoracotomy i.
  transverse i.
incisura
  i. apicis cordis
  i. cardiaca pulmonis sinistri
  i. pulse
incline
  treadmill i.
inclusion
  Rocha-Lima i.
  i. technique of Bentall
incognitus
  Mycoplasma i.
incompetence, incompetency
  aortic i. (AI)
  cardiac valvular i.

chronotropic i.
  mitral i. (MI)
  muscular i.
  pulmonary i.
  pulmonic i.
  pyloric i.
  relative i.
  tricuspid i. (TI)
  valvular i.
incomplete
  i. atrioventricular block
  i. atrioventricular dissociation
  i. A-V dissociation
  i. bilateral bundle branch block
  (IBBBB)
  i. left bundle branch block
  (ILBBB)
  i. right bundle branch block
  (IRBBB)
  i. thrombosis
incongruens
  pulsus i.
incontinentia pigmenti syndrome
increase
  blood pressure i. (BPI)
increased
  i. afterload
  i. contractility
  i. markings emphysema
  i. permeability pulmonary edema
increment
  work rate i.
incremental
  i. atrial pacing
  i. cost-effectiveness ratio (ICER)
  i. shuttle walking test (ISWT)
  i. threshold loading
  i. ventricular pacing
incrementation
  couch i.
incrementing response
incretin mimetic
IND
  investigational new drug
  IND status
Indacrinone
indanyl carbenicillin
indapamide
indecainide
Indeflator Plus 20
independence
  loss of i.
Inderal LA
Inderide
indeterminate single ventricle
index, pl. **indices, indexes**
  airways reactivity i. (ARI)
  ankle-arm i.
  ankle-brachial i. (ABI)

induced
- i. hypertension
- i. pneumothorax

inducibility

inducible
- i. arrhythmia
- i. ischemia
- i. nitric oxide synthase (iNOS)
- i. nitric oxide synthetase (iNOS)
- i. polymorphic ventricular fibrillation
- i. polymorphic ventricular tachycardia

induction
- rapid sequence i. (RSI)
- sputum i.

induration
- brown i.
- essential brown i.
- gray i.
- idiopathic brown i.
- pigment i.
- red i.

indurative
- i. myocarditis
- i. pleurisy
- i. pneumonia

industrial
- i. anthrax
- i. bronchitis

indux
- rale i.

indwelling
- i. central venous catheter
- i. line

inelastic load

inert gas narcosis

inertia

inertial effect

In-Exsufflator respiratory device

InfaMyst aerosol spray device

infancy
- idiopathic arterial calcification of i. (IACI)

infant
- i. airflow and effort sensor
- i. Ambu resuscitator
- continuous noninvasive monitoring of ventilated i.'s
- I. Flow noninvasive nasal CPAP system
- i. nasal cannula assembly (INCA)
- i. respiratory distress syndrome (IRDS)
- I. Resuscitation system
- I. Star 100, 200 ventilator
- I. Star ventilator 500/950

infantile
- i. arteritis

- i. beriberi
- i. lobar emphysema

infarct (*See also* infarction)
- acute multiple brain i.'s (AMBI)
- anterior lateral myocardial i. (ALMI)
- anterolateral wall myocardial i. (ALWMI)
- i. artery
- i. artery patency
- brain i. (BI)
- i. bulging
- caudate i.
- cerebral i.
- embolic i.
- i. expansion
- i. extension
- healed myocardial i. (HMI)
- insular i.
- internal borderzone i. (IBI)
- internal capsule i.'s
- lacunar i.
- partial anterior circulation i. (PACI)
- perforating artery i. (PAI)
- pontine i. (PI)
- posterior circulation i. (POCI)
- posterior wall i. (PWI)
- pulmonary i.
- red i.
- i. scar
- silent cerebral i. (SCI)
- i. size index (ISI)
- subcortical junctional i.
- i. thinning
- total anterior circulation i. (TACI)
- watershed i.
- i. zone wall motion

infarct-avid
- i.-a. hot-spot scintigraphy
- i.-a. imaging
- i.-a. myocardial scintigraphy

infarction (*See also* infarct)
- acute coronary i. (ACI)
- acute diaphragmatic myocardial i.
- acute myocardial i. (AMI)
- age-undetermined myocardial i.
- anterior myocardial i.
- anterior wall i. (AWI)
- anterior wall myocardial i. (AWMI)
- anteroinferior myocardial i.
- anterolateral myocardial i.
- anteroseptal myocardial i. (ASMI)
- apical i.
- atherothrombotic brain i. (ABI)
- atrial myocardial i.
- cardiac i.
- cerebral i.

infarction *(continued)*
    cerebrovascular i. (CVI)
    coitus-induced myocardial i.
    completed myocardial i.
    complicated myocardial i.
    diaphragmatic myocardial i. (DMI)
    ERNA after acute myocardial i.
    evolving myocardial i.
    exercise training in anterior
      myocardial i. (EAMI)
    family history of myocardial i.
    hemorrhagic i. (HI)
    H-form myocardial i.
    impending myocardial i. (IMI)
    inferior myocardial i. (IMI)
    inferior wall i. (IWI)
    inferior wall myocardial i. (IWMI)
    inferolateral myocardial i.
    inferoposterior myocardial i.
    ischemic cerebral i.
    juvenile myocardial i.
    lacunar i. (LI)
    large-vessel i. (LVI)
    lateral medullary i. (LMI)
    lateral myocardial i. (LMI)
    malignant middle cerebral artery i.
      (mMCAI)
    medial medullary i. (MMI)
    mesenteric i.
    myocardial i. (MI)
    National Registry of Myocardial I.
      (NRMI)
    non-Q-wave myocardial i. (NQMI,
      NQWMI)
    non-ST-segment elevation
      myocardial i. (NSTEMI)
    non-ST-segment myocardial i. (non-
      STEMI)
    nontransmural myocardial i. (NTMI)
    old myocardial i. (OMI)
    perioperative myocardial i. (PMI)
    posterior myocardial i.
    postmyocardial i.
    predictive index for myocardial i.
      (PIMI)
    primary i. (PI)
    pulmonary i. (PI)
    Q-wave myocardial i. (QMI)
    recent myocardial i. (RMI)
    recurrent myocardial i.
    right ventricle i. (RVI)
    right ventricular i. (RVI)
    rule out myocardial i. (ROMI)
    silent brain i. (SBI)
    silent cerebral i. (SCI)
    silent myocardial i. (SMI)
    small vessel i. (SVI)
    ST elevation acute myocardial i.
      (STEAMI)
    ST elevation myocardial i.
    striatocapsular i.
    ST-segment elevation myocardial i.
      (STEMI)
    stuttering myocardial i.
    subacute myocardial i.
    subendocardial i. (SEI)
    subendocardial myocardial i.
      (SEMI)
    threatened myocardial i. (TMI)
    thrombolysis in myocardial i.
      (TIMI)
    thrombotic brain i. (TBI)
    through-and-through myocardial i.
    transmural anterior myocardial i.
      (TAMI)
    transmural inferior myocardial i.
      (TIMI)
    transmural myocardial i. (TMI)
    unstable angina/non-Q-wave
      myocardial i. (UA/NQMI)
    watershed i.
    i. with shock

infarctlet
    myocardial i.

infarct-related
    i.-r. artery (IRA)
    i.-r. vessel

Infasurf

infected
    i. aneurysm
    i. myxoma
    i. secretion

infection
    acute lower respiratory tract i.
      (ALRI)
    adenovirus type 40/41 i.
    bacterial respiratory tract i.
    bloodstream i. (BSI)
    catheter-associated bloodstream i.
      (CA-BSI)
    catheter-related i. (CRI)
    catheter-related bloodstream i. (CR-
      BSI)
    community-acquired i.
    coronavirus i.
    deep driveline i.
    driveline i.
    endemic fungal i.
    endobronchial i.
    fascioperitoneal i.
    filarial i.
    fungal i.
    hospital-acquired i.
    human herpesvirus 8 i.
    intracardiac i. (ICI)
    laryngeal i.
    laryngotracheal i.
    latent tuberculosis i. (LTBI)

lung parenchymal i.
MAC i.
MAI i.
miliary i.
Mycobacterium avium complex i.
Mycobacterium avium-intracellulare i.
mycoplasmal i.
mycotic i.
nosocomial i.
nosocomial pulmonary i. (NPI)
opportunistic i.
pleuropulmonary i.
primary i.
pyogenic i.
recurrent respiratory i. (RRI)
respiratory tract i.
rhinocerebral i.
rickettsial i.
secondary i.
spirochetal i.
staphylococcal i.
streptococcal i.
Streptococcus pyogenes i.
subacute suppurative i.
surgical site i. (SSI)
systemic i.
upper respiratory i. (URI)
varicella-zoster i.
viral respiratory i.

infectious
i. asthmatic bronchitis
i. bronchiolitis
I. Diseases Society of America
i. endocarditis
i. esophagitis
i. mononucleosis

infective
i. aneurysm
i. asthma
i. edema
i. embolism
i. endocarditis (IE)
i. exacerbation
i. pericarditis
i. thrombosis
i. thrombus

INFeD injection
inferior
i. accessory fissure
arteria glutealis i.
i. axis flutter
i. border
i. border of lung
i. constrictor muscle
i. constrictor muscle of pharynx
i. costal facet
i. costal pit
i. epigastric artery (IEA)

i. epigastric artery graft
i. esophageal sphincter
fovea costalis i.
i. frontal gyrus (IFG)
i. frontal lobe (IFL)
i. ganglion
i. ganglion of glossopharyngeal nerve
i. laryngeal artery
i. laryngeal cavity
i. laryngeal vein
i. lingular bronchopulmonary segment
i. lobe of left/right lung
macular arteriole i.
i. mesenteric artery (IMA)
i. mesenteric artery retractor
i. mesenteric vascular occlusion
i. myocardial infarction (IMI)
i. parietal/superior temporal lobe (IPSTL)
i. phrenic lymph node
i. temporal artery (ITA)
i. thyroid artery
i. thyroid vein
i. tracheobronchial lymph node
i. triangle sign
i. vena cava (IVC)
i. vena cava occlusion
i. vena cava plethora
i. vena cava pressure (IVCP)
i. vena cava reconstruction (IVCR)
i. vena cava thrombosis (IVCT)
i. venacavography (IVCV)
vena laryngea i.
i. wall infarction (IWI)
i. wall myocardial infarction (IWMI)

inferiores
nodi lymphoidei phrenici i.
nodi lymphoidei tracheobronchiales i.

inferioris
rami esophageales arteriae thyroideae i.

inferius
tuberculum thyroideum i.

inferoapical
inferobasal wall
inferobasilar
inferolateral
i. myocardial infarction
i. segment

inferoposterior myocardial infarction
inferoseptal segment
infestans
Triatoma i.
infestation
parasitic i.

infiltrate
> alveolar i.
> Assmann tuberculous i.
> bronchiolar inflammatory i.
> bronchopneumonic i.
> cellular i.
> diffuse interstitial i.
> fibrous i.
> fleeting i.
> fluffy alveolar i.
> ground-glass i.
> hazy i.
> inflammatory cellular i.
> infraclavicular i.
> interstitial i.
> linear i.
> lobar i.
> migratory pulmonary i.
> nodular i.
> patchy i.
> periadventitial eosinophil-
> predominant i.
> peribronchial lymphocytic i.
> peribronchiolar inflammatory i.
> perivascular eosinophilic i.
> perivascular lymphocytic i.
> pulmonary i.
> reticulonodular i.
> strandy i.
> streaky i.
> Wasserman-positive pulmonary i.
> wedge i.

infiltrating lobular carcinoma
infiltration
> cardiac i.
> epituberculous i.
> gelatinous i.
> gray i.
> inflammatory cell i.
> lymphoplasmacytic i.
> patchy i.
> perivascular i. (PVI)
> plasmacytoid i.
> subepicardial fatty i.

infiltrative cardiomyopathy
Infiltrator local drug delivery device
Infiniti diagnostic catheter
Infinix
> I. DP-i dual C-arm system
> I. NB-i vascular x-ray

Infinnium Paclitaxel system drug-eluting stent
inflammation
> adhesive i.
> aerodigestive tract mucosal i.
> cap i.
> caseating granulomatous i.
> I. Defense Softgels
> granulomatous i.

> lymphocytic alveolar i.
> lymphoplasmacytic i.
> neutrophilic i.
> neutrophil-induced pulmonary i.
> peribronchiolar granulomatous i.
> polymorphonuclear neutrophil-
> dominated i.

inflammatoria
> dysphagia i.
inflammatory
> i. abdominal aortic aneurysm
> (IAAA)
> i. adhesion
> i. airway disease
> i. autobullectomy
> i. cardiomyopathy
> i. cell infiltration
> i. cellular infiltrate
> i. cytokine
> i. marker
> i. mediator
> i. myofibroblastic tumor
> i. pericarditis
> i. pseudotumor (IPT)
> i. reaction

inflation
> balloon i.
> lung i.
> oscillating balloon i.
> i. pressure
> i. reflex

inflatum
> *Tolypocladium i.*
inflection point
infliximab
inflow
> i. propagation velocity
> i. tract
> turbulent diastolic mitral i.

influenza, pl. **influenzae**
> i. A, B, C virus
> Asian i.
> i. bacillus
> endemic i.
> Hong Kong i.
> pandemic i. A
> Port Charles i.
> Russian i.
> Texas i.
> i. tracheobronchitis
> Victoria i.
> i. virus pneumonia
> i. virus vaccine

influenzae
> *Haemophilus i.*
> nontypeable *Haemophilus i.* (NTHI)
influenzal pneumonia
Influenzavirus A, B, C

influx
 calcium i.
 transsarcolemmal calcium i.
infraclavicular
 i. infiltrate
 i. triangle
infracristal
infradiaphragmatic
 i. portion
 i. venous flow
infrahisian
 i. block
 i. conduction system
infrainguinal bypass graft
infranodal extrasystole
infrared
 near i.
 i. thermography
 i. thermometer
infrared-pulsed laser
infrarenal abdominal aortic aneurysm
infrasegmental vein
infratentorial ICH
infrequens
 pulsus i.
infundibula (*pl. of* infundibulum)
infundibular
 i. atresia
 i. obstruction
 i. pulmonary stenosis (IPS)
 i. septal defect
 i. wedge resection
infundibulectomy
 Brock i.
infundibulum, pl. **infundibula**
 i. of lung
 right ventricular i.
 RV i.
 tendo infundibuli
 tendon of i.
Infusaid infusion pump
InfusaSleeve
 I. II catheter
 Kaplan-Simpson I.
 LocalMed I.
Infuse-A-Port pump
infuser
infusion
 Adenoscan i.
 adrenomedullin i.
 brain-heart i.
 bretylium i.
 cardioplegia i.
 CH i.
 continuous intravenous i. (CIV)
 i. device
 ergonovine i.
 heart i. (HI)
 heparin i.

 intracoronary acetylcholine i.
 IO i.
 isoproterenol i.
 nitroprusside i.
 volume i.
ingestion
 superwarfarin i.
ingravescent apoplexy
inguinalis
 regio i.
INH
 isoniazid
inhalant
 i. allergen
 antifoaming i.
 i. antigen
inhalation
 i. agent
 Atrovent Aerosol I.
 i. bronchography
 i. challenge test
 formoterol fumarate powder for i.
 hypertonic saline i.
 isoproterenol sulfate i.
 NebuPent I.
 oral triamcinolone i.
 oxygen i.
 i. pneumonia
 i. powder
 i. therapy
 tobramycin solution for i.
 toxic fume i.
 i. tuberculosis
inhalational
 i. anesthesia
 i. anesthetic
 i. anthrax
inhaled
 i. antibiotic
 i. beta agonist
 i. bronchodilator
 i. corticosteroid (ICS)
 i. glucocorticoid
 i. nitric oxide (INO)
 i. radioaerosol technique
 i. recombinant DNAse
Inhale deep lung delivery system
inhaler
 AeroBid Oral Aerosol I.
 Aerodose insulin i.
 AERx i.
 Azmacort Oral I.
 Beclovent Oral I.
 Beconase AQ Nasal I.
 breath-actuated i. (BAI)
 CFC-free metered-dose i.
 Combivent i.
 Diskhaler i.
 Diskus i.

inhaler *(continued)*
> dry powder i. (DPI)
> Flovent HFA metered-dose i.
> Intal Oral I.
> ipratropium i.
> metered-dose i. (MDI)
> metered-solution i. (MSI)
> Modulite i.
> nicotine i.
> Nicotrol I.
> pressurized metered-dose i. (pMDI)
> Spiros dry powder i.

Inhibace

inhibited
> atrial i. (AAI)
> atrial demand i. (AAI)
> atrial synchronous ventricular i. (VDD)
> both ventricles i. (VDI)
> i. pacing
> ventricular i. (VVI)

inhibition
> antifactor Xa i.
> calpain i.
> leukotriene i.
> magnet i.
> neurohormonal i.
> neutral endopeptidase i. (NEP-I, NEPi)
> PDE4 isoenzyme i.
> phosphodiesterase 3 i. (PDE3I)
> potassium i.

inhibitor
> ACE i.
> acyl-CoA:cholesterol acyltransferase i.
> alpha-2-plasmin i.
> alpha-1 proteinase i.
> angiotensin-converting enzyme i. (ACEI, ACEi)
> atriopeptidase i.
> beta-lactamase i.
> bronchial mucus i.
> calcineurin i.
> carbonic anhydrase i.
> caspase i.
> cholesterol crystallization i. (CCI)
> cholinesterase i.
> complement i.
> converting enzyme i.
> cyclooxygenase i.
> cyclooxygenase-1 i.
> direct thrombin i.
> endopeptidase i.
> farnesyl transferase i.
> glycoprotein IIb/IIIa i.
> HIV fusion i.
> HMG-CoA-reductase i.

> human menopausal gonadotropin coenzyme A reductase i.
> hydroxymethylglutaryl coenzyme A reductase i.
> 3-hydroxy-3-methylglutaryl coenzyme A reductase i.
> Kunitz-type i.
> leukotriene i.
> lipoprotein-associated coagulation i.
> MAO i.
> mast cell i.
> matrix metalloproteinase i. (MMPI)
> metalloproteinase i.
> monoamine oxidase i. (MAOI)
> mucus i.
> Na^+/H^+ exchange i. (NHEI)
> neuraminidase i.
> neutral endopeptidase i.
> nonnucleoside reverse transcriptase i.
> oxysterol i.
> PDE4 i.
> PDE isoenzyme i.
> phosphodiesterase i. (PDE, PDE-I)
> phosphodiesterase 4 i.
> phosphodiesterase isoenzyme i.
> plasminogen activator i. (PAI)
> platelet aggregation i.
> platelet glycoprotein IIb/IIIa i.
> platelet IIb/IIIa i.
> protease i. (PI)
> proteinase i. (Pi)
> proton pump i.
> recombinant human C1 i. (rhC1INH)
> reductase i.
> renin i.
> reversible i.
> RhoGDP-dissociation i. 1
> secretory leukocyte protease i. (SLPI)
> secretory leukoprotease i. (SLPI)
> secretory leukoproteinase i. (SLPI)
> serine elastase i.
> serine protease i.
> small-molecule FXa i.
> thromboxane synthetase i.
> tissue factor pathway i. (TFPI)
> tissue plasminogen activator i. (tPAI)
> vasopeptidase i. (VPI)

inhibitor-1
> plasminogen activator i.-1 (PAI-1)

inhibitory M2 muscarinic receptor
in-home unattended polysomnography
inhomogeneity
initial apnea

initiative
> ischemic heart disease quality enhancement research I. (IHD QUERI)
> NIH *Xenopus* I.
> quality enhancement research I. (QUERI)
> Women's Health I. (WHI)

injectable

injection
> Abbokinase i.
> Activase i.
> Adenocard i.
> Adrucil i.
> A-hydroCort i.
> A-methaPred i.
> Amikin i.
> Apresoline i.
> Aristocort Forte i.
> Aristocort Intralesional i.
> Aristospan Intraarticular i.
> Aristospan Intralesional i.
> Arixtra subcutaneous i.
> Baci-IM i.
> balloon-protected selective thrombin i.
> Benadryl i.
> Bicillin L-A i.
> blood patch i.
> bolus intravenous i.
> bone marrow i.
> Brethine i.
> Brevibloc i.
> Cafcit i.
> i. catheter
> Caverject i.
> Celestone Phosphate i.
> Cel-U-Jec i.
> Ceredase i.
> Chlor-Trimeton i.
> Cipro i.
> Cleocin Phosphate i.
> Compazine i.
> Cortrosyn i.
> Corvert i.
> Cyklokapron i.
> Cytoxan i.
> dalteparin sodium i.
> daptomycin for i.
> DDAVP i.
> Decadron i.
> Delatestryl i.
> Demadex i.
> Depo-Medrol i.
> Depopred i.
> Depo-Provera i.
> D.H.E. 45 i.
> Diflucan i.
> Diprivan i.

> Dopram i.
> Duo-Trach i.
> dye i.
> Edecrin Sodium i.
> Enlon i.
> epoprostenol sodium for i.
> ergonovine i.
> Ethamolin i.
> Flolan i.
> Floxin i.
> Foscavir i.
> Fragmin i.
> gadoteridol i.
> hand i.
> heparin i.
> hep-lock i.
> Hylutin i.
> Indocin IV i.
> INFeD i.
> iopromide i.
> isosorbide dinitrate i.
> Kenalog i.
> Key-Pred i.
> Key-Pred-SP i.
> Lasix i.
> lepirudin rDNA i.
> Levophed i.
> Lincocin i.
> Lincorex i.
> Lovenox i.
> meropenem for i.
> mycophenolate mofetil intravenous for i.
> Narcan i.
> negative-contrast i.
> Neosar i.
> Neutrexin i.
> Normodyne i.
> Oncovin i.
> Osmitrol i.
> Pentam-300 i.
> Permapen i.
> Phenergan i.
> Pitressin i.
> Prednisol TBA i.
> Prodrox i.
> Prostin VR Pediatric i.
> Refludan i.
> Retrovir i.
> Reversol i.
> Rifadin i.
> root i.
> selective septal branch i.
> Solu-Cortef i.
> Solu-Medrol i.
> Sublimaze i.
> Tac-3 i.
> Tensilon i.
> Terramycin IM i.

injection *(continued)*
    tinzaparin sodium i.
    Toposar i.
    Trandate i.
    Triam-A i.
    Triam Forte i.
    Triamonide i.
    Triostat i.
    Ultravist i.
    Ureaphil i.
    Vancoled i.
    VePesid i.
    Vibramycin i.
    Vistaril i.
    Vumon i.
    Wycillin i.
    Zinacef i.
injector
    flow i.
    Medrad Mark IV angiographic i.
    Mill-Rose esophageal i.
    modified Mark IV R-wave-triggered power i.
    power i.
    pressure i.
    Viamonte-Hobbs dye i.
injury, pl. **injuries**
    acute chemical i.
    acute lung i. (ALI)
    aortic i.
    aspiration lung i.
    blunt chest i.
    blunt pulmonary i.
    blunt torso i.
    brachial plexus i.
    chemical inhalation i.
    chest wall i.
    chronic recurrent chemical i.
    contrecoup i.
    i. current
    i. diameter
    diastolic current of i.
    diffuse lung i.
    early lung i.
    early pulmonary i.
    electrical i.
    femoral vascular i.
    immune-mediated i.
    intrathoracic i.
    ischemic/reperfusion i.
    late lung i.
    late pulmonary i.
    lipid-induced lung i.
    lipopolysaccharide-induced lung i.
    lung i.
    macromolecular cell i.
    median nerve i.
    mesangial immune i.
    myocardial i.

    i. pattern
    penetrating chest i.
    phrenic nerve crush i.
    pulmonary parenchymal i.
    radiation-induced lung i.
    radionecrosis i.
    reperfusion i.
    I. Severity Score (ISS)
    systolic current of i.
    thermal inhalation i.
    thoracic i.
    thoracic crush i.
    transfusion-related acute lung i. (TRALI)
    vascular i.
    ventilator-associated lung i. (VALI)
    ventilator-induced lung i. (VILI)
    ventricular i.
    i. VSD
inlet
    i. diameter
    thoracic i.
    ventricular i.
    i. VSD
in-memory gating
inner
    i. city asthma
    i. tube
    i. wall (IW)
Innervasc
    I. expandable vascular access system
    I. percutaneous vascular access device
innervation
    autonomic sensory i.
    parasympathetic i.
Innervision ventricular catheter
innocent
    i. heart murmur
    i. murmur (IM)
    i. murmur of elderly
Innohep
INNO-LiPA Rif.TB assay
innominate
    i. aneurysm
    i. artery
    i. vein
InnoPran XL
Innovace
INO
    inhaled nitric oxide
inoculation
inodilator therapy
inogatran
INOmax
inorganic
    i. acid
    i. acid vapor

i. dust
i. dust disease
i. murmur
iNOS
inducible nitric oxide synthase
inducible nitric oxide synthetase
inosine
inositol triphosphate
inotrope
negative i.
inotropic
i. agent
i. arrhythmia
i. effect
i. parameter
i. support
inotropy
Inoue
I. balloon catheter
I. balloon mitral valvotomy
I. balloon technique
I. endovascular stent-graft
I. self-guiding balloon
I. single-balloon technique
I. triple-branched stent graft
INOvent delivery system
inpatient exercise center (IEC)
INR
international normalized ratio
INR home anticoagulation blood
monitoring system
target INR
in-segment stenosis
insert
AirSep Ultimate nasal seal gel i.
EverGrip clamp i.
Koala vascular i.
insertable loop recorder (ILR)
insertion
catheter i.
homograft i.
percutaneous catheter i.
retrograde catheter i.
route of i.
wire i.
insert/mask
Nasal-Aire ventilator nasal i./m.
insipidus
nephrogenic diabetes i.
insomnia
insomniac
insonation
angle of i.
insonified
Inspector large-bore in-line hemostasis valve
InSpectra tissue spectrometer
inspiration
crowing i.

duration of i. (T$_I$)
sustained maximal i. (SMI)
inspirator
inspiratory
i. airflow
i. breath
i. breathhold
i. capacity (IC)
i. center
i. crackle
i. dyspnea
i. effort
expiratory to i. (E:I)
i. to expiratory (I:E)
i. to expiratory ratio
i. flow rate
i. limb
i. limb flattening
i. loading
i. murmur
i. muscle endurance
i. muscle fatigue
i. muscle training (IMT)
i. narrowing of glottis
i. occlusion pressure
i. positive airway pressure (IPAP)
i. rale
i. reserve capacity (IRC)
i. reserve volume (IRV)
i. resistance and positive expiratory
pressure (IR-PEP)
i. rhonchus
i. stridor
i. threshold load (ITL)
i. time (T$_I$)
i. view
i. vital capacity (IVC)
InspirEase device
inspired
i. gas
i. oxygen
inspirometer
Inspiron
I. device
I. incentive spirometer
inspissated
inspissation
mucous i.
Inspra
instability
catheter i.
circulatory i.
hemodynamic i.
microsatellite i.
instantaneous
i. electrical axis
i. spectral peak velocity
i. vector
Insta-Pulse heart rate monitor

in-stent
    i.-s. neointimal proliferation
    i.-s. restenosis (ISR)
    i.-s. stenosis
    i.-s. thrombosis
InStent VascuCoil stent
instillation
    intracavitary i.
    lavage i.
institute
    Cardiopulmonary Research I.
      (CAPRI)
    National Heart I. (NHI)
    National Heart, Lung, and
      Blood I. (NHLBI)
    Texas Heart I. (THI)
instrument
    activating adjusting i. (AAI)
    bipolar radiofrequency surgical
      ablation i.
    blood sampling i.
    Cooley neonatal i.'s
    Diamond-Lite titanium i.'s
    EndoWrist i.
    ERBE surgical i.
    KinetiX i.'s
    K x-ray fluorescence i.
    Matsuda titanium surgical i.'s
    Micrins microclamp i.
    Multi-Dop X/TCD transcranial
      Doppler i.
    Pneumo-Needle reusable i.
    thrombolytic predictive i. (TPI)
    ultrasound i.
    United States Catheter and I., Inc.
    URx Sonotherapy i.
instrumental activities of daily living (IADL)
instrumentation
    angiographic i.
insudate
insufficiency
    acute coronary i. (ACI)
    aortic i. (AI)
    aortic valvular i.
    arterial i.
    atrial i. (AI)
    atrioventricular valve i.
    cardiac i. (CI)
    cardiovascular i. (CVI)
    cerebrovascular i. (CVI)
    chronic coronary i. (CCI)
    chronic pulmonary i.
    chronic venous i. (CVI)
    coronary i. (CI)
    deep venous i. (DVI)
    distal vascular i.
    energetic dynamic cardiac i.
      (EDCI)

    left ventricular i. (LVI)
    mitral i. (MI)
    mitral valve i. (MVI)
    multivalve i.
    myocardial i.
    Osaka Acute Coronary I. (OACIS)
    periprosthetic valve aortic i.
    pulmonary i. (PI)
    pulmonic i.
    renal i.
    respiratory i.
    rheumatic mitral i.
    Sternberg myocardial i.
    tricuspid i. (TI)
    valvular i.
    velopharyngeal i.
    venous valvular i.
insufflation
    gastric i.
    thoracoscopic talc i.
    tracheal gas i. (TGI)
insufflator
    Endoflator i.
Insuflon device
insula, pl. insulae
insular infarct
insulation
    i. failure
    lead i.
insulin
    beef i.
    glucose, potassium, i. (GKI)
    Humulin L, N, R, U i.
    Lente Iletin I, II i.
    NPH Iletin i.
    pork i.
    i. preparation
    regular purified pork i.
    i. resistance
    i. resistance syndrome
    I. Riabead II radioimmunoassay
    i. shock
insulin-dependent diabetes mellitus (IDDM)
insulin-like growth factor (IGF)
insulin-mediated glucose uptake (IMGU)
insult
    cardiac i.
    vascular i.
InSync
    I. Biventricular Cardiac Pacing
      System
    I. cardiac resynchronization system
    I. cardioverter-defibrillator
    I. III atriobiventricular pacemaker
    I. III CRT-P device
    I. II Marquis CRT-D device
    I. II Marquis remote monitoring
      CRT-ICD

I. implantable cardioverter defibrillator
I. Maximo CRT-D device
I. multisite cardiac stimulator
I. Sentry CRT-D device

intact valve
Intal
I. Nebulizer Solution
I. Oral Inhaler

Intec
I. AID cardioverter-defibrillator generator
I. implantable defibrillator

Integra
I. catheter
I. II balloon

integral
aortic-time-velocity i.
diastolic velocity i. (DVI)
paced depolarization i.
i. pulse frequency modulation (IPFM)
i. pulse frequency modulation/Smith delay compensatory (IPFM/SDC)
systolic velocity i. (SVI)
velocity time i.

integrated
i. backscatter
i. bipolar sensing
i. lead system

integration
digital color Doppler velocity profile i.
vertical i.

integrator
Medical Graphics pneumotachograph with volume i.

integrin
i. blocker
i. signaling

integrin-dependent pathway
Integris
I. cardiac imaging system
I. cardiovascular imaging
I. 3D RA
I. H5000 digital x-ray imaging system

integrity
I. AFx AutoCapture pacing system
I. AFx DR model 5346 pacemaker
I. Micro AutoCapture pacing system
microvascular i.

intellectual dysfunction
Intellicath pulmonary artery catheter
intelligence quotient (IQ)
intelligent
i. cardiovascular monitor (ICM)
i. CPAP

Intellitemp EP energy management device
intensifier
image i.

intensity, pl. **intensities**
echo i.
intravascular signal i.
peak myocardial video i. (PMVI)
point of maximum i.
pulse average i. (Ipa)
reduced signal i.
spatial average i. (I_{sa})
spatial average, temporal average i. (I_{sata})
spatial peak i. (I_{sp})
spatial peak pulse average i. (I_{sppa})
spatial peak, temporal average i. (I_{sapt})
temporal average i. (I_{ta})
temporal peak i. (I_{tp})
waxing and waning in i.

intensive
i. coronary care (ICC)
i. coronary care unit (ICCU)

intensivist
intentionem
per primam i.
per secundum i.

intention to treat (ITT)
interaction
adhesin-receptor i.
blood-surface i.
leukocyte-endothelial cell i.
lung-liver i.

interalveolar
i. communication
i. septa

interarterial
i. communication
i. shunt

interarytenoid
i. edema
i. notch
i. pachyderma

interatrial
i. block
i. conduction time
i. foramen primum
i. pressure gradient (IAPG)
i. septal aneurysm (IASA)
i. septal defect (IASD)
i. septum (IAS)
i. shunting (IAS)

interauricular septal defect
intercadence
intercadent
intercalary
intercellular
i. adhesion molecule (ICAM)

intercellular *(continued)*
  i. adhesion molecule-1 (ICAM-1)
  i. coupling
intercept
  i. angle
interceptor
  I. emboli protection device
  I. Plus filter system
  I. wire distal protection device
intercidens
  pulsus i.
intercompartmental
  1,2 i. supraretinacular artery
intercostal
  i. catheter
  external i.
  internal i.
  i. mammary vessel
  i. nerve block
  i. retraction
  i. space (ICS)
intercostale
  spatium i.
intercurrens
  pulsus i.
interdependence
  ventricular i.
interdigitating dendritic cell
interectopic interval
interelectrode
  i. distance
  i. space
interest
  region of i. (ROI)
interface
  I. arterial blood filter
  electrode-skin i.
  lumen-intima i.
  lung-wall i.
  Monarch Mini Mask nasal i.
  sputum-epithelium i.
  Ultimate Seal gel i.
interfascicular fibrous tissue
interference
  i. beat
  dissociation by i.
  i. dissociation
  electromagnetic
    interference/radiofrequency i.
    (EMI/RFI)
interferon (IFN)
  i. alfa-2a
  i. alfa-2b
  i. alfa-2b and ribavirin combination
    pack
  i. alpha
  alpha-i.

  i. gamma
  i. gamma-1b
interferon-gamma (IFN-gamma)
InterGard heparin vascular graft
interior muscle
interlaced scanning
interlead
  i. QT dispersion
  i. QT variability
interleukin (IL)
  i.-1-11
  i. 4 receptor (IL-4R)
  i. receptor antagonist
interleukin-1-11
interleukin-2
  PEG interleukin-2
interleukin-6
  circulating interleukin-6
interleukin D (ILD)
interlobar
  i. effusion
  i. empyema
  i. pleurisy
  i. surface
  i. surface of lung
interlobular
  i. emphysema
  i. pleurisy
interlobularis
  pneumonia i.
intermediary vesicle
intermediate
  i. bronchus
  i. circumflex artery (ICXA)
  i. coronary syndrome
  i. endpoint biomarker (IEB)
  i. heart
  i. laryngeal cavity
  i. probability
intermediate-density
  i.-d. lipoprotein (IDL)
  i.-d. lipoprotein-cholesterol complex
    (IDL-C, IDL-c)
intermediate-stiffness steerable guidewire
Intermedics
  I. atrial antitachycardia pacemaker
  I. lead
  I. Marathon dual-chamber rate-
    responsive pacemaker
  I. Marathon VVI single-chamber
    pacemaker
  I. Res-Q implantable cardioverter-
    defibrillator
  I. Stride pacemaker
Intermed Inter 3 ventilator
intermedius
  bronchus i.
  ramus i.
intermesenteric arterial anastomosis

intermittence, intermittency
intermittens
    dyskinesia i.
    pulsus respiratione i.
intermittent
    i. aortic occlusion (IAO)
    i. claudication
    i. coronary sinus occlusion (ICSO)
    i. demand ventilation (IDV)
    i. heparinization (IH)
    i. mandatory ventilation (IMV)
    i. mechanical ventilation (IMV)
    i. percussive ventilation (IPV)
    i. pneumatic compression (IPC)
    i. positive airway pressure (IPAP)
    i. positive pressure (IPP)
    i. positive pressure breathing
      (IPPB)
    i. positive pressure ventilation
      (IPPV)
    i. pulse
    i. sinus arrest
interna
    lamina elastica i.
internal
    i. adhesive pericarditis
    i. borderzone infarct (IBI)
    i. branch
    i. branch of superior laryngeal
      nerve
    i. capsule
    i. capsule infarcts
    i. cardioversion
    i. carotid artery (ICA)
    i. cerebral vein (ICV)
    i. diameter
    i. elastic lamina (IEL)
    i. elastic membrane (IEM)
    i. elastic membrane rupture
    i. energy
    i. intercostal
    i. jugular (IJ)
    i. jugular vein
    i. mammary (IM)
    i. mammary artery (IMA)
    i. mammary artery bypass (IMAB)
    i. mammary artery catheter
    i. mammary artery graft
    i. mammary artery graft
      angiography
    i. mammary artery implant (IMAI)
    i. mammary vessel
    i. maxillary artery (IMAX)
    i. orifice diameter (IOD)
    i. pneumatic stabilization
    i. pudendal vein
    i. reed switch
    i. respiration
    i. thoracic artery (ITA)

    i. thoracic artery graft
    i. thoracic vein
    i. work rate
international
    Cardiovascular Credentialing I.
      (CCI)
    I. Classification of Diseases, Ninth
      Revision (ICD-9)
    I. Classification of Sleep Disorders
      (ICSD)
    I. Cooperative Pulmonary Embolism
      Registry (ICOPER)
    I. Early Lung Cancer Action
      Program (I-ELCAP)
    I. Labor Office (ILO)
    I. Labor Office Classification
    I. Liaison Committee on
      Resuscitation (ILCOR)
    i. normalized ratio (INR)
    I. Registry of Acute Aortic
      Dissection (IRAD)
    I. Society for Adult Congenital
      Cardiac Disease (ISACCD)
    I. Society of Cardiology (ISC)
    I. Society and Federation of
      Cardiology (ISFC)
    I. Society for Heart and Lung
      Transplantation (ISHLT)
    I. Society for Heart Transplantation
      (ISHT)
    I. Society of Hypertension (ISH)
    I. Society on Thrombosis and
      Haemostasis (ISTH)
    I. Staging System for Lung Cancer
      (ISSLC)
    I. Standards Organization (ISO)
internet
    i. ICD monitoring
    i. monitoring of ICD
internodal
    i. conduction
    i. pathway
    i. tract
    i. tract of Bachmann
internum
    pericardium i.
interobserver variability
interpleural space
interpolated
    i. beat
    i. extrasystole
    i. premature complex
interposed
    i. abdominal compression
    i. abdominal compression
      cardiopulmonary resuscitation (IAC
      CPR)
interposition of Dacron tube
interpulmonary septum

interpulse
    i. interval (IPI)
    i. potential (Ipp)
interquartile range
interrater sequence
interrogation
    i. device
    Doppler i.
    pacemaker i.
    stereoscopic i.
interrupted
    i. aortic arch (IAA)
    i. inferior vena cava
    i. pledgeted suture
    i. respiration
interruption
    aortic arch i.
intersegmental
    i. artery
    i. part
    i. part of pulmonary vein
intersegmentales
    partes i.
Intersept cardiotomy reservoir
Inter-Society Commission for Heart Diseases (ICHD)
interstitial
    i. distribution
    i. emphysema
    i. fluid
    i. granuloma
    i. infiltrate
    i. lung disease (ILD)
    i. marking
    i. nodule
    i. pattern
    i. and perivascular collagen network
    i. plasma cell pneumonia
    i. pneumonitis
    i. pulmonary edema
    i. pulmonary fibrosis (IPF)
    i. space
interstitium
    axial i.
    cardiac i.
    lung i.
    peripheral i.
intersystole
intersystolic period
Intertach II pacemaker
Intertech anesthesia breathing circuit
InterTherapy intravascular ultrasound
intertrabecular recess
interval
    A-A i.
    A_1-A_2 i.
    a-c i.
    AH i.

A_2 incisural i.
AN i.
A_2 to opening snap i.
atrial escape i.
atriocarotid i.
atrioventricular i.
auriculoventricular i.
automatic capacitor formation i.
A-V i.
A-V delay i.
Bazett corrected QT i.
BH i.
B-H i.
c-a i.
cardioarterial i.
conduction i.
confidence i. (CI)
coupling i.
critical coupling i.
defibrillation response i. (DRI)
electrode replacement i.
electromechanical i.
escape i.
fetal PR i.
f-f i.
filtered atrial rate i. (FARI)
flutter R i.
H-Ae i.
hangout i.
H_1-H_2 i.
His-ventricle i.
H'P i.
H-Q i.
H-QRS i.
HV i.
interectopic i.
interpulse i. (IPI)
isoelectric i.
isometric i.
isovolumic i.
JT i.
long PP i.
long QT i.
magnet pacing i.
NN i.
PA i.
pacemaker escape i.
passive i.
P-H i.
PJ i.
postsphygmic i.
P-P i.
PQ i.
PR i.
presphygmic i.
prolongation of PR i.
Q-H i.
Q-M i.
QR i.

QRB i.
QRS i.
QRS-T i.
QS$_2$ i.
QT i.
QTc i.
QU i.
right ventricular systolic time i.
R-P i.
R-R i.
R-R' i.
RS-T i.
short coupling i.
shortening of PR i.
sphygmic i.
S-QRS i.
S$_1$-S$_2$ i.
ST i.
stimulus-T i.
symptom-free i.
systolic time i. (STI)
TP i.
VA i.
V-H i.

interval-dependent potentiation
interval-strength relation
intervalvular fibrosa
Inter 3 ventilator
intervention
　　cardioreparative drug agent i.
　　coronary sinus i. (CSI)
　　direct percutaneous coronary i. (d-
　　　PCI)
　　elective percutaneous coronary i.
　　fetal i.
　　Kiemeneij percutaneous coronary i.
　　myocardial infarction triage and i.
　　　(MITI)
　　percutaneous coronary i. (PCI)
　　Society for Cardiac Angiography
　　　and I.'s (SCAI)
　　staged percutaneous coronary i.
　　vagomimetic i.
interventional
　　i. cardiac catheterization
　　i. cardiac center (ICC)
　　i. cardiologist
　　i. cardiology
　　i. dilation
　　i. echocardiography
　　i. procedure
　　i. radiology
　　i. reference point
　　i. therapy
intervention-induced myonecrosis
interventricular (IV)
　　i. foramen (IVF)
　　i. septal defect (ISD, IVSD)
　　i. septal motion

i. septal rupture
i. septal thickness (IVS)
i. septum (IVS)
i. septum aneurysm
i. sulcus
i. vein
intervertebral disc
interview
　　Alexithymia Provoked Response I.
　　structured I.
intestinal
　　i. anthrax
　　i. emphysema
　　i. ischemia
　　i. lipodystrophy
intima
　　aortic tunica i.
intimal
　　i. atheroma
　　i. defect
　　i. erosion
　　i. fibrous proliferation (IFP)
　　i. flap
　　i. hyperplasia (IH)
　　i. proliferation
　　i. tear
　　i. thickening
intimal-medial
　　i.-m. thickening
　　i.-m. thickness (IMT)
intolerance
　　carbohydrate i.
　　exercise i.
　　glucose i.
intoxication
　　alcohol i.
　　digitalis i.
　　digoxin i.
intraabdominal adiposity (IAA)
intraacinar vessel
intraalveolar
　　i. deposit
　　i. fibrosis
　　i. pressure
intraaortic (IA)
　　i. balloon (IAB)
　　i. balloon assistance (IABA)
　　i. balloon catheter
　　i. balloon counterpulsation (IABC,
　　　IABCP)
　　i. balloon device
　　i. balloon pulsation (IABP)
　　i. balloon pump (IABP, IBP)
　　i. balloon pumping (IABP)
　　i. counterpulsation (IACP)
intraarterial (IA)
　　i. catheter
　　i. chemotherapy
　　i. conduction defect

intraarterial (*continued*)
  i. counterpulsation
  i. digital subtraction angiography (IADSA, IA-DSA)
  i. gene transfer
  i. line
  i. thrombosis
  i. vasopressin (IAV)
intraatrial (IA)
  i. activation sequence
  i. baffle
  i. block
  i. conduction
  i. conduction time
  i. reentrant tachycardia
  i. reentry
  i. reentry tachycardia (IART)
  i. shunting
intraauricular (IA)
intrabronchial
intracardiac (IC)
  i. accelerometer
  i. amobarbital sodium procedure
  i. atrial activation sequence
  i. catheter
  i. catheter recording (ICR)
  i. ECG
  i. echocardiography (ICE)
  i. electrogram
  i. electrophysiology
  i. event
  i. gas gangrene
  i. infection (ICI)
  i. lead
  i. mapping
  i. mass
  i. navigation
  i. pacing
  i. pressure
  i. pressure curve
  i. shunt
  i. stimulation
  i. sucker
  i. thrombus (ICT)
  i. tumor
intracaval
  i. device
  i. endovascular ultrasonography (ICEUS)
intracavitary
  i. air meniscus
  i. echodensity
  i. electrocardiography
  i. hemorrhage
  i. instillation
  i. mass
  i. pressure-electrogram dissociation
  i. pressure gradient

intracellular
  i. calcium concentration
  i. caveolae
  i. lipid
  i. magnesium
  i. organism (ICO)
  i. pressure
  i. protein
  i. trafficking
  i. tyrosine protein kinase
intracellulare
  Mycobacterium i.
intracellular-like, calcium-bearing crystalloid solution (ICS)
intracerebral hemorrhage (ICH)
IntraCoil
  I. self-expanding nitinol stent
  I. self-expanding peripheral stent
intracoronary
  i. acetylcholine infusion
  i. angioscopy
  i. aqueous oxygen
  i. artery radiation
  i. aspiration thrombectomy (ICAT)
  i. beta-radiation
  i. brachytherapy
  i. Doppler flow wire
  i. phentolamine
  i. pressure
  i. radiation therapy (ICRT, IRT)
  i. sonicated meglumine
  i. stent implantation (ICSI)
  i. stenting
  i. stenting of de novo narrowing
  i. stent placement
  i. streptokinase (ICSK)
  i. thrombolysis balloon valvoplasty
  i. ultrasonography
  i. ultrasound (ICUS)
  i. vascular ultrasound (IVUS)
intracorporeal
  i. heart
  i. ventricular assist device
intracranial
  i. atherosclerotic disease (IAD)
  i. fusiform aneurysm
  i. hemorrhage (ICH)
  i. hypertension (ICH)
  i. microembolic signal
  i. pressure (ICP)
intractable
  i. aspiration
  i. hiccups
  i. hypotension
intragraft thrombus
intrahisian block
intralesion restenosis
Intralipid
intralobar

intralobular line
intraluminal
    i. dissection
    i. fibromyxoid lesion
    i. flap
    i. plaque
    i. thrombus
    i. ultrasound (ILUS)
intramucosal pH
intramural
    i. coronary artery
    i. hematoma (IH, IMH)
    i. hemorrhage (IMH)
    i. thrombosis
    i. thrombus
intramuscular (IM)
intramyocardial
    i. conduction delay
    i. function
    i. hematoma
    i. pressure
    i. sinusoid
intraobserver variability
intraoperative
    i. cell salvage
    i. digital subtraction (IDIS)
    i. digital subtraction angiography (IDISA)
    i. echocardiography (IOE)
    i. hemodynamics
    i. hypoxemia
    i. intraarterial fibrinolytic therapy (IIFT)
    i. mapping
    i. transesophageal echocardiography (IOTEE)
    i. vascular angiography (IVA)
intraosseous (IO)
intraparenchymal
    i. hematoma
    i. hemorrhage
intraparietal sulcus (IPS)
intrapericardial
    i. echo
    i. hemorrhage
    i. pressure (IPP)
    i. sign
intraperitoneal rupture
intraplaque LDL oxidation
intrapleural
    i. catheter
    i. catheter analgesia
    i. loculation
    i. oncotic pressure
    i. rupture
    i. sealed drainage unit
    i. space
intraprocedural stent thrombosis (IPST)

intrapulmonary
    i. percussive ventilation (IPV)
    i. rheumatoid nodule
    i. shunt
    i. shunt fraction (Q_s/Q_t)
    i. shunting
    i. vascular dilation
    i. vein (IPV)
intrapulmonic
intrarectal
intrastent
    i. minimal lumen cross-sectional area (ISMLCSA)
    i. recurrent disease
    i. restenosis (IR)
IntraStent DoubleStrut stent
intrathecal papaverine
intrathoracic
    i. gas
    i. gas compression
    i. hypertension
    i. injury
    i. pressure
    i. PTLPD
    i. thyroid
intratrabecular recess
intratracheal tube
intrauterine
    i. pneumonia
    i. respiration
intravariability
intravasation
    venous i.
intravascular (IV)
    i. aggregate
    i. blood coagulation (IVBC)
    i. brachytherapy
    i. brachytherapy system
    i. bronchoalveolar tumor
    i. catheter electrode
    i. coagulation (IVC)
    i. consumption coagulopathy (IVCC)
    i. Doppler
    i. Doppler-tipped guidewire
    i. elastogram
    i. fetal air sign
    i. fluid (IVF)
    i. foreign body retrieval
    i. gene transfer
    i. mass (IVM)
    i. MRI
    i. oxygenator (IVOX)
    i. papillary endothelial hyperplasia (IPEH)
    i. perfluorochemical emulsion
    i. pressure (IVP)
    i. pressure measurement
    i. procoagulant factor

intravascular *(continued)*
  i. red light therapy (IRLT)
  i. signal intensity
  i. sonotherapy (IST)
  i. stent
  i. thrombus
  i. ultrasound (IVUS)
  i. ultrasound catheter
  i. volume
intravenous (IV)
  i. accurate control (IVAC)
  i. analgesia
  CellCept I.
  i. cholangiogram (IVC)
  i. cholangiography (IVC, IVCh)
  i. digital subtraction angiography
    (IVDSA)
  i. fluid (IVF)
  Fungizone I.
  i. gamma globulin (IVGG)
  i. glucose tolerance test (IVGTT)
  i. hyperalimentation (IVH)
  i. immune globulin
  i. immunoglobulin therapy
  i. inotropic support
  mycophenolate mofetil i.
  i. myocardial contrast
    echocardiography (IMCE)
  i. polyspecific immunoglobulin G
    (IVIG)
  Saventrine I.
  i. vasopressin (IVV)
**intravenously enhanced computed
  tomography (IVCT)**
intraventricular (IV, IVT)
  i. aberration
  i. block (IVB)
  i. catheter (IVC)
  i. conduction
  i. conduction defect (IVCD)
  i. conduction delay
  i. conduction disease (IVCD)
  i. conduction pattern
  i. hemorrhage (IVH)
  i. pressure gradient (IVPG)
intravital capillary video microscopy
intravoxel phase dispersion
intrepid
  I. balloon catheter
  I. PTCA catheter
intrinsic
  i. airway narrowing
  i. asthma
  i. deflection
  i. depolarization
  i. heart rate (IHR)
  i. positive end-expiratory pressure
    (PEEPi)
  i. pulmonary vascular disease

  i. sympathomimetic activity
  i. tenase complex
intrinsicoid deflection
intrinsic PEEP *(var. of* autoPEEP)
introduced
  percutaneously i.
introducer
  Angestat hemostasis i.
  Angetear tearaway i.
  aortic assist balloon i.
  Avanti i.
  Check-Flo i.
  Ciaglia percutaneous
    tracheostomy i.
  Cook Shuttle Flexor i.
  Desilets-Hoffman catheter i.
  Fast-Cath Duo i.
  Flexor i.
  gum elastic bougie i.
  Hemaquet i.
  I. II sheath
  LPS Peel-Away i.
  Maximum hemostasis i.
  Micropuncture Peel-Away i.
  Mullins catheter i.
  Nottingham i.
  PD Access with Peel-Away
    needle i.
  i. sheath
  i. sheath removal
  split-sheath i.
  Tuohy-Borst i.
  Ultimum hemostasis i.
  UMI transseptal Cath-Seal
    catheter i.
  USCI i.
introducer/endoscope
  Czaja-McCaffrey rigid stent i./e.
intron
  i. 16
  i. A
intubate
  do not d. (DNI)
intubated patient
**intubating laryngeal airway mask
  (ILMA)**
intubation
  catheter-guided endoscopic i.
    (CAGEIN)
  endotracheal i.
  i. guide
  lighted stylet i.
  mainstem i.
  nasotracheal i.
  O'Dwyer i.
  orotracheal i.
  rapid-sequence i.
  retrograde translaryngeal i.
  RSI orotracheal i.

i. time
tracheal i.
intubator
intussusception
Invacare
I. nasal prongs
I. Venture HomeFill complete
home oxygen system
Invanz
invasion
blood vessel i. (BVI)
invasive
i. assessment
i. candidiasis
i. filamentous fungus
i. management
i. mechanical ventilation
i. monitoring
i. positive pressure mechanical
ventilation
i. pressure measurement
i. pulmonary aspergillosis (IPA)
in-vein ablation
inventory
Beck Depression i.
Cloninger Temperament and
Character i.
Edinburgh Handedness i. (EHI)
State-Trait Anxiety i. (STAI)
inversa
angina i.
inverse-ratio ventilation (IRV)
Inversine
inversion
right atrial i. (RAI)
shallow T wave i.
i. spin-echo pulse sequence (ISE)
T-wave i.
U-wave i.
ventricular i.
inversus
atrial situs i.
dextrocardia with situs i.
levocardia with situs i.
situs i.
visceroatrial situs i.
inverted
i. buttoned device
i. crush technique
i. T wave
i. V, Y technique
investigation
coronary artery bypass
revascularization i. (CABRI)
investigational
i. new drug (IND)
i. new drug status
investigator
atrial fibrillation i.

Invirase
INVM
isolated noncompaction of ventricular
myocardium
involvement
right atrial i. (RAI)
systemic ischemic branch vessel i.
(SIBVI)
inward-going rectification
INX stent
IO
intraosseous
IO infusion
Iobid DM
IOD
internal orifice diameter
iodide
metocurine i.
potassium i.
saturated solution of potassium i.
(SSKI)
iodine
lithium i. (LiI)
radiolabeled i.
iodine-123 (^{123}I, I-123)
i.-123 heptadecanoic acid
radioactive tracer
i.-123 metaiodobenzylguanidine
i.-123 metaiodobenzylguanidine
uptake
iodine-125 (^{125}I, I-125)
i.-125 isotope
iodine-127
iodine-131 (^{131}I, I-131)
i.-131 MIBG scintigraphy
iodine-132
iodophenyl pentadecanoic acid
iodopovidone
iodoquinol
IOE
intraoperative echocardiography
IOH
idiopathic orthostatic hypotension
Iohexol contrast
Iomeron
ion
calcium i.
i. channel
chloride i.
potassium i.
i. pump
sodium i.
Ionescu
I. method
I. trileaflet valve
Ionescu-Shiley
I.-S. pericardial patch
I.-S. pericardial valve
I.-S. pericardial xenograft

Ionescu-Shiley *(continued)*
I.-S. valve prosthesis
I.-S. vascular graft
ionic mechanism
ionizing radiation (IR)
ionophore
calcium i. A23187
ion-selective electrode (ISE)
iopamidol
Iopamiro
iopromide injection
I-orthoiodohippurate
IOTEE
intraoperative transesophageal
echocardiography
iothalamate meglumine contrast medium
ioversol
ioxaglate
i. meglumine
i. meglumine contrast medium
i. sodium
sodium meglumine i.
ioxilan
IPA
invasive pulmonary aspergillosis
Ipa
pulse average intensity
IPAH
idiopathic pulmonary arterial
hypertension
IPAP
inspiratory positive airway pressure
intermittent positive airway pressure
IPC
intermittent pneumatic compression
ischemic preconditioning
IPC boots
IPEH
intravascular papillary endothelial
hyperplasia
IPF
idiopathic pulmonary fibrosis
interstitial pulmonary fibrosis
IPFM
integral pulse frequency modulation
IPFM/SDC
integral pulse frequency
modulation/Smith delay compensatory
IPG
impedance plethysmography
IPH
idiopathic portal hypertension
idiopathic pulmonary hemosiderosis
idiopathic pulmonary hypertension
IPI
interpulse interval
IPLVAS
implantable left ventricular assist system

IPO
4-ipomeanol
4-ipomeanol (IPO)
IPP
intermittent positive pressure
intrapericardial pressure
Ipp
interpulse potential
IPPB
intermittent positive pressure breathing
IPPV
intermittent positive pressure ventilation
ipratropium
i. and albuterol
i. bromide
i. inhaler
IPS
idiopathic pneumonia syndrome
infundibular pulmonary stenosis
intraparietal sulcus
ipsilateral
i. hilar lymphadenopathy
i. stroke
IPST
intraprocedural stent thrombosis
IPSTL
inferior parietal/superior temporal lobe
IPT
inflammatory pseudotumor
IPV
intermittent percussive ventilation
intrapulmonary percussive ventilation
intrapulmonary vein
IQ
intelligence quotient
IQ nasal mask
iQ200 analysis system
IQmark Digital Spirometer
IR
intrastent restenosis
ionizing radiation
I/R
ischemia/reperfusion
IRA
infarct-related artery
IRAD
International Registry of Acute Aortic
Dissection
irANP
immunoreactive atrial natriuretic peptide
irAVP
immunoreactive arginine vasopressin
IRBBB
incomplete right bundle branch block
irbesartan and hydrochlorothiazide
IRC
inspiratory reserve capacity
IRD
immune restoration disease

IRDS
infant respiratory distress syndrome
I-receptor
imidazoline receptor
Ireland
Cardiac Society of Great Britain and I. (CSGBI)
Iressa
Irex Exemplar ultrasound
iridium-192 seed
iridium strand
iridodonesis
irinotecan
irinotecan
IRIS
immune reconstitution inflammatory reaction
iris
I. coronary stent
I. II stent
IRLT
intravascular red light therapy
IRMA
immunoradiometric assay
IRMA blood gas analysis system
IRMA SL blood glucose strip tester
iron (Fe)
i. chelator
colloidal i. (CI)
i. dextran complex
i. lung
serum i.
i. storage disease
Ironman guidewire
IR-PEP
inspiratory resistance and positive expiratory pressure
irradiation
curative i.
endovascular i. (EI)
prophylactic cranial i. (PCI)
thoracic i.
total axial node i. (TANI)
total body i. (TBI)
total lymphoid i. (TLI)
irregular
i. discrete lesion
i. emphysema
i. hematoma
i. rhythm
irregularis
pulsus i.
irregularly
i. irregular cardiac rhythm
i. irregular pulse
irrespirable

irreversible
i. airway obstruction
i. shock
Irri-Cath suction system
irrigated
i. catheter ablation
i. coiled catheter
irrigated-tip
i.-t. ablation
i.-t. quadripolar ablation catheter
irrigation ablation catheter
irritable
i. heart
i. larynx syndrome
irritant
environmental i.
nonspecific i.
i. receptor
respiratory i.
i. rhinitis
i. sinusitis
irritant-associated vocal cord dysfunction
irritant-induced asthma
irritation
direct diaphragmatic i.
IRT
intracoronary radiation therapy
IRV
inspiratory reserve volume
inverse-ratio ventilation
Isaacs-Ludwig arteriole
ISACCD
International Society for Adult Congenital Cardiac Disease
Isambert disease
ISC
International Society of Cardiology
ischemia
acute cardiac i. (ACI)
acute limb i.
asymptomatic cardiac i. (ACI)
brachiocephalic i.
cardiac i.
cerebral i.
clandestine myocardial i.
colonic i.
critical limb i.
delayed cerebral i. (DCI)
dobutamine-induced i.
end-organ i.
exercise-induced silent myocardial i.
extremity i.
global cerebral i. (GCI)
inducible i.
intestinal i.
left ventricular i. (LVI)
left ventricular subendocardial myocardial i. (LVSEMI)

ischemia *(continued)*
>limb i.
>limb-threatening i.
>low-flow i.
>manifest i.
>mental stress-induced i.
>mesenteric i.
>mucosal i.
>myocardial i. (MI)
>nonocclusive mesenteric i.
>periinfarction i.
>procedural-related myocardial i.
>provocable myocardial i.
>psychophysiological interventions in myocardial i. (PIMI)
>recurrent mesenteric i.
>regional i.
>silent myocardial i.
>subendocardial i.
>transient focal cerebral i. (TFCI)
>transient mesenteric i.
>transmural myocardial i.
>vertebrobasilar territory i. (VBI)

ischemia-driven revascularization
ischemia-guided medical therapy
ischemia-induced
>i.-i. intracellular acidosis
>i.-i. intramyocardial conduction delay

ischemia/reperfusion (I/R)
ischemia/reperfusion-induced apoptosis
ischemic
>i. burden
>i. cardiomyopathy
>i. cascade
>i. cerebral infarction
>i. contracture
>i. contracture of left ventricle
>i. core
>i. coronary disease (ICD)
>i. dysfunction
>i. ECG change
>i. event
>i. heart disease (IHD)
>i. heart disease index (IHDI)
>i. heart disease life stress monitoring program
>i. heart disease quality enhancement research initiative (IHD QUERI)
>i. hypoxia
>i. leukoaraiosis
>i. mitral regurgitation
>i. myocardium
>i. necrosis
>i. paralysis
>i. penumbra
>i. pericarditis
>i. preconditioning (IPC)

>i. rest angina
>i. steel syndrome
>i. stroke
>i. sudden death
>i. threshold
>i. tolerance
>i. zone

ischemic/reperfusion injury
ischemic-type preconditioning stimulus
ischiadic nerve
ISD
>interventricular septal defect

ISDN
>isosorbide dinitrate

ISE
>inversion spin-echo pulse sequence
>ion-selective electrode

iseganan HCl oral solution
isethionate
>aerosolized pentamidine i.
>pentamidine i.
>piritrexim i.

ISFC
>International Society and Federation of Cardiology

ISH
>International Society of Hypertension
>isolated septal hypertrophy

ISHLT
>International Society for Heart and Lung Transplantation

ISHT
>International Society for Heart Transplantation

ISI
>infarct size index

ISMLCSA
>intrastent minimal lumen cross-sectional area

IS-5-MN
>isosorbide-5-mononitrate

Ismo
ISO
>International Standards Organization

isoactin switch
isobutyl 2-cyanoacrylate
isocapnia
isocapnic
>i. condition
>i. hyperpnea
>i. hyperventilation

isocenter system
isochoric
isocratic elution
isocyanate
>methyl i.
>methylene diphenyl i.

isocyanate-induced asthma
isodiphasic complex

isoechoic
isoelectric
    i. interval
    i. line
    i. period
    i. point
    i. ST segment
isoenzyme
    CPK i.
    i. of lactate dehydrogenase found in the heart, erythrocytes, kidneys (LD1)
    myocardial muscle creatine kinase i.
isoetharine
    Dey-Lute I.
    i. HCl
    I. Inhalation Solution USP 1%
isoflavone
    soy i.
isoflurane
isoform
    Apo E3 i.
    CYP1A2 i.
    CYP3A i.
    CYP3A4 i.
    CYP2C9 i.
    CYP2C19 i.
    CYP2D6 i.
    cytochrome P450-3A4 i.
    titin i.
isoglycemia
isointense heterogeneous signal
isolated
    i. cardiovascular malformation (ICM)
    i. cerebral thromboangiitis obliterans disease
    i. chest trauma
    i. conduction defect (ICD)
    i. CTAO
    i. dextrocardia
    i. dysarthria
    i. ectopic beat
    i. heat perfusion
    i. left ventricular noncompaction (IVNC)
    i. low HDL
    i. low high-density lipoprotein (ILHDL)
    i. noncompaction of ventricular myocardium (INVM)
    i. parietal endocarditis
    i. septal hypertrophy (ISH)
    i. systolic hypertension
    i. T wave
    i. volume responder (IVR)
isolation
    electrical i.

    ostial i.
    percutaneous i.
    segmental pulmonary vein i.
isoleucyl-tRNA synthetase
isomer
    dextro i.
isomerism
    atrial i.
isometric
    i. contraction
    i. contraction period
    i. exercise
    i. handgrip
    i. handgrip test
    i. interval
    i. period of cardiac cycle
    i. relaxation period
    i. sports
    i. systolic tension (IST)
isometrically contracting myocardial preparation
isomyosin switch
isoniazid (INH)
    rifampin and i.
isonitrile
    carbomethoxyisopropyl i.
    2-methoxyisobutyl i. (MIBI)
    technetium-99m hexakis 2-methoxyisobutyl i.
    technetium-99m 2-methoxyisobutyl i.
Isopaque
isopentenyl pyrophosphate
isoprenaline
    i. hydrochloride
    i. sulfate
isoprenoid level
isoprenylated protein
isoprophenamine hydrochloride
isopropylarterenol hydrochloride
isoprostane
isoproterenol
    i. hydrochloride
    i. infusion
    i. and phenylephrine
    i. stress test
    i. sulfate
    i. sulfate inhalation
    i. tilt-table test
isoproterenol-induced vasovagal syncope
isoproteronol HCl
Isoptin SR
Isopto Atropine
Isordil
isorhythmic dissociation
isosorbide
    i. dinitrate (ISDN)
    i. dinitrate/hydralazine hydrochloride

isosorbide *(continued)*
  i. dinitrate injection
  i. mononitrate
isosorbide-5-mononitrate (IS-5-MN)
Isospora belli
isothiocyanate
  fluorescein i. (FITC)
isotime
  i. analysis
  dyspnea at i.
isotonic
  i. contraction
  i. exercise
  i. fluid
isotope
  iodine-125 i.
isotypic
isovelocity surface
Isovex
isovolemic hemodilution
isovolume
  i. flow
  i. pressure flow curve (IVPF)
  i. shifting
isovolumetric
  i. contractility
  i. phase index
  i. relaxation
  i. relaxation period (IVRP)
  i. relaxation time (IVRT)
  i. time (IVT)
isovolumic
  i. acceleration (IVA)
  i. contraction
  i. index
  i. interval
  i. phase
  i. pressure decay
  i. relaxation
  i. relaxation period
  i. relaxation time (IVRT)
  i. systole
Isovue contrast medium
isoxsuprine hydrochloride
ISR
  in-stent restenosis
isradipine
israelii
  Actinomyces i.
ISS
  immunostimulatory sequence
  Injury Severity Score
  ISS therapy
ISSLC
  International Staging System for Lung
  Cancer
IST
  inappropriate sinus tachycardia

  intravascular sonotherapy
  isometric systolic tension
i-STAT handheld analyzer
ISTH
  International Society on Thrombosis and
  Haemostasis
isthmectomy
isthmic hypoplasia
isthmus, pl. **isthmi**
  aortic i.
  cavotricuspid i. (CTI)
  Krönig i.
  i. line
  mitral i.
  noncavotricuspid i.
  posterior i.
  reentry circuit i.
  septal i.
  shared i.
  subeustachian i.
  thyroid i.
  tricuspid-inferior vena cava i.
isthmus-dependent atrial flutter
Isuprel Mistometer
ISWT
  incremental shuttle walking test
IT
  implantation test
ITA
  inferior temporal artery
  internal thoracic artery
  ITA graft
ITC balloon catheter
ITD
  impedance threshold device
iterative presyncope
ITL
  inspiratory threshold load
ITP
  idiopathic thrombocytopenic purpura
ITPA index
itraconazole
ITT
  intention to treat
ITV
  impedance threshold valve
IV
  interventricular
  intravascular
  intravenous
  intraventricular
  Avelox IV
  Gammar-P IV
  Hyperstat IV
  Merrem IV
  Vasotec IV
IVA
  intraoperative vascular angiography
  isovolumic acceleration

IVAC
  intravenous accurate control
    IVAC device
    IVAC pump
IVAD
  implantable ventricular assist device
    Thoratec IVAD
Ivalon
  I. plug
  I. sponge
IVB
  intraventricular block
IVBC
  intravascular blood coagulation
IVC
  inferior vena cava
  inspiratory vital capacity
  intravascular coagulation
  intravenous cholangiogram
  intravenous cholangiography
  intraventricular catheter
    IVC thrombosis
IVCC
  intravascular consumption coagulopathy
IVCD
  intraventricular conduction defect
  intraventricular conduction disease
IVCh
  intravenous cholangiography
IVCP
  inferior vena cava pressure
IVCR
  inferior vena cava reconstruction
IVCT
  inferior vena cava thrombosis
  intravenously enhanced computed
    tomography
IVCV
  inferior venacavography
IVDSA
  intravenous digital subtraction
    angiography
Ivemark syndrome
ivermectin
IVF
  interventricular foramen
  intravascular fluid
  intravenous fluid
IVGG
  intravenous gamma globulin
IVGTT
  intravenous glucose tolerance test
IVH
  intravenous hyperalimentation
  intraventricular hemorrhage

IV-Heart nebulizer
IVIG
  intravenous polyspecific immunoglobulin
    G
IVM
  intravascular mass
IVNC
  isolated left ventricular noncompaction
IVOX
  intravascular oxygenator
IVP
  intravascular pressure
IVPF
  isovolume pressure flow curve
IVPG
  intraventricular pressure gradient
IVR
  idioventricular rhythm
  isolated volume responder
IVRP
  isovolumetric relaxation period
IVRT
  isovolumetric relaxation time
  isovolumic relaxation time
IVS
  interventricular septal thickness
  interventricular septum
IVSD
  interventricular septal defect
IVT
  idiopathic ventricular tachycardia
  intraventricular
  isovolumetric time
IVUS
  intracoronary vascular ultrasound
  intravascular ultrasound
    IVUS catheter
    coronary IVUS
    3D IVUS
IVUS-guided balloon angioplasty
IVV
  intravenous vasopressin
Ivy bleeding time
IW
  inner wall
IWI
  inferior wall infarction
IWMI
  inferior wall myocardial infarction
Ixolaris

J

joule
J curve
J exchange wire
J guidewire
J & J stent
J junction
J point
J point electrical axis
J retention wire
J retention wire fracture
J wave

J5 lipopolysaccharidase

JA

juxtaarticular
JA lesion

Jaa Amp
Jaa-Prednisone
Jabaley-Stille Super Cut Scissors
Jaccoud

J. dissociated fever
J. sign

jacket

cardiac cooling j.
heart j.
Medtronic cardiac cooling j.

Jackman

J. coronary sinus electrode catheter
J. orthogonal catheter

Jackson

J. bistoury
J. safety triangle
J. sign
J. syndrome

Jackson-Huber classification
Jacobaeus procedure
Jacobson

J. microbulldog clamp
J. modified vessel clamp

Jacobson-Potts clamp
Jacquet apparatus
Jaeger body test
Jaffe method
jail

stent j.

jailed

j. side branch
j. side branch lesion

Jak

Janus kinase

Jako laryngoscope
Jak/STAT pathway
Jamar

J. hand dynamometer
J. model 0030J4 dynamometer

James

J. accessory tracts
J. bundle
J. exercise protocol
J. fiber

Jamshidi needle
Janeway

J. lesion
J. sphygmomanometer

Janus

J. kinase (Jak)
J. kinase/signal transducer and
activator of transcription
J. syndrome

Janz formula
japonicum

Schistosoma j.

Jarvik

J. 7-70 artificial heart
J. 2000 artificial heart

Jarvik-7 artificial heart
Jatene

J. arterial switch procedure
J. operation
J. technique

Javid

J. carotid artery bypass clamp
J. shunt

jaw reflex (JR)
jaw-thrust/head-tilt maneuver
Jawz disposable biopsy forceps
Jebsen Hand Function Test
jeikeium

Corynebacterium j.

jejunal artery
jejunostomy

percutaneous endoscopic j.

jelly

cardiac j.
electrode j.

Jenkins Activity Survey
Jenner emphysema
jeopardized myocardium
jeopardy

myocardial j.
j. score

JER

junctional escape rhythm

jerk

myoclonic j.

jerky

j. pulse
j. respiration

Jervell and Lange-Nielsen syndrome
Jesberg esophagoscope

J

JET
junctional ectopic tachycardia
jet
anteriorly directed j.
aortic stenosis j.
Doppler color j.
eccentric stenotic j.
j. effect
j. humidifier
j. lesion
mitral regurgitant j.
mosaic j.
j. nebulizer
patent ductus arteriosus flow j.
regurgitant j.
residual j.
saline j.
signal-void j.
stenotic j.
tricuspid regurgitant j.
turbulent j.
j. velocity
j. ventilation
Jeune syndrome
jewel
J. AF implantable arrhythmia management device
J. AF implantable cardioverter-defibrillator
J. AF implantable defibrillator
J. atrial fibrillation dual chamber device
J. pacer-cardioverter-defibrillator
J. PCD
JF
jugular foramen
Jinotti closed suctioning system
jiroveci
Pneumocystis j.
JL4
Judkins left 4
JL4 catheter
JL5
Judkins left 5
JL5 catheter
J-loop technique
JNK
c-Jun N-terminal kinase
Jobst
J. extremity pump
J. pressure garment
J. Vairox gradient compression vascular stockings
Job syndrome
Jocath Maestro coronary balloon catheter
Jography angiographic catheter
Joguide coronary guiding catheter

Johnson
J. & Johnson coronary stent
J. & Johnson Hemopump
J. & Johnson Interventional Systems
J. & Johnson Interventional Systems stent
joint
j. deformity
J. National Committee on Prevention, Detection, Evaluation, and Treatment of High Blood Pressure
tuberculosis of bones and j.'s
Joklik medium
Jomed Jostent coronary stent graft
Jonas
J. modification
J. modification of Norwood procedure
Jones criteria
Jonnson maneuver
jordanis
Legionella j.
Jorgenson thoracic scissors
josamycin
Josephson
J. quadripolar catheter
J. Tip Arrow QuadPolar electrode catheter
Jostent
J. coronary stent
J. coronary stent graft
J. GraftMaster
Jostra
J. arterial blood filter
J. cardiotomy reservoir
J. catheter
joule (J)
Joule-Thompson effect
JPB
junctional premature beat
JPC
junctional premature contraction
JR
jaw reflex
junctional rhythm
JR4
Judkins right 4
JR4 catheter
JR5
Judkins right 5
JR5 catheter
JRT
junctional recovery time
JS
junctional slowing

J-shaped
>   J-s. pacemaker electrode
>   J-s. tube

JT
>   junctional tachycardia
>   JT interval

J-tip guidewire

JTV519 1,4-benzothiazepine derivative

Judkins
>   J. coronary catheter
>   J. curve LAD catheter
>   J. curve LCX catheter
>   J. curve STD catheter
>   J. 4 diagnostic catheter
>   J. guiding catheter
>   J. left 4 (JL4)
>   J. left 5 (JL5)
>   J. pigtail left ventriculography
>   catheter
>   J. right 4 (JR4)
>   J. right 5 (JR5)
>   J. selective coronary arteriography
>   J. technique
>   J. torque control catheter

Judkins-Sones technique

jugular
>   j. bulb catheter placement
>   assessment
>   j. embryocardia
>   external j. (EJ)
>   j. foramen (JF)
>   internal j. (IJ)
>   j. vein (JV)
>   j. vein pulse (JVP)
>   j. venous arch
>   j. venous catechol spillover
>   j. venous catheter (JVC)
>   j. venous distention (JVD)
>   j. venous pressure (JVP)
>   j. venous pulsation (JVP)
>   j. venous pulse
>   j. venous pulse tracing (JVPT)

jugulodigastric lymph node

juice
>   Minute Maid Premium Heart Wise
>   orange j.
>   purple grape j.

Julian thoracic forceps

Jumonji gene

jump graft

jumping thrombosis

junction
>   adherens j.
>   aorto-ostial j.
>   atrioventricular j. (AVJ)
>   A-V j.
>   cardioesophageal j.
>   costochondral j.
>   esophagogastric j.

>   gap j.
>   J j.
>   left atrium-pulmonary vein j.
>   loose j.
>   QRS-ST j.
>   saphenofemoral j.
>   sinotubular j.
>   ST j.
>   sternochondral j.
>   tight j.
>   tracheoesophageal j.
>   triadic j.
>   venoatrial j.
>   xiphosternal j.

junctional
>   atrioventricular j.
>   j. axis
>   j. bigeminy
>   j. bradycardia
>   j. complex
>   j. depression
>   j. ectopic tachycardia (JET)
>   j. escape
>   j. escape beat
>   j. escape rhythm (JER)
>   j. extrasystole
>   j. parasystole
>   j. premature beat (JPB)
>   j. premature contraction (JPC)
>   j. reciprocating tachycardia
>   j. recovery time (JRT)
>   j. rhythm (JR)
>   j. slowing (JS)
>   j. tachycardia (JT)

***Jun* gene**

Junod procedure

Juquitiba virus

Jurkat T cell

jute worker's lung

juvenile
>   j. arrhythmia
>   j. myocardial infarction
>   j. pattern
>   j. rheumatoid arthritis

juvenum
>   cor j.

juxtaarticular (JA)
>   j. lesion

juxtacapillary receptor

juxtacardiac pleural pressure

juxtaductal coarctation

juxtaesophageal lymph node

juxtaluminal
>   j. hemorrhage
>   j. thrombus

juxtapulmonary-capillary receptor

Juzo
>   J. hose

Juzo *(continued)*
  J. shrinker
  J. stockings
JV
  jugular vein
JVC
  jugular venous catheter
JVD
  jugular venous distention

JVP
  jugular vein pulse
  jugular venous pressure
  jugular venous pulsation
JVPT
  jugular venous pulse tracing
J-wire lead

K
 potassium
  K current
  K 54 lead
  K stylet
  K x-ray fluorescence instrument
K4
 fourth Korotkoff sound
K5
 fifth Korotkoff sound
KAAT II Plus intraaortic balloon pump
KabiVitrum
Kahler bronchial biopsy forceps
Kairos pacemaker
Kales scoring method
kaliuresis
kallidinogenase inactivator unit
kallikrein
  k. 1 (KLK1)
  k. gene
  k. inactivating unit (KIU)
kallikrein-bradykinin system
kallikrein-kinin (KK)
Kallmann syndrome
Kaltostat
  K. wound packing dressing
  K. wound packing material
Kampmeier foci
Kampo medicine
kanamycin
kangaroo
  k. care
  K. pump
  K. Web device
kansasii
  Mycobacterium k.
Kantor-Berci video laryngoscope
Kantrowitz
  K. pacemaker
  K. thoracic clamp
kaolin
  k. partial thromboplastin time (KPTT)
  k. pneumoconiosis
kaolin-cephalin clotting time (KCCT)
kaolinosis
Kaon
Kaopectate
Kaplan-Simpson InfusaSleeve
kapok asthma
Kaposi
  K. neoplasm
  K. sarcoma (KS)
Kappa 400 Series pacemaker

karaya asthma
Karell
  K. diet
  K. treatment
Karhunen-Loéve
  K.-L. procedure
  K.-L. transform (KLT)
Karl Storz D-LIGHT AF autofluorescence system
Karmen units
Karmody venous scissors
Karnofsky rating scale
Karolinska quality of life questionnaire
Karplus sign
Kartagener
  K. syndrome
  K. triad
Kasabach-Merritt syndrome
Kasser-Kennedy method
Katayama fever
Kattus
  K. exercise stress test
  K. treadmill protocol
Katz activities of daily living score
Katzen
  K. infusion wire
  K. long balloon dilation catheter
Katz-Wachtel phenomenon
Kaufman pneumonia
Kawai
  K. bioptome
  K. flexible endomyocardial biopsy catheter
Kawasaki
  K. disease
  K. syndrome
Kawashima
  K. intraventricular tunnel
  K. procedure
Kay
  K. annuloplasty
  K. balloon
Kayak hydrophilic guidewire
Kayexalate enema
Kay-Shiley caged-disc valve
KC
 cathodal closing
KCC
 cathodal closing contraction
KCCT
 kaolin-cephalin clotting time
KCG
 kinetocardiogram
K^+ channels

KCl
> potassium chloride

Kd
> distribution coefficient

KDA
> Kennedy's Disease Association

kDa, kd
> kilodalton

Kearns-Sayre syndrome

keel
> McNaught k.

keeled chest

keep vein open (KVO)

Keflex

Keftab

Kefzol

Keith
> K. bundle
> K. node

Keith-Flack node

Keith-Wagener-Barker (KWB)

Kellner questionnaire

Kellock sign

Kelly
> K. clamp
> K. hemostat

keloidal

Kempner diet

Kenalog injection

Kendall sequential compression device

Kennedy
> K. area-length method
> K. disease

Kennedy's Disease Association (KDA)

Kensey rotation atherectomy extrusion

Kent
> K. bundle
> K. bundle ablation
> bundle of Stanley K.
> K. fiber
> K. pathway
> K. potential

Kent-His bundle

Kentrox
> K. RV 65, 75 lead

keratinocyte growth factor (KGF)

keratin pearls

Kerberos
> K. Rinspiration catheter
> K. Rinspiration system
> K. Rinspirator

Kerley A, B, C lines

Kerlone Oral

Kernan-Jackson bronchoscope

Kern technique

kerosene pneumonitis

Keshan
> K. cardiomyopathy
> K. disease

ketamine

ketanserin

Ketek

ketoacidosis

ketoconazole

ketone
> D-Phe-L-Pro-L-Arg-chloromethyl k. (PPACK)

ketoprofen

ketorolac

ketotifen

Kety-Schmidt method

keV
> kiloelectron volt
> 511-keV collimator

keyhole-limpet hemocyanin

keyhole surgery

Key-Pred Injection

Key-Pred-SP injection

key pulse rate (KPR)

Keystone PF analyzer

kg
> kilogram

KGF
> keratinocyte growth factor

kg/m²
> kilogram per meter squared

KI antigen

kick
> atrial k.
> k. count
> idioventricular k.

kidney
> arteriolosclerotic k.
> arteriosclerotic k.
> flea-bitten k.
> Goldblatt k.
> 2-k. Goldblatt
> heart, liver, k.'s (H-L-K)
> isoenzyme of lactate dehydrogenase found in the heart, erythrocytes, k.'s (LD1)
> polycystic k.

Kiel
> K. classification of lymphoma
> K. lymphoma classification

Kiemeneij percutaneous coronary intervention

Kienböck
> K. disease
> K. phenomenon

Kifa catheter material

Kikuchi disease

killer
> natural k. (NK)

Killian bundle

Killian-Jamieson area

Killian-Lynch laryngoscope

Killip
  K. heart disease classification
  K. heart failure classification
Killip-Kimball heart failure classification
kilodalton (kDa, kd)
  45-k. protein
kiloelectron volt (keV)
kilogram (kg)
  milliliter per k. (mL/kg)
  k. per meter squared (kg/m^2)
kilohm (kOhm)
kilojoule (kJ)
kilopascal (kPa)
kilopond (kp)
kilopond-meter (kpm)
kilovolt (kV)
kilowatt (kW)
Kimmelstiel-Wilson syndrome
Kimny
  K. guiding catheter
  K. radial guide catheter
  K. Wiseguide catheter
Kim-Ray
  K.-R. Greenfield caval filter
  K.-R. thermodilution
Kimura cartilage graft
kinase
  adrenergic receptor k. (ARK)
  adrenergic receptor k. 1 (ARK-1)
  beta-adrenergic receptor k. (BARK)
  c-*Jun* N-terminal k. (JNK)
  conserved helix-loop-helix
    ubiquitous k. (CHUK)
  creatine k. (CK)
  extracellularly responsive k. (ERK)
  extracellular-regulated k. (ERK)
  extracellular signal-regulated k.
  focal adhesion k. (FAK)
  intracellular tyrosine protein k.
  Janus k. (Jak)
  mitogen-activated protein k.
    (MAPK)
  P13 k.
  phosphorylase k.
  protein k. (PKase)
  protein k. A (PKA)
  protein k. C (PKC)
  protooncogenic protein k.
  Ras mitogen-activated protein k.
  serine k.
  serum creatine k.
  Src k.
  stress-activated protein k. (SAPK)
  threonine protein k.
Kindt carotid artery clamp
kinesiological electromyogram
kinesis
  color k. (CK)

kinetics
  first-order k.
  zero-order k.
kinetic therapy
KinetiX
  K. instrument
  K. ventilation monitor
kinetocardiogram (KCG)
kinetocardiograph
King
  K. ASD umbrella closure
  K. biopsy method
  K. bioptome
  K. cardiac device
  K. double umbrella closure system
  K. guiding catheter
  K. of Hearts Express 3X cardiac
    event recorder
  K. of Hearts Holter monitor
  K. interlocking device
  K. multipurpose catheter
kingae
  Haemophilus aphrophilus,
    Actinobacillus
    actinomycetemcomitans,
    Cardiobacterium hominis,
    Eikenella corrodens, Kingella k.
    (HACEK)
kinin
  endogenous k.
kininogen
kinked aorta
kinky-hair disease
Kinsey
  K. atherectomy
  K. rotation atherectomy extrusion
    angioplasty
Kinyoun stain
Kirklin fence
Kirstein method
Kisch reflex
kissing
  k. balloon angioplasty
  k. balloon technique
  k. stenting
  k. stent lesion
  k. stents
  k. tonsils
kit
  ACE k.
  AeroGear asthma action k.
  Alatest Latex-specific IgE allergen
    test k.
  AlphaTest k.
  ApopTag k.
  Arrow pneumothorax k.
  AsthmaPACK personal asthma
    care k.

K

kit *(continued)*
    BiPort hemostasis introducer
      sheath k.
    Ciaglia Blue Rhino single-step
      dilator k.
    Ciaglia sequential dilator k.
    cyanide antidote k.
    Enzygnost F1+2 ELISA k.
    Enzygnost TAT complex k.
    Euro-Collins multiorgan
      perfusion k.
    Fergus percutaneous introducer k.
    Gore Eze-Sit valvulotome k.
    Imulyse tPA ELISA k.
    MDI k.
    Myoview k.
    No Pour Pak suction catheter k.
    Oncor ApopTag k.
    percutaneous access k. (PAK)
    percutaneous catheter introducer k.
    Per-fit percutaneous tracheostomy k.
    Pleura-Seal thoracentesis k.
    Portex Per-fit tracheostomy k.
    Pro-Vent arterial blood gas k.
    Pro-Vent arterial blood sampling k.
    Pulsator dry heparin arterial blood
      gas k.
    RNeasy Mini k.
    Tag-It cystic fibrosis k.
    TintElize PAI-1 ELISA k.
    TriPort hemostasis introducer
      sheath k.
    Vari-Lase endovenous laser
      procedure k.
    Vaxcel Mini Stick vascular
      entry k.
    Virgo anticardiolipin screening
      ELISA test k.
KIU
    kallikrein inactivating unit
kJ
    kilojoule
KK
    kallikrein-kinin
    KK system
KL-6
    KL-6 protein antigen
    serum KL-6
Klebsiella
    K. oxytoca
    K. pneumonia
    K. pneumoniae
    K. pneumoniae subsp. *ozaenae*
    K. rhinoscleromatis
Klebs-Loeffler bacillus
Kleihauer-Betke test
Kleihauer test
Klein transseptal introducer sheath
Klein-Waardenburg syndrome

Klenz
    HPB-Artery K.
Klinefelter syndrome
Klippel-Feil syndrome
Klippel-Trenaunay-Weber syndrome
KLK1
    kallikrein 1
KLT
    Karhunen-Loéve transform
knee
    k. extension
    medial inferior artery of k.
    medial superior artery of k.
knife, pl. **knives**
    A-K diamond k.
    Beaver k.
    k. blade
    gamma k.
    Lebsche sternal k.
    roentgen k.
    UltraCision ultrasonic k.
    valvotomy k.
    k. wound
KnightStar
    K. 335 respiratory-support system
    K. 330 ventilator
knitted
    k. polyester crimped graft
    k. sewing ring
    k. vascular prosthesis
knives (*pl. of* knife)
knob
    aortic k.
    thoracic aortic k.
knock
    pericardial k. (PK)
Knoll gland
knuckle
    aortic k.
    B k.
    cervical aortic k.
    k. sign
Ko-Airan bleeding control procedure
koala
    K. vascular clamp
    K. vascular insert
Koate-HP
KOC
    cathodal opening contraction
Koch
    K. bacillus
    K. node
    K. old tuberculin
    K. phenomenon
    triangle of K.
    K. triangle
Kocher-Cushing reflex
Koch-Weeks bacillus
Koffex DM Children

Kogenate
KOH
    potassium hydroxide
Kohlmeier-Degos syndrome
Kohlrausch vein
kOhm
    kilohm
Kohn pore
KoKo Moe pulmonary function filter
Kolephrin GG/DM
Kolmogorov-Smirnov procedure
Kommerell
    diverticulum of K.
    K. diverticulum
    retroesophageal diverticulum of K.
Kondoleon-Sistrunk elephantiasis
  procedure
Konica KFDR-S laser film scanner
Konigsberg catheter
Konno
    K. biopsy method
    K. bioptome
    K. operation
    K. procedure
Kontron
    K. balloon
    K. balloon catheter
    K. intraaortic balloon pump
Konyne 80
Koplik spot
Kopp asthma
Korányi
    K. auscultation
    K. sign
Korean hemorrhagic fever
Korotkoff
    K. phase I–V
    K. sound
    K. test
Kostmann syndrome
Kotonkan virus
Kozak sequence
kp
    kilopond
kPa
    kilopascal
kpm
    kilopond-meter
KPR
    key pulse rate
KPTT
    kaolin partial thromboplastin time
^{81m}Kr
    krypton-81m
Krankenhausarzte
    Arbeitsgemeinschaft Leitende
    Kardiologische K. (ALKK)

Krebs
    K. cycle
    K. solution
Krebs-Henseleit
    K.-H. buffer
    K.-H. solution
Kreiselman unit
Kreysig sign
kringle
Krishaber disease
Krogh apparatus spirometer
Kronecker center
Krönig
    K. area
    K. isthmus
    K. steps
Krukenberg vein
krusei
    Candida k.
krypton-81m (^{81m}Kr)
    k.-81m ventilation imaging
KS
    Kaposi sarcoma
K-space segmentation
K-Sponge
Kubicek equation
Kugel
    K. anastomosis
    K. anastomotic artery
Kugelberg-Welander
    K.-W. disease
    K.-W. syndrome
Kuhn
    K. mask
    K. tube
Kuhnt postcentral vein
Kulchitsky cell
Kunitz-type inhibitor
Kuntz
    nerve of K.
Kupffer cell
kurroa
    Picrorhiza k.
Kurten vein stripper
Kussmaul
    K. breathing
    K. disease
    K. paradoxical pulse
    K. respiration
    K. respiration pattern
    K. sign
    K. symptom
    K. syndrome
Kussmaul-Kien respiration
Kussmaul-Maier disease
kV
    kilovolt
    kV fluoroscopy

K

Kveim
  K. antigen skin test
  K. reaction
Kveim-Siltzbach test
KVO
  keep vein open
kW
  kilowatt
Kwai garlic
kwashiorkor-like malnutrition

KWB
  Keith-Wagener-Barker
    KWB hypertension classification
Kwelcof
kymogram
kymograph
kymography
kymoscope
kyphoscoliosis

L

L 67 lead
L loop

LA

left atrium
left auricle
long acting
    Dexone LA
    Guaifenex LA
    Inderal LA
    Westrim LA

L.A.

long acting
    Dexasone L.A.
    Solurex L.A.

LAA

left atrial appendage
left atrial area
    LAA contraction
    LAA filling
    LAA thrombi

La:A

La:A ratio

LA/Ao

left atrial/aortic
LA/Ao ratio

LABA

laser-assisted balloon angioplasty
long-acting beta-2 agonist bronchodilator

LABBB

left anterior bundle branch block

Labbe neurocirculatory syndrome
Labcor Synergy valve
label

open l. (OL)

labeled

l. FFA scintigraphy
open l. (OL)

labeling

TdT-mediated dUTP nick-end l.
    (TUNEL)

labetalol hydrochloride
labile

l. blood pressure
l. hypertension
l. pulse

lability

transient pulmonary vascular l.
    (TPVL)

laboratory, pl. **laboratories**

Advanced Technology Laboratories,
    Inc. (ATL)
Core Exercise Testing L.
Venereal Disease Research L.
    (VDRL)

Laborde method
labored respiration
Labrador lung
Labtron stethoscope
LABV

left atrial ball valve

LAC

left atrial circumflex
left atrial contraction
low-amplitude contraction
    LAC artery

laceration

parenchymal l.

lacidipine
lacrimalis

fossa glandulae l.

lacrymans

Serpula l.

LACS

lacunar syndrome

lactamase

beta l.

lactate

amrinone l.
l. dehydrogenase
l. extraction
milrinone l.
Ringer l.
sodium l.
l. threshold

lactea

macula l.

lactic

l. acid
l. acid concentration
l. acid dehydrogenase
l. acidosis
l. acid transport
l. dehydrogenase (LDH)

LactiCare-HC
Lactobacillus
lactone

macrocyclic l.

lacuna, pl. **lacunae**

l. pharyngis

lacunar

l. angina
l. infarct
l. infarction (LI)
l. stroke
l. syndrome (LACS)

LAD

left anterior descending
left axis deviation

LAD *(continued)*
LAD coronary artery
native LAD
LADA
left anterior descending artery
LADB
left anterior descending branch
LADCA
left anterior descending coronary artery
LADD
left anterior descending diagonal
LADD coronary artery
ladder
l. diagram
l. incision
L. of Life score
LADP
left anterior descending arterial pressure
Lady Windermere syndrome
LAE
left atrial enlargement
LAEDV
left atrial end-diastolic volume
LAEI
left atrial emptying index
Laënnec
L. catarrh
L. cirrhosis
L. pearl
L. sign
Laerdal resuscitator
LAESV
left atrial end-systolic volume
laevis
Xenopus l.
LAFS
long-axis fractional shortening
lag
homeostatic l.
l. time (LT)
Lagrangian strain
Laguna Negra virus
LAH
left anterior hemiblock
left atrial hypertrophy
laid-back
l.-b. balloon occlusion aortography
l.-b. view
laidlawii
Acholeplasma l.
LAIS laser
laiteuse
tache l.
lake
venous l.'s
LAM
left atrial myxoma
lymphangioleiomyomatosis

LAMA
laser-assisted microanastomosis
LAMB
lentigines, atrial myxoma, mucocutaneous myxoma, blue nevi
LAMB syndrome
Lambert
L. aortic clamp
canal of L.
channels of L.
Lambert-Beer law
Lambert-Eaton myasthenic syndrome
Lambert-Kay aortic clamp
lambertosis
Lambl excrescence
lamella, pl. **lamellae**
dissecting l.
elastic l.
lamifiban
lamina, pl. **laminae**
l. densa
elastic l.
l. elastica interna
external elastic l. (EEL)
internal elastic l. (IEL)
proliferation of elastic l.
laminar blood flow
laminated
l. clot
l. connective tissue
l. thrombus
laminin antibody
laminography
lamivudine (3TC)
zidovudine and l.
lamp
Wood l.
Lamprene
Lam procedure
Lanaphilic topical
lanata
Digitalis l.
lanatoside C
Lancisi sign
landmark
moustache angiographic l.
pitchfork angiographic l.
whale's tail angiographic l.
Landolfi sign
Landouzy-Dejerine
L.-D. dystrophy
facioscapulohumeral dystrophy of L.-D.
L.-D. syndrome
Landry-Guillain-Barré syndrome
LANE
lidocaine, atropine, naloxone, epinephrine [drugs that may be administered via endotracheal tube]

Lange calipers
Langendorff
    L. apparatus
    L. heart preparation
Langer axillary arch
Langerhans
    L. cell granulomatosis
    L. cell histiocytosis
    L. giant cell
Langevin updating procedure
Langhans cell
Langhans-type giant cell
Lannelongue foramen
lanoteplase
Lanoxicaps
Lanoxin
lanreotide
lansingensis
    Legionella l.
LANV
    left atrial neovascularization
Lanz low-pressure cuff endotracheal
  tube
LAO
    left anterior oblique
    left atrial overload
    LAO position
LAP
    laser-assisted palatoplasty
    left atrial pressure
laparoscopic Nissen fundoplication
laparotomy sponge
Laplace
    L. law
    L. mechanism
    L. principle
    L. relationship
Laplacian mapping
lapping murmur
Lap Sac
LAPW
    left atrial posterior wall
LAR
    late asthmatic response
    Sandostatin LAR
Largactil
large-annulus prosthesis
large-bore
    l.-b. angiocatheter
    l.-b. catheter
    l.-b. chest tube
    l.-b. slotted aspirating needle
    l.-b. trocar
    l.-b. Tuohy-Borst side-arm adapter
large-caliber chest tube
large-cell
    l.-c. carcinoma with rhabdoid
      phenotype

    l.-c. neuroendocrine carcinoma
      (LCNEC)
    l.-c. undifferentiated carcinoma
large-tip electrode
large vessel
large-vessel infarction (LVI)
large-volume aspiration
L-arginine
Lariam
Larmor frequency
Laron syndrome (LS)
Larrey
    L. hernia
    L. space
larva migrans
laryngalgia
laryngea
    angina l.
    arteria l.
    prominentia l.
    protuberantia l.
laryngeae
    glandulae l.
laryngeal
    l. aperture
    l. atresia
    l. bursa
    l. cleft
    l. cough reflex (LCR)
    l. cough reflex test
    l. crisis
    l. edema
    l. gland
    l. infection
    l. mask airway (LMA)
    l. nerve
    l. part of pharynx
    l. pouch
    l. prominence
    l. rale
    l. reflex
    l. stridor
    l. syncope
    l. tonsil
    l. vein
    l. ventricle
    l. vertigo
    l. web
    l. wheezing
laryngectomee
larynges (*pl. of* larynx)
laryngeus
    Syngamus l.
laryngis
    cartilago sesamoidea l.
    cavitas l.
    membrana fibroelastica l.
    musculi l.
    sacculus l.

L

laryngis *(continued)*
    tunica mucosa l.
    ventriculus l.
    vestibulum l.
laryngismus
    l. paralyticus
    l. stridulus
laryngitis
    atrophic l.
    catarrhal l.
    chronic catarrhal l.
    croupous l.
    diphtheritic l.
    membranous l.
    phlegmonous l.
    l. sicca
    l. stridulosa
    subglottic l.
    syphilitic l.
    tuberculous l.
    vestibular l.
Laryngoflex reinforced endotracheal tube
laryngomalacia
laryngopharynx
laryngoscope
    Benjamin binocular l.
    Benjamin pediatric l.
    Bullard intubating l.
    Dedo-Pilling l.
    Foregger l.
    Garfield-Holinger l.
    Holinger anterior commissure l.
    Jako l.
    Kantor-Berci video l.
    Killian-Lynch l.
    Lindholm operating l.
    Machida fiberoptic l.
    Macintosh l.
    Magill l.
    Ossoff-Karlan l.
    shadow-free l.
    Shapshay-Healy l.
    Storz-Hopkins l.
laryngoscopy
    direct l.
    mirror-image l.
    suspension l.
laryngospasm
laryngotracheal
    l. diverticulum
    l. groove
    l. infection
laryngotracheitis
laryngotracheobronchitis
larynx, pl. **larynges**
    artificial l.
    cartilage of l.
    cavity of l.

Cooper-Rand intraoral artificial l.
Nu-Vois artificial l.
saccule of l.
tuberculosis of l.
ventricular band of l.
vestibule of l.
LASEC
    left atrial spontaneous echo contrast
laser
    l. ablation
    alexandrite l.
    ArF excimer l.
    argon ion l.
    argon pumped tuneable dye l.
    l. balloon angioplasty (LBA)
    l. bronchoscopy
    l. capture microdissection (LCM)
    carbon dioxide TMR l.
    cool-tip l.
    CO2 TMR Heart L. 2
    coumarin pulsed dye l.
    l. delivery catheter
    l. Doppler flowmeter
    dye l.
    Eclipse holmium l.
    Eclipse TMR l.
    erbium:YAG l.
    excimer cool l.
    excimer gas l.
    l. fiber
    l. firing
    flashlamp-pulsed Nd:YAG l.
    fluorescence-guided smart l.
    free-beam l.
    Heart L.
    HF infrared l.
    high-energy l.
    high-powered l.
    holmium l.
    Ho:YAG l.
    infrared-pulsed l.
    LAIS l.
    low-energy l.
    Lumonics YAG l.
    l. maze operation
    microsecond pulsed flashlamp pumped dye l.
    mid-infrared pulsed l.
    Nd:YAG l.
    neodymium:yttrium-aluminum-garnet l.
    PhotoGenica V-Star l.
    ProYellow+ l.
    pulsed dye l.
    Q-switched Nd:YAG l.
    l. revascularization
    ruby l.
    Spectranetics l.
    spectroscopy-directed l.

Surgilase 150 l.
THC:YAG l.
l. thermal angioplasty
thulium-holmium-chromium:yttrium-
  aluminum-garnet l.
thulium-holmium:YAG l.
l. transluminal angioplasty catheter
  (LASTAK)
transmyocardial revascularization
  with l.
l. tube
tunable pulsed dye l.
ultraviolet l.
Vbeam pulsed dye l.
XeCl excimer l.
xenon chloride excimer l.
YAG l.

laser-assisted
l.-a. balloon angioplasty (LABA)
l.-a. internal fabrication technique
  (LIFT)
l.-a. microanastomosis (LAMA)
l.-a. palatoplasty (LAP)
l.-a. uvulopalatopharyngoplasty
  (LAUPPP)
l.-a. uvulopalatoplasty (LAUP)
laser-cut, self-expanding nitinol stent
Laserdish
L. electrode
L. pacing lead
laser-Doppler flowmetry
laser-induced
l.-i. arterial fluorescence (LIAF)
l.-i. thrombosis
Laserpor pacing lead
Laserprobe catheter
Laserprobe-PLR Flex catheter
laser-sculpted implant
LASH
left anterior superior hemiblock
Lasix
L. injection
L. Oral
L. Special
Lassa
L. fever
L. virus
Lasso catheter
LASTAK
laser transluminal angioplasty catheter
LAT
left atrial thrombus
late
l. afterdepolarization
l. angioplasty complication
l. apical systolic murmur
l. apnea
l. arterial switch
l. asthmatic response (LAR)

l. cyanosis
l. deceleration
l. diastole
l. diastolic murmur
l. diastolic potential (LDP)
l. lung injury
l. potential parameter
l. potential parameter index
l. proarrhythmic effect
l. progressing stroke (LPS)
l. pulmonary injury
l. R in aVR
l. reperfusion
l. silhouette
l. sudden death
l. systole
l. systolic click (LSC)
l. systolic murmur (LSM)
l. tracheostomy
latent
l. cardiomyopathy (LCM)
l. empyema
l. membrane protein-1 (LMP1)
l. pleurisy
l. tuberculosis infection (LTBI)
late-peaking systolic murmur
lateral
l. basal bronchopulmonary segment
l. basal segmental artery
l. basal segmental artery of right
  lung
l. cephalometry
l. flail chest
l. jugular lymph node
l. medullary infarction (LMI)
l. mesocardium
l. myocardial infarction (LMI)
l. pharyngeal space
l. projection
l. sac
l. thrombus
l. ventricular nerve (LVN)
l. view
l. wall (LW)
laterale
segmentum bronchopulmonale
  basale l.
spatium pharyngeum l.
laterales
venae circumflexae femoris l.
lateralis
arteria genus superior l.
ramus anterior l.
vastus l.
laterality index (LI)
lateropharyngeum
spatium l.
laterosporus
Bacillus l.

latex balloon
lathyrogen
Lathyrus odoratus
Latino
latissimus
    l. dorsi
    l. dorsi muscle
    l. dorsi procedure
LATP
    left atrial transmural pressure
LATPT
    left atrial transesophageal pacing test
Latrodectus Mactans
Laubry-Soulle syndrome
laudanosine
LAUP
    laser-assisted uvulopalatoplasty
LAUPPP
    laser-assisted uvulopalatopharyngoplasty
Laurell
    L. method
    rocket immunoelectrophoretic
      method of L.
Laurence-Moon-Bardet-Biedl syndrome
Laurence-Moon-Biedl syndrome
laurentii
    Cryptococcus l.
lauryl dimethyl benzyl ammonium chloride
lavage
    bronchial l.
    bronchoalveolar l. (BAL)
    continuous pericardial l.
    diagnostic peritoneal l. (DPL)
    l. hydroxyproline
    iced saline l.
    l. instillation
    pericardial l.
    pleural l.
    tracheobronchial l.
LAW
    left atrial wall
law
    all or none l.
    Beer L.
    Bowditch l.
    Charles l.
    Dalton l.
    Dalton-Henry l.
    Du Bois-Reymond l.
    Einthoven l.
    Frank-Starling l.
    Graham l.
    l. of the heart
    Henry l.
    Hooke l.
    Lambert-Beer L.
    Laplace l.
    Louis l.
    Marey l.
    Ohm l.
    Poiseuille l.
    Starling l.
    Sutton l.
    Torricelli l.
Lawton
    L. IADL
    L. Instrumental Activities of Daily
      Living scale
LAX
    long axis
laxa
    cutis l.
LAX-DSS
    long axis-discrete subaortic stenosis
layer
    adventitial l.
    fascial l.
    fascioperitoneal l.
    half-value l.
    hypertrophic smooth muscle l.
    M cell l.
    mucous l.
    peribronchiolar l.
    subendocardial l.
lazaroid
LB
    left bundle
LBA
    laser balloon angioplasty
LBB
    left bundle branch
LBBsB
    left bundle branch system block
LBCD
    left border of cardiac dullness
LBD
    left border of dullness
    left brain damage
LBNP
    lower body negative pressure
LBP
    low blood pressure
LBT
    loaded breathing test
LBV
    lung blood volume
LC
    left circumflex
    lymphangitic carcinomatosis
      LC artery
      LC Plus reusable nebulizer
      LC Star reusable nebulizer
LCA
    left circumflex artery
    left coronary artery
LCAD
    lipid coronary artery disease

LCAT
lecithin cholesterol acyltransferase
LCATA
lecithin cholesterol acyltransferase alpha
LCC
left circumflex coronary
left coronary cusp
LCC artery
LCCA
left common carotid artery
LCCE
length contraction compensation element
LCD
liquid crystal display
LCF
left circumflex
lymphocyte chemoattractant factor
LCF coronary artery
LCL
Levinthal-Coles-Lillie
LCL bodies
LCM
laser capture microdissection
latent cardiomyopathy
LCNEC
large-cell neuroendocrine carcinoma
LCO
left coronary ostium
low cardiac output
LCOS
low cardiac output syndrome
LCR
laryngeal cough reflex
ligase chain reaction
LCS
left coronary sinus
LCVA
left hemisphere stroke
LCWI
left cardiac work index
LCX
left circumflex
left circumflex artery
left circumflex coronary artery
LCX coronary artery
LCXB
left coronary circumflex branch
LD1
isoenzyme of lactate dehydrogenase
found in the heart, erythrocytes, kidneys
LDH
lactic dehydrogenase
low-dose heparin
LDH flip
LDL
low-density lipoprotein
LDL direct blood test
native LDL (n-LDL)

oxidative modification of LDL
(oxLDL, ox-LDL)
oxidized LDL
LDL pattern B
LDLA
low-density lipoprotein apheresis
LDL-C, LDL-c
low-density lipoprotein-cholesterol
complex
LDL/HDL
low-density lipoprotein/high-density
lipoprotein
LDL/HDL radio
LDLP
low-density lipoprotein
LDLR, LDL-R
low-density lipoprotein receptor
low-density lipoprotein receptor mutation
database
LDP
late diastolic potential
LDUH
low-dose unfractionated heparin
LE
lupus erythematosus
LEAD
lower extremity arterial disease
lead
3.3 l.
A 67 l.
ABC l.
Accufix II DEC pacing l.
Accufix pacemaker l.
active fixation pacemaker l.
Aescula left ventricular l.
Aescula LV l.
American Pacemaker Corporation l.
Angeflex defibrillation l.
augmented l.
aVF l.
aVL l.
aVR l.
Biocontrol Technology/Coratomic l.
Biotronik l.
bipolar l.
Brilliant l.
capped l.
CapSure cardiac pacing l.
CapSureFix l.
CapSure SP l.
CapSure VDD l.
Cardiac Control Systems l.
CB l.
CF l.
chest l.
CL l.
Cordis Ancar pacing l.
coronary sinus l.

L

lead *(continued)*

CPI endocardial defibrillation/rate-sensing/pacing l.
CPI/Guidant l.
CR l.
dedicated bipolar l.
direct l.
l. dislodgment
dual-coil transvenous l.
Easytrak coronary venous steroid-eluting single-electrode pace/sense l.
Einthoven l.
16-l. electrocardiogram
electrocardiographic l.'s
Elema l.'s
Encor l.
endocardial bipolar l.
Endotak C tripolar transvenous l.
Endotak DSP l.
Endotak Picotip defibrillation l.
Endotak Reliance endocardial l.
epicardial l.
esophageal l.
l. extraction system
finned pacemaker l.
fishhook l.
fixed l.
Flextend pacing l.
Flextend steroid-eluting, transvenous pace/sense l.
floating l.
l. fracture
Frank XYZ orthogonal l.
Hi-Flex l.
ICD l.
l. impedance
implantable cardioverter-defibrillator l.
indirect l.
l. insulation
Intermedics l.
intracardiac l.
J-wire l.
K 54 l.
Kentrox RV 65, 75 l.
L 67 l.
Laserdish pacing l.
Laserpor pacing l.
left ventricular transvenous l.
Lewis l.
Lifeline l.
limb l.
l. locking device (LLD)
Low-Flex l.
Mason-Likar placement of ECG l.
Medtronic l.'s
Medtronic Model 4965 steroid-eluding l.

Medtronic Sprint l.
Microtip l.
modified chest l. (MCL)
monitor l.'s
MR l.
myocardial l.
Myopore l.
nonintegrated transvenous defibrillation l.
Oscor pacing l.
Osypka atrial l.
over-the-wire pacing l.
pacemaker l.'s
Pacesetter/St. Jude l.
Pacesetter Tendril DX steroid-eluting active-fixation pacing l.
pacing l.
pediatric l.
permanent cardiac pacing l.
Pisces l.
l. placement
l. poisoning
Polyflex l.
PolySafe A-track l.
Precept l.
precordial l.
retractable, radiopaque, screw-in pacing l.
l. reversal
reversed arm l.'s
scalar l.'s
screw-in l.
screw-on l.
segmented ring tripolar l.
semidirect l.
silicone l.
single-pass l.
Sorin l.
Sprint Model 6942, 6943 tachyarrhythmia l.
Sprint Quattro quadripolar defibrillator l.
SRT l.
standard limb l.
Stelid II steroid eluting endocardial pacing l.
Stelix II steroid eluting endocardial pacing l.
steroid-eluting pacemaker l.
straight-tined pacing l.
SVC l.
Sweet Tip bipolar l.
Synox fractal pacemaker l.
Target Tip l.
Telectronics Accufix pacing l.
temporary pervenous l.
Tendril DX implantable pacing l.
Tendril DX steroid-eluting active-fixation pacing l.

Tendril SDX model 1688 active-fixation pacing l.
ThinLine EZ bipolar pacemaker l.
ThinLine EZ pacing l.
l. threshold
TIJ l.
transcutaneous l.
Transvene l.
transvenous defibrillator l.
tripolar l.
2-turn epicardial l.
3-turn epicardial l.
unipolar limb l.
unipolar precordial l.
Uni-Silicone l.
V l.
ventral l. 1–6 (V1-V6)
ventricular l.
Vitatron l.
V-Pace transluminal pacing l.
V1-V6 EKG l.'s
Wilson l.

12-lead
12-l. electrocardiogram
12-l. electrocardiography
12-l. voltage-duration product criteria

leading
l. circle concept
l. circle hypothesis
l. edge
l. edge enhancement

lead-letter marker
lead/zirconium/titanium (LZT)
leaflet
adherent l.
l. angle
anterior l. (AL)
anterior mitral l. (AML)
anterior mitral valve l. (aMVL)
anterior pulmonary l.
anterior tricuspid l. (ATL)
aortic valve l.
l. approximation
bowing of mitral valve l.
bridging l.'s
calcified mitral l.
cleft anterior l.
cleft of aortic l.
C valvular l.
doming of l.
dysplastic mitral valvar l.
flail l.
flail mitral l. (FML)
hammocking of posterior mitral l.
mitral l.
mitral valve l. (MVL)
l. motion
posterior l.

posterior mitral l. (PML)
posterior mitral valve l. (pML, PMVL, pMVL)
posterior pulmonary l. (PPL)
posterior tricuspid l. (PTL)
prolapsed middle scallop of posterior l.
prolapsing mitral l. (PML)
prolapsing mitral valvar l.
tethered l.
l. thickening
tricuspid valvular l.
valvular l.
l. vegetation

leak
air l.
alveolar l.
baffle l.
continuous air l.
paraprosthetic l.
perivalvular l.
shunt l.
silent trace l.

leakage
perivalvular l. (PVL)
spectral l.

LEAP
low energy all-purpose
LEAP collimator

Lebsche sternal knife
lecithin
cardiolipin natural l. (CNL)
cardiolipin synthetic l. (CSL)
l. cholesterol acyltransferase (LCAT)
l. cholesterol acyltransferase alpha (LCATA)

lecithin/sphingomyelin (L/S)
Lecompte maneuver
LED
light-emitting diode
LEDC
low energy direct current
ledge
eccentric l.
limbic l.

Leeuwenhoek disease
Lee-White method
left
l. anterior bundle branch block (LABBB)
l. anterior descending (LAD)
l. anterior descending arterial pressure (LADP)
l. anterior descending artery (LADA)
l. anterior descending branch (LADB)

L

left *(continued)*

l. anterior descending coronary artery (LADCA)
l. anterior descending diagonal (LADD)
l. anterior hemiblock (LAH)
l. anterior oblique (LAO)
l. anterior oblique position
l. anterior oblique projection
l. anterior superior hemiblock (LASH)
l. aortic angiography
l. apical cap
apicoposterior branch of l.
l. arm electrode for electrocardiogram (VL)
l. atrial abnormality
l. atrial active emptying fraction
l. atrial active emptying volume
l. atrial angiography
l. atrial to aortic
l. atrial/aortic (LA/Ao)
l. atrial appendage (LAA)
l. atrial appendage area
l. atrial appendage flow velocity
l. atrial appendage function
l. atrial appendage stunning
l. atrial area (LAA)
l. atrial ball valve (LABV)
l. atrial circumferential ablation
l. atrial circumflex (LAC)
l. atrial contraction (LAC)
l. atrial diameter
l. atrial dimension
l. atrial emptying index (LAEI)
l. atrial end-diastolic volume (LAEDV)
l. atrial end-systolic volume (LAESV)
l. atrial enlargement (LAE)
l. atrial hypertension
l. atrial hypertrophy (LAH)
l. atrial isolation procedure
l. atrial maximal volume
l. atrial minimal volume
l. atrial myxoma (LAM)
l. atrial neovascularization (LANV)
l. atrial overload (LAO)
l. atrial partitioning
l. atrial posterior wall (LAPW)
l. atrial pressure (LAP, PLa, Pla)
l. atrial spontaneous echo contrast (LASEC)
l. atrial thrombus (LAT)
l. atrial transesophageal pacing test (LATPT)
l. atrial transmural pressure (LATP)
l. atrial wall (LAW)
l. atrium (LA)

l. atrium-pulmonary vein junction
l. auricle (LA)
l. auricle of heart
l. axis deviation (LAD)
l. border of cardiac dullness (LBCD)
l. border of dullness (LBD)
l. brain damage (LBD)
l. bundle (LB)
l. bundle branch (LBB)
l. bundle branch block
l. bundle branch rhythm
l. bundle branch system block (LBBsB)
l. cardiac work index (LCWI)
l. circumflex (LC, LCF, LCX)
l. circumflex artery (LCA, LCX)
l. circumflex coronary (LCC)
l. circumflex coronary artery (LCX)
l. common carotid artery (LCCA)
l. coronary artery (LCA)
l. coronary artery of stomach
l. coronary catheter
l. coronary circumflex branch (LCXB)
l. coronary cusp (LCC)
l. coronary ostium (LCO)
l. coronary sinus (LCS)
l. crus of diaphragm
l. dominant coronary circulation
l. foot electrode in vectorcardiography
l. gastric artery
l. heart (LH)
l. heart blood volume (LHBV)
l. heart bypass
l. heart catheter
l. heart catheterization (LHC)
l. heart contour
l. heart failure (LHF)
l. heart strain (LHS)
l. hemisphere (LH)
l. hemisphere damage (LHD)
l. hemisphere stroke (LCVA)
l. inferior pulmonary vein
l. inferior vena cava (LIVC)
l. internal jugular vein
l. internal mammary artery (LIMA)
l. internal mammary artery graft
l. internal thoracic artery (LITA)
l. internal thoracic artery graft
l. interventricular coronary (LIC)
l. Judkins catheter
l. lateral projection
l. lateral ventricular preexcitation (LLVP)
l. leg electrode for electrocardiogram (VF)

l. lower lobe (LLL)
l. lower pulmonary vein (LLPV)
l. lung
l. main (LM)
l. main artery (LMA)
l. main bronchus
l. main coronary (LMC)
l. main coronary artery (LMCA)
l. main coronary artery disease (LMCAD)
l. main coronary disease
l. main coronary occlusion
l. main coronary stenosis
l. main disease (LMD)
l. main equivalency
l. main stem (LMS)
l. main stem coronary artery disease (LMS-CAD)
l. marginal (LM)
l. marginal coronary artery occlusion (LMCAO)
l. margin of heart
l. median (LM)
l. median vein
l. middle hemiblock
l. portal view (LPV)
l. posterior hemiblock
l. posterior inferior hemiblock (LPIH)
l. posterior ventricular preexcitation (LPVP)
l. pulmonary artery (LPA)
l. pulmonary vein (LPV)
l. recurrent laryngeal nerve
l. septal flutter
l. septal hemiblock
l. septum (LS)
l. stellate ganglion
l. stellate ganglionic blockade (LSGB)
l. subclavian artery (LSCA)
l. superior pulmonary vein
l. superior vena cava (LSVC)
l. upper lobe (LUL)
l. upper pulmonary vein (LUPV)
l. ventricle (LV)
l. ventricle assist system
l. ventricle outflow (LVO)
l. ventricle outflow height (LVOH)
l. ventricular (LV)
l. ventricular aneurysm (LVA)
l. ventricular angiography
l. ventricular apex
l. ventricular assist device (LVAD)
l. ventricular assist system (LVAS)
l. ventricular assist system implantable pump
l. ventricular bypass pump (LVBP)

l. ventricular cardiac tamponade (LVCT)
l. ventricular cavity dilation
l. ventricular cavity obstruction ring
l. ventricular chamber compliance
l. ventricular contractility
l. ventricular developed pressure (LVDP)
l. ventricular diastolic phase index
l. ventricular diastolic pressure (LVDP)
l. ventricular diastolic relaxation
l. ventricular diastolic volume (LVDP, LVDV)
l. ventricular dimension (LVDI)
l. ventricular dimension in end-diastole (LVDd)
l. ventricular dysfunction (LVD)
l. ventricular dyskinesis
l. ventricular dyssynchrony
l. ventricular ejection (LVE)
l. ventricular ejection fraction (LVEF)
l. ventricular ejection time (LVEJT, LVET)
l. ventricular ejection time index (LVETI)
l. ventricular end-diastole (LVED)
l. ventricular end-diastolic area (LVEDA)
l. ventricular end-diastolic circumference (LVEDC)
l. ventricular end-diastolic diameter (LVEDD)
l. ventricular end-diastolic dimension (LVEDD)
l. ventricular end-diastolic pressure (LVEDP, LVEP)
l. ventricular end-diastolic volume (LVEDV)
l. ventricular end-systolic circumferential wall stress
l. ventricular end-systolic dimension (LVESD)
l. ventricular end-systolic volume (LVESV)
l. ventricular end-systolic wall stress (LVESWS)
l. ventricular enlargement (LVE)
l. ventricular epicardium
l. ventricular failure (LVF)
l. ventricular filling pressure (LVFP)
l. ventricular force
l. ventricular function (LVF)
l. ventricular geometry
l. ventricular hypertrophy (LVH)

L

left *(continued)*

l. ventricular infarct volume (LVIV)
l. ventricular inflow tract obstruction
l. ventricular insufficiency (LVI)
l. ventricular internal diastolic diameter (LVIDD)
l. ventricular internal diastolic dimension (LVIDD)
l. ventricular internal dimension (LVID)
l. ventricular ischemia (LVI)
l. ventricular-left atrial crossover dynamics
l. ventricular mass (LVM)
l. ventricular mass index (LVMI)
l. ventricular minute flow (LVMF)
l. ventricular muscle compliance
l. ventricular myxoma
l. ventricular noncompaction
l. ventricular opacification (LVO)
l. ventricular outflow tract (LVOT)
l. ventricular outflow tract obstruction (LVOTO)
l. ventricular outflow tract tachycardia
l. ventricular outflow tract velocity
l. ventricular output
l. ventricular peak filling rate (LVPFR)
l. ventricular posterior wall (LVPW)
l. ventricular power
l. ventricular pressure (LVP, PLV)
l. ventricular pressure-volume curve
l. ventricular puncture
l. ventricular reduction (LVR)
l. ventricular reduction surgery
l. ventricular-right atrial communication murmur
l. ventricular strain (LVS)
l. ventricular stroke volume (LVSV)
l. ventricular stroke volume index (LVSVI)
l. ventricular stroke work (LVSW)
l. ventricular stroke work index (LVSWI)
l. ventricular subendocardial myocardial ischemia (LVSEMI)
l. ventricular sump catheter
l. ventricular systolic/diastolic function
l. ventricular systolic dimension (LVSD)
l. ventricular systolic dysfunction
l. ventricular systolic index (LVSI)
l. ventricular systolic output (LVSO)
l. ventricular systolic performance
l. ventricular systolic pressure (LVSP)
l. ventricular tension (LVT)
l. ventricular transvenous lead
l. ventricular unloading
l. ventricular volume (LVV)
l. ventricular wall (LVW)
l. ventricular wall motion (LVWM)
l. ventricular wall motion abnormality
l. ventricular wall stress
l. ventricular wall thickness (LVWT)
l. ventricular work (LVW)
l. ventricular work index (LVWI)
l. ventriculogram (LV-gram)
l. ventriculography
l. ventrolateral gluteal (LVLG)
l. vertebral artery (LVA)

left/right lung

left-sided

l.-s. heart failure
l.-s. innominate trunk

left-to-right shunt

leftward ventricular septal bowing (LVSB)

leg

peripheral pulses palpable both l.'s (PPPBL)

legged

4-l. cage valve

Legionella

L. anisa
L. birminghamensis
L. bozemanii
L. cincinnatiensis
L. dumoffii
L. feeleii
L. gormanii
L. jordanis
L. lansingensis
L. longbeachae
L. micdadei
L. oakridgensis
L. pneumonia
L. pneumoniae
L. pneumophila
L. urinary antigen
L. urine antigen
L. wadsworthii
L. waltersii

legionellosis

Legionnaire

L. disease
L. pneumonia

Lehman
    L. cardiac device
    L. ventriculography catheter
leiomyoma, pl. **leiomyomata**
leiomyosarcoma
Leishmania
leishmaniasis
leisure time physical activity (LTPA)
Leitner syndrome
lemakalim
Lemierre
    L. disease
    L. syndrome
Lemmon sternal elevator
LemonPrep
Lenègre
    L. disease
    L. syndrome
length
    antegrade block cycle l.
    atrial fibrillation cycle l. (AFCL)
    atrial-paced cycle l.
    basic cycle l. (BCL)
    basic drive cycle l.
    block cycle l.
    chordal l.
    l. contraction compensation element
        (LCCE)
    cycle l. (CL)
    drive cycle l.
    end-diastolic l. (EDL)
    end-systolic l. (ESL)
    flutter cycle l.
    lesion l. (LL)
    paced cycle l.
    pacing cycle l. (PCL)
    sinus cycle l. (SCL)
    sinus node cycle l. (SNCL)
    l. of stay (LOS)
    tachycardia cycle l.
    ventricular tachycardia cycle l.
        (VTCL)
    Wenckebach cycle l.
length-active tension curve
length-dependent activation
length-resting tension relation
length-tension
    l.-t. curve (LT)
    l.-t. relation
LENI
    lower extremity noninvasive
Lennert lymphoma
lenta
    endocarditis l.
Lente Iletin I, II insulin
lenticulostriate artery
lentigines
    l., atrial myxoma, mucocutaneous
        myxoma, blue nevi (LAMB)

l., electrocardiographic
    abnormalities, ocular hypertelorism,
    pulmonary stenosis, abnormalities
    of genitalia, retardation of
    growth, deafness (LEOPARD)
lentiginosis
lentigo, pl. **lentigines**
lentis
    ectopia l.
Lenz syndrome
Leocor hemoperfusion system
LEOPARD
    lentigines, electrocardiographic
    abnormalities, ocular hypertelorism,
    pulmonary stenosis, abnormalities of
    genitalia, retardation of growth,
    deafness
    LEOPARD syndrome
LEP
    lipoprotein electrophoresis
lepidic growth
lepirudin
    l. rDNA
    l. rDNA injection
leprae
    Mycobacterium l.
lepromin test
leptin
leptospiral pneumonia
leptospirosis
Leptotrichia buccalis
lercanidipine
Leredde syndrome
Leriche syndrome
lesion
    aorto-ostial l.
    Baehr-Lohlein l.
    bifurcation l. (BL)
    bifurcational coronary l.
    bird's nest l.
    Blumenthal l.
    Bracht-Wächter l.
    braid-like l.
    branch l.
    calcified l.
    catheter-induced linear l.
    cavitary l.
    cavitating l.
    coin l.
    colander-like l.
    complex l.
    connective tissue l.
    continuous full-thickness linear l.
    coronary artery l.
    cryoablation l.
    culprit l.
    cystic l.
    deep white matter l. (DWML)
    dendritic l.

L

lesion *(continued)*
    de novo native coronary artery l.
    dilatable l.
    discrete coronary l.
    dottering of l.
    eccentric l.
    enhancing l.
    epicardial radiofrequency atrial l.
    fibrocalcific l.
    fibromusculoelastic l.
    fibromyxoid l.
    fibrous cap l.
    full-thickness linear l.
    Ghon primary l.
    hazy l.
    honeycomb l.
    index l.
    intraluminal fibromyxoid l.
    irregular discrete l.
    JA l.
    jailed side branch l.
    Janeway l.
    jet l.
    juxtaarticular l.
    kissing stent l.
    l. length (LL)
    Libman-Sacks l.
    linear l.
    Lohlein-Baehr l.
    long l.
    macrovascular coronary l.
    l. marking system
    monotypic l.
    mucocutaneous l.
    multifocal l.
    native coronary artery l.
    nonbacterial thrombotic
      endocardial l.
    obstructive l.
    onion scale l.
    ostial l.
    parenchymal l.
    plexiform l.
    polypoidal l.
    pulmonary coin l.
    punctate mucosal l.
    radiofrequency l.
    restenosis l.
    restenotic native coronary artery l.
    rigid core-out of l.'s
    satellite l.
    shunt-dependent l.
    smooth l.
    space-occupying l.
    spot l.
    stenotic l.
    synchronous airway l.'s
    tandem l.
    target l.

    type I, Ia, Ib, Ic, II, III l.
    type Va, Vb, Vc l.
    ulcerated l.
    vegetative l.
    wear-and-tear l.
    wire-loop l.
lesser
    l. circulation
    l. resection
LET
    lidocaine, epinephrine, tetracaine
    LET solution
lethal arrhythmia
letrozole
Letterer-Siwe disease
leucine
leucocidin
    Panton-Valentine l. (PVL)
leucovorin
Leudet
leukemia
    acute lymphocytic l. (ALL)
    acute myelocytic l. (AML)
leukemic cell lysis pneumopathy
Leukeran
leukoaraiosis
    ischemic l.
leukocidin
leukocyte
    l. chemotaxis
    l. elastase
    polymorphonuclear l. (PMN)
leukocyte-endothelial
    l.-e. cell adhesion cascade
    l.-e. cell adhesion molecule
    l.-e. cell interaction
leukocytoblastic vasculitis
leukocytoclastic angiitis
leukocytosis
    transient l.
leukoencephalopathy
    cerebral autosomal dominant
      arteriopathy with subcortical
      infarct and l. (CADASIL)
    l. disease
    progressive multifocal l. (PML)
leukomalacia
    cystic periventricular l.
LeukoNet Filter
leukostasis
    pulmonary l.
leukotactin-1
Leukotrap red cell storage system
leukotriene
    l. A_4
    l. B_4 (LTB_4)
    l. biosynthesis
    l. C_4, D_4, E, E_4
    cysteinyl l. (cys-LT)

l. inhibition
l. inhibitor
l. modifier
l. receptor antagonist
l. synthesis
leumedin
leuprolide acetate
Lev
L. disease
L. syndrome
levalbuterol
l. HCl
l. HCl inhalation solution
levamisole hydrochloride
Levaquin
Levatol
levator muscle of thyroid gland
LeVeen
L. peritoneovenous shunt
L. plaque-cracker
L. valve (LVV)
level
airborne fiber l.
air-fluid l.
anti-Xa l.
beta-thromboglobulin l.
blood oxygen l.
CK19 l.
digoxin l.
ELF l.'s
Health l. 7 (HL7)
isoprenoid l.
malondialdehyde l.
melatonin l.
microvolt l.
multiple shunt l.'s
myofibrillar calcium l.
nocturnal plasma ghrelin l.
peak and trough l.'s
plasma leptin l.
plasma nicotine l.
plasma thyroxine l. (PTL)
plasma triglyceride l.
predose l.
reflecting l.
renin l.
sarcolemmal l.
serum lipid l.
serum renin l.
soluble TREM-1 l.
sublingual carbon dioxide l.
sulfhemoglobin l.
total homocysteine l.
toxic l.
triglyceride l.
trough and peak l.'s
level-dependent
blood oxygenation l.-d. (BOLD)
Levenberg-Marquardt algorithm

Levin catheter
Levine
L. grade 1–6 cardiac murmur
L. sign
Levine-Harvey classification
Levinson-Durbin recursion
Levinthal-Coles-Lillie (LCL)
levoatriocardinal vein
levobupivacaine hydrochloride
levocardia
l. malposition
mixed l.
l. with situs inversus
levocardiogram
levocetirizine
levodopa
Levo-Dromoran
levofloxacin
levogram
levoisomerism
Levophed injection
levoposition
levorphanol
levosimendan
Levothroid
levothyroxine
levotransposition
levoversion
Levovist
L. contrast
L. echocontrast agent
Levoxyl
Levy Chimeric Faces Test
Lewis
L. index
L. lead
L. lines
P substance of L.
L. thoracotomy
L. upper limb cardiovascular disease
Lewis-Pickering test
Lewis-Tanner procedure
Lewy chest holder
Lewy-Rubin needle
Lexxel
Leyden crystal
LFB
low-flow cardiopulmonary bypass
LFC
low fat and cholesterol
LFC diet
LFCT
lung-to-finger circulation time
LFT
liver function test
LGAS
low-gradient aortic stenosis

L

LGV
lymphogranuloma venereum
LH
left heart
left hemisphere
L/H
lung-to-heart
L/H ratio
LHBV
left heart blood volume
LHC
left heart catheterization
LHD
left hemisphere damage
LHF
left heart failure
LHMT
low-range heparin management test
LHS
left heart strain
LI
lacunar infarction
laterality index
LI single coronary artery anomaly
LIAF
laser-induced arterial fluorescence
liberation
Liberator locking stylet
Liberté stent
Libman-Sacks
L.-S. disease
L.-S. endocarditis
L.-S. lesion
L.-S. syndrome
library, pl. **libraries**
Cochrane L.
human cosmid l.
LIC
left interventricular coronary
local intravascular coagulation
LIC artery
licheniformis
Bacillus l.
lichenoides
tuberculosis l.
licorice
Chinese l.
Liddle
L. aorta clamp
L. syndrome
lidocaine
l., atropine, naloxone, epinephrine [drugs that may be administered via endotracheal tube] (LANE)
buffered l. (BL)
l., epinephrine, tetracaine (LET)
l. hydrochloride
Lidodan ointment
lidoflazine

Liebermann-Burchard test
Liebermeister
L. rule
L. sign
Liebow
L. classification
usual interstitial pneumonia of L.
lienis
extremitas anterior l.
porta l.
lifarizine
LIFE
lifestyle intervention, food and exercise program
lung imaging fluorescence endoscope
life, pl. **lives**
L. Care Pump
l. change unit
l. force
health-related quality of l. (HRQL, HRQOL)
Mini Asthma Quality of L. (MAQOL)
quality of l.
stroke-specific quality of l. (SS-QOL)
L. Suit
l. support
Lifecare PLV-100 portable ventilator
Lifecor wearable cardioverter-defibrillator
lifeguard lung
Lifeline lead
LIFE-Lung System
Lifepak
L. defibrillator
L. 5, 7 monitor/defibrillator
Lifepath
L. AAA endovascular graft system
L. stent-graft
LifePort endotracheal tube holder
Lifesaver disposable resuscitator bag
life-saving defibrillation
LifeShirt
L. monitor
L. noninvasive ambulatory system
LifeStent self-expanding stent
Lifestream coronary dilation catheter
lifestyle
l. intervention, food and exercise program (LIFE)
sedentary l.
LifeSync
L. system
L. wireless ECG
life-threatening
l.-t. cardiac event
l.-t. heart rhythm
l.-t. hemoptysis

LifeValve central venous catheter
LifeVest wearable defibrillator
life-year
  quality-adjusted l.-y.'s (QALY)
LIFT
  laser-assisted internal fabrication
  technique
lift
  parasternal systolic l.
  tongue-jaw l.
ligament
  anular l.
  Cooper l.
  costoclavicular l.
  Marshall l.
  pericardiosternal l.
  pulmonary l.
  suspensory l.
  Teutleben l.
  ventricular l.
  vestibular l.
ligamenta anularia trachealia
ligamentum
  l. arteriosum
  l. hepatoesophageum
  l. latum pulmonis
  l. phrenicocolicum
  l. pulmonale
  l. teres cardiopexy
ligand
  l. binding
  Fas l. (FasL)
  macromolecular l.
  l. plus 1, 2, 3
  P-selectin glycoprotein l. 1 (PSGL-1)
ligase chain reaction (LCR)
ligation
  l. clip
  Doppler-guided hemorrhoidal
  artery l.
  Linton radical vein l.
  thoracic duct l.
  variceal l.
  varicose vein stripping and l.
ligature
  Stannius l.
light
  l. chain
  l. criteria
  l. microscopy
  l. pen
  l. pen-determined ejection fraction
  Questran L.
  l. reflection rheography
  l. stroke
  l. Talker device
  l. wand

lighted
  l. stylet
  l. stylet intubation
light-emitting diode (LED)
lighthouse tip
lightwire
lignan
Lignieres test
lignocaine
  M l.
LIhFE
  living with heart failure
  LIhFE questionnaire
LiI
  lithium iodine
  LiI battery
Likert
  L. 5-point scale
  L. scale (LS)
Lilienthal-Sauerbruch
  L.-S. retractor
  L.-S. rib spreader
Lillehei-Kaster
  L.-K. cardiac valve prosthesis
  L.-K. mitral valve prosthesis
  L.-K. pivoting-disc prosthetic valve
Lillehei-Nakib toroidal valve
Lilliput oxygenator
LIMA
  left internal mammary artery
  LIMA graft
LIMA-Lift tool
LIMA-Loop tool
limb
  anacrotic l.
  l. blood flow
  claudicant l.
  expiratory l.
  inspiratory l.
  l. ischemia
  l. lead
  l. salvage
  thoracic l.
limb-girdle
  l.-g. dystrophy of Erb
  l.-g. muscular dystrophy
limb-heart
  cleft l.-h. (CLH)
limbic ledge
limb-kinetic apraxia
limb-threatening ischemia
lime
  bruit de l.
limit
  Nyquist l.
limitation
  airflow l.
  chronic airflow l. (CAL)
  expiratory flow l.

L

limitation (*continued*)
    flow l. (FL)
    permissive flow l.
limited
    l. Doppler examination
    l. peak inspiratory pressure
    l. treadmill test (LTT)
    l. ventricular reserve
limonite pneumoconiosis
Lincocin
    L. injection
    L. Oral
lincomycin hydrochloride
Lincorex injection
lincosamide
Linctus With Codeine phosphate
Lindbergh pump
Lindesmith operation
Linde Walker Oxygen Program
Lindholm
    L. operating laryngoscope
    L. tracheal tube
line
    anterior axillary l. (AAL)
    anterior junction l.
    arterial l. (A-line)
    arterial mean l.
    Beau l.
    Cantlie l.
    central venous l.
    Conradi l.
    Correra l.
    costophrenic septal l.
    CVP l.
    Fleischner l.
    indwelling l.
    intraarterial l.
    intralobular l.
    isoelectric l.
    isthmus l.
    Kerley A, B, C l.'s
    Lewis l.'s
    Linton l.
    M l.'s
    midaxillary l.
    midclavicular l. (MCL)
    paraspinal l.
    pleural l.
    pleuroesophageal l.
    posterior junction l.
    L. Probe Assay
    l. sepsis
    septal l.
    tram l.
    white l.
    Z l.
    Zahn l.'s
    zero velocity l.

linear
    l. atrial ablation
    l. echo
    l. echodensity
    l. infiltrate
    L. KGT tonometer
    l. lesion
    l. local shortening map
    l. phonocardiograph
    l. stenosis
linearity
    amplitude l.
    count-rate l.
linear-phased radiofrequency catheter ablation
linezolid
Lingraphica
    L. aphasic treatment
    L. system treatment technology
linguae
    corpus l.
    dorsum l.
    radix l.
    raphe l.
    septum l.
    tunica mucosa l.
    venae dorsales l.
    vena profunda l.
    vinculum l.
lingual
    l. artery
    l. bone
    l. branch
    l. branch of facial nerve
    l. plexus
    l. quinsy
    l. thyroid
    l. tonsil
    l. vein
lingualis
    arteria l.
    plexus periarterialis arteriae l.
    rami isthmi faucium nervi l.
    tonsilla l.
lingualplasty
lingula, pl. **lingulae**
    l. of left lung
    l. pulmonis sinistri
lingular
    l. bronchus
    l. pneumonia
lingularis
    vena l.
linguofacialis
    truncus l.
linoleic acid
linsidomine
Linton
    L. flap

L. line
L. radical vein ligation
L. vein stripper
Linx
L. exchange guidewire
L. extension guidewire
L. extension wire
L. guidewire extension
L. guidewire extension cardiac
device
LionHeart left ventricular assist system
liothyronine
liotrix
Liotta-BioImplant low-profile
bioprosthesis prosthetic valve
Liotta total artificial heart
LIP
lower inflection point
lymphocytic interstitial pneumonitis
lymphoid interstitial pneumonia
lymphoid interstitial pneumonitis
lipase
diacylglycerol l.
hepatic lipoprotein l.
lipoprotein l. (LL, LPL)
secretin-stimulated serum l. (SSSL)
lipedema
lipemia
postprandial l. (PPL)
lipid
l. A
l. accumulation
antihypertensive neutral
renomedullary l. (ANRL)
atherogenic l.
bumetanide and furosemide on l.
(BUFUL)
cholesterol-lowering l. (CLL)
l. core
l. core density
l. coronary artery disease (LCAD)
l. disorder
endogenous l.
exogenous l.
extracellular l.
fasting plasma l. (FPL)
l. hypothesis
intracellular l.
neutral l. (NL)
l. panel
l. peroxidation
l. peroxidation product
l. peroxide
l. pneumonia
l. raft
renomedullary l.
l. research clinic (LRC)
l. risk factor
sarcolemma l.

l. solubility
l. triad
vasodepressor l. (VDL)
lipidic stria
Lipidil
L. Micro
L. Supra
lipid-induced lung injury
lipid-laden
l.-l. macrophage
l.-l. macrophage index
l.-l. plaque
lipid-lowering
l.-l. agent
l.-l. therapy
lipidosis, pl. **lipidoses**
lipid-rich plaque
Lipitor
lipoarabinomannan
lipocardiac
lipodystrophy
intestinal l.
lipofuscinosis
neuronal ceroid l.
lipogenic theory of atherosclerosis
lipohyalinosis
lipoides
arcus l.
lipoid pneumonia
lipolysis
lipoma, pl. **lipomata**
lipomatous hypertrophy
lipoparticle
lipoperoxidation end product
lipoperoxide
lipophilic drug
lipophilicity
properties of l.
lipopolysaccharidase
J5 l.
lipopolysaccharide (LPS)
l. vaccine
lipopolysaccharide-induced
l.-i. lung injury
l.-i. thrombocytopenia
lipoprotein (LP, Lp)
l. A (LPA, Lp(a))
l. (a) assay
alpha l.
l. apheresis
l. B (LPB, Lp(b))
beta l.
l. electrophoresis (LEP, LPE)
high-density l. (HDL, HDLP)
intermediate-density l. (IDL)
isolated low high-density l.
(ILHDL)
l. lipase (LL, LPL)
l. lipase activity (LPLA)

L

lipoprotein *(continued)*
  low-density l. (LDL, LDLP)
  low-density lipoprotein/high-
    density l. (LDL/HDL)
  malondialdehyde modified low-
    density l. (MDA-LDL)
  microsomal l. (MLP)
  native low-density l.
  non-high-density l. (NHDL)
  normal low-density l. (NLDL)
  oxidized low-density l. (OxLDL)
  l. particle
  pre-beta l.
  l. receptor-related protein (LRP)
  remnant l. (RLP)
  remnant-like particle l.
  RLP l.
  small, dense, low-density l. (SD-
    LDL)
  small low-density l.
  total cholesterol/high-density l.'s
    (TC/HDL)
  triglyceride-rich l. (TRL, TRLP)
  very high density l. (VHDL)
  very low density l. (VLDL)
  l. X (LPX, Lp-X)
lipoprotein-associated
  l.-a. coagulation inhibitor
  l.-a. phospholipase
  l.-a. phospholipase 2
lipoprotein-deficient fraction (LPDF)
lipoproteinemia
liposarcoma
liposomal
Liposorber LA-15 system
Liposyn
lipothymia
lipotoxicity
lipotropin
  human l. (HLT)
Lipovnik virus
5-lipoxygenase
lipoxygenase pathway
LIP/PLH
  lymphoid interstitial
    pneumonia/pulmonary lymphoid
    hyperplasia
    LIP/PLH complex
lip pursing
Liprostin
**Lipton classification (LI, LII-A, LII-B,
  LII-P, RII-A, RII-B)**
Liquaemin
liquefaciens
  Serratia l.
liquefaction necrosis
Liquibid
liquid
  Brontex L.
  l. crystal display (LCD)
  free l.
  Hayfebrol l.
  Histussin D l.
  Hycotuss Expectorant L.
  l. nitrous oxide-filled balloon
  oxygen-carrying perfluorochemical l.
  Rhinosyn l.
  Rhinosyn-PD l.
  l. scintillation spectrophotometer
  l. ventilation
liquifying expectorant
Liqui-Gels
  Alka-Seltzer Plus Flu & Body
    Aches Non-Drowsy L.-G.
  Robitussin Severe Congestion L.-G.
LiquiVent
LIS
  lung injury score
lisinopril
  hydrochlorothiazide and l.
  l. and hydrochlorothiazide
Lissajou loop
Listeria monocytogenes
listeriolysin
list mode
LITA
  left internal thoracic artery
  LITA graft
LITE
  low-intensity treadmill exercise
  LITE protocol
Lite Blade
liter
  millimoles per l. (mmol/L)
  l. per minute (Lpm)
  l. per minute per meter squared
    (Lpm/m^2)
lithium
  l. carbonate
  l. hydride
  l. iodine (LiI)
  l. iodine battery
lithium-powered pacemaker
lithomyxoma
  cardiac l.
Litten
  L. diaphragm sign
  L. phenomenon
Little disease
Littman
  L. class II pediatric stethoscope
  L. defibrillation pad
Litwak left atrial-aortic bypass
LIVC
  left inferior vena cava
livedo
  l. reticularis
  l. vasculitis

livedoid dermatitis
liver
> cardiac l.
> cirrhosis of l.
> cyanotic atrophy of l.
> l. flap
> l. function test (LFT)
> l. palm
> right triangular ligament of l.
> l. shadow
> l. X receptor

lives (*pl. of* life)
Livewire
> L. TC Compass ablation catheter
> L. TC steerable electrophysiology
> catheter

livida
> asphyxia l.

Livierato
> L. reflex
> L. sign
> L. test

living
> activities of daily l.
> impairment of activities of daily l.
> (IADL)
> instrumental activities of daily l.
> (IADL)
> l. related transplant (LRT)
> l. with heart failure (LIhFE)

lixivaptan
LL
> lesion length
> lipoprotein lipase

LLD
> lead locking device

LLL
> left lower lobe

L-looping of ventricle
LLPV
> left lower pulmonary vein

LLVP
> left lateral ventricular preexcitation

LM
> left main
> left marginal
> left median
> LM coronary artery

LMA
> laryngeal mask airway
> left main artery
> LMA CTrach mask
> LMA Fastrach

LMA-Unique laryngeal mask
LMC
> left main coronary
> LMC artery
> LMC disease

LMCA
> left main coronary artery

LMCAD
> left main coronary artery disease

LMCAO
> left marginal coronary artery occlusion

LMD
> left main disease
> low molecular weight dextran

LMI
> lateral medullary infarction
> lateral myocardial infarction

LMP1
> latent membrane protein-1

LMS
> left main stem
> LMS coronary artery

LMS-CAD
> left main stem coronary artery disease

LMWH
> low molecular weight heparin

L-NAME
> N^G-nitro-L-arginine methyl ester

L-NMMA
> N^G-monomethyl-L-arginine

LNOP YI Multisite SpO$_2$ reusable sensor
load
> chronic volume l.
> elastic l.
> electronic pacemaker l.
> end-diastolic l. (EDL)
> exercise l.
> heat l.
> inelastic l.
> inspiratory threshold l. (ITL)
> whole-body amyloid l.

loaded breathing test (LBT)
load-induced cardiac hypertrophy
loading
> bretylium l.
> discontinuous incremental
> threshold l.
> glycogen l.
> incremental threshold l.
> inspiratory l.
> methionine l.
> rapid fluid l.
> relaxation l.
> saline l.
> volume l.

lobar
> l. atelectasis
> l. bronchus
> l. collapse
> l. emphysema
> l. infiltrate
> l. pneumonia
> l. torsion

L

lobares
    bronchi l.
lobe
    azygos l.
    dependent l.
    inferior frontal l. (IFL)
    inferior parietal/superior temporal l. (IPSTL)
    left lower l. (LLL)
    left upper l. (LUL)
    lower l.
    middle l.
    nonprimary l.
    right lower l. (RLL)
    right middle l. (RML)
    right upper l. (RUL)
    side l.
    superior l.
    upper l.
lobectomize
lobectomy
    sleeve l.
    video-assisted thoracic surgical non-rib-spreading l. (VNSSL)
lobeline sulfate
lobular
    l. capillary hemangioma
    l. consolidation
    l. hematoma
    l. pneumonia
lobule
    pulmonary l.
    secondary pulmonary l.
    superior parietal l. (SPL)
lobus
    l. azygos pulmonis dextri
    l. dexter
    l. medius pulmonis dextri
local
    l. anesthetic
    l. asphyxia
    l. intravascular coagulation (LIC)
    l. organ procurement area
    l. reaction
    l. syncope
    l. thrombotic response
LocaLisa technique
localization
    anatomic l.
    sonomicrometry array l.
localized
    l. mediastinal lymph node hyperplasia
    l. obstructive emphysema
    l. pericarditis
    l. sacculation
LocalMed
    L. catheter infusion sleeve
    L. InfusaSleeve

location
    anteroposterior paddle l.
loci (*pl. of* locus)
lock
    L. Clamshell device
    heparin l. (HL)
    l. pericardiocentesis set and tray
Lock-A-Card
locking
    l. device
    l. stylet
LOCM
    low osmolality contrast material
    low osmolality contrast media
locoregional radiotherapy
locular cyst
loculated
    l. cyst
    l. emphysema
    l. empyema
    l. pericardial effusion
    l. pericardial hematoma
loculation
    intrapleural l.
locus, pl. **loci**
    l. ceruleus
    chymase gene l.
    genetic l.
    quantitative trait l. (QTL)
Lode BV Excalibur braked cycle ergometer
Loeffler (*var. of* Löffler)
Loesche classification
lofexidine
Löffler, Loeffler
    L. bacillus
    L. disease
    L. endocardial fibrosis
    L. parietal fibroplastic endocarditis
    L. pneumonia
    L. syndrome
Löfgren syndrome
Lo-Fold balloon
logarithm
    natural l.
logarithmic
    l. dynamic range
    l. phonocardiograph
logic
    L. coronary stent
    L. drug-eluting stent
Lohlein-Baehr lesion
Lombardi sign
lomefloxacin hydrochloride
lomustine
London
    L. School of Hygiene Cardiovascular Rose Questionnaire

L. School of Hygiene and Tropical medicine sphygmomanometer

lone atrial fibrillation

long

l. ACE fixed-wire balloon catheter
l. acting (LA, L.A.)
l. axial oblique view
l. axis (LAX)
l. axis-discrete subaortic stenosis (LAX-DSS)
L. Bare Stent Registry
L. Brite Tip guiding catheter
l. dissection
l. iliac artery occlusion
l. lesion
l. PP interval
l. pulse
l. QT (LQT)
l. QT1 (LQT1)
l. QT2 (LQT2)
l. QT arrhythmia
l. QT interval
l. QT syndrome (LQTS)
l. QTU syndrome
l. skinny over-the-wire balloon catheter
l. taper/stiff shaft Glidewire

long-acting

l.-a. beta-2 agonist bronchodilator (LABA)
l.-a. beta-antagonist
l.-a. nitrate
l.-a. quaternary ammonium antimuscarinic agent
Sinex L.-a.

long-axis

l.-a. fractional shortening (LAFS)
l.-a. parasternal view echocardiogram
l.-a. shortening velocity
l.-a. view

longbeachae

Legionella l.

Longdwel Teflon catheter

long-echo-train-length fast-spin-echo imaging

long-ETL FSE imaging

longitudinal

l. analysis
l. arteriography
l. dissociation
l. midline incision
l. narrowing
l. relaxation time

long-leg venography technique

Longmire valvotomy

long-term

l.-t. care (LTC)
l.-t. care facility

l.-t. electrocardiography (LT-ECG)
l.-t. oxygen therapy (LTOT)

long-time recording

Loniten Oral

loop

atrial vector l.
bulboventricular l.
cine l.
clockwise l.
D l.
l. diuresis
l. diuretic
elliptical l.
exercise tidal flow-volume l. (ETFVL)
flow volume l. (FVL)
Gerdy intraauricular l.
guidewire l.
heart l.
Henle l.
L l.
Lissajou l.
maximum flow-volume l. (MFVL)
maxi-vessel l.'s
memory l.
l. monitor
P l.
postexercise flow volume l.
pressure-volume l.
QRS l.
reentrant l.
rigid monopolar l.
sewing ring l.
T l.
tidal l.
tidal flow volume l. (TFVL)
T-wave l.
U l.
Uresil radiopaque silicone band vessel l.'s
U-shaped catheter l.
vector l.
ventricular pressure-volume l.
video l.
volume l.

loose

l. connective tissue
l. elephant trunk
l. junction

Lopid

Lopressor

Lo-Profile II catheter

Lo-Pro tracheal tube

Lorabid

loracarbef

loratadine

lorazepam

lorcainide

Lorcet Plus

Lore-Lawrence trachea tube
Lortat-Jacob approach
LOS
　　length of stay
　　low cardiac output syndrome
losartan
　　l. and hydrochlorothiazide
　　l. potassium
　　l. potassium/hydrochlorothiazide
loss, pl. **losses**
　　age-related bone l.
　　bone l.
　　l. of capture
　　l. of consciousness
　　cortical volume l.
　　l. of future plans
　　l. of independence
　　l. of role
　　signal l.
　　succession of losses
　　volume l.
Lotensin HCT
lotion
　　reactive skin decontamination l.
　　(RSDL)
lotrafiban
Lotrel
Louis
　　L. angle
　　L. law
Louisiana pneumonia
lovastatin
Lovenox injection
Loven reflex
low
　　l. blood pressure (LBP)
　　l. cardiac output (LCO)
　　l. cardiac output syndrome (LCOS,
　　LOS)
　　l. cholesterol
　　l. energy all-purpose (LEAP)
　　l. energy direct current (LEDC)
　　l. fat and cholesterol (LFC)
　　l. molecular weight dextran (LMD)
　　l. molecular weight heparin
　　(LMWH)
　　l. osmolality contrast material
　　(LOCM)
　　l. osmolality contrast media
　　(LOCM)
　　L. Profile Port vascular access
　　l. right atrium (LRA)
　　l. salt syndrome
　　l. septal atrium
　　l. septal right atrium (LSRA)
　　l. setting
　　l. sodium diet
　　l. sodium syndrome

low-amplitude
　　l.-a. cardiac signal
　　l.-a. contraction (LAC)
low-chloride St. Thomas solution
low-density
　　l.-d. lipoprotein (LDL, LDLP)
　　l.-d. lipoprotein apheresis (LDLA)
　　l.-d. lipoprotein-cholesterol complex
　　(LDL-C, LDL-c)
　　l.-d. lipoprotein/high-density
　　lipoprotein (LDL/HDL)
　　l.-d. lipoprotein receptor (LDLR,
　　LDL-R)
　　l.-d. lipoprotein receptor mutation
　　database (LDLR, LDL-R)
low-dose
　　l.-d. bile-acid sequestrant
　　l.-d. dobutamine cine MRI
　　l.-d. heparin (LDH)
　　l.-d. unfractionated heparin (LDUH)
Lowell pleural needle
Löwenberg cuff sign
low-energy
　　l.-e., high-penetration gamma
　　emitter
　　l.-e. intracardiac cardioversion
　　l.-e. laser
　　l.-e. shock
　　l.-e. synchronized cardioversion
Löwenstein-Jensen medium
Löwenstein medium
lower
　　l. airway
　　l. body negative pressure (LBNP)
　　l. chamber
　　l. extremity arterial disease
　　(LEAD)
　　l. extremity bypass graft
　　l. extremity noninvasive (LENI)
　　l. inflection point (LIP)
　　l. lobe
　　l. lobe bronchus
　　l. lobe of lung
　　l. nodal extrasystole
　　l. nodal rhythm
　　l. respiratory tract
　　l. respiratory tract smear
　　l. ribs
　　L. rings
　　l. tubule
lowering
　　antihypertensive and lipid l. (ALL)
Lower-Shumway cardiac transplant
low-esophageal pH probe
low-fat diet
Low-Flex lead
low-flow
　　l.-f. breathing exerciser
　　l.-f. cardiopulmonary bypass (LFB)

l.-f. ischemia
l.-f. rate
low-frequency murmur
low-gradient aortic stenosis (LGAS)
low-intensity treadmill exercise (LITE)
low-methionine diet
low-molecular
Lown
  L. arrhythmia
  L. class 4a, 4b ventricular ectopic beat
  L. classification
  L. grading system
  L. technique
  L. and Woolf method
Lown-Edmark waveform
Lown-Ganong-Levine syndrome
low-output heart failure
low-pass filter
low-pitched murmur
low-plaque coarctation
low-pressure tamponade
low-prime circuitry
low-profile
  l.-p., balloon-expandable stent
  l.-p. balloon-positioning catheter
  l.-p. semi-compliant balloon
low-ramp protocol
low-range heparin management test (LHMT)
low-reflow phenomenon
low-renin essential hypertension (LREH)
low-risk chest pain (LRCP)
low-salt diet
low-speed rotation angioplasty catheter
low-viscosity mucus
lozenge
  horehound l.
Lozide
Lozol
LP, Lp
  lipoprotein
  lung perfusion
  LP stent
LPA
  left pulmonary artery
  lipoprotein A
Lp(a)
  lipoprotein A
LPB, Lp(b)
  lipoprotein B
LPDF
  lipoprotein-deficient fraction
LPE
  lipoprotein electrophoresis
L-phenylalanine mustard
LPIH
  left posterior inferior hemiblock

LPL
  lipoprotein lipase
LPLA
  lipoprotein lipase activity
Lpm
  liter per minute
Lpm/m²
  liter per minute per meter squared
LPS
  late progressing stroke
  lipopolysaccharide
    LPS Peel-Away introducer
LPV
  left portal view
  left pulmonary vein
LPVP
  left posterior ventricular preexcitation
LPX, Lp-X
  lipoprotein X
LQT
  long QT
    LQT syndrome
LQT1
  long QT1
LQT2
  long QT2
LQTS
  long QT syndrome
LRA
  low right atrium
LRC
  lipid research clinic
LRCP
  low-risk chest pain
LREH
  low-renin essential hypertension
LRP
  lipoprotein receptor-related protein
LRT
  living related transplant
LS
  Laron syndrome
  left septum
  Likert scale
L/S
  lecithin/sphingomyelin
    L/S ratio
LSC
  late systolic click
LSCA
  left subclavian artery
L-selectin
LSGB
  left stellate ganglionic blockade
LSM
  late systolic murmur
LSRA
  low septal right atrium

L

LSVC
    left superior vena cava
LT
    lag time
    length-tension curve
    lung transplant
LTB₄
    leukotriene B₄
LTBI
    latent tuberculosis infection
LTC
    long-term care
        LTC facility
LT-ECG
    long-term electrocardiography
LTOT
    long-term oxygen therapy
LTPA
    leisure time physical activity
LTT
    limited treadmill test
LTx
    lung transplant
L-type calcium blocker
lubeluzole
lubricant
        Rotaglide l.
lubricity
Lucas-Championnière disease
lucency
lucent defect
Luciani-Wenckebach atrioventricular block
luciferase reporter phages
lucigenin chemiluminescence assay
Ludwig
        L. angina
        L. angle
Luer-Lok
        L.-L. connector
        L.-L. needle
        L.-L. needle tip
        L.-L. port
Luer tracheal tube
lues
luetic
        l. aneurysm
        l. aortitis
        l. disease
Lufyllin
Lugol solution
Lukens thymus retractor
Luke procedure
LUL
    left upper lobe
Lumax Flex guiding catheter
lumbar
        l. part of diaphragm
        l. sympathectomy

lumbricoides
        Ascaris l.
lumen, pl. **lumina**
        airway l.
        aortic l.
        l. of artery
        bronchial l.
        capillary l.
        conduit l.
        diastolic l.
        double l. (DL)
        esophageal l.
        false l.
        l. finder
        8-l. manometry catheter
        l. mapping
        pharyngeal tracheal l. (PTL)
        pharyngotracheal l. (PTL)
        plaque l.
        single l.
        true l.
        vessel l.
LuMend Frontrunner X39, XP catheter
lumen-intima interface
lumi-aggregometer
        Chrono-log l.-a.
lumina (*pl. of* lumen)
luminal
        l. diameter
        l. encroachment
        l. narrowing
        l. obstruction
        l. recoil
        L. Sodium
        l. widening
luminescence
Luminexx self-expanding stent
luminogram
luminology
        coronary l.
luminometer
lumiracoxib
Lumonics YAG laser
Lunar DPX total body scanner
lunata
        Curvularia l.
Lunderquist
        L. exchange wire
        L. extra-stiff wire guide
lung
        l. abscess
        l. acinus
        aerated l.
        AIDS-related lymphoma of l. (ARLL)
        air conditioner l.
        aluminum l.
        anterior border of l.

anterior descending segmental artery
  of right l.
apex of l.
l. architecture
artificial l.
atrium of l.
azygos lobe of right l.
base of l.
bible printer's l.
l. biopsy
bird breeder's l.
bird fancier's l.
bird handler's l.
black l.
blast l.
l. blood volume (LBV)
book l.
brown induration of l.
l. bud
cadmium l.
l. carcinoma
cardiac impression on l.
cardiac notch of left l.
cheese handler's l.
cheese washer's l.
cheese worker's l.
l. clearance index
coal miner's l.
cobalt l.
coin lesion of l.'s
collapsed l.
collier's l.
l. compliance
consolidation of l.
l. contusion
costal surface of l.
crack l.
cystic disease of l.
decortication of l.
detergent worker's l.
diffusing capacity of l. (DL)
l. diffusion
dirty l.
drowned l.
dynamic compliance of l.
l. dysfunction
edema of l.
l. edema
l. elasticity
l. elastic recoil
l. elastic recoil pressure (Pel)
end-stage l.
l. entrapment
eosinophilic l.
esophageal l.
essential brown induration of l.
farmer's l.
l. fever
fibrocystic l.

fibroid l.
l. fibrosis
l. field
fish meal l.
fissure of l.
flock worker's l.
l. fluke
l. function
furrier's l.
gastric l.
grain handler's l.
harvester's l.
heart and l. (H&L)
hilum of l.
honeycomb l.
honeycombing of l.
horseshoe l.
humidifier l.
hyperlucent l.
l. imaging fluorescence endoscope
  (LIFE)
inferior border of l.
inferior lobe of left/right l.
l. inflation
infundibulum of l.
l. injury
l. injury score (LIS)
interlobar surface of l.
l. interstitium
iron l.
jute worker's l.
Labrador l.
lateral basal segmental artery of
  right l.
left l.
left/right l.
lifeguard l.
lingula of left l.
lower lobe of l.
machine operator's l.
malt-worker's l.
l. marking
mason's l.
l. mass
meat worker's l.
l. mechanics
medial surface of l.
mediastinal part of l.
mesentery of l.
middle lobe of right l.
miller's l.
miner's l.
mold worker's l.
l. morphometry
l. mucociliary clearance
mushroom worker's l.
l. nodule
oblique fissure of l.
paprika splitter's l.

L

lung *(continued)*
l. parenchymal disease
l. parenchymal infection
l. perfusion (LP, Lp)
pigeon breeder's l.
pigeon fancier's l.
pigment induration of l.
pizza l.
polycystic l.
popcorn worker's l.
posterior basal segmental artery of right l.
postperfusion l.
l. protection
pump l.
quiet l.
l. reduction surgery
l. reexpansion
l. region
respirator l.
l. retractor
rheumatoid l.
right l.
right/left l.
root of l.
l. scan
l. scanning
scleroderma l.
shock l.
silo filler's l.
silver finisher's l.
silver polisher's l.
l. sliding
stiff l.
l. stone
superior lobe of right/left l.
thresher's l.
l. tissue destruction
l. transfer capacity
l. transplant (LT, LTx)
transverse fissure of right l.
trapped l.
trench l.
tuberculosis of l.'s
unilateral hyperlucency of l.
unilateral hyperlucent l.
unilateral nonfunctioning l.
l. unit
upper lobe of l.
l. uptake
uremic l.
vanishing l.
vernal edema of l.
vertebral part of costal surface of l.
vineyard sprayer's l.
l. volume
l. volume recruitment
l. volume reduction
l. volume reduction surgery (LVRS)
l. volume strategy
l. washing
l. water
welder's l.
wet l.
white l.
wood pulp worker's l.
LungAlert test
lunger
chronic l.
lung-liver interaction
Lungmotor
lung-to-finger circulation time (LFCT)
lung-to-heart (L/H)
lung-wall interface
lungworm
lunula, pl. **lunulae**
lupoid
Lupron
L. Depot
L. Depot-Ped
lupus
l. anticoagulant
l. anticoagulant disorder
cerebral l.
l. erythematosus (LE)
l. pernio
l. pleuritis
lupus-associated valve disease
lupus-like syndrome
LUPV
left upper pulmonary vein
Lurselle
Luschka
L. cartilage
foramen of L.
L. tonsil
lusitaniae
Candida l.
lusitropic
l. abnormality
l. effect
lusitropy
lusoria
dysphagia l.
Lutembacher
L. complex
L. syndrome
lutetium
motexafin l.
l. texaphyrin
Lutz-Splendore-Almeida disease
Luxtec fiberoptic system
LV
left ventricle
left ventricular
LV end-diastolic diameter

LVA
  left ventricular aneurysm
  left vertebral artery
LVAD
  left ventricular assist device
    HeartMate LVAD
    Novacor LVAD
    vented-electric HeartMate LVAD
LVAS
  left ventricular assist system
    HeartMate SNAP-VE LVAS
LVBP
  left ventricular bypass pump
LVCT
  left ventricular cardiac tamponade
LVD
  left ventricular dysfunction
LVDd
  left ventricular dimension in end-diastole
LVDI
  left ventricular dimension
LVDP
  left ventricular developed pressure
  left ventricular diastolic pressure
  left ventricular diastolic volume
LVDV
  left ventricular diastolic volume
LVE
  left ventricular ejection
  left ventricular enlargement
LVED
  left ventricular end-diastole
LVEDA
  left ventricular end-diastolic area
LVEDC
  left ventricular end-diastolic
    circumference
LVEDD
  left ventricular end-diastolic diameter
  left ventricular end-diastolic dimension
LVEDP
  left ventricular end-diastolic pressure
LVEDV
  left ventricular end-diastolic volume
LVEF
  left ventricular ejection fraction
LVEJT
  left ventricular ejection time
LVEP
  left ventricular end-diastolic pressure
LVESD
  left ventricular end-systolic dimension
LVESV
  left ventricular end-systolic volume
LVESWS
  left ventricular end-systolic wall stress
LVET
  left ventricular ejection time

LVETI
  left ventricular ejection time index
LVF
  left ventricular failure
  left ventricular function
LVFP
  left ventricular filling pressure
LV-gram
  left ventriculogram
LVH
  left ventricular hypertrophy
LVI
  large-vessel infarction
  left ventricular insufficiency
  left ventricular ischemia
LVID
  left ventricular internal dimension
LVIDD
  left ventricular internal diastolic diameter
  left ventricular internal diastolic
    dimension
LVIV
  left ventricular infarct volume
LVLG
  left ventrolateral gluteal
LVM
  left ventricular mass
LVMF
  left ventricular minute flow
LVMI
  left ventricular mass index
LVN
  lateral ventricular nerve
LVO
  left ventricle outflow
  left ventricular opacification
LVOH
  left ventricle outflow height
LVOT
  left ventricular outflow tract
LVOTO
  left ventricular outflow tract obstruction
LVP
  left ventricular pressure
LVPFR
  left ventricular peak filling rate
LVPmax
  maximum left ventricular pressure
LVPmin
  minimum left ventricular pressure
LVPW
  left ventricular posterior wall
LVR
  left ventricular reduction
LVRS
  lung volume reduction surgery
LVS
  left ventricular strain

L

LVSB
    leftward ventricular septal bowing
LVSD
    left ventricular systolic dimension
LVSEMI
    left ventricular subendocardial
        myocardial ischemia
LVSI
    left ventricular systolic index
LVSO
    left ventricular systolic output
LVSP
    left ventricular systolic pressure
LVSV
    left ventricular stroke volume
LVSVI
    left ventricular stroke volume index
LVSW
    left ventricular stroke work
LVSWI
    left ventricular stroke work index
LVT
    left ventricular tension
LVV
    left ventricular volume
    LeVeen valve
LVW
    left ventricular wall
    left ventricular work
LVWI
    left ventricular work index
LVWM
    left ventricular wall motion
LVWT
    left ventricular wall thickness
LW
    lateral wall
lwoffi
    Acinetobacter l.
lycopene
Lycoperdon
lycoperdonosis
lycopodium asthma
LYG
    lymphomatoid granulomatosis
Lyme
    L. borreliosis
    L. disease
    L. titer
lymph
    l. node
    l. node hyperplasia
lymphadenitis
    tuberculous l.
lymphadenopathy
    fixed l.
    hilar l.
    ipsilateral hilar l.
    matted l.

lymphangiectasis
    chronic pulmonary cystic l.
lymphangioendothelioma
lymphangioleiomyomatosis (LAM)
    pulmonary l.
lymphangioma
lymphangiomatosis
    diffuse pulmonary l.
    pulmonary l.
lymphangiomyomatosis
    pulmonary l.
lymphangitic
    l. carcinoma
    l. carcinomatosis (LC)
    l. spread
lymphangitis carcinomatosa
Lymphapress compression therapy
lymphatic
    l. channel
    l. dilation
    l. edema
    obtuse marginal l.
    subclavian l.
lymphatici
    hilum nodi l.
lymphedema praecox
lymphocyte
    l. chemoattractant factor (LCF)
    l. concentration
    effusion-associated l.
    l. immune globulin
    T l.
    l. transformation test
lymphocytic
    l. alveolar inflammation
    l. alveolitis
    l. infiltrative disorder
    l. interstitial pneumonitis (LIP)
    l. tracheobronchitis
lymphoepithelioma-like carcinoma
lymphogranuloma venereum (LGV)
lymphohematogenous drainage system
lymphoid
    l. alveolitis
    l. hyperplasia
    l. interstitial pneumonia (LIP)
    l. interstitial pneumonia/pulmonary
        lymphoid hyperplasia (LIP/PLH)
    l. interstitial pneumonitis (LIP)
lymphokine
lymphoma
    African Burkitt l.
    AIDS-related l. (ARL)
    B cell l.
    Burkitt l.
    Hodgkin l.
    Kiel classification of l.
    Lennert l.
    mediastinal l.

nodular sclerosing Hodgkin l.
noncleaved cell l.
non-Hodgkin l.
primary effusion l. (PEL)
primary pulmonary non-Hodgkin l.
pulmonary l.
pyothorax-associated l.
lymphomatoid granulomatosis (LYG)
lymphoplasma
lymphoplasmacytic
  l. infiltration
  l. inflammation
lymphoreticular granulomatous vasculitis
lymphosarcoma
lymphotoxin
Lyo-Ject
  Cardizem L.-J.
  L.-J. syringe
Lyon-Horgan procedure
Lyon hypothesis
lyophilization
lyophilize
lyophilized powder
Lyra
  L. 2020 implantable cardioverter
  L. 2020 implantable cardioverter-
    defibrillator
  L. laser system

lysate
lyse
lysed artery
lysine acetylsalicylate
lysine-binding site
lysis
  clot l.
  dilute blood clot l. (DBCL)
  euglobin clot l. (ECL)
  myofibrillar l.
  spontaneous l.
  l. time
Lysodren
lysophosphatidic acid
lysophosphatidylcholine scavenger
lysophospholipase
lysosomal
  l. enzyme
  l. hydrolase
lysosome
lysozyme
lys-plasminogen
  recombinant l.-p.
Lyssavirus
lysyl-bradykinin
lytic bend
LZT
  lead/zirconium/titanium

L

M
  murmur
    M cell layer
    Hemofil M
    M lignocaine
    M lines
    M pattern on right atrial waveform
    M protein
M1
  mitral component
M₁
  mitral first sound
M2
  marked dullness
    M2 receptor dysfunction
M₂
  mitral second sound
M3
  absolute dullness
M6/C cylinder carrying case
M6 oxygen cylinder
m7E3 Fab
MA
  malignant arrhythmia
  mixed apnea
  mounting area
mA
  milliampere
MAA
  macroaggregated albumin
  mandibular advancement appliance
    MAA perfusion lung scintigraphy
MABP
  mean arterial blood pressure
MAC
  malignancy-associated change
  membrane attack complex
  minimal alveolar concentration
  mitral anular calcification
  multiaccess catheter
  Mycobacterium avium complex
    MAC infection
MAC-1
  beta-2 integrin MAC-1
MacCallum patch
MACE
  main adverse coronary event
  major adverse cardiac event
Macewen sign
Mach
    M. band
    M. effect
Machado-Guerreiro test
Machida fiberoptic laryngoscope

machine
    Apogee CX 100 Interspec
      ultrasound m.
    Burdick ECG m.
    bypass m.
    cardiac ultrasound m.
    Century heart-lung m.
    Cobe-Stöckert heart-lung m.
    Corometrics-Aloka
      echocardiograph m.
    echocardiograph m.
    G5 massage and percussion m.
    heart-lung m.
    Hewlett-Packard 500, 1000 Echo-
      Doppler m.
    May-Gibbon heart-lung m.
    m. operator's lung
    Opticon real-time PCR m.
    Respironics CPAP m.
    Respitrace m.
    Sullivan V Elite Real Time Clock
      CPAP m.
    Toshiba electrocardiography m.
    ultrasound m.
    Vivid 7 cardiac ultrasound m.
machinery murmur
Macintosh
    M. blade
    M. laryngoscope
Mackenzie polygraph
Mackler tube
Macleod syndrome
macroaggregated
    m. albumin (MAA)
    m. albumin perfusion lung
      scintigraphy
macroangiopathy
    coronary m.
Macrobid
macrocardia
macrocyclic lactone
Macrodantin
macroembolus, pl. **macroemboli**
macroglobulin
    alpha-2 m.
macroglobulinemia
    Waldenström m.
macroglossia
macrolide
    m. antibiotic
    m. antimicrobial
    m. antimicrobial agent
macromolecular
    m. cell injury
    m. ligand

M

macromolecule
macrophage
    alveolar m.
    foamy m.
    hemosiderin-laden m.
    m. inflammatory protein (MIP)
    m. inflammatory protein-1 (MIP-1)
    lipid-laden m.
    monocyte-derived m.
    tissue-infiltrating m. (TIM)
macrophage-derived foam cell
macroreentrant
    m. atrial tachycardia
    m. circuit
macrosteatosis
macrovascular
    m. artery disease
    m. coronary lesion
MACS
    maximum aortic cusp separation
Mac stent
macula, pl. **maculae**
    m. albida
    m. lactea
    m. tendinea
macular arteriole inferior
maculopapular rash
MAC-VU electrocardiograph
MAD
    mandibular advancement device
MadCAM-1
    mucosal addressin cell adhesion
    molecule-1
MADIT II criteria
MADRS
    Montgomery-Asberg Depression Rating
    Scale
Maestro implantable cardiac pacemaker
MAF
    maximum atrial fragmentation
MAG
    Minnesota antilymphocyte globulin
Magellan monitor
magic
    M. Torque guidewire
    M. Wallstent
    M. Wallstent stent
Magill
    M. forceps
    M. laryngoscope
    M. Safety Clear Plus endotracheal
    tube
magna
    arteria anastomotica auricularis m.
    auricularis m.
Magnascanner
    Picker M.
magnesium
    m. carbonate ($MgCO_3$)

    m. deficiency
    intracellular m.
    m. oxide
    m. salicylate
    serum m.
    m. sulfate
    m. sulfate heptahydrate
    m. supplementation
magnet
    m. application over pulse generator
    m. check
    m. inhibition
    m. pacing interval
    Philips Medical Systems 1.5-T
    Intera m.
    m. rate
    m. wire
magnetic
    m. heart vector (MHV)
    m. moment
    m. relaxation time
    m. resonance angiography (MRA)
    m. resonance coil
    m. resonance coronary angiography
    (MRCA)
    m. resonance flowmetry (MRF)
    m. resonance imaging (MRI)
    m. resonance signal
    m. resonance spectography
    m. resonance spectroscopy (MRS)
    m. resonance venography (MRV)
    m. source imaging (MSI)
    m. valve resistor
magnetite pneumoconiosis
magnetization
    spatial modulation of m. (SPAMM)
    m. technique
magnetocardiogram (MCG)
    vector m. (VMCG)
magnetocardiograph (MC)
magnetocardiography (MC)
    fetal m. (FMCG)
Magnevist
magnification
magnitude
    average pulse m.
    peak m.
Magnolia biondii
Magnum guidewire
magnus
    pulsus m.
Mag-Ox 400
Mahaim
    M. bundle
    M. fiber
Mahaim-type tachycardia
Mahalanobis distance
Maharishi Vedic medicine

Mahler
  M. Baseline Dyspnea Index
    questionnaire
  M. sign
mahogany flush
MAI
  movement arousal index
  Mycobacterium avium-intracellulare
  MAI complex
  MAI infection
MAIC
  Mycobacterium avium-intracellulare
    complex
Maillard reaction
Mailman coronary guidewire
main
  m. adverse coronary event (MACE)
  m. bundle
  left m. (LM)
  m. portal vein (MPV)
  m. pulmonary artery (MPA)
  m. renal vein
  unprotected left m. (ULM)
mainstem
  m. bronchus
  m. coronary artery
  m. intubation
mainstream smoke (MS)
maintained
  adequate hemostasis m.
maintenance
  m. regimen
  m. of wakefulness test (MWT)
major
  m. adverse cardiac event (MACE)
  m. aortopulmonary collateral artery
    (MAPCA)
  Babesia m.
  m. coronary artery (MCA)
  ductus sublingualis m.
  m. fissure
  pectoralis m.
malabsorption
maladie de Roger
malaise
malar flush
malaria
malariae
  Plasmodium m.
malarial pneumonitis
malayi
  Brugia m.
maleate
  azatadine m.
  chlorpheniramine m.
  dexchlorpheniramine m.
  enalapril m.
  ergonovine m.
  methysergide m.

  nomifensine m.
  timolol m.
  trimipramine m.
male pattern obesity
malformation
  angiographically occult intracranial
    vascular m. (AOIVM)
  arteriovenous m. (AVM)
  atrioventricular m. (AVM)
  cardiac m.
  congenital adenomatoid m.
  congenital cardiovascular m.
    (CCVM)
  congenital cystic adenomatoid m.
  conotruncal heart m. (CTHM)
  cystic adenomatoid m.
  dancer's foot m.
  dural arteriovenous m. (DAVM)
  Ebstein m.
  isolated cardiovascular m. (ICM)
  Mondini pulmonary
    arteriovenous m.
  neural crest m.
  pulmonary arteriovenous m.
    (PAVM)
  Taussig-Bing m.
  Uhl m.
malfunction
  pacemaker m.
Malgaigne fossa
malignancy, pl. **malignancies**
  cutaneous m.
  de novo m.
  m. and low molecular weight
    heparin therapy (MALT)
  mesenchymal m.
  non-AIDS-defining m.
  posttransplantation m.
  primary cardiac m.
malignancy-associated
  m.-a. change (MAC)
  m.-a. phlebitis
malignant
  m. arrhythmia (MA)
  m. beat
  m. carcinoid syndrome
  m. endocarditis
  m. fibrous histiocytoma (MFH)
  m. hypertension (MH)
  m. melanoma
  m. middle cerebral artery infarction
    (mMCAI)
  m. pleural effusion (MPE)
  m. pleural mesothelioma (MPM)
  m. superior vena caval syndrome
  m. SVC syndrome
  m. thrombocytopenia
  m. thymoma
  m. vasovagal syndrome

M

malignant *(continued)*
    m. ventricular arrhythmia (MVA)
    m. ventricular tachyarrhythmia
    m. ventricular tachycardia
malinger
malingerer
Mallampati
    M. airway classification I-IV
    M. score
Mallampati-Samsoon airway classification I-IV
mall asthma
malleable retractor
Mallergan-VC with Codeine
Mallinckrodt
    M. angiographic catheter
    M. cuffed endotracheal tube
    M. Hi-Care Pulmonary Hygiene system
    M. radioimmunoassay
Mallory stain
Mallory-Weiss
    M.-W. syndrome
    M.-W. tear
malmoense
    Mycobacterium m.
malnutrition
    alcoholic m.
    kwashiorkor-like m.
    myocardial m.
    protein-calorie m.
malondialdehyde (MDA)
    m. level
    m. modified low-density lipoprotein (MDA-LDL)
Maloney mercury-filled esophageal dilator
malonylaldehyde
malonyl-CoA
    malonylcoenzyme A
malonylcoenzyme A (malonyl-CoA)
malperfused segment
malperfusion phenomenon
malpighian vesicle
malposition
    crisscross heart m.
    double-outlet left ventricle m.
    double-outlet right ventricle m.
    m. of great arteries (MGA)
    levocardia m.
    mesocardia m.
    single ventricle m.
MALT
    malignancy and low molecular weight heparin therapy
maltase deficiency
Malteno valve
maltophilia
    Pseudallescheria m.

    Pseudomonas m.
    Stenotrophomonas m.
    Xanthomonas m.
malt-worker's lung
malum cordis
MAM-B
    mammaglobin B
mammaglobin B (MAM-B)
mammary
    m. artery
    m. artery graft
    internal m. (IM)
    m. souffle
    m. souffle murmur
    m. souffle sound
    m. vessel
man, pl. **men**
    radiation equivalent in m. (rem)
management
    invasive m.
    postprocedural m.
    real-time position m. (RPM)
    ventilator m.
manager
    cardiological workspace m. (CWM)
mandatory
    m. minute ventilation
    m. minute volume (MMV)
    synchronized intermittent m.
mandibular
    m. advancement appliance (MAA)
    m. advancement device (MAD)
    m. plane
    m. plane to hyoid (MP-H)
mandibulopharyngeal
mandrel, mandril
    m. graft
mandrin
maneuver
    Addison m.
    Adson m.
    breathhold m.
    cold pressor testing m.
    costoclavicular m.
    Ejrup m.
    forced expiratory m.
    head-tilt, chin-lift m.
    Heimlich m.
    hemodynamic m.
    Hillis-Müller m.
    hyperventilation m.
    jaw-thrust/head-tilt m.
    Jonnson m.
    Lecompte m.
    Mattox m.
    Miller m.
    modified Miller m. (MM)
    Müller m.
    nonpanting m.

panting m.
peak expiratory m.
Sellick m.
submaximal m.
Valsalva m. (VM)
maneuverability
manganese superoxide dismutase (Mn-SOD)
manidipine
manifest
m. ischemia
Morse m.
m. vector
manifold
manipulation
catheter m.
manmade vitreous fiber (MMVF)
mannequin
manner
Creech m.
m. of Creech
m. of DeBakey
DeBakey-Creech m.
Mannkopf sign
manofluorography (MFG)
manometer
aneroid m.
Dinamap ultrasound blood
pressure m.
Hürthle m.
Mercury medical airway
pressure m.
Posey Cufflator tracheal cuff
inflator and m.
single-patient use m.
manometer-tipped catheter
manometry
esophageal m.
Mansfield
M. balloon
M. bioptome
M. orthogonal electrode catheter
M. Polaris electrode
M. Scientific dilation balloon
catheter
M. Valvoplasty Registry
Mansfield-Webster catheter
mansoni
Schistosoma m.
Mantoux test
manual
M. defibrillator
M. edge detection
M. resuscitation baffle
M. resuscitation bag
M. ventilation
manubrium

MAO
monoamine oxidase
MAO inhibitor
MAOI
monoamine oxidase inhibitor
MAP
mean airway pressure
mean aortic pressure
mean arterial pressure
minimum audible pressure
mitogen-activated protein
monophasic action potential
map
electroanatomical m.
linear local shortening m.
maximum voltage m.
polar coordinate m.
MAPC
multipotent adult progenitor cell
MAPCA
major aortopulmonary collateral artery
MAPD
monophasic action potential duration
MAPK
mitogen-activated protein kinase
MAPK pathway
maple bark disease
mapping
m. and ablation electrophysiology
catheter
activation sequence m.
advanced cardiac m.
atrial activation m.
Biosense left ventricular m.
body surface Laplacian m. (BSLM)
bull's-eye polar coordinate m.
cardiac m.
Carto electroanatomical m.
m. catheter
catheter m.
cavotricuspid isthmus m.
color-coded flow m.
color flow m.
digital phase m. (DPM)
Doppler color flow m. (DCFM)
electrically unexcitable scar m.
electroanatomical m.
electromagnetic m.
electromechanical left ventricular m.
electrophysiologic m.
endocardial m.
endoepicardial m.
entrainment m.
EP m.
flow m.
high-density electroanatomical and
entrainment m.
ice m.
intracardiac m.

M

447

mapping *(continued)*
    intraoperative m.
    Laplacian m.
    lumen m.
    moving slice velocity m.
    MRI velocity m.
    multisite m.
    noncontact endocardial m.
    pulsed myocardial Doppler m.
    pulsed-wave Doppler m.
    retrograde atrial activation m.
    Revelation microcatheter for EP m.
    simultaneous catheter m.
    sinus rhythm m.
    spectral temporal m.
    spectral turbulence m.
    tachycardia pathway m.
    ventricular m.
mapping/ablation catheter
maprotiline
MAQOL
    Mini Asthma Quality of Life
    MAQOL questionnaire
Maquet Servoi ventilator
MAR
    mean atrial rate
    MAR algorithm
marantic
    m. endocarditis
    m. thrombosis
    m. thrombus
marasmic
    m. thrombosis
    m. thrombus
marasmus
Marathon guiding catheter
Marax bronchodilator
Marbach-Weil technique
Marburg virus
marcescens
    Serratia m.
Marcillin
Marek disease
Marey law
Marfan syndrome
margarine
    Benecol m.
    sitostanol ester m.
Margesic H
margin
    costal m.
    dotuse m.
    rib m.
    right costal m. (RCM)
    safety m.
marginal
    m. artery of colon
    m. artery of Drummond
    m. branch #1

    m. branch of circumflex artery
    first obtuse m. (OM1)
    left m. (LM)
    obtuse m.
    m. rale
    second obtuse m. (OM2)
marginatum
    erythema m.
margo
    m. anterior pulmonis
    m. inferior pulmonis
Marie-Bamberger syndrome
Marie syndrome
marine oil
Marinol
marinum
    Mycobacterium m.
Marion-Clatworthy side-to-end vena caval shunt
mark
    alignment m.
    M. IV respiratory pacemaker
    M. VII cooling vest
    M. V ProVis injection system
marked dullness (M2)
marker
    m. annotation
    breath m.
    cardiac m.
    m. catheter
    CD63 platelet activation m.
    CD62p (p-selectin) platelet activation m.
    m. channel
    CYFRA 21-1 tumor m.
    dual m.
    gold m.
    inflammatory m.
    lead-letter m.
    neuroendocrine m.
    plaque m.
    platinum radiopaque m.
    predictive survival m.
    radiopaque end m.
    serum m.
    tantalum myocardial m.
    tumor m.
    vein graft ring m.
marking
    bronchial m.
    bronchovesicular m.
    interstitial m.
    lung m.
    perihilar m.
    pulmonary vascular m.
    vascular m.
Markov process
Marlex mesh

marmorata
    cutis m.
marneffei
    Penicillium m.
Maroteaux-Lamy syndrome
Marpres
Marquest Respirgard II nebulizer
Marquette
    M. 3-channel laser Holter
    M. Case-12 electrocardiographic
      system
    M. Case-12 exercise system
    M. electrocardiograph
    M. 8000 Holter monitor
    M. Holter recorder
    M. Responder 1500 multifunctional
      defibrillator
    M. Series 8000 Holter analyzer
    M. treadmill
Marriott method
Marshall
    M. bundle
    M. fold
    M. ligament
    M. oblique vein
marsupialization
Marsupial Pouch postsurgical drain
  holder
Martorell syndrome
Mary Allen Engle ventricle
MAS
    meconium aspiration syndrome
    mesoatrial shunt
    Motor Assessment Scale
Masimo Set
mask
    Accurox m.
    ACE detachable m.
    AeroChamber m.
    aerosol m.
    air entrainment m.
    AirMed m.
    Ambu Res-Cue m.
    Bili m.
    BLB oxygen m.
    Boothby-Lovelace-Bulbulian
      oxygen m.
    ComfortSeal m.
    EasiVent valved holding
      chamber m.
    ecchymotic m.
    GoldSeal nasal m.
    high-concentration oxygen m.
    intubating laryngeal airway m.
      (ILMA)
    IQ nasal m.
    Kuhn m.
    LMA CTrach m.
    LMA-Unique laryngeal m.

    meter m.
    MiniMe nasal m.
    Mirage nasal m.
    Nasal-Aire ventilator nasal
      insert m.
    Nic the Asthmatic Dragon pediatric
      aerosol m.
    nonrebreather m.
    nonrebreathing m.
    oxygen m.
    partial rebreathing m.
    PEP m.
    Phantom nasal m.
    rebreathing m.
    Rendell-Baker face m.
    Rudolph Full Face m.
    SCRAM face m.
    Series 7900 mouth breathing
      face m.
    Series 8900 nasal and mouth
      breathing face m.
    shovel m.
    SleepNet IQ nasal m.
    Sullivan Mirage nasal m.
    thermoplastic head m.
    Ultimate nasal m.
    ventilation m.
    Venturi m.
masked hypertension
mask-mode
    m.-m. cardiac imaging
    m.-m. subtraction
Mason-Likar
    M.-L. 12-lead ECG system
    M.-L. limb lead modification
    M.-L. placement of ECG lead
mason's lung
Mason Sones transbrachial technique
masquerader
mass
    achromatic m.
    cardiac m.
    echodense m.
    echogenic m.
    m. effect
    false m.
    fat-free m. (FFM)
    fibrotic m.
    fungating m.
    intracardiac m.
    intracavitaryy m.
    intravascular m. (IVM)
    left ventricular m. (LVM)
    lung m.
    m. median aerodynamic diameter
      (MMAD)
    mediastinal m.
    myocardial m.
    pleural m.

M

mass *(continued)*
    posterior mediastinal m.
    ventricular m.
massage
    cardiac m.
    carotid sinus m.
    closed chest cardiac m.
    direct cardiac m.
    external cardiac m. (ECM)
    heart m.
    open chest cardiac m.
    vapor m.
mass-flow anemometer
Massier solution
massive
    m. aspiration
    m. collapse
    m. hemoptysis
    m. pneumonia
    m. thrombus
Masson
    M. body
    M. trichrome stain
MAST
    military antishock trousers
    MAST suit
mast
    m. cell
    m. cell high-affinity Fc receptor
    m. cell inhibitor
    m. cell protease
    m. cell stabilizer
Mastadenovirus
master
    change description m. (CDM)
    M. exercise stress test
    M. Flow Pumpette pump
    M. 2-step exercise test
MasterLab Pro pneumotachograph
    spirometer
MasterScreen BabyBody plethysmograph
mastocytosis syndrome
MAT
    multifocal atrial tachycardia
Matas
    M. aneurysmectomy
    M. test
match defect
matching
    afterload m.
    ventilation/perfusion m.
material
    antimicrobial polymer m.
    bioabsorbable polymeric m. (BPM)
    Carbo-Seal graft m.
    contrast m.
    Duralyn balloon m.
    embolized foreign m.
    fibrinohematic m.

    Fulcrum balloon m.
    Haynes 25 m.
    Hexabrix contrast m.
    Kaltostat wound packing m.
    Kifa catheter m.
    low osmolality contrast m.
     (LOCM)
    Myoview contrast m.
    nonionic contrast m.
    Solutrast contrast m.
    vasodepressor m. (VDEM, VDM)
    vasoexcitor m. (VEM)
    Zenotech graft m.
maternal heart rate (MHR)
maternally inherited cardiomyopathy
matrices (*pl. of* matrix)
Matrigel
matrilysin (MMP 7)
matrix, pl. **matrices**
    biological fibrous m.
    m. collagen
    extracellular m. (ECM)
    m. metalloproteinase (MMP)
    m. metalloproteinase activity
    m. metalloproteinase-9 assay
    m. metalloproteinase inhibitor
     (MMPI)
    m. mode
    myocardial collagen m.
    subendothelial m.
    m. synthesis
    vascular m.
    M. VSG sealing device
    M. VSG system
matrix-array ultrasound
matrix-degrading
    m.-d. neutral metalloproteinase
    m.-d. neutral MMP
Matson-Alexander rib stripper
Matson rib elevator
Matsuda titanium surgical instrument
matted lymphadenopathy
matter
    Patient-Oriented Evidence that M.'s
     (POEM)
    respirable particular m.
    white m. (WM)
Mattox
    M. aorta clamp
    M. maneuver
mattress
    eggcrate m.
    hypothermia m.
    Roho m.
    m. suture
    TheraKair m.
maturation
    affinity m.

MAVD
    mixed aortic valve disease
maverick
    M. balloon
    M. balloon dilation catheter
    m. 2 Monorail m.
    M. OTW catheter
Mavik
MAVIS
    mobile artery and vein imaging system
MAVR
    mitral and aortic valve replacement
max
    maximum
Maxair Inhalation Aerosol
Maxaquin Oral
MaxEPA
MaxForce balloon dilation catheter
Maxi LD PTA dilation catheter
Maxilith pacemaker pulse generator
maxillomandibular
    m. advancement (MMA)
    m. advancement procedure
    m. osteotomy (MMO)
maximal
    m. breathing capacity
    m. exercise systolic pressure (MESP)
    m. exercise test (MET)
    m. expiratory flow rate (MEFR)
    m. expiratory flow volume (MEFV)
    m. expiratory mouth pressure (P_{Emax})
    m. expiratory pressure (MEP)
    m. flow-volume envelope
    m. forced expiratory flow (FEFmax)
    m. heart rate (Hrmax, MHR)
    m. inspiratory flow rate (MIFR)
    m. inspiratory mouth pressure (P_{Imax})
    m. inspiratory pressure (MIP)
    m. midexpiratory flow (MMEF, MMF)
    m. midexpiratory flow rate (MMEFR)
    m. resistive exercise (MRE)
    m. response plateau (MRP)
    m. sniff-induced esophageal pressure
    m. sniff-induced gastric pressure
    m. sniff-induced transdiaphragmatic pressure
    m. sustainable ventilatory capacity (MSVC)
    m. treadmill stress test (MTST)
    m. treadmill testing (MTT)
    m. velocity (V_{MAX}, Vmax)

    m. ventilation (MV)
    m. ventilation rate (MVR)
    m. vital capacity (MVC)
Maxima Plus plasma resistant fiber oxygenator
maximum (max)
    m. aerobic capacity
    m. aortic cusp separation (MACS)
    m. atrial fragmentation (MAF)
    m. breathing capacity (MBC)
    m. closure pressure (MCP)
    m. contraction pattern (MCP)
    m. determined heart rate (MDHR)
    m. diastolic potential (MDP)
    m. digital pulse (MDP)
    m. exercise tolerance test (METT)
    m. expiratory airflow-static lung elastic recoil pressure
    m. expiratory flow at 50% vital capacity (MEF_{50})
    m. expiratory pressure (MEP)
    m. flow rate
    m. flow static recoil (MFSR)
    m. flow-volume loop (MFVL)
    M. hemostasis introducer
    m. inspiratory pressure (MIP)
    m. left ventricular pressure (LVPmax)
    m. medical therapy
    m. midexpiratory flow rate (MMEF, MMF)
    m. negative potential
    m. oxygen consumption
    m. oxygen uptake
    m. predicted heart rate (MPHR)
    m. pulse rate (MPR)
    m. sensory rate
    m. tolerated dose
    m. transverse thoracic dimension
    m. velocity (V_{MAX}, Vmax)
    m. venous outflow (MVO)
    m. ventricular elastance (Emax)
    m. voltage map
    m. voluntary contraction (MVC)
    m. voluntary ventilation (MVV)
    m. walking time
Maxi-Myst vaporizer
Maxipime
maxi-vessel loops
Maxtec Handi oxygen analyzer
Maxzide
Mayaro virus
Mayer wave
May-Gibbon heart-lung machine
May-Grünwald-Giemsa stain
maynei
    Euroglyphus m.
Mayo
    M. classification

M

Mayo *(continued)*
>   M. exercise treadmill protocol
>   M. hemostat

maze
>   m. ablation
>   m. III surgery
>   m. procedure

Mazicon
mazindol
>   hydrogen-3 m.

MB
>   microbubble
>   myocardial band
>   myocardial bridging
>   MB band
>   MB enzymes of CPK
>   MB fraction
>   MB index

MBA hemostasis valve
MBAR
>   myocardial beta adrenergic receptor

MBC
>   maximum breathing capacity

MBF
>   myocardial blood flow

MBG
>   myocardial blush grade

MBIP
>   model-based image processing

MBP
>   mean arterial blood pressure
>   mean blood pressure

MBq
>   megabecquerel

MBTS
>   modified Blalock-Taussig shunt

MBV
>   mitral balloon valvotomy

MC
>   magnetocardiograph
>   magnetocardiography
>   microcirculation
>   mitral commissurotomy
>   myocardial channeling
>   myocarditis

Mc
>   mitral closure

MCA
>   major coronary artery
>   middle cerebral artery

MCAF
>   monocyte chemotactic and activating
>   factor

MCAO
>   middle cerebral artery occlusion

McArdle
>   M. disease
>   M. syndrome

MCAS modular clip application

MCC
>   microcalcification cluster
>   mucociliary clearance

MCCD
>   minimum cumulative cardiotoxic dose

McCort sign
MCCU
>   mobile coronary care unit

MCD
>   molecular coincidence detection
>   MCD imaging

McDowall reflex
MCE
>   myocardial contrast echocardiography

MCES
>   multiple cholesterol emboli syndrome

MCF
>   myocardial contraction force

MCFSR
>   mean circumferential fiber-shortening
>   rate

MCG
>   magnetocardiogram

McGill
>   M. forceps
>   M. Pain Questionnaire

McGill-Melzack Pain Questionnaire
McGinn-White sign
McGoon
>   M. guidelines
>   M. ratio
>   M. technique

McHenry protocol
MCI
>   mean cardiac index

mCi
>   millicurie

MCICU
>   medical coronary intensive care unit

MCL
>   midclavicular line
>   modified chest lead

McNamara
>   M. protocol
>   M. renal exchange wire guide

McNaught keel
MCP
>   maximum closure pressure
>   maximum contraction pattern
>   monocyte chemoattractant protein
>   mucin clot prevention

MCP-1
>   monocyte chemoattractant protein-1
>   monocyte chemotactic protein-1

McPheeters treatment
MC4-R
>   melanocortin-4 receptor

MCRI
>   multifactorial cardiac risk index

MCSD
   mechanical circulatory support device
MCT
   methylcholine challenge testing
     MCT Oil
MCTD
   mixed connective tissue disease
MCV
   mean corpuscular volume
MD
   mitral disease
   myocardial damage
   myocardial disease
MDA
   malondialdehyde
MDA-LDL
   malondialdehyde modified low-density
     lipoprotein
MDBP
   mean resting diastolic blood pressure
MDCM
   mildly dilated congestive cardiomyopathy
MDCT
   multidetector computed tomography
M/D 4 defibrillator system
MDE
   minimum defibrillation energy
MDEBP
   mean daily erect blood pressure
MDF
   myocardial depressant factor
MDG
   mean diastolic gradient
MDHR
   maximum determined heart rate
MDI
   metered-dose inhaler
   methylene diphenyl diisocyanate
     MDI kit
     MDI spacer
MDILog
   M. microelectronic monitor
   M. therapy monitoring device
MDM
   middiastolic murmur
MDP
   maximum diastolic potential
   maximum digital pulse
   methylene diphosphonate
MDPA
   mean daily physical activity
MDR
   multidrug-resistant
MDRSP
   multidrug-resistant *Streptococcus*
     pneumoniae
MDR-TB
   multidrug-resistant tuberculosis

MDS
   minimum data set
   myocardial depressant substance
     MDS system
MDSBP
   mean daily supine blood pressure
MDUO
   myocardial disease of unknown origin
MDV
   myocardial Doppler velocity
MDW
   monophasic defibrillation waveform
mEAD
   monophasic action potential early
     afterdepolarization
Meadows syndrome
Meadox
   M. graft
   M. graft sizer
   M. Teflon felt pledget
   M. woven velour prosthesis
meal
   high-fat m.
mean
   m. age
   m. airway pressure (MAP, Paw)
   m. aortic pressure (MAP)
   arterial m.
   m. arterial blood pressure (MABP,
     MBP)
   m. arterial pressure (MAP)
   m. atrial rate (MAR)
   m. atrial rate algorithm
   m. blood pressure (MBP)
   m. cardiac index (MCI)
   m. circumferential fiber-shortening
     rate (MCFSR)
   m. contrast enhancement
   m. corpuscular volume (MCV)
   m. daily erect blood pressure
     (MDEBP)
   m. daily physical activity (MDPA)
   m. daily supine blood pressure
     (MDSBP)
   m. diastolic gradient (MDG)
   m. diastolic left ventricular
     pressure
   m. electrical axis
   m. forced midexpiratory flow
   m. inspiratory flow (MIF)
   m. intravascular pressure (MIP)
   m. left atrial pressure (MLAP)
   m. luminal diameter (MLD)
   m. manifest vector
   m. maternal arterial blood pressure
     (MMAP)
   m. midexpiratory flow rate (FEF$_{25\text{-}75\%}$)
   m. nocturnal saturation

mean (*continued*)
    m. normalized systolic ejection rate
    m. pressure (PM)
    m. pulmonary arterial (MPA)
    m. pulmonary artery pressure
      (MPAP, PAPm)
    m. pulmonary artery wedge
      pressure (MPAWP)
    m. pulmonary venous pressure
      (MPVP)
    m. QRS axis
    m. rate ejection index (MREI)
    m. reference diameter (MRD)
    m. resting diastolic blood pressure
      (MDBP)
    m. right atrial pressure (MRAP)
    right ventricular m. (RVM)
    m. right ventricular pressure
      (MRVP)
    m. systemic arterial pressure
      (MSAP)
    m. systolic ejection rate (MSER)
    m. systolic left ventricular pressure

MEANS
    modular electrocardiogram analysis
    system

Means-Lerman scratch

measles pneumonia

measure
    adjunctive m.
    ancillary m.
    CD4+ m.
    Cobb m.
    functional independence m. (FIM)

measured
    m. data
    m. output

measurement
    absolute m.
    angiographic m.
    automated cardiac flow m. (ACM)
    automated cardiac output m.
      (ACOM)
    automatic systolic blood
      pressure m. (ABP)
    blood flow m.
    cardiac output m.
    continuous noninvasive m.
    coronary blood flow m.
    Doppler m.
    gas clearance m.
    hemodynamic m.
    intravascular pressure m.
    invasive pressure m.
    M-mode m.
    morphometric m.
    nonpanting m.
    physiologic m.
    PR-AC m.

    pressure m.
    pressure-volume curve m.
    quantitative coronary angiography
      caliper m.
    Reid index m.
    spectral Doppler velocity m.
    splenic perfusion m.
    TDCO m.
    thermodilution m.
    transstenotic pressure gradient m.
    venous flow m.

measuring
    sinus node recovery time,
      direct m. (SNRTd)
    sinus node recovery time,
      indirect m. (SNRTi)

meat
    m., eggs, dairy, invisible fat,
      condiments, snacks (MEDICS)
    m. worker's lung

meat-wrapper's asthma

mebendazole

mec
    meconium

mecamylamine hydrochloride

mechanical
    m. alternation
    m. alternation of heart
    m. cardiopulmonary resuscitation
    m. circulatory support device
      (MCSD)
    m. contractile function
    m. cough
    m. debulking
    m. dyssynchrony
    m. heart
    m. heart valve
    m. lap counter
    m. myocardial channeling (MMC)
    m. obstruction
    m. pleurodesis
    m. prosthesis
    m. thrombectomy
    m. trauma
    m. VAS
    m. ventilation (MV)
    m. ventilator
    m. ventilatory support
    m. ventricular assistance (MVA)
    m. ventricular assist device
      (MVAD)
    m. visual analogue scale

mechanics
    fluid m.
    lung m.
    thoracopulmonary morphology
      and m.

mechanic's bronchitis

mechanism
    m. of action
    blood-clotting m. (BCM)
    compensatory m.
    coronary steal m.
    deglutition m.
    fixation m.
    Frank-Starling m.
    gating m.
    5-HT receptor m.
    ionic m.
    Laplace m.
    nitric oxide-dependent m.
    peeling-back m.
    pinchcock m.
    postsynaptic cholinergic m.
    reentrant m.
    sinus m.
    Starling m.
    steal m.
    subcellular m.
    triggering m.
    vertical deceleration m.
    wave-speed m.
mechanocardiography
mechanoelectrical feedback
mechanoreceptor
mechanoreflex
mechanosensor
mechanotransduction
mechlorethamine hydrochloride
meclofenamate sodium
meconium (mec)
    m. aspiration
    m. aspiration syndrome (MAS)
    m. ileus
Medex
    M. coronary C1 stent
    M. transducer
MedGraphics
    M. Breeze PF software
    M. Cardio O2 system
    M. CPX/D metabolic cart
media (*pl. of* medium)
medial
    m. basal branch of pulmonary
      artery
    m. inferior artery
    m. inferior artery of knee
    m. medullary infarction (MMI)
    m. necrosis
    m. superior artery
    m. superior artery of knee
    m. surface
    m. surface of lung
    m. tear
mediale
    segmentum bronchopulmonale
      basale m.

medialis
    arteria genus superior m.
median
    left m. (LM)
    m. nerve
    m. nerve injury
    m. sternotomy
    m. sternotomy incision
    m. survival time (MST)
medianus
    ramus m.
mediastinal
    m. adenopathy
    m. amyloidosis
    m. crunch
    m. emphysema
    m. fibrosis
    m. flutter
    m. goiter
    m. lymph node
    m. lymph node biopsy
    m. lymphoma
    m. mass
    m. part
    m. part of lung
    m. pleura
    m. pleurisy
    m. seminoma
    m. shadow
    m. shift
    m. space
    m. sump filter
    m. thickening
    m. wedge
    m. widened
    m. widening
mediastinale
    septum m.
mediastinalis
    pleura m.
mediastinitis
    acute m.
    descending necrotizing m. (DNM)
    fibrosing m.
    fibrous m.
    granulomatous m.
    hemorrhagic m.
    vacuum-assisted closure treated m.
mediastinoscope
    Goldberg-MPC m.
mediastinoscopy
    anterior m.
    Chamberlain m.
mediastinotomy
    anterior m.
mediastinum
    superior vascular m.
media-to-media diameter

M

mediator
> inflammatory m.
> pyrogenic m.
> m. receptor antagonist
> vasoactive m.

MedicAIR Plus spirometer

medical
> m. coronary intensive care unit (MCICU)
> M. Graphics Cardiopulmonary Exercise System 2001
> M. Graphics pneumotachograph with volume integrator
> m. intensive care unit (MICU)
> M. Research Council questionnaire
> St. Jude M. (SJM)
> m. therapy
> m. thoracoscopy (MT)

medically refractory atrial fibrillation

medicamentosa
> rhinitis m.

medication
> antiarrhythmic m.
> bolus of m.
> m. monitoring event system (MEMS)
> mucoactive m.
> presyncopal m.
> m. use evaluation (MUE)

medicinalis
> *Hirudo m.*

medicine
> American College of Sports M. (ACSM)
> digital imaging and communications in m. (DICOM)
> evidence-based m. (EBM)
> Kampo m.
> Maharishi Vedic m.
> Society of Nuclear M. (SNM)
> United States Air Force School of Aerospace M.

Medicon rib spreader

Medicopaste bandage

MEDICS
> meat, eggs, dairy, invisible fat, condiments, snacks

Medi-Facts system

Medigraphics 2000 analyzer

Medihaler-150

Medilog 4000 ambulatory ECG recorder

Medinol NIR stent

mediolysis

medionecrosis
> m. of aorta
> m. aortae
> m. aortae idiopathica cystica

meditation

Medi-Tech
> M.-T. balloon catheter
> M.-T. catheter system
> M.-T. multipurpose basket
> M.-T. steerable catheter
> M.-T. wire

Mediterranean
> M. anemia
> M. diet
> M. Diet Pyramid
> M. fever

medium, pl. **media**
> Adenoscan contrast m.
> Amipaque contrast m.
> Angio-Conray contrast m.
> aortic tunica media
> arterial media
> m. chain triglycerides
> Conray contrast m.
> contrast m.
> Eagle m.
> fibrinolytic m.
> iothalamate meglumine contrast m.
> ioxaglate meglumine contrast m.
> Isovue contrast m.
> Joklik m.
> Löwenstein m.
> Löwenstein-Jensen m.
> low osmolality contrast media (LOCM)
> metrizamide contrast m.
> Middlebrook 7H9 m.
> nonionic contrast m.
> Optiray contrast m.
> SHU-454 contrast m.
> SonoVue ultrasound contrast media
> media thickness
> Urografin-76 contrast m.

Medivent
> M. RTX respirator
> M. self-expanding coronary stent
> M. vascular stent

Medlar body

MedNova
> M. CardioShield
> M. filter
> M. NeuroShield cerebral protection system

Medos mechanical circulatory support system

medoxomil
> olmesartan m.

Medrad Mark IV angiographic injector

Medrol
> M. Dosepak
> M. Oral

medroxyprogesterone
> m. acetate (MPA)
> estrogen and m.

Medtronic

M. Activa tremor control therapy device

M. Activitrax rate-responsive unipolar ventricular pacemaker

M. Adapta pacemaker

M. AneuRx stent graft

M. Attain guide catheter set

M. AVE products

M. AVE S660 coronary stent

M. BeStent stent

M. bipolar pacemaker

M. cardiac cooling jacket

M. CardioRhythm Atakr II RF ablation system

M. connector

M. defibrillator implant support device

M. Driver stent

M. Elite DDDR pacemaker

M. Elite II pacemaker

M. EnPulse DR pacemaker

M. Evergreen balloon

M. Export aspiration catheter

M. external cardioverter-defibrillator

M. external tachyarrhythmia control device

M. GEM automatic implantable defibrillator

M. GEM III AT implantable cardioverter-defibrillator

M. Hancock II tissue valve

M. Hemopump

M. Hemopump cardiac assist device

M. Hemopump system

M. Inspire implantable device

M. InSync ICD

M. InSync Maximo CRT-D device

M. InSync Sentry cardiac resynchronization therapy defibrillator

M. InSync Sentry CRT-D device

M. Intact bioprosthetic valve

M. Intact porcine bioprosthesis

M. Interactive Tachycardia Terminating system

M. Interceptor Plus filter system

M. interventional vascular stent

M. Jewel AF 7250 dual-chamber implantable cardioverter-defibrillator

M. Jewel AF implantable arrhythmia management device

M. Jewel 7219D and C device

M. Kappa 400 pacemaker

M. lead

M. MicroDriver coronary stent

M. Micro Jewel II implantable defibrillator

M. Model 4965 steroid-eluding lead

M. Mosaic bioprosthetic valve

M. Mosaic stented prosthesis

M. Octopus tissue stabilizing device

M. Octopus 2+ tissue stabilizing system

M. PCD implantable cardioverter-defibrillator

M. pulse generator

M. Pulsor Intrasound pain reliever

M. radiofrequency receiver

M. Sprint lead

M. 57 stent

M. SynchroMed pump

M. temporary pacemaker

M. Thera DR pacemaker

M. Thera i-series cardiac pacemaker

M. tip

M. Zuma guiding catheter

Medtronic-Hall

M.-H. device

M.-H. heart valve prosthesis

M.-H. monocuspid tilting disc valve

M.-H. prosthetic heart valve

M.-H. tilting disc valve prosthesis

Medtronic-Hancock device

medulla, pl. **medullae**

adrenal m.

m. oblongata

rostral ventrolateral m. (RVLM)

rostral ventromedial m. (RVMM)

ventrolateral m. (VLM)

medullary collecting duct

medusae

caput m.

MEF$_{50}$

maximum expiratory flow at 50% vital capacity

mef(A) **gene**

mefenamic acid

mefloquine hydrochloride

Mefoxin

MEFR

maximal expiratory flow rate

MEFV

maximal expiratory flow volume

megabecquerel (MBq)

megacardia

Megace

megaelectron volt (MeV)

megaesophagus

megahertz (MHz)

megaloblastic anemia

megalocardia

MegaSonics PTCA catheter

M

megaterium
    Bacillus m.
megaunit (MU)
megestrol acetate
meglitinide
meglumine
    intracoronary sonicated m.
    ioxaglate m.
Meier-Magnum system
Meigs syndrome
meizothrombin
melaninogenica
    Prevotella m.
melaninogenicus
    Bacteroides m.
melanocortin-4 receptor (MC4-R)
melanoderma cachecticorum
melanoma
    Clark classification of malignant m.
    m. inhibitory activity (MIA)
    m. inhibitory activity protein
    malignant m.
melanotic carcinoma
melatonin level
melena
melenic stool
melioidosis
melitensis
    Brucella m.
mellitus
    diabetes m. (DM)
    insulin-dependent diabetes m.
    (IDDM)
    non-insulin-dependent diabetes m.
    (NIDDM)
melphalan
Melrose solution
Meltzer
    M. method
    M. sign
Melzack-Wall gate theory
membranacea
    angina m.
    pars m.
membranaceous
membrana fibroelastica laryngis
membrane
    adventitious m.
    alveolar basement m.
    alveolar-capillary m.
    alveolar hyaline m.
    alveolocapillary m.
    antibasement m.
    m. attack complex (MAC)
    basement m.
    Biopore m.
    bronchial mucous m.
    brush border m. (BBM)
    cell m.

    m. channel
    cricothyroid m.
    cuprophane m.
    m. current
    Debove m.
    m. diffusing capacity (Dm)
    ePTFE polymer m.
    external elastic m. (EEM)
    Gore-Tex surgical m.
    Henle elastic m.
    Henle fenestrated m.
    Hybond ECL nitrocellulose m.
    internal elastic m. (IEM)
    polyacrylonitrile m.
    m. potential
    Preclude pericardial m.
    reticular basement m.
    m. rupture
    sarcolemmal m.
    schneiderian respiratory m.
    serous m.
    m. stabilization
    suprapleural m.
membrane-bound membrane-type
    metalloproteinase (MT-MMP)
membrane-stabilizing activity
membranotomy
    transatrial m. (TM)
membranous
    m. bronchitis
    m. croup
    m. laryngitis
    m. obstruction of inferior vena
    cava (MOIVC, MOVC)
    m. pharyngitis
    m. pulmonary atresia
    m. septum
    m. wall
    m. wall of trachea
memory, pl. **memories**
    cardiac m.
    m. catheter
    m. impairment
    m. loop
Memotherm stent
MEMS
    medication monitoring event system
men (*pl. of* man)
Menadol
mendelian disorder
Mendelson syndrome
Menghini needle
Ménière syndrome
meningeal coccidioidomycosis
meningitic respiration
meningitidis
    Neisseria m.
meningitis, pl. **meningitides**
    anthrax m.

coccidioidal m.
HSV m.
Mollaret m.
meningococcal
    m. pericarditis
    m. vaccine
meningococcemia
meningococcus
meningoencephalitis
meningothelial-like nodule
meniscus, pl. menisci
    intracavitary air m.
    m. sign
menopause
MEN 2 syndrome
mental
    m. clouding
    m. status
    m. stress
    m. stress-induced ischemia
MEP
    maximal expiratory pressure
    maximum expiratory pressure
    motor evoked potential
meperidine hydrochloride
mephentermine
Mephyton Oral
mepivacaine hydrochloride
Mepron
mEq
    milliequivalent
MER
    murmur/energy ratio
meralluride
mercaptoacetyltriglycine
    technetium-99m m.
mercaptomerin sodium
6-mercaptopurine
Mercator atrial high-density array
  catheter
Mercedes-Benz sign
Merci retriever
Mercuhydrin
mercury (Hg)
    M. medical airway pressure
      manometer
    millimeter of m. (mmHg)
    m. poisoning
    m. vapor
mercury-in-rubber strain gauge
  plethysmograph
mercury-in-Silastic strain gauge
mercury-195m (^{195m}Hg)
Merendino technique
Meridia
meridian
    m. echocardiogram
    m. echocardiography
    M. pacemaker

meridional wall stress
merodiastolic
meromyosin
meropenem for injection
merosystolic
Merrem IV
Mersilene braided nonabsorbable suture
Mersilk black silk suture
MES
    microembolic signal
mesangial
    m. cell
    m. immune injury
    m. proliferative glomerulonephritis
mesangium
mesaortitis
mesarteritis
    Mönckeberg m.
mesenchymal
    m. cap
    m. intimal cell
    m. malignancy
    m. stem cell (MSC)
mesenchymal-derived tumor
mesenchyme
mesenteric
    m. angiography
    m. arteritis
    m. artery
    m. artery occlusion
    m. bypass graft
    m. infarction
    m. ischemia
    m. vascular occlusion
mesentery of lung
mesh
    Marlex m.
    m. stent
    tantalum m.
mesna
mesoatrial shunt (MAS)
mesocardia malposition
mesocardium
    arterial m.
    dorsal m.
    lateral m.
mesocaval shunt
mesoderm
    precardiac m.
mesodermal tumor
mesodiastolic
mesophlebitis
mesopneumonium
mesopulmonum
mesosystolic
mesothelial
    m. cell
    m. tumor

M

mesothelioma
> benign fibrous m.
> biphasic m.
> desmoplastic m.
> diffuse malignant m. (DMM)
> diffuse malignant pleural m.
> (DMPM)
> epithelioid m.
> malignant pleural m. (MPM)
> pleural m.
> sarcomatoid m.

MESP
> maximal exercise systolic pressure

messenger
> m. ribonucleic acid (mRNA)
> second m.

Messerklinger endoscope
Mestinon
mesylate
> bitolterol m.
> deferoxamine m.
> Desferal M.
> dihydroergotamine m.
> doxazosin m.
> gemifloxacin m.
> phentolamine m.
> saquinavir m.
> tirilazad m.

MET
> maximal exercise test
> metabolic equivalent
> metabolic equivalent of task
> multistage exercise test
> estimated MET

Meta
> M. DDDR pacemaker
> M. MV pacemaker
> M. rate-responsive pacemaker

metaanalysis
metabolator
metabolic
> m. acidosis
> m. alkalosis
> m. cart
> m. encephalopathy
> m. equivalent (MET)
> m. equivalent of task (MET)
> m. parameter determination
> m. rate meter
> m. syncope
> m. syndrome
> m. vasodilatory capacity

metabolism
> aerobic m.
> anaerobic m.
> arachidonate m.
> cerebral rate of glucose m.
> (CMR_{gic})

cerebral rate of oxygen m.
> ($CMRO_2$)
> extracellular matrix m.
> glucose m.
> myocardial m.
> oxidative m.
> oxygen m.
> respiratory m.
> skeletal muscle m.
> substrate m.

metabolite
> arachidonic acid m.
> bilirubin oxidative m.
> m. correction
> prostacyclin m.

metaboreceptor
metaboreflex
> muscle m.
> m. response

metachronous lung cancer
metadata
metaiodobenzylguanidine (MIBG)
> ^{123}I m.
> ^{125}I m.

metal
> m. fume fever (MFF)
> heavy m.
> sensitizing m.
> m. sewing ring
> trace m.

metallic
> m. breath sounds
> m. click
> m. echo
> m. oxide fumes
> m. rale
> m. stent
> m. tinkle

metalloproteinase
> m. inhibitor
> matrix m. (MMP)
> matrix-degrading neutral m.
> membrane-bound membrane-type m.
> (MT-MMP)
> tissue inhibitor of m. (TIMP)

metalloproteinase-3
> tissue inhibitor of m.-3 (TIMP-3)

metamorphosing respiration
metam sodium
metamyelocyte
MetaPhor agarose
metaplasia
> cellular m.
> goblet cell m.
> peribronchiolar m.

metaplastic mucus-secreting cell
metapneumonic
> m. empyema
> m. pleurisy

metapneumonovirus
    human m. (hMPV)
metaproterenol
    m. sulfate
metaraminol bitartrate
metarteriole
metastasectomy
    pulmonary m.
metastasis, pl. metastases
    cannonball metastases
    cardiac m.
    contact m.
    hematogenous m.
    implantation m.
    pleuropulmonary m.
    tumor, node, m. (TNM)
metastatic
    m. calcification
    m. carcinoid syndrome
    m. carcinoma
    m. disease
    m. nodule
    m. phenotype
    m. pneumonia
    m. sarcoma
metazoal myocarditis
Metenix
metenkephalin
meter
    Deltatrac II metabolic rate m.
    ExacTech blood glucose m.
    m. mask
    metabolic rate m.
    m. per second (m/s, m/sec)
    m. per second squared (m/s^2)
    pH M.
    ventilation m.
metered-dose
    m.-d. inhaler (MDI)
    m.-d. spray
metered-solution inhaler (MSI)
metformin
methacholine
    m. bronchoprovocation challenge
    m. challenge test
    m. chloride
    m. reaction
    m. reactivity
    m. response
    reversal speed of
      bronchoconstriction in response
      to m. (r-Sm)
    speed of bronchoconstriction in
      response to m. (Sm)
methamphetamine hydrochloride
methanesulfonanilide derivative
methanesulfonate
    phentolamine m.
methemoglobin

methemoglobinemia
methenamine silver stain
methicillin-sensitive right-sided
   endocarditis
methicillin sodium
methimazole
methionine loading
method
    Alfieri m.
    Allain m.
    Anderson-Keys m.
    Antyllus m.
    area-length m.
    Arvidsson dimension-length m.
    atrial extrastimulus m.
    biplane area-length m.
    Björk m.
    Bland-Altman m.
    body box m.
    Bohr isopleth m.
    Bonferroni m.
    Brasdor m.
    Brisbane m.
    Brown-Dodge m.
    Burow quantitative m.
    Carrel m.
    catheter introduction m.
    Cavalieri m.
    Celermajer m.
    centerline m.
    chromogenic m.
    Clauss m.
    closed-circuit m.
    conductance catheter m.
    constant-flow m.
    Cribier m.
    Cutler-Ederer m.
    cyanmethemoglobin m.
    cyanogen bromide m.
    Danielson m.
    DBCL m.
    Defares rebreathing m.
    Devereux-Reichek m.
    digital color Doppler velocity
      integration m.
    digitized caliper m.
    Dodge area-length m.
    Douglas bag collection m.
    Dow m.
    downstream sampling m.
    dye-dilution m.
    dynamic m.
    edge-detection m.
    Eggleston m.
    Eicken m.
    estimated Fick m.
    Eve m.
    fatigue testing m.
    Fick oxygen m.

M

method *(continued)*
    flow convergence m.
    forward-backward Prony m.
      (FBPM)
    forward triangle m.
    Galanti-Giusti colorimetric m.
    Gärtner m.
    gas clearance m.
    gold-standard m.
    Gräupner m.
    half-time m.
    Hanley-McNeil m.
    Hatle m.
    head-tilt m.
    Heinecke m.
    helium dilution m.
    heparin assay rapid m. (HARM)
    heparin assay rapid easy m.
      (HAREM)
    Howard m.
    immunometric sandwich m.
    indicator dilution m.
    indocyanine green m.
    Ionescu m.
    Jaffe m.
    Kales scoring m.
    Kasser-Kennedy m.
    Kennedy area-length m.
    Kety-Schmidt m.
    King biopsy m.
    Kirstein m.
    Konno biopsy m.
    Laborde m.
    Laurell m.
    Lee-White m.
    Lown and Woolf m.
    Marriott m.
    Meltzer m.
    Monte Carlo multiway sensitivity
      analysis m.
    Murphy m.
    Narula m.
    Ogata m.
    Oliver-Rosalki m.
    open circuit m.
    Orsi-Grocco m.
    oxygen step-up m.
    Pachon m.
    Penaz volume-clamp m.
    Penn m.
    phenylephrine ramp m.
    planimetry m.
    polarographic m.
    prick-test m.
    prism m.
    Prony m. (PM)
    proximal flow convergence m.
    pulse m.
    Purmann m.

    pyramid m.
    m. of Quinones
    Rackley m.
    Raff-Glantz derivative m.
    rebreathing m.
    Rechtschaffen scoring m.
    Roche-Microwell plate
      hybridization m.
    root inclusion m.
    Sandler-Dodge area-length m.
    Satterthwaite m.
    Scarpa m.
    Schafer m.
    Schiller m.
    Schüller m.
    Shimazaki area-length m.
    Sigma m.
    Silvester m.
    Simpson modified m.
    sliding scale m.
    Stanford biopsy m.
    steady-state m.
    Stegemann-Stalder m.
    Strauss m.
    testing m.
    Theden m.
    thermodilution m.
    Thom flap laryngeal
      reconstruction m.
    Thompson-Hatina m.
    Thrombo-Wellcotest m.
    m. of Towbin
    triphenyl tetrazolium staining m.
    TUNEL m.
    Van Slyke m.
    von Claus chronometric m.
    V-slope m.
    Wardrop m.
    Weir m.
    Weiss logarithmic m.
    Welcker m.
    Westergren m.
    Willett-Stampfer m.
    Wilson-White m.
methohexital
methotrexate
methoxamine hydrochloride
methoxsalen
2-methoxyisobutyl
    2-m. isonitrile (MIBI)
    2-m. isonitrile single-photon
      emission computed tomography
      (MIBI-SPECT)
methoxyphenamine hydrochloride
8-methoxypsoralen
methyclothiazide
    m. and cryptenamine tannates
    m. and deserpidine
    m. and pargyline

methyl
- m. bromide
- m. isocyanate
- m. prednisolone

methylase *erm*(B) **gene**
methylcholine challenge testing (MCT)
methyldichloroarsine
methyldopa
- chlorothiazide and m.
- m. and hydrochlorothiazide

methylene
- m. blue
- m. diphenyl diisocyanate (MDI)
- m. diphenyl diisocyanate asthma
- m. diphenyl isocyanate
- m. diphosphonate (MDP)

methylenetetrahydrofolate
- m. reductase (MTHFR)
- m. reductase gene
- m. reductase genotype

methylergonovine
methylisocyanate
methylphenidate
5-methyl-1-phenyl-2(1H)-pyridone
methylprednisolone (MTP)
- m. acetate
- sodium m.
- m. succinate

methyltestosterone
methylxanthine
methylxanthines
methysergide maleate
metoclopramide hydrochloride
metocurine iodide
metolazone
metoprolol
- m. CR
- m. succinate
- m. tartrate

Metras catheter
Metricath
- M. 1000 console catheter
- M. measurement catheter

metrics
Metrix
- M. atrial defibrillation system
- M. Atrioverter
- M. IAD
- M. implantable atrial defibrillator

metrizamide contrast medium
metrocyte
metronidazole
METT
- maximum exercise tolerance test

metyrosine
Metzenbaum scissors
MeV
- megaelectron volt

Mevacor lovastatin tablet

mevalonate
- m. acid
- m. pyrophosphate

mevinolin
Mewi-5 sidehole infusion catheter
Mewissen infusion catheter
Mexican bean weevil asthma
mexiletine hydrochloride
Mexitil
Meyer cartilage
Meyerding retractor
mezlocillin sodium
MF
- modifying factor
- myocardial fibrosis

MFAT
- multifocal atrial tachycardia

MFF
- metal fume fever

MFG
- manofluorography
- middle frontal gyrus

MFH
- malignant fibrous histiocytoma

MFSR
- maximum flow static recoil

MFT
- multifocal atrial tachycardia

MFVL
- maximum flow-volume loop

mg
- milligram

MGA
- malposition of great arteries

Mgb
- myoglobulin

MgCO$_3$
- magnesium carbonate

MGIT
- mycobacterial growth indicator tube

MGMT
- O$_6$-methylguanine-DNA-methyl-transferase

MH
- malignant hypertension

MHA-TP test
MHHP
- Minnesota Heart Health Program

MHR
- maternal heart rate
- maximal heart rate

MHV
- magnetic heart vector

MHz
- megahertz
  - 2-MHz pulsed-wave Doppler transducer

MI
- mitral incompetence

M

MI *(continued)*
   mitral insufficiency
   myocardial infarction
   myocardial ischemia
     elevation MI
MIA
   melanoma inhibitory activity
     MIA protein
mibefradil
MIBG
   metaiodobenzylguanidine
     ^{123}-I MIBG
     ^{125}I MIBG
MIBI
   2-methoxyisobutyl isonitrile
     MIBI SPECT
     MIBI stress test
     technetium-99m MIBI
MIBI-SPECT
   2-methoxyisobutyl isonitrile single-
     photon emission computed tomography
     ^{99m}Tc MIBI-SPECT
MIC
   minimum inhibitory concentration
   mitomycin, ifosfamide, cisplatin
MICAB
   minimally invasive coronary artery
   bypass
     MICAB surgery
MICABG
   minimally invasive coronary bypass
   grafting
mica pneumoconiosis
Micardis
micdadei
   Legionella m.
   Tatlockia m.
Michelson bronchoscope
miconazole
MICRhoGAM
Micrins
   M. microclamp instrument
   M. microsurgical suture
micro
   M. Delta/Max Delta system
   M. DiaryCard spirometer
   M. Guide catheter
   Lipidil M.
   M. Minix pacemaker
   M. Mist nebulizer
   M. Plus spirometer
microaerosol
MicroAir
   M. handheld nebulizer
   M. ultrasonic nebulizer system
microalbuminuria
microanastomosis
   laser-assisted m. (LAMA)

microaneurysm
   Charcot-Bouchard m.
microangiopathic anemia
microangiopathy
   cerebral m. (CMA)
   coronary m.
   thrombotic m. (TMA)
microarousal
   m. detection
   m. scoring
   m. scoring device
microarray
   m. analysis
   oligonucleotide m.
microaspiration
microatelectasis
microatheroma
microballoon
microbiologic brushing
microbleed
microbubble (MB)
   m. persistence
   saline m.
microbulldog clip
microcalcification cluster (MCC)
Microcap handheld capnograph
microcardia
microcatheter
   end-hole Tracker m.
   Excelsior 1018 m.
   Pathfinder mapping m.
   Pathfinder mini mapping m.
   Progreat coaxial m.
   Rebar-18 m.
   Revelation endocardial m.
   Tracer over-the-wire mapping m.
   Tracker m.
microcavitation
microcentrum
MicroChamber
microcirculation (MC)
microcirculatory
   m. adaptation
   m. vasoconstriction
MicroCO carbon monoxide monitor
Micrococcus
microcoil
   Hilal embolization m.
microcontaminant
microcrystal
microdialysis
MicroDigitrapper-S apnea screening device
microdissection
   laser capture m. (LCM)
MicroDriver coronary stent
microelectrode
   tungsten m.

microemboli (*pl. of* microembolus)
microembolic signal (MES)
microembolism
microembolization
microembolus, pl. microemboli
    gaseous m. (GME)
MicroFerret-18 infusion catheter
microfibril
microfibrillar collagen hemostat
microfilaria
microfilter
    OmniFilter percutaneous
      guidewire m.
microflora
    bronchial m.
microfocus, pl. microfoci
MicroGard filter
MicroGas 7650 transcutaneous
  monitoring system
micrognathia
microhemagglutination *Treponema*
  pallidum
Micro-Induction 1000 electrocardiograph
microinfarct
microinvasive
microjoule
Micro-K
Microknit
    M. arterial graft
    M. patch graft
MicroLab ML3500 desktop diagnostic
  spirometer
microlaryngoscope
microlaryngoscopy
    Thornell m.
microlithiasis
    alveolar m.
    pulmonary alveolar m. (PAM)
MicroLoop
    M. II spirometer
    M. pocket spirometer
MicroLysUS system
micromanometer
    m. catheter
    m. catheter system
    catheter-tip m. system
micromanometer-tipped
    5-Fr MPC500 m.-t. catheter
micromanometry
MicroMed DeBakey ventricular assist
  device
micrometastasis
MicroMewi multiple sidehole infusion
  catheter
Micromonospora
Micronase
micronebulizer
microneurography
microneutralization test

micronized progesterone
micron needle
micronodular dissemination
micronutrient balance
Microny
    M. II K pediatric pacemaker
      (models 3500 & 3510)
    M. II SR+ AutoCapture pacing
      system
    M. II SR+ pacemaker
    M. II SR+ pulse generator
    M. K SR pacemaker
    M. SR+ cardiac pacemaker
microorganism
microparticle
    apoptotic endothelial m.
microphage
    fat-laden m.
Micropolyspora faeni
micropuncture
    M. guidewire
    M. introducer needle
    M. introducer set
    M. Peel-Away introducer
microreentry
MicroRint module
microsatellite instability
microscope
    acoustic m.
    electron m.
    epi-illuminated m.
    Nikon Eclipse E400 m.
    scanning electron m. (SEM)
microscopic polyangiitis (MPA)
microscopy
    auramine smear m.
    confocal m.
    darkfield m.
    immunofluorescence m.
    intravital capillary video m.
    light m.
    sputum m.
    transmission electron m. (TEM)
microsecond pulsed flashlamp pumped
  dye laser
MicroSelectron-HDR afterloader
Micro+ Smokerlyzer
microsnare
    Amplatz gooseneck m.
microsomal
    m. lipoprotein (MLP)
    m. triglyceride transfer protein
    (MTP)
microsome
    calf aortic m. (CAM)
Microspacer
microsphere
    EmboGold m.
    perflexane lipid m.

M

microsphere *(continued)*
    perflutren lipid m.
    m. perfusion scintigraphy
    polystyrene latex m.
    radiolabeled m.
    Ultrasound Contrast M.
microsphygmy
microsphyxia
Micross
    M. dilation catheter
    M. SL balloon
microsteatosis
Microstream capnograph
Microsulfon
microsurgical
    m. blade
    m. dilation catheter system
microthromboembolism
    pulmonary m.
microthrombosis
microthrombus
microti
    Babesia m.
    Mycobacterium m.
Microtip lead
microtome
    Cryo-Cut m.
    Stadie-Riggs m.
Micro-Tracer portable ECG
microtransducer
    high-fidelity m.
microvascular
    M. Anastomotic Coupler System
    m. angina
    m. angiopathy (MVA)
    m. artery disease
    m. bleeding (MVB)
    m. clamp
    m. decompression (MVD)
    m. dysfunction
    m. flow distribution
    m. free flap
    m. integrity
    m. permeability
microvasculopathy
    pulmonary m.
Microvasive
    M. Glidewire
    M. Rigiflex TTS balloon
    M. stiff piano wire guidewire
MicroVein Vascular system
Microvel double velour graft
Microvena nitinol guidewire
MicroVent ventilator
microvessel
microvolt
    m. level
    m. T-wave alternans (MTWA)
microwave cardiac ablation system

Microzide
micturition syncope
MICU
    medical intensive care unit
MIDA
    myocardial ischemia dynamic analysis
Midamor
midaxillary line
midazolam
MIDCAB
    minimally invasive direct coronary artery
    bypass
        MIDCAB procedure
        MIDCAB saloon door approach
        MIDCAB surgery
        MIDCAB system
MIDCABG
    minimally invasive direct coronary artery
    bypass graft
midclavicular line (MCL)
midcoronary
    m. artery
    m. artery bypass
    m. segment
middiastolic
    m. murmur (MDM)
    m. rumble
middle
    m. capsular artery
    m. cerebral artery (MCA)
    m. cerebral artery occlusion
     (MCAO)
    m. constrictor muscle
    m. constrictor muscle of pharynx
    m. frontal gyrus (MFG)
    m. lobe
    m. lobe bronchus
    m. lobe of right lung
    m. lobe syndrome
    m. lobe vein ostium
    m. ribs
Middlebrook 7H9 medium
midepigastric bruit
midexpiratory phase
mid-infrared pulsed laser
midinspiratory flow
midline shift
midlung zone
midnodal
    m. extrasystole
    m. rhythm
midodrine
midriff
midsagittal plane
midsystolic
    m. buckling
    m. buckling of mitral valve
    m. click (MSC)
    m. click syndrome

m. closure of aortic valve
m. dip
m. murmur (MSM)
m. notching

midventricle
midventricular (MV)
midwall shortening
MIF
mean inspiratory flow
MIFR
maximal inspiratory flow rate
miglitol
migraine
m. headache
m. stroke
syncopal m.
m. syncope
migrans
erythema m.
larva m.
thrombophlebitis m. (TPM)
visceral larva m.
migrated tumor
migrating
m. pacemaker
m. phlebitis
migration
free liquid m.
neural crest m.
stent m.
migratory
m. bronchiolitis obliterans
organizing pneumonia
m. pulmonary infiltrate
m. thrombus
MIH
minimal intermittent heparin
MIH dose
Mikity-Wilson disease
Mikro-Tip
M.-T. micromanometer-tipped
catheter
M.-T. transducer
Mikulicz-type esophagoscope
mild-intensity exercise
mildly dilated congestive
cardiomyopathy (MDCM)
Miles vena cava clip
miliary
m. coccidioidomycosis
m. embolism
m. infection
m. pattern
m. tuberculosis
milieu
military
m. antishock trousers (MAST)
m. pattern

milk
m. scan
m. scintigraphy
m. spots
milk-alkali syndrome
mill
m. house murmur
m. wheel murmur
Millar
M. asthma
M. Doppler catheter
2F M. Instrument catheter
M. Mikro-Tip catheter pressure
transducer
M. MPC-500 catheter
M. TCB-500 transducer
mille feuilles effect
miller
M. blade
M. elastic stain
M. Fisher variant
M. Fisher variant of Guillain-Barré
syndrome
M. index
M. maneuver
M. septostomy catheter
milleri
Streptococcus m.
miller's
m. asthma
m. lung
milliamperage
milliampere (mA)
millicurie (mCi)
milliequivalent (mEq)
milligram (mg)
m. per kilogram per day
millijoule (mJ)
Milliknit
M. Dacron prosthesis
M. vascular graft prosthesis
milliliter (mL)
nanograms per m. (ng/mL)
m. per kilogram (mL/kg)
millimeter of mercury (mmHg)
millimole (mmol)
m.'s per liter (mmol/L)
million
m. international unit (MIU)
part per m. (ppm)
milliosmole (mOsm)
Millipore filter
millisecond (ms, msec)
milliunit (mU)
millivolt (mV)
Mill-Rose
M.-R. esophageal injector
M.-R. protected specimen
microbiology brush

M

milrinone lactate
Miltex rib spreader
Miltner constraint compliance device
Milton edema
Mima-Herellea
mimetic
  incretin m.
mineral-induced lung disease
mineralocorticoid hormone
mineralocorticoid-induced hypertension
miner's
  m. asthma
  m. lung
  m. phthisis
Mingograf
  M. 62 6-channel electrocardiograph
  M. 82 recorder
Mingograph
mini
  m. arousal
  M. Asthma Quality of Life
    (MAQOL)
  M. Crown stent
  21 M. device
  26 M. II device
  m. profile
  M. Pulse oximeter
  m. stroke
Mini2 Smokerlyzer
minicoil
MiniHEART low-flow nebulizer
Minilith pacemaker pulse generator
minimae
  venae cardiacae m.
  venae cordis m.
minimal
  m. alveolar concentration (MAC)
  m. intermittent heparin (MIH)
  m. leak technique
  m. luminal diameter (MLD)
  m. vascular resistance (MVR)
minimally
  m. invasive combined mitral valve
    repair and direct coronary artery
    bypass
  m. invasive coronary artery bypass
    (MICAB)
  m. invasive coronary bypass
    grafting (MICABG)
  m. invasive direct coronary artery
    bypass (MIDCAB)
  m. invasive direct coronary artery
    bypass graft (MIDCABG)
  m. invasive direct coronary artery
    bypass procedure
  m. invasive procedure (MIP)
  m. invasive valve repair (MIVR)
  m. invasive valve replacement
    (MIVR)

MiniMe nasal mask
Mini-Motionlogger Actigraph
minimum
  m. audible pressure (MAP)
  m. bactericidal concentration
  m. cumulative cardiotoxic dose
    (MCCD)
  m. data set (MDS)
  m. data set system
  m. defibrillation energy (MDE)
  m. inhibitory concentration (MIC)
  m. left ventricular pressure
    (LVPmin)
  m. lumen diameter (MLD)
MiniOX
  M. IA oxygen analyzer
  M. 1000 oxygen analyzer
  M. 3000 oxygen monitor
Minipress
Mini-Profile catheter
Miniscope MS-3 pocket ECG
ministernotomy
Mini-Torr Plus NIPB monitor
minitracheostomy
  prophylactic m.
Minitran Patch
Minizide
Minnesota
  M. antilymphocyte globulin (MAG)
  M. classification of ECG
  M. criteria
  M. criteria for high R wave
  M. ECG classification
  M. Heart Health Program (MHHP)
  M. Impedance Cardiograph
  M. Leisure Time Physical Activity
    Questionnaire
  M. Living with Heart Failure
    questionnaire
  M. Q-QS code
minocycline hydrochloride
minor
  m. fissure
  pectoralis m.
minores
  ductus sublinguales m.
minoxidil
Minoxigaine
Mintezol
minute
  alveolar ventilation per m. (V_A)
  beats per m. (BPM, bpm)
  counts per m. (C/M)
  liter per m. (Lpm)
  M. Maid Premium Heart Wise
    orange juice
  m. output
  oxygen consumption per m.
    (VO_2max)

physiological dead space ventilation per m. (V_D)

pulses per m. (ppm)

10-m. supine/30-minute tilt test

m. ventilation (V_E)

m. volume

6-minute

6-m. corridor walk test

6-m. walk distance (6MWD)

6-m. walking test (6MWT, 6-MWT)

minute-gun cough

Miochol-E

miosis

miosphygmia

MIP

macrophage inflammatory protein

maximal inspiratory pressure

maximum inspiratory pressure

mean intravascular pressure

minimally invasive procedure

MIP-1

macrophage inflammatory protein-1

mirabilis

Proteus m.

mirage

M. hydrophilic guidewire

M. nasal mask

M. over-the-wire balloon catheter

Mirostipen

MIRP

myocardial infarction rehabilitation program

mirror

m. movement

van Helmont m.

mirror-image

m.-i. brachiocephalic branching

m.-i. dextrocardia

m.-i. laryngoscopy

m.-i. lung syndrome

Mirsky

formula of M.

M. thick wall model

MIRU

myocardial infarction research unit

misery perfusion

mismatch

prosthesis-patient m. (PPM)

ventilation/perfusion m.

$\dot{V}/\dot{Q}$ m.

mismatching

afterload m.

missed

m. beat

m. ostium sequence (MOS)

missense mutation

missile emboli

miss rate

mist

Ayr Saline m.

child-adult m. (CAM)

cool m.

Primatene M.

m. tent

Mistogen

M. nebulizer

M. passover humidifier

Mistometer

Isuprel M.

mite

dust m.

house dust m. (HDM)

MITI

myocardial infarction triage and intervention

mitis

Streptococcus m.

mitochondrial

m. apoptotic pathway

m. biogenesis

m. calcium deposition

m. cardiomyopathy

m. enzyme

m. function

m. genotype

m. oxidative phosphorylation

m. respiration

mitochondrion, pl. **mitochondria**

mitogen-activated

m.-a. kinase pathway

m.-a. protein (MAP)

m.-a. protein kinase (MAPK)

mitogenic radiation

mitomycin

m. C-induced interstitial pneumonitis

m., ifosfamide, cisplatin (MIC)

m., vinblastine, cisplatin (MVP)

mitotane

mitoxantrone hydrochloride

mitral

m. anular area

m. anular calcification (MAC)

m. anular calcium

m. anular Z score

m. anulus flutter

m. anulus motion

m. and aortic valve replacement (MAVR)

m. apparatus

m. arcade

m. atresia

m. balloon commissurotomy

m. balloon valvotomy (MBV)

m. buttonhole

m. click

m. closure (Mc)

M

mitral *(continued)*
    m. commissurotomy (MC)
    m. component (M1)
    m. disease (MD)
    m. E-to-F slope
    m. E velocity curve
    m. E-wave transmission
    m. facies
    m. first sound (M_1)
    m. funnel
    m. incompetence (MI)
    m. insufficiency (MI)
    m. isthmus
    m. leaflet
    m. leaflet remodeling
    m. leaflet tip
    m. opening (Mo)
    m. opening snap (MOS)
    m. orifice (MO)
    posterior m. (PM)
    m. prolapse murmur
    m. prosthesis
    m. redo surgery
    m. reflux (MR)
    m. regurgitant flow (MRF)
    m. regurgitant jet
    m. regurgitation (MR)
    m. regurgitation artifact
    m. regurgitation murmur
    m. restenosis
    m. ring annuloplasty
    m. second sound (M_2)
    m. sounds (MS)
    m. stenosis (MS)
    m. stenosis murmur
    m. tap
    m. valve aneurysm
    m. valve anulus
    m. valve area (MVA)
    m. valve billowing
    m. valve closure index
    m. valve commissurotomy
    m. valve dilator
    m. valve disease (MVD)
    m. valve echo (MVE)
    m. valve echocardiogram
    m. valve endocarditis
    m. valve excursion (MVE)
    m. valve flow (MVF)
    m. valve gradient (MVG)
    m. valve homograft
    m. valve hypoplasia
    m. valve insufficiency (MVI)
    m. valve leaflet (MVL)
    m. valve opening (MVO)
    m. valve orifice (MVO)
    m. valve orifice area (MVOA)
    m. valve prolapse (MVP)
    m. valve prolapse syndrome (MVPS)
    m. valve prolapse-systolic click (MVP-SC)
    m. valve regurgitation
    m. valve replacement (MVR)
    m. valve valvotomy
    m. valvoplasty
    m. valvulitis
    m. velocity

mitrale
    P m.

mitralis
    facies m.

mitralism

mitralization

mitral-septal apposition

Mitroflow Synergy PC stented pericardial valve

mitrotricuspid facies

MIU
    million international unit

Mivacron

mivacurium

mivazerol

MIVR
    minimally invasive valve repair
    minimally invasive valve replacement

mix
    oncology m.

mixed
    m. alveolar-interstitial pneumonitis
    m. aneurysm
    m. angina
    m. aortic valve disease (MAVD)
    m. apnea (MA)
    m. asthma
    m. beat
    m. connective tissue disease (MCTD)
    m. connective tissue disorder
    m. expired gas
    m. flora
    m. germ cell tumor
    m. hematopoietic chimerism
    m. levocardia
    m. mitral valve disease (MMVD)
    m. neurally mediated syncope
    m. obstructive and restrictive pattern
    m. thrombus
    m. venous blood
    m. venous oxygen saturation (SvO_2)

mixed-dust pneumoconiosis

mixing
    cardiogenic m.
    convective gas m.
    gas m.

mixture
  helium-oxygen m. (heliox)
mizoribine
mJ
  millijoule
mL
  milliliter
MLAP
  mean left atrial pressure
MLD
  mean luminal diameter
  minimal luminal diameter
  minimum lumen diameter
MLH
  multiple lobar hemorrhage
M-line protein
mL/kg
  milliliter per kilogram
MLP
  microsomal lipoprotein
MLR
  myocardial laser revascularization
    MLR procedure
MLS$_B$ phenotype
MM
  modified Miller maneuver
MMA
  maxillomandibular advancement
MMAD
  mass median aerodynamic diameter
MMAP
  mean maternal arterial blood pressure
MMC
  mechanical myocardial channeling
mMCAI
  malignant middle cerebral artery
    infarction
MME
  M-mode echocardiography
MMEF, MMF
  maximal midexpiratory flow
  maximum midexpiratory flow rate
MMEFR
  maximal midexpiratory flow rate
MMF
  mycophenolate mofetil
mmHg
  millimeter of mercury
MMI
  medial medullary infarction
MMO
  maxillomandibular osteotomy
M-mode
  motion mode
    M-mode echocardiogram
    M-mode echocardiography (MME)
    M-mode measurement
    omnidirectional M-mode

M-mode strip chart recording
M-mode transducer
mmol
  millimole
mmol/L
  millimoles per liter
MMP
  matrix metalloproteinase
  matrix-degrading neutral MMP
MMP 7
  matrilysin
MMP 8
  neutrophil collagenase
MMPI
  matrix metalloproteinase inhibitor
MMR
  myocardial metabolic rate
MMV
  mandatory minute volume
MMVD
  mixed mitral valve disease
MMVF
  manmade vitreous fiber
Mn-SOD
  manganese superoxide dismutase
MO
  mitral orifice
MO$_2$
  myocardial oxygen
Mo
  mitral opening
MO2 utilization
mobile
  m. artery and vein imaging system
    (MAVIS)
  carina sharp and m.
  cor m.
  m. coronary care unit (MCCU)
  m. myxoma
  m. thrombus
  m. vegetation
mobilization
  secretion m.
mobilizer
  AMD3100 stem cell m.
Mobin-Uddin
  M.-U. filter system
  M.-U. sieve
  M.-U. vena cava filter
Mobitz
  M. first-degree block
  M. second-degree block
  M. type I, II atrioventricular block
  M. types of atrioventricular block
modafinil
modality
  pacing m.
  therapeutic m.

M

mode

A m.
AAI rate-responsive m.
AAT m.
autodecremental m.
AutoPilot operational m.
curved M m.
DDDR m.
demand m.
dual-helical slice m.
dual-slice m.
fixed-rate m.
gated list m.
harmonic imaging m.
histogram m.
list m.
mask m.
matrix m.
motion m. (M-mode)
noise-reversion m.
OOO m.
overdrive m.
pacing m.
passive m.
patient activator m.
rate-drop response m.
RDR m.
m. switch
m. switching
triggered m.
VDD m.
VDI pacing m.
VVD m.
VVIR m.
VVT m.

model

M. 700 aggregometer
AIS m.
health behavior m.
Hodgkin-Huxley m.
Impact portable aspirator m. 326
Mirsky thick wall m.
Torricelli m.
Tracheostomy TOM anatomical m.
Weisfeldt and Becker 3-phase m.
windkessel m.

model-based image processing (MBIP)
modeling

electrocardiographic m.
genetic m.

moderate hypothermia
moderate-ramp protocol
moderator band
modification

A-V nodal m.
Cooley m.
Fontan m.
Jonas m.
Mason-Likar limb lead m.

Mullins m.
Rossetti m.
Sade m.
Samsoon-Young m.
Sano m.
slow-pathway m.

modified

m. Blalock-Taussig shunt (MBTS)
m. brachial technique
m. Bruce protocol
m. chest lead (MCL)
m. David reimplantation operation
m. elephant trunk staged procedure
m. Ellestad protocol
m. Fontan procedure
m. human graft umbilical vein graft
m. Mark IV R-wave-triggered power injector
m. Miller maneuver (MM)
m. multifactorial index
m. multifactorial index of cardiac risk
m. Rashkind PDA occluder
m. Seldinger technique
m. shuttle test
m. treadmill exercise test (MTET)
m. ultrafiltration (MUF)

modifier

leukotriene m.

modifying factor (MF)
MODS

multiple-organ dysfunction syndrome

modular electrocardiogram analysis system (MEANS)
modulated

pulse position m. (PPM)

modulation

autonomic m.
brightness m.
integral pulse frequency m. (IPFM)
pulse amplitude m. (PAM)
pulse time m. (PTM)
pulse with m. (PWM)
rate m.
spatial m.

modulator

neurohormonal m.
positive airway pressure gas m.
selective estrogen receptor m. (SERM)

module

BioZ ICG M.
Cartomerge image integration m.
CO-Oximeter m.
MicroRint m.
Omnicell catheter m.
Research Pneumotach System instrumentation m.

Modulite inhaler
modulus
>impedance m.
>Peterson elastic m.
>Young m.

Moduretic
Moe
>multiple reentrant wavelet
>hypothesis of M.
>M. multiple wavelet hypothesis
>M. multiple wavelet hypothesis of
>atrial defibrillation

Moersch bronchoscope
moexipril
>m. hydrochloride
>m. and hydrochlorothiazide

mofetil
>mycophenolate m. (MMF)

Mogul 3-French steerable decapolar
electrophysiology diagnostic catheter
moiety-conserved cycle
moist
>Nasal M.
>m. rale

moisturizer
>Cann-Ease nasal m.
>RoEzIt skin m.

MOIVC, MOVC
>membranous obstruction of inferior vena
>cava

mold worker's lung
molecular
>m. chemotherapy
>m. coincidence detection (MCD)
>m. diffusion
>m. imaging
>m. sieve bed

molecule
>antiadhesion m.
>cell adhesion m. (CAM)
>chemoattracting m.
>circulating adhesion m. (CAM)
>endothelial cell adhesion m.
>endothelium-leukocyte adhesion m.
>(E-LAM)
>E-selectin cell adhesion m.
>fluoropolymer m.
>glycosaminoglycan m.
>intercellular adhesion m. (ICAM)
>leukocyte-endothelial cell
>adhesion m.
>proapoptotic m.
>proatherothrombogenic m.
>P-selectin cell adhesion m.
>soluble adhesion m.
>soluble intracellular adhesion m.
>(sICAM)

molecule-1
>intercellular adhesion m.-1 (ICAM-
>1)
>mucosal addressin cell
>adhesion m.-1 (MadCAM-1)
>vascular cell adhesion m.-1
>(VCAM-1)

Molina needle catheter
Mol-Iron
Mollaret meningitis
mollis
>pulsus m.

molluscum contagiosum
Molnar disc
Moloney murine leukemia virus
(MoMLV)
molsidomine
molybdenum
moment
>magnetic m.

Momentum DR pacemaker
mometasone furoate
MoMLV
>Moloney murine leukemia virus

Monaghan
>M. respirator
>M. 300 ventilator

Monaldi drainage system
monarch
>M. 25 inflation device
>M. Mini Mask nasal interface

Monark bicycle ergometer
Mönckeberg
>M. arrhythmia
>M. arteriosclerosis
>M. calcification
>M. degeneration
>M. mesarteritis
>M. sclerosis
>M. syndrome

Monday
>M. dyspnea
>M. fever

Mondini pulmonary arteriovenous
malformation
Mondor
>M. disease
>M. syndrome

Monge disease
Monilia albicans
monilial esophagitis
moniliasis
>chronic mucocutaneous m.

moniliformis
>*Streptobacillus m.*

Monitan
monitor
>Accucap CO_2/O_2 m.
>Accucom cardiac output m.

M

monitor *(continued)*

Accutorr multiparameter m.

Accutracker II ambulatory blood pressure m.

Acuson V5M transesophageal echocardiographic m.

aerosol inhalation m. (AIM)

AID-Check m.

ambulatory Holter m.

AMI infant apnea m.

antepartum m. (APM)

APM-2000 vital signs m.

apnea m.

Arrhythmia Net arrhythmia m.

atrial fibrillation m. (AFm)

automatic oscillometric blood pressure m.

AvoSure PT m.

Bedfont carbon monoxide m.

bedside m.

bioimpedance m.

Biotrack coagulation m.

BioZ.com cardiac output m.

BioZ ICG M.

blood perfusion m. (BPM)

CA m.

Capintec nuclear VEST m.

Capnocheck II hand-held CO2/SpO2 m.

Capnocheck Plus capnograph m.

cardiac apnea m.

CardioBeeper CB 12L cardiac m.

Cardiocap/5 m.

cardiovascular m. (CVM)

CareLink m.

3-channel Holter m.

Chronicle implantable hemodynamic m.

CoaguChek Pro DM m.

Corometrics material fetal m.

CO Sleuth carbon monoxide m.

CO$_2$SMO Plus! respiratory profile m.

Datascope Accutorr bedside m.

Deltatrac II metabolic m.

Digitrapper pH 400 m.

Dinamap Accutorr A1, A3 blood pressure m.

Doppler-Cavin m.

Doppler fetal heart m.

DynaPulse 5000A blood pressure m.

ecg@home heart m.

EcoCheck oxygen m.

EC50 ToxCO breath carbon monoxide m.

electrocardiographic transtelephonic m.

electronic fetal m.

endotracheal cardiac output m. (ECOM)

event recorder m.

Finapres blood pressure m.

Gastrolyzer breath hydrogen m.

HBT Sleuth portable hydrogen m.

HeartCard m.

HEM780 blood pressure m.

Hemochron m.

HemoTec activated clotting time m.

Holter m.

home m.

HomMed m.

Insta-Pulse heart rate m.

intelligent cardiovascular m. (ICM)

KinetiX ventilation m.

King of Hearts Holter m.

m. leads

LifeShirt m.

loop m.

Magellan m.

Marquette 8000 Holter m.

MDILog microelectronic m.

MicroCO carbon monoxide m.

MiniOX 3000 oxygen m.

Mini-Torr Plus NIPB m.

MRM-2 oxygen consumption m.

nDx m.

Nellcor Symphony blood pressure m.

Neotrend multiparameter blood gas m.

NICO$_2$ noninvasive cardiac output m.

noninvasive m.

NOxBOX m.

NOxBOX+ m.

Ohmeda 6200, 6300 CO$_2$ m.

One Touch blood glucose m.

OptiVol fluid m.

OSD m.

PAM2, PAM3 m.

Paratrend 7 continuous blood gas m.

Paratrend 7+ multiparameter blood gas m.

patient m.

Physios CTM 01 cardiac transplant m.

Pick and Go m.

Polar Vantage XL heart rate m.

portable oxygen m.

Porta-Resp m.

Pressurometer blood pressure m.

PrinterNOx nitric oxide/nitrogen dioxide m.

Propaq Encore vital signs m.

Pulse Pro heart rate m.

Puritan Bennett 7250 metabolic m.
Q-TRAK IAQ m.
RIP portable sleep m.
Smokerlyzer breath carbon
    monoxide m.
STAN S31 fetal heart m.
TCM30 transcutaneous oxygen m.
Tensys T-line blood pressure m.
ToxCO+ breath carbon
    monoxide m.
transcutaneous oxygen m. (TCOM)
transtelephonic exercise m. (TEM)
Vasotrac blood pressure m.
VentCheck handheld respiratory m.
VenTrak respiratory mechanics m.
ventricular arrhythmia m. (VAM)
Veris MR vital signs
    physiological m.
VEST ambulatory ventricular
    function m.
video m.
Vigilance CCO/SvO$_2$/CEDV m.
V.I.P. Bird volume m.
Vitalograph BreathCO M.
Vitalograph pulmonary m.
V-Tam T shirt m.

monitor/defibrillator
Lifepak 5, 7 m./d.

monitoring
ambulatory m.
ambulatory blood pressure m.
    (ABPM)
ambulatory electrocardiographic m.
    (AEM)
ambulatory Holter m. (AHM)
ambulatory oximetry m. (AOM)
beat-by-beat hemodynamic m.
capnography ventilation m.
cardiac m. (CM)
CareLink network for patient m.
Doptone m.
endotracheal cardiac output m.
    (ECOM)
hemodynamic m. (HM)
Holter m. (HM)
internet ICD m.
invasive m.
NIBP m.
on-demand m.
OptiVol fluid status m.
physiologic m.
physiological m.
pleural space m.
precordial electrocardiographic m.
    (PEM)
pulse oximetry m. (POM)
train-of-4 m.
transcutaneous pCO$_2$ m.
transtelephonic m. (TTM)

transtelephonic ambulatory m.
    (TAM)
transtelephonic arrhythmia m.
transtelephonic cardiac event m.
transthoracic intracardiac m. (TIM)
ultrasonic cardiac output m.
    (USCOM)
Monneret pulse
monoamine
m. oxidase (MAO)
m. oxidase inhibitor (MAOI)
monobactam
monocarboxylate
m. proton cotransporter
m. transporter
monocardiogram
Mono-Cedocard
monochloramine
Monoclate-P
monoclonal
m. antibody 3G4
m. antifibronectin antibody
m. anti-IgE antibody
m. antimyosin antibody
m. hypothesis
m. immunoglobulin M gammopathy
m. theory of atherogenesis
MonoClone immunoenzymetric assay
monocrotaline
monocrotic pulse
monocrotism
monocrotus
pulsus m.
monocyte
m. chemoattractant protein (MCP)
m. chemoattractant protein-1 (MCP-
    1)
m. chemotactic and activating
    factor (MCAF)
m. chemotactic protein-1 (MCP-1)
surface adherent m. (SAM)
transcardiac m.
monocyte-derived macrophage
monocytic leukemoid reaction
monocytogenes
Listeria m.
monodisperse
Monodox Oral
monofilament
m. absorbable suture
m. polypropylene suture
Semmes-Weinstein m.
monoform tachycardia
Mono-Gesic
monohydrate
cefadroxil m.
cephalexin m.
Monojector
Monoket

M

Monolithic fetal pacemaker
Monolyth oxygenator
monomer
    actin m.
    fibrin m. (FM)
    transthyretin m.
N^G-monomethyl-L-arginine (L-NMMA)
monomorphic ventricular tachycardia
  (MVT)
mononeuritis multiplex
Mononine
mononitrate
    isosorbide m.
mononuclear
    m. alveolitis
    m. cell
mononucleosis
    infectious m.
monophasic
    m. action potential (MAP)
    m. action potential duration
      (MAPD)
    m. action potential early
      afterdepolarization (mEAD)
    m. complex
    m. contour of QRS complex
    m. defibrillation waveform (MDW)
    m. negative QRS complex
    m. pulse
    m. shock therapy
monophonic wheeze
monophosphate
    adenosine m. (AMP)
    cyclic adenosine m. (cAMP)
    cyclic guanosine m. (cGMP)
    cyclic nucleotide adenosine m.
    guanosine m. (GMP)
monoplace chamber
monopolar temporary electrode
Monopril
monopropionate
    beclomethasone m. (BMP)
Monorail
    M. angioplasty catheter
    M. delivery system
    M. guidewire
    M. imaging catheter
    M. Speedy balloon
monoresistance
monosaturated
    m. fat
    m. fatty acid
Monostrut cardiac valve prosthesis
monosulfate
    guanethidine m.
monotest
    R-lactate enzyme m.
monotherapy

monotypic lesion
monounsaturated fatty acid (MUFA)
Mono-Vacc
Monovial
    Cardizem M.
    M. drug delivery system
monoxide
    carbon m. (CO)
    corrected diffusing capacity for
      carbon m. ($DLCO_c$)
    diffusing capacity of lung for
      carbon m. (DLCO)
    partial pressure of carbon m.
      (PCO)
monoxide-oximetry
monoxime
    butanedione m.
Monro
    foramen of M.
Monte Carlo multiway sensitivity
  analysis method
montelukast
    m. sodium
Montgomery
    M. Safe-T Tube
    M. speaking valve
    M. tracheostomy
Montgomery-Asberg Depression Rating
  Scale (MADRS)
Moody friction factor
moon face
Moore
    M. procedure
    M. tracheostomy button
Moraxella
    M. catarrhalis
    M. nonliquefaciens
morbidity
morbid obesity
Morbillivirus
morcellation
Morch respirator
More-Flow long-term high-flow catheter
Morestin syndrome
Moretz clip
Morgagni
    M. disease
    foramen of M.
    M. hernia
    M. nodule
Morgagni-Adams-Stokes
    M.-A.-S. syncope
    M.-A.-S. syndrome
Morganella morganii
morganii
    Morganella m.
moribund
moricizine

moriens
    ultimum m.
morphine
morphogenesis
morphologic
morphology
    flutter wave m.
    hills-and-valley m.
    P-wave m.
    QRS m.
    skeletal muscle m.
    valvular m.
    windsock m.
morphometric measurement
morphometry
    aerosol-derived airway m. (ADAM)
    airway m.
    lung m.
Morph steerable and deflectable vascular catheter
Morquio-Brailsford disease
Morquio syndrome
morrhuate sodium
Morrow procedure
Morse manifest
mortality rate (MR)
mortis
    myocardial rigor m.
Morton cough
MOS
    missed ostium sequence
    mitral opening snap
mosaic
    M. cardiac bioprosthesis
    m. jet
    m. jet signals
    m. pattern
    m. perfusion
    M. porcine bioprosthetic heart valve
Moschcowitz
    M. disease
    M. sign
    M. test
Mosher life-saving tracheal tube
mOsm
    milliosmole
mosquito
    m. clamp
    m. hemostat
moss-agate sputum
Mosso sphygmomanometer
motexafin lutetium
motility
    esophageal m.
    receptor for hyaluronan-mediated m. (RHAMM)
motion
    abnormal wall m. (AWM)

    m. artifact
    atrioventricular junction m.
    chest wall m.
    circulation. sensation, m. (CSM)
    cusp m.
    diastolic m.
    m. display echo
    endocardial m.
    fetal atrial wall m.
    fetal ventricular wall m.
    gated wall m.
    infarct zone wall m.
    interventricular septal m.
    leaflet m.
    left ventricular wall m. (LVWM)
    mitral anulus m.
    m. mode (M-mode)
    paradoxic wall m.
    plaque m.
    precordial m.
    regional wall m. (RWM)
    right ventricular wall m.
    segmental wall m. (SWM)
    septal wall m.
    systolic m. (SM)
    systolic anterior m. (SAM)
    thoracoabdominal wall m.
    tricuspid anular m. (TAM)
    ventricular wall m. (VWM)
    wall m. (WM)
    whorl m.
motoneuron
motor
    M. Assessment Scale (MAS)
    M. Club Assessment test of motor activity
    m. evoked potential (MEP)
    m. neglect
motor-exploratory hemineglect
motoricity
motorized transducer pullback device
MOTT
    mycobacteria other than tuberculosis
mottled
mottling
    m. of extremities
    quantum m.
Moulaert
    muscle of M.
moulin
    bruit de la roue de m.
Mounier-Kuhn syndrome
mountain sickness
mounting area (MA)
Mount-Mayfield forceps
mouse
    pleural m.
mousetail pulse

M

moustache
> m. angiographic landmark
> m. angiographic landmark of left anterior descending coronary artery bifurcation

mouth of aneurysm
mouthguard
> Snorex m.

mouthpiece
> Pneumotach disposable m.
> SafeTway pediatric m.

mouth-to-face shield ventilation
mouth-to-mask ventilation
mouth-to-mouth
> m.-t.-m. respiration
> m.-t.-m. resuscitation
> m.-t.-m. ventilation

mouth-to-nose ventilation
mouth-to-stoma ventilation
mouthwash
> chlorhexidine gluconate m.

movable
> m. core straight safety wire guide
> m. heart
> m. pulse

Movat
> M. pentachrome
> M. stain

MOVC (*var. of* MOIVC)
movement
> air m.
> ameboid m.
> anomalous m.
> m. arousal index (MAI)
> chest wall m.
> ciliary m.
> circus m.
> m. disorder
> mirror m.
> nonrapid eye m. (NREM)
> periodic limb m. (PLM)
> precordial m.
> quality of m. (QOM)
> rapid eye m. (REM)
> m. science physiotherapy
> sleep-onset rapid eye m. (SOREM)
> sustained outward m. (SOM)
> vessel wall m.

moving slice velocity mapping
moxalactam
moxibustion
moxifloxacin HCl
moxonidine
moyamoya
> m. disease
> m. of heart

Moynahan syndrome
MPA
> main pulmonary artery

> mean pulmonary arterial
> medroxyprogesterone acetate
> microscopic polyangiitis
> > MPA pressure

MPAP
> mean pulmonary artery pressure

MPatch vascular closure system
MPAWP
> mean pulmonary artery wedge pressure

MPE
> malignant pleural effusion

MP-H
> mandibular plane to hyoid

MPHR
> maximum predicted heart rate

MPI
> myocardial perfusion imaging

MPIF
> myeloid progenitor inhibitory factor

MPM
> malignant pleural mesothelioma

MPO
> myeloperoxidase

MPR
> maximum pulse rate

M-protein serotype
MPS
> myocardial perfusion scintigraphy
> myocardial protection system

MPT
> multiple-parameter telemetry

MPV
> main portal vein

MPVP
> mean pulmonary venous pressure

MR
> mitral reflux
> mitral regurgitation
> mortality rate
> myocardial revascularization
> > MR cine imaging
> > MR 290 humidification chamber
> > MR lead

MRA
> magnetic resonance angiography
> > 3D TOF MRA
> > TOF MRA

MRAP
> mean right atrial pressure

MRCA
> magnetic resonance coronary angiography
> > respiratory gated MRCA

MRD
> mean reference diameter

MRE
> maximal resistive exercise

MREI
> mean rate ejection index

MRF
  magnetic resonance flowmetry
  mitral regurgitant flow
MRI
  magnetic resonance imaging
    CASL-PI MRI
    cine gradient-echo MRI
    diffusion MRI
    diffusion-weighted MRI
    DSC MRI
      dynamic susceptibility contrast-enhanced MRI
    dynamic susceptibility contrast-enhanced MRI (DSC MRI, DSC MRI)
    FLASH MRI
    functional MRI
    Gd-DTPA-enhanced MRI
    GE Signa 1.5-T MRI
    gradient echo-cine MRI
    GRASS MRI
    hemodynamically weighted MRI (HW)
    intravascular MRI
    low-dose dobutamine cine MRI
    perfusion imaging MRI
    Philips ACS NT 1.5 Gyroscan MRI
    Siemens Magnetom 1.5-T MRI
    spin-echo MRI
    Toshiba MRT 200 MRI
    T2-weighted MRI
    MRI velocity mapping
MRI-identified stroke
MRL Pacette
MRM-2 oxygen consumption monitor
mRNA
  messenger ribonucleic acid
    osteopontin mRNA
    skeletal alpha-actin mRNA
MRP
  maximal response plateau
MRS
  magnetic resonance spectroscopy
MRV
  magnetic resonance venography
MRVP
  mean right ventricular pressure
MS
  mainstream smoke
  mitral sounds
  mitral stenosis
    MS Classique balloon dilation catheter
m/s
  meter per second
m/s^2
  meter per second squared

ms
  millisecond
MSAP
  mean systemic arterial pressure
MSC
  mesenchymal stem cell
  midsystolic click
MSCT
  multislice spiral computed tomography
MSD Enteric Coated ASA
m/sec
  meter per second
msec
  millisecond
MSER
  mean systolic ejection rate
MSI
  magnetic source imaging
  metered-solution inhaler
MSLT
  multiple sleep latency test
MSM
  midsystolic murmur
MSNA
  muscle sympathetic nerve activity
MSOF
  multisystem organ failure
MSPECT
  myocardial single photon emission tomography
MSPS
  myocardial stress perfusion scintigraphy
MSS
  muscular subaortic stenosis
MST
  median survival time
MSU
  myocardial substrate uptake
MSVC
  maximal sustainable ventilatory capacity
MT
  medical thoracoscopy
  mural thrombosis
  mural thrombus
MT-100 ECG Holter system
MTB
  Mycobacterium tuberculosis
MTBC LightCycler assay
MTC catheter
MTD
  Mycobacterium Tuberculosis Direct
    MTD test
MTET
  modified treadmill exercise test
Mt. Fuji sign
MTHFR
  methylenetetrahydrofolate reductase
    MTHFR gene
    MTHFR genotype

M

MT-MMP
> membrane-bound membrane-type
> metalloproteinase

MTP
> methylprednisolone
> microsomal triglyceride transfer protein
> MTP gene

MTST
> maximal treadmill stress test

MTT
> maximal treadmill testing

MTWA
> microvolt T-wave alternans

M-type alpha-1 antitrypsin

MU
> megaunit

mU
> milliunit

much
> M. bacillus
> M. granules

mucicarmine stain

mucin
> m. antisense oligonucleotide
> m. clot prevention (MCP)
> epithelial m.

mucinous
> m. adenocarcinoma
> m. carcinoma

mucoactive
> m. medication
> m. therapy

mucociliary
> m. clearance (MCC)
> m. efficiency
> m. escalator
> m. system
> m. transport

mucocutaneous
> m. lesion
> m. lymph node syndrome

mucoepidermoid carcinoma

mucoepithelial dysplasia

Muco-Fen DM, LA

mucogenicum
> *Mycobacterium m.*

mucoid
> m. exopolysaccharide
> m. impaction
> m. medial degeneration
> m. sputum

mucokinetic

mucolipidosis, pl. **mucolipidoses**

mucolytic
> classic m.
> peptide m.

mucomembranous

Mucomyst

mucopolysaccharide
> acid m. (AMP)

mucopolysaccharidosis,
> pl. **mucopolysaccharidoses**

mucopurulent sputum

mucopus

Mucor

Mucoraceae

mucoregulatory agent

mucoretention cyst

mucormycosis
> primary pulmonary m.
> pulmonary m.
> rhinocerebral m.

mucosa
> airway m.
> m. of bronchus
> cardia m. (CM)
> esophageal m.
> region of respiratory m.
> respiratory m.
> tracheal m.
> tunica m.

mucosal
> m. addressin cell adhesion
> molecule-1 (MadCAM-1)
> m. edema
> m. ischemia

mucoserous

mucous
> m. cell
> m. desiccation
> m. gel
> m. gland hyperplasia
> m. gland hypertrophy
> m. inspissation
> m. layer
> m. plugging
> m. rale
> m. retention cyst
> m. sheets
> m. thread

mucoviscidosis

mucus
> m. clearance device
> m. hypersecretion
> m. inhibitor
> low-viscosity m.
> oyster mass of m.
> m. plug
> m. production
> m. retention
> m. secretion
> tenacious m.
> thick and sticky m.
> m. transport
> viscid m.
> m. viscosity

mucus-producing respiratory condition

MUE
medication use evaluation
Muerto Canyon virus
MUF
modified ultrafiltration
MUFA
monounsaturated fatty acid
muffled heart sounds
MUGA
multiple gated acquisition
MUGA cardiac blood pool scan
MUGA exercise stress test
MUGA scanning
Müller
M. banding
M. catheter guide
M. experiment
M. maneuver
M. sign
M. test
M. vena caval clamp
Mullins
M. blade and balloon septostomy
M. blade technique
M. cardiac device
M. catheter introducer
M. dilator
M. modification
M. modification of transseptal
catheterization
M. sheath/dilator
M. sheath system
M. transseptal catheter
M. transseptal catheterization sheath
multiaccess catheter (MAC)
multiaxis accelerometer
multibreath nitrogen washout technique
multicellular stent
multi-chamber stimulation device
Multicor II cardiac pacemaker
multicrystal gamma camera
multidetector
m. computed tomography (MDCT)
m. row helical computed
tomography
multidetector-row chest CT
**multidisciplinary pulmonary
rehabilitation program**
**Multi-Dop X/TCD transcranial Doppler
instrument**
multidrug resistance
multidrug-resistant (MDR)
m.-r. *Streptococcus pneumoniae*
(MDRSP)
m.-r. tuberculosis (MDR-TB)
multielectrode
m. basket catheter
m. impedance catheter
m. probe

multielement linear array
multifactorial
m. cardiac risk index (MCRI)
m. cough
**MULTIFIT computer-based chronic
illness management system**
multifocal
m. atrial tachycardia (MAT,
MFAT, MFT)
m. lesion
m. micronodular pneumocyte
hyperplasia
m. supraventricular tachyarrhythmia
multiform
m. premature ventricular complex
m. tachycardia
multiforme
erythema m.
glioblastoma m. (GBM)
recurrent glioblastoma m. (RGM)
multigated angiography
multihead detector
multiinfarct dementia
multikringle glycoprotein
multilamellar body
multilesion angioplasty
multilimb catheter
Multi-Link
M.-L. Ascent stent
M.-L. Duet coronary stent
M.-L. Frontier coronary stent
system
M.-L. Penta coronary stent
M.-L. Penta coronary stent system
M.-L. Pixel coronary stent
M.-L. Pixel stent system
M.-L. Solo stent
M.-L. Tetra coronary stent
M.-L. Tetra coronary stent system
M.-L. Tristar balloon
M.-L. Tristar stent system
M.-L. Ultra coronary stent
M.-L. Vision RX and OTW
coronary stent system
M.-L. Zeta coronary stent system
multilobar disease
multilocular cyst
multilocularis
Echinococcus m.
multimer assay
multinucleated giant cell
multiplace chambers
multiplanar reconstruction technique
**multiplane transesophageal
echocardiography**
multiple
m. antimycobacterial agents
m. cholesterol emboli syndrome
(MCES)

M

multiple *(continued)*
    m. CVIs
    m. embolisms
    m. gated acquisition (MUGA)
    m. gated acquisition cardiac blood pool scan
    m. lentigines syndrome
    m. lipoprotein-type hyperlipidemia
    m. lobar hemorrhage (MLH)
    m. point electrode
    m. reentrant wavelet hypothesis of Moe
    m. sclerosis
    m. shunt levels
    m. sleep latency test (MSLT)
    m. system atrophy
    m. wavelet hypothesis
multiple-balloon valvoplasty
multiple-dilator technique
multiple-organ
    m.-o. dysfunction
    m.-o. dysfunction syndrome (MODS)
    m.-o. failure
multiple-parameter telemetry (MPT)
multiple-trauma patient
multiplex
    mononeuritis m.
    m. neuropathy
multipolar
    m. catheter electrode
    m. electrode catheter
multipotent adult progenitor cell (MAPC)
multiprogrammable pulse generator
multisensor catheter
multiseptate cyst
multi-sideport catheter infusion set
multisite
    m. biventricular pacing
    m. mapping
multislab technique
multislice spiral computed tomography (MSCT)
multispine catheter
MultiSPIRO
    M. Clear Advantage pulmonary function filter
    M. Series SX/DX computerized spirometry
multistage
    m. exercise test (MET)
    m. maximal effort exercise stress test
multisystem
    m. disease
    m. organ failure (MSOF)
multisystemic inflammatory disorder
multitargeted antifolate

Multitest cell-mediated immunity system
multivalve
    m. disease
    m. endocarditis
    m. insufficiency
    m. operation
    m. pathology
multivalvular
    m. disease
    m. disease murmur
multivariate regression analysis
Multi-Vent
    Hudson M.-V.
multivessel (MV)
    m. coronary artery disease
    m. coronary artery obstruction
    m. disease (MVD)
multivorans
    Burkholderia m.
multiwire gamma camera
multocida
    Pasteurella m.
Münchausen stridor
MUO
    myocardiopathy of unknown origin
mupirocin
mural
    m. aneurysm
    m. endocarditis
    m. endocardium
    m. nodule
    m. thrombosis (MT)
    m. thrombus (MT)
Murat sign
Murgo pressure contour
mu rhythm
murine cardiac myosin
murmur (M)
    accidental m.
    amphoric m.
    anemic m.
    aneurysmal m.
    aortic-left ventricular tunnel m.
    aortic-mitral combined disease m.
    aortic regurgitation m.
    aortic sclerotic m.
    aortic stenosis m.
    apex m.
    apical mid diastolic heart m.
    apical systolic heart m.
    arterial m.
    atriosystolic m.
    atrioventricular flow rumbling m.
    attrition m.
    Austin Flint m.
    basal diastolic m.'s
    bellows m.
    blood m.
    blowing m.

blubbery diastolic m.
brain m.
Bright m.
bronchial collateral artery m.
Cabot-Locke m.
carcinoid m.
cardiac m. (CM)
cardiopulmonary m.
cardiorespiratory m.
Carey Coombs short mid-
  diastolic m.
carotid artery m.
click m.
coarse m.
Cole-Cecil m.
congenital m.
continuous m. (CM)
continuous heart m.
cooing m.
Coombs m.
crescendo m.
crescendo-decrescendo diamond-
  shaped systolic ejection m.
Cruveilhier-Baumgarten m.
decrescendo m.
deglutition m.
diamond ejection m.
diamond-shaped ejection m.
diastolic m. (DM)
diastolic decrescendo m.
direct m.
Docke m.
dove coo musical m.
Duroziez m.
dynamic m.
early diastolic m. (EDM)
early-peaking systolic m.
ejection m. (EM)
ejection systolic m. (ESM)
end-diastolic m.
endocardial m.
end-systolic m.
Eustace Smith m.
exit block m.
exocardial m.
expiratory m.
extracardiac m.
Fisher m.
Flint m.
flow m.
Fräntzel m.
friction m.
functional m.
Gallavardin m.
Gibson m.
goose-honk m.
grade 1-6 m.
Graham Steell m.
groaning m.

Hamman m.
harsh m.
heart m. (HM)
hemic m.
high-frequency m.
high-pitched m.
Hodgkin-Key m.
holodiastolic decrescendo m.
holosystolic m. (HSM)
honking m.
hourglass m.
humming m.
humming-top m.
incidental m.
indirect m.
innocent m. (IM)
innocent heart m.
inorganic m.
inspiratory m.
lapping m.
late apical systolic m.
late diastolic m.
late-peaking systolic m.
late systolic m. (LSM)
left ventricular-right atrial
  communication m.
Levine grade 1–6 cardiac m.
low-frequency m.
low-pitched m.
machinery m.
mammary souffle m.
middiastolic m. (MDM)
midsystolic m. (MSM)
mill house m.
mill wheel m.
mitral prolapse m.
mitral regurgitation m.
mitral stenosis m.
multivalvular disease m.
muscular m.
musical m.
noninvasive m.
nun's venous hum m.
obstructive m.
organic m.
outflow m.
pansystolic m.
Parrot m.
patent ductus arteriosus m.
pathologic m.
pericardial m.
physiologic m.
pleuropericardial m.
PPS m.
prediastolic m.
presystolic m. (PM, PSM)
primary pulmonary hypertension m.
protodiastolic m.
pulmonary m., pulmonic m.

M

murmur *(continued)*
  rasping m.
  reduplication m.
  regurgitant m.
  respiratory m.
  Roger m.
  rubs, gallops, m.'s
  rumbling diastolic m.
  scratchy m.
  seagull m.
  seesaw m.
  Steell m.
  stenosal m.
  Still m.
  subclavian m.
  subclavicular m.
  systolic m. (SM)
  systolic apical m.
  systolic ejection m. (SEM)
  systolic regurgitant m.
  to-and-fro m.
  transmitted m.
  Traube m.
  tricuspid m.
  vascular m.
  venous m.
  ventricular septal defect m.
  vesicular m.
  waterwheel m.
  whooping m.
murmur/energy ratio (MER)
Muromonab-CD3
Murphy
  M. method
  M. percussion
Murray score
muscarinic
  m. agonist
  m. receptor
  m. stimulation
muscle
  accessory inspiratory m.
  airways smooth m. (ASM)
  anterior papillary m. (APM)
  m. artifact
  m. bridge
  bronchial smooth m.
  bronchoesophageal m.
  cardiac m. (CM)
  Chassaignac axillary m.
  constrictor m.
  elevator m.
  m. ergoreceptor
  m. fraction enzyme of CPK (CPK-
    MM, CPK-3)
  glottic constrictor m.'s
  human aortic smooth m. (HASMC)
  inferior constrictor m.
  interior m.

latissimus dorsi m.
m. metaboreflex
middle constrictor m.
m. of Moulaert
Oehl m.
overrecruitment of glottic
  constrictor m.'s
papillary m. (PM)
pectinate m.
pleuroesophageal m.
posterior cricoarytenoid m.
posterior papillary m. (PPM)
rectus abdominis m.
Reisseisen m.
m. relaxant
ribbon m.
semispinal m.
serratus anterior m.
short-axis plane, papillary m.
  (SAX-PM)
skeletal m.
spinal m.
m. stiffness
strap m.
m. sympathetic nerve activity
  (MSNA)
m. of thorax
m. trabeculation
trachealis m.
transverse m.
transversus nuchae m.
venous smooth m.
muscle-sparing thoracotomy
muscular
  m. bridging
  m. coat
  m. coat of bronchus
  m. coat of esophagus
  m. coat of trachea
  m. contraction
  m. dystrophy
  m. incompetence
  m. murmur
  m. subaortic stenosis (MSS)
  m. venous pump
  m. ventricular septal defect
    (MVSD)
musculoskeletal
  m. intervention center (MUSIC)
  m. pain
musculus, pl. **musculi**
  m. bronchoesophageus
  m. diaphragma
  musculi laryngis
  m. levator glandulae thyroideae
  m. pleuroesophageus
mushroom
  m. dust

m. worker's disease
m. worker's lung

MUSIC
musculoskeletal intervention center

musical
m. bruit
m. chest
m. cough
m. murmur
m. rale

Musset sign

mustard
M. atrial baffle
M. atrial repair
M. atrial switch operation
L-phenylalanine m.
nitrogen m.
M. procedure

Mustard-Senning procedure

Mustargen Hydrochloride

mutagenicity

Mutamycin

mutant allele

mutation
factor V Leiden m.
missense m.
nonsense m.
sarcomeric protein m.
SCN5A m.
thrombophilic factor V Leiden m.
Z m.

mute
m. reflex
m. toe sign

muzolimine

MV
maximal ventilation
mechanical ventilation
midventricular
multivessel

mV
millivolt

MVA
malignant ventricular arrhythmia
mechanical ventricular assistance
microvascular angiopathy
mitral valve area

MVAD
mechanical ventricular assist device

MVB
microvascular bleeding

MVC
maximal vital capacity
maximum voluntary contraction
myocardial vascular capacity

MVD
microvascular decompression
mitral valve disease

multivessel disease
myocardial vasodilation

MVE
mitral valve echo
mitral valve excursion

MVF
mitral valve flow

MVG
mitral valve gradient
myocardial velocity gradient

MVI
mitral valve insufficiency

MVL
mitral valve leaflet

MVO
maximum venous outflow
mitral valve opening
mitral valve orifice

MVO₂
myocardial oxygen consumption

MVOA
mitral valve orifice area

MVP
mitomycin, vinblastine, cisplatin
mitral valve prolapse
MVP catheter

MVPS
mitral valve prolapse syndrome

MVP-SC
mitral valve prolapse-systolic click

MVR
maximal ventilation rate
minimal vascular resistance
mitral valve replacement

MVSD
muscular ventricular septal defect

MVT
monomorphic ventricular tachycardia

MVV
maximum voluntary ventilation

6MWD
6-minute walk distance

MWT
maintenance of wakefulness test
myocardial wall thickness

6MWT, 6-MWT
6-minute walking test

myalgia gravis

Myambutol

myasthenia
m. cordis
m. gravis
m. gravis pseudoparalytica

myasthenic crisis

MyBP-C
myosin-binding protein C
MyBP-C gene

mycetoma

MycoAKT latex bead agglutination test

M

mycobacteria
    nontuberculous m. (NTM)
    m. other than tuberculosis (MOTT)
mycobacterial
    m. disease
    m. growth indicator tube (MGIT)
mycobacteria testing
Mycobacterium
    M. abscessus
    M. africanum
    M. avium
    M. avium complex (MAC)
    M. avium complex infection
    M. avium-intracellulare M. (MAIC)
    M. avium-intracellulare (MAI)
    M. avium-intracellulare infection
    M. bovis
    M. chelonae
    M. fortuitum
    M. fortuitum-chelonae complex
    M. gastri
    M. genavense
    M. gordonae
    M. haemophilum
    M. intracellulare
    M. kansasii
    M. leprae
    M. malmoense
    M. marinum
    M. microti
    M. mucogenicum
    M. peregrinum
    M. phlei
    M. pneumoniae
    M. scrofulaceum
    M. simiae
    M. smegmatis
    M. szulgai
    M. terrae
    M. thermoresistibile
    M. tuberculosis (MTB)
    M. Tuberculosis Direct (MTD)
    M. Tuberculosis Direct Test
    M. ulcerans
    M. vaccae
    M. xenopi
Mycobutin Oral
mycology
mycophenolate
    m. mofetil (MMF)
    m. mofetil capsule
    m. mofetil intravenous
    m. mofetil intravenous for injection
    m. mofetil oral suspension
    m. mofetil tablet
Mycoplasma
    M. faucium
    M. hominis
    M. incognitus

    M. pneumoniae
    M. xenopi
mycoplasmal
    m. infection
    m. pneumonia
mycoplasmosis
mycosis, pl. **mycoses**
    m. fungoides
    Posadas m.
    pulmonary m.
Mycostatin Topical
mycotic
    m. aortic aneurysm
    m. aortography
    m. endocarditis
    m. infection
MycroMesh Plus biomaterial
MycroPhylax implantable cardioverter-defibrillator
mydriatic
myectomy
    septal m.
myelinolysis
    extrapontine m.
    pontine m.
myelodysplasia
myelofibrosis
myeloid progenitor inhibitory factor (MPIF)
myeloma
myelonecrosis
myeloperoxidase (MPO)
myelosuppression
Myers Solution
MYHC
    heavy chain cardiac myosin
MYHCA
    heavy chain cardiac myosin alpha
Myleran
myoblast
    skeletal m. (SKMB)
myocardia (*pl. of* myocardium)
myocardial
    m. abscess
    m. adrenergic signaling
    m. angiogenesis
    m. anoxia
    m. band (MB)
    m. band enzymes of CPK (CPK-MB, CPK-2)
    m. band index
    m. bed
    m. beta adrenergic receptor (MBAR)
    m. blood flow (MBF)
    m. blush
    m. blush grade (MBG)
    m. border zone
    m. bridge

m. bridging (MB)
m. cell
m. cell hypertrophy
m. channeling (MC)
m. clamp
m. cold-spot perfusion scintigraphy
m. collagen matrix
m. concussion
m. contractility
m. contraction force (MCF)
m. contraction state
m. contrast echocardiography (MCE)
m. contusion
m. creatine phosphate
m. damage (MD)
m. deformation
m. depolarization
m. depressant factor (MDF)
m. depressant substance (MDS)
m. depression
m. disarray
m. disease (MD)
m. disease of unknown origin (MDUO)
m. Doppler velocity (MDV)
m. dysfunction
m. edema
m. electrocardiography
m. electrode
m. endothelin
m. energy
m. failure
m. fiber shortening
m. fibrosis (MF)
m. fibrous scar
m. fractional flow reserve (FFR$_{myo}$)
m. free wall rupture
m. function
m. hamartoma
m. heterogeneity
m. hibernation
m. hypoperfusion
m. indirect calorimetry
m. infarction (MI)
M. Infarction Data Acquisition System
m. infarction in dumbbell form
m. infarction frame count
m. infarction rehabilitation program (MIRP)
m. infarction research unit (MIRU)
m. infarction triage and intervention (MITI)
m. infarctlet
m. infiltrative process
m. infundibular stenosis
m. injury
m. insufficiency

m. ischemia (MI)
m. ischemia dynamic analysis (MIDA)
m. ischemic syndrome
m. jeopardy
m. jeopardy index
m. lactate extraction
m. laser revascularization (MLR)
m. laser revascularization procedure
m. lead
m. long-chain fatty acid uptake defect
m. malnutrition
m. mass
m. metabolic rate (MMR)
m. metabolism
m. muscle creatine kinase isoenzyme
m. necrosis
m. oxygen (MO$_2$)
m. oxygen consumption (MVO$_2$)
m. oxygen demand
m. oxygen supply
m. oxygen uptake
m. perforation
m. performance
m. performance index
m. perfusion
m. perfusion imaging (MPI)
m. perfusion scan
m. perfusion scintigraphy (MPS)
m. protection
m. protection pouch
m. protection system (MPS)
m. remodeling
m. repolarization
m. reserve
m. revascularization (MR)
m. rigor mortis
m. salvage
m. scar tissue
m. single photon emission tomography (MSPECT)
m. sinusoid
m. sleeves
m. sparing
m. stiffness
m. stress perfusion scintigraphy (MSPS)
m. stunning
m. substrate uptake (MSU)
m. syncytium
m. tension
m. tissue
m. tissue reperfusion
m. vascular capacity (MVC)
m. vasodilation (MVD)
m. velocity gradient (MVG)
m. velocity pattern

M

myocardial *(continued)*
    m. viability
    m. viability scintigraphy
    m. VIDA
    m. wall thickness (MWT)
myocardiograph
myocardiopathy
    alcoholic m.
    chagasic m.
    congestive m. (CM)
    m. of unknown origin (MUO)
myocardiorrhaphy
myocarditic
myocarditis (MC)
    acute isolated m.
    asymptomatic m.
    atrial m.
    bacterial m.
    burned out viral m.
    cardiac sarcoidosis m.
    Chagas m.
    chronic m.
    clostridial m.
    coxsackievirus m.
    cryptococcal m.
    diphtheritic m.
    ECHO virus m.
    echovirus m.
    experimental autoimmune m.
     (EAM)
    Fiedler m.
    fragmentation m.
    fulminant m.
    giant cell m.
    helminthic m.
    Histoplasma m.
    hypersensitivity m.
    idiopathic m.
    indurative m.
    metazoal m.
    parenchymatous m.
    peripartum m.
    protozoal m.
    rheumatic m.
    rickettsial m.
    spirochetal m.
    syphilitic m.
    toxic m.
    tuberculoid m.
    viral m. (VM)
myocardium, pl. **myocardia**
    border zone m.
    dysfunctional m.
    dyssynergic m.
    fragmentation of m.
    hibernating m.
    hypertrophied m.
    hypoperfused m.
    idiopathic disease of m. (IDM)

    ischemic m.
    isolated noncompaction of
     ventricular m. (INVM)
    jeopardized m.
    necrotic m.
    postischemic m.
    reperfused m.
    senescent m.
    sleeve of m.
    spongy m.
    stunned m.
    underperfused m.
    viable m.
    vulnerable m.
myocardosis
    Reisman m.
myoclonic jerk
myocyotosis
    focal m.
myocyte
    amplifying m.
    Anitschkow m.
    m. apoptosis
    cardiac m.
    m. deenergization
    m. hypertrophy
    m. hypoxia
    m. magnesium stores
    m. metabolic activity
    m. necrosis
    ventricular m.
myocytolysis
    coagulative m.
    m. of heart
myoendocarditis
myofascial
myofibrillar
    m. ATPase
    m. calcium level
    m. disarray
    m. lysis
myofibril pellet
myofibroblast
myofibrosis cordis
myofilament
    m. calcium responsiveness
    m. contractile activation
myogenic theory
myoglobin
    m. assay
    serum m.
myoglobinuria
myoglobulin (Mgb)
    m. cardiac diagnostic test
myoglobulinuria
myoinositol
myointimal plaque
myolysis
    cardiotoxic m.

myomalacia cordis
myomectomy
myonecrosis
    intervention-induced m.
myopathia cordis
myopathy
    centronuclear m.
    myotubular m.
    nemaline m.
    skeletal muscle m.
    tachycardia-induced m.
myopericarditis
myoplasmic calcium
myoplasty
myopleuropericarditis
Myopore lead
myopotential oversensing
myorhythmia
Myoscint
MyoSIGHT dedicated nuclear cardiology
   camera system
myosin
    antibody to murine cardiac m.
     (AMM)
    anticardiac m. (ACM)
    cardiac m.
    m. filament
    m. heavy chain
    heavy chain cardiac m. (MYHC)
    m. light chain
    murine cardiac m.
myosin-binding
    m.-b. protein C (MyBP-C)
    m.-b. protein C gene
myosin-specific antibody
myositis
Myosplint
    M. device
    M. procedure
MYOtherm XP cardioplegia delivery
   system
myotomy
    hyoid m.
    septal m.
myotomy-myectomy-septal resection

myotonia congenita
myotonic muscular dystrophy
Myotrace Plus electromyography unit
myotubular myopathy
Myoview
    M. contrast material
    M. kit
MyoVive
myringoplasty
    venous graft m. (VGM)
myrtillus
    Vaccinium m.
Mytussin
    M. AC
    M. DAC
    M. DM
myurous pulse
myurus
    pulsus m.
myxedema
    m. heart
    pretibial m.
myxedematous
myxoid fibroblastic tissue
myxoma, pl. myxomata
    atrial m.
    cardiac m.
    familial atrial m.
    infected m.
    left atrial m. (LAM)
    left ventricular m.
    mobile m.
    petrified cardiac m.
    right atrial m.
    right ventricular m.
    stone-like m.
    m. tumor
    ventricular m.
myxomatous
    m. change
    m. degeneration
    m. proliferation
    m. pulmonary embolism
    m. valve disease

N
   N cell
   N High Sensitivity CRP assay
   N region
N₂
   nitrogen-13
   N₂ oximetry
N-13
   nitrogen-13
      N-13 ammonia
      N-13 ammonia positron emission
         tomography
      N-13 ammonia uptake
N-20 terminal peptide
N/2 artifact
N-395 pulse oximeter
n-3 fatty acid
n-6 fatty acid
N95-Companion accessory
NAA
   nucleic acid amplification
N-acetylcysteine
***N*-acetylneuraminic acid**
***N*-acetyl procainamide (NAPA)**
Nachlas tube
nacre dust asthma
NACT
   National Alliance of Cardiovascular
      Technologists
NAD
   nicotinamide adenine dinucleotide
NADC
   non-AIDS-defining cancer
nadir of QRS complex
nadolol
Nadopen-V
NADPH
   nicotinamide adenine dinucleotide
      phosphate
nadroparin calcium
Naegleria gruberi
NAEP
   National Asthma Education Program
NAEPP
   National Asthma Education and
      Prevention Program
naeslundii
   Actinomyces n.
nafamostat
nafazatrom
nafcillin sodium
naftidrofuryl
Nagle exercise stress test

Na⁺/H⁺
   Na⁺/H⁺ exchange inhibitor (NHEI)
   Na⁺/H⁺ exchanger (NHE)
NAHC
   National Advisory Heart Council
nail
   n. bed
   hippocratic n.'s
   n. pulse
nail-fold skin
nail-patella disease
nail-to-nail bed angle
Na+/K+
   sodium-potassium
   Na+/K+ pump
Nakata index
Na+/K+-ATPase
   sodium-potassium pump
Nakayama
   N. anastomosis
   N. anastomosis apparatus
nalbuphine hydrochloride
Naldecon Senior EX
Nalfon
nalidixic acid
nalmefene hydrochloride
naloxone hydrochloride
naltrexone
NAME
   nevi, atrial myxoma, myxoid
      neurofibromas, ephelides
   NAME syndrome
Namic
   N. angiographic syringe
   N. catheter
NANC
   nonadrenergic, noncholinergic
nandrolone decanoate
NANIPER
   nonallergic, noninfectious perennial
      rhinitis
nanograms per milliliter (ng/mL)
nanomedicine
nanomole (nmol)
nanoparticle
   paramagnetic n.
nanoporous
Nanos 01 pacemaker
nanotechnology
NAPA
   N-acetyl procainamide
nape
   transverse muscle of n.
napkin-ring
   n.-r. calcification

N

napkin-ring *(continued)*
    n.-r. defect
    n.-r. stenosis
Naprosyn
naproxen
NAPSE
    North American Society for Pacing and
    Electrophysiology
Naqua
Narcan injection
Narco
    N. Biosystems recorder
    N. Physiograph-6B recorder
narcolepsy
Narcomatic flowmeter
narcosis
    inert gas n.
    nitrogen n.
narcotic
NARES
    nonallergic rhinitis with eosinophilia
narrow communication
narrow-complex tachycardia
narrowed pulse pressure
NarrowFlex intraaortic balloon catheter
narrowing
    atherosclerotic n.
    concentric n.
    de novo n.
    eccentric n.
    intracoronary stenting of de
        novo n.
    intrinsic airway n.
    longitudinal n.
    luminal n.
    nonatheromatous arterial n.
    ostial n.
    restenotic n.
    systolic coronary artery n. (SCAN)
Narula method
NAS
    no added salt
Nasabid
Nasacort AQ
nasal
    n. airways
    n. asthma
    n. cannula
    n. continuous positive airway
        pressure (NCPAP, nCPAP)
    n. CPAP
    n. CPAP system
    DDAVP N.
    Drixoral N.
    n. flaring
    n. lavage fluid
    N. Moist
    N. Moist Gel
    n. nocturnal ventilation (NNV)

n. part
n. part of pharynx
n. pillow
n. polyposis
n. pool technique
n. positive pressure ventilation
    (NPPV)
n. potential difference
n. prongs
n. steroid (NS)
n. strip
triamcinolone inhalation, n.
n. trumpet
Nasal-Aire
    N.-A. ventilator nasal insert mask
    N.-A. ventilator nasal insert/mask
NasalCrom Nasal Solution
Nasalide Nasal Aerosol
nasalis
    regio n.
Nasarel
nascent HDL
nasi
    ala n.
    regio respiratoria tunicae
        mucosae n.
nasobronchial reflex
nasogastric (NG)
    n. tube
    n. tube feeding (NTF)
nasopharyngeal (NP)
    n. carcinoma
    n. groove
    n. reflux
    n. secretion
    n. wash
nasopharyngitis
nasopharyngoscopy
nasopharynx
nasotracheal
    n. intubation
    n. suction
    n. tube
nateglinide
Nathan test
national
    N. Advisory Heart Council
        (NAHC)
    N. Alliance of Cardiovascular
        Technologists (NACT)
    N. Asthma Education and
        Prevention Program (NAEPP)
    N. Asthma Education Program
        (NAEP)
    N. Board for Respiratory Care
        (NBRC)
    N. Cardiovascular Data Registry
        (NCDR)
    N. Cardiovascular Network (NCN)

N. Cholesterol Education Panel guidelines
N. Cholesterol Education Program (NCEP)
N. Cholesterol Education Program of the American Heart Association
N. Death Index
N. Health Interview Survey (NHIS)
N. Health and Medical Research Council
N. Health and Nutrition Examination Survey (NHANES)
N. Health and Nutrition Examination Survey I
N. Health Service (NHS)
N. Heart Foundation (NHF)
N. Heart Institute (NHI)
N. Heart, Lung, and Blood Institute (NHLBI)
N. Heart, Lung, and Blood Institute/National Asthma Education Prevention Program (NHLBI/NAEPP)
N. High Blood Pressure Education Program (NHBPEP)
N. Home Oxygen Patients Association
N. Hospital Network
N. Institute for Clinical Excellence (NICE)
N. Institute of Occupational Safety and Health (NIOSH)
N. Institutes of Health (NIH)
N. Institutes of Health left ventriculography catheter
N. Institutes of Health marking catheter
N. Institutes of Health mitral valve-grasping forceps
N. Institutes of Health Stroke Scale (NIHSS)
N. Institutes of Neurological Disorders and Stroke (NINDS)
N. Lung Health Education Program (NLHEP)
N. Nosocomial Infection Surveillance
N. Registry of Myocardial Infarction (NRMI)
N. Society of Cardiovascular Technologists (NSCT)

native
n. arterial circulation
n. coarctation
n. coronary anatomy
n. coronary artery
n. coronary artery disease
n. coronary artery lesion
n. LAD
n. LDL (n-LDL)
n. low-density lipoprotein
n. tissue harmonic imaging
n. valve
n. valve endocarditis (NVE)
n. valve fibroplastic endocarditis
n. vessel

Natrecor
Natrilix
natriuresis
natriuretic
n. hormone
n. peptide

natural
n. anatomy
n. failing heart
n. frequency
n. heart transplant
n. history
n. killer (NK)
n. logarithm
n. resistance macrophage-associated protein (Nramp)
n. strain

1-natural-log-unit elevation
Naughton
N. cardiac exercise treadmill test
N. graded exercise stress test
N. treadmill protocol

Nauheim
N. bath
N. treatment

NavAblator catheter
Navelbine
Navidrex
Navier-Stokes equation
navigation
intracardiac n.

navigator echo signal
Naviport
N. deflectable tip guiding catheter
N. hollow-lumen guiding catheter

NaviStar
N. Celsius DS diagnostic/ablation catheter
N. diagnostic/ablation deflectable tip catheter
N. DS diagnostic/ablation catheter
N. mapping/ablation catheter

Naxos disease
n-BCA
n-butyl cyanoacrylate

NBRC
National Board for Respiratory Care

NBTE
nonbacterial thrombotic endocarditis

n-butyl cyanoacrylate (n-BCA)

N

NC
noncardiac
NC balloon
NC Bandit ball
NC Bandit catheter
NC Raptor over-the-wire coaxial
  PTCA dilation balloon catheter
NCA
noncontractile area
normal coronary arteries
NCC
noncoronary cusp
NCDR
National Cardiovascular Data Registry
NCEP
National Cholesterol Education Program
NCEP guidelines
NCEP Step-One Diet
NCEP-II guidelines
NCN
National Cardiovascular Network
NCPAP, nCPAP
nasal continuous positive airway pressure
Aladdin^{II} NCPAP
NCPAP therapy
NCPE
noncardiac pulmonary edema
NCR
no cardiopulmonary resuscitation
NCV
nerve conduction velocity
NDA
new device angioplasty
nDx monitor
Nd:YAG laser
NE
norepinephrine
near
n. field
n. infrared
n. patient test (NPT)
n. syncope
near-fainting
near-fatal asthma (NFA)
near-field visualization
near-gain
near-infrared
n.-i. cerebral oximetry
n.-i. spectroscopy (NIRS, NIS)
near-syncope
nebacumab
nebivolol
NebuChamber
Nebuhaler
Nebules
Ventolin N.
nebulization
aqueous solution for n.

continuous albuterol n. (CAN)
wet n.
nebulized
n. bronchodilator
n. Ig therapy
n. tobramycin
nebulizer
Acorn II n.
AeroEclipse breath actuated n.
AeroNeb InLine n.
AeroNeb portable n.
aerosol n.
AeroSonic personal ultrasonic n.
AeroTech II n.
air-powered n.
Babington-type n.
baffled jet n.
Bestneb n.
Centimist n.
n. chronolog
compact silent n.
compressor-generated n. (CGN)
Compu-Neb ultrasonic n.
DeVilbiss n.
handheld n.
Heart n.
heliox n.
Hope continuous & Heliox n.
IV-Heart n.
jet n.
LC Plus reusable n.
LC Star reusable n.
Marquest Respirgard II n.
MicroAir handheld n.
Micro Mist n.
MiniHEART low-flow n.
Mistogen n.
Pari LC Plus reusable n.
Pari LC Star reusable n.
Pari Proneb Ultra n.
PermaNeb reusable n.
Proneb Ultra n.
Pulmo-Aide n.
PulmoSonic n.
Respirgard II n.
Schuco n.
Sidestream high-efficiency n.
small-volume n. (SVN)
Sonix 2000 ultrasonic n.
Twin Jet n.
ultrasonic n. (USN)
UniHeart IV universal n.
Updraft handheld n.
Ventstream n.
VixOne small-volume n.
NebuPent Inhalation
NEC
nonesterified cholesterol
Necator americanus

necessitatis
    empyema n.
neck
    transverse artery of n.
necrobacillosis
necrobiosis lipoidica diabeticorum
necrobiotic nodule
necrolysis
    toxic epidermal n.
necrophorum
    Fusobacterium n.
necrophorus
    Sphaerophorus n.
necropsy
necrosis, pl. **necroses**
    avascular n.
    coagulation n.
    contraction band n.
    cystic medial n. (CMN)
    digital n.
    dirty n.
    electrolyte and steroid cardiopathy
      with n. (ESCN)
    embolic n.
    Erdheim cystic medial n.
    n. factor
    fibrinoid n.
    ischemic n.
    liquefaction n.
    medial n.
    myocardial n.
    myocyte n.
    pressure n.
    renal cortical n.
    tissue n.
    tubular n.
necrotic
    n. cyst
    n. myocardium
necrotisans
    phlebitis nodularis n.
necrotizing
    n. angiitis
    n. arterial disease
    n. arteriolitis
    n. aspergillosis
    n. bronchopneumonia
    n. granuloma
    n. granulomatous vasculitis
    n. pneumonia
    n. sarcoid granulomatosis
nedocromil sodium
need
    perfusion n.'s
needle
    Abrams n.
    Adson aneurysm n.
    Aldrete n.
    arachnophlebectomy n.

    argon n.
    arterial n.
    n. aspirate
    aspirating n.
    Atraloc n.
    atraumatic n.
    Becton-Dickinson Teflon-sheathed n.
    BRK series transseptal n.
    Brockenbrough curved n.
    butterfly n.
    Cardiopoint n.
    Chiba n.
    Cope pleural biopsy n.
    Cournand n.
    Cournand-Grino angiography n.
    Cournand-Potts n.
    Curry n.
    disposable percutaneous entry
      thinwall n.
    DLP cardioplegic n.
    Dos Santos n.
    ergonomic vascular access n.
      (EVAN)
    Ethalloy n.
    eyeless n.
    Fergie n.
    Ferguson n.
    Fischer pneumothoracic n.
    27G n.
    n. guide
    n. holder
    hollow-core n.
    Hustead n.
    Jamshidi n.
    large-bore slotted aspirating n.
    Lewy-Rubin n.
    Lowell pleural n.
    Luer-Lok n.
    Menghini n.
    micron n.
    Micropuncture introducer n.
    O'Brien airway n.
    olive-tipped n.
    PercuCut biopsy n.
    percutaneous cutting n.
    pericardiocentesis n.
    pilot n.
    polytef-sheathed n.
    Potts n.
    Potts-Cournand n.
    Ranfac n.
    Riley n.
    Rochester n.
    Ross n.
    Rotex n.
    Safe Step blood-collection n.
    scalp vein n.
    Seldinger n.
    N.'s Eye snare

N

needle *(continued)*
    slotted n.
    standard n.
    steel-winged butterfly n.
    Stifcore aspiration n.
    Stifcore biopsy injection n.
    THI n.
    thin-walled n.
    thoracentesis n.
    n. thoracostomy
    TMC n.
    transbronchial n.
    transseptal n.
    Tru-Cut biopsy n.
    Tuohy n.
    Venflon n.
    Vim-Silverman n.
    Wang transbronchial n.
    Wasserman n.
    Zavala lung biopsy n.
needlepoint electrocautery
Needle-Pro needle protection device
NEEP
    negative end-expiratory pressure
nefazodone
Neff percutaneous access set
negative
    n. chronotropism
    n. contrast
    n. contrast echocardiography
    n. deflection
    n. deflection that follows R wave
    (S)
    n. end-expiratory pressure (NEEP)
    n. expiratory pressure (NEP)
    false n.
    n. inotrope
    n. inspiratory force
    n. intrapleural pressure
    n. predictive value (NPV)
    n. pressure pulmonary edema
    (NPPE)
    n. pressure ventilation (NPV)
    n. remodeling
    n. treppe
    n. T, U wave
negative-contrast
    n.-c. injection
    n.-c. intravascular ultrasound
NegGram
neglect
    motor n.
    perceptual-sensory n.
    unilateral spatial n. (USN)
    visuospatial n.
Negri body
Negus bronchoscope
Neisseria
    N. catarrhalis

    N. gonorrhoeae
    N. meningitidis
neisserial
nelfinavir
Nellcor
    N. N200 pulse oximeter
    N. N-395 pulse oximeter
    N. Puritan Bennett (NPB)
    N. Puritan-Bennett ventilator
    N. Puritan Bennett 840 ventilator
    system
    N. Symphony blood pressure
    monitor
    N. Symphony pulse oximeter
nemaline myopathy
Nembutal
neoadjuvant chemotherapy
neoangiogenesis
neocapillarization
neocarzinostatin
Neo-Codema
neodymium:yttrium-aluminum-garnet
    laser
neoendothelium
NEO-fit
    NEO-f. endotracheal tube grip
    NEO-f. neonatal endotracheal tube
    holder
neoformans
    Cryptococcus n.
neoglottis
neointima
neointimal
    n. generation
    n. hyperplasia
    n. hyperplastic response
    n. proliferation
    n. ridge
    n. tear
    n. thickening
    n. tissue
neolumen
NeoMend arterial closure device
neomycin sulfate
neonatal
    Exosurf N.
    N. respiratory distress syndrome
    (NRDS)
    N. Y TrachCare
neonatorum
    anoxia n.
    apnea n.
    asphyxia n.
neoplasia
    pericardial n.
neoplasm
    extrathoracic n.
    Kaposi n.
    primary bronchogenic n.

neoplastic
- n. airway obstruction
- n. cavity
- n. cell
- n. disease
- n. pericardial effusion
- n. pericarditis

neopterin
- serum n.

Neoral cyclosporine capsule
Neosar injection
Neo-Sert umbilical vessel catheter insertion set
Neo-Synephrine 12 Hour Nasal Solution
NeoTect imaging agent
Neo-Therm neonatal skin temperature probe
Neothylline
Neotrend
- N. multiparameter blood gas monitor
- N. system

neovascularity
- plaque n.

neovascularization
- left atrial n. (LANV)

NeoVO2R infant volume control resuscitator
NEP
- negative expiratory pressure
- neutral endopeptidase

nephelometry
nephritis, pl. **nephritides**
- familial n.
- immune-mediated membranous n.
- tuberculous n.

Nephro-Fer
nephrogenesis
nephrogenic diabetes insipidus
nephrogram
nephron
nephropathic cardiomyopathy
nephropathy
- analgesic n.
- contrast n.
- diabetic n.
- hypertensive n. (HTN)
- hyperuricemic n.

nephrosclerosis
- arteriolar n.

nephrostolithotomy
nephrotic syndrome
nephrotoxicity
NEP-I, NEPi
- neutral endopeptidase inhibition

neprilysin

Neptune
- N. high-pressure PTCA balloon catheter
- N. Pad

Nernst equation
nerve
- accelerator n.
- accompanying artery of ischiadic n.
- accompanying artery of median n.
- n. action potential
- aortic n.
- aortic depressor n. (ADN)
- axillary n.
- brachial n.
- cardiac sensory n.
- cardiac sympathetic n. (CSN)
- cardiopulmonary splanchnic n.'s
- carotid sinus n.
- n. conduction velocity (NCV)
- cranial n.'s I–XII
- esophageal branch of vagus n.
- external branch of superior laryngeal n.
- facial n.
- faucial branches of lingual n.
- n. fiber
- glossopharyngeal n.
- n. of Hering
- hypoglossal n.
- inferior ganglion of glossopharyngeal n.
- internal branch of superior laryngeal n.
- ischiadic n.
- n. of Kuntz
- laryngeal n.
- lateral ventricular n. (LVN)
- left recurrent laryngeal n.
- lingual branch of facial n.
- median n.
- pharyngeal branch of glossopharyngeal n.
- pharyngeal branch of vagus n.
- phrenic n.
- recurrent laryngeal n.
- right recurrent laryngeal n.
- sensory n.
- n. sheath tumor
- superior laryngeal n.
- sympathetic n.
- thoracic n.
- trigeminal n.
- ulnar n.
- vagus n.

nervi
- ganglion inferius n.
- ganglion superius n.

nervorum
- vasa n.

nervosa
> anorexia n.
> dysphagia n.

nervous
> n. asthma
> n. plexus
> n. respiration
> n. system
> n. tachypnea

nesiritide citrate
nest of veins
net
> n. absorption
> Health On the N. (HON)

Netherton syndrome
netilmicin sulfate
network
> acromial arterial n.
> advanced heart failure shared
>   clinical experience n. (AHF
>   SCENE)
> CareLink patient monitoring n.
> Chiari n.
> Encompass cardiac n.
> fibrillar collagen n.
> hypertension genetic
>   epidemiology n.
> interstitial and perivascular
>   collagen n.
> National Cardiovascular N. (NCN)
> National Hospital N.
> Organ Procurement and
>   Transplantation N. (OPTN)
> Purkinje n.

Neubauer artery
neuf
> bruit de cuir n.

NeuGene
Neumovent Bebé infant ventilator
Neupogen
neural
> n. cardioesophageal reflex
> n. crest malformation
> n. crest migration
> n. plasticity
> n. substrate

neuralgia
> glossopharyngeal n.

neuralgic amyotrophy
neurally
> n. mediated syncopal syndrome
> n. mediated syncope (NMS)
> n. mediated vasovagal syncope
>   (NMVS)

neuraminidase inhibitor
neurapraxia
neurenteric cyst
neurilemmoma

neuritis
> optic n.

neuroblastoma
neurocardiac syncope
neurocardiogenic syncope
neurocirculatory asthenia
neurocognitive decline
neurodegenerative disease
neurodiagnostics
neuroectodermal tumor
neuroendocrine
> n. drive
> n. marker
> n. theory
> n. tumor

neuroendovascular
neuroenteric cyst
neuroepithelial body
neurofibroma
neurofibromatosis
**Neuroform microdelivery stent delivery
  system**
neurogenic
> n. abnormality
> n. fibrosarcoma
> n. pulmonary edema
> n. theory
> n. tumor

neurohormonal
> n. arterial constriction
> n. function
> n. inhibition
> n. modulator
> n. perturbation
> n. stimulation

neurohormone
neurohumeral cascade
neurohumoral
> n. factors
> n. stimulus

neurokinin A (NKA)
neuroleptic
neurologic
> n. DCS
> n. deficit
> n. examination
> n. status
> n. syncope

neurological disorder
neuromediated syncope
neuromuscular
> n. blockade
> n. blocking agent (NMBA)
> n. coupling
> n. disease
> n. disorder
> n. function
> n. hypertension

neuromyopathic disorder

neuromyopathy
 carcinomatous n.
neuronal ceroid lipofuscinosis
neuron-specific enolase (NSE)
neuropathy
 angiopathic n.
 axonal n.
 cardiac autonomic n. (CAN)
 diabetic n.
 diabetic autonomic n. (DAN)
 IgA n.
 immunoglobulin A n. (IgAN)
 multiplex n.
 peripheral n.
 vasculitic n.
neuropeptide
 human n.
 n. Y
Neuroperfusion pump
neuroprotection
neuroprotective
 n. agent
 n. drug
NeuroShield
 N. cerebral protection device
 N. emboli protection device
neurosis, pl. **neuroses**
 anxiety n.
 cardiac n.
Neurostar angiography system
neurosyphilis
neuroticism
neurotoxic effect
neurotransmission
 sympathetic n.
neurotransmitter substance
neurotrophic effect
neurovascular bundle
NeuroVasx submicroinfusion catheter
neutral
 n. endopeptidase (NEP)
 n. endopeptidase inhibition (NEP-I, NEPi)
 n. endopeptidase inhibitor
 n. lipid (NL)
Neutrexin injection
neutron activation analysis
neutropenia
 febrile n.
neutropenic angina
neutrophil
 n. chemotaxis
 n. collagenase (MMP 8)
 n. elastase
 polymorphonuclear n. (PMN)
 segmented n.'s
neutrophil-derived serine protease
neutrophilia
 pleural fluid n.

neutrophilic inflammation
neutrophil-induced pulmonary inflammation
NEV
 noninvasive extrathoracic ventilator
nevi (*pl. of* nevus)
Neville
 N. stent
 N. tracheal prosthesis
nevirapine (NVP)
nevus, pl. **nevi**
 n. araneus
 nevi, atrial myxoma, myxoid neurofibromas, ephelides (NAME)
 lentigines, atrial myxoma, mucocutaneous myxoma, blue nevi (LAMB)
new
 n. device angioplasty (NDA)
 N. York catheter exchange wire guide
 N. York Heart Association (NYHA)
 N. York Heart Association functional classification I–IV
newborn
 hyaline membrane disease of the n.
 persistent pulmonary hypertension of n. (PPHN)
 respiratory distress syndrome of the n.
 transient tachypnea of n. (TTNB)
NewLife
 N. Elite concentrator
 N. oxygen concentrator
Newport
 N. E100M ventilator
 N. Wave V200 ventilator
Newton
 N. catheter
 N. guidewire
NexStent carotid stent
NextStitch cardiovascular valve suture
Nexus
 N. coronary stent
 N. 2 linear ablation catheter
NF
 Nissen fundoplication
NFA
 near-fatal asthma
NF-ATc protein
NF-kappa-B
 nuclear factor-kappa B
NG
 nasogastric
 NG tube
N-geneous automated HDL cholesterol test

N

ng/mL
  nanograms per milliliter
NH
  nodal-His
    NH region
    NH region of A-V node
NHANES
  National Health and Nutrition
    Examination Survey
NHBPEP
  National High Blood Pressure Education
    Program
NHDL
  non-high-density lipoprotein
NHE
  Na^+/H^+ exchanger
NHEI
  Na^+/H^+ exchange inhibitor
NHF
  National Heart Foundation
NHI
  National Heart Institute
NHIS
  National Health Interview Survey
NHLBI
  National Heart, Lung, and Blood Institute
NHLBI/NAEPP
  National Heart, Lung, and Blood
    Institute/National Asthma Education
    Prevention Program
NHS
  National Health Service
N-[8-(2-hydroxybenzoyl)amino]caprylate
  sodium N-[8-(2-
    hydroxybenzoyl)amino]caprylate
    (SNAC)
niacin
niacinamide
niacinate
  xanthinol n.
niacin/lovastatin
  extended-release n./l.
Niaspan
NIBP
  noninvasive blood pressure
    NIBP monitoring
NiCad
  nickel-cadmium
nicardipine hydrochloride
Nic the Asthmatic Dragon pediatric
  aerosol mask
NICE
  National Institute for Clinical Excellence
    NICE group
nickel
  salt of n.
nickel-cadmium (NiCad)
  n.-c. battery
Nickerson-Kveim test

nicking
  arteriovenous n.
Nicks procedure
NicoDerm Patch
nicofuranose
Nicoladoni-Branham sign
Nicoladoni sign
Nicolet
  N. Vascular Pocket-Dop II
    handheld Doppler probe
  N. VersaLab APM
$NICO_2$ noninvasive cardiac output
  monitor
nicorandil
Nicorette
  N. Gum
  N. Plus
Nicostatin
nicotinamide
  n. adenine dinucleotide (NAD)
  n. adenine dinucleotide phosphate
    (NADPH)
nicotinamidoethyl
  2-n. nitrate
nicotinate
  aluminum n.
nicotine
  n. by-product
  crystalline n.
  n. dependence
  n. fading
  n. gum
  n. inhaler
  n. nasal spray (NNS)
  n. replacement therapy (NRT)
  n. staining
  n. transdermal patch
Nicotinex
nicotinic acid
Nicotrol
  N. Inhaler
  N. NS nasal spray
  N. Patch
nicoumalone
NIDCM
  nonischemic dilated cardiomyopathy
NIDDM
  non-insulin-dependent diabetes mellitus
nidulans
  Aspergillus n.
nidus
Niemann-Pick disease
nifedipine enzyme immunoassay
Niferex
niger
  Aspergillus n.
night
  N. Owl pocket polygraph

n. sweats
n. terrors
nigra
cardiopathia n.
nigricans
Acanthosis n.
nigrum
Epicoccum n.
NIH
National Institutes of Health
NIH Cardiomarker catheter
NIH mitral valve-grasping forceps
NIH *Xenopus* Initiative
Nihon
N. Kohden polygraph system
N. Kohden polysomnogram
NIHSS
National Institutes of Health Stroke Scale
Nikaidoh-Bex technique
Nikaidoh translocation
nikethamide
Nikon Eclipse E400 microscope
Nilandron
nilutamide
Nimbex
Nimbus Hemopump
nimesulide
nimodipine
Nimotop
NINDS
National Institutes of Neurological
Disorders and Stroke
Ninja FX series over-the-wire coaxial PTCA dilation balloon catheter
NI-NR
no infection-no rejection
niobium
NIOSH
National Institute of Occupational Safety
and Health
NIOX nitric oxide breath test system
NIP
nonspecific chronic interstitial
pneumonitis
Nipah virus (NiV)
nipple
aortic n.
NIPPV
noninvasive positive pressure ventilation
NIPS
noninvasive programmed stimulation
NIRflex
N. coronary stent
N. stent system
NIRoyal Elite Monorail coronary stent system
NIRS, NIS
near-infrared spectroscopy
NIR stent

Nisocor
nisoldipine
Nissen
N. 360-degree wrap fundoplication
N. fundoplication (NF)
niter paper
nitinol
n. cage
n. filter
n. hypotube
n. mesh stent
n. petal
n. polymeric compound
n. self-expandable stent
n. self-expanding coil stent
n. snare
n. thermal memory stent
Nit-Occlud device
nitrate
long-acting n.
2-nicotinamidoethyl n.
peroxyacetyl n.
n. reductase assay (NRA)
n. resistance
nitrendipine
nitric
n. acid
n. oxide (NO)
n. oxide analyzer (NOA)
n. oxide bioavailability
n. oxide-dependent mechanism
n. oxide-mediated relaxation
n. oxide synthase (NOS)
n. oxide synthase 1 (NOS1)
n. oxide synthase gene therapy
n. oxide system
nitrite
amyl n.
sodium n.
Nitro-Bid Ointment
nitroblue tetrazolium
Nitrocap
Nitro-Dial
Nitro-Dur Patch
nitrofurantoin
Nitrogard Buccal
nitrogen
blood urea n. (BUN)
n. curve
n. dioxide (NO_2)
n. mustard
n. narcosis
n. oxide
urea n.
n. washout technique
nitrogen-13 (N-13, N_2)
n.-13 ammonia
nitroglycerin (NTG)
n. ointment (NTGO)

N

nitroglycerin *(continued)*
    oral n. (ONTG)
    n. paste
nitroglycerin-induced dilation
nitroglycerol
Nitroglyn Oral
nitroimidazole
nitroimidazopyran
Nitrolin
Nitrolingual Translingual Spray
Nitrol Ointment
Nitropress
nitroprusside
    n. infusion
    sodium n.
    n. sodium
NitroQuick sublingual tablets
nitrosative stress
nitrosopnea
    childhood n.
nitrosothiol
Nitrospan
Nitrostat Sublingual
nitrothiol
nitrotyrosine
nitrous oxide
nitrovasodilator
NIV
    noninvasive ventilation
NiV
    Nipah virus
NIVS
    noninvasive ventilatory support
Nizoral Oral
NK
    natural killer
        NK cell
NKA
    neurokinin A
NL
    neutral lipid
NL63
NLDL
    normal low-density lipoprotein
n-LDL
    native LDL
NLHEP
    National Lung Health Education Program
NMBA
    neuromuscular blocking agent
NMDA receptor
N-methyl-D-aspartate
nmol
    nanomole
NMR
    nuclear magnetic resonance
        NMR diffusometry
        NMR LipoProfile analysis
        NMR relaxometry

    NMR spectroscopy
    NMR topography
NMRI
    nuclear magnetic resonance imaging
NMS
    neurally mediated syncope
NMVS
    neurally mediated vasovagal syncope
NN
    normal-to-normal
        NN interval
N^G**-nitro-L-arginine methyl ester (L-NAME)**
NNMT Medical CardioSEAL septal occlusion system
NNS
    nicotine nasal spray
NNT
    number needed to treat
NNV
    nasal nocturnal ventilation
NO
    nitric oxide
NO₂
    nitrogen dioxide
no
        no added salt (NAS)
        no atrial pacing
        no cardiopulmonary resuscitation (NCR)
        no infection-no rejection (NI-NR)
        No Pour Pak suction catheter kit
NOA
    nitric oxide analyzer
Nocardia
        N. asteroides
        N. brasiliensis
        N. transvalensis
nocardiosis
nociceptive threshold
no-clamp technique
nocturia
nocturnal
        n. angina
        n. asthma
        n. cardiovascular blunting
        n. desaturation
        n. dyspnea
        n. hypoventilation
        n. oximetry
        n. oximetry screening
        n. oxygenation
        n. plasma ghrelin level
        n. polysomnogram (NPSG)
        n. polysomnography
        n. ventilation
        n. walking
nod
        bishop's n.

nodal
  n. arrhythmia
  n. artery
  n. bigeminy
  n. bradycardia
  n. contracture
  enhanced atrioventricular n.
    (EAVN)
  n. escape
  n. escape rhythm
  n. extrasystole
  n. paroxysmal tachycardia
  n. premature beat (NPB)
  n. premature contraction (NPC)
  n. reentrant tachycardia
  n. tissue
nodal-His (NH)
node
  Aschoff-Tawara n.
  atrioventricular n. (AVN)
  A-V n.
  axillary lymph n.'s
  azygos n.
  bifurcation lymph n.
  bronchopulmonary lymph n.
  carinal lymph n.
  compact A-V n.
  Cruveilhier n.'s
  Delphian n.
  dual atrioventricular n.
  Flack n.
  Fraenkel n.
  Heberden n.
  hilar lymph n.
  hilum of lymph n.
  His-Tawara n.
  homolateral lymph n.
  inferior phrenic lymph n.
  inferior tracheobronchial lymph n.
  jugulodigastric lymph n.
  juxtaesophageal lymph n.
  Keith n.
  Keith-Flack n.
  Koch n.
  lateral jugular lymph n.
  lymph n.
  mediastinal lymph n.'s
  NH region of A-V n.
  Osler n.
  paratracheal lymph n.
  perihilar lymph n.'s
  prelaryngeal lymph n.
  pretracheal lymph n.
  pulmonary lymph n.
  n. of Ranvier
  retropharyngeal lymph n.
  S-A n.
  sentinel n.
  shotty n.'s

  singer's n.
  sinoauricular n. (SAN)
  sinuatrial n. (SAN, SN)
  sinus n. (SN)
  subaortic lymph n.
  subcarinal n.
  superior phrenic lymph n.
  superior tracheobronchial lymph n.
  supraclavicular lymph n.
  Tawara atrioventricular n.
  teacher's n.
  tracheal lymph n.
node-His-Purkinje system
nodi
  n. lymphoidei bronchopulmonales
  n. lymphoidei juxtaesophageales
    pulmonales
  n. lymphoidei paratracheales
  n. lymphoidei phrenici inferiores
  n. lymphoidei phrenici superiores
  n. lymphoidei prelaryngeales
  n. lymphoidei pretracheales
  n. lymphoidei retropharyngeales
  n. lymphoidei tracheobronchiales
    inferiores
  n. lymphoidei tracheobronchiales
    superiores
nodofascicular
nodohisian bypass tract
nodosa
  arteritis n.
  periarteritis n.
  polyarteritis n.
nodose arteriosclerosis
nodosum
  erythema n.
nodoventricular
  n. fiber
  n. tract
nodular
  n. aortic stenosis
  n. arteriosclerosis
  n. infiltrate
  n. interlobular septal thickening
  n. lymphoid hyperplasia
  n. opacity
  n. pulmonary amyloidosis
  n. sarcoidosis
  n. sclerosing Hodgkin lymphoma
  n. sclerosis
  n. vasculitis
nodularity
nodule
  acinar n.
  Albini n.
  Arantius n.
  Aschoff n.
  Bianchi n.
  calcified n.

N

nodule *(continued)*
    Caplan n.
    centrilobular n.
    cold n.
    hematogenous n.
    hemorrhage pulmonary n.
    interstitial n.
    intrapulmonary rheumatoid n.
    lung n.
    meningothelial-like n.
    metastatic n.
    Morgagni n.
    mural n.
    necrobiotic n.
    peribronchiolar n.
    perilymphatic n.
    pulmonary n.
    random n.
    rheumatoid n.
    round pneumonia n.
    solitary pulmonary n. (SPN)
    subcutaneous n.
    warm n.
    Wegener n.
nodus
    n. atrioventricularis
    n. sinuatrialis
    n. sinuatrialis echo
NOGA cardiac navigation system
noise
    perceived n. (PN)
    n. reversion
noise-canceling technique
noise-reversion mode
noisy chest
no-leak technique
Nolvadex tablet
nomifensine maleate
nomogram
    Radford n.
nonacute total coronary occlusion
nonadrenergic, noncholinergic (NANC)
nonagenarian
non-AIDS-defining
    n.-A.-d. cancer (NADC)
    n.-A.-d. malignancy
nonallergic
    n., noninfectious perennial rhinitis (NANIPER)
    n. rhinitis with eosinophilia (NARES)
nonarticulated stent
nonasthmatic eosinophilic bronchitis
nonatheromatous
    n. arterial narrowing
    n. arteriosclerosis
    n. artery

nonatopic
    n. asthma
    n. wheezing
nonatrial fibrillation
nonbacteremic
nonbacterial
    n. thrombotic endocardial lesion
    n. thrombotic endocarditis (NBTE)
    n. verrucous endocarditis
nonballoon therapy
nonbronchioalveolar adenocarcinoma
nonbullous
noncalcified valve
noncardiac (NC)
    n. angiography
    n. pulmonary edema (NCPE)
    n. surgery
    n. syncope
noncardiogenic pulmonary edema
noncaseating granuloma
noncavitary
noncavotricuspid isthmus
noncholinergic
    nonadrenergic, n. (NANC)
noncleaved cell lymphoma
noncollagenous pneumoconiosis
noncommitted biphasic shock therapy
noncommunicating air space
noncompaction
    isolated left ventricular n. (IVNC)
    left ventricular n.
noncompensatory pause
noncompliant
    n. balloon
    n. ventricle
noncontact endocardial mapping
noncontractile area (NCA)
noncoronary
    n. cusp (NCC)
    n. sinus
noncrushing vascular clamp
non-CTI dependent
nonculprit coronary artery disease
nondecremental retrograde ventriculoatrial conduction
nondepolarizing drug
nondihydropyridine calcium blocker
nondisjunction
nondominant vessel
none
    all or n.
nonejection systolic click
noneosinophilic atopic asthma
nonessential
nonesterified
    n. cholesterol (NEC)
    n. fatty acid
nonexcitatory signal
nonexertional angina

nonexpansional dyspnea
nonfasting state
nonfatal
    n. cardiac event
    n. heart attack
nonfenestrated endothelium
nonfluent aphasia
nongenomic
nonglycoside inotropic agent
nonhemodynamic effect
non-high-density lipoprotein (NHDL)
non-Hodgkin lymphoma
nonhomogeneous pulmonary time-
   constant distribution
nonhypercapnic respiratory failure
non-IgE-mediated reaction
nonimmunocompromised host
nonimplantable system
noninducible
noninfectious complication
noninfective valve endocarditis
noninhalation
Nonin Onyx pulse oximeter
non-insulin-dependent diabetes mellitus
   (NIDDM)
nonintegrated transvenous defibrillation
   lead
nonintubated patient
noninvasive
    n. assessment
    n. blood pressure (NIBP)
    n. detection
    n. electrical energy
    n. evaluation
    n. extrathoracic ventilator (NEV)
    n. face mask ventilation
    lower extremity n. (LENI)
    n. mechanical ventilation
    n. monitor
    n. murmur
    n. positive pressure ventilation
    (NIPPV, NPPV)
    n. positive pressure ventilatory
    support
    n. programmed stimulation (NIPS)
    n. temporary pacemaker
    n. test
    n. transcutaneous cardiac pacing
    (NTCP)
    n. ventilation (NIV)
    n. ventilation with positive pressure
    n. ventilatory support (NIVS)
    n. visualization
nonionic
    n. contrast material
    n. contrast medium
nonischemic dilated cardiomyopathy
   (NIDCM)

nonliquefaciens
    Moraxella n.
nonmalignant tissue
nonmassive hemoptysis
nonnecrotizing angiitis
nonnucleoside reverse transcriptase
   inhibitor
nonobstructive
    n. atelectasis
    n. valve thrombosis
nonocclusive mesenteric ischemia
nonoperative closure
nonostial plaque
nonpanting
    n. maneuver
    n. measurement
nonparametric data
nonparoxysmal atrioventricular
   junctional tachycardia (NPJT)
nonpenetrating rupture
nonpharmacologic measure of treatment
nonphasic sinus arrhythmia
nonpitting edema
nonpolymer-based
    n.-b. paclitaxel-eluting stent
    n.-b. rapamycin-eluting stent
nonpressor dose
nonprimary
    n. cardiac arrest
    n. lobe
    n. pulmonary hypertension
    n. ventricular fibrillation
nonpulmonary complication
nonpyramidal hemimotor syndrome
nonquinolone antibiotic
non-Q-wave myocardial infarction
   (NQMI, NQWMI)
nonrapid eye movement (NREM)
nonrebreather mask
nonrebreathing
    n. mask
    n. valve
nonreset nodus sinuatrialis
nonreversibility
nonrheumatic
    n. AF
    n. stenotic aortic valve
    n. valvular aortic stenosis
nonsegmental
    n. disease
    n. perfusion defect
nonselective coronary angiography
nonseminomatous germ cell tumor
nonsense mutation
nonsensing
    atrial n.
nonsinusoidal waveform

N

505

non-small-cell
n.-s.-c. lung cancer (NSCLC)
n.-s.-c. lung carcinoma (NSCLC)
nonspecific
n. bronchial hyperreactivity
n. challenge test
n. chronic interstitial pneumonitis (NIP)
n. climatic change
n. idiopathic pulmonary fibrosis
n. interstitial pneumonia (NSIP)
n. interstitial pneumonitis (NSIP)
n. intraventricular block
n. intraventricular conduction delay (NSIVCD)
n. irritant
n. lung fibrosis
n. ST and T (NSSTT)
n. T-wave aberration
n. T-wave abnormality
non-STEMI
non-ST-segment myocardial infarction
nonsteroidal
n. antiinflammatory agent
n. antiinflammatory drug (NSAID)
non-ST-segment
n.-ST-s. elevation myocardial infarction (NSTEMI)
n.-ST-s. myocardial infarction (non-STEMI)
nonsuppressible
n. arrhythmia
n. ventricular tachycardia
nonsurgical
n. bypass without anesthesia
n. septal reduction therapy (NSRT)
nonsustained ventricular tachycardia (NSVT)
nonthoracotomy
n. defibrillation lead system
n. lead implantable cardioverter-defibrillator
n. system antitachycardia device (NTS-AICD)
nonthrombogenic
nontissue density
nontransmural
n. fibrosis
n. myocardial infarction (NTMI)
nontransplanted
nontuberculous mycobacteria (NTM)
nontypeable *Haemophilus influenzae* **(NTHI)**
nonuniform
n. direct cardiac compression
n. rotational defect (NURD)
nonvalved graft
nonvalvular atrial fibrillation (NVAF)
nonvenereal syphilis

nonventilated patient
nonwheezing bronchial asthma
noodle wire
Noonan syndrome
Noon A-V fistula clamp
no-phase wrap
noradrenaline
Nordach treatment
No-React
N.-R. detoxification process
N.-R. pericardial patch
no-reflow
n.-r. phenomenon
n.-r. syndrome
norepinephrine (NE)
n. bitartrate
fasting plasma n.
plasma n.
n. uptake 1
norethindrone
norfloxacin
norimbergensis
Pandoraea n.
Norisodrine
normal
n. coronary arteries (NCA)
n. electrical axis
n. geometry
n. intravascular pressure
n. low-density lipoprotein (NLDL)
n. saline
n. sinus rhythm (NSR)
n. transvalvular regurgitation (NTVR)
n. triglyceridemia (NTG)
n. vital capacity (NVC)
normalization of inverted T wave
normalized systemic vascular resistance (NSVR)
normal-to-normal (NN)
normobaric environment
normocapnia
normocapnic hyperpnea
normocholesterolemic
Normodyne
N. injection
N. Oral
normokinesia
normolipidemic
normomagnesemia
normonatremic
normoperfused
normotensive (NT)
n. pneumothorax
normothermic cardioplegia
normovolemia
normovolemic (NV)
n. hemodilution
normoxia

Normozide
Noroxin Oral
Norpace CR
Norpramin
Nor-QD
Norris
  N. score
  N. test
north
  N. American blastomycosis
  N. American Inoue Balloon
    registry
  N. American Society for Pacing
    and Electrophysiology (NAPSE)
northern
  N. blot
  N. hybridization analysis
Norton flow-directed Swan-Ganz
  thermodilution catheter
nortriptyline hydrochloride
Norvasc
norvegicus
  Rattus n.
norverapamil
Norvir
Norwalk agent
Norwood
  N. operation
  N. operation for hypoplastic left-
    sided heart
  N. repair
  N. univentricular heart procedure
NOS
  nitric oxide synthase
nose
  alar artery of n.
  n. clip
  respiratory region of tunica mucosa
    of n.
Nosema connori
NOSI
  nitric oxide synthase 1
no-sigh period
nosocomial
  n. aspiration
  n. disease
  n. endocarditis
  n. infection
  n. pathogen
  n. pneumonia (NP)
  n. pulmonary infection (NPI)
nosology
  Berlin n.
Nostrilla
notatum
  Penicillin n.
notch
  anacrotic n.
  aortic n.

atrial n.
cardiac n.
dicrotic n. (DN)
interarytenoid n.
Sibson n.
sternal n.
suprasternal n. (SN)
thyroid n.
notched
  n. P, S wave
  n. ST-segment elevation
notching
  midsystolic n.
  rib n.
note
  percussion n. (PN)
notha
  angina n.
  peripneumonia n.
  pneumonia n.
no-touch technique
Nottingham
  N. Extended Activities of Daily
    Living scale
  N. Health profile
  N. introducer
  N. Sensory Assessment test
Novacode serial ECG classification
Novacor
  N. Diasys cardiac device
  N. heart pump
  N. left ventricular assist device
  N. left ventricular assist system
  N. LVAD
  N. mechanical circulatory support
    system
Nova II pacemaker
Novametrix
  N. NICO cardiopulmonary
    management system
  N. pulse oximeter
  N. Tidal Wave handheld
    capnograph
Novamoxin
Novantrone
Novartis
Novasen
Novastan
novel
  N. device
  n. high magnification
    bronchovideoscope
  organic cation transporter n. type
    2 (OCTN2)
novo
  de n.
Novo-Atenol
Novo-AZT
Novo-Captopril

N

Novo-Chlorpromazine
Novo-Clonidine
Novo-Cloxin
Novo-Cromolyn
Novo-Digoxin
Novo-Diltazem
Novo-Dipiradol
Novo-Hydrazide
Novo-Hydroxyzine
Novo-Hylazin
Novo-Lexin
Novolin 70/30
Novomedopa
Novo-Metoprolol
Novo-Nifedin
Novo-Pen-VK
Novo-Pindol
Novo-Prazin
Novo-Prednisolone
Novo-Prednisone
Novo-Reserpine
Novo-Rythro Encap
Novo-Salmol
Novo-Semide
NovoSeven
Novo-Spiroton
Novoste
    N. Beta-Cath system
    N. catheter
Novo-Tamoxifen
Novo-Thalidone
Novo-Timol
Novo-Triamzide
Novo-Trimel
Novo-Veramil
NOxBOX
    N. mobile nitric oxide delivery
      and monitoring system
    N. monitor
NOxBOX+ monitor
Nozovent nasal valve dilator
NP
    nasopharyngeal
    nosocomial pneumonia
NPB
    Nellcor Puritan Bennett
    nodal premature beat
NPB-40 handheld pulse oximeter
NPB-75 handheld capnograph/pulse
  oximeter
NPC
    nodal premature contraction
NPH Iletin insulin
NPI
    nosocomial pulmonary infection
NPJT
    nonparoxysmal atrioventricular junctional
      tachycardia
NPM cells

NPPE
    negative pressure pulmonary edema
NPPV
    nasal positive pressure ventilation
    noninvasive positive pressure ventilation
N-propanol
NPSG
    nocturnal polysomnogram
NPT
    near patient test
NPV
    negative predictive value
    negative pressure ventilation
NQMI
    non-Q-wave myocardial infarction
NQWMI
    non-Q-wave myocardial infarction
NR
      Organidin NR
      Tussi-Organidin DM NR
NRA
    nitrate reductase assay
Nramp
    natural resistance macrophage-associated
     protein
NRDS
    neonatal respiratory distress syndrome
NREM
    nonrapid eye movement
     NREM sleep
NRMI
    National Registry of Myocardial
     Infarction
NRT
    nicotine replacement therapy
NS
    nasal steroid
     NS echo
NSAID
    nonsteroidal antiinflammatory drug
NSCLC
    non-small-cell lung cancer
    non-small-cell lung carcinoma
NSCT
    National Society of Cardiovascular
     Technologists
NSE
    neuron-specific enolase
NSIP
    nonspecific interstitial pneumonia
    nonspecific interstitial pneumonitis
NSIVCD
    nonspecific intraventricular conduction
     delay
NSR
    normal sinus rhythm
NSRT
    nonsurgical septal reduction therapy

NSSTT
  nonspecific ST and T
    NSSTT wave
NSTEMI
  non-ST-segment elevation myocardial
    infarction
NSVR
  normalized systemic vascular resistance
NSVT
  nonsustained ventricular tachycardia
NT
  normotensive
NTCP
  noninvasive transcutaneous cardiac
    pacing
N-terminal
    N-t. proANF
    N-t. proatrial natriuretic factor
    N-t. pro brain natriuretic peptide
      (NT-proBNP)
N-terminus
    extracellular N-t.
NTF
  nasogastric tube feeding
NTG
  nitroglycerin
  normal triglyceridemia
NTGO
  nitroglycerin ointment
NTHI
  nontypeable *Haemophilus influenzae*
NTM
  nontuberculous mycobacteria
NTMI
  nontransmural myocardial infarction
NT-proBNP
  N-terminal pro brain natriuretic peptide
    NT-proBNP ELISA enzyme
      immunoassay
NTS-AICD
  nonthoracotomy system antitachycardia
    device
NTVR
  normal transvalvular regurgitation
Nu-Amoxi
Nu-Ampi
Nu-Atenol
Nu-Capto
Nu-Cephalex
nuchal rigidity
nuclear
    n. factor-kappa B (NF-kappa-B)
    n. magnetic resonance (NMR)
    n. magnetic resonance imaging
      (NMRI)
    n. pacemaker
    n. perfusion imaging
    n. probe
    n. stent

nucleatum
    Fusobacterium n.
nuclei (*pl. of* nucleus)
nucleic
    n. acid amplification (NAA)
    n. acid direct amplification test
nucleotide
    total adenine n. (TAN)
nucleus, pl. **nuclei**
    apoptotic n.
    caudate n.
    paraventricular n. (PVN)
    suprachiasmatic n.
    vein of caudate n.
Nu-Clonidine
Nu-Cloxi
Nucofed Pediatric Expectorant
Nu-Cotrimox
Nucotuss
Nu-Diltiaz
Nuhn gland
Nu-Hydral
Nu-Iron
null
    n. hypothesis
    n. point
number
    n. needed to treat (NNT)
    representative CT (Hounsfield) n.
    Reynolds n.
    Strouhal n.
    Wasserman n.
    wave n.
Nu-Medopa
Nu-Metop
nummiform
nummular
    n. aortitis
    n. sputum
nummulation
Nu-Nifedin
nun's venous hum murmur
Nu-Pen-VK
Nu-Pindol
Nu-Prazo
Nu-Propranolol
NURD
  nonuniform rotational defect
Nurolon suture
nursing
    coronary care n. (CCN)
    n. home pneumonia
nutcracker
    n. esophagus
    n. phenomenon
Nu-Timolol
nutraceutical, nutriceutical
Nutracort
Nutraplus topical

N

Nu-Triazide
nutriceutical (*var. of* nutraceutical)
nutrient cardioplegia
Nu-Trim dietary fat substitute
nutrition
    enteral n.
    parenteral n.
Nuvance
Nu-Verap
Nu-Vois artificial larynx
Nuvolase 660 laser system
NV
    normovolemic
NVAF
    nonvalvular atrial fibrillation
NVC
    normal vital capacity
NVE
    native valve endocarditis

NVP
    nevirapine
Nycore pigtail catheter
NYHA
    New York Heart Association
    NYHA classification of congestive
      heart failure
    NYHA class I-IV symptoms
    NYHA functional classification
      I–IV
Nylex diagnostic catheter
nylon
    n. fiber
    Xcelon n.
Nyman pigtail catheter
Nyquist limit
nystatin
Nystat-Rx

O

oxygen
O antigen
antistreptolysin O (ASO)
O point
O point of cardiac apex pulse

O₂

oxygen
O_2 Advantage oxygen conserving device
ambulatory O_2
O_2 radical
O_2 via nasal cannula

OA

occipital artery
occupational asthma
oral appliance

OACIS

Osaka Acute Coronary Insufficiency

OAD

obstructive airway disease

oakridgensis

Legionella o.

OARS

Older Americans Resources and Services

Oasis thrombectomy system

oat

o. cell
o. cell carcinoma

OB

obliterative bronchiolitis

obesity

android o.
exogenous o.
female pattern o.
gynoid o.
o. hypertension
o. hypoventilation syndrome (OHS)
male pattern o.
morbid o.
Roux-en-Y o.
WHR for upper body o.

objective

o. bronchodilator reversibility
ventilatory o.

obligatory differential diagnosis

oblique

anterior o. (AO)
o. fissure
o. fissure of lung
left anterior o. (LAO)
right anterior o. (RAO)
o. sinus

obliterans

arteriosclerosis o.

arteritis o.
bronchiolitis o. (BO)
bronchiolitis fibrosa o.
cerebral thromboangiitis o. (CTAO)
endarteritis o.
pericarditis o.
phlebitis o.
thromboangiitis o.

obliterating

o. pericarditis
o. phlebitis

obliteration

coil o.

obliterative

o. bronchiolitis (OB)
o. bronchitis
o. cardiomyopathy
o. pericarditis
o. pleuritis
o. pulmonary hypertension (OPH)
o. vascular disease

oblongata

medulla o.

O'Brien

O. airway needle
O. stentless porcine heart valve

obscuration

aortic o.

Observer's Assessment of Alertness/Sedation Scale

obstructed

obstruction

airflow o.
airways o. (AO)
aortic arch vessel o.
baffle o.
chronic airflow o. (CAO)
chronic thrombotic pulmonary vascular o. (CTPVO)
chronic upper respiratory o.
coronary artery o. (CAO)
cricopharyngeal o.
dynamic intracavitary o.
embolic o.
endobronchial o.
extracranial carotid o.
extrathoracic airway o.
fixed airflow o.
fixed upper airway o.
foreign body airway o. (FBAO)
hypopharyngeal o.
infundibular o.
irreversible airway o.
left ventricular inflow tract o.

O

obstruction *(continued)*

left ventricular outflow tract o. (LVOTO)
luminal o.
mechanical o.
multivessel coronary artery o.
neoplastic airway o.
outflow tract o.
predilated polytetrafluoroethylene o.
pulmonary vascular o. (PVO)
retropalatal o.
reversible airway o.
right ventricular inflow o.
right ventricular outflow o.
right ventricular outflow tract o. (RVOTO)
static o.
stop-valve airway o.
subaortic o.
subpulmonary o.
subvalvar o.
subvalvar aortic o. (SAO)
superior vena cava o. (SVCO)
symptomatic airway o.
total o. (TO)
upper airway o. (UAO)
variable extrathoracic o.
variable intrathoracic o.
vena cava o.
vena caval o.
ventricular inflow tract o.
ventricular outflow tract o.

obstructive

o. airway disease (OAD)
o. atelectasis
o. edema
o. emphysema
o. hypertrophic cardiomyopathy (OHC)
o. hypopnea
o. lesion
o. lung disease (OLD)
o. murmur
o. pattern
o. pneumonia
o. shock
o. sleep apnea (OSA)
o. sleep apnea-hypopnea syndrome (OSAHS)
o. sleep apnea-induced cardiovascular change
o. sleep apnea syndrome (OSAS)
o. thrombus
o. valve thrombosis
o. ventilatory defect (OVD)
o. ventilatory dysfunction

obturating embolism
obturator

Check-Flo sheath o.

Fitch o.
Hemaflex PTCA sheath with o.
Hemaquet PTCA sheath with o.
Thora-Port o.

obtuse

o. marginal
o. marginal artery (OMA)
o. marginal branch (OMB)
o. marginal coronary artery
o. marginal lymphatic
o. margin of heart

OC

open cell
optimized conformability

occipital artery (OA)
occipitalis

basilaris ossis o.

occluded

o. area
o. artery

occluder

air clamp inflatable vessel o.
Amplatzer duct o.
Amplatzer PFO o.
Amplatzer septal o. (ASO)
ASDOS umbrella o.
o. balloon wash-out technique
Bard Clamshell septal o.
CardioSEAL septal o.
catheter-tip o.
clamshell septal o.
Crile tip o.
double-disc o.
Flo-Rester vascular o.
Helex septal o.
Hunter detachable balloon o.
modified Rashkind PDA o.
Pediatric Cardiology Devices Sideris Buttoned device o.
percutaneous left atrial appendage transcatheter o. (PLAATO)
PFO-Star o.
septal o.
square-shaped o.
tilting disc o.
tip o.

occludin
occluding thrombus
occlusion

acute coronary o. (ACO)
angioplasty-related vessel o.
arterial o.
balloon o.
balloon coronary o. (BCO)
balloon test o. (BTO)
basilar artery o. (BAO)
bradycardia after arteriovenous fistula o. (BAVFO)
branch retinal artery o. (BRAO)

branch retinal vein o. (BRVO)
branch vein o.
branch vessel o. (BVO)
central retinal artery o. (CRAO)
central vein o. (CVO)
chronic coronary O.'s
chronic total o. (CTO)
circumflex o.
coronary artery o.
coronary branch o.
o. device
femoral artery o.
femoral vein o.
graft o.
iliac artery o.
inferior mesenteric vascular o.
inferior vena cava o.
intermittent aortic o. (IAO)
intermittent coronary sinus o.
  (ICSO)
left main coronary o.
left marginal coronary artery o.
  (LMCAO)
long iliac artery o.
mesenteric artery o.
mesenteric vascular o.
middle cerebral artery o. (MCAO)
nonacute total coronary o.
ostial o.
percutaneous left atrial appendage
  transcatheter o. (PLAATO)
peripheral arterial o. (PAO)
pressure-controlled intermittent
  coronary sinus o. (PICSO)
pulmonary artery o. (PAO)
recurrent mesenteric vascular o.
side-branch o.
snare-assisted coil o.
superior mesenteric vascular o.
temporary unilateral pulmonary
  artery o.
thrombotic o. (TO)
transcatheter coil o.
transient spastic o. (TSO)
venous mesenteric vascular o.
occlusive
o. disease
o. thromboaortopathy
o. thrombosis
o. thrombus
OCCPR
open chest cardiopulmonary resuscitation
occult
o. bronchogenic carcinoma
o. cardiogenic shock
o. cystic fibrosis
o. pericardial constriction
o. pericarditis

occupational
o. asthma (OA)
o. asthmogen
o. formalin asthma
o. health and safety (OHS)
o. lung disease
**occupational-environmental lung disease
  (OELD)**
OCG
omnicardiogram
Ochrobactrum anthropi
ochrometer
ochronosis
Ochsner-Mahorner
O.-M. echocardiogram
O.-M. test
OCR
oculocardiac reflex
OCT
optical coherence tomography
orthotopic cardiac transplantation
octafluoropropane
octapolar catheter
OCTN2
organic cation transporter novel type 2
Octocaine
octopus
O. 2+, 3 tissue stabilization
  system
O. tissue stabilizer
O. tissue stabilizing device
octreotide
oculocardiac reflex (OCR)
oculocraniosomatic disease
oculomucocutaneous syndrome
oculopharyngeal reflex
oculoplethysmography (OPG)
oculopneumoplethysmography
oculovagal reflex
OD
outer diameter
odansetron hydrochloride
odds ratio (OR)
ODI
oxygen desaturation index
ODISsey tissue oximeter
ODN
oligodeoxynucleotide
odorans
Alcaligenes o.
odoratus
Lathyrus o.
odor-triggered panic attack
ODTS
organic dust toxic syndrome
O'Dwyer intubation
odynophagia
OEF
oxygen extraction fraction

Oehler symptoms
Oehl muscle
OELD
    occupational-environmental lung disease
O₂ER
    oxygen extraction ratio
Oertel treatment
off-axis
office
    o. angina
    o. hypertension
    International Labor O. (ILO)
off-pump
    o.-p. beating heart surgery
    o.-p. CABG
    o.-p. coronary artery bypass
      (OPCAB)
    o.-p. coronary artery bypass graft
      (OPCABG)
    o.-p. vascular surgery
ofloxacin
Ogata method
OGTT
    oral glucose tolerance test
OHC
    obstructive hypertrophic cardiomyopathy
OHCA
    out-of-hospital cardiac arrest
OHD
    organic heart disease
OHDC
    oxyhemoglobin disassociation curve
OHI
    operative hypertension indicator
ohm
Ohmeda
    O. 6200, 6300 CO₂ monitor
    O. handheld oximeter
    O. pulse oximeter
    O. thoracic suction regulator
ohmic heating
Ohm law
ohmmeter
Ohnell
    X wave of O.
OHS
    obesity hypoventilation syndrome
    occupational health and safety
    open heart surgery
OHT
    orthotopic heart transplant
OIA
    osmotically induced asthma
oil
    canola o.
    o. embolism
    emu o.
    fish o.
    flaxseed o.

    marine o.'s
    MCT O.
    o. mist asthma
    progesterone O.
    rapeseed o.
    o. red O stain
    trypsin, balsam peru, castor o.
oil-aspiration pneumonia
ointment
    Cellegesic o.
    Lidodan o.
    Nitro-Bid O.
    nitroglycerin o. (NTGO)
    Nitrol O.
    Whitfield o.
    Xylocaine Topical O.
OKT3
    OKT3 antibody
    Orthoclone OKT3
OL
    open label
    open labeled
OLB
    open lung biopsy
Olbert
    O. balloon
    O. balloon catheter
OLBI
    overlapping biphasic impulse
Olcott torque device
OLD
    obstructive lung disease
**Older Americans Resources and
   Services (OARS)**
old myocardial infarction (OMI)
Olean
oleate
    ethanolamine o.
oleogomenol
olestra
Oligella urethralis
oligemia
    pulmonary o.
oligemic shock
oligodeoxynucleotide (ODN)
    antisense o.
oligonucleotide
    o. microarray
    mucin antisense o.
oliguria
Oliver-Rosalki method
Oliver sign
olive-tipped
    o.-t. Magnum wire
    o.-t. needle
olivopontocerebellar
    o. atrophy
    o. degeneration
olmesartan medoxomil

olprinone
Olympix II PTCA dilation catheter
Olympus
    O. bioptome
    O. echoendoscope
    O. One-Step Button tube
    O. XBF-UC40P bronchoscope
OM1
    first obtuse marginal
OM2
    second obtuse marginal
OMA
    obtuse marginal artery
Omacor
omalizumab
omapatrilat
OMB
    obtuse marginal branch
OM coronary artery
omega
    O. NV angioplasty catheter
    O. stent
omega-3 unsaturated fatty acid
omental wrap
omentopexy
omeprazole
O_6-methylguanine-DNA-methyl-transferase (MGMT)
OMI
    old myocardial infarction
Omni
    O. analyzer
    O. Flush catheter
    O. Flush shape
Omnicarbon
    O. cardiac valve prosthesis
    O. heart valve prosthesis
    O. prosthetic heart valve
omnicardiogram (OCG)
OmniCath atherectomy catheter
Omnicef
Omnicell
    O. catheter module
    O. supply system
omnidirectional M-mode
OmniFilter percutaneous guidewire microfilter
Omnilink balloon-expandable stent
Omnipaque
Omniplane TEE
Omniscience single leaflet cardiac valve prosthesis
Omni-Stanicor pacemaker
Omni-Tract system
omnivore
omotracheale
    trigonum o.
omphalitis
omphalocele

Omsk hemorrhagic fever
OMVC
    open mitral valve commissurotomy
Oncaspar
Onchocerca volvulus
oncology mix
Onconase
Oncor ApopTag kit
oncostatin M
oncotic pressure
Oncovin injection
ondansetron
on-demand monitoring
Ondine
    O. breathing
    O. curse
One Touch blood glucose monitor
onion
    o. bulb dilation
    o. scale lesion
on-pump
ON-Q PainBuster postoperative pain relief system
onset
    sudden rate o.
Ontak
ONTG
    oral nitroglycerin
On-X
    O.-X aortic valve
    O.-X mechanical bi-leaflet prosthetic heart valve
onychograph
Onyx liquid embolic system
oocyte
    Xenopus o.
OOH/CA
    out-of-hospital cardiac arrest
OOH-SCD
    out-of-hospital sudden cardiac death
OOO mode
opacification
    alveolar o.
    amorphous parenchymal o.
    faint o.
    ground-glass o.
    left ventricular o. (LVO)
    selective graft o.
opacify
opacity
    ground-glass o.
    nodular o.
    p/q o.
    vitreous o.
opalescent sputum
OPCAB
    off-pump coronary artery bypass
OPCABG
    off-pump coronary artery bypass graft

O

open
- o. atrial disc
- o. bronchus sign
- o. cell (OC)
- o. chest cardiac massage
- o. chest cardiac resuscitation
- o. chest cardiopulmonary resuscitation (OCCPR)
- o. chest surgery
- o. circuit method
- o. heart CABG
- o. heart surgery (OHS)
- keep vein o. (KVO)
- o. label (OL)
- o. labeled (OL)
- o. lung approach
- o. lung biopsy (OLB)
- o. mitral valve commissurotomy (OMVC)
- O. Pivot heart valve
- o. pleural biopsy
- o. pneumothorax
- o. surgery (OS)
- o. surgical valvotomy
- o. technique
- o. tuberculosis

Open-Cath
- Abbokinase O.-C.

opener
- adenosine triphosphate-sensitive potassium channel o.
- potassium channel o.

opening
- anodal o. (AO)
- aortic o. (AO)
- aortic valve o. (AVO)
- atrioventricular o. (AVO)
- atrioventricular valve o. (AO)
- esophageal o.
- fistulous o.
- mitral o. (Mo)
- mitral valve o. (MVO)
- o. pressure
- o. snap (OS)
- tricuspid o. (To)

open-label ACE-inhibitor therapy

OpenSail
- O. balloon dilation catheter
- O. coronary dilation catheter

operation (*See also* procedure)
- Abbe o.
- Anel o.
- arterial switch o.
- atrial baffle o.
- Babcock o.
- Baffes o.
- Barnard o.
- Beck I, II o.
- Bentall o.
- Berger o.
- bidirectional Glenn o.
- Blalock-Hanlon o.
- Blalock-Taussig o.
- Brock o.
- cautery-assisted palatal stiffening o. (CAPSO)
- Cox maze o.
- Damus-Kaye-Stansel o.
- David reimplantation o.
- DKS o.
- electrode catheter ablation o.
- encircling endocardial ventriculotomy o.
- endocardial to epicardial resection o.
- Estlander o.
- extracardiac Fontan o.
- fenestrated Fontan o.
- Fontan o.
- Freund o.
- Glenn o.
- Goldsmith o.
- Grondahl-Finney o.
- Guiraudon corridor o.
- Heller-Belsey o.
- Heller-Nissen o.
- hemi-Fontan o.
- Hunter o.
- Ilbawi o.
- Jatene o.
- Konno o.
- laser maze o.
- Lindesmith o.
- modified David reimplantation o.
- multivalve o.
- Mustard atrial switch o.
- Norwood o.
- Palma o.
- Potts o.
- Ransohoff o.
- Rastan o.
- Rastelli o.
- Sawyer o.
- Schede o.
- second-look o.
- Senning and Mustard o.
- switch o.
- talc o.
- Tanner o.
- transcatheter closure of atrial septal defect o.
- Trendelenburg o.
- triangular resection of leaflet o.
- valve-conserving o.
- Waterston o.

operative hypertension indicator (OHI)

operculum, pl. **opercula**

OPG
    oculoplethysmography
OPH
    obliterative pulmonary hypertension
opiate
opioid
Opisthorchis
Opitz syndrome
OPO
    organ procurement organization
opportunistic
    o. fungal pneumonia
    o. infection
opsoclonia
opsonin
opsonization
opsonophagocytic receptor
Opta
    O. 5 catheter
    O. Pro PTA dilation catheter
Opti
    O. 1 pH/blood gas analyzer
    O. 1 portable blood analyzer
optic
    o. atrophy
    o. disc
    o. neuritis
    o. tweezers
optical
    o. aggregometer
    o. coherence tomography (OCT)
    o. fiber catheter
    O. Sensors stand-alone arterial
      blood gas monitoring system
Opticath oximeter catheter
OptiChamber valved holding chamber
Opticon real-time PCR machine
OptiCor digital cardiac communication
    and storage system
Opti-Flow catheter
Optiform mitral valve
OptiHaler drug delivery system
Optima pacemaker
optimized conformability (OC)
Opti-Plast XT balloon catheter
Optiray
    O. 320
    O. contrast
    O. contrast medium
Optison
    O. contrast
    O. contrast agent
    O. injectable suspension
OptiVol
    O. fluid index
    O. fluid monitor
    O. fluid status
    O. fluid status monitoring

OPTN
    Organ Procurement and Transplantation
    Network
Optochin
    O. disc test
    O. test for *Streptococcus*
      pneumoniae
optoelectronic plethysmography
Optrin
opus
    O. cardiac troponin I assay
    O. RM single chamber pacemaker
OR
    odds ratio
oracle
    O. Focus imaging catheter
    O. Focus PTCA catheter
    O. Micro Plus
    O. Micro Plus PTCA catheter
oral
    Achromycin V O.
    o. airflow in liters per second
      (V_O)
    Aller-Chlor O.
    AllerMax O.
    Altace O.
    o. anticoagulant therapy
    o. appliance (OA)
    Apresoline O.
    Aristocort O.
    Atarax O.
    Banophen O.
    Benadryl O.
    Betapace O.
    Betapen-VK O.
    Blocadren O.
    Brethine O.
    Calm-X O.
    o. candidiasis
    Cartrol O.
    Catapres O.
    CeeNU O.
    Ceftin O.
    Celestone O.
    Chlor-Trimeton O.
    Cipro O.
    Cleocin HCl O.
    Cleocin Pediatric O.
    Compazine O.
    o. contraceptive-induced
      hypertension
    Cortef O.
    Cyklokapron O.
    Cytomel O.
    Cytoxan O.
    Decadron O.
    Delta-Cortef O.
    Deltasone O.
    Demadex O.

O

oral *(continued)*
>Diflucan O.
>Dormin O.
>Doryx O.
>Doxychel O.
>Dramamine O.
>Dynacin O.
>Edecrin O.
>E.E.S. O.
>E-Mycin O.
>Eryc O.
>EryPed O.
>Ery-Tab O.
>Erythrocin O.
>Eryzole O.
>Flagyl O.
>o. flecainide therapy
>o. flora
>Floxin O.
>Flumadine O.
>Genahist O.
>o. glucose tolerance test (OGTT)
>Indocin O.
>o. inhalation dexamethasone
>Kerlone O.
>o. L-arginine system
>Lasix O.
>Lincocin O.
>Loniten O.
>Maxaquin O.
>Medrol O.
>Mephyton O.
>Monodox O.
>Mycobutin O.
>o. nitroglycerin (ONTG)
>Nitroglyn O.
>Nizoral O.
>Normodyne O.
>Noroxin O.
>o. part
>o. part of pharynx
>PCE O.
>PediaCare O.
>Pediapred O.
>Pediazole O.
>poliovirus vaccine, live, trivalent, o.
>Prelone O.
>Proglycem O.
>Provera O.
>Retrovir O.
>Rifadin O.
>Rimactane O.
>Sporanox O.
>Sterapred O.
>Sumycin O.
>Trandate O.
>o. triamcinolone inhalation
>o. tuberculosis
>Vancocin O.
>Vasotec O.
>Veetids O.
>VePesid O.
>Vibramycin O.
>Videx O.
>Vistaril O.
>Xylocaine O.

oralis
>*Bacteroides o.*

Orbenin
orbofiban
orciprenaline sulfate
order
>anodal opening o. (AOO)

Ordrine AT Extended Release Capsule
Oretic
organ
>Golgi tendon o.
>o. procurement organization (OPO)
>O. Procurement and Transplantation Network (OPTN)
>o. system failure
>o. transplantation system

organelle
>vesicular-vacuolar o. (VVO)

organic
>o. anion
>o. cation transporter novel type 2 (OCTN2)
>o. dust
>o. dust pneumoconiosis
>o. dust toxic syndrome (ODTS)
>o. heart disease (OHD)
>o. murmur
>o. phosphorus
>o. thiophosphate

Organidin NR
organism
>Cox o.
>encapsulated o.
>gram-negative o.
>gram-positive o.
>intracellular o. (ICO)
>pleuropneumonia-like o. (PPLO)

organization
>Extracorporeal Life Support O. (ELSO)
>International Standards O. (ISO)
>organ procurement o. (OPO)
>World Health O. (WHO)

organized thrombus
organizing
>o. empyema
>o. pneumonia
>o. thrombus

organoid pattern
organophosphate
oriental hemoptysis

orifice
    aortic o.
    aortic valve o. (AVO)
    atrioventricular o.
    cardiac o.
    common atrioventricular o. (CAVO)
    effective regurgitant o. (ERO)
    esophagogastric o.
    flow across o.
    mitral o. (MO)
    mitral valve o. (MVO)
    pulmonary o.
    o. of pulmonary trunk
    regurgitant o.
    stent-jail o.
    o. of superior vena cava
    tricuspid o.
    valvular o.
orificial
    o. stenosis
    o. tuberculosis
origin
    anomalous o.
    anomalous coronary o. (ACO)
    myocardial disease of unknown o. (MDUO)
    myocardiopathy of unknown o. (MUO)
original
    Doan's O.
    O. Pink Tape waterproof adhesive tape
Orimune
orlistat
Ornish
    O. diet
    O. theory
ornithosis
oroendotracheal tube
oropharyngeal
    o. colonization
    o. tularemia
oropharynx
    crowded o.
orotracheal
    o. intubation
    o. tube
orphan
    enteric cytopathogenic human o. (ECHO)
    enterocytopathogenic human o. (ECHO)
    respiratory and enteric o. (REO)
Orsi-Grocco method
ORT
    orthodromic reciprocating tachycardia
orthoarteriotony
orthocardiac reflex
Orthoclone OKT3

orthodeoxia
orthodox sleep
orthodromic
    o. atrioventricular reciprocating tachycardia
    o. A-V reentrant tachycardia
    o. circus movement tachycardia
    o. conduction
    o. reciprocating tachycardia (ORT)
orthogonal
    o. electrocardiogram
    o. lead system
    o. plane
    o. view
orthograde conduction
Orthomyxoviridae virus
orthomyxovirus
orthopercussion
ortho-phthalaldehyde
orthopnea
    2-pillow o.
    3-pillow o.
orthopneic
orthosis
    ankle-foot o. (AFO)
orthostasis autoregulation
orthostatic
    o. dyspnea
    o. hypertension
    o. hypopiesis
    o. hypotension
    o. syncope
    o. tachycardia
orthostatism
    vasovagal o.
orthotopic
    o. cardiac transplant
    o. cardiac transplantation (OCT)
    o. heart transplant (OHT)
    o. univentricular artificial heart
Ortner syndrome
Oruvail
oryzae
    Aspergillus o.
    Rhizopus o.
OS
    opening snap
    open surgery
OSA
    obstructive sleep apnea
OSAHS
    obstructive sleep apnea-hypopnea syndrome
Osaka Acute Coronary Insufficiency (OACIS)
OSAP appliance
OSAS
    obstructive sleep apnea syndrome
Osborne (J) wave

Osciflator balloon inflation syringe
oscillating
    o. balloon inflation
    o. dilation
    o. paraboloid
    o. saw
oscillation
    external chest wall o.
    forced o. (FO)
    high-frequency o. (HFO)
    high-frequency chest wall o.
      (HFCWO)
    o. technique
oscillator
    Hayek o.
oscillatory
    o. afterpotential
    o. response
oscillometer
oscillometric signal
oscilloscope
Oscor pacing lead
OSD
    OSD monitor
    Profilate OSD
oseltamivir phosphate
OSF
    outlet strut fracture
Osler
    O. node
    O. sign
    O. triad
Osler-Weber-Rendu
    O.-W.-R. disease
    O.-W.-R. syndrome
Osmitrol injection
osmolality
osmolarity
osmometer
osmoregulation
osmoregulatory
osmotaxis
osmotic
    o. challenge
    o. demyelination syndrome
    o. diuretic
    o. pressure
osmotically induced asthma (OIA)
ossification
    diffuse pulmonary o.
    pulmonary o.
ossifying pneumonitis
Ossoff-Karlan laryngoscope
osteitis
    caseous o.
    o. deformans
    o. tuberculosa multiplex cystica
osteoarthritis
    hyperplastic o.

osteoarthropathy
    hypertrophic pulmonary o.
    pneumogenic o.
    pulmonary hypertrophic o.
osteochondroma
osteogenesis imperfecta
Osteomark test
osteonecrosis
    dysbaric o.
osteoplastica
    tracheobronchopathia o.
    tracheopathia o.
osteopontin
    o. messenger ribonucleic acid
    o. mRNA
osteoradionecrosis
osteosarcoma
osteosynthesis
    exit surgical o.
    plastic surgical o.
    surgical o.
osteotomy
    anterior inferior mandibular o.
      (AIMO)
    maxillomandibular o. (MMO)
ostial
    o. isolation
    o. lesion
    o. narrowing
    o. occlusion
    o. stenosis
    o. stent
ostium, pl. **ostia**
    coronary o.
    o. of coronary sinus (CSO)
    left coronary o. (LCO)
    middle lobe vein o.
    o. primum
    o. primum defect
    right coronary o. (RCO)
    o. secundum
    o. secundum defect
    solitary coronary o.
    o. trunci pulmonalis
    ostia venarum pulmonalium
    venous o.
Ostwald viscometer
Osypka
    O. atrial lead
    O. rotational angioplasty
otopharyngeal tube
Ototemp 3000
ototoxicity
OTW
  over-the-wire
    OTW HighSail coronary dilation
      catheter
    OTW perfusion catheter

SV OTW
OTW thrombolytic brush
O-Two
    O-T. ALS handheld resuscitator
    O-T. BLS handheld resuscitator
    O-T. CAREvent BLS+ resuscitator
ouabain
Outback re-entry catheter
outer diameter (OD)
outflow
    o. cardiac patch
    left ventricle o. (LVO)
    maximum venous o. (MVO)
    o. murmur
    o. reconstruction
    right ventricular o. (RVO)
    subcostal o.
    o. tract
    o. tract obstruction
outlet
    o. strut
    o. strut fracture (OSF)
    o. VSD
out-of-hospital
    o.-o.-h. cardiac arrest (OHCA, OOH/CA)
    o.-o.-h. sudden cardiac death (OOH-SCD)
output
    biliary cholesterol o. (BCO)
    cardiac o. (CO, Q, QT, Q-T)
    cardiac minute o. (CMO)
    cardiac power o. (CPO)
    o. circuit
    continuous cardiac o. (CCO)
    Fick cardiac o.
    heart minute o. (HMO)
    impedance cardiac o. (ICO)
    left ventricular o.
    left ventricular systolic o. (LVSO)
    low cardiac o. (LCO)
    measured o.
    minute o.
    pacemaker o.
    postoperative low cardiac o. (PLCO)
    predicted cardiac o. (PCO)
    respiratory system motoneural o.
    right ventricular stroke o. (RVSO)
    stroke o.
    thermodilution cardiac o. (TDCO)
    ultrasonic cardiac o. (UCO)
outside-in signaling
ovale
    foramen o. (FO)
    patent foramen o. (PFO)
    Plasmodium o.
    probe-patent foramen o.
oval foramen

ovalis
    anulus o.
    fossa o.
Ovatio implantable cardioverter-defibrillator
OVD
    obstructive ventilatory defect
over-and-under ventricles
overdilation
overdistention, overdistension
    alveolar o.
    end-inspiratory o.
overdrive
    o. atrial pacing
    o. mode
    o. suppression
overexpressed protein
overexpression
    beta-2 AR o.
    cardiac-specific o.
    IGF-1 o.
    TIMP-3 o.
    tissue inhibitor of metalloproteinase-3 o.
overflow wave
Overholt procedure
overhydration
overinflation
    congenital lobar o.
overlap
    stent o.
    o. syndrome
    o. vasculitis
overlapping biphasic impulse (OLBI)
overlay
    psychogenic o.
overload
    circulatory o.
    diastolic o.
    left atrial o. (LAO)
    pressure o.
    right ventricular diastolic o. (RVDO)
    right ventricular volume o. (RVVO)
    volume o.
overnight
    o. polysomnography
    o. pulse oximetry
overreactivity
    physiological o.
overrecruitment of glottic constrictor muscles
override
    aortic o.
overriding
    o. aorta
    o. valve
oversampling

O

oversedation
oversensing
    afterpotential o.
    myopotential o.
    o. pacemaker
oversewing
overshoot phenomenon
over-the-needle catheter
over-the-wire (OTW)
    o.-t.-w. balloon dilation catheter
    o.-t.-w. balloon dilation catheter
      system
    o.-t.-w. pacing lead
    o.-t.-w. PTCA balloon catheter
overt rupture
overventilation
Owens
    O. balloon
    O. balloon catheter
    O. Lo-Profile dilation catheter
Owren
    O. disease
    O. factor V deficiency
oxacillin sodium
oxalate
    calcium o.
oxalosis
oxamniquine
oxandrolone
oxazepam
oxazolidinone
Oxford
    O. Handicap Scale
    O. technique
ox heart
oxidant stress
oxidase
    cytochrome c o. (COX)
    diamine o. (DO)
    monoamine o. (MAO)
    postheparin plasma diamine o.
      (PHD)
    xanthine o.
oxidation
    intraplaque LDL o.
oxidative
    o. metabolism
    o. modification of LDL (oxLDL,
      ox-LDL)
    o. phosphorylation
    o. stress
oxide
    cadmium o.
    endothelium-derived nitric o.
      (EDNO)
    ethylene o. (ETO)
    exhaled nitric o. (eNO, ENO)
    exogenous nitric o.
    expired nitric o. (eNO, ENO)

    inhaled nitric o. (INO)
    magnesium o.
    nitric o. (NO)
    nitrogen o.
    nitrous o.
    stannic o.
    tin o.
    total exhaled nitric o. (FENO)
    tributyltin o.
oxidized
    o. cellulose
    o. LDL
    o. low-density lipoprotein (OxLDL)
oxidoreductase
    dopachrome o. (DCOR)
OxiFirst fetal oxygen saturation
  monitoring system
Oxilan
OxiLink oximeter probe cover
OxiMax
    O. pulse oximeter
    O. pulse oximetry device
oximeter
    Armstrong handheld pulse o.
    Autocorr Plus pulse o.
    Autocorr portable pulse o.
    AVOXimeter 1000E whole
      blood o.
    BI-OX III ear o.
    CO o.
    CO_2SMO capnograph/pulse o.
    Cricket pulse o.
    Criticare pulse o.
    Datascope pulse o.
    Dinamap pulse o.
    ear o.
    FingerPrint handheld pulse o.
    8500 handheld pulse o.
    Hewlett-Packard ear o.
    Mini Pulse o.
    920M Plus pulse o.
    Nellcor N200 pulse o.
    Nellcor N-395 pulse o.
    Nellcor Symphony pulse o.
    Nonin Onyx pulse o.
    Novametrix pulse o.
    NPB-40 handheld pulse o.
    NPB-75 handheld
      capnograph/pulse o.
    N-395 pulse o.
    ODISsey tissue o.
    Ohmeda handheld o.
    Ohmeda pulse o.
    OxiMax pulse o.
    Oxypleth pulse o.
    OxySat pulse o.
    OxyTemp handheld pulse o.
    Oxytrak pulse o.

Palco Laboratories Model 300, 400
  pulse o.
pulse o.
3800 pulse o.
Pulsox-5 pulse o.
Respironics 920P handheld pulse o.
Respironics 930 pulse o.
SensorMedics SAT-TRAK pulse o.
SET carbon monoxide pulse o.
Tidal Wave Sp capnometer/pulse o.
VitalSAT pulse o.
oximetric catheter
Oximetrix 3 System
oximetry
  ambulatory pulse o.
  carbon monoxide o. (CO-oximetry)
  central venous o.
  cerebral o.
  CO o.
  CO_2 o.
  continuous pulse o.
  finger o.
  Hb o.
  HbO_2 o.
  N_2 o.
  near-infrared cerebral o.
  nocturnal o.
  overnight pulse o.
  OxiScan overnight pulse o.
  oxygen saturation measured by
    pulse o. (SpO_2)
  pCO_2 o.
  pO_2 o.
  pulse o. (PO)
  reflectance o.
  spectrophotometric o.
OxiScan
  O. overnight pulse oximetry
  O. oximetry program
  O. oximetry recording and
    reporting system
Oxisensor II adult sensor
**Oxismart advanced signal processing
  and alarm technology**
Oxis Turbuhaler
oxitropium bromide
OxLDL
  oxidized low-density lipoprotein
oxLDL, ox-LDL
  oxidative modification of LDL
oxolamine
oxothiazolidine
oxotremorine
oxprenolol
Oxsoralen Topical
oxtriphylline
OxyALERT device
oxybate
  sodium o.

Oxycel
Oxyfill oxygen refilling system
oxygen (O, O_2)
  aqueous o.
  blood o.
  blow-by o.
  o. capacity
  central venous o. (CVO)
  o. challenge test
  o. concentrator
  o. consumption (VO_2max)
  o. consumption index
  o. consumption per minute
    (VO_2max)
  o. content
  o. cost
  o. cost of breathing
  O. Cost Diagram questionnaire
  o. cylinder
  cytotoxic singlet o.
  o. debt
  o. delivery (DO_2)
  o. dependence
  o. desaturation index (ODI)
  o. dissociation curve
  o. entrainment
  o. exchange
  o. extraction
  o. extraction fraction (OEF)
  o. extraction ratio (O_2ER)
  fraction of inspired o. (FIO_2, FiO_2)
  o. free radical release
  humidified o.
  hyperbaric o. (HBO)
  o. inhalation
  inspired o.
  intracoronary aqueous o.
  o. mask
  o. metabolism
  myocardial o. (MO_2)
  o. paradox
  partial pressure of o. (pO_2)
  partial pressure of inspiratory o.
    (PIO_2)
  o. poisoning
  o. pulse
  o. radical
  o. radical scavenger
  o. reservoir
  o. saturation (SO_2)
  o. saturation of hemoglobin of
    arterial blood
  o. saturation measured by pulse
    oximetry (SpO_2)
  o. step-up method
  supplemental o.
  o. supply
  o. tension
  o. tent

O

oxygen *(continued)*
    o. therapy
    o. toxicity
    T-piece o.
    o. transport
    transtracheal o. (TTO)
    o. uptake (oxygen uptake peak VO_2)
oxygen-15
oxygenated
    o. blood
    o. hemoglobin
oxygenation
    apneic o.
    bubble o.
    disc o.
    enhanced o.
    extracorporeal membrane o.
     (ECMO)
    fetal o.
    film o.
    hyperbaric o.
    nocturnal o.
    pump o.
    rotating disc o.
    screen o.
    venoarterial extracorporeal
     membrane o. (VA-ECMO)
oxygenator
    Affinity o.
    Biocor 200 high performance o.
    bubble o.
    disc o.
    extracorporeal membrane o.
    extracorporeal pump o.
    Gambro o.
    intravascular o. (IVOX)
    Lilliput o.
    Maxima Plus plasma resistant
     fiber o.
    Monolyth o.
    o. Optima o.
    pump o.
    Sarns membrane o. (SMO)
oxygen-binding capacity
oxygen-carrying
    o.-c. capacity
    o.-c. perfluorochemical liquid

oxygen-conserving
    o.-c. nasal cannula
    o.-c. pendant
oxygen-derived free radical
oxygen-diffusing capacity
oxygen-free radical
oxygen-induced
    o.-i. hypercapnia
    o.-i. hypercarbia
oxyhemodynamic index
oxyhemoglobin (HbO₂)
    o. disassociation curve (OHDC)
    o. dissociation curve
    o. saturation
Oxy-Hood pressurizer
**Oxylator-EM 100 automatic
  resuscitation and inhalation system**
OxyLead interconnect cable
Oxylite ambulatory oxygen system
Oxymatic
    O. 411 electronic conserver
    O. 401 electronic oxygen conserver
oxymetazoline
oxymetolazone
Oxymizer
Oxypleth pulse oximeter
oxypurinol
OxySat pulse oximeter
oxysterol inhibitor
OxyTemp handheld pulse oximeter
oxytetracycline hydrochloride
OxyTip sensor
oxytoca
    Klebsiella o.
oxytocin
Oxytrak pulse oximeter
**Oxy-Ultra-Lite ambulatory oxygen
  system**
oyster mass of mucus
ozaenae
    Klebsiella pneumoniae subsp. *o.*
ozone
    ambient o.

P
electrocardiographic wave corresponding
to wave of depolarization crossing atria
partial pressure
pressure
P cell
P congenitale
P duration
factor P
P loop
P mitrale
P pulmonale
P pulmonale syndrome
P substance of Lewis
P synchronous pacing
P terminal force
P vector
P wave

p
pulse

P2
pulmonic second heart sound

2500P
Edwards Prima Plus Stentless
Bioprosthesis Model 2500P

P50
hemoglobin .

P$_A$
arterial pressure of arterial fluid

P$_{atm}$
atmospheric pressure

P$_{Emax}$
maximal expiratory mouth pressure

P$_{Imax}$
maximal inspiratory mouth pressure

P$_{IO_2}$
partial pressure of inspiratory oxygen

P$_T$
total pressure

p24
p24 antigen
p24 antigen test

P13 kinase
p22^{phox} protein
P2y12 Plavix assay
p47^{phox} protein
p53-dependent signaling system
p67^{phox} protein
PA
atrial pressure
partial pressure of arterial fluid
pressure augmentation
pulmonary angiography
pulmonary arterial
pulmonary artery

pulmonary atresia
pulmonary autograft
Adalat CC, PA
PA banding
PA conduction time
PA filling pressure
PA interval
PA pressure

P&A
percussion and auscultation

Pa
pascal
pulmonary arterial

pAAT
plasma alpha-1 antitrypsin

PAB
premature atrial beat

PABP
pulmonary artery balloon pump

PABV
percutaneous aortic balloon valvoplasty

PAC
pericarditis. arthropathy, camptodactyly
phenacetin, aspirin, caffeine
premature atrial beat
premature atrial contraction
pulmonary artery catheterization
PAC syndrome

**Paceart complete pacemaker patient
testing system**
Pace bipolar pacing catheter
paced
p. beat
p. cycle length
p. depolarization integral
p. rhythm
p. ventricular evoked response

pacemaker (PM)
AAI p.
AAI/AAIR p.
AAT p.
Accufix p.
Activitrax II p.
Activitrax single-chamber
responsive p.
Activitrax variable rate p.
activity-guided p.
activity-sensing p.
Actros p.
p. adaptive rate
adaptive-rate p.
AddVent atrioventricular p.
Aequitron p.
Affinity p.
AFP II p.

P

pacemaker *(continued)*
    p. afterpotential
    Alcatel p.
    p. amplifier refractory period
    antitachycardia p. (ATP)
    AOO p.
    artificial p.
    Arzco p.
    Astra T4, T6 p.
    atrial asynchronous p.
    atrial-based p.
    atrial demand inhibited p.
    atrial demand triggered p.
    atrial synchronous
      noncompetitive p.
    atrial synchronous ventricular
      inhibited p.
    atrial triggered noncompetitive p.
    atrial VOO p.
    atriobiventricular p.
    atrioventricular sequential p.
    p. augmentor
    Autima II dual-chamber p.
    automatic p.
    p. automaticity
    A-V sequential p.
    A-V synchronous p.
    Axios 04 p.
    Betacel-Biotronik p.
    bifocal demand DVI p.
    Biorate p.
    Biotronik p.
    bipolar p.
    breathing p.
    p. burst pacing
    p. can
    p. capture
    cardiac p.
    p. catheter
    Chardack-Greatbatch p.
    Chardack Medtronic p.
    Circadia dual-chamber rate-
      adaptive p.
    circadian p.
    p. circus movement tachycardia
      (PCMT)
    p. code system
    committed mode p.
    Contak CD ventricular
      resynchronization p.
    Cook p.
    Coratomic R wave inhibited p.
    Cosmos 283 DDD p.
    Cosmos II DDD p.
    CPI/Guidant p.
    crosstalk p.
    p. current (I_F)
    Cyberlith p.
    Cybertach automatic-burst atrial p.

    Cybertach 60 bipolar p.
    Cylos p.
    Dash single-chamber rate-adaptic p.
    DDD p.
    DDI mode p.
    demand p.
    Devices, Ltd. p.
    Dialog p.
    Discovery DDDR p.
    Dromos p.
    DSI-III screw-in lead p.
    dual-chamber p. (DCP)
    dual-chamber Medtronic Kappa
      400 p.
    dual-demand p.
    Durapulse p.
    DVI p.
    Ectocor p.
    ectopic p.
    electric cardiac p.
    p. electrode
    Electrodyne p.
    electronic p.
    Elema p.
    Elema-Schonander p.
    Elite dual-chamber rate-
      responsive p.
    Encor p.
    p. endocarditis
    end-of-life p.
    Endotak p.
    Enertrax 7l00 p.
    EnRhythm p.
    Entity p.
    escape p.
    p. escape interval
    external p.
    p. failure
    fixed-rate p.
    fully automatic p.
    Guardian p.
    Guidant CRM p.
    Hancock bipolar balloon p.
    p. hysteresis
    Identity DR model 5370 p.
    Identity SR model 5172 p.
    Identity XL DR model 5376 p.
    p. impedance
    InSync III atriobiventricular p.
    Integrity AFx DR model 5346 p.
    Intermedics atrial antitachycardia p.
    Intermedics Marathon dual-chamber
      rate-responsive p.
    Intermedics Marathon VVI single-
      chamber p.
    Intermedics Stride p.
    p. interrogation
    Intertach II p.
    Kairos p.

Kantrowitz p.
Kappa 400 Series p.
p. lead
p. lead fracture
lithium-powered p.
Maestro implantable cardiac p.
p. malfunction
Mark IV respiratory p.
Medtronic Activitrax rate-responsive
  unipolar ventricular p.
Medtronic Adapta p.
Medtronic bipolar p.
Medtronic Elite DDDR p.
Medtronic Elite II p.
Medtronic EnPulse DR p.
Medtronic Kappa 400 p.
Medtronic temporary p.
Medtronic Thera DR p.
Medtronic Thera i-series cardiac p.
Meridian p.
Meta DDDR p.
Meta MV p.
Meta rate-responsive p.
Micro Minix p.
Microny II K pediatric p. (models
  3500 & 3510)
Microny II SR+ p.
Microny K SR p.
Microny SR+ cardiac p.
migrating p.
Momentum DR p.
Monolithic fetal p.
Multicor II cardiac p.
Nanos 01 p.
noninvasive temporary p.
Nova II p.
nuclear p.
Omni-Stanicor p.
Optima p.
Opus RM single chamber p.
p. output
p. output reprogramming
p. output voltage
oversensing p.
Pacesetter Regency SC+ p.
Pacesetter Trilogy DR p.
Paragon II p.
permanent p. (PPM)
pervenous p.
phantom p.
Philos DR-T p.
physiologic p.
piezoelectric crystal-based p.
Pinnacle p.
p. pocket
p. potential
primary p.
Programalith A-V p.
Programalith II, III p.

programmable p.
programmer p.
Pulsar DDD p.
Pulsar NI implantable p.
P-wave triggered ventricular p.
QT interval sensing p.
Quantum p.
rate-adaptive p.
rate-modulated p.
reedswitch of p.
p. reedswitch
Reflex 8220 p.
reflex p.
refractory period of electronic p.
runaway p.
p. sensitivity
Sensor p.
Sequicor III p.
shifting p.
Siemens p.
Siemens-Elema p.
single-chamber, rate-responsive p.
smart p.
Sorin p.
p. sound
p. spike
standby p.
p. stimulus artifact
subsidiary atrial p.
Symbios 7006 p.
Synchrocor p.
p. syndrome (PS)
Synergyst DDD p.
Synergyst II p.
Telectronics p.
p. telemetry
temperature-sensing p.
temporary p. (TPM)
p. threshold
tined lead p.
transcutaneous p. (TCP)
transmural antitachycardia p.
transthoracic p.
transvenous p. (TVP)
Ultra p.
p. undersensing
unipolar atrial p.
unipolar sequential p.
universal p.
VAT p.
VDD p.
Ventak AICD p.
Ventak PRx p.
Ventricor p.
ventricular asynchronous p.
ventricular demand-inhibited p.
ventricular demand-triggered p.
Versatrax II 7000A p.
Vigor DR p.

P

pacemaker *(continued)*
    Vista 4, T, TRS p.
    Vitatron Diamond II p.
    VOO p.
    VVD p.
    VVI p.
    VVIR p.
    VVT p.
    wandering p.
    wandering atrial p. (WAP)
    p. wire (PMW)
    Zoll NTP 1000 noninvasive p.
pacemaker-mediated tachycardia (PMT)
pacemapping
Paceport catheter
pacer-cardioverter-defibrillator (PCD)
    Jewel p.-c.-d.
Pacerone tablet
Pacesetter
    P. APS II 3004 programmer
    P. APS pacemaker programmer
    P. Regency SC+ pacemaker
    P. Tendril DX steroid-eluting active-fixation pacing lead
    P. Trilogy DR pacemaker
Pacesetter/St. Jude lead
pace-terminable
pace-terminate
Pacette
    MRL P.
Pachon
    P. method
    P. test
pachyderma
    interarytenoid p.
pachypleuritis
PACI
    partial anterior circulation infarct
pacing
    AAI p.
    AAI-RR p.
    AAT p.
    acceleration-guided activity p.
    activity-guided p.
    antitachycardia p. (ATP)
    AOO p.
    asynchronous p.
    atrial p. (AP)
    atrial-based p.
    atrial incremental p.
    atrial overdrive p.
    atrial septum septal p.
    atrial train p.
    atrioventricular sequential p.
    atrioventricular synchronous p.
    autodecremental p.
    A-V sequential p.
    biatrial p.
    biventricular p.

burst atrial p.
burst of rapid atrial p. (BRAP)
burst of ventricular p. (BVP)
cardiac p. (CP)
p. in cardiomyopathy (PIC)
cardioventricular p. (CVP)
p. catheter
closed-loop p.
p. code
p. counter
coupled atrial p. (CAP)
p. cycle length (PCL)
DDD p.
DDDR p.
DDI p.
DDIR p.
decremental atrial p.
demand p.
p. device
diaphragmatic p.
direct His bundle p. (DHBP)
dual-chamber p.
dual-site right atrial p.
p. duration
DVI p.
endocardial p.
epicardial p.
external high-output ramp p.
high-frequency burst p.
p. hysteresis
implantable cardioverter-defibrillator/atrial tachycardia p. (ICD-ATP)
p. impulse (PI)
incremental atrial p.
incremental ventricular p.
inhibited p.
intracardiac p.
p. lead
p. lead impedance
p. modality
p. mode
multisite biventricular p.
no atrial p.
noninvasive transcutaneous cardiac p. (NTCP)
overdrive atrial p.
pacemaker burst p.
permanent p.
P synchronous p.
RAMP p.
rapid p.
rapid atrial p. (RAP)
rapid-burst p.
rate modulated p. (RAMP)
rate-responsive ventricular p.
right atrial p.
right ventricular outflow tract p.
right ventricular septal p.

RVOT p.
sequential p.
shock p.
p. spike
p. stimulus
subthreshold p.
suprathreshold p.
SVA p.
p. system analyzer
temporary p.
p. threshold
threshold p.
trains of ventricular p.
transatrial p.
transcutaneous p. (TCP)
transesophageal p. (TEP)
transesophageal atrial p. (TAP, TEAP)
transesophageal echocardiography with p. (TEEP)
triggered p.
underdrive p.
univentricular p.
VAT p.
VDD p.
VDI p.
ventricular p. (VP)
ventricular-based p.
ventricular safety p.
VOO p.
VVD p.
VVI p.
VVIR p.
VVI-RR p.
VVI/VVIR p.
VVT p.

pacing-induced
p.-i. angina
p.-i. heart failure
p.-i. tachycardia (PIT)

Pacis
pack
AeroGear fanny p.
interferon alfa-2b and ribavirin combination p.

packer
body p.

pack-year smoking history
paclitaxel
paclitaxel-coated coronary stent
paclitaxel-eluting stent (PES)
PaCO$_2$
arterial carbon dioxide tension
arterial partial pressure of CO_2

PACP
pulmonary artery counterpulsation

PACS
partial anterior circulation syndrome

postoperative atrial fibrillation in cardiac surgery

PACT
Philadelphia Association of Clinical Trials
Prescription Analyses and Cost

PACU
postanesthesia care unit

PACWP
pulmonary arterial capillary wedge pressure

PAD
peripheral arterial disease
phenacetin, aspirin, desoxyephedrine
pressure applied dressing
public access to defibrillation
public access defibrillation
public access defibrillator
pulmonary artery diastolic
pulsatile assist device
Clo-Sur P.A.D.

P.A.D.
peripheral arterial disease
phenacetin, aspirin, desoxyephedrine
pressure applied dressing
public access to defibrillation
public access defibrillation
public access defibrillator
pulmonary artery diastolic
pulsatile assist device

pad
Chito-Seal topical hemostasis p.
digitizing p.
electrode p.
Heartstream FR2 AED with attenuated defibrillation p.
Littman defibrillation p.
Neptune P.
pericardial fat p.
pharyngoesophageal p.'s
p. sign
Signa P.
SomaSensor p.

PADCAB
perfusion-assisted direct coronary artery bypass

paddle
anteroposterior p.
cardioversion p.
defibrillation p.
defibrillator p.
electrode p.

PADP
pulmonary artery diastolic pressure

PAE
postantibiotic effect

Paecilomyces variotii
PAEDP
pulmonary artery end-diastolic pressure

P

PAF
  paroxysmal atrial fibrillation
  platelet activating factor
  pulmonary arteriovenous fistula
PAFD
  pulmonary artery filling defect
PAFIB
  paroxysmal atrial fibrillation
PAG
  pulmonary angiography
PAGE
  perfluorocarbon-associated gas exchange
Page episodic hypertension
Paget disease of bone
Paget-von
    P.-v. Schrötter syndrome
    P.-v. Schrötter venous thrombosis
PAGOD
  pulmonary hypoplasia, hypoplasia of
    pulmonary artery, agonadism,
    omphalocele/diaphragmatic defect,
    dextrocardia
    PAGOD syndrome
PAH
  polycyclic aromatic hydrocarbon
  pulmonary alveolar hypoventilation
  pulmonary artery hypertension
  pulmonary artery hypotension
PAHVC
  pulmonary alveolar hypoxic
    vasoconstrictor
PAI
  perforating artery infarct
  plasminogen activator inhibitor
PAI-1
  plasminogen activator inhibitor-1
pain
    anginal p.
    atypical chest p.
    burning p.
    calf p.
    chest p. (CP)
    crushing chest p.
    dream p.
    dull p.
    functional p.
    low-risk chest p. (LRCP)
    musculoskeletal p.
    p., pallor, pulselessness, paresthesia,
      paralysis, prostration (PPPPPP)
    phantom p.
    pleuritic chest p.
    psychogenic p.
    pulmonary p.
    respirophasic p.
    rest p.
    staccato p.
    vasoocclusive p. (VOP)
    waxing and waning chest p.

paired
    p. beats
    p. electrical stimulation
    p. stimulus
PAK
  percutaneous access kit
pal
    Vital-Port Infusion P.
palatal surgery
palate
    high arched p.
palatina
    tonsilla p.
palatine tonsil
palatini
    tensor p.
palatopharyngeal sphincter
palatoplasty
    laser-assisted p. (LAP)
palatovaginal canal
**Palco Laboratories Model 300, 400
  pulse oximeter**
pale
    p. hypertension
    p. thrombus
paleopneumoniae
    Peptostreptococcus p.
palestinensis
    Acanthamoeba p.
palisading histiocyte
palivizumab
palliation
    Fontan p.
palliative
    p. prognostic index
    p. surgery
pallida
    asphyxia p.
pallidum
    microhemagglutination *Treponema* p.
    Treponema p.
pallor
    elevation p.
palm
    liver p.
    tripe p.
Palma operation
palmar
    p. arch
    carpal arch p.
    p. click
    p. erythema
    p. xanthoma
palmare
    xanthoma striatum p.
Palmaz
    P. balloon-expandable stent for
      renal arteries

P. Genesis stent
P. vascular stent
Palmaz-Schatz (PS)
    P.-S. balloon-expandable stent
    P.-S. coronary stent
    P.-S. Crown stent
    P.-S. PS-204 stent
    P.-S. stent (PSS)
palmi (*pl. of* palmus)
palmic
palmitate
    clofazimine p.
    colfosceril p.
palmitic acid
palmitoylcarnitine
palmodic
palmoscopy
palmus, pl. **palmi**
palpable A wave
palpation
    bimanual precordial p.
palpitatio cordis
palpitation
    fleeting p.'s
    heart p.'s
    paroxysmal p.
    premonitory p.
PALS
    pediatric life support
palsy
    cerebral p. (CP)
    pseudobulbar p.
    suprabulbar p.
Palv
    alveolar pressure
PAM
    pulmonary alveolar microlithiasis
    pulse amplitude modulation
2-PAM
    2-pralidoxime
PAM2, PAM3 monitor
Pamelor
p-**aminosalicylic acid**
pamoate
    pyrantel p.
PAMP
    pulmonary artery mean pressure
Panacet
panacinar emphysema
panbronchiolitis
    diffuse p. (DPB)
pANCA
    perinuclear antineutrophil cytoplasmic
    antibody
pancarditis
panchamber enlargement
Pancoast
    P. syndrome
    P. tumor

panconduction defect
pancreas
    fibrocystic disease of p.
    Starling curve of p.
pancreatic
    p. acinar cell
    p. dornase
    p. enzyme
    p. extract
    p. polypeptide (PP)
pancreaticopleural fistula
pancreatin asthma
pancreatitis
pancreatopleural fistula
pancuronium bromide
pandemic influenza A
pandiastolic
Pandoraea
    P. apista
    P. norimbergensis
    P. pnomenusa
    P. pulmonicola
    P. sputorum
panel
    cardiac laboratory p. (CLP)
    lipid p.
    RAST p.
    p. of reactive antibodies (PRA)
    thyroid p.
    Triage Cardio ProfilER p.
panel-reactive antibody (PRA)
pang
    breast p.
Panhematin
panhyperemia
panhypogammaglobulinemia
panic disorder
Panje voice button
panlobular emphysema
panniculitis
panniculus
panning
panophthalmitis
pansystolic
    p. flow
    p. murmur
pantaloon
    p. embolism
    p. patch
Panther balloon
panting maneuver
Panton-Valentine
    P.-V. leucocidin (PVL)
    P.-V. leucocidin gene
pantoprazole sodium
pantothenate synthetase
pantyhose
    Glattelast compression p.
panvascular thrombosis

P

panzerherz
PAO
  peripheral arterial occlusion
  pulmonary artery occlusion
PAO$_2$
  alveolar oxygen partial pressure
PAo
  ascending aortic pressure
  pulmonary artery occlusion pressure
PaO$_2$
  arterial oxygen partial pressure
  arterial oxygen tension
PAOD
  peripheral arterial occlusive disease
  peripheral arteriosclerotic occlusive
    disease
PAOP
  pulmonary artery occlusion pressure
PAP
  positive airway pressure
  pulmonary artery pressure
  pulmonary artery pseudoaneurysm
papain
Papanicolaou solution
papaverine
    p. hydrochloride
    intrathecal p.
    preservative-free intrathecal p.
paper
    asthma p.
    niter p.
papilla, pl. **papillae**
    Bergmeister p.
papillary
    p. adenocarcinoma
    p. carcinoma
    p. fibroelastoma (PFE)
    p. frond
    p. muscle (PM)
    p. muscle abscess
    p. muscle of conus arteriosus
    p. muscle dysfunction
    p. muscle rupture (PMR)
    p. muscle sling
    p. muscle syndrome
    p. muscle tip
    p. muscle traction
    p. tumor
papilledema
papillitis
papillomatosis
    recurrent respiratory p.
papillomavirus
    human p. (HPV)
papillotome
    Wilson-Cook p.
PAPm
    mean pulmonary artery pressure
Pappenheim stain

paprika splitter's lung
papule
    Gottron p.
papulonecrotic tuberculosis
papulosis
    atrophic p.
pa-pv
    pulmonary arterial pressure, pulmonary
    venous pressure
PAPVC
    partial anomalous pulmonary venous
    connection
PAPVD
    partial anomalous pulmonary venous
    drainage
PAPVR
    partial anomalous pulmonary venous
    return
Paq
    SPY P.
PAR
    posterior wall of aortic root
    primary angioplasty research
    pulmonary arteriolar resistance
    pulse amplitude ratio
paraaminobenzoic acid
paraaminosalicylate sodium
paraaminosalicylic acid (PAS, PASA)
paraaortic bodies
paraboloid
    oscillating p.
paracentesis
    pericardial p.
    thoracic p.
    p. thoracis
paracetamol sensitivity
parachute
    p. deformity
    p. mitral valve
paracicatricial emphysema
Paracoccidioides brasiliensis
paracoccidioidin skin test
paracoccidioidomycosis
paracorporeal heart
paracrine
    p. factor
    p. signaling
paradigm
paradox
    calcium p.
    early systolic p. (ESP)
    French p.
    p. image
    oxygen p.
    thoracoabdominal p.
paradoxic
    p. embolism
    p. pulse
    p. rocking impulse

p. split of S$_2$
p. wall motion
paradoxical
  p. aberrancy
  p. bronchospasm
  p. cerebral embolism
  p. embolization
  p. embolus
  p. hypotension
  p. inspiratory closure
  p. inspiratory closure of vocal
    cords
  p. pulse (PP)
  p. reaction
  p. respiration
  p. split
  p. systolic expansion (PSE)
  p. vasoconstriction
  p. vocal cord adduction
  p. worsening
  p. worsening of tuberculosis
paradoxically split S$_2$ sound
paradoxus
  pulsus p. (PP)
paraesophageal hernia
paraffin block
paraffinoma
PARAFlow circulatory support system
paraganglioma tumor
paragon
  P. coronary stent
  P. II pacemaker
  P. nitinol stent
  P. PAS stent
paragonimiasis
Paragonimus westermani
parahaemolyticus
  Haemophilus p.
  Vibrio p.
parahilar
  p. fibrosis
  p. region
parahisian accessory pathway
parainfluenza
  p. virus (PIV)
  p. virus type 1 (PIV-1)
  p. virus type 2 (PIV-2)
  p. virus type 3 (PIV-3)
  p. virus type 4 (PIV-4)
parainfluenzae
  Haemophilus p. (HPI)
parallel shunt
paralysis, pl. **paralyses**
  depth of p.
  diaphragmatic p.
  diphtheric p.
  diphtheritic p.
  hemidiaphragm p.
  hypokalemic periodic p.

ischemic p.
periodic p.
phrenic nerve p.
respiratory p.
sleep p.
tick p.
vasomotor p.
Volkmann ischemic p.
paralytica
  dysphagia p.
paralytic chest
paralyticus
  laryngismus p.
  thorax p.
paramagnetic
  p. nanoparticle
  p. substance
paramedic
parameter
  flow p.
  hemodynamic p.
  ICD p.'s
  inotropic p.
  late potential p.
  portable monitor of respiratory p.'s
    (PMRP)
  respiratory p.
  systemic hemodynamic p.'s
  velocity p.
  ventricular inotropic p. (VIP)
parameterized diastolic filling (PDF)
paramethasone acetate
parametric
  p. image
  p. imaging
Paramyxoviridae virus
Paramyxovirus
paraneoplastic
  p. pemphigus
  p. syndrome
paraoxonase polymorphism
paraPAC ventilator
parapharyngeum
  spatium p.
paraplane echocardiography
Paraplatin
parapneumonic
  p. effusion
  p. space
paraprosthetic leak
paraproteinemia
parapsilosis
  Candida p.
paraquat
pararrhythmia
parasagittal plane
paraseptal
  p. emphysema
  p. pathway

P

parasitic
- p. cardiomyopathy
- p. infestation

paraspinal line

parasternal
- p. examination
- p. heave
- p. long axis
- p. long-axis view
- p. long-axis view echocardiogram
- p. short axis
- p. short-axis view
- p. short-axis view echocardiogram
- p. systolic lift
- p. systolic thrill
- p. window

parasympathetic
- p. function
- p. innervation
- p. nerve fibers
- p. nervous system

parasympathomimetic

parasynapsis

parasyndesis

parasystole
- atrial p.
- junctional p.
- pure p.
- ventricular p.

parasystolic
- p. beat
- p. ventricular tachycardia

parathyroid
- p. adenoma
- p. hormone (PTH)

paratracheal
- p. chain
- p. lymph node
- p. region

paratracheales
- nodi lymphoidei p.

Paratrend
- P. 7 continuous blood gas monitor
- P. 7+ multiparameter blood gas monitor

paravalvular regurgitation

paraventricular nucleus (PVN)

ParCA
- Parodi catheter for angiography
- ParCA catheter

parchemin
- bruit de p.

parchment
- p. heart
- p. right ventricle

parecoxib

parenchyma
- pulmonary p.

parenchymal
- p. amyloidosis
- p. asbestosis
- p. aspergillosis
- p. disease
- p. fibrosis
- p. hematoma (PH)
- p. hemorrhage (PH)
- p. laceration
- p. lesion
- p. sarcoidosis

parenchymatous
- p. myocarditis
- p. pneumonia

parenteral
- Coly-Mycin M P.
- P. nutrition
- P. vasodilator

parent radionuclide

paresis

pargyline
- methyclothiazide and p.

Pari
- P. LC Plus reusable nebulizer
- P. LC Star reusable nebulizer
- P. Proneb Ultra nebulizer

paries membranaceus tracheae

parietal
- p. ball
- p. band
- p. endocarditis
- p. pericardiectomy
- p. pericardium (PP)
- p. pleura
- p. pleural damage
- p. pulse (PP)
- p. thrombus

parietalis
- pleura p.

parietooccipital artery

park
- P. aneurysm
- P. blade septostomy

Parks 800 bidirectional Doppler flowmeter

Parlodel

Parodi
- P. Anti-Embolism System
- P. balloon catheter
- P. catheter for angiography (ParCA)

paromomycin sulfate

paroxetine

paroxysmal
- p. atrial fibrillation (PAF, PAFIB)
- p. atrial tachycardia (PAT)
- p. atrial tachycardia with aberrancy
- p. atrioventricular nodal reciprocal tachycardia (PAVNRT)

p. burst
p. cough
p. dyspnea on exertion (PDE)
p. hypertension
p. junctional tachycardia (PJT)
p. nocturnal dyspnea (PND)
p. nocturnal hemoglobinuria (PNH)
p. nodal tachycardia
p. palpitation
p. pulmonary edema
p. reentrant supraventricular
  tachycardia
p. sinus tachycardia
p. sleep
p. supraventricular arrhythmia
p. supraventricular tachycardia
  (PST, PSVT)
p. tachycardia (PT)
p. ventricular tachycardia (PVT)
paroxysm of coughing
parrot
p. fever
P. murmur
pars
p. abdominalis esophagi
p. basalis arteriae pulmonalis
p. cervicalis esophagi
p. costalis diaphragmatis
p. intralobaris intersegmentalis
  venae posterioris lobi superioris
  pulmonis dextri
p. lumbalis diaphragmatis
p. mediastinalis pulmonis
p. membranacea
p. nasalis pharyngis
p. oralis pharyngis
p. pharyngea hypophyseos
p. thoracica esophagi
part
abdominal p.
central apical p. (CAP)
certified distinct p. (CDP)
cervical p.
intersegmental p.
mediastinal p.
nasal p.
oral p.
p. per million (ppm)
thoracic p.
vertebral p.
partes intersegmentales
partial
p. anomalous pulmonary veins
p. anomalous pulmonary venous
  connection (PAPVC)
anomalous pulmonary venous
  connections, total or p.
p. anomalous pulmonary venous
  drainage (PAPVD)

p. anomalous pulmonary venous
  return (PAPVR)
p. anterior circulation infarct
  (PACI)
p. anterior circulation syndrome
  (PACS)
p. artificial heart
p. atrioventricular canal
p. autobullectomy
p. A-V canal defect
p. chordal-sparing mitral valve
  replacement
p. clamping
p. confluens sinuum thrombosis
p. CVID
p. encircling endocardial
  ventriculotomy
p. heart block
p. ileal bypass (PIB)
p. intermixed fibrosis
p. liquid ventilation (PLV)
p. occlusion clamp
p. occlusion inferior vena cava
  clip
p. pressure (P, PP)
p. pressure of arterial fluid (PA)
p. pressure of carbon dioxide
  (pCO_2)
p. pressure of carbon monoxide
  (PCO)
p. pressure of end-tidal CO_2
  ($PETCO_2$)
p. pressure of inspiratory oxygen
  (P_{IO_2})
p. pressure of oxygen (pO_2)
p. rebreathing mask
p. thromboplastin time (PTT)
p. volume effect
partially coagulated effusion
particle
Amberlite p.'s
Dane p.
embolization p.
lipoprotein p.
PVA foam embolization p.
remnant-like lipoprotein p. (RLP)
particulate
p. matter less than 10 micrometers
  in diameter (PM10)
p. respirator
partition
atrial p.
partitioning
left atrial p.
Parvolex
parvovirus human bocavirus (HBoV)
parvula
Veillonella p.

535

parvus
    pulsus p.
PAS
   paraaminosalicylic acid
   peripheral access system
   persistent atrial standstill
   posterior airway space
   premature atrial stimulus
   pulmonary arterial stenosis
   pulmonary artery systolic
PASA
   paraaminosalicylic acid
pascal (Pa)
    P. principle
PASE
   Physical Activity Scale for the Elderly
   Evaluation
PASG
   pneumatic antishock garment
PASP
   pulmonary artery systolic pressure
passage
    adiabatic fast p.
    P. hemostasis valve
Passager stent-graft
passivation
    pharmacologic plaque p.
    plaque p.
passive
    p. clot
    p. congestion
    p. edema
    p. girdle effect
    p. hyperemia
    p. interval
    p. mode
    p. postnatal smoking
    p. prenatal smoking
    p. tilting
    p. vascular exercise (pavex)
passover humidifier
Passy-Muir
    P.-M. O2 Adapter
    P.-M. tracheostomy speaking valve
paste
    electrode p.
    nitroglycerin p.
Pasteurella
    P. aerogenes
    P. multocida
pasteurellosis
PASVR
   pulmonary anomalous superior venous
   return
PAT
   paroxysmal atrial tachycardia
   peripheral arterial tone
    PAT signal
patch, pl. **patches**

Acuseal cardiovascular p.
Adcon-C resorbable liquid p.
p. angioplasty
atrial septal defect p.
autologous blood p.
autologous pericardial p.
BioGlue surgical p.
buspirone transdermal p.
cardiac p.
CardioFix pericardium p.
chest wall p.
p. closure
CorRestore implantable p.
Dacron intracardiac p.
defibrillation p.
electrodispersive skin p.
epicardial defibrillator p.
extrapericardial p.
Fluoropassiv thin-wall carotid p.
Gore-Tex Acuseal cardiovascular p.
Gore-Tex soft tissue p.
p. graft reconstruction
Habitrol P.
Ionescu-Shiley pericardial p.
MacCallum p.
Minitran P.
NicoDerm P.
nicotine transdermal p.
Nicotrol P.
Nitro-Dur P.
No-React pericardial p.
outflow cardiac p.
pantaloon p.
pericardial p.
Peyer p.
polypropylene intracardiac p.
p. repair
retropectoral p.
sandwich p.
Silastic p.
SJM pericardial p.
soldier's patches
subcutaneous p.
SyvekPatch topical hemostasis p.
2-p. technique
Teflon felt p.
Teflon intracardiac p.
transanular p.
transcatheter p.
Transderm-Nitro P.
patch-coil system
patch-graft
    p.-g. angioplasty
    Dacron onlay p.-g.
patchplasty
patchwork fibrosis
patchy
    p. atelectasis
    p. consolidation

p. hyperintensity
p. infiltrate
p. infiltration

PATE
pulmonary artery thromboembolism

patency
artery p.
catheter p.
coronary bypass graft p.
epicardial artery p.
epicardial vessel p.
graft p.
heparin and early p.
infarct artery p.
probe p.
p. rate
stent p.
TIMI p.
vein graft p.
venous coronary graft p.

patent
p. bronchus sign
p. ductus (PD)
p. ductus arteriosus (PDA)
p. ductus arteriosus flow jet
p. ductus arteriosus murmur
p. ductus arteriosus umbrella
p. foramen ovale (PFO)

Pathfinder
P. mapping microcatheter
P. mini mapping microcatheter

pathogen
nosocomial p.

pathogenesis
pathogenicity
pathognomonic
pathologic
p. complete response
p. criteria
p. murmur
p. postsystolic shortening
p. QT (QTU)
p. Q wave
p. trigger

pathological cascade
pathology, pl. **pathologies**
coexistent p.
multivalve p.

pathomechanism
pathophysiology
pathostimulation
pathway
accessory p. (AP)
angiotensin II-independent p.
antegrade internodal p.
anterior internodal p.
apoptotic p.
atrio-His p.
atrioventricular p. (AP)

atrioventricular node p.
Bachmann p.
concealed accessory p.
conduction p.
diacylglycerate p.
electrical p.
Fas-Fas ligand p.
FasL p.
fast p.
final common p.
Fontan p.
free-wall accessory p.
integrin-dependent p.
internodal p.
Jak/STAT p.
Kent p.
lipoxygenase p.
MAPK p.
mitochondrial apoptotic p.
mitogen-activated kinase p.
parahisian accessory p.
paraseptal p.
reentrant p.
retinohypothalamic p.
retrograde fast p.
scavenger cell p.
selective past p.
septal p.
shunt p.
slow A-V node p.
slow and fast A-V nodal p.
stress signaling p.
surgical ablation of p.
Thorel p.

patient
ABCDE in trauma p.
p. activator mode
p. compliance
intubated p.
p. monitor
multiple-trauma p.
nonintubated p.
nonventilated p.
postinfarct p.
Postural Assessment Scale for
Stroke P.
trauma p.

patient-controlled
p.-c. analgesia (PCA)
p.-c. analgesic (PCA)

patient-driven protocol
**Patient-Oriented Evidence that Matters
(POEM)**
patient-triggered
p.-t. recording
p.-t. ventilation

Patil stereotactic system
Patriot moderate support guidewire

P

pattern
  abdominal paradox breathing p.
  airspace-filling p.
  airway p.
  alveolar p.
  alveolar-filling p.
  ballerina-foot p.
  bat wing p.
  butterfly p.
  candle flame p.
  cephalization of pulmonary flow p.
  circadian blood pressure p.
  concave p.
  contraction p.
  crazy paving p.
  crochetage EKG p.
  cyclic alternating p. (CAP)
  deer-antler vascular p.
  diastolic filling p.
  dip-and-plateau p.
  dipper p.
  disturbed circadian blood
    pressure p.
  eggshell p.
  electrocardiographic strain p.
  embryonic phenotype p.
  fishnet p.
  F-wave p.
  ground-glass p.
  honeycomb p.
  hourglass p.
  impaired relaxation mitral flow p.
  injury p.
  interstitial p.
  intraventricular conduction p.
  juvenile p.
  Kussmaul respiration p.
  maximum contraction p. (MCP)
  miliary p.
  military p.
  mixed obstructive and restrictive p.
  mosaic p.
  myocardial velocity p.
  obstructive p.
  organoid p.
  physiological p.
  pseudoinfarction p.
  pulmonary venous drainage p.
  pulmonray flow p.
  QR, QS p.
  respiratory alternans breathing p.
  restrictive filling p.
  restrictive physiology mitral
    flow p.
  reticular p.
  reticulonodular p.
  salt and pepper p.
  sawtooth p.
  scintillating speckle p.
  scooped p.
  sine wave p.
  sinusoidal strut p.
  S_1Q_3 p.
  $S_1Q_3T_3$ p.
  torpedo-shaped p.
  upstroke p.
  uptake-mismatch p.
  vascular p.
  ventricular contraction p.
  VPW p.
  W p.
  watershed p.

patty
  cottonoid p.

PAU
  penetrating aortic ulcer
  penetrating atherosclerotic ulcer

pauciimmune glomerulonephritis

pause
  apneic p.
  compensatory p.
  full compensatory p.
  noncompensatory p.
  postectopic p.
  postextrasystolic p.
  preautomatic p.
  sinus exit p.
  ventricular p.

pause-dependent arrhythmia

PAV
  percutaneous aortic valvoplasty
  proportional assist ventilation

Pavcnik Monodisk device

pavementing

Paveral Stanley Syrup With Codeine
  Phosphate

pavex
  passive vascular exercise

PAVF
  pulmonary arteriovenous fistula

Pavlov reflex

PAVM
  pulmonary arteriovenous malformation

PAVNRT
  paroxysmal atrioventricular nodal
    reciprocal tachycardia

pAVP
  plasma arginine vasopressin

PAVSD
  pulmonary atresia with ventricular septal
    defect

PAW
  pulmonary artery wedge

Paw
  mean airway pressure

PAWP
  pulmonary artery wedge pressure

Paykel scale

PB
>premature beat

PBC
>perfusion balloon catheter

PBF
>peripheral blood flow
>pulmonary blood flow

PBMC
>percutaneous balloon mitral
>commissurotomy
>peripheral blood mononuclear cell

PBMV
>pulmonary blood mixing volume

PBP
>percutaneous balloon pericardiotomy

PBPV
>percutaneous balloon pulmonary
>valvoplasty

PBS
>phosphate-buffered saline
>pulmonary branch stenosis

PBV
>percutaneous balloon valvoplasty
>pulmonary balloon valvoplasty
>pulmonary blood volume

PBZ
>pyribenzamine

PC
>phosphorylcholine
>plasma cell
>portacaval
>posterior circulation
>posterior circumflex artery
>precordial
>pressure control
>pulmonary circulation
>pulmonary compliance
>pulmonic closure

PCA
>patient-controlled analgesia
>patient-controlled analgesic
>portacaval anastomosis
>posterior cerebral artery
>precoronary care area
>prehospital cardiac arrest
>>fetal-type PCA
>>PCA system

PCAD
>progression of coronary artery disease

PCB
>portacaval bypass
>protected catheter brushing

PCBS
>percutaneous cardiopulmonary bypass
>support

PCC
>precoronary care

PC-coated stent

PCCU
>postcoronary care unit

PCD
>pacer-cardioverter-defibrillator
>primary ciliary dyskinesia
>programmable cardioverter-defibrillator
>>PCD ICD generator
>>Jewel PCD
>>PCD Transvene implantable
>>cardioverter-defibrillator system

PCDC
>plasma clot diffusion chamber

PCE Oral

PCF
>peak cough flow

PCG
>phonocardiogram
>pneumocardiogram

PCI
>percutaneous coronary intervention
>prophylactic cranial irradiation

PCIRV
>pressure-controlled inverse ratio
>ventilation

PCIS
>postcardiac injury syndrome

PCL
>pacing cycle length

PC-MRA
>phase-contrast magnetic resonance
>angiography

PCMT
>pacemaker circus movement tachycardia

PCNA
>proliferating cell nuclear antigen

PCO
>partial pressure of carbon monoxide
>predicted cardiac output

pCO$_2$
>partial pressure of carbon dioxide
>>pCO$_2$ oximetry

PcomA
>posterior communicating artery

P-congenitale

PCP
>peripheral coronary pressure
>*Pneumocystis carinii* pneumonia
>postoperative constrictive pericarditis
>pulmonary capillary pressure

PCPB
>percutaneous cardiopulmonary bypass

PCPS
>percutaneous cardiopulmonary support

PCR
>polymerase chain reaction
>>PCR assay
>>PCR test

PCr
>phosphocreatine

PCRA
percutaneous coronary rotational atherectomy
PCS
portacaval shunt
postcardiotomy syndrome
proximal coronary sinus
PCT
percutaneous tracheostomy
portacaval transposition
balloon-facilitated PCT
PCTI
penetrating cardiac trauma index
PCV
pressure-controlled ventilation
PCW
pulmonary capillary wedge
PCWP
pulmonary capillary wedge pressure
PD
patent ductus
postural drainage
pulsed diastolic
pulse duration
pure dysarthria
PD Access with Peel-Away needle introducer
PD 123319 AT receptor agonist
PD 2000 defibrillator
Duotan PD
P/D
proximal-to-distal
P/D vessel
Pd
diastolic pressure
PDA
patent ductus arteriosus
posterior descending artery
snare-assisted coil occlusion of PDA
PDA umbrella
PD-AB-SAAP
pulsed diastolic autologous blood selective aortic arch perfusion
PDB
preperitoneal dilator balloon
PDB preperitoneal distention balloon system
PDC, PdC
pediatric cardiology
PD-CSE
pulsed Doppler cross-sectional echocardiography
PDE
paroxysmal dyspnea on exertion
phosphodiesterase inhibitor
pulsed Doppler echocardiography
PDE isoenzyme inhibitor

PDE4
phosphodiesterase 4
PDE4 inhibitor
PDE4 isoenzyme inhibition
PDE-I
phosphodiesterase inhibitor
PDE3I
phosphodiesterase 3 inhibition
P-dextrocardiale
PDF
parameterized diastolic filling
probability density function
PDGF
platelet-derived growth factor
PDGF-AB
platelet-derived growth factor-AB
PD-GXT
postdischarge graded-exercise test
PDH
progressive disseminated histoplasmosis
pyruvate dehydrogenase
PDHRF
platelet-derived histamine-releasing factor
PDP
peak diastolic pressure
PD&P
postural drainage and percussion
PDPV
postural drainage, percussion, vibration
PDR
proliferative diabetic retinopathy
PDT
percutaneous dilational tracheostomy
photodynamic therapy
PDUFA
Prescription Drug User Fee Act
PDV
peak diastolic velocity
PE
cisplatin and etoposide
pericardial effusion
preexcitation
pulmonary edema
pulmonary embolism
pulmonary emphysema
PE balloon
PE-60-I-2 implantable pronged unipolar electrode
PE-60-K-10 implantable unipolar endocardial electrode
PE-60-KB implantable unipolar endocardial electrode
PE-85-I-2 implantable pronged unipolar electrode
PE-85-K-10 implantable unipolar endocardial electrode
PE-85-KB implantable unipolar endocardial electrode

PE-85-KS-10 implantable unipolar endocardial electrode
PEA
   pulseless electrical activity
peak
   p. A, E velocity
   p. airway pressure (Ppeak)
   atrial filling p.
   p. cough flow (PCF)
   p. diastolic filling rate
   p. diastolic pressure (PDP)
   p. diastolic velocity (PDV)
   p. ejection rate (PER)
   p. ejection time (PET)
   p. ejection velocity (V_{pe})
   p. emptying rate
   p. exercise
   p. exercise oxygen consumption
      (VO_2max)
   p. exercise ventilation (V_E)
   p. expiratory flow (PEF)
   p. expiratory flow rate (PEFR)
   p. expiratory maneuver
   p. filling rate (PFR)
   p. flow (PF)
   p. flowmeter (PFM)
   p. flow variability
   h p.
   p. heart rate (PHR)
   p. incidence
   p. inspiratory flow (PIF)
   p. inspiratory flow rate (PIFR)
   p. inspiratory pressure (PIP)
   p. instantaneous Doppler gradient
   p. jet flow rate
   p. left ventricular pressure (PLVP)
   p. lengthening rate
   p. magnitude
   p. myocardial video intensity
      (PMVI)
   p. negative pressure (P-min, PNP)
   p. oxygen uptake
   p. positive pressure (P+max)
   p. pulmonary artery pressure
   p. shortening rate
   p. systolic aortic pressure (PSAP)
   p. systolic gradient (PSG)
   p. systolic gradient pressure
   p. systolic pressure (PSP)
   p. systolic velocity (PSV)
   p. of thrombin generation (PTG)
   p. tidal expiratory flow (PTEF)
   p. tidal inspiratory flow (PTIF)
   time to p. (TTP)
   p. transaortic flow velocity
   p. transaortic valve gradient
   p. and trough
   p. and trough levels
   p. twitch force

   p. workload
   p. work rate (Wmax)
peaked P wave
peak-to-peak gradient
PEAP
   positive end-airway pressure
pearl
   keratin p.
   Laënnec p.
   p. sign
   string of p.'s
pear-shaped heart
peau d'orange
PEC
   pulmonary ejection click
pecorum
   Chlamydia p.
pectinate muscle
pectoral
   ectopia cordis p.
   p. emulation
   p. fascia
   p. fremitus
   p. heart
   p. tea
pectoralgia
pectoralis
   fascia p.
   p. major
   p. minor
   regio p.
pectoriloquous bronchophony
pectoriloquy
   aphonic p.
   whispered p.
   whispering p.
pectoris
   angina p. (AP)
   angor p.
   stable angina p. (SAP)
   unstable angina p. (UAP)
   variant angina p. (VAP)
   vasospastic angina p.
pectorophony
pectus
   p. carinatum
   p. deformity
   p. excavatum
   p. gallinatum
   p. recurvatum
pedal
   p. edema
   p. pulse
pedal-mode ergometer
PediaCare Oral
Pediacof
PediaFlow system
Pediapred Oral

pediatric
    Benylin P.
    p. cardiology (PDC, PdC)
    P. Cardiology Devices Sideris
      Buttoned device occluder
    p. cardiomyopathy
    Cleocin P.
    p. finger clip sensor
    p. hypertension
    P. Jarvik 2000 FlowMaker
    p. lead
    P. LifeShirt system
    p. life support (PALS)
    p. pigtail catheter
    Robitussin P.
    p. vascular clamp
Pediazole Oral
pedicle graft
Pedi-Dri
PediPump ventricular assist device
Pedituss
Pedoff continuous wave transducer
pedunculated thrombus
PedvaxHIB
peel
    pericardial p.
    pleural p.
    visceral p.
peel-away
    P.-a. banana catheter
    P.-a. introducer set
    p.-a. sheath
peeling-back mechanism
PEEP
    positive end-expiratory pressure
    PEEP valve
PEEPi
    intrinsic positive end-expiratory pressure
PEEP-related alveolar recruitment
PEF
    peak expiratory flow
    pulmonary edema fluid
%PEF
    percent predicted peak expiratory flow
pefloxacin
PEFR
    peak expiratory flow rate
PEG
    polyethylene glycol
    PEG interleukin-2
    PEG tube
pegademase bovine
pegaspargase
PEG-LES
    polyethylene glycol electrolyte lavage
      solution
pegvisomant
PEJ tube

PEL
    primary effusion lymphoma
Pel
    lung elastic recoil pressure
PELA
    peripheral excimer laser angioplasty
PELCA
    percutaneous excimer laser coronary
      angioplasty
      PELCA Registry
Pelger-Huet cell
pellagra
pellet
    myofibril P.
pellucidum
    pineal p.
    septum p.
Pelorus stereotactic system
Pel-V
    elastic pressure-volume
PEM
    precordial electrocardiographic
      monitoring
pemetrexed
pemphigus
    paraneoplastic p.
PE-MT balloon dilation catheter
pen
    Cardioblate surgical ablation p.
    Cardioblate XL p.
    light p.
Penaz volume-clamp method
penbutolol sulfate
PenChant coronary stent delivery
  system
penciclovir
pencil-beam total body scanner
pencil percussion
pendant
    oxygen-conserving p.
pendelluft
    p. effect
    p. phenomenon
pendulous heart
pendulum
    cor p.
    p. rhythm
    p. test
penetrance
penetrating
    p. aortic ulcer (PAU)
    p. atherosclerotic ulcer (PAU)
    p. cardiac trauma index (PCTI)
    p. chest injury
    p. rupture
    p. thoracic trauma
penetration
penetrator artery

penicillin
    benzathine benzyl p.
    p. G
    p. G benzathine
    p. G benzathine and procaine
      combined
    p. G procaine
    penicillinase-resistant p.
    p. phenoxymethyl
    semisynthetic p.
    p. VK
    p. V potassium
penicillinase-resistant penicillin
Penicillin notatum
penicillin-resistant *Streptococcus*
   pneumoniae **(PRSP)**
penicilliosis
Penicillium marneffei
penicilloyl polylysine (PPL)
penile-brachial pressure index
penis
    cavernous vein of p.
Penn
    P. Convention criteria
    P. formula
    P. method
    P. State TAH
pentachloride
    antimony p.
pentachrome
    Movat p.
pentaerythritol tetranitrate (PETN)
pentagastrin
pentalogy
    Cantrell p.
    Fallot p.
    p. of Fallot
Pentalumen catheter
pentamidine
    p. in aerosol form
    aerosolized p.
    p. isethionate
Pentam-300 injection
pentane
pentasaccharide
Penta stent
Pentatrichomonas hominis
Pentax bronchoscope
pentazocine
pentetate
    imciromab p.
Penthalaris
pentobarbital
Pentothal Sodium
pentoxifylline
pentraxin
pentraxin 3 (PTX3)
penumbra
    ischemic p.

PEP
    positive expiratory pressure
    preejection period
      PEP mask
PEPA
    peptidase A
PEPc
    corrected preejection period
PEPI
    preejection period index
pepper
    P. Medical Antidisconnect Device
      strap
    P. Medical tube neck band
peppermint test
peptic
    p. aspiration pneumonitis
    p. esophagitis
    p. ulcer
peptidase
    p. A (PEPA)
    dipeptidyl p.
peptide
    adrenomedullin p.
    atrial natriuretic p. (ANP)
    atrial natriuretic p. A (ANP-A)
    atrial natriuretic p. B (ANP-B)
    atrial natriuretic p. C (ANP-C)
    brain natriuretic p. (BNP)
    B-type natriuretic p. (BNP)
    calcitonin gene-related p. (CGRP)
    cerebrovascular amyloid p. (CVAP)
    C-terminal p.
    C-type natriuretic p. (CNP)
    Dendroaspis natriuretic p. (DNP)
    human atrial natriuretic p. (hANP)
    immunoreactive atrial natriuretic p.
      (iANP, irANP)
    p. mucolytic
    natriuretic p.
    N-20 terminal p.
    N-terminal pro brain natriuretic p.
      (NT-proBNP)
    proadrenomedullin N-terminal 20 p.
    procollagen type III
      aminoterminal p. (PIIIP)
    protegrin antimicrobial p.
    rat atrial natriuretic p. (rANP)
    TFF-domain p.
    thrombin receptor activating p.
      (TRAP)
    tick anticoagulant p.
    vasoactive intestinal p. (VIP)
    vasoconstrictor p.
    vasoinhibitory p. (VIP)
    vasorelaxant p.
peptidoglycan
peptidomimetic
Peptococcus constellatus

P

Peptostreptococcus
>P. anaerobius
>P. asaccharolyticus
>P. evolutus
>P. paleopneumoniae
>P. prevotii
>P. productus

PER
>peak ejection rate

per
>p. primam healing
>p. primam intentionem
>p. secundum healing
>p. secundum intentionem

peracetic acid
Per-C-Cath
perceived
>p. exertion
>p. noise (PN)

percent
>p. diameter stenosis (%DS)
>p. of maximum predicted heart rate
>p. predicted peak expiratory flow (%PEF)

perceptual-sensory neglect
perchloric acid
Perclose
>P. vascular closure device
>P. vascular surgical closure system

Percor Stat-DL intraarotic balloon catheter
PercuCut biopsy needle
PercuQuick tracheostomy cannula
percussion
>auscultation and p. (A&P)
>p. and auscultation (P&A)
>auscultatory p.
>chest p.
>coin p.
>p. dullness
>fist p.
>Goldscheider p.
>high-frequency p.
>Murphy p.
>p. note (PN)
>pencil p.
>piano p.
>Plesch p.
>p. and postural drainage (P&PD)
>postural drainage and p. (PD&P)
>slapping p.
>p. sound
>strip p.
>tangential p.
>threshold p.
>p. wave

percussor
>G5 Neocussor p.
>Vibracare p.

PercuSurge
>P. Export aspiration catheter
>P. GuardWire
>P. Guardwire Plus distal protection system

percutaneous
>p. access
>p. access kit (PAK)
>p. alcohol septal reduction
>p. aortic balloon valvoplasty (PABV)
>p. aortic valvoplasty (PAV)
>p. approach
>p. balloon angioplasty
>p. balloon aortic valvoplasty
>p. balloon mitral commissurotomy (PBMC)
>p. balloon mitral valvoplasty
>p. balloon pericardiotomy (PBP)
>p. balloon pulmonary valvoplasty (PBPV)
>p. balloon pulmonic valvoplasty
>p. balloon valvoplasty (PBV)
>p. brachial sheath
>p. cannulated screw
>p. cardiopulmonary bypass (PCPB)
>p. cardiopulmonary bypass support (PCBS)
>p. cardiopulmonary support (PCPS)
>p. catheter insertion
>p. catheter introducer kit
>p. coronary intervention (PCI)
>p. coronary intervention myocardial blush
>p. coronary rotational atherectomy (PCRA)
>p. cutting needle
>p. dilational tracheostomy (PDT)
>p. edge-to-edge technique
>p. embolotherapy
>p. endocoronary sinus catheter
>p. endoscopic jejunostomy
>p. excimer laser coronary angioplasty (PELCA)
>p. extrapleural analgesia
>p. femoral
>p. in situ bypass
>p. in situ coronary venous arterialization (PICVA)
>p. intraaortic balloon counterpulsation (PIBC)
>p. intraaortic balloon counterpulsation catheter
>p. intracoronary angioscopy
>p. intrapericardial fibrin-glue infusion therapy

p. isolation
p. isolation of multiple pulmonary veins
p. laser angioplasty
p. left atrial appendage transcatheter occluder (PLAATO)
p. left atrial appendage transcatheter occlusion (PLAATO)
p. left heart bypass (PLHB)
p. mechanical mitral commissurotomy (PMMC)
p. mechanical thrombectomy (PMT)
p. mechanical thrombectomy system
P. Mitral Annuloplasty System
p. mitral anular reduction
p. mitral balloon commissurotomy (PMBC)
p. mitral balloon valvoplasty (PMBV)
p. mitral balloon valvotomy (PMBV)
p. mitral commissurotomy (PMC)
p. mitral valvoplasty (PMV)
p. mitral valvotomy (PMV)
p. myocardial channeling (PMC)
p. myocardial laser revascularization
p. myocardial revascularization (PMR)
p. myocardial revascularization procedure
p. needle aspiration biopsy
p. occlusion of ductus
p. patent ductus arteriosus closure
p. pericardiocentesis
p. radiofrequency catheter
p. radiofrequency catheter ablation
p. rotational thrombectomy (PRT)
p. rotational thrombectomy catheter
p. technique
p. thrombolytic device (PTD)
p. tracheostomy (PCT)
p. tracheotomy
p. transatrial mitral commissurotomy
p. transhepatic cardiac catheterization
p. transluminal
p. transluminal angioplasty (PTA)
p. transluminal angioscopy (PTAS)
p. transluminal balloon angioplasty (PTBA)
p. transluminal balloon dilation (PTBD)
p. transluminal balloon valvoplasty
p. transluminal coronary
p. transluminal coronary angioplasty (PTCA)
p. transluminal coronary recanalization (PTCR)

p. transluminal coronary revascularization (PTCR)
p. transluminal coronary rotational ablation (PTCRA)
p. transluminal dilation (PTD)
p. transluminal myocardial revascularization (PTMR)
p. transluminal renal angioplasty (PTRA)
p. transluminal rotational atherectomy (PTRA)
p. transluminal septal myocardial ablation (PTSMA)
p. transmyocardial laser revascularization (PMR)
p. transmyocardial revascularization (PTMR)
p. transseptal ventricular assist (PTVA)
p. transthoracic needle biopsy (PTNB)
p. transtracheal bronchography
p. transtracheal jet ventilation (PTJV)
p. transtracheal needle ventilation
p. transvenous mitral commissurotomy (PTMC)
p. transverse mitral annuloplasty (PTMA)
p. tunnel
p. ventricular assist device (pVAD)
percutaneously introduced
PercuTwist tracheostomy
PerDUCER percutaneous pericardial access device
peregrinum
  Mycobacterium p.
perennial allergic rhinitis
Pérez sign
Per-fit percutaneous tracheostomy kit
perflenapent injectable emulsion
perflexane lipid microsphere
perflubron
perfluorocarbon (PFC)
perfluorocarbon-associated gas exchange (PAGE)
perfluorocarbon-exposed sonicated dextrose albumin (PESDA)
perfluoropolyether agent
perflutren
  Definity p.
  p. lipid microsphere
perforating
  p. artery
  p. artery infarct (PAI)
perforation
  cardiac p.
  coronary artery p. (CAP)
  esophageal p.

P

perforation *(continued)*
    guidewire p.
    myocardial p.
    septal p.
    ventricular p.
perforator
    gaiter p.
    septal p.
Performa diagnostic catheter
performance
    cardiac p. (CP)
    p. index (PI)
    left ventricular systolic p.
    myocardial p.
    Tei index of myocardial p.
    ventricular p.
Performer cardiopulmonary bypass system
perfringens
    Clostridium p.
PerfTrak
    P. display
    P. perfusion waveform display
perfuse
perfusing rhythm
perfusion
    American Academy of Cardiology P. (AACP)
    antegrade brain p.
    autologous blood selective aortic arch p. (AB-SAAP)
    p. balloon catheter (PBC)
    p. balloon PTCA
    p. bed
    blood p.
    bradykinin p.
    cardiac p.
    p. catheter
    cerebral p.
    cool head-warm body p.
    p. defect
    iced saline p.
    p. imaging MRI
    isolated heat p.
    lung p. (LP, Lp)
    misery p.
    mosaic p.
    myocardial p.
    p. needs
    p. pressure
    pulsed diastolic autologous blood selective aortic arch p. (PD-AB-SAAP)
    regional p.
    relative p.
    remote access p. (RAP)
    retrograde brain p.
    root p.
    p. scan
    p. scintigraphy
    selective p.
    selective aortic arch p. (SAAP)
    splanchnic bed p.
    stuttering of p.
    p. technology
    transcardiac vein p.
    p. via collateral
perfusion-assisted direct coronary artery bypass (PADCAB)
perfusionist
    Australasian Society of Cardiology P.'s (ASCVP)
    Certified Cardiology P. (CCP)
perfusion-weighted
    p.-w. imaging
    p.-w. magnetic resonance imaging (PWI)
periaccretio pericardii
periadventitial eosinophil-predominant infiltrate
periaortic
    p. abscess
    p. hematoma
periapical
periarteriolar fibrosis
periarteritis nodosa
peribronchial
    p. cuffing
    p. desquamation
    p. fibrosis
    p. lymphocytic infiltrate
    p. pneumonia
    p. sheath
peribronchiolar
    p. airspace consolidation
    p. granulomatous inflammation
    p. inflammatory infiltrate
    p. layer
    p. metaplasia
    p. nodule
peribronchiolitis
peribronchitis
peribronchovascular
    p. disease
    p. distortion
    p. hemorrhage
    p. thickening
pericarbon
    p. bioprosthesis
    P. Freedom
    P. More valve
    p. pericardial prosthesis
pericardectomy
pericardia (*pl. of* pericardium)
pericardiaca
    pleura p.
pericardiacophrenica
    arteria p.

pericardiac tumor
pericardial
    p. baffle
    p. basket
    p. biopsy
    p. calcification
    p. constraint
    p. constriction
    p. cyst
    p. disease
    p. echinococcosis
    p. echo
    p. effusion (PE)
    p. fat pad
    p. flap
    p. fluid (PF)
    p. fluid culture (PFC)
    p. fremitus
    p. friction rub
    p. friction sound
    p. knock (PK)
    p. lavage
    p. murmur
    p. neoplasia
    p. paracentesis
    p. patch
    p. peel
    p. poudrage
    p. pressure
    p. reflex
    p. sac
    p. sling
    p. symphysis
    p. synechia
    p. tamponade (PT)
    p. tap
    p. teratoma
    p. valve
    p. well
    p. window
pericardiectomy
    parietal p.
    visceral p.
pericardii (*gen. of* pericardium)
pericardiocentesis, pericardicentesis
    echo-guided p.
    p. needle
    percutaneous p.
pericardiology
pericardiophrenic artery
pericardioplasty
pericardiorrhaphy
pericardioscopy
pericardiosternal ligament
pericardiostomy
pericardiotomy
    balloon p.
    percutaneous balloon p. (PBP)

    p. scissors
    subxiphoid limited p.
pericarditic
pericarditis
    acute fibrinous p.
    acute idiopathic p. (AIP)
    acute lupus p. (ALP)
    adhesive p.
    amebic p.
    p., arthropathy, camptodactyly
      (PAC)
    bacterial p.
    calcific p.
    p. calculosa
    p. callosa
    carcinomatous p.
    cholesterol p.
    chronic constrictive p.
    constrictive p. (CP)
    drug-associated p.
    drug-induced p.
    dry p.
    effusive-constrictive p.
    epistenocardiac p.
    p. epistenocardica
    fibrinous p.
    fibrous p.
    gram-negative p.
    hemorrhagic p.
    histoplasmic p.
    idiopathic p.
    infective p.
    inflammatory p.
    internal adhesive p.
    ischemic p.
    localized p.
    meningococcal p.
    neoplastic p.
    p. obliterans
    obliterating p.
    obliterative p.
    occult p.
    postinfarction p.
    postmyocardial injury p.
    postoperative p.
    postoperative constrictive p. (PCP)
    purulent p. (PP)
    radiation-induced p.
    rheumatic p.
    serofibrinous p.
    serous p.
    p. sicca
    Sternberg p.
    subacute p.
    suppurative p.
    transient p.
    traumatic p.
    tuberculous p.
    uremic p.

P

pericarditis *(continued)*
> p. villosa
> viral p.
> p. with effusion

pericarditis-myocarditis syndrome

pericardium, gen. **pericardii,**
> pl. **pericardia**
>> absent p.
>> adherent p.
>> bread-and-butter p.
>> calcified p.
>> concretio p.
>> congenital absence of left p. (CALP)
>> congenitally absent p.
>> diaphragmatic p.
>> dropsy of p.
>> empyema of p.
>> p. externum
>> p. fibrosum
>> fibrous p.
>> hydrops p.
>> p. internum
>> parietal p. (PP)
>> periaccretio p.
>> p. serosum
>> shaggy p.
>> synechia p.
>> thickened p.
>> ventricular p. (VP)
>> visceral p.

pericardium-coated prosthetic anuloplasty ring

pericardotomy

pericentriolar

periciliary fluid

pericostal suture

pericyte

perielectrode fibrosis

periesophageal

Periflow balloon dilation catheter

Periflux PF 1 D blood-flowmeter

perigraft
> p. flow
> p. thrombosis

perihilar
> p. adenopathy
> p. haze
> p. lymph node
> p. marking

periinfarction
> p. block
> p. conduction defect (PICD)
> p. ischemia
> p. zone

perilymphatic
> p. distribution
> p. nodule

perimembranous ventricular septal defect

perimetric
> p. distribution
> p. distribution of radiofrequency energy

Perimount RSR pericardial bioprosthesis

perimuscular plexus

perimyocarditis

perimyocytic fibrosis

perimyoendocarditis

perindoprilat

perindopril erbumine

perineal artery

perinodal tissue

perinuclear
> p. antineutrophil cytoplasmic antibody (pANCA)
> p. cisterna

period
> absolute refractory p. (ARP)
> accessory pathway effective refractory p. (APERP)
> p. of accommodation
> alveolar p.
> antegrade refractory p.
> atrial effective refractory p. (AERP)
> atrial refractory p.
> atrioventricular node functional refractory p. (AVNFRP)
> atrioventricular refractory p. (AVRP)
> blanking p.
> canalicular p.
> corrected preejection p. (PEPc)
> diastolic filling p. (DFP)
> effective conduction p. (ECP)
> effective refractory p. (ERP)
> ejection p.
> functional conduction p. (FCP)
> functional refractory p. (FRP)
> heartbeat p. (HBP)
> intersystolic p.
> isoelectric p.
> isometric contraction p.
> isometric relaxation p.
> isovolumetric relaxation p. (IVRP)
> isovolumic relaxation p.
> no-sigh p.
> pacemaker amplifier refractory p.
> postinfarction p.
> postsphygmic p.
> postventricular atrial refractory p. (PVARP)
> preejection p. (PEP)
> presphygmic p.
> pulse p.
> pulse repetition p. (PRP)

refractory p.
relative refractory p. (RRP)
relaxation p.
right ventricular preejection p.
  (RVPEP)
right ventricular refractory p.
  (RVERP)
saccular p.
sigh p.
systolic ejection p. (SEP)
TAB p.
total atrial blanking p.
total atrial refractory p. (TARP)
ventricular effective refractory p.
  (VERP)
p. of ventricular filling
ventriculoatrial effective
  refractory p.
vulnerable p.
washout p.
Wenckebach p.
periodic
  p. breathing
  p. edema
  p. limb movement (PLM)
  p. limb movement disorder
    (PLMD)
  p. paralysis
  p. polyserositis
  p. respiration
  p. short pulse (PSP)
periodicity
  A-V node Wenckebach p.
  circadian p.
  Wenckebach p.
perioperative
  p. antibiotic
  p. blood transfusion
  p. myocardial infarction (PMI)
  p. platelet transfusion
periorbital edema
periosteotome
  Alexander-Farabeuf p.
periosteum
peripartal
  p. cardiomyopathy
  p. heart disease
  p. heart failure
peripartum
  p. cardiac failure (PPCF)
  p. cardiomyopathy
  p. myocarditis
peripharyngeal space
peripharyngeum
peripheral
  p. access system (PAS)
  p. airspace
  P. AngioJet system

p. arterial disease (PAD, P.A.D.)
p. arterial occlusion (PAO)
p. arterial occlusive disease
  (PAOD)
p. arterial tone (PAT)
p. arteriosclerosis
p. arteriosclerotic occlusive disease
  (PAOD)
p. artery
p. artery bypass
p. artery tonometry
p. atherectomy system
p. atherosclerotic disease
p. blood eosinophilia
p. blood flow (PBF)
p. blood mononuclear cell (PBMC)
p. blood smear
p. chemoreceptor
p. circulation
p. conduction disease
p. coronary pressure (PCP)
p. cyanosis
p. edema
p. excimer laser angioplasty
  (PELA)
p. hyperemia
p. interstitial disease
p. interstitium
p. laser angioplasty (PLA)
p. muscle strength
p. neuropathy
p. paracicatricial emphysema
p. pulmonary artery stenosis
  (PPAS)
p. pulmonic stenosis (PPS)
p. pulse present
p. pulses palpable both legs
  (PPPBL)
p. resistance
p. resistance unit (PRU)
p. stigmata
p. transluminal angioplasty
p. vascular disease (PVD)
p. vascular resistance (PVR)
p. vasoconstriction
p. vasodilation
p. vasodilator effect
p. venous pressure (PVP)
p. zone radioaerosol clearance
peripherally
  p. inserted catheter (PIC)
  p. inserted central catheter (PICC)
peripneumonia notha
periprosthetic
  p. mitral regurgitation
  p. valve abscess
  p. valve aortic insufficiency
peripylephlebitis

P

peristalsis
    high-altitude p.
    high-amplitude p. (HAP)
peristaltic wave (PW)
peristasis
peristatic hyperemia
Peri-Strips
perisystole
perisystolic
perithelium
    Eberth p.
peritoneal
    continuous cyclic p.
    p. dialysis
peritracheal
peritubular capillary (PTC)
perivalvular
    p. leak
    p. leakage (PVL)
perivascular
    p. calcium
    p. canal
    p. edema
    p. eosinophilic infiltrate
    p. epithelioid cell
    p. fibrosis
    p. foam cell
    p. infiltration (PVI)
    p. lymphocytic infiltrate
    p. rupture
    p. sheath
    p. spaces
periventricular hyperintensity (PVH, PVHI)
Perles
    Tessalon P.
Perma-Flow coronary bypass graft
PermaNeb reusable nebulizer
permanent
    p. atrial tachycardia
    p. cardiac pacing lead
    p. junctional reciprocating tachycardia (PJRT)
    p. occlusion device
    p. pacemaker (PPM)
    p. pacemaker placement
    p. pacing
Permapen injection
permeability
    airway p.
    alveolar p. (AP)
    endothelial p.
    microvascular p.
permissive
    p. hypercapnia (PHC)
    p. hypercapnia (PHC)
    p. hypercapnic ventilation
permutation

pernio
    lupus p.
peroneal
    p. artery
    p. muscular atrophy
peroxidase
    avidin-biotin p.
peroxidation
    lipid p.
peroxide
    hydrogen p.
    lipid p.
peroxisome
    p. proliferator-activated receptor (PPAR)
    p. proliferator-activated receptor gamma (PPAR-gamma)
    p. proliferator response element (PPRE)
peroxyacetyl nitrate
peroxyl radical-trapping potential
peroxynitrite
perpetual arrhythmia
perpetuus
    pulsus irregularis p.
Per-Q-Cath percutaneously inserted central venous catheter
Persantine
    P. myocardial perfusion study
    P. thallium stress test
Persantine-isonitrile stress test
persistence
    microbubble p.
persistent
    p. atrial standstill (PAS)
    p. common atrioventricular canal
    p. ductus arteriosus
    p. fetal circulation (PFC)
    p. hiccups
    p. left superior vena cava (PLSVC)
    p. ostium primum
    p. pulmonary hypertension of newborn (PPHN)
    p. shunt
    p. truncus arteriosus (PTA)
personal
    P. Best peak flowmeter
    p. heart device (PHD)
personalized aerobics for cardiovascular enhancement
person-year
Perspex block
persulfate salt
pertechnetate sodium
Perthes
    P. syndrome
    P. test

perturbation
> autonomic p.
> neurohormonal p.

perturbed
> p. autonomic nervous system function
> p. carotid baroreceptor

pertussis
> *Bordetella p.*
> *Haemophilus p.*
> p. toxin

peruana
> verruga p.

pervenous
> p. catheter
> p. pacemaker

PES
> paclitaxel-eluting stent
> postextrasystolic
> preexcitation syndrome
> programmed electrical stimulation

PESDA
> perfluorocarbon-exposed sonicated dextrose albumin

PESP
> postextrasystolic potentiation

pestis
> *Yersinia p.*

PET
> peak ejection time
> polyethylene terephthalate
> poor exercise tolerance
> positron emission tomography
> progressive exercise test
> > PET balloon atherectomy device
> > PET scan
> > PET scanning
> > PET with C-11 acetate

petal
> nitinol p.

petal-fugal flow
PETCO$_2$
> partial pressure of end-tidal CO_2

petechia, pl. **petechiae**
petechial hemorrhage
Peterson elastic modulus
pethidine
Petit sinus
PETN
> pentaerythritol tetranitrate

Petriellidium boydii
petrified cardiac myxoma
Petrillium
petrosal ganglion
pexelizumab
Peyer patch
Peyrot thorax
PF
> peak flow

> pericardial fluid
> pulmonary function

PFA
> platelet function analyzer
> profunda femoris artery

PFA-100
PFC
> perfluorocarbon
> pericardial fluid culture
> persistent fetal circulation

PFE
> papillary fibroelastoma

PFF
> polymer fume fever

PFM
> peak flowmeter
> > TruZone PFM

PFO
> patent foramen ovale

PFO-Star occluder
PFR
> peak filling rate

PFS
> preservative-free solution
> > Idamycin PFS
> > Vincasar PFS

PFSDQ
> Pulmonary Functional Status and Dyspnea Questionnaire

PFSS
> pulmonary functional status scale

PFT
> pulmonary function test

PG
> post graft

PGCMS
> Philadelphia Geriatric Center Morale Scale

PGF
> primary graft failure

PGF2-alpha
> prostaglandin 2 alpha

PGI$_2$
> prostacyclin

P-glycoprotein
Pg-Ppl
> gastric-intrapleural pressure

PGVS
> postganglionic vagal stimulation

PH
> parenchymal hematoma
> parenchymal hemorrhage
> pulmonary hypertension

pH
> hydrogen ion concentration
> > pH conduction time
> > intramucosal pH
> > pH Meter
> > scalp pH

P

phacoma
phage
  luciferase reporter p.
phagocyte
phagocytic
  p. function
  p. natural killer cell
  p. pneumonocyte
phagocytose
phagocytosis
phalangis
  corpus p.
phalanx, pl. **phalanges**
  body of p.
Phalen stress test
Phanatuss Cough Syrup
phantom
  p. aneurysm
  p. flow artifact
  P. guidewire
  P. nasal mask
  P. nasal mask CPAP
  p. pacemaker
  p. pain
  p. sponge
  p. tumor
  P. V Plus catheter
pharmacodynamics
pharmacoeconomics
pharmacogenetic biomarker
pharmacokinetics
pharmacologic
  p. environment
  p. plaque passivation
  p. stress
  p. stress echocardiography
  p. stress perfusion imaging
pharmacological
  p. cardioversion
  p. challenge
  p. intervention in atrial fibrillation
    (PIAF)
pharmacology
  in vitro p.
pharmacomechanical thrombolysis
pharmacopeia
  British P. (BP)
  United States P. (USP)
pharmacotherapy
pharyngalgia
pharyngea, pl. **pharyngeae**
  arteria p.
  venae pharyngeae
pharyngeal
  p. arch
  p. branch
  p. branch of descending palatine
    artery

p. branch of glossopharyngeal
  nerve
p. branch of inferior thyroid artery
p. branch of pterygopalatine
  ganglion
p. branch of vagus nerve
p. canal
p. collapsibility
p. crisis
p. gland
p. lymphatic ring
p. nervous plexus
p. pouch
p. pouch syndrome
p. raphe
p. reflex
p. ridge
p. space
p. speculum
p. tonsil
p. tracheal lumen (PTL)
p. vein
pharyngeales
  glandulae p.
pharyngealis
  tonsilla p.
pharynges (*pl. of* pharynx)
pharyngeus
  plexus nervosus p.
  recessus p.
pharyngis
  cavitas p.
  cavum p.
  globus p.
  pars nasalis p.
  pars oralis p.
  raphe p.
  tunica mucosa p.
  tunica muscularis p.
pharyngitis
  acute p.
  arcanobacterial p.
  atrophic p.
  catarrhal p.
  chronic p.
  croupous p.
  diphtheric p.
  diphtheritic p.
  follicular p.
  gangrenous p.
  glandular p.
  granular p.
  herpangina p.
  membranous p.
  phlegmonous p.
  plague p.
  p. sicca
  p. ulcerosa
pharyngobranchial duct

pharyngoconjunctival fever
pharyngoepiglottic
pharyngoesophageal
    p. cushions
    p. pads
    p. sphincter
pharyngoglossal
pharyngoglossus
pharyngolaryngeal
pharyngomaxillary space
pharyngometer
    acoustic p.
    Eccovision acoustic p.
pharyngonasal cavity
pharyngooral
pharyngopalatine
pharyngopalatinus
pharyngoparalysis
pharyngoplasty
    Hynes p.
pharyngoscopy
pharyngospasm
pharyngostaphylinus
pharyngotracheal
    p. lumen (PTL)
    p. lumen airway (PTLA)
pharyngotympanic groove
pharynx, pl. **pharynges**
    constrictor muscle of p.
    inferior constrictor muscle of p.
    lacuna pharyngis
    laryngeal part of p.
    middle constrictor muscle of p.
    nasal part of p.
    oral part of p.
    raphe of p.
phase
    p. angle
    convalescent p.
    ejection p.
    fibrinopurulent p.
    fibroproliferative p.
    harmonic p. (HARP)
    p. heterophony
    p. image
    p. image analysis
    p. imaging
    isovolumic p.
    Korotkoff p. I–V
    4-p. Lifestick CPR
    midexpiratory p.
    plateau p.
    recovery p.
    relaxation p.
    single-breath wash-in p.
    supernormal recovery p.
    terminal p.
    upstroke p.
    venous p.

    vulnerable p.
    washout p.
phase-contrast magnetic resonance angiography (PC-MRA)
phased
    p. array receiver coil
    p. array sector scanner
    p. array sector transducer
    p. array system
    p. array technology
    p. array ultrasonographic device
phase-encoded velocity image
phasic
    p. excursion
    p. intragraft flow velocity
    p. sinus arrhythmia
PHAVER
    pterygia, heart defects, autosomal recessive inheritance, vertebral defects, ear anomalies, radial defect
    PHAVER syndrome
PHC
    permissive hypercapnia
PHD
    personal heart device
    postheparin plasma diamine oxidase
Phemister elevator
phenacetin
    p., aspirin, caffeine (PAC)
    p., aspirin, desoxyephedrine (PAD, P.A.D.)
phenazopyridine
    sulfisoxazole and p.
Phenergan
    P. injection
    P. With Codeine
Phenhist Expectorant
phenindamine tartrate
phenindione sensitivity
phenobarbital
    theophylline, ephedrine, p.
phenolformaldehyde
phenomenon, pl. **phenomena**
    AFORMED p.
    Anrep p.
    Aschner p.
    Ashley p.
    Ashman p.
    Austin Flint p.
    black hole p.
    blush p.
    Bowditch p.
    cascade p.
    cogwheel p.
    coronary steal p.
    diaphragm p.
    diaphragmatic p.
    dip p.
    Duckworth p.

P

phenomenon *(continued)*
    Ehret p.
    embolic p.
    Friedreich p.
    Gallavardin p.
    gap conduction p.
    Gärtner vein p.
    Goldblatt p.
    Gregg p.
    Hering p.
    Hill p.
    Katz-Wachtel p.
    Kienböck p.
    Koch p.
    Litten p.
    low-reflow p.
    malperfusion p.
    no-reflow p.
    nutcracker p.
    overshoot p.
    pendelluft p.
    preconditioning p.
    Raynaud p.
    recoil p.
    reentry p.
    R-on-T p.
    Schellong-Strisower p.
    Splendore-Hoeppli p.
    staircase p.
    steal p.
    treppe p.
    Venturi p.
    warmup p.
    washout p.
    Wenckebach p.
    Williams p.
    Woodworth p.
    zone 1 p.
phenothiazine
phenotype
    high-risk p.
    large-cell carcinoma with
      rhabdoid p.
    metastatic p.
    MLS_B p.
    Pi p.
    Pi MM, MZ, SS, SZ, ZZ p.
    priapism p.
    proteinase inhibitor p.
    rhabdoid p.
    skeletal muscle p.
phenoxybenzamine hydrochloride
phenoxymethyl
    penicillin p.
phenprocoumon
phentermine
    fenfluramine and p. (fen-phen)
phentolamine
    p. hydrochloride

    intracoronary p.
    p. mesylate
    p. methanesulfonate
phenyl
    p. aminosalicylate
    p. salicylate
phenylalanine
    formyl methionyl leucyl p. (FMLP)
phenylalkylamine
phenylbutazone sensitivity
phenylephrine
    guaifenesin, phenylpropanolamine, p.
    p. hydrochloride
    isoproterenol and p.
    p. ramp method
phenylpropanolamine
    caramiphen and p.
    guaifenesin and p.
    p. hydrochloride
    hydrocodone and p.
    p. toxicity
phenytoin
pheochromocytoma
PHI
    pontine hyperintensity
Phialophora verrucosa
Philadelphia
    P. Association of Clinical Trials
      (PACT)
    P. Geriatric Center Morale Scale
      (PGCMS)
Philip gland
Philips
    P. ACS NT 1.5 Gyroscan MRI
    P. Electronics' HeartStart Home
      Defibrillator
    P. HeartStart Home OTC
      defibrillator
    P. Integris 3000 biplane digital
      subtraction angiography device
    P. Medical Systems 1.5-T Intera
      magnet
    P. Medical Systems Tomoscan
      AVE1 CT spiral scanner
    P. Medical Systems Tomoscan SR
      7000 CT spiral scanner
    P. Tomoscan 310 CT scanner
Philos DR-T pacemaker
P-H interval
PHLA
    postheparin lipolytic activity
phlebarteriectasia
phlebectasia
phlebectomy
    transilluminated powered p. (TIPP)
phlebemphraxis
phlebitis
    adhesive p.
    blue p.

chlorotic p.
descending p.
gouty p.
malignancy-associated p.
migrating p.
p. nodularis necrotisans
p. obliterans
obliterating p.
plastic p.
puerperal p.
sclerosing p.
superficial p.
phlebodynamics
phlebogenous
phlebogram
phlebograph
phlebography
phlebolithiasis
phlebomanometer
phlebostasis
phlebotomize
phlebotomy
bloodless p.
phlegm
phlegmasia
p. alba dolens
p. cerulea dolens
phlegmonosa
angina p.
phlegmonous
p. laryngitis
p. pharyngitis
phlei
Mycobacterium p.
phonarteriogram
phonarteriography
Phonate speaking valve
phonoangiography
carotid p.
phonocardiogram (PCG)
phonocardiograph
linear p.
logarithmic p.
spectral p.
stethoscopic p.
phonocardiographic transducer
phonocardiography
spectral p. (SPCG)
phonocatheter
phonoscope
phonoscopy
phorbol ester
phosducin
phosgene
phosphatase
acid p.
alkaline p. (AP)
alkaline phosphatase antialkaline p.
(APAAP)

phosphate
Aralen P.
azapetine p.
chloroquine p.
Cleocin P.
codeine p.
dexamethasone sodium p. (DSP)
disopyramide p.
etoposide p.
glyceraldehyde 3-p.
Hexadrol P.
histamine acid p.
hydrocortisone sodium p.
Linctus With Codeine p.
myocardial creatine p.
nicotinamide adenine dinucleotide p.
(NADPH)
oseltamivir p.
Paveral Stanley Syrup With
Codeine P.
polyribosylribitol p. (PRP)
primaquine p.
sodium p.
triciribine p. (TCN-P)
phosphate-buffered saline (PBS)
phosphatidylcholine (PtdCho)
dipalmitoyl p. (DPPC)
phosphatidylinositol
phosphatidylserine
phosphine
phosphinic acid
phosphocreatine (PCr)
phosphodiesterase
p. 4 (PDE4)
p. enzyme
p. 3 inhibition (PDE3I)
p. inhibitor (PDE, PDE-I)
p. 4 inhibitor
p. isoenzyme inhibitor
sphingomyelin p.
phosphofructokinase
phosphoinositide
phosphoinositol
phosphokinase
brain isoenzymes of creatine p.
(CPK-BB)
creatine p. (CPK)
phospholamban
phospholipase
lipoprotein-associated p.
lipoprotein-associated p. 2
postheparin p. (PHP)
phospholipid
surfactant p.
**phospholipid-bound activated factor X
(Fxa)**
phospholipidosis
alveolar p.
phosphomonoesterase

P

phosphorus
  organic p.
  p. tribromide
phosphorus-31 magnetic resonance spectroscopy (^{31}P-MRS)
phosphorylase
  glycogen p.
  p. kinase
  thymidine p.
phosphorylation
  mitochondrial oxidative p.
  oxidative p.
phosphorylcholine (PC)
Phospho-Soda
  Fleet P.-S.
photoablation
photoaffinity
photoangioplasty
photobiological response
photochemical air pollution
photochemotherapy
  extracorporeal p.
photocoagulation
PhotoDerm VL device
photodiode
photodisruption
photodynamic therapy (PDT)
Photofrin
PhotoGenica
  P. V-Star
  P. V-Star laser
photohemotachometer
photometer
  HemoCue p.
photometry
  emission flame p.
photomicrography
photomultiplier
photon
  annihilation p.
  P. DR dual-chamber ICD
  P. DR implantable cardioverter-defibrillator
  P. Micro DR/VR implantable cardioverter-defibrillator
photopeak
photoplethysmography (PPG)
photoprotection
photoreactivation
photoresection
photosensitizing reaction
photostethoscope
pHOx CO-oximeter
PHP
  postheparin phospholipase
PHR
  peak heart rate
phrenic
  p. artery

  p. nerve
  p. nerve crush injury
  p. nerve paralysis
  p. pleura
phrenica
  pleura p.
phrenicocolic
phrenicocolicum
  ligamentum p.
phrenicocostal sinus
phrenicogastric
phrenicoglottic
phrenicohepatic
phrenicosplenic
phrenocardia
phrenocolic
phrenogastric
phrenohepatic
PHRT
  Public Health Response Team
  PHRT protocol
pH-stat
PHT
  portal hypertension
  pressure half-time
  pulmonary hypertension
  PHT eSense PiKo
phthalic anhydride irritant-induced asthma
phthinoid
  p. bronchitis
  p. chest
phthisis
  aneurysmal p.
  bacillary p.
  black p.
  collier's p.
  diabetic p.
  fibroid p.
  grinder's p.
  miner's p.
  potter's p.
  pulmonary p.
  stone cutter's p.
phycoerythrin
phycomycosis
Phylax
  P. AV dual-chamber implantable cardioverter-defibrillator
  P. AV implantable ICD
  P. 06 implantable cardioverter-defibrillator
phylaxis
phyllosilicate
physical
  P. Activity Scale for the Elderly Evaluation (PASE)
  p. inactivity
  p. stimulus

p. therapy
P. Work Capacity exercise stress test

physician
American College of P.'s
American College of Chest P.'s (ACCP)

physiochemical

Physio-Control Lifestat sphygmomanometer

physiologic
p. congestion
p. dead space
p. dead space fraction
p. dead space/tidal volume ratio (V_D/V_T)
p. dead space ventilation (V_D/V_T)
p. measurement
p. monitoring
p. murmur
p. pacemaker
p. pattern release (PPR)
p. shunt fraction
p. third heart sound

physiological
p. dead space ventilation per minute (V_D)
p. monitoring
p. overreactivity
p. pattern
p. provocation
p. split of S_2
p. stress

physiologically split S_2 sound

physiology
constrictive p.
Damus-Kaye-Stansel procedure for single ventricle p.
Eisenmenger p.
restrictive right ventricular p.
single-ventricle p.

Physios
P. CTM 01 cardiac transplant monitor
P. CTM 01 noninvasive cardiac transplant monitoring system

physiotherapy
chest p. (CPT)
movement science p.

phytanic acid accumulation

Phytis stent

phytoestrogen
soy p.

phytohemagglutinin

phytonadione

phytopneumoconiosis

phytosterol

PI
pacing impulse
performance index
pontine infarct
primary infarction
protease inhibitor
pulmonary infarction
pulmonary insufficiency
pulsatility index
alpha-1 PI
PI MRI technique

Pi
proteinase inhibitor
Pi MM, MZ, SS, SZ, ZZ phenotype
Pi phenotype

PIA
preinfarction angina

PIAF
pharmacological intervention in atrial fibrillation
prognosis in atrial fibrillation

pial collateralization

piano percussion

piaulement
bruit de p.

PIB
partial ileal bypass

PIBC
percutaneous intraaortic balloon counterpulsation
PIBC catheter

PIC
pacing in cardiomyopathy
peripherally inserted catheter

PICA
posterior inferior cerebellar artery
posterior inferior communicating artery

PICC
peripherally inserted central catheter

Piccolino
P. balloon
P. Monorail catheter

PICD
periinfarction conduction defect

PICH
primary intracerebral hemorrhage

pick
P. and Go monitor
P. syndrome

picker
P. CS scanner
P. Edge 1.5-T scanner
P. Magnascanner
P. PQ 2000 CT scanner
P. Voxel image analysis system

pickwickian syndrome

Picornaviridae virus

piCO+ Smokerlyzer

Picrorhiza kurroa

picrosirius red stain

P

PICSO
>> pressure-controlled intermittent coronary sinus occlusion

picture
>> anodal opening p. (AOP)

PICVA
>> percutaneous in situ coronary venous arterialization
>> PICVA treatment

PID
>> preimplantation diagnosis

PIE
>> prosthetic infectious endocarditis
>> pulmonary infiltrate with eosinophilia
>> pulmonary infiltration with eosinophilia
>> pulmonary interstitial emphysema
>> PIE syndrome

piece
>> Ayers T p.
>> 2-p. bifurcated intraluminal graft

piechaudii
>> *Alcaligenes p.*

Pie Medical CAAS II analysis system
Pierce-Donachy Thoratec ventricular assist device
Pierre Robin syndrome
piesimeter
>> Hales p.

piesis
piezoelectric
>> p. crystal
>> p. crystal-based pacemaker
>> p. snore sensor
>> p. ultrasound transducer

piezo film sensor
PIF
>> peak inspiratory flow

PIFR
>> peak inspiratory flow rate

pigeon
>> p. breast deformity
>> p. breeder's disease
>> p. breeder's lung
>> p. chest
>> p. fancier's lung

piggyback
pigment
>> p. induration
>> p. induration of lung

pigmented treatment
pigskin
pigtail
>> p. angiographic catheter
>> p. rotation catheter

PIH
>> pregnancy-induced hypertension

PIIIP
>> procollagen type III aminoterminal peptide

PI3-kinase
PiKo
>> PHT eSense P.
>> P. spirometer

pilin
pill
>> birth control p.

pillar
>> tonsillar p.

Pilling
>> P. bronchoscope
>> P. Weck Y-stent forceps

pillow
>> nasal p.
>> 2-p. orthopnea
>> 3-p. orthopnea

pillow-shaped balloon
pilocarpine iontophoresis test
pilot
>> P. guidewire
>> p. needle

PILP
>> postinfarction late potential

pilsicainide
Pima
PIMI
>> predictive index for myocardial infarction
>> psychophysiological interventions in myocardial ischemia

pimobendan
PIMS
>> programmable implantable medication system

pinacidil
pinchcock mechanism
pincushion distortion
pindolol
pineal pellucidum
pine resin
pinhole
>> p. balloon rupture
>> 7-p. tomography
>> p. VSD

pink
>> p. puffer
>> p. sputum
>> p. tetralogy of Fallot

pinked up
Pinkerton .018 balloon catheter
pinnacle
>> P. introducer sheath
>> P. pacemaker

pinocytosis
pinocytotic
pinosome
Pins
>> P. sign
>> P. syndrome

pioglitazone

PIOPED
  Prospective Investigation of Pulmonary
    Embolism Diagnosis
PIP
  peak inspiratory pressure
  plasma cell interstitial pneumonitis
  positive inspiratory pressure
pipecuronium bromide
piperacillin and tazobactam sodium
piperazine citrate
pipobroman
pirbuterol
  p. acetate
  p. acetate inhalation aerosol
pirenzepine
piretanide
pirfenidone
piriform, pyriform
  p. sinus
  p. thorax
piritrexim isethionate
pirmenol
pirodavir
Pirogoff angle
pirolazamide
piroximone
Pirquet reaction
PIRS
  postinfarction risk stratification
PIS
  preinfarction syndrome
PISA
  proximal isovelocity surface area
Pisces lead
pistol
pistol-shot
  p.-s. femoral sound
  p.-s. sound
piston pulse
PIT
  pacing-induced tachycardia
pit
  inferior costal p.
pitavastatin
pitchfork
  p. angiographic landmark
  p. angiographic landmark of left
    anterior descending coronary
    artery bifurcation
Pitressin injection
pitting edema
Pittman IMA retractor system
Pittsburgh
  P. pneumonia
  P. pneumonia agent
PIV
  parainfluenza virus
PIV-1
  parainfluenza virus type 1

PIV-2
  parainfluenza virus type 2
PIV-3
  parainfluenza virus type 3
PIV-4
  parainfluenza virus type 4
pivampicillin
pivot point
pivoxil
  cefditoren p.
pixel
pizza lung
Pizzolatto stain
PJC
  premature junctional contraction
PJ interval
PJP
  Pneumocystis jiroveci pneumonia
PJRT
  permanent junctional reciprocating
    tachycardia
PJT
  paroxysmal junctional tachycardia
PK
  pericardial knock
PKA
  protein kinase A
PKase
  protein kinase
PKC
  protein kinase C
PLA
  peripheral laser angioplasty
PLa
  left atrial pressure
PlA, Pla
  platelet antigen
PLAATO
  percutaneous left atrial appendage
    transcatheter occluder
  percutaneous left atrial appendage
    transcatheter occlusion
placebo
placement
  anteroposterior paddle p.
  carotid angioplasty and stent p.
  catheter-directed thrombolysis and
    endovascular stent p.
  conduit p.
  endotracheal tube p.
  intracoronary stent p.
  lead p.
  permanent pacemaker p.
  prophylactic filter p.
  stent p.
  stent-graft p.
  temporary pacemaker p.
  Thoracoport p.

placental
  p. barrier
  p. 11 b-hydroxysteroid
    dehydrogenase type 2
  p. circulation
  p. respiration
plague
  bubonic p.
  p. pharyngitis
  p. pneumonia
  pneumonic p.
plain old balloon angioplasty (POBA)
PLA-I platelet antigen
plakoglobin
plan
  loss of future p.'s
planar
  p. myocardial imaging
  p. myocardial scintigraphy
  p. thallium imaging
  p. thallium scintigraphy
  p. thallium test
  p. xanthoma
plane
  Addison p.
  anular p.
  apical 4-chamber p. (Ap4CH)
  axial p.
  circular p.
  coronal p.
  cove p.
  mandibular p.
  midsagittal p.
  orthogonal p.
  parasagittal p.
  sagittal p.
  short-axis p.
  sternal p.
  sternoxiphoid p.
  transaxial p.
planigraphy
planimeter
planimetry
  p. method
  TapeMeasure computerized p.
  p. volume
planithorax
plant
  p. stanol
  p. sterol
  p. toxicity
plantar ischemia test
plaque
  amorphous p.
  p. area
  atheromatous p.
  atherosclerotic p. (AP)
  p. burden
  calcified p.

carcinoid p.
carotid p.
complex p.
coronary p.
p. destabilization
disrupted p.
p. disruption
echogenic p.
echolucent p.
p. embolization
fibrofatty p.
fibrous p.
p. fissure
p. fissuring
p. fracture
glistening yellow coronary p.
heterogeneous p.
Hollenhorst p.
homogeneous p.
hypoechoic p.
intraluminal p.
lipid-laden p.
lipid-rich p.
p. lumen
p. marker
p. motion
myointimal p.
p. neovascularity
nonostial p.
p. passivation
pleural p.
p. prolapse
protuberant p.
p. rupture
senile p.
shelf of p.
p. shift
p. stabilization
p. stabilization therapy
p. strutting
submucosal p.
thoracic aortic atherosclerotic p.
ulcerated p.
unstable p.
p. volume
p. vulnerability
vulnerable p.
white p.
yellow p.
plaque-cracker
  LeVeen p.-c.
Plaquenil
plaque-trapping device
plaquing
plasma
  p. aldosterone
  p. alpha-1 antitrypsin (pAAT)
  p. arginine vasopressin (pAVP)
  p. beta-thromboglobulin

p. catecholamine
p. cell (PC)
p. cell interstitial pneumonitis (PIP)
p. cell pneumonia
p. cell-type variant of Castleman disease (CD-PC)
p. clot diffusion chamber (PCDC)
p. coagulation system
p. colloid osmotic pressure
p. endothelin
p. endothelin concentration
p. erythropoietin
p. exchange column
p. extravasation
p. fibrinogen
fresh frozen p. (FFP)
p. glycocalicin
p. homocysteine
p. homocysteine concentration
p. leptin level
p. nicotine level
p. norepinephrine
platelet-poor p. (PPP)
platelet-rich p. (PRP)
p. protein exudation
p. renin
p. renin activity (PRA)
p. retinol
p. skimming
p. thromboplastin antecedent (PTA)
p. thromboplastin component (PTC, PTH)
p. thromboplastin factor (PTF)
p. thyroxine level (PTL)
p. triglyceride level
p. viscosity (PV)
p. volume
p. volume expander
zoster immune p. (ZIP)

plasmacytoid infiltration
plasmacytoma
extramedullary p.
plasmagel
plasmahaut
plasmakinin
plasmalemma
Plasma-Lyte A
Plasmanate
plasmapheresis
plasmatic vascular destruction
plasmin
plasminemia
plasminogen
p. activator
p. activator inhibitor (PAI)
p. activator inhibitor-1 (PAI-1)
plasminogen-streptokinase complex
Plasmodium
P. embolism
P. falciparum
P. malariae
P. ovale
P. vivax

plastic
p. bronchitis
p. endocarditis
p. phlebitis
p. pleurisy
p. polymer
p. sewing ring
p. surgical osteosynthesis
plasticity
cortical p.
neural p.
skeletal muscle p.
plasty
endoventricular circular patch p.
FAA p.
sliding p.
plate
polar p.
Strasburger cell p.
tantalum p.
p. thrombosis
p. thrombus
trach p.
tracheostomy p.
plateau
h p.
maximal response p. (MRP)
p. phase
p. pressure (Pplat)
p. pulse
p. response
ventricular p.
plateauing
plateau-pressure target
platelet
p. activating factor (PAF)
p. activation
p. activity
p. aggregation
p. aggregation inhibitor
p. antibody
p. antigen (PlA)
p. consumption
p. factor 4
p. function
p. function analyzer (PFA)
gel-filtered p. (GFP)
p. glycoprotein IIb/IIIa blockade
p. glycoprotein IIb/IIIa blocker
p. glycoprotein IIb/IIIa inhibitor
hemolysis, elevated liver enzymes, low p.'s (HELLP)
p. IIb/IIIa inhibitor
p. imaging
p. membrane glycoprotein

platelet *(continued)*
    p. receptor glycoprotein
    p. thrombosis
    p. thrombus
platelet-aggregating factor
platelet-derived
    p.-d. growth factor (PDGF)
    p.-d. growth factor-AB (PDGF-AB)
    p.-d. growth factor-AB assay
    p.-d. histamine-releasing factor
    (PDHRF)
platelet-mediated thrombosis
plateletpheresis
platelet-poor plasma (PPP)
platelet-rich plasma (PRP)
platelike atelectasis
platform
    Complete stent delivery p.
    stabilization p.
    TomTec echo p.
Platinol-AQ
platinum
    p. coil
    P. Plus guidewire
    p. radiopaque marker
    salt of p.
    p. wire
platinum-iridium electrode
platypnea
platypnea-orthodeoxia syndrome
platysma
Plavix
PLB
    pursed lip breathing
PLCO
    postoperative low cardiac output
PLCx
    posterolateral circumflex branch
        PLCx coronary artery
PLE
    protein-losing enteropathy
pledget
    Meadox Teflon felt p.
    p.-supported
    Teflon p.
pledgeted mattress suture
Plegiaguard pressure relief valve
pleiotropic cytokine
pleiotropy
Plendil
plenus
    pulsus p.
pleomorphic
    p. adenoma
    p. premature ventricular complex
    p. tachycardia
Plesch
    P. percussion
    P. test

Pletal
plethora
    inferior vena cava p.
plethoric
plethysmograph
    air p.
    body p.
    BPXG body p.
    MasterScreen BabyBody p.
    mercury-in-rubber strain gauge p.
    pressure p.
    pressure-compensated flow p.
    respiratory inductance p. (RIP)
    Respitrace p.
    volume-displacement p.
plethysmography
    cuff p.
    digital pulse p. (DPP)
    impedance p. (IPG)
    optoelectronic p.
    respiratory inductance p. (RIP)
    serial impedance p.
    servocontrolled p.
    strain-gauge p.
    thermistor p.
    venous impedance p. (VIP)
    venous occlusion p. (VOP)
pleura, pl. **pleurae**
    adipose folds of p.
    black p.
    cavum pleurae
    cervical p.
    costal p.
    p. costalis
    costodiaphragmatic recess of p.
    costomediastinal recess of p.
    cupula of p.
    cupula pleurae
    diaphragmatic p.
    p. diaphragmatica
    discission of p.
    fibrin bodies of p.
    mediastinal p.
    p. mediastinalis
    parietal p.
    p. parietalis
    p. pericardiaca
    phrenic p.
    p. phrenica
    p. pulmonalis
    pulmonary p.
    solitary fibrous tumor of p.
    (SFTP)
    visceral p.
    p. visceralis
pleuracentesis *(var. of* pleurocentesis)
    (*See also* thoracentesis)
pleuracotomy

pleural
- p. abrasion
- p. adhesion
- p. amyloidosis
- p. aspergillosis
- p. biopsy
- p. bleb
- p. calculus
- p. cap
- p. carcinomatosis
- p. cavity
- p. crackle
- p. cupula
- p. disease
- p. effusion shunt
- p. empyema
- p. fibrin ball
- p. fluid
- p. fluid neutrophilia
- p. fremitus
- p. friction rub
- p. lavage
- p. line
- p. mass
- p. meniscus sign
- p. mesothelioma
- p. mouse
- p. peel
- p. plaque
- p. poudrage
- p. pressure (Ppl)
- p. rale
- p. reaction
- p. recess
- p. rings
- p. sac
- p. scarring
- p. sclerosant
- p. shock
- p. sinus
- p. sliding
- p. space
- p. space elastance
- p. space evacuation
- p. space monitoring
- p. suction
- p. surface
- p. tag
- p. tap
- p. tent
- p. thickening
- p. toilet
- p. tube
- p. villi

pleurales
- recessus p.
- villi p.

pleuralgia

pleuralis
- cavitas p.

pleural-pleural apposition
Pleura-Seal thoracentesis kit
pleurectomy
- thoracoscopic apical p.

Pleur-evac
- P.-e. autotransfusion system
- P.-e. device
- P.-e. suction

pleurisy
- acute p.
- adhesive p.
- blocked p.
- cholesterol p.
- chronic p.
- chyliform p.
- chylous p.
- circumscribed p.
- costal p.
- diaphragmatic p.
- diffuse p.
- double p.
- dry p.
- encysted p.
- exudative p.
- fibrinous p.
- hemorrhagic p.
- ichorous p.
- indurative p.
- interlobar p.
- interlobular p.
- latent p.
- mediastinal p.
- metapneumonic p.
- plastic p.
- primary p.
- productive p.
- proliferating p.
- pulmonary p.
- pulsating p.
- purulent p.
- sacculated p.
- secondary p.
- serofibrinous p.
- serous p.
- single p.
- suppurative p.
- tuberculous p.
- typhoid p.
- visceral p.
- wet p.
- p. with effusion

pleuritic
- p. chest pain
- p. pneumonia
- p. rub

pleuritis
- fibrinous acute p.

pleuritis *(continued)*
    lupus p.
    obliterative p.
    rheumatoid p.
    tuberculous p.
pleuritogenous
pleurocentesis, pleuracentesis
pleurodesis
    chemical p.
    doxycycline p.
    mechanical p.
    talc p.
    thoracoscopic talc p.
    thorascopic talc p.
pleurodynia
pleuroesophageal
    p. fistula
    p. line
    p. muscle
pleuroesophageus
    musculus p.
pleurogenic pneumonia
pleurogenous
pleurography
pleurolith
pleuroparenchymal abnormality
pleuroparietopexy
pleuropericardial
    p. cyst
    p. incision
    p. murmur
    p. rub
    p. window
pleuropericarditis
pleuroperitoneal
    p. canal
    p. cavity
    p. fold
    p. shunt
    p. shunting
pleuropneumonectomy
pleuropneumonia-like organism (PPLO)
pleuropulmonary
    p. blastoma
    p. infection
    p. metastasis
pleuroscopy
pleurovisceral
PleurX long-term intercostal catheter
Pleurx pleural catheter
plexectomy
plexiform lesion
PlexiPulse compression device
plexogenic pulmonary arteriopathy
plexopathy
    brachial p.
plexus, pl. **plexuses**
    acromial p.
    ascending pharyngeal p.

    Batson p.
    brachial p.
    esophageal nervous p.
    Gelweave 3-branch P.
    p. gulae
    Haller p.
    lingual p.
    p. nervosus esophageus
    p. nervosus pharyngeus
    nervous p.
    p. periarterialis arteriae lingualis
    p. periarterialis arteriae pharyngeae ascendentis
    perimuscular p.
    pharyngeal nervous p.
    p. pulmonalis
    pulmonary nervous p.
    superior vascular p. (SVP)
PLHB
    percutaneous left heart bypass
pliability
PLIC
    posterior limb of internal capsule
plicamycin
plicatic acid
plication
    Spencer p.
PLLA
    poly-L-lactic acid
PLM
    periodic limb movement
    PLM sensor
PLMD
    periodic limb movement disorder
PLMV
    posterior leaf mitral valve
plombage
plop
    cardiac tumor p.
    tumor p.
plot
    box p.
    box-and-whisker p.
    bull's-eye p.
    whisker p.
PLSA
    posterolateral segment artery
    posterolateral segment [coronary] artery
PLSVC
    persistent left superior vena cava
plug
    collagen p.
    Dittrich p.
    Ivalon p.
    mucus p.
    polypoid connective tissue p.
    Shiley decannulation p.
    Teflon Bardic p.
    Traube p.

plugged telescoping catheter
plugging
  mucous p.
plumb-line sign
Plummer disease
Plummer-Vinson syndrome
plunging goiter
plurilocular
plus
  CO_2SMO P.
  Duramist P.
  Indeflator P. 20
  ligand p. 1, 2, 3
  Lorcet P.
  920M P. pulse oximeter
  Nicorette P.
  Oracle Micro P.
2010 Plus Holter system
PLV
  left ventricular pressure
  partial liquid ventilation
  posterior left ventricle
PLVP
  peak left ventricular pressure
PM
  mean pressure
  pacemaker
  papillary muscle
  posterior mitral
  presystolic murmur
  Prony method
PM10
  particulate matter less than 10
    micrometers in diameter
P+max
  peak positive pressure
PMBC
  percutaneous mitral balloon
    commissurotomy
PMBV
  percutaneous mitral balloon valvoplasty
  percutaneous mitral balloon valvotomy
PMC
  percutaneous mitral commissurotomy
  percutaneous myocardial channeling
  premature mitral closure
  premotor cortex
PMD
  primary myocardial disease
  pulsed myocardial Doppler
pMDI
  pressurized metered-dose inhaler
PM-DM
  polymyositis-dermatomyositis
PMF
  progressive massive fibrosis
PMH
  pure motor hemiparesis

PMHR
  predicted maximal heart rate
PMI
  perioperative myocardial infarction
  point of maximal impulse
  point of maximum impulse
P-min
  peak negative pressure
PMIS
  postmyocardial infarction syndrome
PML
  posterior mitral leaflet
  progressive multifocal
    leukoencephalopathy
  prolapsing mitral leaflet
pML
  posterior mitral valve leaflet
    anterior tracking of pML
PMMC
  percutaneous mechanical mitral
    commissurotomy
PMN
  polymorphonuclear leukocyte
  polymorphonuclear neutrophil
PMR
  papillary muscle rupture
  percutaneous myocardial
    revascularization
  percutaneous transmyocardial laser
    revascularization
PMRP
  portable monitor of respiratory
    parameters
^{31}P-MRS
  phosphorus-31 magnetic resonance
    spectroscopy
PMS-Amantadine
PMS-Erythromycin
PMS-Hydroxyzine
PMS Isoniazid
PMS-Levothyroxine Sodium
PMS-Methylphenidate
PMS-Progesterone
PMS-Pyrazinamide
PMS-Sodium Cromoglycate
PMT
  pacemaker-mediated tachycardia
  percutaneous mechanical thrombectomy
    PMT AccuSpan tissue expander
    Thrombex PMT
PMV
  percutaneous mitral valvoplasty
  percutaneous mitral valvotomy
  prolapse of mitral valve
    PMV 2000 series speaking valve
PMVI
  peak myocardial video intensity
PMVL, pMVL
  posterior mitral valve leaflet

P

PMW
  pacemaker wire
PN
  perceived noise
  percussion note
PNB
  premature nodal beat
PNC
  premature nodal contracture
PND
  paroxysmal nocturnal dyspnea
  postnasal drip
PND-Rh
  postnasal drip due to rhinitis
PNDS
  postnasal drainage syndrome
  postnasal drip syndrome
PND-Si
  postnasal drip due to sinusitis
pneocardiac reflex
pneopneic reflex
PNET
  primitive neuroectodermal tumor
pneumatic
    p. antishock garment (PASG)
    p. compression stockings
    p. cuff
    p. hammer disease
    p. peripheral circulation
      improvement device
    p. tourniquet
    p. trousers
pneumatics
pneumatocardia
pneumatocele
pneumatohemia
pneumatonometer
    Digibind p.
pneumectomy
pneumobacillus
    Friedländer p.
pneumobulbar
pneumocardial
pneumocardiogram (PCG)
pneumocentesis
pneumococcal
    p. bacteremia
    p. empyema
    p. pneumonia
    p. vaccine
pneumococcosis
pneumococcus, pl. **pneumococci**
    Fraenkel p.
pneumoconiosis
    antimony p.
    arc welder's p.
    asbestos p.
    bauxite p.
    China clay p.

  coal miner's p.
  coal worker's p. (CWP)
  cobalt p.
  collagenous p.
  fuller's earth p.
  graphite p.
  hard metal p.
  kaolin p.
  limonite p.
  magnetite p.
  mica p.
  mixed-dust p.
  noncollagenous p.
  organic dust p.
  rheumatoid p.
  shale p.
  p. siderotica
  silicotic p.
  talc p.
  tungsten carbide p.
pneumocystic
Pneumocystis
    P. carinii
    P. carinii pneumonia (PCP)
    P. choroidopathy
    P. jiroveci
    P. jiroveci pneumonia (PJP)
    P. pneumonitis
pneumocystosis
pneumocyte
    type II p.
Pneumo disposable pneumotachometer
pneumodynamics
pneumogastric
pneumogenic osteoarthropathy
pneumogram
pneumograph
pneumohemia
pneumohemothorax
pneumohydropericardium
pneumohydrothorax
pneumomediastinography
pneumomediastinum
    spontaneous p.
pneumomycosis
pneumonectomy
    extrapleural p. (EPP)
    simultaneously stapled p. (SSP)
pneumoneedle
Pneumo-Needle reusable instrument
pneumonia (*See also* pneumonitis)
    abortive p.
    acute eosinophilic p.
    acute interstitial p. (AIP)
    adenoviral p.
    p. alba
    alcoholic p.
    amebic p.
    anaerobic p.

anthrax p.
antimicrobial-resistant hospital-
  acquired p.
apex p.
apical p.
p. aposthematosa
aspiration p.
atypical p.
avian influenza p.
bacillary p.
bacterial pneumococcal p.
bilious p.
bronchial p.
bronchiolitic interstitial p. (BIP)
bronchiolitis obliterans with
  organizing p. (BOOP)
Buhl desquamative p.
Candida p.
Carrington p.
caseous p.
catarrhal p.
central p.
cerebral p.
cheesy p.
chemical p.
Chlamydia p.
chronic eosinophilic p. (CEP)
chronic fibrous p.
cold agglutinin p.
community-acquired p. (CAP)
congenital aspiration p.
contusion p.
core p.
Corrigan p.
croupous p.
cryptogenic organizing p. (COP)
deglutition p.
desquamative interstitial p. (DIP)
p. dissecans
double p.
Eaton agent p.
embolic p.
Enterobacter p.
eosinophilic p.
ephemeral p.
ether p.
exogenous lipid p.
fibrinous acute lobar p.
fibrous p.
Friedländer bacillus p.
gangrenous p.
gelatinous acute p.
giant cell p.
group A streptococcal p.
healthcare-associated p. (HCAP)
Hecht p.
hematogenous p.
herpes simplex p.
hospital-acquired p. (HAP)

HSV p.
hypersensitivity p.
hypostatic p.
idiopathic acute eosinophilic p.
idiopathic interstitial p. (IIP)
indurative p.
influenzal p.
influenza virus p.
inhalation p.
p. interlobularis
p. interlobularis purulenta
interstitial plasma cell p.
intrauterine p.
Kaufman p.
Klebsiella p.
Legionella p.
Legionnaire p.
leptospiral p.
lingular p.
lipid p.
lipoid p.
lobar p.
lobular p.
Löffler p.
Louisiana p.
lymphoid interstitial p. (LIP)
massive p.
measles p.
metastatic p.
migratory bronchiolitis obliterans
  organizing p.
mycoplasmal p.
necrotizing p.
nonspecific interstitial p. (NSIP)
nosocomial p. (NP)
p. notha
nursing home p.
obstructive p.
oil-aspiration p.
opportunistic fungal p.
organizing p.
parenchymatous p.
peribronchial p.
Pittsburgh p.
plague p.
plasma cell p.
pleuritic p.
pleurogenic p.
pneumococcal p.
Pneumocystis carinii p. (PCP)
Pneumocystis jiroveci p. (PJP)
polymicrobial p.
postobstructive p.
primary atypical p.
primary eosinophilic p.
primary influenza p.
progressive p.
Proteus p.
purulent p.

P

pneumonia *(continued)*
    Reisman p.
    retrocardiac p.
    rheumatic p.
    rickettsial p.
    Scopulariopsis p.
    secondary p.
    segmental p.
    septic p.
    Serratia p.
    P. Severity Index (PSI)
    spherical p.
    staphylococcal p.
    steroid-resistant bronchiolitis
      obliterans organizing p.
    Stoll p.
    streptococcal p.
    superficial p.
    suppurative p.
    terminal p.
    toxemic p.
    transplant p.
    traumatic p.
    Trichosporon beigelii p.
    tuberculous p.
    tularemic p.
    TWAR p.
    typhoid p.
    unilateral p.
    unresolved p.
    uremic p.
    usual interstitial p. (UIP)
    vagus p.
    varicella p.
    ventilator-acquired p. (VAP)
    ventilator-associated p. (VAP)
    viral p.
    walking p.
    wandering p.
    white p.
    woolsorter's p.
pneumoniae
    Bacillus p.
    Chlamydia p.
    Diplococcus p.
    Klebsiella p.
    Legionella p.
    multidrug-resistant *Streptococcus* p.
      (MDRSP)
    Mycobacterium p.
    Mycoplasma p.
    Optochin test for *Streptococcus* p.
    penicillin-resistant *Streptococcus* p.
      (PRSP)
    Streptococcus p.
pneumonic
    p. fever
    p. plague
pneumonic-type adenocarcinoma

pneumonitis *(See also* pneumonia)
    acute interstitial p. (AIP)
    acute lupus p. (ALP)
    acute radiation p.
    aspiration p.
    blood p.
    bronchiolitis with interstitial p.
      (BIP)
    chemical p.
    cholesterol p.
    CMV p.
    cryptogenic organizing p. (COP)
    cytomegalovirus p.
    desquamative interstitial p. (DIP)
    eosinophilic p.
    giant cell interstitial p. (GIP)
    granulomatous p.
    herpes simplex p.
    hypersensitivity p. (HP)
    interstitial p.
    kerosene p.
    lymphocytic interstitial p. (LIP)
    lymphoid interstitial p. (LIP)
    malarial p.
    mitomycin C-induced interstitial p.
    mixed alveolar-interstitial p.
    nonspecific chronic interstitial p.
      (NIP)
    nonspecific interstitial p. (NSIP)
    ossifying p.
    peptic aspiration p.
    plasma cell interstitial p. (PIP)
    Pneumocystis p.
    radiation p.
    uremic p.
    usual interstitial p. (UIP)
    varicella p.
pneumonoconiosis
    bauxite p.
    rheumatoid p.
pneumonocyte
    phagocytic p.
pneumonopathy
    eosinophilic p.
pneumonoresection
pneumonotherapy
pneumoparotid
pneumopathy
    leukemic cell lysis p.
    seropositive nonsyphilitic p.
Pneumopent
pneumopericardium (PPC)
    tension p.
    ventilator-induced p.
pneumopexy
pneumophila
    Legionella p.
pneumoplethysmography
pneumopleuritis

pneumopleuroparietopexy
pneumoprotein
 serum p.
pneumoresection
pneumorrhachis
pneumoscope
pneumosilicosis
pneumosintes
 Bacteroides p.
PneumoSleeve
Pneumotach
 P. disposable mouthpiece
 P. spirometer
pneumotachogram
pneumotachograph
 Fleisch p.
 flow-sensing p.
 Silverman-Lilly p.
pneumotachometer
 disposable p.
 hot-wire p.
 Pneumo disposable p.
pneumotaxic center
pneumotherapy
pneumothorax, pl. **pneumothoraces**
 artificial p.
 catamenial p.
 clicking p.
 closed chest p.
 extrapleural p.
 iatrogenic p.
 induced p.
 normotensive p.
 open p.
 pressure p.
 primary spontaneous p. (PSP)
 pure p.
 secondary spontaneous p.
 simultaneous bilateral
  spontaneous p. (SBSP)
 spontaneous p. (SP)
 tension p.
 therapeutic p.
 traumatic p.
 unilateral p.
 valvular p.
 ventilator-induced p.
pneumotomy
Pneumovax 23
pneumovirus
Pneupac resuscitator
pneuPAC ventilator
PneuView ventilator testing and
 training system
PNH
 paroxysmal nocturnal hemoglobinuria
pnomenusa
 Pandoraea p.

PNP
 peak negative pressure
PNPB
 positive-negative pressure breathing
PNS
 posterior nasal spine
  PNS Unna boot
^{31}P nuclear magnetic resonance
 spectroscopy
PO
 pulse oximetry
pO$_2$
 partial pressure of oxygen
  pO$_2$ oximetry
POBA
 plain old balloon angioplasty
POC
 point-of-care
 polyolefin copolymer
  POC Bandit catheter
  POC blood gas test
POCD
 postoperative cognitive deficit
POCI
 posterior circulation infarct
pocket
 abdominal p.
 generator p.
 pacemaker p.
 regurgitant p.
 retropectoral p.
 p. shot
 p. of Zahn
Pocket-Dop II
Pockethaler
Pocketpeak peak flowmeter
PocketView ECG
POCS
 posterior circulation syndrome
POCT
 point-of-care testing
  POCT device
pod
 rigid p.
podagra
POEM
 Patient-Oriented Evidence that Matters
POEMS
 polyneuropathy, organomegaly,
  endocrinopathy, monoclonal
  gammopathy, skin changes
  POEMS syndrome
POET
 pulse oximeter/end tidal CO$_2$
pogonion
 gonion to p. (GO-POG)
POH
 postoperative hemorrhage
poikilocytosis

P

poikilothermy
point
>A p.
>Addison p.
>p. of Arrhigi
>Boyd p.
>C p.
>p. of care test
>Castellani p.
>p. of critical stenosis
>cut p.
>D p.
>de Mussy p.
>dose at the interventional
> reference p. (DIRP)
>E p.
>equal pressure p. (EPP)
>Erb p.
>exit p.
>F p.
>Guéneau de Mussy p.
>hinge p.
>inflection p.
>interventional reference p.
>isoelectric p.
>J p.
>lower inflection p. (LIP)
>p. of maximal impulse (PMI)
>p. of maximum impulse (PMI)
>p. of maximum intensity
>null p.
>O p.
>pivot p.
>reference p.
>sella nasion p. A (SNA)
>sella nasion p. B (SNB)
>p. tenderness
>upper infection p.
>Z p.

pointes
>quinidine-induced torsade de p.
>torsade de p. (TDP, TdP)

point-of-care (POC)
>p.-o.-c. analysis
>p.-o.-c. testing (POCT)
>p.-o.-c. testing device

Poiseuille
>P. equation
>P. law
>P. resistance formula

poisoning
>arsenic p.
>arsine gas p.
>fluorocarbon p.
>lead p.
>mercury p.
>oxygen p.

Poisson regression

pokkuri sudden arrhythmia-death
> **syndrome**
polacrilex chewing gum
polar
>p. coordinate map
>P. Electro sport tester
>p. plate
>P. Vantage XL heart rate monitor

Polaramine
polarcardiography computing system
PolarCath
>P. Peripheral Dilation System
>P. peripheral transluminal
> angioplasty system

Polaris CPAP system
Polaris-DX steerable diagnostic catheter
polarity
>reverse p.

polarization
>electrochemical p.
>fluorescence p.

polarographic method
pole
>4-p. Butterworth filtering
>20-p. steerable mapping catheter

Polhemus-Schafer-Ivemark syndrome
Polichinelle
>voix de P.

policy, pl. **policies**
>chest pain p. (CPP)

poliomyelitis
poliovirus vaccine, live, trivalent, oral
polixus
>*Rhodnius p.*

pollen asthma
pollution
>air p.
>photochemical air p.

poloxamer 188
polyacrylamide gel electrophoresis
polyacrylonitrile membrane
polyamide
polyamidoamine
polyamine
>aliphatic p.

polyangiitis
>microscopic p. (MPA)

polyanion precipitation procedure
polyarteritis
>disseminated p.
>hypertensive pulmonary p.
>p. nodosa

polyarthritis
polyblennia
polycarbonate urethane
polycardia
polychondritis
>relapsing p. (RP)

Polycitra-K

polyclonal gammopathy
polycrotic
polycrotism
polycyclic aromatic hydrocarbon (PAH)
polycystic
    p. kidney
    p. kidney disease
    p. lung
    p. tumor
polycythemia
    compensatory p.
    p. hypertonica
    p. vera
polydactyly
polyene
polyestradiol
polyether alcohol asthma
polyethylene
    p. glycol (PEG)
    p. glycol electrolyte lavage solution
     (PEG-LES)
    p. terephthalate (PET)
    p. terephthalate balloon
Polyflex
    P. lead
    P. stent
Polygam S/D
polygenic
    p. hypercholesterolemia
    p. hyperlipidemia
polyglandular autoimmune syndrome
  type II
polyglycolic acid
polygonal arcade
polygraph
    Mackenzie p.
    Night Owl pocket p.
polyharmonic
polyhedral surface reconstruction
PolyHeme blood substitute
polyhydroxybutyrate polymer
poly-L-lactic
    p.-L-l. acid (PLLA)
    p.-L-l. acid stent
polylysine
    benzylpenicilloyl p. (PPL)
    penicilloyl p. (PPL)
polymer
    p. fume fever (PFF)
    hyaluronic acid p.
    plastic p.
    polyhydroxybutyrate p.
    polyphosphate esters p.
polymerase
    p. chain reaction (PCR)
    Taq DNA p.
polymeric endoluminal paving stent
polymetabolic syndrome
polymicrobial pneumonia

polymorphic
    p. premature ventricular complex
    p. slow wave
    p. ventricular tachycardia
polymorphism
    ACE deletion/insertion p.
    adducin p.
    angiotensin-converting enzyme
     deletion/insertion p.
    beta-receptor p.
    gene p.
    paraoxonase p.
    restriction fragment length p.
     (RFLP)
    single-nucleotide p. (SNP)
    TNF-alpha promotor p.
    tumor necrosis factor-alpha
     promotor p.
polymorphonuclear
    p. leukocyte (PMN)
    p. neutrophil (PMN)
    p. neutrophil-dominated
     inflammation
polymorphous ventricular tachycardia
polymyalgia rheumatica syndrome
polymyositis-dermatomyositis (PM-DM)
polymyxa
    Bacillus p.
polyneuritiformis
    heredopathia atactica p.
polyneuropathy
    amyloid p.
    ascending p.
    familial amyloid p. (FAP)
    idiopathic p.
    p., organomegaly, endocrinopathy,
     monoclonal gammopathy, skin
     changes (POEMS)
    Roussy-Lévy p.
    synthesis p.
polyolefin
    p. copolymer (POC)
    p. copolymer balloon
polyorganophosphazene-coated stent
polyostotic fibrous dysplasia
polyp
    bronchial p.
    bronchial inflammatory p.
    cardiac p.
polypeptide
    atrial natriuretic p. (ANP)
    gastric inhibitory p. (GIP)
    pancreatic p. (PP)
polyphaga
    Acanthamoeba p.
polyphenol
    red wine p.
polyphosphate esters polymer
polyphosphoinositide

P

571

polypill
polyploidy
polypoid
    p. bronchitis
    p. connective tissue plug
polypoidal lesion
polyposis
    nasal p.
polypous endocarditis
polypropylene
    p. intracardiac patch
    p. stent
polyribosylribitol
    p. phosphate (PRP)
    p. phosphate-diphtheria toxoid
      conjugate
polysaccharide-iron complex
polysaccharide storage disease
PolySafe A-track lead
polyserositis
    familial paroxysmal p.
    periodic p.
polysomatic
polysome
polysomnogram (PSG)
    Nihon Kohden p.
    nocturnal p. (NPSG)
polysomnographic index
polysomnography (PSG)
    attended p.
    full-night attended p.
    home unattended p.
    in-home unattended p.
    nocturnal p.
    overnight p.
    telemonitored p.
    unattended p.
polysplenia
    p. syndrome
Polystan
    P. cardiotomy reservoir
    P. perfusion cannula
    P. venous return catheter
polystyrene latex microsphere
polytef
    p. artificial vessel
    p. implant
polytef-sheathed needle
polytetrafluoroethylene (PTFE)
    p. covered stent
    expanded p. (ePTFE)
    predilated p.
    p. prosthesis
    p. stent graft
polytetrafluoroethylene-covered coronary stent graft
polythiazide
    prazosin and p.

polyunsaturated
    p. fat
    p. fatty acid (PUFA)
polyurethane
    p. foam
    p. foam embolus
polyuria
polyvinyl
    p. alcohol (PVA)
    p. chloride (PVC)
    p. chloride balloon
    p. chloride tube
    p. prosthesis
POM
    pulse oximetry monitoring
Pompe disease
Ponceau S staining
ponderal index
ponderance
    ventricular p.
Pondocillin
ponopalmosis
Ponstel
Pontiac fever
pontine
    p. hyperintensity (PHI)
    p. infarct (PI)
    p. ischemic rarefaction
    p. myelinolysis
Pontocaine
P-on-T wave
pool
    blood p.
pooling
poor
    p. exercise tolerance (PET)
    p. expiratory effort
    p. R-wave progression
poorly
    p. differentiated carcinoma
    p. reversible asthma
POPC
    postoperative pulmonary complication
popcorn
    p. calcification
    p. worker's lung
popliteal
    p. aneurysm
    p. artery
    p. pulse
pop-off valve
poppet
    prosthetic p.
    Silastic p.
popping sensation
POPS
    postoperative pacing study
POR
    postocclusive oscillatory response

porcelain aorta
porcine
    p. aortic valve
    p. bioprosthesis
    p. coronary artery
    p. factor VIII
    p. gelatin sponge
    p. heterograft
    p. prosthesis
    p. prosthetic valve
    p. xenograft
pore
    alveolar p.
    Kohn p.
porfimer
pork
    p. insulin
    p. NPH Iletin II
    p. Regular Iletin II
porphyria
    acute intermittent p. (AIP)
porphyrin
Porphyromonas gingivalis
Porstmann technique
PORT
    postoperative radiotherapy
port
    p. access technique
    CathLink 20 implanted p.
    P. Charles influenza
    chest p.
    entrainment p.
    Import vascular access p.
    Luer-Lok p.
    Q P.
    SEA p.
    side-arm pressure p.
    titanium p.
    Triumph VTX p.
porta, pl. **portae**
    p. hepatis
    p. lienis
    P. Pulse 3 defibrillator
portable
    p. aerosol delivery device
    p. chest radiograph
    p. monitoring device
    p. monitor of respiratory
      parameters (PMRP)
    p. oxygen cylinder
    p. oxygen device
    p. oxygen monitor
    p. volume ventilator
Port-A-Cath
    P.-A-C. device
    P.-A-C. implantable catheter system
portacaval (PC)
    p. anastomosis (PCA)
    p. bypass (PCB)

    p. H graft
    p. shunt (PCS)
    p. transposition (PCT)
port-access
    P.-a. coronary artery bypass
      grafting
    P.-a. minimally invasive cardiac
      surgery
    St. Jude Medical P.-a.
portae (*pl. of* porta)
Portagen diet
portal
    p. circulation
    p. hypertension (PHT)
    p. perfusion pressure (PPP)
    p. pressure gradient (PPG)
    p. pyemia
    p. systemic hypertension
    p. vein (PV)
    p. vein dilation (PVD)
    p. vein thrombosis (PVT)
    p. venous flow (PVF)
Porta-Resp monitor
Porter sign
Portex
    P. Per-fit tracheostomy kit
    P. Per-fit tracheostomy tube
    P. Soft-Seal cuff system
portion
    infradiaphragmatic p.
    p. of segment between end of S
      wave and beginning of T wave
      (ST)
    stenotic p.
portogram
portography
    arterial p.
    computed tomography
      angiographic p. (CTAP)
    computed tomography in arterial p.
      (CTAP)
    splenic p.
    transthoracic p. (THP)
portoportal anastomosis
portopulmonary
    p. hypertension
    p. shunt
portosystemic anastomosis
portovenography
Porvidx early lung cancer screening
PORxin technology
Posadas mycosis
Posadas-Wernicke disease
Posey Cufflator tracheal cuff inflator and manometer
position
    Andral decubitus p.
    anteroposterior paddle p.
    body p.

position *(continued)*
    electrical heart p.
    good lung down p.
    heart p.
    LAO p.
    left anterior oblique p.
    RAO p.
    RA-RV p.
    recovery p.
    right anterior oblique p.
    scalloped subcoronary p.
    semilateral supine p.
    shock p.
    sniffing p.
    Trendelenburg p.
    tricuspid p.
positional obstructive sleep apnea syndrome
positioner
    CAS-8000V general angiography p.
    Thornton anterior p. (TAP)
positioning
    anteroposterior paddle p.
    prone p.
positive
    p. afterpotential
    p. airway pressure (PAP)
    p. airway pressure gas modulator
    p. airway. pressure ventilation
    p. arterial remodeling
    p. chronotropism
    p. end-airway pressure (PEAP)
    p. end-expiratory pressure (PEEP)
    p. end-expiratory pressure-related alveolar recruitment
    p. expiratory pressure (PEP)
    false p.
    p. inspiratory pressure (PIP)
    p. predictive value (PPV)
    p. pressure
    p. pressure mechanical ventilation
    p. pressure ventilation (PPV)
    p. support ventilator (PSV)
    P. Symptom Distress Index (PSDI)
    p. symptom total (PST)
    p. treppe
positive-negative pressure breathing (PNPB)
Positrol II catheter
positron
    p. emission tomography (PET)
    p. emitter
Possis AngioJet
post
    p. balloon angioplasty restenosis
    p. bypass spasm
    p. graft (PG)
    p. hoc analysis
postabsorptive state

postanesthesia
    p. care unit (PACU)
    p. pulmonary edema
    p. respiratory depression
postanginal
postangioplasty
postantibiotic effect (PAE)
postbronchodilator
postbypass
postcapillary hypertension
postcardiac injury syndrome (PCIS)
postcardiotomy
    p. psychosis syndrome
    p. shock
    p. syndrome (PCS)
postcardioversion pulmonary edema
postcatheterization
postcoital asthma
postcommissurotomy syndrome
postcontrast echocardiogram
postcoronary care unit (PCCU)
postdiastolic
postdicrotic
postdiphtheritic stenosis
postdischarge graded-exercise test (PD-GXT)
postdiuresis scan
postdrive depression
postductal
POSTEC
postectopic pause
posterior
    p. airway space (PAS)
    p. approach
    p. basal segmental artery
    p. basal segmental artery of right lung
    p. branch of right superior
    p. cerebral artery (PCA)
    p. circulation (PC)
    p. circulation infarct (POCI)
    p. circulation syndrome (POCS)
    p. circumflex artery (PC)
    p. communicating artery (PcomA)
    p. cricoarytenoid muscle
    p. descending artery (PDA)
    p. descending branch
    p. diamond-shaped chink
    p. inferior cerebellar artery (PICA)
    p. inferior communicating artery (PICA)
    p. isthmus
    p. junction line
    p. leaflet
    p. leaf mitral valve (PLMV)
    p. left ventricle (PLV)
    p. left ventricular wall motion on echocardiogram
    p. limb of internal capsule (PLIC)

p. margin of pulmonary artery (PPA)
p. mediastinal mass
p. mitral (PM)
p. mitral leaflet (PML)
p. mitral valve leaflet (pML, PMVL, pMVL)
p. myocardial infarction
p. nasal spine (PNS)
p. papillary muscle (PPM)
p. pulmonary artery (PPA)
p. pulmonary leaflet (PPL)
p. Q wave
regio p.
regio cruris p.
p. rib fracture
p. right coronary artery (pRCA)
p. tibial pulse
p. tricuspid leaflet (PTL)
p. upper lung zone
p. wall (PW)
p. wall of aortic root (PAR)
p. wall excursion (PWE)
p. wall infarct (PWI)
p. wall of left ventricle (PWLV)
p. wall thickness
posterius
segmentum bronchopulmonale p.
segmentum bronchopulmonale basale p.
posteroinferior dyskinesis
posterolateral
p. circumflex branch (PLCx)
p. descending branch
p. segment artery (PLSA)
p. segment [coronary] artery (PLSA)
p. thoracotomy
posteroseptal wall
postesophageal
postexercise
p. echocardiogram
p. flow volume loop
p. scan
postextrasystolic (PES)
p. aberrancy
p. beat
p. pause
p. potentiation (PESP)
p. T wave
postganglionic vagal stimulation (PGVS)
postheparin
p. lipolytic activity (PHLA)
p. phospholipase (PHP)
p. plasma diamine oxidase (PHD)
posthyperventilation apnea
postictal state
postinfarct
p. cardiosclerosis

p. patient
p. ventricular remodeling
postinfarction
p. angina
p. late potential (PILP)
p. pericarditis
p. period
p. risk stratification (PIRS)
p. syndrome
p. ventricular septal defect
postinfectious bradycardia
postinfective bradycardia
postinflammatory
postinfluenza asthenia
postinjury
p. empyema
p. immunosuppression
postinterventional followup
postintervention hemodynamic index
postischemic
p. dysfunction
p. heart
p. myocardium
postmenopausal
postmicturition syncope
postmitotic
postmortem
p. clot
p. thrombus
postmyocardial
p. infarction
p. infarction syndrome (PMIS)
p. injury pericarditis
postnasal
p. catarrh
p. drainage syndrome (PNDS)
p. drip (PND)
p. drip due to rhinitis (PND-Rh)
p. drip due to sinusitis (PND-Si)
p. drip syndrome (PNDS)
postobstructive
p. atelectasis
p. pneumonia
postocclusion hyperemia
postocclusive oscillatory response (POR)
postoperative
p. atrial fibrillation
p. atrial fibrillation in cardiac surgery (PACS)
p. chest radiograph
p. cognitive deficit (POCD)
p. constrictive pericarditis (PCP)
p. endocarditis
p. hemorrhage (POH)
p. hypertension
p. low cardiac output (PLCO)
p. pacing study (POPS)
p. pericarditis

P

postoperative *(continued)*
    p. pulmonary complication (POPC)
    p. radiotherapy (PORT)
postparalytic syndrome
postpartum
    p. cardiomyopathy (PPCM)
    p. hypertension
postperfusion
    p. arrhythmia
    p. lung
    p. psychosis
    p. syndrome
postpericardiotomy syndrome (PPS)
postpharyngeal space
postphlebitic syndrome
postpneumonectomy tuberculous empyema
postpneumonic
postprandial
    p. angina
    p. blood sugar
    p. hypotension
    p. lipemia (PPL)
postprimary tuberculosis
postprocedural management
postpump
    p. image
    p. syndrome
postrandomization
postrema
postrenal azotemia
postresuscitation
postresuscitative death
postrheumatic cusp retraction
postsphygmic
    p. interval
    p. period
poststenotic (PST)
    p. dilation (PSD)
post-stenting restenosis
poststreptococcal
    p. glomerulonephritis
    p. inflammatory process
poststroke pruritus
postsynaptic cholinergic mechanism
postsystolic shortening
posttest
    Tukey-Kramer p.
postthrombolytic therapy
posttransfusion syndrome
posttransplantation
    p. lymphoproliferative disorder (PTLPD, PTLD)
    p. malignancy
    p. survival
posttransplant lymphoproliferative disorder
posttraumatic
    p. ARDS

    p. pseudoaneurysm
    p. pulmonary pseudocyst
posttussive
    p. emesis
    p. syncope
postural
    P. Assessment Scale for Stroke Patient
    p. drainage (PD)
    p. drainage of infected secretion
    p. drainage and percussion (PD&P)
    p. drainage, percussion, vibration (PDPV)
    p. hypotension
    p. orthostatic tachycardia syndrome (POTS)
    p. syncope
posture
    Stern p.
    p. technique
posturing
    decerebrate p.
    posturing decerebrate p.
postventricular
    p. atrial blanking (PVAB)
    p. atrial refractory period (PVARP)
Potain sign
potassium (K)
    p. aminosalicylate
    amoxicillin and clavulanate p.
    canrenoate p.
    p. channel opener
    p. chloride (KCl)
    p. chloride cardioplegia
    p. citrate and citric acid
    p. gluconate
    glucose, insulin, p. (GIK, GIP)
    p. hydroxide (KOH)
    p. inhibition
    p. iodide
    p. ion
    losartan p.
    penicillin V p.
    ticarcillin and clavulanate p.
    p. wasting
potassium/hydrochlorothiazide
    losartan p./h.
potassium-sparing diuretic
potassium-wasting diuretic
potential
    action p.
    bioelectric p.
    cardiac action p.
    compound motor action p. (CMAP)
    diastolic p.
    electrical p.
    endocardial p. (ECP)
    endogenous thrombin p. (ETP)
    fast induction steady state p.

fibrillation p.
heart synchronized evoked p.
   (HSEP)
His bundle p.
interpulse p. (Ipp)
Kent p.
late diastolic p. (LDP)
maximum diastolic p. (MDP)
maximum negative p.
membrane p.
monophasic action p. (MAP)
motor evoked p. (MEP)
nerve action p.
pacemaker p.
peroxyl radical-trapping p.
postinfarction late p. (PILP)
putative slow pathway p.
resting membrane p.
right ventricular endocardial p
   (RVECP)
sensory nerve action p. (SNAP)
sinus node p. (SNP)
somatosensory evoked p. (SSEP)
spike-and-dome p.
total peroxyl radical-trapping
   antioxidant p. (TRAP)
transmembrane p.
ventricular late p. (VLP)
potentiated twitch force
potentiation
   interval-dependent p.
   postextrasystolic p. (PESP)
   twitch p.
potentiator
POTS
   postural orthostatic tachycardia syndrome
Pott aneurysm
Pottenger sign
potter's
   p. asthma
   p. phthisis
Potts
   P. anastomosis
   P. bronchial forceps
   P. needle
   P. operation
   P. procedure
   P. shunt
Potts-Cournand needle
Potts-Smith anastomosis
pouch
   Cardio-Cool myocardial
      protection p.
   p. hematoma
   laryngeal p.
   myocardial protection p.
   pharyngeal p.
poudrage
   Beck epicardial p.

epicardial p.
pericardial p.
pleural p.
talc p.
pound
   p.'s per square inch (psi)
   p.'s per square inch gauge (psig)
Pourcelot index
POV
   pulmonary occlusive venopathy
povidone-iodine
powder
   Acarosan dust mite p.
   budesonide inhalation p.
   dust mite p.
   fluticasone propionate and
      salmeterol inhalation p.
   formoterol fumarate p.
   inhalation p.
   lyophilized p.
powdered tantalum
power
   cardiac p.
   p. Doppler ultrasound
   exercise cardiac p. (ECP)
   p. failure
   P. Grip Over the Wire Stent
      Delivery system
   P. Grip stent
   p. infusion device
   p. injector
   left ventricular p.
   p. M-mode transcranial Doppler
   p. motion imaging
   P. Pulse spray (PPS)
   resolving p.
   spectral p.
   p. spectral analysis
   p. spectral density (PSD)
   p. spectrum of HRV
   ventricular p.
Powerflex
   P. angioplasty balloon
   P. Extreme PTA balloon catheter
   P. P3 high pressure balloon
      catheter
Powerheart
   P. AECD
   P. AED
   P. automated external defibrillator
   P. automatic external cardioverter-
      defibrillator
   P. defibrillator-monitor
PowerLine catheter
Powerlink
   P. endovascular graft
   P. system

P

PowerSail
P. balloon
P. coronary dilation catheter
PP
pancreatic polypeptide
paradoxical pulse
parietal pericardium
parietal pulse
partial pressure
pulse pressure
pulsus paradoxus
purulent pericarditis
PPA
posterior margin of pulmonary artery
posterior pulmonary artery
pure pulmonary atresia
Ppa
pulmonary artery pressure
PPACK
D-Phe-L-Pro-L-Arg-chloromethyl ketone
PPAR
peroxisome proliferator-activated receptor
PPAR-gamma
peroxisome proliferator-activated receptor
gamma
PPAS
peripheral pulmonary artery stenosis
Ppaw
pulmonary artery wedge pressure
PPC
pneumopericardium
PPCF
peripartum cardiac failure
PPCID
PPCID sequential foot compression
device
PPCID slippers
PPCM
postpartum cardiomyopathy
PPD
purified protein derivative
PPD skin test
P&PD
percussion and postural drainage
Ppeak
peak airway pressure
PPG
photoplethysmography
portal pressure gradient
PPH
primary pulmonary hypertension
PPHN
persistent pulmonary hypertension of
newborn
P-P interval
PPL
benzylpenicilloyl polylysine
penicilloyl polylysine
posterior pulmonary leaflet

postprandial lipemia
PPL skin test
Ppl
pleural pressure
Pplat
plateau pressure
PPLO
pleuropneumonia-like organism
PPM
permanent pacemaker
posterior papillary muscle
prosthesis-patient mismatch
pulse position modulated
ppm
part per million
pulses per minute
PPP
platelet-poor plasma
portal perfusion pressure
PPPBL
peripheral pulses palpable both legs
PPPPPP
pain, pallor, pulselessness, paresthesia,
paralysis, prostration
PPR
physiologic pattern release
PPR verapamil
PPRE
peroxisome proliferator response element
PPS
peripheral pulmonic stenosis
postpericardiotomy syndrome
Power Pulse spray
PPS murmur
pPTCA
primary percutaneous transluminal
coronary angioplasty
PPV
positive predictive value
positive pressure ventilation
Ppw
pulmonary wedge pressure
P-Q, PQ
pressure flow
PQ interval
P-Q segment depression
p/q opacity
P:QRS ratio
PR
pulmonary regurgitation
pulse rate
pulse repetition
time between P wave and beginning of
QRS complex
PR duration to diastolic duration
(PRi)
PR interval
PR segment

P&R
    pulse and respiration
PRA
    panel of reactive antibodies
    panel-reactive antibody
    plasma renin activity
PR-AC measurement
practitioner
    respiratory care p. (RCP)
practolol
^{32}**P radioactive stent**
praecox
    ascites p.
    lymphedema p.
2-pralidoxime (2-PAM)
pranayama breathing technique
pranlukast
prasugrel
Pravachol
pravastatin sodium
prawn asthma
praxis
praziquantel
prazosin
    p. hydrochloride
    p. and polythiazide
pRCA
    posterior right coronary artery
preacinar vessel
preamplifier
    Arzco p.
preanesthetic
prearteriolar vessel
preatheroma
preautomatic pause
pre-beta 1 HDL
precapillary
    p. anastomosis
    p. arteriole
    p. pulmonary hypertension
    p. sphincter
precardiac mesoderm
precatheterization
Precedex
Precept lead
precipitation
    heparin-induced extracorporeal low-
        density lipoprotein p. (HELP)
precipitin
precipitous drop in blood pressure
Precise self-expanding stent
Preclude pericardial membrane
preconditioning
    ischemic p. (IPC)
    p. phenomenon
    p. signal
    p. stimulus
precordial (PC)
    p. A wave

    p. bulge
    p. catch syndrome
    p. electrocardiographic monitoring
        (PEM)
    p. electrocardiography
    p. heave
    p. honk
    p. lead
    p. motion
    p. movement
    p. pulse
    p. ST depression
    p. ST segment
    p. thrill
    p. thump
    p. thumpversion
    p. whoop
precordialgia
precordium
    quiet p.
precoronary
    p. angioplasty
    p. care (PCC)
    p. care area (PCA)
Precose
Predator PTCA catheter
predeposit autologous donation
prediastole
prediastolic murmur
predicrotic
predicted
    p. cardiac output (PCO)
    p. maximal heart rate (PMHR)
prediction
    code excited linear p. (CELP)
predictive
    p. index
    p. index for myocardial infarction
        (PIMI)
    p. survival marker
    p. value
predictor
    APACHE CV Risk P.
    Corazonix P.
    univariate p.
predilated
    p. polytetrafluoroethylene
    p. polytetrafluoroethylene graft
    p. polytetrafluoroethylene obstruction
    p. polytetrafluoroethylene stent
predischarge test
prednisolone
    methyl p.
    systemic p.
Prednisol TBA injection
prednisone
predominance
    zonal p.
predominant emphysema

P

predose level
preductal
preeclampsia
preejection
p. period (PEP)
p. period index (PEPI)
preexcitation (PE)
left lateral ventricular p. (LLVP)
left posterior ventricular p. (LPVP)
right posterior ventricular p. (RPVP)
p. syndrome (PES)
ventricular p.
preexcited atrial fibrillation
preexisting condition
preexposure prophylaxis
preganglionic tumor
pregnancy, pl. **pregnancies**
anaphylactoid syndrome of p.
dyspnea of p.
pregnancy-induced hypertension (PIH)
prehospital cardiac arrest (PCA)
prehypertensive
preimplantation diagnosis (PID)
preinfarction
p. angina (PIA)
p. syndrome (PIS)
preinterventional high-grade stenosis
prekallikrein
prelaryngeales
nodi lymphoidei p.
prelaryngeal lymph node
preload
cardiac p.
p. reduction
p. reserve
ventricular p.
Prelone Oral
premature
p. atherosclerosis
p. atrial beat (PAB, PAC)
p. atrial complex
p. atrial contraction (PAC)
p. atrial extrastimulus
p. atrial stimulus (PAS)
p. atrioventricular junctional complex
p. beat (PB)
p. contraction
p. diastolic distention
p. excitation
p. junctional beat
p. junctional contraction (PJC)
p. mitral closure (PMC)
p. nodal beat (PNB)
p. nodal contracture (PNC)
p. systole
p. valve closure
ventricular p. (VP, Vp)

p. ventricular beat (PVB)
p. ventricular complex
p. ventricular complex-trigger hypothesis
p. ventricular contraction (PVC)
p. ventricular depolarization (PVD)
p. ventricular extrasystole (PVE)
p. ventricular systole (PVS)
prematurity
chronic pulmonary insufficiency of p.
retinopathy of p. (ROP)
premedication
premonitory
p. palpitation
p. syndrome
premotor cortex (PMC)
premounted stent
prenalterol hydrochloride
prenylamine
preoperative antibiotic
preparation
antilymphocyte antibody p.
insulin p.
isometrically contracting myocardial p.
Langendorff heart p.
preperitoneal
p. dilator balloon (PDB)
p. fat
preprandial
prepump image
prerenal azotemia
presacral edema
presaturation pulse
presbycardia
presbyesophagus
presbylaryngia
prescription
P. Analyses and Cost (PACT)
P. Drug User Fee Act (PDUFA)
exercise p.
present
peripheral pulse p.
presentation
reciprocal p.
roentgenographic p.
preservation
tissue p.
preservative-free
p.-f. intrathecal papaverine
p.-f. solution (PFS)
preserved left ventricular systolic function
preshaped catheter
presphygmic
p. interval
p. period
Press-mate SAT

pressor
    p. drug
    p. effect
pressoreceptive
pressoreceptor reflex
pressosensitive
pressosensitivity
    reflexogenic p.
pressure (P)
    absolute p.
    active p. (AP)
    adjustable dilation p.
    airway p.
    airway-esophageal balloon p.
    alveolar p. (Palv)
    alveolar-capillary intravascular p.
    alveolar carbon dioxide p.
    alveolar oxygen partial p. (PAO_2)
    ambient p.
    ambulatory blood p. (ABP)
    ambulatory venous p. (AVP)
    aortic p. (AOP, AoP, AP)
    aortic blood p. (AoBP)
    aortic dicrotic notch p.
    aortic mean p. (AOMP, AoMP)
    aortic pullback p.
    aortic systolic p. (ASP)
    p. applied dressing (PAD, P.A.D.)
    area diastolic p. (ADP)
    area systolic p. (ASP)
    arterial p. (AP)
    arterial blood p. (ABP, aBP)
    arterial carbon dioxide p.
    arterial dicrotic notch p.
    arterial oxygen partial p. (PaO_2)
    ascending aortic p. (PAo)
    ascending aortic blood p.
    assisted peak systolic p. (APSP)
    atmospheres of p.
    atmospheric p. (P_{atm})
    atrial p. (PA)
    atrial filling p.
    p. augmentation (PA)
    automatic positive airway p.
     (APAP)
    average diastolic p. (AVDP)
    average mean p. (AMP)
    back p.
    balloon aortic end-diastolic p.
     (BAEDP)
    balloon inflation p.
    barometric p.
    beat-to-beat finger arterial p.
    bilevel positive airway p. (BiPAP)
    blood p. (BP, B/P)
    brachial artery p. (BrAP)
    capillary p. (CP)
    capillary hydrostatic p. (CHP)
    capillary wedge p.

carbon dioxide p.
cardiovascular p.
central venous p. (CVP)
cerebral perfusion p. (CPP)
chest wall elastic recoil p. (Pth)
coaxial p.
colloidal osmotic p. (COP)
colloid oncotic p. (COP)
colloid osmotic p.
compliance, rate, oxygenation, p.
 (CROP)
continuous positive airway p.
 (CPAP)
p. control (PC)
p. controller
p. control ventilation
p. conversion
coronary perfusion p. (CPP)
coronary sinus occlusion p. (CSOP)
coronary venous p.
cricoid p.
p. cycled ventilator
p. decay
deep venous p. (DVP)
delta p. (delta P)
diastolic p. (DP, Pd)
diastolic aortic p. (DAP)
diastolic blood p. (DBP)
diastolic filling p. (DFP)
diastolic pulmonary artery p.
differential blood p.
dilation p.
distal coronary occlusion p.
 (DCOP)
distal coronary perfusion p.
Donders p.
Doppler p.
downstream venous p. (DSVP)
dynamic p.
effective systolic p. (ESP)
elastic recoil p.
end-diastolic p. (EDP)
end-diastolic left ventricular p.
end-expiratory esophageal p.
endocardial p.
end-systolic p. (ESP)
end-systolic left ventricular p.
erect diastolic blood p. (EDBP)
expiratory positive airway p.
 (EPAP)
external cardiac p. (ECP)
extreme p. (EP)
femoral artery p.
femoral blood p. (FBP)
filling p. (FP)
finger systolic blood p. (FSBP)
p. flow (P-Q, PQ)
p. garment
gastric-intrapleural p. (Pg-Ppl)

P

pressure *(continued)*
    p. gradient
    p. guide pressure wire
    p. half-time (PHT)
    p. half-time technique
    high blood p. (HBP)
    hyperbaric p.
    inferior vena cava p. (IVCP)
    inflation p.
    p. injector
    inspiratory occlusion p.
    inspiratory positive airway p. (IPAP)
    inspiratory resistance and positive expiratory p. (IR-PEP)
    intermittent positive p. (IPP)
    intermittent positive airway p. (IPAP)
    intraalveolar p.
    intracardiac p.
    intracellular p.
    intracoronary p.
    intracranial p. (ICP)
    intramyocardial p.
    intrapericardial p. (IPP)
    intrapleural oncotic p.
    intrathoracic p.
    intravascular p. (IVP)
    intrinsic positive end-expiratory p. (PEEPi)
    Joint National Committee on Prevention, Detection, Evaluation, and Treatment of High Blood P.
    jugular venous p. (JVP)
    juxtacardiac pleural p.
    labile blood p.
    left anterior descending arterial p. (LADP)
    left atrial p. (LAP, PLa, Pla)
    left atrial transmural p. (LATP)
    left ventricular p. (LVP, PLV)
    left ventricular developed p. (LVDP)
    left ventricular diastolic p. (LVDP)
    left ventricular end-diastolic p. (LVEDP, LVEP)
    left ventricular filling p. (LVFP)
    left ventricular systolic p. (LVSP)
    limited peak inspiratory p.
    low blood p. (LBP)
    lower body negative p. (LBNP)
    lung elastic recoil p. (Pel)
    maximal exercise systolic p. (MESP)
    maximal expiratory p. (MEP)
    maximal expiratory mouth p. (P_{Emax})
    maximal inspiratory p. (MIP)
    maximal inspiratory mouth p. (P_{Imax})
    maximal sniff-induced esophageal p.
    maximal sniff-induced gastric p.
    maximal sniff-induced transdiaphragmatic p.
    maximum closure p. (MCP)
    maximum expiratory p. (MEP)
    maximum expiratory airflow-static lung elastic recoil p.
    maximum inspiratory p. (MIP)
    maximum left ventricular p. (LVPmax)
    mean p. (PM)
    mean airway p. (MAP, Paw)
    mean aortic p. (MAP)
    mean arterial p. (MAP)
    mean arterial blood p. (MABP, MBP)
    mean blood p. (MBP)
    mean daily erect blood p. (MDEBP)
    mean daily supine blood p. (MDSBP)
    mean diastolic left ventricular p.
    mean intravascular p. (MIP)
    mean left atrial p. (MLAP)
    mean maternal arterial blood p. (MMAP)
    mean pulmonary artery p. (MPAP, PAPm)
    mean pulmonary artery wedge p. (MPAWP)
    mean pulmonary venous p. (MPVP)
    mean resting diastolic blood p. (MDBP)
    mean right atrial p. (MRAP)
    mean right ventricular p. (MRVP)
    mean systemic arterial p. (MSAP)
    mean systolic left ventricular p.
    p. measurement
    minimum audible p. (MAP)
    minimum left ventricular p. (LVPmin)
    MPA p.
    narrowed pulse p.
    nasal continuous positive airway p. (NCPAP, nCPAP)
    p. necrosis
    negative end-expiratory p. (NEEP)
    negative expiratory p. (NEP)
    negative intrapleural p.
    noninvasive blood p. (NIBP)
    noninvasive ventilation with positive p.
    normal intravascular p.
    oncotic p.
    opening p.

osmotic p.
p. overload
p. overload-induced aortic valve
  calcific thickening
PA p.
PA filling p.
partial p. (P, PP)
peak airway p. (Ppeak)
peak diastolic p. (PDP)
peak inspiratory p. (PIP)
peak left ventricular p. (PLVP)
peak negative p. (P-min, PNP)
peak positive p. (P+max)
peak pulmonary artery p.
peak systolic p. (PSP)
peak systolic aortic p. (PSAP)
peak systolic gradient p.
perfusion p.
pericardial p.
peripheral coronary p. (PCP)
peripheral venous p. (PVP)
plasma colloid osmotic p.
plateau p. (Pplat)
p. plethysmograph
pleural p. (Ppl)
p. pneumothorax
portal perfusion p. (PPP)
positive p.
positive airway p. (PAP)
positive end-airway p. (PEAP)
positive end-expiratory p. (PEEP)
positive expiratory p. (PEP)
positive inspiratory p. (PIP)
precipitous drop in blood p.
PSG p.
pullback p.
pulmonary arterial capillary
  wedge p. (PACWP)
pulmonary arterial end-diastolic p.
pulmonary arterial pressure,
  pulmonary venous p. (pa-pv)
pulmonary arterial wave p.
pulmonary artery p. (PAP, Ppa)
pulmonary artery diastolic p.
  (PADP)
pulmonary artery end-diastolic p.
  (PAEDP)
pulmonary artery mean p. (PAMP)
pulmonary artery occlusion p.
  (PAo, PAOP)
pulmonary artery occlusive
  wedge p.
pulmonary artery systolic p.
  (PASP)
pulmonary artery wedge p.
  (PAWP, Ppaw)
pulmonary capillary p. (PCP)
pulmonary capillary wedge p.
  (PCWP)

pulmonary hypertension p.
pulmonary vascular p.
pulmonary venous p. (PVP)
pulmonary wedge p. (Ppw, PWP)
pulse p. (PP)
p. pulse
p. pulse differentiation
PW p.
radial artery systolic p. (RASP)
p. range
p. recovery
resting pulmonary vein-left
  atrium p.
resting venous p. (RVP)
right atrial p. (RAP)
right atrial mean p. (RAMP)
right ventricular p. (RVP)
right ventricular diastolic p.
right ventricular end-diastolic p.
  (RVEDP)
right ventricular filling p. (RVFP)
right ventricular peak systolic p.
right ventricular systolic p. (RVSP)
RVED p.
seated diastolic blood p. (SDBP)
segmental limb p. (SLP)
segmental limb systolic p. (SLP)
shunt p. (SP)
p. sling
sniff nasal inspiratory p.
standing diastolic blood p. (SDBP)
standing venous p. (SVP)
p. stasis
stopped flow p. (SFP)
stump p.
supersystemic pulmonary artery p.
supine diastolic blood p. (SDBP)
p. support ventilation (PSV)
p. support ventilator (PSV)
systemic arterial p. (SAP)
systemic blood p. (Psa)
systemic mean arterial p. (SMAP)
systolic p. (Ps, SP)
systolic arterial blood p. (SABP)
systolic atrial p. (SAP)
systolic blood p. (BPS, SBP, SYS-
  BP)
systolic left ventricular p.
systolic pulmonary artery p. (sPAP)
p. time product (PTP)
torr p.
total p. (P_T)
p. tracing
transdiaphragmatic p.
p. transducer
p. transducer airflow sensor
transesophageal p.
transmural p.
transmyocardial perfusion p.

P

pressure *(continued)*
> transpulmonary p. (Ptp)
> transthoracic p.
> twitch esophageal p.
> twitch gastric p.
> twitch transdiaphragmatic p.
> unintended positive end-expiratory p. (autoPEEP, intrinsic PEEP)
> upper airway closing p. (UACP)
> upper airway opening p. (UAOP)
> p. urticaria
> variable positive airway p. (VPAP)
> venous p. (VP)
> venous blood p. (VBP)
> venous stop flow p. (VSFP)
> ventricular p. (PV)
> ventricular diastolic p.
> ventricular filling p.
> p. volume (PV)
> water vapor p.
> p. wave (PW)
> p. waveform
> wedge p. (WP)
> widening of pulse p.
> zero diastolic blood p.
> zero end-expiratory p. (ZEEP)
> zero end-inspiratory p.
> zero-flow p. (Pzf, ZFP)

pressure-compensated
> p.-c. flow
> p.-c. flow plethysmograph

pressure-controlled
> p.-c. intermittent coronary sinus occlusion (PICSO)
> p.-c. inverse ratio ventilation (PCIRV)
> p.-c. respirator
> p.-c. ventilation (PCV)
> p.-c. ventilation technique

pressure-cycled ventilation

pressure-flow
> p.-f. relation
> p.-f. relationship

pressure-like
> p.-l. sensation
> p.-l. sensation in chest

pressure-natriuresis curve

pressure-overload hypertrophy

pressure-regulated
> p.-r. volume control (PRVC)
> p.-r. volume control ventilation

pressure-volume
> p.-v. analysis
> p.-v. curve
> p.-v. curve measurement
> p.-v. curve measurement using syringe technique
> p.-v. data

> p.-v. diagram
> elastic p.-v. (Pel-V)
> p.-v. loop
> p.-v. relation

PressureWire3 sensor

PressureWire5 sensor

PressureWire guidewire

pressurized metered-dose inhaler (pMDI)

pressurizer
> Oxy-Hood p.

Pressurometer blood pressure monitor

PresTab
> Glynase P.

presternalis
> regio p.

Presto-Flash spirometry system

Presto spirometry system

presyncopal
> p. episode
> p. medication
> p. spell

presyncope
> iterative p.

presystole

presystolic
> p. gallop (PSG)
> p. murmur (PM, PSM)
> p. pressure and volume
> p. pulsation
> p. thrill

pretibial
> p. edema
> p. myxedema

pretracheales
> nodi lymphoidei p.

pretracheal lymph node

pretransplant cachexia

pretreatment
> icatibant p.

Pretz-D

prevalence

Prevel sign

prevention
> Centers for Disease Control and P. (CDC)
> mucin clot p. (MCP)
> primary p.
> secondary p.

preventive allergy treatment

preventricular stenosis

Preveon

prevertebral space

Prevotella melaninogenica

prevotii
> *Peptostreptococcus p.*

PreVue III digitizing system

PREVU(x) skin sterol test

PRF
  pulse repetition frequency
PRHHP
  Puerto Rico Heart Health Program
PRi
  PR duration to diastolic duration
priapism phenotype
prickle cell carcinoma
prick-test method
Priftin
Prima
  P. laser guidewire
  P. Plus porcine tissue valve
  P. Plus stentless valve
  P. total occlusion device
  P. total occlusion system
Primacor
primaquine
  p. phosphate
  p. phosphate antimalarial
primary
  p. alveolar hypoventilation
  p. angioplasty research (PAR)
  p. atelectasis
  p. atypical pneumonia
  p. bronchogenic neoplasm
  p. bronchus
  p. cardiac arrhythmia
  p. cardiac malignancy
  p. ciliary dyskinesia (PCD)
  p. closure
  p. coccidioidomycosis
  p. complex
  p. donor (d(A))
  p. effusion lymphoma (PEL)
  p. electrical disease
  p. endocardial fibroelastosis
  p. eosinophilic pneumonia
  p. fibroproliferative pulmonary
    vasculopathy
  p. graft failure (PGF)
  p. hyperlipidemia
  p. hypertension
  p. idiopathic chylopericardium
  p. infarction (PI)
  p. infection
  p. influenza pneumonia
  p. intracerebral hemorrhage (PICH)
  p. isolated chylopericardium
  p. lung carcinoma
  p. myocardial disease (PMD)
  p. pacemaker
  p. percutaneous transluminal
    coronary angioplasty (pPTCA)
  p. pleural aspergillosis
  p. pleurisy
  p. pleuropulmonary disease
  p. prevention
  p. prophylaxis

  p. pulmonary histiocytosis X
  p. pulmonary hypertension (PPH)
  p. pulmonary hypertension murmur
  p. pulmonary Langerhans cell
    histiocytosis
  p. pulmonary mucormycosis
  p. pulmonary non-Hodgkin
    lymphoma
  p. pulmonary parenchymal disease
  p. restrictive cardiomyopathy
  p. sensorimotor cortex (SM1)
  p. spontaneous pneumothorax (PSP)
  p. systemic amyloidosis
  p. systemic vasculitis
  p. thrombus
  p. tuberculosis
  p. ventricular fibrillation (PVF)
  p. ventricular tachycardia (PVT)
Primatene Mist
Primaxin
prime
  crystalloid p.
  P. ECG electrocardiac mapping
    system
  RR p.
  rsr p.
primed lymphocyte test
priming
  p. dose
  retrograde autologous p.
primitive
  p. aorta
  p. neuroectodermal tumor (PNET)
**Primo noninvasive blood pressure
  measurement system**
primordial catheter tube
primum
  p. atrial septal defect
  interatrial foramen p.
  ostium p.
  persistent ostium p.
  septum p.
Principen
principle
  Beer-Lambert p.
  Castaneda p.
  Fick p.
  Frank-Straub-Wiggers-Starling p.
  hemodynamic p.
  Huygens p.
  Laplace p.
  Pascal p.
Prinivil
PrinterNOx
  P. nitric oxide/nitrogen dioxide
    monitor
  P. nitric oxide with MKII analyzer
Prinzide

P

Prinzmetal
   P. effect
   P. variant angina
prion disease
priori
   a p.
prism method
privet cough
Prizm defibrillator
proaccelerin
proadrenomedullin N-terminal 20 peptide
Pro-Air
ProAmatine
Pro-Amox
Pro-Ampi
proANF
   proatrial natriuretic factor
   N-terminal proANF
proapoptotic molecule
proarrhythmia
proarrhythmic effect
proatherosclerotic factor
proatherothrombogenic molecule
proatrial natriuretic factor (proANF)
probability, pl. **probabilities**
   Cooperman event p.
   p. density function (PDF)
   intermediate p.
Pro-Bal Protected balloon-tipped catheter
proband
probe
   acoustic impedance p.
   acridinium ester labeled nucleic
      acid p.
   ambulatory ventricular function p.
   AngeLase combined mapping-
      laser p.
   p. balloon catheter
   4-beam laser Doppler p.
   bilateral circumactive p. (BICAP)
   bipolar circumactive p.
   blood flow p.
   cardiac p.
   Cardiac View P.
   Chandler V-pacing p.
   coronary artery p.
   cryotherapy p.
   digoxigenin-labeled DNA p.
   DNA p.
   Doppler flow p.
   Doppler velocity p.
   Hewlett-Packard biplane 5-MHz p.
   Hewlett-Packard Omniplane 5-
      MHz p.
   high-esophageal pH p.
   hot-tip laser p.
   low-esophageal pH p.

   multielectrode p.
   Neo-Therm neonatal skin
      temperature p.
   Nicolet Vascular Pocket-Dop II
      handheld Doppler p.
   nuclear p.
   p. patency
   Radiometer p.
   Robicsek vascular p.
   scintillation p.
   p. shield
   Siemens-Elema AB pulse
      transducer p.
   Silverstein stimulator p.
   surgical ablation p.
   transesophageal echo p.
probe-patent foramen ovale
Probeta
probing sheath exchange catheter
probiotic
problem
   ventilatory p.
proBNP test
probucol
procainamide
   N-acetyl p. (NAPA)
   p. hydrochloride
procaine
   p. hydrochloride
   penicillin G p.
Procanbid
Procan SR
procarbazine
   cyclophosphamide, doxorubicin,
      methotrexate, p. (CAMP)
   p., hydroxyurea, radiotherapy
      protocol
Procardia XL
procaterol
Procath electrophysiology catheter
procedural-related myocardial ischemia
procedure (*See also* operation)
   ad hoc p.
   Alfieri p.
   Anderson p.
   Aquapheresis advance
      ultrafiltration p.
   arachnophlebectomy p.
   arterial switch p.
   atrial maze p.
   atrial switch p.
   Batista left ventricular reduction p.
   Batista left ventriculectomy p.
   beating-heart bypass p.
   Bentall p.
   Bernstein p.
   bidirectional Glenn p. (BDG)
   Bing-Taussig heart p.
   biochemical assay p.

Björk method of Fontan p.
Blalock-Park p.
Blalock-Taussig p.
Bolling p.
Brock p.
cardiac hybrid revascularization p.
catheterization p.
Chamberlain p.
Charles p.
cherry-picking p.
Clagett p.
Cockett p.
compartment p.
corridor p.
Daggett p.
Damian graft p.
Damus-Kaye-Stansel p.
deairing p.
debubbling p.
debulking p.
diagnostic electrophysiology p.
domino p.
Dor p.
Dotter p.
double switch p.
elephant trunk p.
esophageal sling p.
extracardiac Fontan p.
fenestrated Fontan p.
Flex-4 p.
Fontan-Baudet p.
Fontan-Kreutzer p.
Fontan modification of Norwood p.
genioglossal advancement p.
Gill-Jonas modification of
    Norwood p.
Glenn anastomosis p.
hemi-Fontan p. (HFP)
high-risk staged p.
His-Hass p.
Ilbawi p.
interventional p.
intracardiac amobarbital sodium p.
Jacobaeus p.
Jatene arterial switch p.
Jonas modification of Norwood p.
Junod p.
Karhunen-Loéve p.
Kawashima p.
Ko-Airan bleeding control p.
Kolmogorov-Smirnov p.
Kondoleon-Sistrunk elephantiasis p.
Konno p.
Lam p.
Langevin updating p.
latissimus dorsi p.
left atrial isolation p.
Lewis-Tanner p.
Luke p.

Lyon-Horgan p.
maxillomandibular advancement p.
maze p.
MIDCAB p.
minimally invasive p. (MIP)
minimally invasive direct coronary
    artery bypass p.
MLR p.
modified elephant trunk staged p.
modified Fontan p.
Moore p.
Morrow p.
Mustard p.
Mustard-Senning p.
myocardial laser revascularization p.
Myosplint p.
Nicks p.
Norwood univentricular heart p.
Overholt p.
percutaneous myocardial
    revascularization p.
polyanion precipitation p.
Potts p.
Quaegebeur p.
RA-RV Fontan p.
Rashkind p.
Rastan-Konno p.
Rastelli p.
revascularization p.
Ross aortic valve replacement p.
Ross-Konno pediatric
    aortoventriculoplasty p.
Sade modification of Norwood p.
salting-out p.
Schenk-Eichelter vena cava plastic
    filter p.
Schonander p.
second-stage p.
Senning-Rastelli p.
Senning transposition p.
septation p.
shunt p. (SP)
Simplate p.
skeletal muscle morphologic p.
Somnoplasty p.
Sondergaard p.
Stansel p.
Sterling Edwards p.
Sugiura p.
switch p.
Thal p.
tonsillar Somnoplasty p.
transjugular balloon valvoplasty p.
Vineberg cardiac
    revascularization p.
Waterston-Cooley p.
Womack p.
process, pl. **processes**
    consolidative p.

P

587

process *(continued)*
  costal pit of transverse p.
  Grip Technology stent crimping p.
  Markov p.
  myocardial infiltrative p.
  No-React detoxification p.
  poststreptococcal inflammatory p.
  quality improvement p. (QIP)
  vocal p.
  xiphisternal p.
  xiphoid p.
process-based criteria
processing
  film p.
  model-based image p. (MBIP)
  signal p.
processor
prochlorperazine
procoagulant
procollagen
  p. type III aminoterminal peptide
    (PIIIP)
  type I, III p.
proconvertin
  p. blood coagulation factor
  p. prothrombin conversion
    accelerator
Procort
Procrit
ProCross
  P. Rely balloon
  P. Rely over-the-wire balloon
    catheter
Procytox
Prodose AAD system
prodromal symptom
prodrome
Prodrox injection
prodrug
  combretastatin A4 p. (CA4P)
product
  Ad5FGF-4 gene therapy p.
  Autoplex Factor VIII inhibitor
    bypass p.
  BioBypass gene-based drug
    delivery p.
  calcium p.
  CFC-free p.
  digoxin reduction p. (DRP)
  double p.
  fibrin degradation p. (FDP)
  fibrinogen degradation p.
  fibrinogen-fibrin degradation p.
  fibrin split p.
  gene therapy p.
  heart rate-pressure p.
  heart rate-systolic blood pressure p.
    (RPP)
  lipid peroxidation p.

  lipoperoxidation end p.
  Medtronic AVE p.'s
  pressure time p. (PTP)
  rate-pressure p. (RPP)
production
  carbon dioxide p.
  energy p.
  IL-10 p.
  mucus p.
  sputum p.
  T-helper 1-type cytokine p.
  venous carbon dioxide p. (VCO_2)
  ventilation/carbon dioxide p.
    (VE/VCO_2)
productive
  p. bronchitis
  p. cough
  p. pleurisy
  p. sputum
  p. tuberculosis
productus
  Peptostreptococcus p.
profibrinolytic
profibrotic factor
Profilate OSD
profile
  aortic valve velocity p.
  Astra p.
  BUFUL p.
  coronary risk p.
  deflated p.
  flow p.
  hemodynamic p.
  Hospital Admission Risk P.
    (HARP)
  mini p.
  Nottingham Health p.
  P. Plus balloon dilation catheter
  risk factor p.
  serum lipid p.
  Sickness Impact P. (SIP)
  sound intensity p.
  ultra low p. (ULP)
profilin
profiling
  vascular p. (VP)
Profilnine heat-treated
Proflex 5 catheter
profound systemic vasodilation
profunda
  p. femoris artery (PFA)
  p. femoris vein
  reconstitution via p.
  vena circumflexa iliaca p.
profundaplasty
profusion
progenitor cell
progeria
Progestasert

progestational agent
progesterone
    continuous p.
    cyclic p.
    micronized p.
    p. oil
progestin
Proglycem Oral
prognosis in atrial fibrillation (PIAF)
Prograf
program
    Air Wise p.
    APT p.
    azimilide supraventricular
      arrhythmia p.
    cardiac rehabilitation and
      prevention p.
    conditioning p.
    coronary care training p. (CCTP)
    coronary rehabilitation p. (CRP)
    expedited recovery p.
    International Early Lung Cancer
      Action P. (I-ELCAP)
    ischemic heart disease life stress
      monitoring p.
    lifestyle intervention, food and
      exercise p. (LIFE)
    Linde Walker Oxygen P.
    Minnesota Heart Health P.
      (MHHP)
    multidisciplinary pulmonary
      rehabilitation p.
    myocardial infarction
      rehabilitation p. (MIRP)
    National Asthma Education P.
      (NAEP)
    National Asthma Education and
      Prevention P. (NAEPP)
    National Cholesterol Education P.
      (NCEP)
    National Heart, Lung, and Blood
      Institute/National Asthma
      Education Prevention P.
      (NHLBI/NAEPP)
    National High Blood Pressure
      Education P. (NHBPEP)
    National Lung Health Education P.
      (NLHEP)
    OxiScan oximetry p.
    Puerto Rico Heart Health P.
      (PRHHP)
    recurrent coronary prevention p.
      (RCPP)
    Sentry antimicrobial surveillance p.
    SleepGen polysomnography data
      entry p.
    SMILE p.
    smoking cessation p. (SCP)

Programalith
    P. A-V pacemaker
    P. II, III pacemaker
programmability
programmable
    p. cardioverter-defibrillator (PCD)
    p. implantable medication system
      (PIMS)
    p. pacemaker
programmed
    p. cut-off rate
    p. electrical stimulation (PES)
    p. ventricular stimulation (PVS)
programmer
    p. pacemaker
    Pacesetter APS II 3004 p.
    Pacesetter APS pacemaker p.
Progreat
    P. coaxial microcatheter
    P. coaxial microcatheter system
progression
    p. of coronary artery disease
      (PCAD)
    poor R-wave p.
    R-wave p. (RWP)
progressive
    p. disseminated histoplasmosis
      (PDH)
    p. dyspnea
    p. exercise test (PET)
    p. interstitial pulmonary fibrosis
    p. massive fibrosis (PMF)
    p. multifocal leukoencephalopathy
      (PML)
    p. multiple hyaloserositis
    p. parenchymal restriction
    p. pneumonia
    p. pulmonary hypertension
    p. pump failure
    p. scanning
    p. systemic sclerosis (PSS)
    p. thrombus
ProHance
proinflammatory
    p. cytokine
    p. disease
    p. effect
    p. factor
    p. substance
proiosystole, proiosystolia
proischemic
project
    bronchoscopy quality
      improvement p.
    coronary drug p. (CDP)
projection
    angiographic area of lateral p.
      (AL)

P

projection *(continued)*
    angiographic area of left anterior oblique p. (ALAO)
    angiographic area of right anterior oblique p. (ARAO)
    anterior oblique p.
    anteroposterior p.
    AP p.
    lateral p.
    left anterior oblique p.
    left lateral p.
    RAO 30 p.
    right anterior oblique p.
    spider p.
    steep left anterior oblique p.
    Waters p.
projector
    Tagarno 3SD cineangiography p.
prolactin-producing decidual cell
prolapse
    aortic valve p.
    bileaflet p.
    p. coil
    cusp p.
    idiopathic mitral valve p. (IMVP)
    p. of mitral valve (PMV)
    mitral valve p. (MVP)
    plaque p.
    tricuspid valve p. (TVP)
    unileaflet p.
    valvular p.
prolapsed
    p. middle scallop of posterior leaflet
    p. mitral valve syndrome
prolapsing
    p. mitral leaflet (PML)
    p. mitral valvar leaflet
Prolastin
Proleukin
proliferans
    endarteritis p.
proliferating
    p. cell nuclear antigen (PCNA)
    p. pleurisy
proliferation
    p. of elastic lamina
    in-stent neointimal p.
    intimal p.
    intimal fibrous p. (IFP)
    myxomatous p.
    neointimal p.
proliferative
    p. bronchiolitis
    p. diabetic retinopathy (PDR)
prolongation
    p. of expiration
    p. of PR interval
    QTc p.

prolonged
    p. pulmonary eosinophilia
    p. QT interval syndrome
Proloprim
promethazine
    p. and dextromethorphan
    p. hydrochloride
    p., phenylephrine, codeine
Promine
prominence
    laryngeal p.
    subcutaneous bursa of laryngeal p.
prominent
    p. pulmonary vein
    p. U wave
prominentia laryngea
Promit
promotor
    p. region
    p. region of endothelial oxide synthase
    p. region of eNOS
promyelocyte
Proneb
    P. Ultra nebulizer
    P. Ultra nebulizer compressor
prone positioning
prong
    Allegiance nasal p.'s
    Invacare nasal p.'s
    nasal p.'s
    Pro-Tech nasal p.'s
proning
Pronova suture
Pronto thrombectomy catheter
Prony method (PM)
propafenone hydrochloride
propagated thrombus
propagating thrombosis
propagation
    impulse p.
    retrograde p.
    p. of R wave
    p. of thrombus
propantheline
Propaq Encore vital signs monitor
Pro/Pel
    P./P. coating
    P./P. coating cardiac device
propellant
    halogenated hydrocarbon p.
propensity
    systemic thrombotic p.
propeptide
    aminoterminal p.
property, pl. **properties**
    chemoattracting p.
    properties of lipophilicity
    vagolytic p.

prophylactic
  p. antibiotic
  p. aspirin regimen
  p. cranial irradiation (PCI)
  p. filter placement
  p. implantable cardioverter-
    defibrillator implantation
  p. minitracheostomy
  p. therapy
  p. thoracostomy
prophylaxis
  antithrombotic p.
  preexposure p.
  primary p.
  SBE p.
propidium iodide stain
propionate
  fluticasone p. (FP)
  salmeterol and fluticasone p.
Propionibacterium acnes
propionyl-L-carnitine
propofol
proportional assist ventilation (PAV)
propranolol
  p. hydrochloride
  p. and hydrochlorothiazide
proprius
Propulsid
propylthiouracil (PTU)
prorenin
ProSom
prospective
  p. gating
  P. Investigation of Pulmonary
    Embolism Diagnosis (PIOPED)
prostacyclin (PGI$_2$)
  p. metabolite
prostaglandin
  p. 2 alpha (PGF2-alpha)
  p. D2, E, E1, G$_2$, H$_2$
  p. therapy
Prostar
  P. 9F, 11F percutaneous vascular
    surgery system
  P. Plus percutaneous vascular
    surgical device
  P. XL hemostatic puncture closure
    device
  P. XL 8, 10 suture mediated
    closure system
PROStent
prosthesis, pl. **prostheses**
  Alvarez p.
  Angelchik antireflux p.
  antireflux p.
  aortic p.
  ball-and-cage p.
  ball valve p.
  Barnard mitral valve p.

Beall disc valve p.
Beall mitral valve p.
bifurcated aortofemoral p.
bifurcation p.
bileaflet mechanical p.
biological p.
Björk-Shiley aortic valve p.
Björk-Shiley convexoconcave 60-
  degree valve p.
Björk-Shiley floating disc p.
blood vessel p. (BVP)
caged ball valve p.
Carbomedics cardiac valve p.
Carbo-Seal ascending aortic p.
cardiac valve p.
Carpentier-Edwards aortic valve p.
Carpentier-Edwards glutaraldehyde-
  preserved porcine xenograft p.
Carpentier-Edwards Perimount PSR
  pericardial p.
collar p.
Cooley-Bloodwell mitral valve p.
Cutter aortic valve p.
Cutter-Smeloff aortic valve p.
DeBakey ball valve p.
DeBakey Vasculour-II vascular p.
Delrin frame of valve p.
duckbill voice p.
Duromedics valve p.
Edwards Lifesciences Perimount
  Magna stented p.
elephant trunk p.
esophageal p.
Golaski-UMI vascular p.
Gott-Daggett heart valve p.
Groningen voice p.
Hammersmith mitral p.
Hancock mitral valve p.
heart valve p.
Hemobahn endovascular p.
Ionescu-Shiley valve p.
knitted vascular p.
large-annulus p.
Lillehei-Kaster cardiac valve p.
Lillehei-Kaster mitral valve p.
Meadox woven velour p.
mechanical p.
Medtronic-Hall heart valve p.
Medtronic-Hall tilting disc valve p.
Medtronic Mosaic stented p.
Milliknit Dacron p.
Milliknit vascular graft p.
mitral p.
Monostrut cardiac valve p.
Neville tracheal p.
Omnicarbon cardiac valve p.
Omnicarbon heart valve p.
Omniscience single leaflet cardiac
  valve p.

P

prosthesis *(continued)*
    pericarbon pericardial p.
    polytetrafluoroethylene p.
    polyvinyl p.
    porcine p.
    Quattro mitral valve p.
    single-disc p.
    Soprano stented p.
    Sorin Bicarbon bileaflet aortic
      valve p.
    Sorin Biomedica Cardio Solo
      stentless p.
    Sorin mitral valve p.
    Starr-Edwards aortic valve p.
    Starr-Edwards ball valve p.
    Starr-Edwards cardiac valve p.
    Starr-Edwards disc valve p.
    Starr-Edwards heart valve p.
    Starr-Edwards mitral p.
    stentless porcine aortic valve p.
    St. Jude heart valve p.
    St. Jude Medical valve p.
    supraanular p.
    Teflon trileaflet p.
    Teflon woven p.
    tilting disc aortic valve p.
    Ultra low resistance voice p.
    valve p.
    vascular graft p.
    Weavenit p.
    woven Teflon p.
    woven-tube vascular graft p.
prosthesis-patient mismatch (PPM)
prosthetic
    p. aortic valve
    p. ball valve
    p. cardiac valve
    p. heart valve
    p. infectious endocarditis (PIE)
    p. mitral valve thrombosis
    p. poppet
    p. ring annuloplasty
    St. Jude composite p.
    p. valve endocarditis (PVE)
    p. valve regurgitation (PVR)
    p. valve sewing ring
    p. valve sound
    p. valve stenosis (PVS)
    p. valve vegetation
Prostin VR Pediatric injection
prostration
    pain, pallor, pulselessness,
      paresthesia, paralysis, p. (PPPPP)
Protg GPS nitinol self-expanding long
  stent
protamine sulfate
protease
    p. inhibitor (PI)

    mast cell p.
    neutrophil-derived serine p.
protease-antiprotease
    p.-a. imbalance
    p.-a. theory of emphysema
Pro-Tech nasal prongs
protected
    p. catheter brushing (PCB)
    p. specimen brush (PSB)
    p. specimen brushing (PSB)
protection
    airway p.
    automated boundary p. (ABP)
    lung p.
    myocardial p.
    second window of p. (SWOP)
    short transitional edge p. (STEP)
protective
    p. block
    p. ventilation
    p. ventilator strategy
    p. zone
protector
    pulse-oximetry p.
Protegra
protegrin antimicrobial peptide
protein
    p. A
    activator p. (AP)
    alpha-B-crystallin p.
    amyloid A p.
    amyloid precursor p. (APP)
    apolipoprotein regulatory p. (ARP)
    p. B
    bone morphogenetic p. type 2
      (BMP-2)
    BvgS p.
    cardiac gap junction p.
    CD45 cell surface p.
    cholesterol ester transfer p. (CETP)
    Clara cell secretory p. (CCSP)
    coagulation p.
    contractile p.
    C-reactive p. (CRP)
    p. C, S deficiency
    CTLA4Ig p.
    cytoskeletal p.
    cytosolic p.
    p. electrophoresis
    enhanced green fluorescent p.
      (eGFP)
    eosinophil cationic p. (ECP)
    fatty acid-binding p. (FABP)
    G p.
    G_i p.
    Gc p.
    glycosylation of intracellular p.'s
    gp100 p.
    gp91^{phox} p.

guanine nucleotide exchange factor p.
heart-type fatty acid binding p. (H-FABP)
heat shock p. (HSP, hsp)
heat shock p. 47 (HSP47)
heat shock p. 70 (HSP70)
heptahelical p. G
heterotrimeric p. G
high-density lipoprotein binding p. (HDLBP)
high-sensitivity C-reactive p. (hs-CRP, hsCRP)
intracellular p.
isoprenylated p.
45-kilodalton p.
p. kinase (PKase)
p. kinase A (PKA)
p. kinase C (PKC)
latent membrane p.-1 (LMP1)
lipoprotein receptor-related p. (LRP)
M p.
macrophage inflammatory p. (MIP)
melanoma inhibitory activity p.
MIA p.
microsomal triglyceride transfer p. (MTP)
mitogen-activated p. (MAP)
M-line p.
monocyte chemoattractant p. (MCP)
myosin-binding p. C (MyBP-C)
natural resistance macrophage-associated p. (Nramp)
NF-ATc p.
overexpressed p.
$p22^{phox}$ p.
$p47^{phox}$ p.
$p67^{phox}$ p.
protooncogenic p.
rat urine p.
recognition p.
redox-sensitive regulatory p.
p. S
p. S-100B
secretory leukoprotease inhibitor p.
serum eosinophilic cationic p.
soy p.
STAT4 p.
STAT6 p.
sterol regulatory element-binding p. (SREBP)
p. sulfuryl group
surfactant p. (SP)
surfactant p. A (SP-A)
surfactant p. A, B, C
surfactant-specific p.
Tamm-Horsfall p.
thrombus precursor p. (TpP)
ToxR p.

p. tyrosine phosphatase-gamma (PTP-gamma)
tyrosine phosphorylated p.
ubiquitin-conjugated p.
underexpressed p.
von Willebrand p. (vWP)
wild-type p.
protein-1
macrophage inflammatory p.-1 (MIP-1)
monocyte chemoattractant p.-1 (MCP-1)
monocyte chemotactic p.-1 (MCP-1)
proteinaceous edema fluid
proteinase
p. inhibitor (Pi)
p. inhibitor phenotype
protein-calorie
p.-c. deficiency
p.-c. malnutrition
protein-losing enteropathy (PLE)
proteinosis
alveolar p.
pulmonary alveolar p.
proteinuria
proteoglycan
proteoglycan-rich tissue
proteoglycans
proteolysis
chemokine p.
quantum p.
proteolytic enzyme
Proteus
P. mirabilis
P. pneumonia
P. syndrome
P. vulgaris
Protex swivel adapter
prothrombin
p. activity (PTA)
p. complex (PTC)
p. G20210A mutated allele
p. time (PTT)
p. time fixing agent (PTFA)
p. time/partial thromboplastin time (PT/PTT)
p. time ratio (PTR)
prothrombinase complex
prothrombosis
systemic p.
prothrombotic state
protionamide
protocol
ABC p.
ACLS p.
Astrand-Rhyming p.
Balke treadmill p.
Balke-Ware treadmill p.
Bruce treadmill p.

P

protocol *(continued)*
cardiac rehabilitation p.
chronotropic exercise assessment p.
 (CEAP)
continuous ramp p.
Cornell exercise p.
Cornell modification of the
 Bruce p.
Ellestad p.
exsanguination p.
Goodwin p.
high-ramp p.
James exercise p.
Kattus treadmill p.
LITE p.
low-ramp p.
Mayo exercise treadmill p.
McHenry p.
McNamara p.
moderate-ramp p.
modified Bruce p.
modified Ellestad p.
Naughton treadmill p.
patient-driven p.
PHRT p.
procarbazine, hydroxyurea,
 radiotherapy p.
RAMP antitachycardia p.
RAMP-based p.
RAMP treadmill p.
Reeves treadmill p.
rehabilitation p.
reinjection p.
resident assessment p. (RAP)
rest metabolism/stress perfusion p.
Sheffield modification of Bruce
 treadmill p.
Sheffield treadmill p.
1-shock p.
3-shock p.
standard Bruce p.
Stanford treadmill exercise p.
step treadmill p.
TAMI p.
therapist-driven p. (TDP)
USAFSAM treadmill exercise p.
weaning p.
Weber-Janicki cardiopulmonary
 exercise p.
Westminster drug-free p.
protodiastolic
p. gallop
p. murmur
p. rumble
protofibril
protokylol hydrochloride
proton
p. density

p. pump inhibitor
p. spectroscopy
proton-beam radiotherapy
Protonix
protooncogene
protooncogenic
p. effect
p. protein
p. protein kinase
protoplasmic block
protoporphyrin
erythrocyte p.
free p.
p. IX
zinc p.
protoveratrine A, B
protozoal myocarditis
protozoan
protracted bacterial bronchitis
protriptyline hydrochloride
protruding atheroma
protrusio acetabuli
protuberantia laryngea
protuberant plaque
prourokinase
recombinant p.
Provasca
Pro-Vent
P.-V. arterial blood gas kit
P.-V. arterial blood sampling kit
Proventil HFA
Provera Oral
Providencia
Provigil
provisional
p. side-branch stenting
p. spot stenting
provocable myocardial ischemia
provocation
bronchial p.
histamine p.
physiological p.
p. test
Provocholine
provoking agent
Provox speaking valve
prowazekii
Rickettsia p.
proxetil
cefpodoxime p.
proximal
p. acinar emphysema
p. convoluted tubule
p. coronary sinus (PCS)
p. and distal portion of vessel
p. entry tear
p. flow convergence method
p. isovelocity surface area (PISA)

p. segment
p. stenosis
proximal-to-distal (P/D)
Proxis
P. catheter
P. Embolic Protection System
ProYellow+ laser
PRP
platelet-rich plasma
polyribosylribitol phosphate
pulse repetition period
PRP-D vaccine
PRP-OMPC vaccine
PRR
pulmonary reimplantation response
pulse repetition rate
PR/RP ratio
PRSP
penicillin-resistant *Streptococcus pneumoniae*
PRS wave
PRT
percutaneous rotational thrombectomy
PRU
peripheral resistance unit
prudent diet
Pruitt-Inahara carotid shunt
prune
p. juice expectoration
p. juice sputum
pruning
branch vessel p.
pruritus
poststroke p.
Prussian helmet sign
PRVC
pressure-regulated volume control
PRVC ventilation
PRx implantable cardioverter-defibrillator
PS
pacemaker syndrome
Palmaz-Schatz
pulmonary sequestration
pulmonary stenosis
pulmonic stenosis
PS 153 stent
Ps
systolic pressure
Psa
systemic blood pressure
psammoma bodies
psammosarcoma
PSAP
peak systolic aortic pressure
PSB
protected specimen brush
protected specimen brushing

PSC
pulse synchronized contraction
PSD
poststenotic dilation
power spectral density
PSDI
Positive Symptom Distress Index
PSE
paradoxical systolic expansion
P-selectin
P-s. cell adhesion molecule
P-s. expression
P-s. glycoprotein ligand 1 (PSGL-1)
P-Series sleep monitoring system
Pseudallescheria
P. boydii
P. maltophilia
P. stutzeri
pseudallescheriasis
pseudangina, pseudoangina
pseudo
p. R′ wave
p. S wave
pseudoalternating current
pseudoaneurysm
apical p.
arterial p.
femoral p.
posttraumatic p.
pulmonary artery p. (PAP)
pseudoangina (*var. of* pseudangina)
pseudoapoplexy
pseudoasthma
pseudo-A-V block
pseudobronchiectasis
pseudobulbar palsy
Pseudo-Car DM
pseudocavitation
pseudocholinesterase deficiency
pseudochylothorax
pseudocirrhosis
pseudocoarctation of aorta
pseudocomplication
pseudocroup
pseudocylindrical bronchiectasis
pseudocyst
posttraumatic pulmonary p.
pulmonary p.
pseudodextrocardia
pseudodiastolic
pseudodiphtheriticum
Bacillus p.
pseudodisappearance criterion
pseudoephedrine
acetaminophen, dextromethorphan, p.
acrivastine and p.
carbinoxamine and p.
chlorpheniramine and p.

P

pseudoephedrine *(continued)*
   p. and dextromethorphan
   guaifenesin and p.
   p. HCl
   hydrocodone and p.
   p. and ibuprofen
   triprolidine and p.
pseudofusion beat
pseudo-heart disease
pseudohypertension
pseudohypoparathyroidism
pseudohypotension
pseudoinfarction pattern
pseudo-Kaposi sarcoma
pseudolumen
pseudolupus
pseudo-Mahaim fiber
pseudomalfunction
pseudomallei
   Pseudomonas p.
pseudomembranous
   p. angina
   p. *Aspergillus* tracheobronchitis
   p. bronchitis
   p. croup
   p. tracheobronchial aspergillosis
pseudomonad
Pseudomonas
   P. aeruginosa
   P. cepacia
   P. elastase
   P. exotoxin
   P. maltophilia
   P. pseudomallei
   P. stutzeri
pseudomucinous
pseudonormalization
   p. of T wave
   T-wave p.
pseudoparalytica
   myasthenia gravis p.
pseudopericarditis
pseudopneumonia
pseudopodia
pseudo-P pulmonale
pseudorosette
pseudo-steroid-resistant asthma
pseudothrombocytopenia
pseudotruncus arteriosus
pseudotuberculosis
   Yersinia p.
pseudotumor
   inflammatory p. (IPT)
pseudotumoral mediastinal amyloidosis
Pseudovent
pseudoxanthoma
   p. elasticum
   p. elasticum syndrome

PSG
   peak systolic gradient
   polysomnogram
   polysomnography
   presystolic gallop
    full PSG
    PSG LOC guidewire extension
    PSG pressure
PSGL-1
   P-selectin glycoprotein ligand 1
PSI
   Pneumonia Severity Index
psi
   pounds per square inch
psig
   pounds per square inch gauge
P-sinistrocardiale
psittaci
   Chlamydia p.
psittacosis inclusion bodies
PSM
   presystolic murmur
PSP
   peak systolic pressure
   periodic short pulse
   primary spontaneous pneumothorax
PSS
   Palmaz-Schatz stent
   progressive systemic sclerosis
   pure sensory syndrome
PST
   paroxysmal supraventricular tachycardia
   positive symptom total
   poststenotic
PSV
   peak systolic velocity
   positive support ventilator
   pressure support ventilation
   pressure support ventilator
PSVT
   paroxysmal supraventricular tachycardia
psychic akinesia
psychocardiac reflex
psychogenic
   p. cough
   p. dyspnea
   p. overlay
   p. pain
   p. stridor
   p. syncope
psychological
   p. factor
   p. stimulus
psychophysiological interventions in myocardial ischemia (PIMI)
psychosis
   postperfusion p.

psychosocial
    P. Adjustment to Illness Scale
    p. factor
psychostimulant
psychotherapy
psychotropic agent
psyllium
PT
    paroxysmal tachycardia
    pericardial tamponade
    pulmonary thrombosis
        PT Graphix guidewire
PTA
    percutaneous transluminal angioplasty
    persistent truncus arteriosus
    plasma thromboplastin antecedent
    prothrombin activity
PTAS
    percutaneous transluminal angioscopy
PTB
    pulmonary tuberculosis
PTBA
    percutaneous transluminal balloon
        angioplasty
PTBD
    percutaneous transluminal balloon
        dilation
PTC
    peritubular capillary
    plasma thromboplastin component
    prothrombin complex
PTCA
    percutaneous transluminal coronary
        angioplasty
        PTCA dilation catheter
        perfusion balloon PTCA
        rescue PTCA
PTCR
    percutaneous transluminal coronary
        recanalization
    percutaneous transluminal coronary
        revascularization
PTCRA
    percutaneous transluminal coronary
        rotational ablation
PTD
    percutaneous thrombolytic device
    percutaneous transluminal dilation
PtdCho
    phosphatidylcholine
PTED
    pulmonary thromboembolic disease
PTEF
    peak tidal expiratory flow
pteridine
pteronyssinus
    Dermatophagoides p.
pterygium, pl. **pterygia**

pterygia, heart defects, autosomal
    recessive inheritance, vertebral
    defects, ear anomalies, radial
    defect (PHAVER)
pterygoid chest
pterygopalatine ganglion
PTF
    plasma thromboplastin factor
PTFA
    prothrombin time fixing agent
PTFE
    polytetrafluoroethylene
        PTFE closure
        PTFE stent graft
PTFE-covered stent
PTG
    peak of thrombin generation
PT^2 guidewire
PTH
    parathyroid hormone
    plasma thromboplastin component
Pth
    chest wall elastic recoil pressure
PTIF
    peak tidal inspiratory flow
PTJV
    percutaneous transtracheal jet ventilation
PTL
    pharyngeal tracheal lumen
    pharyngotracheal lumen
    plasma thyroxine level
    posterior tricuspid leaflet
PTLA
    pharyngotracheal lumen airway
PtL airway
PTLPD, PTLD
    posttransplantation lymphoproliferative
    disorder
        intrathoracic PTLPD
PTM
    pulse time modulation
Ptm
    transmural pressure of collapsible
    segment
Ptm′
    critical closing pressure of collapsible
    segment
PTMA
    percutaneous transverse mitral
        annuloplasty
PTMC
    percutaneous transvenous mitral
        commissurotomy
PTMR
    percutaneous transluminal myocardial
        revascularization
    percutaneous transmyocardial
        revascularization

P

PTNB
　　percutaneous transthoracic needle biopsy
PTP
　　pressure time product
Ptp
　　transpulmonary pressure
PTP-gamma
　　protein tyrosine phosphatase-gamma
PT/PTT
　　prothrombin time/partial thromboplastin
　　time
PTR
　　prothrombin time ratio
PTRA
　　percutaneous transluminal renal
　　　angioplasty
　　percutaneous transluminal rotational
　　　atherectomy
PTSMA
　　percutaneous transluminal septal
　　　myocardial ablation
PTT
　　partial thromboplastin time
　　prothrombin time
　　pulse transmission time
PTU
　　propylthiouracil
PTVA
　　percutaneous transseptal ventricular assist
PTX3
　　pentraxin 3
public
　　p. access defibrillation (PAD,
　　　P.A.D.)
　　p. access to defibrillation (PAD,
　　　P.A.D.)
　　p. access defibrillator (PAD,
　　　P.A.D.)
　　P. Health Response Team (PHRT)
puerile respiration
puerperal
　　p. phlebitis
　　p. thrombosis
Puerto Rico Heart Health Program
　　(PRHHP)
PUFA
　　polyunsaturated fatty acid
puff
　　p. of smoke
　　veiled p.
puffball
puffer
　　pink p.
puffing sound
pullback
　　aortic p.
　　p. atherectomy device
　　p. pressure
　　p. technique

pulley
pull-out endarterectomy
pull-through
　　station p.-t.
Pullularia
Pulmanex resuscitator
Pulmicort
　　P. Respules
　　P. Turbuhaler
Pulminiq
pulmo
　　p. dexter
　　p. sinister
Pulmo-Aide
　　P.-A. aerosol compressor/nebulizer
　　P.-A. nebulizer
　　P.-A. Traveler
pulmoaortic canal
Pulmocare
Pulmo-Graph
pulmolith
PulmoMate aerosol compressor/nebulizer
pulmometry
Pulmo-Mist compressor
pulmonale
　　acute cor p.
　　acutely decompensated cor p.
　　atrium p.
　　chronic cor p.
　　cor p. (CP)
　　glomus p.
　　ligamentum p.
　　P p.
　　pseudo-P p.
pulmonales
　　nodi lymphoidei
　　　juxtaesophageales p.
　　venae p.
pulmonalis
　　arteria p.
　　ostium trunci p.
　　pars basalis arteriae p.
　　pleura p.
　　plexus p.
　　sinus trunci p.
　　sulcus p.
　　truncus p.
　　valva trunci p.
pulmonalium
　　ostia venarum p.
pulmonary
　　p. acid aspiration syndrome
　　p. acinus
　　p. actinomycosis
　　p. adenomatosis
　　p. agenesis
　　p. air embolism
　　p. alveolar hemorrhage
　　p. alveolar hypoventilation (PAH)

p. alveolar hypoxic vasoconstrictor (PAHVC)
p. alveolar microlithiasis (PAM)
p. alveolar proteinosis
p. alveolus
p. amebiasis
p. amyloidosis
p. angiogram
p. angiography (PA, PAG)
p. angioscopy
p. angiotensin I converting enzyme
p. anomalous superior venous return (PASVR)
p. anthrax
p. aplasia
p. arch
p. arterial (PA, Pa)
p. arterial capillary wedge pressure (PACWP)
p. arterial end-diastolic pressure
p. arterial hypertension
p. arterial pressure, pulmonary venous pressure (pa-pv)
p. arterial stenosis (PAS)
p. arterial system
p. arterial wave pressure
p. arterial web
p. arteriolar resistance (PAR)
p. arterioplasty
p. arteriovenous fistula (PAF, PAVF)
p. arteriovenous malformation (PAVM)
p. arteritides
p. artery (PA)
p. artery anastomosis
p. artery atresia
p. artery balloon pump (PABP)
p. artery band
p. artery banding
p. artery catheterization (PAC)
p. artery counterpulsation (PACP)
p. artery diastolic (PAD, P.A.D.)
p. artery diastolic pressure (PADP)
p. artery end-diastolic pressure (PAEDP)
p. artery filling defect (PAFD)
p. artery flotation catheter
p. artery homograft
p. artery hypertension (PAH)
p. artery hypotension (PAH)
p. artery mean pressure (PAMP)
p. artery occlusion (PAO)
p. artery occlusion pressure (PAo, PAOP)
p. artery occlusive wedge pressure
p. artery pressure (PAP, Ppa)
p. artery pseudoaneurysm (PAP)
p. artery rupture

p. artery sling
p. artery steal
p. artery stenosis
p. artery systolic (PAS)
p. artery systolic pressure (PASP)
p. artery thromboembolism (PATE)
p. artery wedge (PAW)
p. artery wedge pressure (PAWP, Ppaw)
p. aspergillosis
p. atresia (PA)
p. atresia with ventricular septal defect (PAVSD)
p. autograft (PA)
p. autograft valve
p. A-V O_2 difference
p. balloon valvoplasty (PBV)
p. barotrauma
basal part of left and right inferior p.
p. bed gradient
p. blastoma
p. blood flow (PBF, Qp)
p. blood mixing volume (PBMV)
p. blood volume (PBV)
p. botryomycosis
p. branch of autonomic
p. branch stenosis (PBS)
p. bulla
p. calcification
p. candidiasis
p. capillaritis
p. capillary blood flow (Qc, Qpc)
p. capillary blood volume (Vc)
p. capillary hemangiomatosis
p. capillary pressure (PCP)
p. capillary wedge (PCW)
p. capillary wedge pressure (PCWP)
p. capillary wedge pressure tracing
p. cavitation
p. cavity
p. circulation (PC)
p. coccidioidomycosis
p. coin lesion
p. compliance (PC)
p. complication
p. component
p. component of second heart sound
p. cone
p. congestion
p. consolidation
p. contusion
p. conus
p. cryptococcosis
p. cyanosis
p. DCS
p. diffusion capacity (D_{CO})

P

pulmonary *(continued)*
- p. disease anemia syndrome
- p. drug delivery
- p. dysmaturity syndrome
- p. dyspnea
- p. edema (PE)
- p. edema fluid (PEF)
- p. effusion
- p. ejection click (PEC)
- p. embolectomy
- p. embolism (PE)
- p. embolization
- p. embolus
- p. emphysema (PE)
- p. epithelium
- p. failure
- p. fat embolism syndrome
- p. fever
- p. fibrosis
- p. function (PF)
- P. Functional Status and Dyspnea Questionnaire (PFSDQ)
- p. functional status scale (PFSS)
- p. function status
- p. function test (PFT)
- p. gas exchange
- p. glomangiosis
- p. hamartoma
- p. heart
- p. hemangioendothelioma
- p. hematoma
- p. hemodynamics
- p. hemosiderosis
- p. hilum
- p. hyalinizing granuloma
- p. hyperinfection syndrome
- p. hypertension (PH, PHT)
- p. hypertension pressure
- p. hypertrophic osteoarthropathy
- p. hypoplasia, hypoplasia of pulmonary artery, agonadism, omphalocele/diaphragmatic defect, dextrocardia (PAGOD)
- p. hypostasis
- p. incompetence
- p. infarct
- p. infarction (PI)
- p. infarction syndrome
- p. infiltrate
- p. infiltrates with eosinophilia syndrome
- p. infiltrate with eosinophilia (PIE)
- p. infiltration with eosinophilia (PIE)
- p. insufficiency (PI)
- p. interstitial edema
- p. interstitial emphysema (PIE)
- p. Langerhans cell histiocytosis
- p. leukostasis
- p. ligament
- p. lobule
- p. lymphangioleiomyomatosis
- p. lymphangiomatosis
- p. lymphangiomyomatosis
- p. lymph node
- p. lymphoma
- p. meniscus sign
- p. metastasectomy
- p. microthromboembolism
- p. microvasculopathy
- p. mucormycosis
- p. murmur
- p. mycosis
- p. nervous plexus
- p. nodule
- p. notch sign
- p. obstruction index
- p. occlusive venopathy (POV)
- p. oligemia
- p. orifice
- p. ossification
- p. outflow tract
- p. pain
- p. parenchyma
- p. parenchymal disease
- p. parenchymal injury
- p. parenchymal tuberculosis
- p. parenchymal window
- p. phthisis
- p. pleura
- p. pleurisy
- p. pseudocyst
- p. pulse
- p. rale
- p. reexpansion
- p. regurgitation (PR)
- p. rehabilitation
- p. reimplantation response (PRR)
- p. resistance
- p. restriction
- p. ridge
- p. sarcoidosis
- p. scintigraphy
- p. secretion
- p. sequestration (PS)
- p. shunt
- p. sinus
- p. sling syndrome
- p. stenosis (PS)
- p. sulcus
- p. surfactant
- p. systemic blood flow ratio
- p. target sign
- p. thromboembolic disease (PTED)
- p. thromboembolism
- p. thrombosis (PT)
- p. toilet
- p. transpiration

p. trunk
p. tuberculosis (PTB)
p. valve (PV)
p. valve anomaly
p. valve area
p. valve disease
p. valve echocardiography
p. valve gradient (PVG)
p. valve repair (PVR)
p. valve replacement (PVR)
p. valve restenosis
p. valve stenosis
p. valve vegetation
p. valvoplasty
p. valvotomy
p. valvular regurgitation
p. valvular stenosis (PVS)
p. vascular bed
p. vascular disease (PVD)
p. vascular marking
p. vascular obstruction (PVO)
p. vascular obstructive disease (PVOD)
p. vascular pressure
p. vascular reactivity
p. vascular redistribution
p. vascular resistance (PVR)
p. vascular resistance index (PVRI)
p. vasculature
p. vasculitis
p. vasoconstriction
p. vasodilation
p. vein (PV)
p. venoocclusive disease (PVOD)
p. venous atrial (PVa)
p. venous atrium
p. venous confluence (PVC)
p. venous congestion (PVC)
p. venous connection
p. venous connection anomaly
p. venous drainage
p. venous drainage pattern
p. venous flow (PVF)
p. venous hypertension (PVH)
p. venous pressure (PVP)
p. venous return
p. venous return anomaly
p. venous systolic (PVs)
p. ventilation
p. wedge (PW)
p. wedge angiography
p. wedge pressure (Ppw, PWP)
pulmonary-to-systemic
p.-t.-s. flow ratio (Qp:Qs)
p.-t.-s. vascular resistance (Rp:Rs)
pulmonic
aortic end p.
p. area
p. closure (PC)

p. endocarditis
p. incompetence
p. insufficiency
p. murmur
p. regurgitation
p. second heart sound (P2)
p. stenosis (PS)
p. tricuspid
p. valve
p. valve closure
p. valve closure sound
p. valve stenosis
pulmonicola
Pandoraea p.
pulmonic-to-systemic flow ratio (Qp:Qs)
pulmonis
alveoli p.
apex p.
basis p.
facies costalis p.
facies interlobares p.
facies medialis p.
facies mediastinalis p.
fissura obliqua p.
hilum p.
impressio cardiaca p.
ligamentum latum p.
margo anterior p.
margo inferior p.
pars mediastinalis p.
pulmonitis
pulmonocoronary reflex
pulmonologist
pulmonray flow pattern
PulmoSonic nebulizer
PulmoSphere
PulmoTrack respiratory sound analyzer
Pulmowrap
Pulmozyme
Pulsar
P. DDD pacemaker
P. Max II pacemaker system
P. Max sensor
P. NI implantable pacemaker
pulsate
pulsatile
p. assist device (PAD, P.A.D.)
p. flow
p. ventricular assist device
pulsatility index (PI)
pulsating
p. empyema
p. pleurisy
pulsation
ascending aorta synchronized p. (AASP)
intraaortic balloon p. (IABP)
jugular venous p. (JVP)

P

pulsation *(continued)*
    presystolic p.
    suprasternal p.
Pulsator
    P. dry heparin arterial blood gas kit
    P. syringe
pulse (p) *(See also* pulsus)
    abdominal p.
    abrupt p.
    alternating p.
    amplitude of p.
    p. amplitude
    p. amplitude modulation (PAM)
    p. amplitude ratio (PAR)
    anacrotic p.
    anadicrotic p.
    apical p. (AP)
    arterial p.
    atrial liver p.
    atrial venous p.
    p. average intensity (Ipa)
    Bamberger bulbar p.
    bigeminal p.
    bigeminal bisferious p.
    bisferious p.
    blood pressure and p. (BP&P)
    blood volume p. (BVP)
    bounding p.
    brachial p.
    bulbar p.
    cannonball p.
    capillary p.
    carotid p.
    catacrotic p.
    catadicrotic p.
    catatricrotic p.
    centripetal venous p.
    collapsing p.
    cordy p.
    Corrigan p.
    coupled p.
    C point of cardiac apex p.
    p. curve
    CV wave of jugular venous p.
    C wave of jugular venous p.
    p. deficit
    p. delivery device
    dicrotic p.
    digitalate p.
    dorsalis pedis p.
    p. duration (PD)
    elastic p.
    entoptic p.
    filiform p.
    formicant p.
    F point of cardiac apex p.
    funic p.
    f wave of jugular venous p.

    gaseous p.
    p. generator
    p. generator change
    guttural p.
    hard p.
    hyperkinetic p.
    hypokinetic p.
    I_{sata} p.
    I_{sapt} p.
    I_{sa} p.
    incisura p.
    intermittent p.
    p. inversion harmonic imaging
    irregularly irregular p.
    jerky p.
    jugular vein p. (JVP)
    jugular venous p.
    Kussmaul paradoxical p.
    labile p.
    long p.
    maximum digital p. (MDP)
    p. method
    Monneret p.
    monocrotic p.
    monophasic p.
    mousetail p.
    movable p.
    myurous p.
    nail p.
    O point of cardiac apex p.
    p. oximeter
    3800 p. oximeter
    p. oximeter/end tidal CO_2 (POET)
    p. oximetry (PO)
    p. oximetry device
    p. oximetry monitoring (POM)
    oxygen p.
    paradoxic p.
    paradoxical p. (PP)
    parietal p. (PP)
    pedal p.
    p. period
    periodic short p. (PSP)
    p.'s per minute (ppm)
    piston p.
    plateau p.
    popliteal p.
    p. position modulated (PPM)
    posterior tibial p.
    precordial p.
    presaturation p.
    p. pressure (PP)
    pressure p.
    P. Pro heart rate monitor
    P. Pro heart rate monitor watch
    pulmonary p.
    quadrigeminal p.
    quick p.
    Quincke p.

radial p. (RP)
p. rate (PR)
p. repetition (PR)
p. repetition frequency (PRF)
p. repetition period (PRP)
p. repetition rate (PRR)
p. and respiration (P&R)
respiratory p.
reversed paradoxical p.
Riegel p.
SF wave of cardiac apex p.
soft p.
spike-and-dome p.
standard temperature and p. (STP)
sustained p.
p. synchronized contraction (PSC)
temperature and p. (T&P, T+P)
tense p.
thready p.
tibial p.
tidal wave p.
p. time modulation (PTM)
p. tracing
p. transmission time (PTT)
trigeminal p.
triphammer p.
triple-humped pressure p.
p. trisection
ulnar p.
undulating p.
unequal p.
vagus p.
venous p.
vermicular p.
p. volume recording (PVR)
V peak of jugular venous p.
water hammer p.
water-hammer p.
p. wave (PW)
p. wave duration
p. wave velocity (PWV)
p. width
wiry p.
p. with modulation (PWM)
X depression of jugular venous p.
X descent of jugular venous p.
Y depression of jugular venous p.
Y descent of jugular venous p.

pulsed

p. diastolic (PD)
p. diastolic autologous blood
  selective aortic arch perfusion
  (PD-AB-SAAP)
p. Doppler cross-sectional
  echocardiography (PD-CSE)
p. Doppler echocardiography (PDE)
p. Doppler flowmetry
p. Doppler tissue imaging
p. dye laser

p. laser ablation
p. myocardial Doppler (PMD)
p. myocardial Doppler mapping
p. spectral Doppler
PulseDose
P. EX2000D oxygen conserver
P. oxygen delivery technology
P. portable compressed oxygen
  system
pulsed-wave
p.-w. Doppler (PWD)
p.-w. Doppler mapping
p.-w. tissue Doppler (PWTD)
pulse-height analyzer
pulseless
p. bradycardia
p. disease
p. electrical activity (PEA)
p. idioventricular rhythm
pulse-oximetry protector
PulseSpray infusion system
pulsimeter, pulsometer
Pulsox-5 pulse oximeter
PulStar pneumatic wrap system
pulsus (*See also* pulse)
p. alternans
p. anadicrotus
p. bigeminus
p. bisferiens
p. caprisans
p. catacrotus
p. catadicrotus
p. celer
p. celerrimus
p. cordis
p. debilis
p. differens
p. duplex
p. durus
p. filiformis
p. fluens
p. formicans
p. fortis
p. frequens
p. heterochronicus
p. inaequalis
p. incongruens
p. infrequens
p. intercidens
p. intercurrens
p. irregularis
p. irregularis perpetuus
p. magnus
p. mollis
p. monocrotus
p. myurus
p. paradoxus (PP)
p. parvus
p. parvus et tardus

P

pulsus *(continued)*
    p. plenus
    p. quadrigeminus
    p. rarus
    p. respiratione intermittens
    p. tardus
    p. tremulus
    p. trigeminus
    p. vacuus
    p. venosus
    p. vibrans
pultaceous debris
Pulvinal
Pulvules
    Cinobac P.
    Seromycin P.
Pumactant
pumilus
    Bacillus p.
pump
    Abbott infusion p.
    abdominothoracic p.
    Acat 1 intraaortic balloon p.
    Affinity blood p.
    antibiotic efflux p.
    AutoCAT intraaortic balloon p.
    AVCO balloon p.
    axial flow p.
    Axiom double sump p.
    balloon p.
    Bio-Medicus p.
    blood p.
    BVS p.
    CADD-Plus intravenous infusion p.
    cardiopulmonary bypass p.
    centrifugal p.
    Cormed ambulatory infusion p.
    p. current
    Datascope System 90 intraaortic
      balloon p.
    DeBakey VAD continuous-axial-
      flow p.
    ECMO p.
    Emerson p.
    p. failure
    p. failure death
    Flowtron DVT p.
    p. function
    Gomco thoracic drainage p.
    Harvard p.
    heart p.
    HeartMate p.
    Imed infusion p.
    impeller p.
    Infusaid infusion p.
    Infuse-A-Port p.
    intraaortic balloon p. (IABP, IBP)
    ion p.
    IVAC p.
    Jobst extremity p.
    KAAT II Plus intraaortic
      balloon p.
    Kangaroo p.
    Kontron intraaortic balloon p.
    left ventricular assist system
      implantable p.
    left ventricular bypass p. (LVBP)
    Life Care P.
    Lindbergh p.
    p. lung
    Master Flow Pumpette p.
    Medtronic SynchroMed p.
    muscular venous p.
    Na+/K+ p.
    Neuroperfusion p.
    Novacor heart p.
    p. oxygenation
    p. oxygenator
    pulmonary artery balloon p.
      (PABP)
    Quest Medical MPS cardioplegia
      fluid delivery p.
    Reitan catheter p.
    respiratory p.
    roller p.
    sodium-potassium p. (Na+/K+-
      ATPase)
    sump p.
    SynchroMed programmable p.
    Thoratec p.
    TransAct intraaortic balloon p.
    Travenol infusion p.
    VentrAssist heart p.
    volumetric infusion p.
pump-assisted coronary hemoperfusion
Pumpette
    Stat 2 P.
pumping
    intraaortic balloon p. (IABP)
    p. rate
    venoarterial bypass p. (VABP)
pumpkin-seeding
pump-oxygenator
punch
    Abrams pleural biopsy p.
    p. biopsy
    Goosen vascular p.
punctate
    p. hyperintensity
    p. mucosal lesion
puncture
    apical left ventricular p.
    computer-assisted pericardial p.
      (CASPER)
    direct cardiac p.
    left ventricular p.
    p. site
    tracheoesophageal p.

transcricothyroid p.
transseptal p.
venous p.
ventricular p.
pup cell
pupil
Argyll Robertson p.
Pura-Vario stent
pure
p. dysarthria (PD)
p. flutter
p. motor hemiparesis (PMH)
p. motor stroke
p. parasystole
p. pneumothorax
p. pulmonary atresia (PPA)
p. sensorimotor stroke
p. sensory stroke
p. sensory syndrome (PSS)
purified
p. histidyl-tRNA synthetase
p. protein derivative (PPD)
p. protein derivative test
p. protein derivative of tuberculin
purifier
Air Supply wearable air p.
Bemis air p.
purine nucleotides adenosine
triphosphate
purinergic action
purinoceptor
endothelial p.
Puritan
P. all purpose compressor
P. Bennett Aeris 590 oxygen
concentrator
P. Bennett 7250 metabolic monitor
P. Bennett ventilator
P. Bennett 840 ventilator system
Purkinje
P. cell
P. conduction
P. disease
P. fiber
P. image tracker
P. network
P. system
P. tumor
Purkinje-His
Purmann method
puromucous
purple grape juice
purpose
purpura
allergy p.
anaphylactoid p.
p. fulminans
Henoch-Schönlein p.

idiopathic thrombocytopenic p.
(ITP)
thrombotic thrombocytopenic p.
(TTP)
purpurea
Digitalis p.
purr
purring thrill
pursed lip breathing (PLB)
pursestring suture
pursing
lip p.
Pursuit balloon angioplasty catheter
purulent
p. effusion
p. pericarditis (PP)
p. pleurisy
p. pneumonia
p. sputum
purulenta
pneumonia interlobularis p.
pushability
pusher wire
putative
p. agent
p. slow pathway potential
putrid
p. bronchitis
p. empyema
p. sputum
PV
plasma viscosity
portal vein
pressure volume
pulmonary valve
pulmonary vein
ventricular pressure
PV curve
PVA
polyvinyl alcohol
PVA foam embolization particle
PVa
pulmonary venous atrial
PVAB
postventricular atrial blanking
pVAD
percutaneous ventricular assist device
TandemHeart pVAD
PVARP
postventricular atrial refractory period
PVB
premature ventricular beat
PVC
polyvinyl chloride
premature ventricular contraction
pulmonary venous confluence
pulmonary venous congestion
PVD
peripheral vascular disease

P

PVD *(continued)*
portal vein dilation
premature ventricular depolarization
pulmonary vascular disease
PVE
premature ventricular extrasystole
prosthetic valve endocarditis
PVF
portal venous flow
primary ventricular fibrillation
pulmonary venous flow
PVG
pulmonary valve gradient
PVH
periventricular hyperintensity
pulmonary venous hypertension
PVHI
periventricular hyperintensity
PVI
perivascular infiltration
PVL
Panton-Valentine leucocidin
perivalvular leakage
PVL gene
PVN
paraventricular nucleus
PVO
pulmonary vascular obstruction
PVOD
pulmonary vascular obstructive disease
pulmonary venoocclusive disease
PVP
peripheral venous pressure
pulmonary venous pressure
PVR
peripheral vascular resistance
prosthetic valve regurgitation
pulmonary valve repair
pulmonary valve replacement
pulmonary vascular resistance
pulse volume recording
PVRI
pulmonary vascular resistance index
PVS
premature ventricular systole
programmed ventricular stimulation
prosthetic valve stenosis
pulmonary valvular stenosis
PVs
pulmonary venous systolic
PVT
paroxysmal ventricular tachycardia
portal vein thrombosis
primary ventricular tachycardia
PV-Tussin
PW
peristaltic wave
posterior wall
pressure wave

pulmonary wedge
pulse wave
PW pressure
P-wave
P-w. amplitude
P-w. axis
P-w. duration
P-w. morphology
P-wave triggered ventricular pacemaker
PWD
pulsed-wave Doppler
PWE
posterior wall excursion
PWI
perfusion-weighted magnetic resonance
imaging
posterior wall infarct
PWLV
posterior wall of left ventricle
PWM
pulse with modulation
PWP
pulmonary wedge pressure
PWTD
pulsed-wave tissue Doppler
PWV
pulse wave velocity
Pycnogenol
pyemia
arterial p.
portal p.
pyemic
p. edema
p. embolism
pyknosis
pylori
Helicobacter p.
pyloric incompetence
pyocyanine
pyoderma gangrenosum
pyogenes
Streptococcus p.
pyogenic infection
Pyopen
pyopneumopericardium
pyopneumothorax
pyothorax-associated lymphoma
PYP
pyrophosphate
PYP imaging
PYP scan
pyramid
Food Guide P.
Mediterranean Diet P.
p. method
pyrantel pamoate
pyrazinamide (PZA)
rifampin, isoniazid, p.

pyrexia
pyribenzamine (PBZ)
pyridazinone dinitrile
pyridoxalated
    stroma-free hemoglobin p. (SFHb)
    p. stroma-free hemoglobin (SFHb)
pyridoxine hydrochloride
pyriform (*var. of* piriform)
pyrimethamine
    sulfadoxine and p.
pyrogenic mediator
pyrogen reaction
pyrolytic
    p. carbon
    p. carbon aortic valve
pyrophosphate (PYP)

    farnesyl p.
    geranyl p.
    p. imaging
    isopentenyl p.
    mevalonate p.
    p. scan
    p. scintigram
    p. scintigraphy
    technetium p.
    technetium-99m p.
pyruvate dehydrogenase (PDH)
pyruvic acid
PZA
    pyrazinamide
Pzf
    zero-flow pressure

P

Q

cardiac output

Q fever

Q Port

Q wave

Q wave regression

QALY

quality-adjusted life-years

QAR

quantitative autoradiography

QAV

quadricuspid aortic valve

Qc

pulmonary capillary blood flow

QCA

quantitative coronary analysis

quantitative coronary angiography

quantitative coronary arteriography

Q-cath catheterization recording system

QC 253 CO-oximetry control

QCS

quick confusion scale

QCT

quantitative computed tomography

QCU

qualitative coronary ultrasound

Q-H interval

QIP

quality improvement process

QMI

Q-wave myocardial infarction

Q-M interval

QOM

quality of movement

Qp

pulmonary blood flow

Qpc

pulmonary capillary blood flow

Q-Plex metabolic cart and pulmonary function unit

Qp:Qs

pulmonary-to-systemic flow ratio

pulmonic-to-systemic flow ratio

Q$_s$/Q$_t$

intrapulmonary shunt fraction

QQ, QR, TT genotype

QR, Q-R

QR interval

QR, QS pattern

QRB interval

QRS

complex of Q, R, S, waves corresponding
to depolarization of ventricles

abnormal ECG rhythm of small R,
bigger R of QRS (rSR′, rsr
prime)

QRS alternans

QRS axis

QRS change

QRS complex

QRS complex configuration

QRS complex duration

QRS contour

fusion QRS

QRS interval

QRS loop

QRS morphology

small R, bigger R of QRS (rSR)

QRS synchronous atrial
defibrillation shocks

QRS vector

QRS-ST junction

QRS-T

QRS-T angle

QRS-T complex

QRS-T interval

QRS-T value

QS

QS complex

QS deflection

QS wave

QS$_2$

total electromechanical systole

QS$_2$ interval

Qs

systemic blood flow

Qs/Qt

shunted blood to total blood flow

Qs/Qt ratio

Q-Stress

Q-S. treadmill

Q-S. treadmill stress test

Q-switched Nd:YAG laser

QT, Q-T

cardiac output

corrected QT

QT dispersion (QTd)

QT interval

QT interval corrected for heart
rate (QTc, Q-Tc)

QT interval dispersion

QT interval duration

QT interval sensing pacemaker

long QT (LQT)

pathologic QT (QTU)

QT syndrome

QT ventilation

QT1
    long QT1 (LQT1)
QT2
    long QT2 (LQT2)
QTc, Q-Tc
    QT interval corrected for heart rate
    QTc interval
    QTc prolongation
QTd
    QT dispersion
QTI:QT index
QTL
    quantitative trait locus
QTp/QTe
    ratio of QTp/QTe
QT/QTc dispersion
Q-TRAK IAQ monitor
QTU
    pathologic QT
    QTU prolongation
QU, Q-U
    QU interval
quad
    q. coughing
    q. screen format
QuaDDS stent
Quad-Lumen catheter
QuadPolar electrode
quadrangular resection
quadratum
    foramen q.
quadrature
    q. birdcage coil
    q. head coil
quadricuspid aortic valve (QAV)
quadrigeminal
    q. pulse
    q. rhythm
quadrigeminus
    pulsus q.
quadrigeminy
quadriparesis
quadriplegia
quadripolar
    q. diagnostic catheter
    q. Itrel 2 pulse generator
    q. pacing catheter
    q. Quad electrode
    q. steerable electrode catheter
    q. steerable mapping/ablation
      catheter
    q. thermocouple-equipped ablation
      catheter
quadruple rhythm
quadruplet
Quaegebeur procedure

Quain
    Q. fatty degeneration
    Q. fatty heart
qualitative coronary ultrasound (QCU)
quality
    q. control
    q. enhancement research initiative
      (QUERI)
    q. improvement process (QIP)
    indoor air q. (IAQ)
    q. of life
    q. of movement (QOM)
    Q. of Well-Being Index
    Q. of Well-Being Scale
      questionnaire
quality-adjusted life-years (QALY)
quality-of-care
    q.-o.-c. evaluation
    q.-o.-c. indicator
Quanam
    Q. QP2 coronary stent
    Q. QuaDDS stent
    Q. QuaDS-QP2 stent system
QuantiFeron-TB test
quantification
    acoustic q. (AQ)
    digital echo q. (DEQ)
    shunt q.
quantify
Quantison contrast agent
quantitative
    q. arteriography
    q. autoradiography (QAR)
    q. computed tomography (QCT)
    q. coronary analysis (QCA)
    q. coronary angiographic analysis
    q. coronary angiography (QCA)
    q. coronary angiography caliper
      measurement
    q. coronary arteriography (QCA)
    q. 2-dimensional echocardiography
    q. Doppler
    q. edge-detection angiography
    q. left ventriculography
    q. trait locus (QTL)
    q. wall motion score (QWMS)
quantum
    q. mottling
    Q. pacemaker
    q. proteolysis
    Q. TTC balloon dilator
Quartet system
quartile range
quartisternal
quartz transducer
quasisinusoidal waveform
quaternary ammonium atropine
  derivative
Quattro mitral valve prosthesis

Queckenstedt sign
Queensland
    Q. fever
    Q. tick typhus
quellung reaction
Quénu-Muret sign
quercetin
QUERI
    quality enhancement research initiative
    IHD QUERI
query fever
quest
    Q. Medical microplegia system
    Q. Medical microplegia system
    Q. Medical MPS cardioplegia fluid delivery pump
    Q. Medical MPS console
    Q. Medical MPS delivery set
    Q. MPS microplegia system
    Q. MPS myocardial protection system
questionnaire
    Asthma Quality of Life Q. (AQLQ)
    Berlin q.
    Childhood Asthma Q. (CAQ)
    Chronic Respiratory Q. (CRQ)
    Chronic Respiratory Disease Q. (CRQ)
    Cognitive Failures Q. (CFQ)
    Coping Strategies q.
    cough-specific quality of life q.
    Dyspnea Scale q.
    Fagerstrom Tolerance Q. (FTQ)
    Functional Outcomes of Sleep Q. (FOSQ)
    Guyatt q.
    Karolinska quality of life q.
    Kellner q.
    LIhFE q.
    London School of Hygiene Cardiovascular Rose Q.
    Mahler Baseline Dyspnea Index q.
    MAQOL q.
    McGill-Melzack Pain Q.
    McGill Pain Q.
    Medical Research Council q.
    Minnesota Leisure Time Physical Activity Q.
    Minnesota Living with Heart Failure q.
    Oxygen Cost Diagram q.
    Pulmonary Functional Status and Dyspnea Q. (PFSDQ)
    Quality of Well-Being Scale q.
    Rose Q.
    Seattle Angina Q.
    Sickness Impact Profile q.
    St. George Respiratory Q. (SGRQ)

    Veterans Specific Activity Q. (VSAQ)
Questran Light
Quetelet index
Quibron
quick
    q. confusion scale (QCS)
    Q. intravenous liver function test
    q. prothrombin time
    q. pulse
QuickDraw venous cannula
QuickFlash arterial catheter
QuickFlow
    Q. DPS
    Q. DPS distal perfusion system
QuickFurl SL balloon
QuicKlamp hemostasis device
QuickSeal
    Q. arterial closure device
    Q. femoral arterial closure system
    Q. sealing device
quiet
    q. breath sounds
    q. chest
    q. heart sounds
    q. lung
    q. precordium
Quik-Chek external pacer tester
Quik-Prep electrode
quinacrine
quinapril
    q. hydrochloride
    q. and hydrochlorothiazide
quinaprilat
Quinatime
Quincke
    Q. disease
    Q. edema
    Q. pulse
    Q. sign
quinestrol
quinethazone
Quinidex Extentabs
quinidine
    q. gluconate
    q. sulfate
    q. syncope syndrome
quinidine-induced torsade de pointes
quinine sulfate
quinolidomicin
quinolone
Quinones
    method of Q.
quinsy
    lingual q.
quintana
    Rochalimaea q.
Quinton
    Q. PermCath catheter

Quinton *(continued)*
    Q. Synergy cardiac information
        management system
Quinton-Scribner shunt
quinupristin
quotient
    intelligence q. (IQ)
    respiratory q. (RQ)
    V̇/Q̇ q.

Qvar
QVAR inhaled corticosteroid
Q-wave myocardial infarction (QMI)
QwikLoad
    CardioSEAL septal occlusion
        system with Q.
QWMS
    quantitative wall motion score

R
first positive deflection during the QRS complex
gas constant
roentgen
R axis
R on T ventricular premature contraction
R unit
R wave

R3
ReoPro Readministration Registry

R'
second positive deflection during QRS complex
R' wave

RA
rheumatoid arthritis
right atrium
right auricle
rotational atherectomy
RA 523 blood gas/CO-oximetry control
RA cell
Integris 3D RA

RAA
right atrial appendage

RAAS
renin-angiotensin-aldosterone system

rAAT
recombinant alpha-1 antitrypsin

rabbit
r. antithymocyte globulin
r. aorta-contracting substance (RCS)
r. ear sign
r. fever

rabies

Rabinov venography technique

RACAT
rapid acquisition computed axial tomography

racemic
r. epinephrine
r. warfarin sodium

racemose aneurysm

racemosum
angioma venosum r.

Racer balloon-expandable stent

Rackley method

racquet incision

RAD
reactive airways disease
regional alveolar damage
right atrium diameter
right axis deviation
RAD airway laryngeal blade

rad
radiation absorbed dose

radarkymography

Radford nomogram

radial
r. approach
r. artery
r. artery graft
r. artery systolic pressure (RASP)
r. pulse (RP)

RadiAnalyzer

radiant heat device (RHD)

radiata
corona r.

radiation
r. absorbed dose (rad)
biological effects of ionizing r.
r. bronchitis
r. burden
r. equivalent in man (rem)
extended field r. (EFR)
r. fibrosis
gamma r.
hyperfractionated r. (HRT)
intracoronary artery r.
ionizing r. (IR)
r. lung disease
mitogenic r.
r. pneumonitis
r. safety
scatter r.
secondary r.
r. therapy

radiation-induced
r.-i. atherosclerosis
r.-i. heart disease (RIHD)
r.-i. lung injury
r.-i. pericarditis

radical
free r.
hydroxyl r.
O_2 r.
oxygen r.
oxygen-derived free r.
oxygen-free r.

radicle

radiculitis
cervical r.

Radifocus
R. catheter guidewire
R. Glidewire
R. wire

radii (*pl. of* radius)

R

Radii-T catheter
radio
    LDL/HDL r.
radioablation
radioactive
    r. iodinated serum albumin (RISA)
    r. stent
    r. tantalum
    r. xenon test
radioallergosorbent test (RAST)
radiocardiogram (RKG)
radiocardiography
radiocontrast dye
radiodense
radiodermatitis
radioelectrocardiography (RECG)
radiofemoral delay
radiofrequency (RF)
    r. ablation (RFA)
    r. ablator
    r. catheter ablation
    r. current (RFC)
    r. electrophrenic respiration
    r. energy
    r. energy ablation
    r. energy area
    r. energy delivery
    r. hot balloon
    r. lesion
    r. percutaneous myocardial
      revascularization (RF-PMR)
    r. tissue ablation (RFTA)
radiofrequency-assisted valvotomy
radiograph (*See also* x-ray)
    chest r. (CXR, CxR)
    portable chest r.
    postoperative chest r.
radiographic
    r. cephalometry
    r. technique
radiography
    computed r. (CR)
    digital r.
    dual-energy digital r.
radioimmunoassay (RIA)
    Coat-a-Count r.
    Insulin Riabead II r.
    Mallinckrodt r.
radioimmunotherapy
radioisotope
radiolabeled
    r. fibrinogen (RLF)
    r. gallium
    r. iodine
    r. microsphere
radioligand binding assay
radiologic scimitar syndrome
radiologist
    thoracic r.

radiology
    interventional r.
    Society of Cardiovascular and
      Interventional R. (SCVIR)
radiolucent
Radiometer probe
radiometry
    BACTEC r.
radionecrosis injury
Radionics radiofrequency generator
radionuclide
    r. angiocardiography
    r. angiography (RNA)
    r. cineangiocardiography
    daughter r.
    r. generator
    gold-195m r.
    r. imaging
    parent r.
    r. superior cavography (RNSC)
    r. technique
    r. venography (RNV)
    r. ventriculography (RNV, RNVG)
radiopacity
radiopaque
    r. end marker
    r. ERCP catheter
    r. tantalum stent
radiopharmaceutical imaging
radiotelemetry
radiotherapy (XRT)
    continuous hyperfractionated
      accelerated r. (CHART)
    locoregional r.
    postoperative r. (PORT)
    proton-beam r.
radiotherapy-induced carotid stenosis
radiotracer
RadiStop radial compression system
radius, pl. **radii**
    R. self-expanding stent
    thrombocytopenia-absent r. (TAR)
radixin
radix linguae
radon
RADS
    reactive airways disease syndrome
    reactive airways dysfunction syndrome
RAE
    right atrial enlargement
    RAE endotracheal tube
Raeder-Harbitz syndrome
RAF
    repetitive atrial firing
Raff-Glantz derivative method
raft
    lipid r.
RAFW
    right atrial free wall

ragpicker's disease
ragsorter's disease
RAH
    right atrial hypertrophy
Rahn-Otis sample
RAI
    right atrial inversion
    right atrial involvement
railroad track sign
raised-volume rapid thoracoabdominal
    compression technique
RAITI
    right atrial inversion time index
rake retractor
rale
        amphoric r.
        atelectatic r.
        basilar r.
        bibasilar r.
        border r.
        bronchial r.
        bronchiectatic r.
        bubbling r.
        cavernous r.
        cellophane r.
        clicking r.
        coarse r.
        collapse r.
        consonating r.
        crackling r.
        crepitant r.
        dry r.
        extrathoracic r.
        gurgling r.
        guttural r.
        r. indux
        inspiratory r.
        laryngeal r.
        marginal r.
        metallic r.
        moist r.
        mucous r.
        musical r.
        pleural r.
        pulmonary r.
        r. redux
        r.'s and rhonchi
        sibilant r.
        Skoda r.
        snoring r.
        sonorous r.
        subcrepitant r.
        tracheal r.
        Velcro r.
        ventricular r. (VR)
        vesicular r.
        wet r.
        whistling r.

Ralstonia
raltitrexed
Raman
        R. spectography
        R. spectroscopy
rami (*pl. of* ramus)
ramipril
Ramond sign
RAMP
        rate modulated pacing
        right atrial mean pressure
        RAMP antitachycardia protocol
        RAMP pacing
        RAMP treadmill protocol
ramp
        R. cardiac marker test
        R. Reader and Ramp Myoglobin
        Test
RAMP-based protocol
Ramsay score
RAMT
        right atrial mobile thrombus
ramus, pl. **rami**
        r. anterior descendens
        r. anterior lateralis
        rami bronchiales
        rami bronchiales segmentorum
        r. communicans cum nervo
        glossopharyngeo
        r. coronary bypass
        rami esophageales
        rami esophageales aortae thoracicae
        rami esophageales arteriae gastricae
        sinistrae
        rami esophageales arteriae
        thyroideae inferioris
        rami esophagei
        rami esophagei nervi laryngei
        recurrentis
        rami esophagei nervi vagi
        r. intermedius
        r. intermedius artery
        r. internus nervi laryngei superioris
        rami isthmi faucium nervi lingualis
        r. lobi medii arteriae pulmonalis
        dextrae
        r. medianus
        r. posterior descendens
        r. posterior venae pulmonalis
        dextrae superioris
        rami pulmonales systematis
        autonomici
Randall-Baker Soucek
Rand appropriateness selection criteria
randomized
        r. clinical trial (RCT)
        R. Intervention Treatment of
        Angina (RITA)

R

randomized *(continued)*
    R. Outpatient Milrinone Evaluation (ROME)
    r. trial
randomized, controlled trial (RCT)
random nodule
random-zero sphygmomanometer
Ranexa
Ranfac needle
range
    D2L OTW balloon dilation catheter with extended pressure r.
    dynamic r.
    extended pressure r.
    heart rate r. (HRR)
    interquartile r.
    logarithmic dynamic r.
    pressure r.
    quartile r.
    R2L rapid exchange balloon dilation catheter with extended pressure r.
range-alternating current
range-gated transducer
ranger
    R. balloon
    R. over-the-wire balloon catheter
ranging
    echo r.
ranine artery
Ranke complex
Rankin Disability Scale
ranolazine
rANP
    rat atrial natriuretic peptide
Ransohoff operation
Ranvier
    node of R.
RAO
    right anterior oblique
    RAO angulation
    RAO position
    RAO 30 projection
    RAO view
RAP
    rapid atrial pacing
    remote access perfusion
    resident assessment protocol
    right atrial pressure
    RAP cannula
RA-PA
    right atrium to pulmonary artery
Rapamune
rapamycin
rape
    bruit de scie ou de r.
rapeseed oil
raphe
    r. linguae

    pharyngeal r.
    r. pharyngis
    r. of pharynx
rapid
    r. acquisition computed axial tomography (RACAT)
    r. antigen-detection test
    r. atrial pacing (RAP)
    r. atrial stimulation (RAS)
    r. depolarization
    r. early action in coronary treatment (REACT)
    r. empiric therapy
    r. exchange (RX)
    r. eye movement (REM)
    r. filling
    r. filling wave
    r. fluid loading
    r. nonsustained ventricular tachycardia
    r. pacing
    r. plasma test
    r. platelet function assay (RPFA)
    r. repolarization
    r. sequence induction (RSI)
    r. shallow breathing index (RSBI)
    r. troponin T
    r. ventricular rate
    r. Y descent
rapid-burst pacing
rapid-exchange catheter
Rapidlab 800 Critical Care system
RapidMist metered dose spray applicator
Rapidpoint
    R. access
    R. Coag Analyzer
rapid-sequence intubation
RapidVUE particle shape and size analyzer
Rappaport-Sprague stethoscope
rappel
    bruit de r.
Raptorail catheter
Raptor PTCA balloon
rarefaction
    pontine ischemic r.
rarus
    pulsus r.
RA-RV
    right atrium to right ventricle
    RA-RV anastomosis
    RA-RV conduit
    RA-RV connection
    RA-RV Fontan procedure
    RA-RV position
RAS
    rapid atrial stimulation
    renal artery stenosis

renin-angiotensin system
rotational atherectomy system

rash
    erythematous maculopapular r.
    Gottron r.
    maculopapular r.

Rashkind
    R. balloon atrial septostomy
    R. balloon technique
    R. double umbrella device
    R. procedure
    R. septostomy balloon catheter

Ras mitogen-activated protein kinase

Rasmussen
    R. aneurysm
    R. syndrome

Rasor blood pumping system (RBPS)

RASP
    radial artery systolic pressure

raspatory
    rib r.

rasping murmur

RAST
    radioallergosorbent test
    RAST panel

Rastan-Konno procedure

Rastan operation

Rastelli
    R. operation
    R. procedure

rat
    r. atrial natriuretic peptide (rANP)
    r. urine protein

rate
    atrial r. (AR)
    atrial heart r. (AHR)
    atrial overdrive stimulation r.
    (AST)
    atrial tachycardia detection r.
    (ATDR)
    basal fetal heart r. (BFHR)
    basal heart r. (BHR)
    basal metabolic r. (BMR)
    baseline variability of fetal heart r.
    beat-to-beat variability of fetal
    heart r.
    beginning-of-life r.
    blood flow r. (BFR)
    blunted heart r.
    body acceleration synchronous with
    heart r. (BASH)
    cerebral r.
    complication r.
    r. control
    count r.
    critical r.
    diastolic descent r. (DDR)
    disintegration r.
    ejection r. (ER)

end-of-life r.
erythrocyte sedimentation r. (ESR)
expiratory flow r.
fetal heart r. (FHR)
flow r.
glomerular filtration r. (GFR)
heart r. (HR, HRT)
highest equivalent heart r. (HEHR)
r. hysteresis
r. immunonephelometry
indocyanine green plasma
    disappearance r. (ICG-PDR)
inspiratory flow r.
internal work r.
intrinsic heart r. (IHR)
key pulse r. (KPR)
left ventricular peak filling r.
    (LVPFR)
low-flow r.
magnet r.
maternal heart r. (MHR)
maximal expiratory flow r.
    (MEFR)
maximal heart r. (Hrmax, MHR)
maximal inspiratory flow r. (MIFR)
maximal midexpiratory flow r.
    (MMEFR)
maximal ventilation r. (MVR)
maximum determined heart r.
    (MDHR)
maximum flow r.
maximum midexpiratory flow r.
    (MMEF, MMF)
maximum predicted heart r.
    (MPHR)
maximum pulse r. (MPR)
maximum sensory r.
mean atrial r. (MAR)
mean circumferential fiber-
    shortening r. (MCFSR)
mean midexpiratory flow r. ($FEF_{25-75\%}$)
mean normalized systolic
    ejection r.
mean systolic ejection r. (MSER)
miss r.
r. modulated pacing (RAMP)
r. modulation
mortality r. (MR)
myocardial metabolic r. (MMR)
pacemaker adaptive r.
patency r.
peak diastolic filling r.
peak ejection r. (PER)
peak emptying r.
peak expiratory flow r. (PEFR)
peak filling r. (PFR)
peak heart r. (PHR)
peak inspiratory flow r. (PIFR)

R

rate *(continued)*
    peak jet flow r.
    peak lengthening r.
    peak shortening r.
    peak work r. (Wmax)
    percent of maximum predicted heart r.
    predicted maximal heart r. (PMHR)
    programmed cut-off r.
    pulse r. (PR)
    pulse repetition r. (PRR)
    pumping r.
    QT interval corrected for heart r. (QTc, Q-Tc)
    rapid ventricular r.
    relative slow sinus r. (RSSR)
    relative survival r.
    repetition r.
    respiratory r. (RR)
    resting heart r. (RHR)
    resting metabolic r. (RMR)
    r. and rhythm (R&R)
    right ventricular peak filling r. (RVPFR)
    slew r. (SR)
    r. smoothing
    spontaneous inspiratory flow r.
    stroke ejection r.
    ST-segment divided by heart r. (ST/HR)
    submaximal heart r.
    submaximum heart r.
    Svedberg flotation r.
    systolic ejection r. (SER)
    target heart r. (THR)
    time forced expiratory r.
    time-to-peak filling r.
    transvalvular flow r.
    vasoconstriction r. (VCR)
    ventilator r.
    ventricular escape r.
    ventricular heart r. (VHR)
    Westergren erythrocyte sedimentation r.
    Wintrobe sedimentation r.
    work r.
rate-adaptive
    r.-a. device
    r.-a. pacemaker
rate-dependent
    r.-d. angina
    r.-d. bundle branch block
rate-drop
    r.-d. response (RDR)
    r.-d. response mode
    r.-d. sensing
rate-modulated pacemaker
rate-pressure product (RPP)

rate-responsive
    dual-chamber r.-r.
    r.-r. pulse generator
    single-chamber r.-r.
    r.-r. ventricular pacing
Rathke pouch tumor
rating
    Borg dyspnea r.
    r. of perceived breathing difficulty (RPBD)
    r. of perceived exertion (RPE)
ratio *(See also* relation)
    AH:HA r.
    ankle-brachial blood pressure r.
    aorta-left atrium r.
    aortic root r.
    balloon to artery r.
    benefit-risk r.
    bur-to-artery r.
    cardiothoracic r. (CTR)
    cell proliferation-to-apoptosis r.
    conduction r.
    contrast r.
    C/P r.
    C/PL r.
    C/TG r.
    dead space gas volume to tidal gas volume r. (V_{DS}/V_T)
    dead space/tidal volume r.
    early to late diastolic filling r. (E:A)
    E/A wave r.
    E:I r.
    embolus-to-blood r. (EBR)
    end-systolic volume r.
    r. of expiration time and total time of breathing cycle (tE/tTOT)
    flow r.
    forced expiratory volume in 1 second to forced vital capacity r. (FEV_1/FVC)
    forced expiratory volume timed to forced vital capacity r. (FEV/FVC)
    I:E r.
    incremental cost-effectiveness r. (ICER)
    r. of ingested saturated fat and cholesterol to calories
    r. of inspiration time and total time of breathing cycle (tI/tTOT)
    inspiratory to expiratory r.
    r. of inspiratory time to total breathing cycle time (T_I/T_{TOT})
    international normalized r. (INR)
    La:A r.
    LA/Ao r.
    L/H r.
    L/S r.

R

McGoon r.
murmur/energy r. (MER)
odds r. (OR)
oxygen extraction r. (O_2ER)
physiologic dead space/tidal
volume r. (V_D/V_T)
P:QRS r.
prothrombin time r. (PTR)
PR/RP r.
pulmonary systemic blood flow r.
pulmonary-to-systemic flow r.
(Qp:Qs)
pulmonic-to-systemic flow r.
(Qp:Qs)
pulse amplitude r. (PAR)
Qs/Qt r.
r. of QTp/QTe
renal vein renin r.
residual volume/total lung
capacity r.
resistance r.
respiratory exchange r. (RER)
respiratory rate to tidal volume r.
(f/VT)
risk-benefit r.
R/Q wave r.
RV/TLC r.
S/A r.
segmental venous capacitance r.
(SVCR)
sex r.
shunt r.
signal-to-noise r.
subendocardial to epicardial resting
perfusion r.
systolic velocity r.
TC/HDL r.
r. of tidal expiratory flow at 25%
of tidal volume and peak tidal
expiratory flow ($TEF_{25}/PTEF$)
r. of tidal expiratory and
inspiratory flow at 50% of tidal
volume (TEF_{50}/TIF_{50})
transmitral Doppler E:A r.
transmitral E:A r.
trough-to-peak r.
V/C r.
velocity r. (VR)
venous diameter r. (VDR)
ventilation/perfusion r.
waist-to-hip r. (WHR)
rationalization
rattle of return
Rattus
R. norvegicus
R. norvegicus allergen
Rauchfuss triangle
Raulerson syringe
Rautaharju ECG criteria

Rauwolfia
R. alkaloid
R. extract
R. serpentina
rauwolscine
RAVC
retrograde atrioventricular conduction
RAW
resistance, airway
right atrial wall
Raw
airways resistance
ray
beta r.
gamma r.
scattered r.'s
secondary r.'s
r. sum
Rayleigh scattering
Raynaud
R. disease
R. gangrene
R. phenomenon
R. sign
R. syndrome
RB
respiratory bronchiolitis
right bundle
Rb
rubidium
Rb-82
rubidium-82
Rb-82 PET
RBA
right brachial artery
RBB
right bundle branch
RBBB
right bundle branch block
RBBsB
right bundle branch system block
RBC
red blood cell
RBC osmotic fragility
RBCD
right border cardiac dullness
RBD
right border of dullness
right brain damage
RB-ILD
respiratory bronchiolitis-interstitial lung
disease
RBPS
Rasor blood pumping system
RBV
right brachial vein
RCA
right coronary artery
rotational coronary atherectomy

RCBF
  renal cortical blood flow
rCBF
  regional cerebral blood flow
RCC
  right coronary cusp
RCCA
  right common carotid artery
RCD
  relative cardiac dullness
RCFR
  relative coronary flow reserve
RCHF
  right congestive heart failure
RCM
  right costal margin
RCO
  right coronary ostium
RCP
  respiratory care practitioner
RCPP
  recurrent coronary prevention program
RCS
  rabbit aorta-contracting substance
  right coronary sinus
RCT
  randomized clinical trial
  randomized, controlled trial
RCVA
  right cerebrovascular accident
RCVR
  renal cortical vascular resistance
RCWI
  right cardiac work index
RDC
  Robert David Cerfolio
    RDC classification
    RDC classification system
RDF
    Adriamycin PFS, RDF
RDI
  respiratory disturbance index
rDNA
  recombinant deoxyribonucleic acid
    lepirudin rDNA
RDPA
  right descending pulmonary artery
RDR
  rate-drop response
RDR mode
RDS
  respiratory distress syndrome
RDX coronary radiation catheter delivery system
reabsorbable suture
reabsorption
    sodium r.
REACT
  rapid early action in coronary treatment

reaction
  allergic r.
  anaphylactoid r.
  antigen-driven inflammatory r.
  Arthus-type r.
  cholera vaccine r.
  egg-yellow r.
  Eisenmenger r.
  Fernandez r.
  fibrinolytic r.
  fight-or-flight r.
  Haber-Weiss r.
  hemoclastic r.
  hexokinase r.
  hunting r.
  immune reconstitution
    inflammatory r. (IRIS)
  inflammatory r.
  Kveim r.
  ligase chain r. (LCR)
  local r.
  Maillard r.
  methacholine r.
  monocytic leukemoid r.
  non-IgE-mediated r.
  paradoxical r.
  photosensitizing r.
  Pirquet r.
  pleural r.
  polymerase chain r. (PCR)
  pyrogen r.
  quellung r.
  reverse transcriptase polymerase
    chain r. (RT-PCR)
  smallpox vaccine r.
  vagal r.
  vasovagal r.
  Weil-Felix r.
  xanthine oxidase r.
reactivation tuberculosis
reactive
  r. airways disease (RAD)
  r. airways disease syndrome
    (RADS)
  r. airways dysfunction syndrome
    (RADS)
  r. dilation
  r. hyperemia
  r. mesothelial hyperplasia
  r. oxygen species (ROS)
  r. skin decontamination lotion
    (RSDL)
  r. upper airways dysfunction
    syndrome (RUDS)
reactivity
  bronchial r.
  cerebrovascular r. (CVR)
  digital vascular r. (DVR)
  methacholine r.

pulmonary vascular r.
vascular r.

reader

ReadMyHeart handheld ECG device

Read test

reagent

Chrono-Lume r.
Chrono-Par aggregation r.

reagin

Rea-Lo

real-time

r.-t. 3-dimensional dobutamine
stress echocardiography
r.-t. endobronchial ultrasound-guided
transbronchial needle aspiration
r.-t. perfusion imaging
r.-t. position management (RPM)
r.-t. position management tracking
system
r.-t. telemetry
r.-t. ultrasound

reassessment

Reaven syndrome

Rebar-18 microcatheter

Rebetron

reblockage

rebound angina

reboxetine

rebreathing

r. bag
r. mask
r. method
r. technique

recainam

recalcitrant

r. hypertension
r. obstructive airways disease

recall antigen

recalled

spoiled gradient r. (SPGR)

recanalization

balloon occlusive intravascular lysis
enhanced r.
chronic total occlusion r.
coronary r.
excimer vascular r.
percutaneous transluminal
coronary r. (PTCR)
x-ray-guided r.

receiver

Medtronic radiofrequency r.

recent myocardial infarction (RMI)

receptive aphasia

receptor

A_{2A} adenosine r.
adrenergic r. (ADR, AR)
A-II r.
alpha r.
alpha-1A adrenergic r. (ADRA1A)

alpha-1-adrenergic r.
alpha-2-adrenergic r. (ADRA2)
alpha-2C adrenergic r. (ADRA2C)
beta r.
beta-1, -2 r.
beta-adrenergic r. (BAR)
beta-1B adrenergic r. (ADRA1B)
r. blocker
bone morphogenetic protein r.
(BMPR)
cholinergic r.
chylomicron remnant r.
cough r.
dopamine D2 r. (DD2R)
endothelin A, B r.'s
epithelial 5′-nucleotide r.
factor II r. (F2R)
Fas r.
Fc r.'s
FMLP r.
G-couple surface r.
glycoprotein IIb/IIIa r.
H1 r.
r. for hyaluronan-mediated motility
(RHAMM)
imidazoline r. (I-receptor)
inhibitory M2 muscarinic r.
interleukin 4 r. (IL-4R)
irritant r.
juxtacapillary r.
liver X r.
low-density lipoprotein r. (LDLR,
LDL-R)
mast cell high-affinity Fc r.
melanocortin-4 r. (MC4-R)
muscarinic r.
myocardial beta adrenergic r.
(MBAR)
NMDA r.
opsonophagocytic r.
peroxisome proliferator-activated r.
(PPAR)
peroxisome proliferator-activated r.
gamma (PPAR-gamma)
ryanodine r.
RyR2 r.
soluble dimeric TNF r.
soluble tumor necrosis factor r.
(sTNFR)
stretch r.
tachykinin r.
toll-like r. (TLR)
tumor necrosis factor r. (TNFR)
very low density lipoprotein r.
(VLDLR)

receptor-operated calcium channel

recess

costodiaphragmatic r.
costomediastinal r.

recess *(continued)*
    intertrabecular r.
    intratrabecular r.
    pleural r.
    Rosenmüller r.
    subphrenic r.
    superior omental r.
    supratonsillar r.
recessed balloon septostomy catheter
recessus
    r. pharyngeus
    r. pleurales
RECG
    radioelectrocardiography
Rechtschaffen scoring method
recidivism
recipient heart
reciprocal
    r. beat
    r. bigeminy
    r. presentation
    r. regulation
    r. rhythm
    r. ST depression
reciprocating
    r. macroreentry orthodromic
      tachycardia
    r. rhythm
    r. tachycardia (RT)
reciprocity
reclosure
recoarctation of aorta
recognition protein
recoil
    elastic r.
    luminal r.
    lung elastic r.
    maximum flow static r. (MFSR)
    r. phenomenon
    systolic r.
    r. wave
recombinant
    r. activated factor VII (rFVIIa)
    r. alpha-1 antitrypsin (rAAT)
    r. alteplase
    r. deoxyribonucleic acid (rDNA)
    r. desulfatohirudin
    r. hirudin (r-hirudin)
    r. human antithrombin III (rhATIII)
    r. human C1 inhibitor (rhC1INH)
    r. human IL-10 (rhuIL-10)
    r. human relaxin
    r. human vascular endothelial
      growth factor (rhVEGF)
    r. lys-plasminogen
    r. polyethylene glycol (r-PEG)
    r. prourokinase
    r. tissue plasminogen activator (rt-PA)

    r. tissue-type plasminogen activator
    r. urokinase (r-UK)
Recombinate
recompression chamber
reconstitution
    r. via collateral
    r. via profunda
**reconstructed pulsed-wave Doppler
  myocardial imaging**
reconstruction
    3-dimensional r.
    aortic r.
    arterial r.
    bifurcated vein graft for
      vascular r.
    endoluminal r.
    inferior vena cava r. (IVCR)
    outflow r.
    patch graft r.
    polyhedral surface r.
    retrospective gated r.
    right ventricular outflow tract r.
    Sheen airway r.
    stent r.
    vascular r.
recorder
    blood pressure r. (BPR)
    Card Guard cardiac event r.
    cardiac event r.
    cardiac output r. (COR)
    circadian event r.
    Del Mar Avionics three-channel r.
    Digitrapper pH 400 ambulatory 24-
      hour pH r.
    DM-400 Holter ECG cassette r.
    EdenTrace II Plus r.
    event r.
    Heart Aide Etd r.
    HeartCard 3X cardiac event r.
    24-hour ambulatory
      electrocardiographic r.
    implantable loop r.
    insertable loop r. (ILR)
    King of Hearts Express 3X cardiac
      event r.
    Marquette Holter r.
    Medilog 4000 ambulatory ECG r.
    Mingograf 82 r.
    Narco Biosystems r.
    Narco Physiograph-6B r.
    Reveal Plus insertable loop r.
    videotape r.
recording
    bipolar esophageal r.
    cardiopneumographic r. (CPG)
    Doppler r.
    intracardiac catheter r. (ICR)
    long-time r.
    M-mode strip chart r.

patient-triggered r.
pulse volume r. (PVR)
2120 R. Spirometer
time-based event r.
transtelephonic r.
X r.'s

recovery
corrected time of sinuatrial node
function r. (CTSNFR)
fluid-attenuated inversion r.
(FLAIR)
r. from inactivation
functional r.
heart rate r. (HRR)
r. phase
r. position
pressure r.

recrudescence
recruit
recruitable collateral vessel
recruitment
alveolar volume r.
capillary r.
eosinophil r.
host-generated neutrophils r.
lung volume r.
PEEP-related alveolar r.
positive end-expiratory pressure-
related alveolar r.

rectification
anomalous r.
inward-going r.

rectilinear
r. biphasic shock
r. biphasic waveform
r. scan
r. ST-segment depression

rectivirgula
Saccharopolyspora r.

rectocardiac reflex
rectus abdominis muscle
recurrence
early ischemic r. (EIR)
familial r.
r. risk

recurrent
r. coronary prevention program
(RCPP)
r. glioblastoma multiforme (RGM)
r. infective exacerbation
r. laryngeal nerve
r. lobar hemorrhage (RLH)
r. mesenteric ischemia
r. mesenteric vascular occlusion
r. myocardial infarction
r. respiratory infection (RRI)
r. respiratory papillomatosis

recurrentis
rami esophagei nervi laryngei r.

recurring
R. Figures Test (for short-term
memory)
r. venous thromboembolism (RVTE)
R. Words Test (for short-term
memory)

recursion
Levinson-Durbin r.

recurvatum
pectus r.

red
r. atrophy
r. blood cell (RBC)
r. blood cell osmotic fragility
r. cedar asthma
r. coronary thrombus
r. hepatization
r. hypertension
r. induration
r. infarct
r. light therapy (RLT)
ruthenium r.
r. soft coral asthma
R. system
r. wine polyphenol

Redha-cut catheter
redilation
redistribution
r. imaging
pulmonary vascular r.
vascular r.

redox-sensitive regulatory protein
red-streaked sputum
reduced
r. afterload
r. hemoglobin
r. signal intensity
r. vascular response (RVR)

reducer
reducing
r. event
r. valve

reductase
3-hydroxy-3-methylglutaryl coenzyme
A r.
r. inhibitor
methylenetetrahydrofolate r.
(MTHFR)

reduction
absolute risk r. (ARR)
afterload r.
alcohol septal r.
gradient r.
left ventricular r. (LVR)
lung volume r.
percutaneous alcohol septal r.
percutaneous mitral anular r.
preload r.

R

reduction *(continued)*
    relative risk r. (RRR)
    stapled lung r.
redundant cusp syndrome
reduplication murmur
redux
    rale r.
REE
    resting energy expenditure
reedswitch
    pacemaker r.
    r. of pacemaker
reelevation
    ST r.
    ST-segment r.
Reel syndrome
reendothelialization
reentrant
    r. atrial tachycardia
    r. circuit
    r. excitation
    r. loop
    r. mechanism
    r. pathway
    r. supraventricular tachycardia
    r. tachycardia (RT)
    r. ventricular arrhythmia (RVA)
    r. ventricular tachyarrhythmia
reentry
    anatomical r.
    anisotropic r.
    atrial r.
    atrioventricular nodal r. (AVNR)
    A-V nodal r.
    bundle branch r. (BBR)
    r. circuit isthmus
    r. circuit site
    dual-loop intraatrial r.
    figure-of-8 intraatrial r.
    intraatrial r.
    r. phenomenon
    Schmitt-Erlanger model of r.
    sinuatrial nodal r.
    sinus nodal r.
    r. theory
    ventricular r.
    r. waveform
    wavelength of r.
Reeves treadmill protocol
reexpansion
    lung r.
    pulmonary r.
    r. pulmonary edema
reexploration
    surgical r.
REF
    ejection fraction at rest
    right ventricular ejection fraction
refeeding syndrome

Refenesen 400
reference
    r. catheter
    r. electrode
    r. phantom CT
    r. point
    r. value
    r. vessel diameter (RVD)
REFI
    regional ejection fraction image
refill
    transcapillary r.
refined grain
reflectance oximetry
reflected pressure waveform
reflecting
    r. chronic hypoxemia
    r. level
reflection
    guidewire r.
reflex, pl. **reflexes**
    R. 8220 pacemaker
    abdominocardiac r.
    Abrams heart r.
    r. angina
    aortic r.
    Aschner r.
    Aschner-Dagnini r.
    r. asthma
    atriopressor r.
    auriculopressor r.
    Babinski r.
    Bainbridge r.
    baroreceptor r.
    Bezold-Jarisch r.
    bregmocardiac r.
    Breuer-Hering inflation r.
    Capps r.
    cardiac depressor r.
    cardioesophageal r.
    carotid sinus r.
    chemoreceptor r.
    Churchill-Cope r.
    coronary r.
    cough r.
    r. cough
    r. cough test
    craniocardiac r.
    Cushing r.
    depressor r.
    diving r.
    Erben r.
    esophagosalivary r.
    exercise pressor r.
    eyeball compression r.
    eyeball-heart r.
    gag r.
    gasp r.
    Head paradoxical r.

heart r.
Hering-Breuer r.
Hoffman r.
hypochondrial r.
inflation r.
jaw r. (JR)
Kisch r.
Kocher-Cushing r.
laryngeal r.
laryngeal cough r. (LCR)
Livierato r.
Loven r.
McDowall r.
mute r.
nasobronchial r.
neural cardioesophageal r.
oculocardiac r. (OCR)
oculopharyngeal r.
oculovagal r.
orthocardiac r.
r. pacemaker
Pavlov r.
pericardial r.
pharyngeal r.
pneocardiac r.
pneopneic r.
pressoreceptor r.
psychocardiac r.
r. pulmonary arterial
    vasoconstriction
pulmonocoronary r.
rectocardiac r.
respiratory r.
RIII r.
sinus r.
sneeze r.
somatic nociceptive flexion r.
spinal nociceptive flexion r.
R. steerable guidewire
r. stimulation
suck r.
r. sympathetic dystrophy
r. sympathoexcitation
r. tachycardia
vagal r.
r. vagal bronchoconstriction
vascular r.
r. vasoconstriction
vasoconstrictive r.
r. vasodilation
vasopressor r.
venorespiratory r.
viscerocardiac r.
Re/Flex filter
reflexogenic pressosensitivity
Reflotron bedside theophylline test
Refludan injection
reflux
abdominojugular r.

cardioesophageal r.
erosive r.
esophageal r.
r. esophagitis
extraesophageal r.
gastroesophageal r. (GER)
hepatojugular r. (HJR)
mitral r. (MR)
nasopharyngeal r.
transvalvular r.
valvular r.
venous r. (VR)
reform
capacitor r.
refractoriness
dispersion of r.
refractory
r. congestive heart failure
r. hypoxemia
r. to medical therapy
r. neurocardiogenic syncope
r. period
r. period of electronic pacemaker
r. shock
r. tachycardia
refrigeration
thermoacoustic r.
Ref-Star EP catheter
Refsum
R. disease
R. syndrome
regadenoson
Regency SR, SR+ pulse generator
**regeneration heat exchanger cycle
    system**
regimen
antithrombotic r.
dosage r.
drug-based r.
exercise r.
maintenance r.
prophylactic aspirin r.
stepped-care antihypertensive r.
titration r.
triple-drug maintenance r.
regio
r. axillaris
r. cruris anterior
r. cruris posterior
r. inguinalis
r. nasalis
r. pectoralis
r. posterior
r. presternalis
r. respiratoria tunicae mucosae nasi
region
AN r.
border zone r.
DiGeorge chromosome r. (DGCR)

R

625

region *(continued)*
    DiGeorge critical r. (DGCR)
    DiGeorge syndrome critical r.
      (DGSCR)
    gas-exchanging r.
    r. of interest (ROI)
    lung r.
    N r.
    NH r.
    parahilar r.
    paratracheal r.
    promotor r.
    respiratory r.
    r. of respiratory mucosa
    watershed r.

regional
    r. alveolar damage (RAD)
    r. cerebral blood flow (rCBF)
    r. dyssynergy
    r. ejection fraction image (REFI)
    r. gas concentration
    r. ischemia
    r. metabolic rate of glucose
      (rMRGlu)
    r. myocardial blood flow (RMBF)
    r. oxygen saturation (rSO$_2$)
    r. perfusion
    r. vasodilation
    r. wall motion (RWM)
    r. wall motion abnormality
      (RWMA)
    r. wall motion index

registration
    flow-time r.

registry
    Acute Decompensated Heart Failure
      National R. (ADHERE)
    ADHERE heart failure r.
    balloon valvoplasty r. (BVR)
    Cardiac Ablation R.
    International Cooperative Pulmonary
      Embolism R. (ICOPER)
    Long Bare Stent R.
    Mansfield Valvoplasty R.
    National Cardiovascular Data R.
      (NCDR)
    North American Inoue Balloon r.
    PELCA R.
    ReoPro Readministration R. (R3)

regression
    arteriographic r.
    CIMT r.
    coronary plaque r.
    r. equation
    Poisson r.
    Q wave r.
    xanthoma r.

regular
    R. Iletin II

    r. purified pork insulin
    r. rate and rhythm (RRR, RR&R)
    r. sinus rhythm (RSR, rSR′)

regularly irregular rhythm

regulation
    reciprocal r.

regulator
    aluminum oxygen r.
    Boehringer suction R.
    CF transmembrane ion r.
    cystic fibrosis transmembrane r.
      (CFTR)
    cystic fibrosis transmembrane
      conductance r.
    Easy Dial Reg oxygen r.
    Ohmeda thoracic suction r.

regulon
    BvgAS r.

regurgitant
    r. fraction
    r. jet
    r. jet area
    r. murmur
    r. orifice
    r. orifice area (ROA)
    r. pocket
    r. volume (RV, RVol)
    r. wave

regurgitation
    aortic r. (AR)
    aortic valve r.
    atrioventricular valve r.
    commissural mitral r.
    faint pulmonary r.
    functional mitral r.
    homograft insertion for
      pulmonary r.
    ischemic mitral r.
    mitral r. (MR)
    mitral valve r.
    normal transvalvular r. (NTVR)
    paravalvular r.
    periprosthetic mitral r.
    prosthetic valve r. (PVR)
    pulmonary r. (PR)
    pulmonary valvular r.
    pulmonic r.
    Sellers classification of mitral r.
    semilunar valve r.
    silent mitral r.
    tricuspid r. (TR)
    tricuspid valve r. (TVR)
    valve r.
    valvular r.

rehabilitation
    American Association of
      Cardiovascular and Pulmonary R.
      (AACVPR)
    cardiac r. (CR)

r. exercise
home-based cardiac r.
r. protocol
pulmonary r.
vocational r.
work r.
rehalation
Reich-Nechtow clamp
Reid
    R. classification
    R. index
    R. index measurement
Reil
    ball of R.
    band of R.
reinfarction
reinfection tuberculosis
reinflation
reinfusion
reinjection protocol
reinnervation in transplanted heart
Reisman
    R. myocardosis
    R. pneumonia
Reisseisen muscle
Reitan catheter Pump
Reiter
    R. disease
    R. syndrome
reject control
rejection
    acute r. (AR)
    acute allograft r.
    acute cellular xenograft r.
    acute lung r.
    allograft r.
    r. cardiomyopathy
    r. cardiomyopathy transplant
    chronic airway r.
    chronic vascular r.
    delayed xenograft r. (DXR)
    graft r.
    hyperacute r.
    no infection-no r. (NI-NR)
rejection-associated pulmonary fibrosis
relapsing
    r. fever
    r. polychondritis (RP)
relation (*See also* ratio)
    concentration-effect r.
    diastolic pressure-volume r.
    end-systolic pressure-volume r.
    end-systolic stress-dimension r.
    force-frequency r.
    force-length r.
    force-velocity r.
    force-velocity-length r.
    force-velocity-volume r.
    interval-strength r.

length-resting tension r.
length-tension r.
pressure-flow r.
pressure-volume r.
resting length-tension r.
tension-length r.
ultrasonic tissue characterization r.
ventilation/perfusion r.
ventricular end-systolic pressure-
    volume r.
relationship
    diastolic pressure-flow r. (DPFR)
    end-systolic force-length r. (ESFL)
    end-systolic pressure-volume r.
    (ESPVR)
    exposure-response r.
    Fick r.
    Laplace r.
    pressure-flow r.
    stress-shortening r.
    ventilation/perfusion r.
relative
    r. cardiac dullness (RCD)
    r. cardiac volume
    r. coronary flow reserve (RCFR)
    r. heart rate variability (RHRV)
    r. humidity (RH)
    r. incompetence
    r. inspiratory effort (RIE)
    r. lymphocyte count
    r. mitral stenosis
    r. perfusion
    r. refractory period (RRP)
    r. risk (RR)
    r. risk reduction (RRR)
    r. slow sinus rate (RSSR)
    r. survival rate
    r. vessel diameter (RVD)
    r. wall thickness (RWT)
relaxant
    muscle r.
    smooth muscle r.
relaxation
    r. atelectasis
    atrial r.
    diastolic r.
    dynamic r.
    early diastolic r. (EDR)
    endothelium-dependent vascular r.
    endothelium-independent vascular r.
    endothelium-mediated r.
    isovolumetric r.
    isovolumic r.
    left ventricular diastolic r.
    r. loading
    nitric oxide-mediated r.
    r. period
    r. phase
    smooth muscle r.

R

relaxation *(continued)*
    stress r.
    r. technique
    r. time
    r. time index
    r. training
    ventricular r.
relaxin
    recombinant human r.
relaxometry
    NMR r.
release
    allergen-induced mediator r.
    catecholamine r.
    controlled r. (C-R)
    extended r. (XL, XR, XT)
    oxygen free radical r.
    physiologic pattern r. (PPR)
    sustained r. (SR)
Relenza
reliever
    Arthritis Foundation Pain R.
    Medtronic Pulsor Intrasound pain r.
REM
    rapid eye movement
    REM sleep
    REM sleep-related hypoxemia
rem
    radiation equivalent in man
Remac system
remedial psychological stressor
remedy
    R. sleep therapy
    R. sleep therapy system
Remicade
remifentanil
remission
remnant
    chylomicron r. (CMR)
    r. lipoprotein (RLP)
    r. lipoprotein cholesterol
    r. lipoprotein triglyceride
remnant-like
    r.-l. lipoprotein particle (RLP)
    r.-l. particle lipoprotein
remodeling
    adverse ventricular r.
    airway r.
    aortic r.
    arterial r.
    atrial reverse r.
    Batista ventricular r.
    cardiac r.
    concentric r.
    coronary r.
    flow-responsive r.
    Glagov r.
    heart chamber r.
    mitral leaflet r.

    myocardial r.
    negative r.
    positive arterial r.
    postinfarct ventricular r.
    reverse r.
    vascular r.
    ventricular r.
Remodulin
remote
    r. access perfusion (RAP)
    r. access perfusion cannula
remotely monitored ICD
removal
    extracorporeal carbon dioxide r.
      (ECCO$_2$R)
    introducer sheath r.
REMstar
    R. auto CPAP
    R. CPAP system
Renaissance spirometry system
renal
    r. angiography
    r. arteriography
    r. artery
    r. artery bypass graft
    r. artery disease
    r. artery forceps
    r. artery-reverse saphenous vein
      bypass
    r. artery stenosis (RAS)
    r. azotemia
    r. blood vessel
    r. cortical blood flow (RCBF)
    r. cortical necrosis
    r. cortical vascular resistance
      (RCVR)
    r. cyst
    r. dialysis
    r. diet
    r. dyspnea
    r. failure
    r. fistula
    r. function
    r. hypertension
    r. insufficiency
    r. juxtaglomerular cell
    r. kallikrein-kinin system
    r. parenchymal disease
    r. plasma flow (RPF)
    r. tuberculosis
    r. vein
    r. vein renin ratio
    r. venography
renal-splanchnic steal
Rendell-Baker face mask
Rendu-Osler-Weber
    R.-O.-W. disease
    R.-O.-W. syndrome
Renese

renin
    r. angiotensin
    r. inhibitor
    r. level
    plasma r.
renin-angiotensin
    r.-a. blocker
    r.-a. system (RAS)
renin-angiotensin-aldosterone
    r.-a.-a. cascade
    r.-a.-a. system (RAAS)
renography
    captopril r.
renomedullary lipid
renoprival hypertension
renopulmonary
Renormax
renovascular
    r. angiography
    r. hypertension (RVH)
Rentamine
Rentrop
    R. catheter
    R. classification
REO
    respiratory and enteric orphan
    REO virus
reocclusion
reoperation
ReoPro Readministration Registry (R3)
Reovirus
reovirus
    respiratory r.
repaglinide
repair
    Alfieri r., Alfieri-plasty
    Allison hiatal hernia r.
    Boerema hernia r.
    Brom r.
    cap r.
    DeBakey-Creech aneurysm r.
    edge-to-edge technique mitral
     valve r.
    Effler hiatal hernia r.
    endovascular r. (EVR)
    endovascular aneurysm r. (EVAR)
    fascioperitoneal patch r.
    Fontan r.
    Hatafuku fundus onlay patch
     esophageal r.
    minimally invasive valve r.
     (MIVR)
    Mustard atrial r.
    Norwood r.
    patch r.
    pulmonary valve r. (PVR)
    Senning atrial baffle r.
reparative cardiac surgery

repeat
    r. balloon mitral valvotomy
    r. revascularization
repeated ultrasound-guided needle
    thoracocentesis
Repel-CV bioresorbable adhesion-barrier
    film
reperfused myocardium
reperfusion (RP)
    r. arrhythmia
    r. catheter
    emergency r.
    facilitated r.
    r. injury
    late r.
    myocardial tissue r.
    r. pulmonary edema
    r. therapy
reperfusion-induced hemorrhage
reperfusion/occlusion
repertoire
    T-cell r.
repetition
    pulse r. (PR)
    r. rate
    r. time (TR)
repetitive
    r. atrial firing (RAF)
    r. monomorphic ventricular
     tachycardia
    r. paroxysmal ventricular
     tachycardia
    r. stunning
    r. ventricular response (RVR)
rephasing
    even-echo r.
replacement
    aortic arch r.
    aortic bioprosthesis stentless
     pericardial aortic heart valve r.
    aortic root r. (ARR)
    aortic valve r. (AVR)
    battery elective r.
    blood r.
    collagen r.
    composite valve graft r.
    double valve r. (DVR)
    extended aortic root r. (EARR)
    minimally invasive valve r.
     (MIVR)
    mitral and aortic valve r. (MAVR)
    mitral valve r. (MVR)
    partial chordal-sparing mitral
     valve r.
    pulmonary valve r. (PVR)
    supraanular mitral valve r. (SMVR)
    total chordal-sparing mitral valve r.
    tricuspid valve r. (TVR)

R

replacement *(continued)*
    valve r. (VR)
    valve-sparing aortic root r.
repletion
replication
repolarization
    atrial r.
    benign early r. (BER)
    early r. (ER)
    early rapid r.
    ECG r.
    final rapid r.
    myocardial r.
    rapid r.
repositionable
representative CT (Hounsfield) number
repression
reprogramming
    pacemaker output r.
reptilase
RER
    respiratory exchange ratio
RERA
    respiratory effort-related arousal
Rescaps-D Capsule
Rescriptor
ReSCU
    respiratory special care unit
rescue
    r. angioplasty
    R. aspiration catheter
    citrovorum r.
    r. PTCA
    r. shock
    r. stent implantation
    r. thrombolysis
    R. thrombus management system
rescuPAC ventilator
research
    Agency for Health Care Policy
      and R. (AHCPR)
    R. Group on Instability in
      Coronary Artery Disease (RISC)
    R. Pneumotach System
      instrumentation module
    primary angioplasty R. (PAR)
resection
    activation map-guided surgical r.
    atrial septal r.
    bronchial sleeve r.
    r. clamp
    endocardial r.
    endocardial-to-endocardial r.
    infundibular wedge r.
    lesser r.
    myotomy-myectomy-septal r.
    quadrangular r.
    segmental lung r.
    septal r.

    sleeve r.
    stapled wedge r.
    Torek r. of thoracic esophagus
    triangular r.
    wedge r.
Resectisol Irrigation Solution
reserpine
    chlorothiazide and r.
    hydralazine, hydrochlorothiazide, r.
    hydrochlorothiazide and r.
    hydroflumethiazide and r.
reserve
    r. air
    blood flow r.
    breathing r. (BR)
    cardiac r.
    cardiopulmonary r. (CPR)
    r. cell carcinoma
    contractile r.
    coronary arterial r.
    coronary flow r. (CFR)
    coronary flow velocity r. (CFVR,
      CVR)
    coronary vascular r.
    coronary vasodilator r.
    diastolic r.
    enzymatic r.
    extraction r.
    flow r.
    fractional flow r. (FFR)
    fractional velocity r. (FVR)
    Frank-Starling r.
    heart rate r. (HRR)
    limited ventricular r.
    myocardial r.
    myocardial fractional flow r.
      (FFR_{myo})
    preload r.
    relative coronary flow r. (RCFR)
    respiratory r.
    stenotic flow r. (SFR)
    systolic r.
    vasodilator r.
    ventricular r.
reservoir
    r. cannula
    cardiotomy r.
    Intersept cardiotomy r.
    Jostra cardiotomy r.
    oxygen r.
    Polystan cardiotomy r.
    venous r.
    William Harvey cardiotomy r.
reset
    r. nodus sinuatrialis
    sinus node r.
resident assessment protocol (RAP)
residua
    embryonic r.

residual
    r. air
    r. deep vein thrombosis
    r. DVT
    r. gradient
    r. jet
    r. lung capacity
    r. pleural thickening
    r. shunt
    r. stenosis
    r. volume (RV)
    r. volume fraction (RVF)
    r. volume/total lung capacity (RV/TLC)
    r. volume/total lung capacity ratio

residue
    fucose r.

resin
    anion exchange r.
    bile acid binding r.
    cholestyramine r.
    epoxy r.
    pine r.
    thermosetting r.
    urea-formaldehyde r.

resistance
    afterload r.
    r., airway (RAW)
    airway r.
    airways r. (Raw)
    aortic valve r.
    cerebrovascular r. (CVR)
    coronary vascular r.
    diaphragmatic fatigue r.
    elastic r.
    expiratory r.
    glucocorticoid r.
    hydraulic r.
    insulin r.
    minimal vascular r. (MVR)
    r. to movement of lung tissue (Rti)
    multidrug r.
    nitrate r.
    normalized systemic vascular r. (NSVR)
    peripheral r.
    peripheral vascular r. (PVR)
    pulmonary r.
    pulmonary arteriolar r. (PAR)
    pulmonary-to-systemic vascular r. (Rp:Rs)
    pulmonary vascular r. (PVR)
    r. ratio
    renal cortical vascular r. (RCVR)
    respiratory r. (Rrs)
    stenosis r.
    systemic arterial r. (Rsa)
    systemic vascular r. (SVR)

    total airway r. (Rtot)
    total peripheral r. (TPR)
    total peripheral vascular r. (TPVR)
    total pulmonary r.
    total pulmonary vascular r. (TPVR)
    total systemic vascular r. (TSVR)
    total vascular r. (TVR)
    r. training (RT)
    valve r.
    vascular r. (VR)
    vascular peripheral r.
    r. to venous return (RVR)
    r. vessel

resistant
    high-altitude pulmonary edema r. (HAPE-r)
    r. hypertension

resistive heating
resistor
    fixed orifice r.
    magnetic valve r.
    spring-loaded r.
    threshold r.
    underwater seal r.
    water column r.
    weighted ball r.

resolution
    energy r.
    high spatial r.
    spatial r.
    spontaneous r.
    ST-segment r.
    temporal r.

resolving power
resonance
    amphoric r.
    bandbox r.
    bellmetal r.
    cardiovascular magnetic r. (CMR, CVMR)
    cough r.
    cracked-pot r.
    delayed contrast-enhanced cardiovascular magnetic r. (DE-CMR)
    nuclear magnetic r. (NMR)
    shoulder-strap r.
    skodaic r.
    tympanitic r.
    whispering r.
    wooden r.

resonant frequency
resorption
    r. atelectasis
    bulla r.

Respa DM
Respaire-60 SR
Respaire-120 SR
Respalor

R

Respa-1st
RESPeRATE interactive breathing
  device
Respihaler
Respipac
  Zagam R.
respirable
  r. aerosol
  r. particular matter
Respiradyne pulmonary function device
respiration
  abdominal r.
  absent r.
  accelerated r.
  accessory muscles of r.
  aerobic r.
  agonal r.
  amphoric r.
  anaerobic r.
  apneustic r.
  artificial r.
  assisted r.
  asthmoid r.
  Austin Flint r.
  Biot r.
  Bouchut r.
  bronchial r.
  bronchocavernous r.
  r. bronchoscope
  bronchovesicular r.
  cavernous r.
  cell r.
  central r.
  cerebral r.
  Cheyne-Stokes r.
  cogwheel r.
  collateral r.
  controlled diaphragmatic r.
  Corrigan r.
  costal r.
  cyclic r.
  decreased r.
  diaphragmatic r.
  diffusion r.
  direct r.
  divided r.
  electrophrenic r.
  external r.
  forced r.
  granular r.
  harsh r.
  internal r.
  interrupted r.
  intrauterine r.
  jerky r.
  Kussmaul r.
  Kussmaul-Kien r.
  labored r.
  meningitic r.

  metamorphosing r.
  mitochondrial r.
  mouth-to-mouth r.
  nervous r.
  paradoxical r.
  periodic r.
  placental r.
  puerile r.
  pulse and r. (P&R)
  radiofrequency electrophrenic r.
  rude r.
  Schafer method of artificial r.
  Seitz metamorphosing r.
  shallow r.
  sighing r.
  slow r.
  sonorous r.
  spontaneous r.
  stertorous r.
  stridulous r.
  supplementary r.
  suppressed r.
  temperature, pulse, r. (TPR)
  thoracic r.
  transitional r.
  tubular r.
  unlabored r.
  vesiculocavernous r.
  vicarious r.
  wavy r.
respiratometer
  Collins r.
respirator
  BABYbird r.
  Bragg-Paul r.
  cuirass r.
  Drinker r.
  elastomeric half-face r.
  Emerson cuirass r.
  r. lung
  Medivent RTX r.
  Monaghan r.
  Morch r.
  particulate r.
  pressure-controlled r.
  tank r.
  volume-controlled r.
  volumetric diffusive r. (VDR)
respiratoria
  glottis r.
  rima r.
respiratorii
  bronchioli r.
respiratorium
  systema r.
respiratorius
  apparatus r.
respiratory
  r. acidosis

r. activity
r. airway
r. alkalosis
r. allergy
r. alternans
r. alternans breathing pattern
r. apparatus
r. arousal scoring
r. arrest
r. arrhythmia
r. artifact
r. bronchiole
r. bronchiolitis (RB)
r. bronchiolitis-interstitial lung
disease (RB-ILD)
r. burst
r. capacity
r. care practitioner (RCP)
r. center
r. collapse
r. compromise
r. cycle
r. dead space
r. depressant action
r. depression
r. distress
r. distress syndrome (RDS)
r. distress syndrome of the
newborn
r. disturbance index (RDI)
r. drive
r. effort
r. effort-related arousal (RERA)
r. embarrassment
r. and enteric orphan (REO)
r. event
r. exchange
r. exchange ratio (RER)
r. excursion
r. extremis
r. failure
r. feedback (RFb)
r. flora
r. frequency (f)
r. function
r. gas analysis
r. gated 3-dimensional gradient-echo
sequence
r. gated MRCA
r. gating
r. glycoconjugate (RGC)
r. inductance plethysmograph (RIP)
r. inductance plethysmography
(RIP)
r. insufficiency
r. irritant
r. metabolism
r. minute volume
r. mucosa

r. murmur
r. muscle fatigue
r. ordered phase encoding (ROPE)
r. paralysis
r. parameter
r. pulse
r. pump
r. quotient (RQ)
r. rate (RR)
r. rate to tidal volume ratio
(f/VT)
r. reflex
r. region
r. region of tunica mucosa of
nose
r. reovirus
r. reserve
r. resistance (Rrs)
r. sinus arrhythmia (RSA)
r. sound
r. special care unit (ReSCU)
r. standstill
r. stridor
r. support
r. swing
r. syncytial virus (RSV)
r. syncytial virus conduit
r. syncytial virus immunoglobulin
(RSV-IG)
r. syncytial virus IV immune
globulin
r. system
r. system motoneural output
Taiwan acute r. (TWAR)
r. therapy
r. toilet
r. tract
r. tract infection
r. tract lining fluid (RTLF)
r. triggering
r. ventilator
r. waveform variation

respiratory-gated 2D segmented-FLASH MRCA image
Respirgard II nebulizer
respirogram
respirometer
Dräger r.
Fraser Harlake r.
Haloscale r.
Wright r.
Respironics
R. BIPAP bilevel ventilator
R. CPAP machine
R. Oasis humidifier
R. 920P handheld pulse oximeter
R. 930 pulse oximeter
respirophasic pain

Respitrace
    R. machine
    R. plethysmograph
responder
    isolated volume r. (IVR)
    r. ventilator
response
    acute r.
    allele-specific T-cell r.
    antigen-specific adaptive immune
      r.
    atrial flutter r. (AFR)
    atrial tachycardic r.
    autonomic r.
    biphasic r.
    blunted exercise r.
    bronchodilator r.
    cardioinhibitory r.
    cell-mediated immune r.
    cephalic vasomotor r. (CVR)
    chemotactic r.
    cholinergic r.
    chronic innate immune r.
    chronotropic r.
    controlled ventricular r.
    Cushing pressure r.
    R. CV catheter system
    depressed cough r.
    double ventricular r. (DVR)
    dynamic frequency r.
    dysfunctional airway immune r.
    early asthmatic r. (EAR)
    electrocardiographic r. (ECR)
    R. electrophysiology catheter
    endothelium-dependent dilator r. to
      substance P
    fetal ventricular myocyte
      proliferative r.
    fight-or-flight r.
    frequency r.
    giving-in/giving-up r.
    Glagov remodeling r.
    hemodynamic mental stress r.
    Henry-Gauer r.
    hypercapnic ventilatory r.
    hyperplastic r.
    hypoxic ventilatory r. (HVR)
    implantation r.
    incrementing r.
    late asthmatic r. (LAR)
    local thrombotic r.
    metaboreflex r.
    methacholine r.
    neointimal hyperplastic r.
    oscillatory r.
    paced ventricular evoked r.
    pathologic complete r.
    photobiological r.
    plateau r.
    postocclusive oscillatory r. (POR)
    pulmonary reimplantation r. (PRR)
    rate-drop r. (RDR)
    reduced vascular r. (RVR)
    repetitive ventricular r. (RVR)
    sensor-driven r.
    sequential vascular r. (SVR)
    slow r.
    square wave r.
    sympathoexcitatory r.
    sympathoinhibitory r.
    tend-and-befriend r.
    thyrotropin-releasing hormone r.
    vagal r.
    vagotonic baroreceptor r.
    vasodilatory r.
    vasomotor r. (VMR)
    ventilatory r.
    ventricular r.
    vigilance r.
    visually evoked flow r. (VEFR)
response-to-injury
    r.-t.-i. hypothesis
    r.-t.-i. hypothesis of atherogenesis
    r.-t.-i. theory
responsiveness
    adenosine airways r.
    bronchial r. (BR)
    myofilament calcium r.
Respules
    Pulmicort R.
Res-Q
    R.-Q ACD implantable cardioverter-
      defibrillator
    R.-Q arrhythmia control device
    R.-Q Micron ICD
    R.-Q Micron implantable
      cardioverter-defibrillator
rest
    r. angina
    r. dyspnea
    r. ejection fraction
    ejection fraction at r. (REF)
    r. and exercise gated nuclear
      angiography
    r. hypoxemia
    r. metabolism/stress perfusion
      protocol
    r. pain
    r. radionuclide angiography
rested state contraction (RSC)
Resten-MP
Resten-NG
restenosed stent
restenosis
    aortic valve r.
    binary angiographic r.
    chronic occlusive in-stent r.
      (COISR)

computer-assisted evaluation of stenosis and r. (CAESAR)
coronary r.
coronary artery descriptors and r. (CADR)
diffuse in-stent r.
in-stent r. (ISR)
intralesion r.
intrastent r. (IR)
r. lesion
mitral r.
post balloon angioplasty r.
post-stenting r.
pulmonary valve r.
r. risk
Rotablator and r. (R&R)
tricuspid r.

restenotic
r. narrowing
r. native coronary artery lesion
r. small coronary vessel

rest-exercise equilibrium radionuclide ventriculography

resting
r. dyspnea
r. energy expenditure (REE)
r. heart rate (RHR)
r. hypertension
r. length-tension relation
r. membrane potential
r. metabolic rate (RMR)
r. parasternal long-axis view
r. parasternal short-axis view
r. pulmonary vein-left atrium pressure
r. sinus tachycardia
r. stroke volume
r. systolic function
r. tidal breathing
r. tidal volume
r. value
r. vascular tone
r. venous pressure (RVP)

Reston subtype of Ebola
restoration
r. of spontaneous circulation (ROSC)
surgical anterior ventricular r. (SAVR)
surgical anterior ventricular endocardial r. (SAVER)
surgical ventricular r. (SVR)

restored cycle
Restoril
rest-redistribution thallium-201 imaging
rest-reinjection thallium tomography
restriction
r. endonuclease
r. endonuclease assay

r. fragment length polymorphism (RFLP)
progressive parenchymal r.
pulmonary r.

restrictive
r. airways defect
r. airways disease
r. cardiomyopathy
r. filling pattern
r. functional impairment
r. heart disease
r. lung disease
r. physiology mitral flow pattern
r. right ventricular physiology
r. ventilatory defect
r. ventilatory dysfunction
r. VSD

restrictus
Aspergillus r.

result
false-positive r.
test r.
true-negative test r.
true-positive test r.

resuscitate
do not r. (DNR)

resuscitation
ACLS protocol r.
active compression-decompression cardiopulmonary r. (ACD-CPR)
albumin r.
bystander cardiopulmonary r. (BCPR, ByCPR)
cardiac r. (CR)
cardiopulmonary r. (CPR)
cardiopulmonary cerebral r. (CPCR)
r. cart
closed chest cardiac r. (CCCR)
closed chest cardiopulmonary r. (CCPR)
crystalloid r.
do not attempt r. (DNAR)
external cardiopulmonary r. (ECPR)
family-witnessed r.
heart-lung r. (HLR)
high-impulse cardiopulmonary r. (HI-CPR)
high-impulse compression cardiopulmonary r. (HIC-CPR)
International Liaison Committee on R. (ILCOR)
interposed abdominal compression cardiopulmonary r. (IAC CPR)
mechanical cardiopulmonary r.
mouth-to-mouth r.
no cardiopulmonary r. (NCR)
open chest cardiac r.
open chest cardiopulmonary r. (OCCPR)

R

resuscitation *(continued)*
    standard cardiopulmonary r. (SCPR)
    volume r.
resuscitator
    active compression-decompression r.
    Ambu Spur disposable r.
    r. bag
    BagEasy disposable manual r.
    First Response manual r.
    Hope r.
    Hudson Lifesaver r.
    infant Ambu r.
    Laerdal r.
    NeoVO2R infant volume control r.
    O-Two ALS handheld r.
    O-Two BLS handheld r.
    O-Two CAREvent BLS+ r.
    Pulmanex r.
resveratrol
resynchronization
    cardiac r.
resynchronize
resynchronizer
    HFCWO ventricular r.
    high-frequency chest wall
      oscillation ventricular r.
    ventricular r.
retained lung fluid (RLF)
retard
    expiratory r.
retardation
    fragile X-mental r. (FRAX-MR)
Retavase
retention
    r. cyst
    mucus r.
    secretion r.
    sodium r.
    sputum r.
    tracer r.
    water r.
reteplase (RPA, r-PA)
reteplase-abciximab
rethoracotomy
reticula (*pl. of* reticulum)
reticular
    r. basement
    r. basement membrane
    r. basement membrane thickening
    r. pattern
reticularis
    livedo r.
reticulation
reticuloendothelial system
reticulonodular
    r. infiltrate
    r. pattern
reticulum, pl. **reticula**
    agranular endoplasmic r. (AER)

    endoplasmic r.
    sarcoplasmic r.
retina, pl. **retinas, retinae**
    cyanosis retinae
retinal
    r. artery
    r. vessel
retinohypothalamic pathway
retinoic acid
retinol
    plasma r.
    serum r.
retinopathy
    arteriosclerotic r.
    cancer-related r.
    diabetic r.
    hypertensive r.
    r. of prematurity (ROP)
    proliferative diabetic r. (PDR)
retractable, radiopaque, screw-in pacing lead
retraction
    cusp r.
    intercostal r.
    postrheumatic cusp r.
    r. wave
retractor
    abdominal vascular r.
    Ablaza-Blanco aortic wall r.
    Adson r.
    Allison lung r.
    Andrews r.
    Bookwalter r.
    Cooley atrial r.
    Cosgrove r.
    Davidson scapular r.
    Davis double-end soft tissue r.
    DeBakey chest r.
    Finochietto r.
    Finochietto-Geissendorfer rib r.
    Gelpi r.
    IMA r.
    inferior mesenteric artery r.
    Lilienthal-Sauerbruch r.
    Lukens thymus r.
    lung r.
    malleable r.
    Meyerding r.
    rake r.
    Rosenkranz pediatric open heart r.
    soft-tissue r.
    Theis rib r.
    Zalkind lung r.
Retract-O-Tape
retraining
    computerized diaphragmatic
      breathing r. (CDBR)
retransplantation

retrieval
    intravascular foreign body r.
retriever
    Merci r.
retrocardiac
    r. pneumonia
    r. space
retroconduction
retrocrural adenopathy
retroesophageal
    r. aorta
    r. diverticulum of Kommerell
retrognathia
retrograde
    r. amnesia
    r. aortography
    r. arterial capture
    r. atrial activation mapping
    r. atrioventricular conduction
       (RAVC)
    r. autologous priming
    r. beat
    r. block
    r. brain perfusion
    r. catheter insertion
    r. catheterization
    r. embolism
    r. fast pathway
    r. femoral approach
    r. filling
    r. hypertension
    r. propagation
    r. P wave
    r. signal
    r. translaryngeal intubation
    r. VA conduction
retrolingual
retropalatal
    r. airways
    r. obstruction
retropectoral
    r. patch
    r. pocket
retroperfusion
    coronary sinus r.
    synchronized r. (SRP)
retroperitoneal
    r. bleed
    r. hematoma
retropharyngeal
    r. abscess
    r. lymph node
    r. space
retropharyngeales
    nodi lymphoidei r.
retropharyngeum
    spatium r.
retropharyngitis
retropharynx

retrospective gated reconstruction
retrosternal
    r. air space
    r. thyroid
retrotracheal space
Retrovir
    R. injection
    R. Oral
retroviral vector
retrovirus
return
    anomalous pulmonary venous r.
    blood pressure r.
    r. extrasystole
    hemianomalous pulmonary
       venous r. (HAPVR)
    partial anomalous pulmonary
       venous r. (PAPVR)
    pulmonary anomalous superior
       venous r. (PASVR)
    pulmonary venous r.
    rattle of r.
    resistance to venous r. (RVR)
    r. of spontaneous circulation
       (ROSC)
    systemic venous r.
    total anomalous pulmonary
       venous r. (TAPVR)
    venous r. (VR)
returning cycle
Retzius veins
reuptake blockade
Reuter tip deflecting wire guide
revascularization
    r. approach
    Biosense-guided laser myocardial r.
    catheter-based r.
    coronary r.
    direct myocardial r. (DMR)
    heart laser r.
    hybrid r.
    ischemia-driven r.
    laser r.
    myocardial r. (MR)
    myocardial laser r. (MLR)
    percutaneous myocardial r. (PMR)
    percutaneous myocardial laser r.
    percutaneous transluminal
       coronary r. (PTCR)
    percutaneous transluminal
       myocardial r. (PTMR)
    percutaneous transmyocardial r.
       (PTMR)
    percutaneous transmyocardial
       laser r. (PMR)
    r. procedure
    radiofrequency percutaneous
       myocardial r. (RF-PMR)
    repeat r.

R

revascularization *(continued)*
    robotic coronary r.
    surgical r.
    r. system
    target lesion r. (TLR)
    target vessel r. (TVR)
    transmyocardial r. (TMR)
    transmyocardial laser r. (TMLR)
Revatio
Reveal Plus insertable loop recorder
revelation
    R. endocardial microcatheter
    R. Helix catheter
    R. microcatheter for EP mapping
    R. T-Flex catheter
    R. Tx linear ablation catheter
    R. Tx microcatheter for RF
    ablation
reverberation
    r. artifact
    echo r.
reversal
    atrial r. (AR)
    holodiastolic flow r.
    lead r.
    r. speed of bronchoconstriction in
    response to methacholine (r-Sm)
    systolic r.
    venous flow r.
reverse
    r. differential cyanosis
    r. polarity
    r. remodeling
    r. saphenous vein
    r. squeeze
    r. transcriptase polymerase chain
    reaction (RT-PCR)
    r. transcriptase polymerase chain
    reaction test
reversed
    r. arm leads
    r. bypass
    r. coarctation
    r. ductus arteriosus
    r. paradoxical pulse
    r. reciprocal rhythm
    r. saphenous vein graft
    r. shunt
    r. 3 sign
reversibility
    objective bronchodilator r.
reversible
    r. airway obstruction
    r. bronchospasm
    r. inhibitor
    r. ischemic neurologic defect
    (RIND)
    r. left ventricular dysfunction
    r. obstructive airways disease
    (ROAD)
reversion
    noise r.
Reversol injection
Revex
reviparin
revision
    International Classification of
    Diseases, Ninth R. (ICD-9)
rewarming
    continuous arteriovenous r. (CAVR)
Reye syndrome
Rey figure copying test
Reynolds number
RF
    radiofrequency
    rheumatic fever
        RF catheter ablation
        RF Marinr catheter
        RF wave
RFA
    radiofrequency ablation
RFb
    respiratory feedback
**RfB System-I for controlled
diaphragmatic breathing**
RFC
    radiofrequency current
RF-generated thermal balloon catheter
RFLP
    restriction fragment length polymorphism
RF-PMR
    radiofrequency percutaneous myocardial
    revascularization
RFTA
    radiofrequency tissue ablation
rFVIIa
    recombinant activated factor VII
RGC
    respiratory glycoconjugate
RGEA
    right gastroepiploic artery
RGM
    recurrent glioblastoma multiforme
RH
    relative humidity
    right heart
Rh
    Rhesus
        Rh antibody
        Rh factor
rhabdoid phenotype
rhabdomyolysis
rhabdomyoma
    cardiac r.
rhabdomyosarcoma
RHAMM
    receptor for hyaluronan-mediated motility

rhamnolipid mucus secretion
rhATIII
    recombinant human antithrombin III
RHB
    right heart bypass
RHC
    right heart catheterization
rhC1INH
    recombinant human C1 inhibitor
RHD
    radiant heat device
    rheumatic heart disease
    right hemisphere damage
rhDNase
rheocardiography
rheography
    light reflection r.
rheologic
    r. change
    r. therapy
rheology
rheolytic
    r. coronary thrombectomy
    r. thrombectomy catheter
Rhesus (Rh)
rheumatic
    r. AF
    r. aortitis
    r. arteritis
    r. carditis
    r. endocarditis
    r. fever (RF)
    r. heart disease (RHD)
    r. mitral insufficiency
    r. mitral stenosis (RMS)
    r. mitral valve stenosis
    r. myocarditis
    r. pericarditis
    r. pneumonia
    r. valvular heart disease (RVHD)
    r. valvulitis
rheumatica
    angina r.
rheumatism
    desert r.
    r. of the heart
    tuberculous r.
rheumatoid
    r. arteritis
    r. arthritis (RA)
    r. factor
    r. lung
    r. nodule
    r. pleuritis
    r. pneumoconiosis
    r. pneumonoconiosis
rheumatology
    American College of R.
Rheumatrex

RHF
    right heart failure
rhinitis
    allergic r.
    irritant r.
    r. medicamentosa
    nonallergic, noninfectious
      perennial r. (NANIPER)
    perennial allergic r.
    postnasal drip due to r. (PND-Rh)
    seasonal allergic r.
    vasomotor r.
rhinocerebral
    r. infection
    r. mucormycosis
rhinoconjunctivitis
Rhinocort Aqua
rhinomanometer
rhinopharyngeal
rhinopharynx
rhinoscleroma
rhinoscleromatis
    Klebsiella r.
rhinoscopy
    fiberoptic r.
rhinosinusitis
    bacterial r.
    viral r.
Rhinosyn-DMX
Rhinosyn Liquid
Rhinosyn-PD Liquid
rhinovirus (RV)
r-hirudin
    recombinant hirudin
Rhizomucor
Rhizopus oryzae
RHMV
    right heart mixing volume
rhodesiense
    Trypanosoma r.
Rho(D) immune globulin
Rhodnius polixus
Rhodococcus equi
RhoGAM
RhoGDP-dissociation inhibitor 1
Rho GTPase
Rho-kinase
rhonchal fremitus
rhonchus, pl. **rhonchi**
    expiratory r.
    inspiratory r.
    rales and rhonchi
    sibilant r.
    sonorous r.
Rhotral
RHR
    resting heart rate
RHRV
    relative heart rate variability

R

rhuIL-10
  recombinant human IL-10
rhVEGF
  recombinant human vascular endothelial
  growth factor
Rhyder diagnostic catheter
rhysodes
  Acanthamoeba r.
rhythm
  accelerated atrioventricular
    junctional r.
  accelerated A-V junctional r.
  accelerated idioventricular r.
    (AIVR)
  accelerated ventricular r. (AVR)
  agonal r.
  artificial pacemaker-induced
    ventricular r. (APIVR)
  atrial escape r.
  atrioventricular junction r.
  atrioventricular junctional r. (AVJR)
  atrioventricular nodal r., A-V
    nodal r.
  A-V atrioventricular junctional r.
  baseline r.
  bigeminal r.
  cantering r.
  cardiac r. (CR)
  R. catheter
  chaotic r.
  circadian r.
  concealed r.
  coronary nodal r.
  coronary sinus r.
  coupled r.
  r. discrimination
  r. disturbance
  diurnal r.
  ectopic r.
  embryocardia r.
  escape r.
  fetal heart r.
  fibrillation r.
  force and r. (F and R)
  gallop r.
  heart r.
  idiojunctional r.
  idionodal r.
  idioventricular r. (IVR)
  irregular r.
  irregularly irregular cardiac r.
  junctional r. (JR)
  junctional escape r. (JER)
  left bundle branch r.
  life-threatening heart r.
  lower nodal r.
  midnodal r.
  mu r.
  nodal escape r.

  normal sinus r. (NSR)
  paced r.
  pendulum r.
  perfusing r.
  pulseless idioventricular r.
  quadrigeminal r.
  quadruple r.
  rate and r. (R&R)
  reciprocal r.
  reciprocating r.
  regularly irregular r.
  regular rate and r. (RRR, RR&R)
  regular sinus r. (RSR)
  reversed reciprocal r.
  right bundle branch r.
  sinus r. (SR)
  slow escape r.
  r. strip
  systolic gallop r.
  tic-tac r.
  trainwheel r.
  trigeminal r.
  triple r.
  underlying heart r. (UHR)
  ventricular r. (VR)
  ventricular paced r. (VPR)
  wide complex r.
rhythmicity
Rhythmin
Rhythmonorm
RI
  Röhrer index
RIA
  radioimmunoassay
rib
  r. approximator
  r. cage
  r. cutter
  r. elevator
  r. fracture
  r. guillotine
  lower r.
  r. margin
  middle r.
  r. notching
  r. raspatory
  r. shears
  r. spreader
  r. stripper
  upper r.
ribavirin
Ribbert thrombosis
ribbon
  r. muscle
  safety r.
ribonucleic acid (RNA)
riboprobe
  CMV IE-2 r.

HIV-1 r.
IE-2 r.
riboside
AICA r.
ribosome
RIC
right interventricular coronary
RIC artery
Richet aneurysm
Richter transformation
ricin
Ricketts-Abrams technique
Rickettsia
R. *australis*
R. *prowazekii*
rickettsial
r. endocarditis
r. infection
r. myocarditis
r. pneumonia
ridge
eustachian r.
neointimal r.
pharyngeal r.
pulmonary r.
supraaortic r. (SAR)
riding
r. embolism
r. embolus
RIE
relative inspiratory effort
Riedel
R. struma
R. thyroiditis
Riegel pulse
Rienhoff-Finochietto rib spreader
Rienhoff thoracic scissors
RIF
rifampin
rifabutin
Rifadin
R. injection
R. Oral
rifalazil
Rifamate
rifampicin
rifampin (RIF)
r. and isoniazid
r., isoniazid, pyrazinamide
rifamycin
rifapentine
Rifater
Rift Valley fever virus
right
r. ankle index
r. anterior oblique (RAO)
r. anterior oblique equivalent
r. anterior oblique position
r. anterior oblique projection

r. aortic arch
r. arm electrode for electrocardiogram (VR)
r. atrial appendage (RAA)
r. atrial enlargement (RAE)
r. atrial free wall (RAFW)
r. atrial hypertrophy (RAH)
r. atrial inversion (RAI)
r. atrial inversion time index (RAITI)
r. atrial involvement (RAI)
r. atrial mean pressure (RAMP)
r. atrial mobile thrombus (RAMT)
r. atrial myxoma
r. atrial pacing
r. atrial pressure (RAP)
r. atrial thrombus
r. atrial wall (RAW)
r. atrium (RA)
r. atrium diameter (RAD)
r. atrium to pulmonary artery (RA-PA)
r. atrium to right ventricle (RA-RV)
r. auricle (RA)
r. auricle of heart
r. axis deviation (RAD)
r. border cardiac dullness (RBCD)
r. border of dullness (RBD)
r. brachial artery (RBA)
r. brachial vein (RBV)
r. brain damage (RBD)
r. bundle (RB)
r. bundle branch (RBB)
r. bundle branch block (RBBB)
r. bundle branch rhythm
r. bundle branch system block (RBBsB)
r. cardiac work index (RCWI)
r. cerebrovascular accident (RCVA)
r. common carotid artery (RCCA)
r. congestive heart failure (RCHF)
r. coronary artery (RCA)
r. coronary catheter
r. coronary cusp (RCC)
r. coronary ostium (RCO)
r. coronary sinus (RCS)
r. costal margin (RCM)
r. crus of diaphragm
r. descending pulmonary artery (RDPA)
r. gastroepiploic artery (RGEA)
r. heart (RH)
r. heart bypass (RHB)
r. heart catheter
r. heart catheterization (RHC)
r. heart failure (RHF)
r. heart mixing volume (RHMV)
r. hemidiaphragm height

R

right (*continued*)

r. hemisphere damage (RHD)
r. hemisphere stroke
r. inferior pulmonary vein
r. inferior vena cava (RIVC)
r. internal mammary artery (RIMA)
r. internal mammary artery graft
r. internal thoracic artery (RITA)
r. internal thoracic artery graft
r. interventricular coronary (RIC)
r. Judkins catheter
r. lower lobe (RLL)
r. lower pulmonary vein (RLPV)
r. lung
r. main bronchus
r. margin of heart
r. middle cerebral artery (R-MCA)
r. middle lobe (RML)
r. parasternal impulse
r. parasternal impulses
r. portal vein (RPV)
r. posterior ventricular preexcitation (RPVP)
r. pulmonary artery (RPA)
r. pulmonary vein (RPV)
r. recurrent laryngeal nerve
r. septum (RS)
r. single lung transplant (RSLTx)
r. superior pulmonary vein
r. superior vena cava (RSVC)
r. triangular ligament of liver
r. upper lobe (RUL)
r. upper pulmonary vein (RUPV)
r. ventricle (RV)
r. ventricle activation (RVA)
r. ventricle afterload
r. ventricle anterior wall (RVAW)
r. ventricle infarction (RVI)
r. ventricular (RV)
r. ventricular apex (RVA)
r. ventricular assist device (RVAD)
r. ventricular cardiomyopathy
r. ventricular copulsation balloon (RVCB)
r. ventricular diastolic collapse (RVDC)
r. ventricular diastolic overload (RVDO)
r. ventricular diastolic pressure
r. ventricular diastolic volume (RVDV)
r. ventricular dimension (RVD)
r. ventricular dysplasia
r. ventricular ejection fraction (REF, RVEF)
r. ventricular ejection time (RVET)
r. ventricular end-diastolic (RVED)
r. ventricular end-diastolic diameter (RVEDD)

r. ventricular end-diastolic pressure (RVEDP)
r. ventricular end-diastolic volume (RVEDV)
r. ventricular end-diastolic volume index (RVEDVI)
r. ventricular end-flow (RVEF)
r. ventricular endocardial potential (RVECP)
r. ventricular end-systolic volume (RVESV)
r. ventricular end-systolic volume index (RVESVI)
r. ventricular enlargement (RVE)
r. ventricular failure (RVF)
r. ventricular filling pressure (RVFP)
r. ventricular function
r. ventricular heave
r. ventricular hypertrophy (RVH)
r. ventricular hypoplasia
r. ventricular infarction (RVI)
r. ventricular inflow obstruction
r. ventricular inflow tract (RVIT)
r. ventricular infundibulum
r. ventricular internal dimension (RVID)
r. ventricular isovolumic relaxation time (RV-IVRT)
r. ventricular mean (RVM)
r. ventricular myxoma
r. ventricular outflow (RVO)
r. ventricular outflow obstruction
r. ventricular outflow tract (RVOT)
r. ventricular outflow tract obstruction (RVOTO)
r. ventricular outflow tract pacing
r. ventricular outflow tract reconstruction
r. ventricular outflow tract tachycardia
r. ventricular peak filling rate (RVPFR)
r. ventricular peak systolic pressure
r. ventricular preejection period (RVPEP)
r. ventricular pressure (RVP)
r. ventricular refractory period (RVERP)
r. ventricular septal pacing
r. ventricular stroke output (RVSO)
r. ventricular stroke volume (RVSV)
r. ventricular stroke work (RVSW)
r. ventricular stroke work index (RVSWI)
r. ventricular systolic pressure (RVSP)
r. ventricular systolic time interval

r. ventricular volume (RVV)
r. ventricular volume overload (RVVO)
r. ventricular wall (RVW)
r. ventricular wall motion
r. ventricular wall thickness (RVWT)
r. vertebral artery (RVA)

right-angle chest tube
right/left lung
right-sided
r.-s. endocarditis
r.-s. heart failure
right-to-left shunt (RLS, RLSh)
rightward axis
rigid
r. bronchoscopy
r. core-out of lesions
r. monopolar loop
r. pod
r. thoracoscope
rigidity
nuchal r.
Rigiflex TTS balloon catheter
rigor
calcium r.
RIHD
radiation-induced heart disease
RIII reflex
Riley-Cournand equation
Riley-Day syndrome
Riley needle
rilmenidine
riluzole
RIMA
right internal mammary artery
free RIMA
RIMA graft
rima
r. respiratoria
r. vestibuli
r. vocalis
Rimactane Oral
rimantadine hydrochloride
rimiterol
RIND
reversible ischemic neurologic defect
Rindfleisch fold
ring
r. abscess
AnnuloFlex flexible annuloplasty r.
AnnuloFlo annuloplasty r.
annuloplasty r.
aortic r.
atrial r.
atrioventricular valve r.
cardiac lymphatic r.
Carpentier-Edwards Physio annuloplasty r.

Carpentier rigid r.
circumaortic venous r.
coronary r.
Cosgrove-Edwards r.
double-flanged valve sewing r.
Duran annuloplasty r.
Edwards IMR ETlogix annuloplasty r.
r. electrode
esophageal contraction r.
fibrous r.
knitted sewing r.
left ventricular cavity obstruction r.
Lower r.'s
metal sewing r.
pericardium-coated prosthetic anuloplasty r.
pharyngeal lymphatic r.
plastic sewing r.
pleural r.'s
prosthetic valve sewing r.
Schatzki esophageal r.
Sculptor anuloplasty r.
Seguin anuloplasty r.
sewing r.
r. shadow
r. sign
SJM Seguin annuloplasty r.
SJM Tailor anuloplasty r.
St. Jude Medical rigid saddle r.
supraanular suture r.
supraaortic r. (SAR)
tantalum r.
tonsillar r.
tracheal r.
vascular r.
Waldeyer throat r.
Waldeyer tonsillar r.
ringer
R. lactate
R. solution
RinoFlow ENT wash unit
Rinspirator
Kerberos R.
Riolan
anastomosis of R.
RIP
respiratory inductance plethysmograph
respiratory inductance plethysmography
RIP portable sleep monitor
RISA
radioactive iodinated serum albumin
RISC
Research Group on Instability in Coronary Artery Disease
rise
impedance r.
r. time

risk
r. calculator
cardiac r.
competing r.'s
r. factor
r. factor profile
Goldman index of r.
r. index
modified multifactorial index of
  cardiac r.
recurrence r.
relative r. (RR)
restenosis r.
Sentinel Event Notification Systems
  for Occupational R. (SENSOR)
stochastic r.
r. stratification
r. stratify
surgical r.
r. threshold
risk-benefit ratio
RITA
Randomized Intervention Treatment of
  Angina
right internal thoracic artery
  RITA graft
Ritalin
Ritalin-SR
Ritchie Articular Index
Rithron-XR
R.-XR coronary stent
R.-XR coronary stent system
ritodrine
ritonavir
Riva-Rocci sphygmomanometer
RIVC
right inferior vena cava
Rivermead
R. Behavioral Memory Test
R. Motor Assessment Arm score
Rivero-Carvallo
R.-C. effect
R.-C. sign
Riviere sign
Rivinus
R. canals
R. gland
RKG
radiocardiogram
R2L
R2L rapid exchange balloon
  dilation catheter
R2L rapid exchange balloon
  dilation catheter with extended
  pressure range
R-lactate enzyme monotest
RLF
radiolabeled fibrinogen
retained lung fluid

RLH
recurrent lobar hemorrhage
RLL
right lower lobe
RLP
remnant-like lipoprotein particle
remnant lipoprotein
  RLP lipoprotein
RLPV
right lower pulmonary vein
RLS, RLSh
right-to-left shunt
R-Lsh
RLT
red light therapy
RMBF
regional myocardial blood flow
R-MCA
right middle cerebral artery
RMI
recent myocardial infarction
  RMI antegrade cardioplegia catheter
RML
right middle lobe
RMR
resting metabolic rate
rMRGlu
regional metabolic rate of glucose
RMS
rheumatic mitral stenosis
RNA
radionuclide angiography
ribonucleic acid
  RNA glycosidase toxin
RNeasy Mini kit
RNSC
radionuclide superior cavography
RNV
radionuclide venography
radionuclide ventriculography
RNVG
radionuclide ventriculography
ROA
regurgitant orifice area
ROAD
reversible obstructive airways disease
Roadmapper
roadmapping
coronary r.
Roadrunner extra-support wire guide
Robafen
R. AC
R. DM
Robert
R. David Cerfolio (RDC)
R. David Cerfolio classification
R. David Cerfolio classification
  system
Robertshaw tube

Robertson sign
Robicsek
    R. technique
    R. vascular probe
Robinson index
Robinul Forte
Robitussin
    R. DM
    R. Pediatric
    R. Severe Congestion Liqui-Gels
robotic
    r. coronary revascularization
    r. heart surgery
Rocephin IM
Rochalimaea
    R. henselae
    R. quintana
Rocha-Lima inclusion
Roche analyzer
Roche-Microwell plate hybridization
  method
Rochester
    R. Kocher clamp
    R. needle
    R. Péan clamp
rocker
rocket immunoelectrophoretic method of
  Laurell
Rockey ventricular cannula
rocking bed
Rocky Mountain spotted fever
rocuronium
Roda Patient Monitoring System
rodhaini
    Babesia r.
Rodrigo equation
Rodriguez aneurysm
roentgen (R)
    r. knife
roentgenogram
    apical lordotic r.
    chest r. (CR)
roentgenographically occult lung cancer
  (ROLC)
roentgenographic presentation
roentgenography
    chest r. (CR)
RoEzIt skin moisturizer
Rofact
rofecoxib
Roferon-A
roflumilast
Rogaine topical
Roger
    R. bruit
    bruit de R.
    R. disease
    maladie de R.
    R. murmur

Rogers sphygmomanometer
Rogitine
Roho mattress
Röhrer
    R. equation
    R. index (RI)
ROI
    region of interest
Rokitansky disease
ROLC
    roentgenographically occult lung cancer
role
    cardioprotective r.
    loss of r.
roller
    r. bottle
    r. pump
Rolleston rule
rolling hernia
Romãna sign
Romano-Ward syndrome
ROME
    Randomized Outpatient Milrinone
    Evaluation
Romhilt-Estes
    R.-E. point score criteria
    R.-E. point scoring system
    R.-E. score
ROMI
    rule out myocardial infarction
Rondamine-DM drops
Rondec
    R. Drops
    R. Filmtabs
    R. Syrup
Rondec-DM
rongeur
    aortic valve r.
    Bailey aortic valve r.
R-on-T
    R-o.-T arrhythmia susceptibility
    R-o.-T phenomenon
    R-o.-T premature ventricular
      complex
R-on-T-initiated
    R-o.-T-i. nonsustained VT
    R-o.-T-i. VF
roof of left atrium
room
    cardiovascular recovery r. (CVRR)
Roos test
root
    anterior wall of aortic r. (AWAR)
    aortic r.
    free r.
    r. inclusion method
    r. injection
    r. of lung
    r. perfusion

R

root *(continued)*
    posterior wall of aortic r. (PAR)
    r. stabilization
    r. tailoring
root-mean-square voltage
ROP
    retinopathy of prematurity
ROPE
    respiratory ordered phase encoding
ropy sputum
ROS
    reactive oxygen species
Rosai-Dorfman disease
Rosalki technique
ROSC
    restoration of spontaneous circulation
    return of spontaneous circulation
rose
    r. hips asthma
    R. Questionnaire
    r. spot
    R. tamponade
Rosenbach syndrome
Rosenberg syndrome
Rosenkranz pediatric open heart retractor
Rosenmüller recess
rosette
    acinar r.
rosiglitazone
Ross
    R. aortic valve replacement procedure
    R. needle
    R. River virus
Rossetti
    R. modification
    R. modification of Nissen fundoplication
Ross-Konno pediatric aortoventriculoplasty procedure
Rostan asthma
rostral
    r. ventrolateral medulla (RVLM)
    r. ventromedial medulla (RVMM)
rosuvastatin
ROTA
    Rotablator atherectomy
rotablator
    R. atherectomy (ROTA)
    R. and restenosis (R&R)
Rotacaps
    Ventolin R.
ROTACS
    rotational angioplasty catheter system
Rotadisk
    Flovent R.
Rotaglide lubricant

Rotahaler
RotaLink rotational atherectomy device
rotary
    r. atherectomy device
    r. ventricular assist device
    r. vertigo
rotastent
rotating
    r. blades
    r. disc oxygenation
rotation
    antibiotic class r.
    cardiac r.
    clockwise r.
    counterclockwise r.
    shoulder r.
rotational
    r. ablation
    r. angioplasty catheter system (ROTACS)
    r. aortogram
    r. atherectomy (RA)
    r. atherectomy device
    r. atherectomy system (RAS)
    r. coronary atherectomy (RCA)
    r. dynamic angioplasty catheter
RotaWire Floppy Gold guidewire
Rotch sign
Rotex needle
Rothia dentocariosa
Rothschild sign
Roth spot
Rotoslide
rotundum
    foramen r.
Roubac
Roubin infusion catheter
Rougnon-Heberden disease
rouleau formation
round
    r. foramen
    r. heart
    r. hematoma
    r. pneumonia nodule
rounded atelectasis
round-robin classification
roundworm
Rous sarcoma virus (RSV)
Roussy-Lévy
    R.-L. disease
    R.-L. polyneuropathy
    R.-L. syndrome
route of insertion
routine
    cardiac ambulation r. (CAR)
Roux-en-Y obesity
Rovamycine
roxithromycin

royal

R. Flush Plus high-flow angiographic flush catheter

r. jelly-induced asthma

RP

radial pulse

relapsing polychondritis

reperfusion

RPA

reteplase

right pulmonary artery

r-PA

reteplase

RPBD

rating of perceived breathing difficulty

RPE

rating of perceived exertion

r-PEG

recombinant polyethylene glycol

RPF

renal plasma flow

RPFA

rapid platelet function assay

R-P interval

RPM

real-time position management

RPM tracking system

RPM tracking system/catheter

RPP

heart rate-systolic blood pressure product

rate-pressure product

Rp:Rs

pulmonary-to-systemic vascular resistance

RPV

right portal vein

right pulmonary vein

RPVP

right posterior ventricular preexcitation

RQ

respiratory quotient

R/Q wave ratio

RR

relative risk

respiratory rate

RR cycle

RR interval dynamics

RR interval stability

RR prime

R&R

rate and rhythm

Rotablator and restenosis

RRI

recurrent respiratory infection

R-R interval

R-R′ interval

RRP

relative refractory period

RRR

regular rate and rhythm

relative risk reduction

RR&R

regular rate and rhythm

Rrs

respiratory resistance

RS

right septum

RS complex

RS deflection

RSA

respiratory sinus arrhythmia

Rsa

systemic arterial resistance

RSBI

rapid shallow breathing index

RSC

rested state contraction

RSDL

reactive skin decontamination lotion

RSI

rapid sequence induction

RSI orotracheal intubation

RSLTx

right single lung transplant

r-Sm

reversal speed of bronchoconstriction in response to methacholine

rSO₂

regional oxygen saturation

RSR, rSR′

regular sinus rhythm

rSR

abnormal rhythm on ECG

small R, bigger R of QRS

rSR (rSR prime)

abberrant condition of supraventricular beat

abnormal ECG rhythm of small R, bigger R of QRS

rSr

RSSR

relative slow sinus rate

R-Stent stent

RS-T interval

RST segment

RSV

respiratory syncytial virus

Rous sarcoma virus

RSVA

ruptured sinus of Valsalva aneurysm

RSVC

right superior vena cava

RSV-IG

respiratory syncytial virus immunoglobulin

RT

reciprocating tachycardia

R

RT *(continued)*
    reentrant tachycardia
    resistance training
RT3D echo
R-Test Evolution
Rti
    resistance to movement of lung tissue
RTLF
    respiratory tract lining fluid
Rtot
    total airway resistance
rt-PA
    recombinant tissue plasminogen activator
        catabolism of rt-PA
        double-chain rt-PA
RT-PCR
    reverse transcriptase polymerase chain
      reaction
rub
    centripetal r. (CPR)
    friction r.
    gallop, murmur, r. (GMR)
    r.'s, gallops, murmurs
    pericardial friction r.
    pleural friction r.
    pleuritic r.
    pleuropericardial r.
    saddle leather friction r.
rubbery sputum
rubella syndrome
rubeola
Rubex
Rubicon
    R. Embolic Filter
    R. filter device
    R. filter system
rubidium (Rb)
rubidium-81
rubidium-82 (Rb-82)
    r.-82 imaging
    r.-82 positron emission tomography
Rubinstein-Taybi syndrome
rubitecan
rubor
    dependent r.
Rubulavirus
ruby laser
rude respiration
rudimentary chamber
Rudolph Full Face mask
RUDS
    reactive upper airways dysfunction
      syndrome
Ruel aorta clamp
r-UK
    recombinant urokinase
RUL
    right upper lobe

rule
    r. of bigeminy
    Gibson r.
    Liebermeister r.
    r. out myocardial infarction
      (ROMI)
    Rolleston r.
    shorthand r.
    Simpson r.
    trapezoidal r.
rumble
    Austin Flint r.
    booming r.
    diastolic r.
    filling r.
    middiastolic r.
    protodiastolic r.
    third sound r.
rumbling diastolic murmur
Rumel
    R. clamp
    R. tourniquet
Rumpel-Leede test
run
    second pump r.
runaway pacemaker
runoff
    aortofemoral arterial r.
    aortogram with distal r.
    arterial r.
    r. arteriogram
    digital r.
    distal r.
    venous r.
rupture
    aortic r.
    balloon r.
    blunt cardiac r.
    cardiac r.
    chamber r.
    chordae tendineae r.
    chordal r.
    contained r.
    coronary plaque r.
    diaphragmatic r.
    esophageal r.
    evolving r.
    IEM r.
    internal elastic membrane r.
    interventricular septal r.
    intraperitoneal r.
    intrapleural r.
    membrane r.
    myocardial free wall r.
    nonpenetrating r.
    overt r.
    papillary muscle r. (PMR)
    penetrating r.
    perivascular r.

pinhole balloon r.
plaque r.
pulmonary artery r.
thoracic aortic r. (TAR)
traumatic r.
r. trigger
valve r.
ventricular septal r.

ruptured
r. aortic aneurysm
r. sinus of Valsalva
r. sinus of Valsalva aneurysm
(RSVA)

RUPV
right upper pulmonary vein

Ruschelit polyvinyl chloride endotracheal tube

Russian influenza

rusty sputum

ruthenium red

Rutherford claudication classification

Ru-Tuss
R.-T. DE
R.-T. Expectorant

RV
regurgitant volume
residual volume
rhinovirus
right ventricle
right ventricular
RV infundibulum

RVA
reentrant ventricular arrhythmia
right ventricle activation
right ventricular apex
right vertebral artery

RVAD
right ventricular assist device

RVAW
right ventricle anterior wall

RVCB
right ventricular copulsation balloon

RVD
reference vessel diameter
relative vessel diameter
right ventricular dimension

RVDC
right ventricular diastolic collapse

RVDO
right ventricular diastolic overload

RVDV
right ventricular diastolic volume

RVE
right ventricular enlargement

RVECP
right ventricular endocardial potential

RVED
right ventricular end-diastolic
RVED pressure

RVEDD
right ventricular end-diastolic diameter

RVEDP
right ventricular end-diastolic pressure

RVEDV
right ventricular end-diastolic volume

RVEDVI
right ventricular end-diastolic volume
index

RVEF
right ventricular ejection fraction
right ventricular end-flow

RVERP
right ventricular refractory period

RVESV
right ventricular end-systolic volume

RVESVI
right ventricular end-systolic volume
index

RVET
right ventricular ejection time

RVF
residual volume fraction
right ventricular failure

RVFP
right ventricular filling pressure

RVH
renovascular hypertension
right ventricular hypertrophy

RVHD
rheumatic valvular heart disease

RVI
right ventricle infarction
right ventricular infarction

RVID
right ventricular internal dimension

RVIT
right ventricular inflow tract

RV-IVRT
right ventricular isovolumic relaxation
time

RVLM
rostral ventrolateral medulla

RVM
right ventricular mean

RVMM
rostral ventromedial medulla

RVO
right ventricular outflow

RVol
regurgitant volume

RVOT
right ventricular outflow tract
RVOT pacing

RVOTO
right ventricular outflow tract obstruction

RVP
resting venous pressure
right ventricular pressure

R

RVPEP
right ventricular preejection period
RVPFR
right ventricular peak filling rate
RVR
reduced vascular response
repetitive ventricular response
resistance to venous return
RVSO
right ventricular stroke output
RVSP
right ventricular systolic pressure
RVSV
right ventricular stroke volume
RVSW
right ventricular stroke work
RVSWI
right ventricular stroke work index
RVTE
recurring venous thromboembolism
RV/TLC
residual volume/total lung capacity
RV/TLC ratio
RVV
right ventricular volume
RVVO
right ventricular volume overload
RVW
right ventricular wall

RVWT
right ventricular wall thickness
R-wave
R-w. amplitude
R-w. gating
R-w. progression (RWP)
R-w. upstroke
RWM
regional wall motion
RWMA
regional wall motion abnormality
RWP
R-wave progression
RWT
relative wall thickness
RX
rapid exchange
RX CrossSail coronary dilation
catheter
Folgard RX
RX Streak balloon catheter
ryanodine receptor
Rynacrom
Rynatan
Rynatuss Pediatric Suspension
RyR2 receptor
Rythmodan
Rythmodan-LA
Rythmol

S
negative deflection that follows R wave
septum
systole
Golden sign of S
S wave
S′ wave
S₁
first heart sound
S100 stain
S₂
second heart sound
S2 allele
S₃
third heart sound
S₃ gallop
S₄
fourth heart sound
S₄ gallop
S₇
summation gallop
S₇ gallop
S7 coronary stent
S660
S660 small vessel coronary stent
S660 with Discrete Technology coronary stent system
S670
S670 coronary stent
S670 with Discrete Technology coronary stent system
SA
salvage angioplasty
secondary arrest
sinuatrial
sinus arrest
sinus arrhythmia
stable angina
S-A
sinuatrial
S-A nodal reentrant tachycardia
S-A node
S/A
stent-to-artery
S/A ratio
SAA
serum amyloid type A
SAAP
selective aortic arch perfusion
SAB
sinuatrial block
saber-sheath trachea
Sabin-Feldman dye test
Sable PTCA balloon catheter

sabot
coeur en s.
s. heart
SABP
systolic arterial blood pressure
Sabulin
sac
air s.
alveolar s.
aneurysmal s.
aortic s.
Hilton s.
Lap S.
lateral s.
pericardial s.
pleural s.
sacchari
Thermoactinomyces s.
Saccharomonospora
Saccharomyces anginae
Saccharopolyspora rectivirgula
Saccomanno
S. fixative
S. morphologic criteria
saccular
s. bronchiectasis
s. false aneurysm
s. period
sacculated
s. empyema
s. pleurisy
sacculation
localized s.
saccule of larynx
sacculus
s. alveolares
s. alveolaris
s. laryngis
saccus endolymphaticus
SAC data acquisition technology
sacral edema
sacrococcygeal aorta
SACS
secondary anticoagulation system
SACT
sinuatrial conduction time
SAD
sinoaortic denervation
saddle
s. embolism
s. embolus
s. leather friction rub
s. thrombus
saddle-backed appearance

Sade
- S. modification
- S. modification of Norwood procedure

SADS
- sudden arrhythmic death syndrome

SAEB
- sinuatrial entrance block

SAECG
- signal-averaged electrocardiogram
- signal-averaged electrocardiography

SAED
- semiautomatic external defibrillator

Safar bronchoscope

safe
- S. Step blood-collection needle
- S. Tussin 30
- s. zone

Safe-Cross guidewire

Safe-Cross-RF guidewire

SafeSheath CSG introducer sheath

Safe-Steer
- S.-S. guidewire
- S.-S. support catheter
- S.-S. Total Occlusion Crossing System

Safe-T Tube

SafeTway pediatric mouthpiece

safety
- s. guidewire
- s. margin
- occupational health and s. (OHS)
- radiation s.
- s. ribbon

sag
- ST s.

sagittal
- s. cut
- s. plane
- s. view

SAH
- subarachnoid hemorrhage

Sahara S1100a Pleur-evac Chest Drainage System

SAHS
- sleep apnea/hypopnea syndrome

sail sound

saint (St.)

Sala cell

salbutamol

Salflex

salicylate
- antipyrine s.
- carbazochrome s.
- choline s.
- magnesium s.
- phenyl s.
- sodium s.

saline
- Broncho S.
- half-normal s.
- heparinized s.
- hypertonic s.
- iced s.
- s. jet
- s. loading
- s. microbubble
- normal s.
- phosphate-buffered s. (PBS)
- s. slush

salivagram

salivaris
- caruncula s.

salivarius
- *Streptococcus s.*

salivation, lacrimation, urination, defecation (SLUD)

Salkowski test

salmeterol
- s. and fluticasone propionate
- s. xinafoate

Salmonella
- *S. choleraesuis*
- S. mycotic aneurysm

salmon skin

salol

saloon door parasternal approach

salsalate

salt
- s. depletion syndrome
- dietary s.
- ethylenediaminetetraacetic acid disodium s.
- gold s.
- s. of nickel
- no added s. (NAS)
- s. and pepper appearance
- s. and pepper pattern
- persulfate s.
- s. of platinum
- s. wasting
- s. and water dependent hypertension

saltans
- thrombophlebitis s.

salt-free diet

salting-out procedure

Salubria biomaterial

saluresis

saluretic agent

salute
- allergic s.

Salutensin-Demi

saluting

salvage
- s. angioplasty (SA)
- s. balloon angioplasty

intraoperative cell s.
limb s.
myocardial s.
salves
tachycardia en s.
salvo
s. of beats
s. of ventricular tachycardia
SAM
surface adherent monocyte
systolic anterior motion
SAM system
Sam Levine sign
sample
end-tidal s.
Haldane-Priestley s.
Rahn-Otis s.
sampler
continuous ambulatory blood s.
(CABS)
sampling
bioptic s.
blood s.
chorionic villus s.
Samsoon-Young modification
Samuels
S. forceps
S. hemoclip
SAN
sinoauricular node
sinuatrial node
San
S. Joaquin Valley disease
S. Joaquin Valley fever
Sanchez-Cascos cardioauditory syndrome
sand
hydatid s.
Sanders bed
Sandhoff disease
Sandifer syndrome
Sandler-Dodge area-length method
Sandman system
Sandoglobulin
Sandostatin LAR
Sandrock test
sandwich
s. enzyme-linked immunosorbent
assay
s. patch
stent s.
Sanfilippo syndrome
sanguinis
fragilitas s.
ictus s.
Sano modification
Sansert
Sansom sign
SANWS
sinuatrial node weakness syndrome

SAO
subvalvar aortic obstruction
SaO$_2$
arterial oxygen saturation
SAP
stable angina pectoris
systemic arterial pressure
systolic atrial pressure
SAPD
signal-averaged P-wave duration
saphenofemoral
s. junction
s. system
saphenous
s. vein (SV)
s. vein bypass (SVB)
s. vein bypass graft angiography
s. vein bypass grafting (SVBG)
s. vein cannula
s. vein cutdown (SVC)
s. vein graft (SVG)
s. vein graft disease
s. vein graft intervention using
AngioGuard (GUARD)
s. vein harvesting (SVH)
s. vein patch closure
s. vein varicosity
SAPHfinder surgical balloon dissector
SAPHtrak balloon dissector
SAPK
stress-activated protein kinase
saprophytic
SAPS
Simplified Acute Physiology Score
SAQLI
Sleep Apnea Quality of Life Index
saquinavir mesylate
SAR
supraaortic ridge
supraaortic ring
saralasin
sarcoglycan
sarcoid
Boeck s.
endobronchial s.
s. granuloma
sarcoid-like pulmonary disorder
sarcoidosis
alveolar s.
bronchial s.
fibrocystic s.
nodular s.
parenchymal s.
pulmonary s.
sarcoidosis-induced pulmonary hypertension
sarcolemmal
s. bleb
s. calcium channel

653

sarcolemmal *(continued)*
  s. glucose
  s. level
  s. membrane
  s. reticular transport
sarcolemma lipid
sarcoma
  cardiac s.
  Kaposi s. (KS)
  metastatic s.
  pseudo-Kaposi s.
  soft tissue s.
  spindle cell s.
  synovial s.
sarcomatoid mesothelioma
sarcomatous tumor
sarcomere
sarcomeric protein mutation
Sarcophaga
sarcoplasmic
  s. reticular transport
  s. reticulum
  s. reticulum-associated glycolytic
    enzymes
sarcosporidiosis
sarcotubular system
Sarns
  S. aortic arch cannula
  S. electric saw
  S. intracardiac suction tube
  S. membrane oxygenator (SMO)
  S. soft-flow aortic cannula
  S. 2-stage cannula
  S. ventricular assist device
  S. wire-reinforced catheter
Sarot bronchus clamp
SARS
  severe acute respiratory syndrome
SARS-CoV
  severe acute respiratory syndrome-
    associated coronavirus
SART
  sinuatrial recovery time
saruplase
SAS
  small aorta syndrome
  subaortic stenosis
  subarachnoid space
  supravalvar aortic stenosis
  synchronous atrial stimulation
SAST
  selective arterial secretin injection test
SAT
  subacute thrombosis
  systolic acceleration time
    Press-mate SAT
satellite lesion
Satinsky clamp

sativa
  Vicia s.
Satterthwaite method
saturated
  s. fatty acid (SFA)
  s. solution
  s. solution of potassium iodide
    (SSKI)
saturation
  arterial s.
  arterial oxygen s. (SaO_2)
  s. index
  mean nocturnal s.
  mixed venous oxygen s. (SvO_2)
  oxygen s. (SO_2)
  oxyhemoglobin s.
  regional oxygen s. (rSO_2)
  step-up in oxygen s.
  s. time
  venous s.
saucerize
Sauerbruch-Herrmannsdorfer-Gerson diet
sausaging of vein
SAV
  sequential atrioventricular
Savary-Gilliard esophageal dilator
Saventrine Intravenous
SAVER
  surgical anterior ventricular endocardial
    restoration
saver
  Cell S.
  Haemonetics Cell S.
SAVR
  surgical anterior ventricular restoration
    SAVR surgical treatment
Savvy PTA dilation catheter
saw
  oscillating s.
  Sarns electric s.
  sternum s.
  Stryker s.
sawtooth
  s. pattern
  s. P wave
Sawyer operation
SAX
  short axis
SAX-MV
  short-axis mitral valve
SAX-PM
  short-axis plane, papillary muscle
SB
  shortness of breath
  sinus bradycardia
SBE
  shortness of breath on exertion
  subacute bacterial endocarditis
    SBE prophylaxis

SBF
systemic blood flow
SBI
silent brain infarction
SBP
systolic blood pressure
SBS
sick building syndrome
SBSE
supine bicycle stress echocardiography
SBSP
simultaneous bilateral spontaneous
pneumothorax
SBT
serum bactericidal titer
SC
systolic click
SC-210 sidestream capnograph
SC-300 portable capnograph
SCA
sudden cardiac arrest
superior cerebellar artery
scabbard trachea
SCABG
single coronary artery bypass graft
SCAD, sCAD
spontaneous coronary artery disease
spontaneous coronary artery dissection
Scadding stage 0-IV
scaffolding
SCAI
Society for Cardiac Angiography and
Interventions
scalar
s. electrocardiogram
s. lead
scale
Abbreviated Injury S. (AIS)
activity s.
ADL s.
Ashworth S.
Behavioral Dyscontrol S. (BDCS)
Berg Balance S.
Borg s. (1-20)
Borg numerical s. (1-20)
Borg rating of perceived
exertion s.
Borg treadmill exertion s.
cardiac adjustment s. (CAS)
Centers for Epidemiologic Studies
Depression s. (CES-D)
Cook-Medley hostility s.
Cook multiple-assessment s.
Delirium Rating S.
dyspnea s.
Epworth Sleepiness S. (ESS)
European Stroke S. (ESS)
Fagerstrom Tolerance S.
French s.

Fugl-Meyer motor test s.
Gaffky s.
Geriatric Depression S.
Glasgow Coma S. (GCS)
gray s.
Grossman s.
Health Locus of Control S.
Holmes-Rahe s.
Hospital Anxiety and Depression S.
(HADS)
Karnofsky rating s.
Lawton Instrumental Activities of
Daily Living s.
Likert s. (LS)
Likert 5-point s.
mechanical visual analogue s.
Montgomery-Asberg Depression
Rating S. (MADRS)
Motor Assessment S. (MAS)
National Institutes of Health
Stroke S. (NIHSS)
Nottingham Extended Activities of
Daily Living s.
Observer's Assessment of
Alertness/Sedation S.
Oxford Handicap S.
Paykel s.
Philadelphia Geriatric Center
Morale S. (PGCMS)
Psychosocial Adjustment to
Illness S.
pulmonary functional status s.
(PFSS)
quick confusion s. (QCS)
Rankin Disability S.
Sickness Impact Profile s.
SIP s.
Spielberger Anger Expression s.
Stroke Impact S. (SIS)
subject's treatment-emergent
symptom s. (STRESS)
Toronto Alexithymia S.
visual analog s. (VAS)
voxel gray s.
Wigle s.
scalene
s. fat pad biopsy
s. lymph node biopsy
scalenectomy
scalenotomy
Adson-Coffey s.
scalenus
s. anterior syndrome
s. anticus syndrome
scalloped
s. commissure
s. subcoronary position
scalloping

S

scalp
  s. electrode
  s. pH
  s. vein needle
SCAN
  systolic coronary artery narrowing
scan
  apical hypoperfusion on thallium s.
  Cardiolite s.
  Cardiotec s.
  carotid duplex s.
  cine s.
  computed tomographic s.
  s. converter
  coronary artery s. (CAS)
  CT s.
  dipyridamole thallium-201 s.
  duplex Doppler s.
  dynamic CT s.
  gallium s.
  gallium-67 s.
  gated cardiac s.
  4-hour s.
  HRCT s.
  lung s.
  milk s.
  MUGA cardiac blood pool s.
  multiple gated acquisition cardiac
    blood pool s.
  myocardial perfusion s.
  perfusion s.
  PET s.
  postdiuresis s.
  postexercise s.
  PYP s.
  pyrophosphate s.
  rectilinear s.
  scintillation s.
  scout s.
  sector s.
  septal hyperperfusion on thallium s.
  sestamibi s.
  spiral CT s.
  TCT s.
  teboroxime s.
  technetium-99m hexamibi s.
  thallium s.
  thin-slice CT s.
  transmission s.
  ultrafast computed tomography s.
  ultrafast CT s.
  ventilation/perfusion lung s.
  V̇/Q̇ lung s.
scanner
  computed tomography s.
  Corometrics Doppler s.
  Del Mar Avionics S.
  Evolution s.
  GE 9800 CT s.
  GE Lightspeed CT s.
  GE Signa Horizon SR 120 whole-
    body s.
  Hewlett-Packard 77020 A phased-
    array sector s.
  Imatron C-150XP electron beam
    CT s.
  Konica KFDR-S laser film s.
  Lunar DPX total body s.
  pencil-beam total body s.
  phased array sector s.
  Philips Medical Systems Tomoscan
    AVE1 CT spiral s.
  Philips Medical Systems Tomoscan
    SR 7000 CT spiral s.
  Philips Tomoscan 310 CT s.
  Picker CS s.
  Picker Edge 1.5-T s.
  Picker PQ 2000 CT s.
  Siemens Somatom DR CT s.
  Siemens Somatom Plus 4A s.
  Site-Rite II ultrasound s.
  SonoHeart s.
  Sonos 1500, 2500 s.
  Toshiba s.
  ultrafast computed tomographic s.
  ultrafast CT s.
scanning
  coronary calcium s.
  duplex s.
  electronic s.
  s. electron microscope (SEM)
  fluorodopamine positron emission
    tomographic s.
  s. format
  gated blood-pool s.
  helical CT s.
  interlaced s.
  lung s.
  MUGA s.
  PET s.
  progressive s.
  radionuclide perfusion lung s.
  thallium s.
  venous duplex s. (VDS)
scanning-beam digital x-ray
scar
  s. cancer
  s. carcinoma
  s. emphysema
  fibrotic s.
  infarct s.
  myocardial fibrous s.
  s. and pulmonary vein-related
    flutter
  zipper s.
scarlatinosa
  angina s.
scarlet fever

Scarpa
S. fascia
S. method
scar-related ventricular tachycardia
scarring
apical s.
pleural s.
scatter
Compton s.
s. radiation
scattered
s. echo
s. rays
scattergram
scattering
Rayleigh s.
scatterplot smoothing technique
scavenger
s. cell pathway
free-radical s.
lysophosphatidylcholine s.
oxygen radical s.
scavenging tube
SCD
sequential compression device
subacute coronary disease
sudden cardiac death
sudden coronary death
SCE
serious cardiac event
Scedosporium apiospermum
SCF
stem cell factor
Schafer
S. method
S. method of artificial respiration
Schapiro sign
Schapiro-Wilks test
Schatzki esophageal ring
Schatz-Palmaz intravascular stent
Schaumann
S. disease
S. syndrome
Schede
S. operation
S. thoracoplasty
Scheie syndrome
Schellong-Strisower phenomenon
Schellong test
schenckii
Sporothrix s.
Schenk-Eichelter vena cava plastic filter procedure
Schepelmann sign
Schick sign
Schiff test
Schiller method
Schindler esophagoscope

Schistosoma
S. *haematobium*
S. *japonicum*
S. *mansoni*
schistosomiasis
hepatosplenic mansonic s.
schistothorax
Schlesinger solution
Schlichter test
Schmidt-Lanterman cleft
Schmidt syndrome
Schmitt-Erlanger model of reentry
Schmitz-Rode catheter
Schmorl furrow
Schneider
S. index
S. Speedy stent
S. Wallstent
schneiderian respiratory membrane
Schneider-Meier-Magnum system
Scholten
S. biopsy forceps
S. endomyocardial bioptome
Schonander
S. procedure
S. technique
Schoonmaker-King single catheter technique
Schott treatment
Schuco nebulizer
Schueler Model 200 Aspirator
Schüller method
Schultz angina
Schultze test
Schumacher aorta clamp
schwannoma
Schwarten LP guidewire
SCI
silent cerebral infarct
silent cerebral infarction
scie
bruit de s.
Scimed
S. angioplasty catheter
S. stent
scimitar
s. sign
s. syndrome
s. vein
scintigram
pyrophosphate s.
scintigraphic
s. criteria
s. perfusion defect
s. variable
scintigraphy
AMA-Fab s.
antimyosin infarct-avid s.
captopril s.

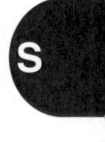

scintigraphy *(continued)*
 diethylenetriaminepentaacetate aerosol
  inhalation lung s.
 dipyridamole thallium-201 s.
 dobutamine perfusion s.
 DTPA aerosol inhalation lung s.
 exercise thallium s.
 exercise thallium-201 s.
 gallium-67 s.
 gastroesophageal s.
 gated blood-pool s.
 GBP s.
 indium-111 s.
 infarct-avid hot-spot s.
 infarct-avid myocardial s.
 iodine-131 MIBG s.
 labeled FFA s.
 MAA perfusion lung s.
 macroaggregated albumin perfusion
  lung s.
 microsphere perfusion s.
 milk s.
 myocardial cold-spot perfusion s.
 myocardial perfusion s. (MPS)
 myocardial stress perfusion s.
  (MSPS)
 myocardial viability s.
 perfusion s.
 planar myocardial s.
 planar thallium s.
 pulmonary s.
 pyrophosphate s.
 single-photon gamma s.
 SPECT s.
 stress perfusion s.
 stress thallium s.
 ^{99m}Tc sestamibi s.
 thallium myocardial s. (TMS)
 thallium-201 perfusion s.
 thallium-201 planar s.
 thallium rest-redistribution s.
 thallium-201 SPECT s.
 ventilation s.
scintillating speckle pattern
scintillation
 s. camera
 s. cocktail
 s. probe
 s. scan
scintiphotography
scintiscan
 technetium-99m stannous
  pyrophosphate s.
scintiscanner
scintiview
scirrhous carcinoma
scissors
 bandage s.
 Beall circumflex artery s.

 Crafoord lobectomy s.
 De Martel s.
 Dennis dissecting s.
 Duffield cardiovascular s.
 Jabaley-Stille Super Cut S.
 Jorgenson thoracic s.
 Karmody venous s.
 Metzenbaum s.
 pericardiotomy s.
 Rienhoff thoracic s.
SCL
 sinus cycle length
SCLC
 small-cell lung carcinoma
sclera, pl. **sclerae**
 blue s.
scleredema
 s. adultorum
 s. of Buschke
sclerodactyly
scleroderma
 diffuse cutaneous s.
 s. lung
ScleroLaser
Scleromate
ScleroPLUS HP laser system
sclerosant
 pleural s.
sclerosing
 s. agent
 s. cholangitis
 s. hemangioma
 s. phlebitis
 variceal s.
sclerosis, pl. **scleroses**
 amyotrophic lateral s. (ALS)
 aortic valve s.
 arterial s.
 arteriocapillary s.
 arteriolar s.
 capillary s.
 coronary s. (CS)
 endocardial s.
 forme fruste of tuberous s.
 Mönckeberg s.
 multiple s.
 nodular s.
 progressive systemic s. (PSS)
 subendocardial s.
 systemic s. (SS, SSc)
 tuberous s.
 valvular s.
 vascular s.
 venous s.
Sclerosol intrapleural aerosol
sclerotherapy
 endoscopic variceal s. (EVS)
 variceal s.
sclerotic

SCN5A mutation
Scoop 1, 2 catheter
scooped pattern
scooping
> ST s.

SCOPA
> South Carolina Organ Procurement
> Agency

scope
> EBUS-TBNA s.

Scopulariopsis **pneumonia**
score
> Acute Physiology and Chronic
> Health Evaluation s.
> Agatston s.
> Aldrich ST elevation s.
> Anderson phasing s.
> Anderson-Wilkins acuteness s.
> angina index s.
> APACHE s.
> asthma severity s. (ASS)
> AW acuteness s.
> Barthel ADL s.
> Berning and Steensgaard-Hansen s.
> Birmingham Vasculitis Activity S.
> (BVAS)
> blush s.
> Brasfield chest radiograph s.
> Brush electrocardiographic s.
> calcium s.
> Califf s.
> Canadian Cardiovascular Society
> angina s. (CCSAS)
> Cardiac Infarction Injury S.
> clinical pulmonary infection s.
> (CPIS)
> coronary calcium s.
> Detsky s.
> Dripps-American Surgical
> Association s.
> Duke myocardial jeopardy s.
> Duke treadmill exercise s.
> Duke treadmill prognostic s.
> Dundee rank factor s. (DRFS)
> echo s.
> Estes s.
> Framingham risk s.
> Fugl-Meyer motor test s.
> Gensini s.
> Goldman cardiac risk index s.
> Hollenberg treadmill exercise s.
> Injury Severity S. (ISS)
> jeopardy s.
> Katz activities of daily living s.
> Ladder of Life s.
> lung injury s. (LIS)
> Mallampati s.
> mitral anular Z s.
> Murray s.

Norris s.
quantitative wall motion s.
> (QWMS)
Ramsay s.
Rivermead Motor Assessment
> Arm s.
Romhilt-Estes s.
Selvester complete 32-point QRS s.
Selvester simplified QRS s.
Shwachman s.
Simplified Acute Physiology S.
> (SAPS)
summed stress s. (SSS)
thrombolysis in myocardial
> infarction risk s.
TIMI blush s.
TIMI risk s.
total coronary s. (TCS)
transition dyspnea index focal s.
treadmill s. (TS)
VAMC prognostic s.
wall motion s.
Wilkins echocardiographic s.
Yesavage s.
Z s.

scoring
> microarousal s.
> respiratory arousal s.

scorpion venom
scotoma, pl. **scotomata**
Scot-Tussin
> S.-T. DM Cough Chasers
> S.-T. Senior Clear

scout
> s. film
> s. scan
> s. view

SCP
> smoking cessation program

SCPR
> standard cardiopulmonary resuscitation

sCRAG
> serum cryptococcal antigen

SCRAM face mask
scratch
> Means-Lerman s.

scratchy murmur
screening
> nocturnal oximetry s.
> Porvidx early lung cancer s.
> spirometric s.

screen oxygenation
screw
> afterloading s.
> percutaneous cannulated s.

screw-in
> s.-i. epicardial electrode
> s.-i. fixation

S

screw-in *(continued)*
    s.-i. lead
    s.-i. sutureless myocardial electrode
screw-on lead
screw-thread stent
scrofula
scrofulaceum
    Mycobacterium s.
scroll reentrant wave
scrub typhus
SCS
    spinal cord stimulation
    systolic click syndrome
Sculptor anuloplasty ring
scurvy
SCV-CPR
    simultaneous compression-ventilation
    CPR
SCVIR
    Society of Cardiovascular and
    Interventional Radiology
SD
    septal defect
    spreading depression
    systolic discharge
S/D
    systolic/diastolic
        Polygam S/D
SDB
    sleep-disordered breathing
SDBP
    seated diastolic blood pressure
    standing diastolic blood pressure
    supine diastolic blood pressure
SDH
    subdural hematoma
SDHD
    sudden death heart disease
SDIHD
    sudden death ischemic heart disease
SD-LDL
    small, dense, low-density lipoprotein
SDS
    stent delivery system
SDS-PAGE
    sodium dodecylsulfate polyacrylamide
    gel electrophoresis
SDS-polyacrylamide gel
SE
    spin-echo
        SE image
SEA
    side-entry access
        SEA port
sea frond
seagull
    s. bruit
    s. murmur

seal
    Asherman chest s.
    Ultimate Seal CPAP mask s.
    watertight s.
sealant
    CoSeal resorbable synthetic s.
    CoSeal surgical s.
    FloSeal Matrix hemostatic s.
    FocalSeal-L surgical s.
seal-bark cough
sealing
    collagen vascular s. (CVS)
Sealy-Laragh technique
searcher
    Allport-Babcock s.
seasonal
    s. allergic rhinitis
    s. allergy
seated diastolic blood pressure (SDBP)
Seattle Angina Questionnaire
SEB
    surrogate endpoint biomarker
Sebastiani syndrome
SEC
    spontaneous echo contrast
SECG
    stress electrocardiography
Sechrist
    S. 500A hyperbaric ventilator
    S. IV-100 infant ventilator
second
    beats per s. (BPS)
    breaths per s. (BPS)
    dyne s.'s
    forced expiratory volume in 1 s.
      (FEV_1)
    s. gas effect
    s. harmonic imaging (SHI)
    s. harmonic imaging ultrasound
      technique
    s. heart sound (S_2)
    s. messenger
    meter per s. (m/s, m/sec)
    s. mitral sound
    s. obtuse marginal (OM2)
    s. obtuse marginal artery
    oral airflow in liters per s. (V_O)
    s. positive deflection during QRS
      complex (R′)
    s. pump run
    s. through fifth shock count
    s. window of protection (SWOP)
secondary
    s. anticoagulation system (SACS)
    s. aortic area
    s. arrest (SA)
    s. asphyxia
    s. atelectasis
    s. bronchitis

s. bronchus
s. cardiomyopathy
s. chemoprophylaxis
s. dextrocardia
s. infection
s. pleurisy
s. pneumonia
s. prevention
s. pulmonary hypertension
s. pulmonary lobule
s. radiation
s. rays
s. septal hypertrophy
s. spontaneous pneumothorax
s. thrombus
s. tuberculosis
s. vasculitis
second-degree
s.-d. A-V block
s.-d. heart block
second-generation cephalosporin
secondhand smoke
second-look operation
second-phase tilt
second-stage procedure
second-wind angina
secretagogue
secretin-stimulated serum lipase (SSSL)
secretion
airway s.
altered airway s.
antidiuretic hormone s.
chloride s.
circadian s.
constitutive s.
continuous aspiration of
subglottic s.'s (CASS)
infected s.
s. mobilization
mucus s.
nasopharyngeal s.
postural drainage of infected s.
pulmonary s.
s. retention
rhamnolipid mucus s.
specialized CC-chemokine s.
subglottic s.
syndrome of inappropriate
antidiuretic hormone s. (SIADH)
secretor
gene s.
secretory
s. leukocyte protease inhibitor
(SLPI)
s. leukoprotease inhibitor (SLPI)
s. leukoprotease inhibitor protein
s. leukoproteinase inhibitor (SLPI)
s. sphingomyelinase (S-SMase)

sector
s. scan
s. scan echocardiography
s. transducer
Sectral
secundum
s. atrial septal defect (ASD2)
foramen s.
ostium s.
septum s.
secundum-type atrial septal defect
Securon SR
sedation
conscious s.
sedative administration
sedative-hypnotic drug
sedentary lifestyle
seed
iridium-192 s.
seeding
cell s.
graft s.
pumpkin-s.
Seeker guidewire
seesaw murmur
segment
abnormal ST s.
akinetic s.
anterolateral s.
anteroseptal s.
apical bronchopulmonary s.
apicoposterior bronchopulmonary s.
bronchopulmonary s.
critical closing pressure of
collapsible s. (Ptm')
depressed ST s.
downsloping ST s.
downstream s.
dyskinetic s.
dyssynergic myocardial s.
flail s.
horizontal ST s.
inferior lingular
bronchopulmonary s.
inferolateral s.
inferoseptal s.
isoelectric ST s.
lateral basal bronchopulmonary s.
s. length, septal (SLS)
s. length, systolic (SLS)
malperfused s.
midcoronary s.
PR s.
precordial ST s.
proximal s.
RST s.
ST s.
subapical s.
subsuperior s.

segment *(continued)*
  Ta s.
  TP s.
  T-P-Q s.
  TQ s.
  transmural pressure of
    collapsible s. (*P*tm)
  tunneled s.
  upsloping ST s.
  upstream s.
segmental
  s. arterial disorganization
  s. arterial Doppler study
  s. atelectasis
  s. bronchus
  s. limb pressure (SLP)
  s. limb systolic pressure (SLP)
  s. lung resection
  s. ostial pulmonary vein ablation
  s. pneumonia
  s. pressure index
  s. pulmonary vein isolation
  s. stenosis
  s. venous capacitance (SVC)
  s. venous capacitance ratio (SVCR)
  s. wall motion (SWM)
  s. wall motion analysis (SWMA)
segmentalis
  bronchus s.
segmentation
  K-space s.
  time-resolved imaging by automatic
    data s. (TRIADS)
segmentectomy
segmented
  s. extracardiac radioactive
    distribution
  s. hyalinizing vasculitis
  s. K-space approach
  s. neutrophils
  s. ring tripolar (SRT)
  s. ring tripolar lead
segmentorum
  rami bronchiales s.
  stratum s.
segmentum
  s. bronchopulmonale
  s. bronchopulmonale apicale
  s. bronchopulmonale basale anterius
  s. bronchopulmonale basale laterale
  s. bronchopulmonale basale mediale
  s. bronchopulmonale basale
    posterius
  s. bronchopulmonale lingulare
    superius
  s. bronchopulmonale posterius
  s. cardiacum
  s. subapicale
  s. subsuperius

Seguin anuloplasty ring
SEI
  subendocardial infarction
Seiler cartilage
seismic wave
seismocardiogram
seismocardiography
Seitz
  S. metamorphosing respiration
  S. sign
seizure
  autonomic s.
SELCA
  smooth excimer laser coronary
    angioplasty
Seldinger
  S. needle
  S. percutaneous technique
  S. sheath
selectin blocker
selective
  s. angiography
  s. aortic arch perfusion (SAAP)
  s. aortography
  s. arterial secretin injection test
    (SAST)
  s. arteriography
  s. cardiac catheterization
  s. chamber compression
  s. estrogen receptor modulator
    (SERM)
  s. graft opacification
  s. intracoronary thrombolysis
    (SICT)
  s. past pathway
  s. perfusion
  s. septal branch injection
  s. septal branch injection of
    ethanol
  s. shunt (SS)
  s. transvenous approach
  s. venous catheterization (SVC)
selenium
  s. compound
  s. deficiency
  s. dioxide
  s. sulfide
self-expandable metallic stent
self-expanding
  s.-e. microporous stent (SEMS)
  s.-e. nitinol stent
  s.-e. stent (SES)
  s.-e. wire mesh stent
self-guiding catheter
self-positioning balloon catheter
self-powered treadmill
self-terminating tachycardia
sella, pl. **sellae**
  foramen diaphragmatis sellae

s. nasion point A (SNA)
s. nasion point B (SNB)
Sellers
S. classification of mitral regurgitation
S. criteria
S. grade
S. mitral regurgitation classification
Sellick maneuver
Selute Picotip steroid-eluting device
Selvester
S. complete 32-point QRS score
S. simplified QRS score
SEM
scanning electron microscope
systolic ejection murmur
sematilide hydrochloride
Semb apicolysis
SEMI
subendocardial myocardial infarction
semiautomatic external defibrillator (SAED)
semidirect lead
semihorizontal heart
semiinvasive aspergillosis
semilateral supine position
semilunar
s. valve
s. valve closure
s. valve regurgitation
s. valve stenosis
seminoma
mediastinal s.
semiquantitation
semiquantitative index
semirigid catheter
semi-skeletonized
semispinal
s. muscle
s. muscle of thorax
semisynthetic penicillin
semivertical heart
Semliki Forest virus
Semmes-Weinstein monofilaments
Semon sign
Semple technique
Semprex-D
SEMS
self-expanding microporous stent
SEMT
specific expiratory muscle training
Sendai virus
SenDx 100 blood gas and electrolyte analysis system
senescent
s. aortic stenosis
s. calcification
s. heart
s. myocardium

senile
s. amyloidosis
s. arrhythmia
s. arteriosclerosis
s. cardiac calcification syndrome
s. emphysema
s. plaque
s. systemic amyloidosis (SSA)
senilis
arcus s.
circus s.
senility
Senning
S. atrial baffle repair
S. and Mustard operation
S. transposition procedure
Senning-Rastelli procedure
Sensaire handheld spirometer
sensation
elephant-on-the-chest s.
S. intraaortic balloon catheter
popping s.
pressure-like s.
thermal s.
sensing
afterpotential s.
s. circuit
far-field R-wave s.
integrated bipolar s.
rate-drop s.
s. spike
sensitivity
s. analysis
atrial s.
aureomycin s.
baroreceptor s.
baroreceptor reflex s. (BRS)
baroreflex s. (BRS)
chlortetracycline s.
digitalis s.
pacemaker s.
paracetamol s.
phenindione s.
phenylbutazone s.
sulfonamide s.
ventricular s.
sensitization
baroreceptor s.
sensitized
beryllium s. (BeS)
s. cell
sensitizer
sensitizing metal
SENSOR
Sentinel Event Notification Systems for Occupational Risk
sensor
activity s.
BioZtect s.

S

sensor *(continued)*
s. blending
blood gas s.
Capnostat CO_2 s.
catheter-based s.
ClipTip reusable s.
CritScan hematocrit s.
Dymedix sleep s.
FilterWatch s.
flat tube pressure s.
Gemini s.
ImPressure s.
infant airflow and effort s.
LNOP YI Multisite SpO_2
  reusable s.
Oxisensor II adult s.
OxyTip s.
S. pacemaker
pediatric finger clip s.
piezoelectric snore s.
piezo film s.
PLM s.
pressure transducer airflow s.
PressureWire3 s.
PressureWire5 s.
S. PTFE-nitinol guidewire with
  hydrophilic tip
Pulsar Max s.
SpiroSense flow s.
VTI oxygen monitor with
  disposable polarographic oxygen s.
sensor-driven response
sensorimotor
s. cortex (SMC)
s. stroke
sensorium, pl. **sensoria**, pl. **sensoriums**
clouded s.
SensorMedics
S. generator
S. mass flow sensor heated wire
  flowmeter
S. 2900 metabolic cart
S. SAT-TRAK pulse oximeter
S. ventilator
sensory
s. cross-checking
s. nerve
s. nerve action potential (SNAP)
s. nerve conduction velocity
  (SNCV)
Sentinal seal pleural drainage unit
sentinel
S. Event Notification Systems for
  Occupational Risk (SENSOR)
S. ICD device
S. 2010 implantable cardioverter-
  defibrillator
s. node
S. self-expanding stent

**Sentry antimicrobial surveillance
  program**
SEP
systolic ejection period
separation
aortic cusp s.
E point to septal s. (EPSS)
maximum aortic cusp s. (MACS)
Sephadex G24 chromatography
Sepracoat coating solution
Sepracor
SEPS
subfascial endoscopic perforator surgery
sepsis
alcoholism, leukopenia,
  pneumococcal s. (ALPS)
Capnocytophaga canimorsus s.
endotoxic s.
line s.
**sepsis-related organ failure assessment
  (SOFA)**
septa (*pl. of* septum)
septal
s. ablation
s. akinesia
s. annuloplasty
s. arcade
s. artery embolization
s. cell
s. collateral
s. defect (SD)
s. dip
s. dropout
s. hyperperfusion
s. hyperperfusion on thallium scan
s. hypertrophy
s. hypoperfusion
s. isthmus
s. line
s. myectomy
s. myotomy
s. occluder
s. pathway
s. perforating artery
s. perforation
s. perforator
s. perforator branch
s. resection
segment length, s. (SLS)
s. thickening
s. wall motion
septation
conotruncal s.
s. of heart
s. procedure
septectomy
atrial s.
Blalock-Hanlon atrial s.
Edwards s.

septi
septic
    s. edema
    s. embolization
    s. endocarditis
    s. fever
    s. pneumonia
    s. pulmonary edema (SPE)
    s. shock
    s. thromboembolism
septicemia
    anthrax s.
    s. sputum
Septi-Check mycobacteria culture system
septicum
    Clostridium s.
septomarginalis
    trabecula s.
septoplasty
    balloon atrial s.
    bedside balloon atrial s.
    Brockenbrough atrial s.
septostomy
    atrial balloon s.
    balloon s.
    balloon atrial s. (BAS)
    blade atrial s.
    Mullins blade and balloon s.
    Park blade s.
    Rashkind balloon atrial s.
Septra DS
septum, pl. **septa (S)**
    alveolar s.
    aneurysm of atrial s. (AAS)
    aneurysm of ventricular portion of
      membranous s.
    atrial s. (AS)
    basal interventricular s.
    conal s.
    deranged fibrotic septa
    interalveolar septa
    interatrial s. (IAS)
    interpulmonary s.
    interventricular s. (IVS)
    left s. (LS)
    s. linguae
    s. mediastinale
    membranous s.
    s. pellucidum
    s. primum
    right s. (RS)
    s. secundum
    sigmoid s.
    s. spurium
    Swiss cheese interventricular s.
    tissue septa
    ventricular s. (VS)
sequela, pl. **sequelae**
Sequel compression system

sequence
    activation s.
    anaplerotic s.
    cine s.
    2D gradient-echo s.
    DiGeorge s. (DGS)
    direct mapping s.
    3D segmented-FLASH imaging s.
    3D time-of-flight magnetic
      resonance angiographic s.
    FLASH s.'s
    immunostimulatory s. (ISS)
    interrater s.
    intraatrial activation s.
    intracardiac atrial activation s.
    inversion spin-echo pulse s. (ISE)
    Kozak s.
    missed ostium s. (MOS)
    respiratory gated 3-dimensional
      gradient-echo s.
    spin-echo imaging s.
sequencing
    DNA s.
sequential
    s. atrioventricular (SAV)
    s. compression device (SCD)
    s. dilation
    s. grafting
    s. organ failure assessment (SOFA)
    s. pacing
    s. vascular response (SVR)
    s. ventriculoatrial (SVA)
sequestrant
    bile acid s.
    low-dose bile-acid s.
Sequestra 1000 system
sequestration
    s. bronchopneumonia
    bronchopulmonary s.
    pulmonary s. (PS)
sequestrectomy
Sequicor III pacemaker
sequoisis
SER
    systolic ejection rate
sera (*pl. of* serum)
Serafini hernia
seratrodast
Seretide
Serevent Diskus
serial
    s. autocorrelation
    s. autocorrelation data acquisition
      technology
    s. blood gas
    s. change
    s. cut films
    s. dilation
    s. ECG tracing

S

serial *(continued)*
    s. electrocardiogram tracing
    s. enzyme determination
    s. impedance plethysmography
    s. thrombin time (STT)
series
    800 s. blood gas and critical analyte system
    s. elastic element
    S. 7900 mouth breathing face mask
    S. 8900 nasal and mouth breathing face mask
serine
    s. elastase inhibitor
    s. kinase
    s. protease inhibitor
serious cardiac event (SCE)
SERM
    selective estrogen receptor modulator
seroconversion
serofibrinous
    s. pericarditis
    s. pleurisy
serological test
Seroma-Cath catheter
Seromycin Pulvules
seronegative
    CMV s.
    s. spondyloarthropathy
seropneumothorax
seropositive
    CMV s.
    HIV s.
    s. nonsyphilitic pneumopathy
serosanguineous effusion
serosum
    pericardium s.
serothorax
serotonin
serotype
    M-protein s.
serotyping
serous
    s. effusion
    s. membrane
    s. pericarditis
    s. pleurisy
serpentina
    Rauwolfia s.
serpentine aneurysm
serpiginosum
    angioma s.
serpiginous
Serpula lacrymans
Serralnyl suture
Serralsilk suture

serrated catheter
Serratia
    S. liquefaciens
    S. marcescens
    S. pneumonia
serraticus
    stridor s.
serratus anterior muscle
sertraline hydrochloride
serum, pl. **sera**
    s. albumin
    s. amylase
    s. amyloid type A (SAA)
    antilymphocyte s.
    s. autoantibody
    s. bactericidal titer (SBT)
    brain-heart infusion and rabbit s. (BHIRS)
    s. cholesterol
    s. creatine kinase
    s. cryptococcal antigen (sCRAG)
    s. eosinophilic cationic protein
    ERIG s.
    s. glutamic-oxaloacetic transaminase (SGOT)
    s. glutamic-pyruvic transaminase (SGPT)
    s. IgE
    s. immunoreactive trypsinogen
    s. iron
    s. KL-6
    s. lipid level
    s. lipid profile
    s. magnesium
    s. marker
    s. myoglobin
    s. neopterin
    s. pneumoprotein
    s. precipitin testing
    s. prothrombin conversion accelerator (SPCA)
    s. renin level
    s. reserve cholesterol binding capacity (SRCBC)
    s. retinol
    s. shock
    s. sickness
    s. thrombotic accelerator (STA)
    s. thromboxane
    s. triglyceride
service
    Centers for Medicare and Medicaid S.'s (CMS)
    National Health S. (NHS)
    Older Americans Resources and s.'s (OARS)
    vascular access s. (VAS)

Servo
    S. Screen 390 ventilator monitoring device
    S. Ventilator 300
servocontrolled plethysmography
SES
    self-expanding stent
    sirolimus-eluting stent
sesquioxide
    germanium s.
sestamibi
    s. gated SPECT
    s. perfusion imaging
    s. scan
    ^{99m}Tc s.
    s. technetium-99m SPECT with dipyridamole stress test
    thallium-201 s.
    ^{201}Tl s.
SET
    shredding embolectomy thrombectomy
    SET carbon monoxide pulse oximeter
    SET catheter
set
    Acland-Banis arteriotomy s.
    Arrow Hi-flow infusion s.
    Borst side-arm introducer s.
    Dotter intravascular retrieval s.
    Elliptosphere cardiac catheter s.
    Flexor Check-Flo introducer s.
    Masimo S.
    Medtronic Attain guide catheter s.
    Micropuncture introducer s.
    minimum data s. (MDS)
    multi-sideport catheter infusion s.
    Neff percutaneous access s.
    Neo-Sert umbilical vessel catheter insertion s.
    Peel-Away introducer s.
    Quest Medical MPS delivery s.
    Shuttle-SL Flexor Tuohy Borst side-arm introducer s.
    Tissomat application device and spray s.
    U-Mid-O_2 Jet S.
    Wylie endarterectomy s.
SetPoint endovascular temperature cooling system
setting
    high s.
    low s.
severe
    s. acute respiratory syndrome (SARS)
    s. acute respiratory syndrome-associated coronavirus (SARS-CoV)
    s. refractory neurocardiogenic syncope
Severinghaus electrode
severity
    stenosis s.
sevoflurane
Sewall technique
sewing
    s. ring
    s. ring area (SRA)
    s. ring loop
sew-on electrode
sex
    s. ratio
    s. steroid
sexual
    s. angina
    s. asthma
    s. syncope
SF
    shunt flow
    spontaneous fibrillation
    SF wave of cardiac apex pulse
SF-36
    Short-Form 36
    SF-36 Health Survey
SF_6
    sulfur hexafluoride
SFA
    saturated fatty acid
    subclavian flap aortoplasty
    superficial femoral artery
    superior femoral artery
SFHb
    pyridoxalated stroma-free hemoglobin
    stroma-free hemoglobin pyridoxalated
SFP
    stopped flow pressure
SFR
    stenotic flow reserve
SFTP
    solitary fibrous tumor of pleura
SG
    stent graft
Sgarbossa criteria
SGOT
    serum glutamic-oxaloacetic transaminase
SGPT
    serum glutamic-pyruvic transaminase
SGRQ
    St. George Respiratory Questionnaire
SGS
    stroke guidance system
SH
    spontaneously hypertensive
    standard heparin
shadow
    acoustic s.
    S. balloon

S

shadow *(continued)*
> bat wing s.
> butterfly s.
> cardiac s.
> liver s.
> mediastinal s.
> S. over-the-wire balloon catheter
> ring s.
> snowstorm s.
> summation s.
> tubular s.

shadow-free laryngoscope
shadowing
> acoustic s.

shaggy pericardium
Shaher-Puddu classification
shake test
shaking sound
shale pneumoconiosis
shallow
> s. breathing
> s. pathologic Q wave
> s. respiration
> s. T wave inversion
> s. water blackout

shallow-water blackout syndrome
shape
> echo-signal s.
> Omni Flush s.
> spheroid left ventricular s.

shaping behavioral technique
Shapshay-Healy laryngoscope
shared isthmus
sharing
> United Network for Organ S.
> (UNOS)

Shaver disease
SHD
> structural heart disease
> sudden heart death

shear
> atrial s.
> s. force
> s. rate of blood
> s. stress
> s. thinning

shears
> Bethune-Coryllos s.
> Coryllos-Bethune rib s.
> Coryllos-Shoemaker rib s.
> Duval-Coryllos rib s.
> Frey-Sauerbruch rib s.
> Giertz-Shoemaker rib s.
> Gluck rib s.
> rib s.
> Shoemaker rib s.

sheath
> Ansel Flexor introducer s.
> armed long s.

> Arrow s.
> arterial s.
> blue Cook s.
> Brite Tip s.
> cardiogenic s.
> carotid s.
> chronic s.
> compensated s.
> Cordis Bioptome s.
> Daig s.
> Desilets-Hoffman s.
> s. and dilator system
> excimer s.
> Fast-Cath s.
> femoral venous s.
> French s.
> 7-F Shuttle s.
> Hemaflex PTCA s.
> Hemaquet introducer s.
> Hemaquet PTCA s.
> hemostatic s.
> introducer s.
> Introducer II s.
> Klein transseptal introducer s.
> Mullins transseptal catheterization s.
> peel-away s.
> percutaneous brachial s.
> peribronchial s.
> perivascular s.
> Pinnacle introducer s.
> SafeSheath CSG introducer s.
> Seldinger s.
> short monorail polyethylene
> imaging s.
> Shuttle s.
> SL1 s.
> sonolucent distal imaging s.
> Spectranetics laser s. (SLS)
> St. Jude s.
> subclavian peel-away s.
> Super ArrowFlex catheterization s.
> Teflon s.
> Terumo Pinnacle s.
> transseptal s.
> vascular s.
> venous s.
> X-Sept transseptal s.

sheath-based IVUS catheter
sheath/dilator
> Mullins s./d.

sheathing
> halo s.

Sheehan and Dodge technique
Sheen airway reconstruction
sheep
> s. antidigoxin Fab antibody
> s. blowfly asthma

sheepskin boot

sheet
    cellular s.
    chest pain order s. (CPOS)
    mucous s.'s
    s. sign
Sheffield
    S. exercise stress test
    S. modification of Bruce treadmill protocol
    S. Screening Test for Acquired Language Disorders (STALD)
    S. treadmill protocol
Shekelton aneurysm
shelf
    apical s.
    s. of plaque
shell
    chest s.
shellfish asthma
shelving edge
Shenstone tourniquet
shepherd's crook deformity
Sherpa guiding catheter
SHF
    systolic heart failure
SHI
    second harmonic imaging
    SHI ultrasound technique
Shibley sign
shield
    Cath-Gard catheter contamination s.
    chest s.
    face s.
    probe s.
shift
    antigenic s.
    axis s.
    baseline s.
    chloride s.
    Doppler s.
    fluid s.
    mediastinal s.
    midline s.
    plaque s.
shifter
    frequency s.
shifting
    isovolume s.
    s. pacemaker
Shigella
shiitake mushroom extract
Shiley
    S. catheter
    S. convexoconcave heart valve
    S. decannulation plug
    S. Phonate speaking valve
    S. tracheostomy tube
Shimadzu
    S. cardiac ultrasound

    S. DAR-2400 coronary arteriographic analyzer
Shimazaki area-length method
shiner
    allergic s.
Shinobi
    S. steerable guidewire
    S. wire
SHJL4 catheter
SHJR4 catheter
SHJR4s
    side-hole Judkins curve right 4 short SHJR4s catheter
shock
    atrial defibrillation s.
    biphasic s.
    s. blocks
    burst s.
    cardiac output s.
    cardiogenic s. (CGS, CS)
    chronic s.
    circulatory s.
    compensated s.
    s. count
    DC electric s.
    declamping s.
    decompensated s.
    defibrillation s.
    diastolic s.
    direct current electric s.
    distributive s.
    double external direct current s.
    electrocardiac s.
    endotoxin s.
    hemodynamic s.
    high-energy defibrillation s.
    high-energy transthoracic s.
    hyperdynamic septic s.
    hypovolemic s.
    s. index
    infarction with S.
    insulin s.
    irreversible s.
    low-energy s.
    s. lung
    obstructive s.
    occult cardiogenic s.
    oligemic s.
    s. pacing
    pleural s.
    s. position
    postcardiotomy s.
    QRS synchronous atrial defibrillation s.'s
    rectilinear biphasic s.
    refractory s.
    rescue s.
    septic s.
    serum s.

S

shock *(continued)*
    synchronized s.
    systolic s.
    s. therapy
    toxic s.
    transthoracic s.
    T-wave s.
    vasodilatory s.
    vasogenic s.
    s. waveform
1-shock
    1-s. defibrillation
    1-s. protocol
3-shock
    3-s. defibrillation
    3-s. protocol
shocky
shoddy fever
Shoemaker rib shears
shone
    S. anomaly
    S. complex
    S. syndrome
short
    s. axis (SAX)
    s. coupling interval
    s. monorail imaging catheter
    s. monorail polyethylene imaging
      sheath
    side-hole Judkins curve right 4 s.
      (SHJR4s)
    s. stent
    s. Taper
    s. transitional edge protection
      (STEP)
short-axis
    s.-a. image
    s.-a. mitral valve (SAX-MV)
    s.-a. parasternal view
    s.-a. plane
    s.-a. plane mitral valve
    s.-a. plane, papillary muscle (SAX-
      PM)
    s.-a. slice
    s.-a. tomogram
shortening
    circumferential fiber s.
    endocardial s.
    fiber s.
    s. fraction
    fractional myocardial s.
    long-axis fractional s. (LAFS)
    midwall s.
    myocardial fiber s.
    pathologic postsystolic s.
    postsystolic s.
    s. of PR interval
    telomeric s.
    s. velocity

    velocity of circumferential fiber s.
      (VCF)
    ventricular wall s.
Short-Form
    S.-F. 36 (SF-36)
    S.-F. 36 Health Survey
shorthand rule
short-long-short cycle
shortness
    s. of breath (SB, SOB)
    s. of breath on exertion (SBE,
      SOBOE)
short-term
    flow-assisted s.-t. (FAST)
short-winded
sho-seiryu-to granule
Shoshin disease
shot
    fast low-angle s. (FLASH)
    pocket s.
    sinus s.
shotgunning
shotty node
shoulder
    s. horizontal flexion
    s. rotation
shoulder-hand syndrome
shoulder-strap resonance
shovel mask
shower
    embolic s.
Shprintzen syndrome
shredding
    s. embolectomy thrombectomy
      (SET)
    s. embolectomy thrombectomy
      catheter
shrinkage
    arterial s.
shrinker
    Juzo s.
shrinking lung syndrome (SLS)
SHU-454 contrast medium
shudder
    carotid s.
shunt
    Allen-Brown s.
    AnastaFlo s.
    aorta to pulmonary artery s.
    aortofemoral artery s.
    aortopulmonary s.
    arteriovenous s. (AVS)
    ascending aorta to pulmonary
      artery s.
    atrial ventricular s.
    atriopulmonary s.
    A-V s.
    balloon s.
    bidirectional cavopulmonary s.

Blalock-Taussig s. (BTS)
BT s.
Buselmeier s.
cardiac s.
carotid artery s.
cavocaval s.
cavopulmonary s.
Cimino arteriovenous s.
ClearView intracoronary s.
ClearView intravascular
  arteriotomy s.
coronary anastomotic s.
s. cyanosis
Denver pleural effusion s.
s. detection
distal splenorenal s.
Drapanas mesocaval s.
emergency portocaval s. (EPCS)
extracardiac s.
Flo-Thru intraluminal s.
s. flow (SF)
Glenn s.
Gore-Tex s.
Gott s.
interarterial s.
intracardiac s.
intrapulmonary s.
Javid s.
s. leak
left-to-right s.
LeVeen peritoneovenous s.
Marion-Clatworthy side-to-end vena
  caval s.
mesoatrial s. (MAS)
mesocaval s.
modified Blalock-Taussig s.
  (MBTS)
parallel s.
s. pathway
persistent s.
pleural effusion s.
pleuroperitoneal s.
portacaval s. (PCS)
portopulmonary s.
Potts s.
s. pressure (SP)
s. procedure (SP)
Pruitt-Inahara carotid s.
pulmonary s.
s. quantification
Quinton-Scribner s.
s. ratio
residual s.
reversed s.
right-to-left s. (RLS, RLSh)
selective s. (SS)
side-to-side portacaval s. (SSPS)
splenorenal s.
Sundt carotid endarterectomy s.

systemic to pulmonary s.
Thomas s.
total cavopulmonary s. (TCPS)
transjugular intrahepatic
  portosystemic s. (TIPS)
Uresil Vascu-Flo carotid s.
USCI s.
Vascu-Flo carotid s.
ventriculoatrial s. (VAS)
Waterston s.
Waterston-Cooley pulmonary
  artery s.

shunt-dependent lesion
shunted
  s. blood
  s. blood to total blood flow
  (Qs/Qt)
shunting
  s. circuit
  interatrial s. (IAS)
  intraatrial s.
  intrapulmonary s.
  pleuroperitoneal s.
  venoarterial s.
shuttle
  7-F S. sheath
  S. sheath
  s. test
  s. test walk
shuttlemaker's disease
Shuttle-SL Flexor Tuohy Borst side-arm
  introducer set
Shwachman
  S. score
  S. score of clinical well-being
  S. syndrome
Shy-Drager syndrome
SI
  stroke index
Si
  silicon
  Si Carbide
SIAD
  syndrome of inappropriate antidiuresis
SIADH
  syndrome of inappropriate antidiuretic
  hormone
  syndrome of inappropriate antidiuretic
  hormone secretion
sialic acid
sialoprotein
  bone s.
SIBD
  silent ischemic brain damage
sibilance
sibilant
  s. rale
  s. rhonchus

S

Sibson
> S. aponeurosis
> S. notch
> S. vestibule

sibutramine

SIBVI
> systemic ischemic branch vessel involvement

sICAM
> soluble intracellular adhesion molecule

Sicar sign

sicca
> bronchiectasia s.
> bronchitis s.
> laryngitis s.
> pericarditis s.
> pharyngitis s.
> s. syndrome

SICH
> spontaneous intracerebral hemorrhage

Sicilian Gambit formulation

sick
> s. building syndrome (SBS)
> s. sinus syndrome (SSS)

sickle
> s. cell anemia
> s. cell crisis
> s. cell disease
> s. cell hemoglobinopathy
> s. cell thalassemia
> s. cell trait

Sickledex test

sicklemia

sickling

sickness
> acute mountain s. (AMS)
> African sleeping s.
> altitude s.
> cardiopulmonary decompression s. (the chokes)
> cave s.
> compressed-air s.
> decompression s. (DCS)
> S. Impact Profile (SIP)
> S. Impact Profile questionnaire
> S. Impact Profile scale
> mountain s.
> serum s.
> sleeping s.

SICOR recording system

SICT
> selective intracoronary thrombolysis

SICU
> surgical intensive care unit

side
> s. branch
> s. lobe
> s. lobe artifact
> s. stretching

side-arm
> s.-a. adapter
> s.-a. pressure port

side-biting clamp

side-branch
> s.-b. compromise
> s.-b. occlusion
> s.-b. stenting

side-entry access (SEA)

side-hole
> s.-h. Judkins curve right 4
> s.-h. Judkins curve right 4 short (SHJR4s)

sideport

Sideris
> S. adjustable buttoned device
> S. clamp

sideropenic dysphagia

siderophage

siderophore

siderosis
> welder's s.

siderotica
> pneumoconiosis s.

sidestream
> s. $ETCO_2$
> S. high-efficiency nebulizer
> s. smoke (SS)

side-to-side portacaval shunt (SSPS)

sidewinder percutaneous intra-aortic balloon catheter

SIDS
> sudden infant death syndrome

Siemens
> S. biplane Neurostar digital subtraction angiography system
> S. Evolution electron beam CT
> S. Magnetom 1.5-T MRI
> S. open heart table
> S. Orbiter gamma camera
> S. pacemaker
> S. SI 400 ultrasound
> S. Somatom DR CT scanner
> S. Somatom Plus 4A scanner
> S. Sonoline CD echograph
> S. ventilator

Siemens-Elema
> S.-E. AB pulse transducer probe
> S.-E. AG bicycle ergometer
> S.-E. pacemaker

SIESTA
> snooze-induced excitation of sympathetic triggered activity

sieve
> Mobin-Uddin s.

Sievers model 280 nitric oxide analyzer

sievert (Sv)

sigh
  s. function
  s. period
sighing
  s. dyspnea
  s. respiration
sigma
  S. II Dualplace hyperbaric oxygen therapy system
  S. I monoplace hyperbaric therapy system
  S. method
  S. Plus monoplace hyperbaric oxygen therapy system
  unipolar Pisces S.
sigmoid septum
sign
  Abrahams s.
  ace of spades s.
  air bronchogram s.
  air crescent s.
  antler s.
  applesauce s.
  Aschner s.
  atrioseptal s.
  Auenbrugger s.
  Aufrecht s.
  auscultatory s.
  Baccelli s.
  bagpipe s.
  Bamberger s.
  Bamberger-Pins-Ewart s.
  Bard s.
  B6 bronchus s.
  Béhier-Hardy s.
  bent bronchus s.
  Bethea s.
  Biermer s.
  Biot s.
  Bird s.
  black pleura s.
  Bouillaud s.
  Boyce s.
  Bozzolo s.
  Branham s.
  Braunwald s.
  bread-and-butter textbook s.
  breathing bag s.
  Broadbent inverted s.
  Brockenbrough s.
  Brockenbrough-Braunwald s.
  Brockenbrough-Braunwald-Morrow s.
  bronchial meniscus s.
  calcium s.
  Carabello s.
  Cardarelli s.
  cardiorespiratory s.
  Carvallo s.
  Castellino s.
  cavitation s.
  Cegka s.
  Charcot s.
  Cheyne-Stokes s.
  Chvostek s.
  clenched fist s.
  comet tail s.
  cooing s.
  Corrigan s.
  crescent s.
  Cruveilhier s.
  Cruveilhier-Baumgarten s.
  cuff s.
  D'Amato s.
  Davis s.
  deep sulcus s.
  Delbet s.
  Delmege s.
  Demarquay s.
  de Musset s. (aortic aneurysm)
  de Mussy s. (pleurisy)
  d'Espine s.
  Dew s.
  Dieuaide s.
  Dorendorf s.
  double-lumen s.
  doughnut s.
  dropped lung s.
  Drummond s.
  Duchenne s.
  Duroziez s.
  E s.
  Ebstein s.
  Ellis s.
  epicardial fat pad s.
  Erni s.
  Ewart s.
  Ewing s.
  Faget s.
  failing lung s.
  fallen lung s.
  Federici s.
  Fischer s.
  fissure s.
  flying W s.
  Friedreich s.
  Glasgow s.
  gloved finger s.
  Golden S s.
  Gowers s.
  Grancher s.
  Greene s.
  Griesinger s.
  Grocco s.
  Grossman s.
  Gunn crossing s.
  Hall s.
  halo s.
  Hamman s.

S

673

sign *(continued)*

    Heim-Kreysig s.
    Heimlich s.
    Hill s.
    hilum convergence s.
    hilum overlay s.
    Homans s.
    Hoover s.
    Hope s.
    Horner s.
    hot nose s.
    Huchard s.
    hyperdense middle cerebral artery s. (HMCAS)
    inferior triangle s.
    intrapericardial s.
    intravascular fetal air s.
    Jaccoud s.
    Jackson s.
    Karplus s.
    Kellock s.
    knuckle s.
    Korányi s.
    Kreysig s.
    Kussmaul s.
    Laënnec s.
    Lancisi s.
    Landolfi s.
    Levine s.
    Liebermeister s.
    Litten diaphragm s.
    Livierato s.
    Lombardi s.
    Löwenberg cuff s.
    Macewen s.
    Mahler s.
    Mannkopf s.
    McCort s.
    McGinn-White s.
    s. mechanism for ventilator breathing
    Meltzer s.
    meniscus s.
    Mercedes-Benz s.
    Moschcowitz s.
    Mt. Fuji s.
    Müller s.
    Murat s.
    Musset s.
    mute toe s.'s
    Nicoladoni s.
    Nicoladoni-Branham s.
    Oliver s.
    open bronchus s.
    Osler s.
    pad s.
    patent bronchus s.
    pearl s.
    Pérez s.

    Pins s.
    pleural meniscus s.
    plumb-line s.
    Porter s.
    Potain s.
    Pottenger s.
    Prevel s.
    Prussian helmet s.
    pulmonary meniscus s.
    pulmonary notch s.
    pulmonary target s.
    Queckenstedt s.
    Quénu-Muret s.
    Quincke s.
    rabbit ear s.
    railroad track s.
    Ramond s.
    Raynaud s.
    reversed 3 s.
    ring s.
    Rivero-Carvallo s.
    Riviere s.
    Robertson s.
    Romãna s.
    Rotch s.
    Rothschild s.
    Sam Levine s.
    Sansom s.
    Schapiro s.
    Schepelmann s.
    Schick s.
    scimitar s.
    Seitz s.
    Semon s.
    sheet s.
    Shibley s.
    Sicar s.
    silhouette s.
    Skoda s.
    Smith s.
    snake-tongue s.
    snowman s.
    square root s.
    steeple s.
    Steinberg thumb s.
    Sterles s.
    Sternberg s.
    stretched bronchus s.
    string s.
    stripe s.
    superior triangle s.
    T s.
    tail s.
    tenting s.
    thumbprint bronchus s.
    tilt vital s.'s
    trapezius ridge s.
    Traube s.
    Trimadeau s.

tripod s.
Troisier s.
Trunecek s.
Unschuld s.
vital s.'s
Walker-Murdoch wrist s.
water lily s.
Weill s.
Wenckebach s.
Westermark s.
Williams s.
Williamson s.
windsock s.
Wintrich s.

Signa
S. EXCITE 3.0T MRI system
S. Pad

signal
s. amplitude
s. averaging
blood-borne s.
cardiac s.
Doppler s.
electrical s.
gating s.
high-intensity transient s. (HITS)
hyperintense heterogeneous s.
intracranial microembolic s.
isointense heterogeneous s.
s. loss
low-amplitude cardiac s.
magnetic resonance s.
microembolic s. (MES)
mosaic jet s.'s
navigator echo s.
nonexcitatory s.
oscillometric s.
PAT s.
preconditioning s.
s. processing
retrograde s.
spin echo s.
terminal filtered QRS s.
s. transducer and activator of transcription (Stat)
s. transducer and activator of transcription protein family
ventricular far-field s.

signal-averaged
s.-a. echocardiogram
s.-a. echocardiography
s.-a. electrocardiogram (SAECG)
s.-a. electrocardiography (SAECG)
s.-a. P-wave duration (SAPD)

signaling
autocrine s.
integrin s.
myocardial adrenergic s.
outside-in s.

paracrine s.
transmembrane s.
signal-loss cloud
signal-to-noise ratio
signal-void jet
signet-ring cell carcinoma
Sigvaris compression stockings
Silafed Syrup
Silastic
S. catheter
S. electrode casing
S. patch
S. poppet
S. strain gauge
S. tape
sildenafil citrate
Sildicon-E
silence
ECG s.
silent
s. angina
s. brain infarction (SBI)
s. cerebral infarct (SCI)
s. cerebral infarction (SCI)
s. coronary artery fistula
s. electrode
s. embolism
s. gap
s. ischemic brain damage (SIBD)
s. mitral regurgitation
s. mitral stenosis
s. myocardial infarction (SMI)
s. myocardial ischemia
S. Night diagnostic and screening device
S. Nite external nasal dilator
s. pericardial effusion
s. postnasal drip
s. stroke
s. trace leak
silhouette
cardiac s.
cardiomediastinal s.
egg-on-a-string s.
immediate s.
late s.
s. sign
s. sign of Felson
silica
amorphous s.
s. tetrahedral crystal
silicatosis
silicoanthracosis
silicon (Si)
silicone
s. embolism syndrome
free liquid s.
s. lead

silicone *(continued)*
    s. stent
    s. suture hole
silicoproteinosis
silicosis
    accelerated s.
    acute s.
    chronic s.
silicotic pneumoconiosis
silicotuberculosis
silk guidewire
silo
    s. filler's disease
    s. filler's lung
Silphen
    S. Cough
    S. DM
Siltussin DM
silver (Ag)
    s. bead electrode
    s. finisher's lung
    Grocott methenamine s.
    s. polisher's lung
    S. Speed hydrophilic guidewire
    s. sulfadiazine
    S. syndrome
SilverHawk
    S. plaque excision system
    S. System plaque excision device
Silverman-Lilly pneumotachograph
silver-methenamine stain
silver-silver chloride electrode
Silverstein stimulator probe
silver-wire effect
silver-wiring of retinal artery
Silvester method
SIMA
    single internal mammary artery
simiae
    Mycobacterium s.
simian virus 40 (SV40)
Simmons II, III catheter
Simmons-type sidewinder catheter
Simon
    S. foci
    S. nitinol inferior vena cava filter
    S. nitinol IVC filter
Simplate
    S. bleeding time
    S. procedure
simple chronic bronchitis
simplex
    angina s.
    carcinoma s.
    herpes s.
Simplicity Spirometer
Simplified Acute Physiology Score (SAPS)
Simplify D-dimer

Simpson
    S. atherectomy catheter
    S. AtheroCath catheter
    S. AtheroCath system
    S. modified method
    S. peripheral AtheroCath
    S. PET balloon
    S. positron emission tomography balloon
    S. rule
    S. rule for ventricular volume
Simpson-Golabi-Behmel syndrome
Simpson-Robert
    S.-R. catheter
    S.-R. vascular dilation system
Simron
SIMT
    specific inspiratory muscle training
simulator
Simulect
simultaneous
    s. bilateral spontaneous pneumothorax (SBSP)
    s. catheter mapping
    s. compression-ventilation CPR (SCV-CPR)
    s. kissing stent (SKS)
simultaneously stapled pneumonectomy (SSP)
SIMV
    synchronized intermittent mandatory ventilation
simvastatin
Sindbis virus
sine
    s. wave
    s. wave pattern
sinensis
    Clonorchis s.
Sinequan
Sinex Long-Acting
singer's node
Singh-Vaughan-Williams arrhythmia classification
single
    s. atrium
    s. breathhold cardiac-synchronized angiography
    s. chain urokinase-type plasminogen activator
    s. coronary artery bypass graft (SCABG)
    s. extrastimulus
    s. internal mammary artery (SIMA)
    s. internal thoracic artery (SITA)
    s. lumen
    s. papillary muscle syndrome
    s. pleurisy
    s. premature atrial beat

s. premature extrastimulation
s. ventricle
s. ventricle malposition

single-balloon
s.-b. valvoplasty
s.-b. valvotomy

single-breath
s.-b. carbon monoxide test
s.-b. diffusion
s.-b. nitrogen curve
s.-b. nitrogen elimination
s.-b. nitrogen washout test
s.-b. wash-in phase

single-chamber
s.-c. cardiac pacing system
s.-c. pulse generator
s.-c. rate-responsive
s.-c., rate-responsive pacemaker

single-crystal gamma camera
single-dilator technique
single-disc prosthesis
single-gene disorder
single-lung transplant (SLT)
single-nucleotide polymorphism (SNP)
single-pass lead
single-patient use manometer
single-photon
s.-p. detection
s.-p. emission
s.-p. emission computed
tomographic imaging
s.-p. emission computed
tomography (SPECT)
s.-p. emission tomography (SPET)
s.-p. emission tomography imaging
s.-p. gamma scintigraphy

single-plane aortography
single-stage exercise stress test
Singleton-Merten syndrome
single-ventricle physiology
single-vessel
s.-v. coronary stenosis
s.-v. disease (SVD)

Singulair
singultus
sinister
bronchus principalis s.
pulmo s.

sinistra
arteria pulmonalis s.
vena obliqua atrii s.
vena pulmonalis inferior s.
vena pulmonalis superior s.

sinistrae
rami esophageales arteriae
gastricae s.

sinistri
incisura cardiaca pulmonis s.
lingula pulmonis s.

sinistrocardia
sinistrum
atrium cordis s.
cor triatriatum s.

Sin Nombre virus (SNV)
sinoaortic
s. baroreflex activity
s. denervation (SAD)

sinoatrial (*var. of* sinuatrial)
sinoauricular
s. block
s. node (SAN)

sinobronchial syndrome
sinobronchitis
sinogram
sinopulmonary
sinospiral fiber
sinotubular junction
sinoventricular
s. conduction
s. tachycardia (SVT)

Sintrom
sinuatrial, sinoatrial (SA, S-A)
s. arrest
s. ball
s. baroreflex
s. block (SAB)
s. bradycardia
s. conduction time (SACT)
s. entrance block (SAEB)
s. exit block
s. nodal artery
s. nodal reentry
s. node (SAN, SN)
s. node dysfunction
s. node weakness syndrome
(SANWS)
s. recovery time (SART)

sinuatrialis
nodus s.
nonreset nodus s.
reset nodus s.

sinus
aortic s.
s. arrest (SA)
s. arrhythmia (SA)
basilar s.
s. bradyarrhythmia
s. bradycardia (SB)
carotid s.
s. catarrh
cavernous s. (CS)
s. coronarius
coronary s. (CS)
costophrenic s.
s. cycle length (SCL)
distal coronary s. (DCS)
s. exit block
s. exit pause

S

sinus *(continued)*
    left coronary s. (LCS)
    s. mechanism
    s. nodal automaticity
    s. nodal reentrant tachycardia
    s. nodal reentry
    s. node (SN)
    s. node artery
    s. node/AV conduction abnormality
    s. node cycle length (SNCL)
    s. node disease
    s. node dysfunction (SND)
    s. node electrogram (SNE)
    s. node formation (SNF)
    s. node function
    s. node potential (SNP)
    s. node recovery time (SNRT, SRT)
    s. node recovery time, direct measuring (SNRTd)
    s. node recovery time, indirect measuring (SNRTi)
    s. node reset
    noncoronary s.
    oblique s.
    ostium of coronary s. (CSO)
    Petit s.
    phrenicocostal s.
    piriform s.
    pleural s.
    proximal coronary s. (PCS)
    pulmonary s.
    s. reflex
    s. rhythm (SR)
    s. rhythm mapping
    right coronary s. (RCS)
    s. shot
    s. standstill
    superior sagittal s. (SSS)
    s. tachycardia (ST)
    s. thrombosis
    transverse s. (TS)
    transverse/sigmoid s. (TS/SS)
    s. trunci pulmonalis
    unroofed coronary s.
    Valsalva s.
    s. of Valsalva
    s. of Valsalva aneurysm
    s. of Valsalva aortography
    s. venosus
    s. venosus atrial septal defect
    s. x-ray
SinuScope system
sinusitis
    irritant s.
    postnasal drip due to s. (PND-Si)
sinusoid
    intramyocardial s.
    myocardial s.

sinusoidal strut pattern
SIP
    Sickness Impact Profile
        SIP scale
siphon
    carotid s.
Siri equation
Sirius red stain
sirolimus-coated stent
sirolimus-eluting stent (SES)
sirolimus-induced pulmonary hypersensitivity
SIRS
    systemic inflammatory response syndrome
SIS
    Stroke Impact Scale
SISA
    stenting in small arteries
SITA
    single internal thoracic artery
sitaxsentan
site
    arrhythmogenic s.
    arterial access s.
    arterial entry s.
    artery puncture s.
    entry s.
    exit s.
    extrapulmonary s.
    femoral artery puncture s.
    gene transfer injection s.
    glycine s.
    lysine-binding s.
    puncture s.
    reentry circuit s.
    target s.
    vascular puncture s.
Site-Rite II ultrasound scanner
site-specific surgery
Sitophilus granarius
sitostanol ester margarine
sitting-up view
situ
    carcinoma in s.
    in s.
situation
    bailout s.
situational syncope
situs
    s. ambiguus
    cardiac s.
    s. inversus
    s. inversus totalis
    s. solitus
    s. transversus
sivelestat
size
    aerodynamic s.

enzymatic infarct s.
histamine equivalent wheal s.
(HEWS)

sizer

Björk-Shiley heart valve s.
graft s.
Meadox graft s.
valve s.

sizing balloon
SJM

St. Jude Medical
SJM Biocor supra valve
SJM Genesis system
SJM Masters Series heart valve
SJM mechanical heart valve
SJM pericardial patch
SJM Quattro mitral valve
SJM Regent mechanical aortic
heart valve
SJM Seguin annuloplasty ring
SJM Tailor anuloplasty ring

Sjögren

S. syndrome
S. syndrome A and B antibody
(SSA/SSB)
S. syndrome-associated interstitial
lung disease

SK

streptokinase

skein
skeletal

s. alpha-actin mRNA
s. muscle
s. muscle biopsy
s. muscle metabolism
s. muscle morphologic procedure
s. muscle morphology
s. muscle myopathy
s. muscle phenotype
s. muscle plasticity
s. muscle strength testing
s. muscle tissue
s. myoblast (SKMB)
s. myopathic disease
s. myopathic disorder

skeleton

cardiac s.
fibrous s.
s. of heart
Teflon-coated wire s.

skeletonization
skewer technique
skilled nursing facility (SNF)
Skimmer laryngeal blade tip
skimming

plasma s.

skin

s. button
s. change

s. cholesterol
s. heart
nail-fold s.
s. prick test (SPT)
salmon s.
tenting of s.
s. test anergy
s. turgor

skin-fold thickness
skip graft
skipped beat
skirt technique
SKMB

skeletal myoblast

Skoda

S. rale
S. sign

skodaic resonance
SKS

simultaneous kissing stent

SL1 sheath
slalom

S. balloon
S. PTA dilation catheter

slant-hole

s.-h. collimator
s.-h. tomography

slapping percussion
**slaved programmed electrical
stimulation**
SLB

surgical lung biopsy

SLD

Spatz-Lindenberg disease

SLE

systemic lupus erythematosus
SLE 2000 neonatal, infant, and
pediatric ventilator

sleep

s. apnea
s. apnea/hypopnea syndrome
(SAHS)
S. Apnea Quality of Life Index
(SAQLI)
s. architecture
s. bruxism
crescendo s.
D s.
deep s.
s. deprivation
desynchronized s.
s. diagnostic
s. diary
s. disorder
s. disturbance
diurnal s.
dreaming s.
fast wave s.
s. fragmentation

S

sleep *(continued)*
    s. hypoxia
    S. Multimedia 2.6 computerized textbook
    NREM s.
    orthodox s.
    s. paralysis
    paroxysmal s.
    REM s.
    slow-wave s. (SWS)
    s. spindle
    synchronized s. (S-sleep)
sleep-disordered
    s.-d. breathing (SDB)
    s.-d. breathing event
SleepGen polysomnography data entry program
sleepiness
    excessive daytime s. (EDS)
sleeping
    s. sickness
    s. tachycardia
SleepNet IQ nasal mask
sleep-onset rapid eye movement (SOREM)
Sleepscan
    S. Airflow Pressure Transducer
    S. Traveler ambulatory polysomnography system
    S. Traveler home monitoring system
sleeve
    s. lobectomy
    LocalMed catheter infusion s.
    myocardial s.'s
    s. of myocardium
    s. resection
sleuth
    carbon monoxide s.
    CO S.
    ETO S.
slew rate (SR)
SL-GXT
    symptom-limited graded exercise test
slice
    canthomeatal s.
    coronal s.
    short-axis s.
    16-s. spiral computed tomography
    transaxial s.
sliding
    s. filament theory
    s. hiatal hernia
    lung s.
    s. plasty
    pleural s.
    s. rail catheter
    s. scale method
slim disease

sling
    cardiac s.
    papillary muscle s.
    pericardial s.
    pressure s.
    pulmonary artery s.
    s. ring complex
    vascular s.
slippers
    PPCID s.
    WalkCare s.
slipping rib syndrome
slit ventricle syndrome (SVS)
SLK-View stent and delivery system
Slo-Niacin
slope
    closing s.
    diastolic s.
    disappearance s.
    D-to-E s.
    E-to-F s.
    flat diastolic s.
    mitral E-to-F s.
    ST/HR s.
slot blot
slotted
    s. needle
    s. tube articulated stent
slough
sloughed bronchial epithelium
slow
    s. A-V node pathway
    s. channel
    s. channel blocker
    s. escape rhythm
    s. and fast A-V nodal pathway
    S. Fe
    s. filling wave
    s. paroxysmal atrial tachycardia (SPAT)
    s. respiration
    s. response
    s. tissue
    s. vital capacity (SVC)
    s. zone
slow-fast tachycardia
slowing
    conduction s.
    diffuse paroxysmal s.
    junctional s. (JS)
slow-pathway
    s.-p. ablation
    s.-p. modification
slow-reacting substance of anaphylaxis (SRS-A)
slow-wave sleep (SWS)
SLP
    segmental limb pressure
    segmental limb systolic pressure

SLPI
    secretory leukocyte protease inhibitor
    secretory leukoprotease inhibitor
    secretory leukoproteinase inhibitor
SLS
    segment length, septal
    segment length, systolic
    shrinking lung syndrome
    Spectranetics laser sheath
SLT
    single-lung transplant
SLUD
    salivation, lacrimation, urination, defecation
sludged blood
sludging
slurred
    s. R wave
    s. speech
slurry
    gelatin sponge s.
    talc s.
slush
    saline s.
Sly disease
SM
    sonomicrometry
    systolic motion
    systolic murmur
SM1
    primary sensorimotor cortex
Sm
    speed of bronchoconstriction in response to methacholine
SMA
    smooth muscle actin
    superior mesenteric artery
    supplemental motor area
small
    s. airways disease
    s. aorta syndrome (SAS)
    s. coronary vessel
    s., dense, low-density lipoprotein (SD-LDL)
    s. low-density lipoprotein
    s. P wave
    s. R, bigger R of QRS (rSR)
    s. vessel (SV)
    s. vessel infarction (SVI)
small-cell
    s.-c. carcinoma
    s.-c. lung carcinoma (SCLC)
small-molecule FXa inhibitor
small-particle aerosol generator (SPAG)
smallpox vaccine reaction
small-volume
    s.-v. aspiration
    s.-v. nebulizer (SVN)

SMAP
    systemic mean arterial pressure
smart
    S. CapnoLine O2 monitoring device
    S. Control self-expanding stent
    s. defibrillator
    S. MAC-Line capnography system
    S. MAC-Line O2 sedation monitoring device
    s. pacemaker
    S. Trigger
    S. Trigger Bear 1000 ventilator
SmartFlow multiple lesion device
SmartMist
    S. asthma management system
    S. respiratory management system
SmartNeedle
SMC
    sensorimotor cortex
    smooth muscle cell
smear
    bronchoscopic s.
    buffy coat s.
    lower respiratory tract s.
    peripheral blood s.
    sputum s.
smearing artifact
smear-negative tuberculosis
smear-positive tuberculosis
Smec balloon catheter
smegmatis
    Mycobacterium s.
Smeloff-Cutter ball-and-cage prosthetic valve
Smeloff heart valve
SMG
    supramarginal gyrus
S-Mgb assay
SMI
    silent myocardial infarction
    sustained maximal inspiration
SMILE
    So Much Improvement with a Little Exercise
    SMILE program
Smith
    S. clip
    S. sign
Smith-Lemli-Opitz syndrome
SMO
    Sarns membrane oxygenator
smoke
    cigarette s. (CS)
    echocardiographic s.
    environmental tobacco s. (ETS)
    mainstream s. (MS)
    puff of s.
    secondhand s.

S

smoke *(continued)*
    sidestream s. (SS)
    wood s.
smokelike echoes
smoker
    chain s.
    s.'s bronchitis
    s.'s cough
    s.'s tongue
Smokerlyzer
    S. breath carbon monoxide monitor
    COmpact S.
    Micro+ S.
    Mini2 S.
    piCO+ S.
smoking
    s. cessation
    s. cessation program (SCP)
    cigarette s.
    s. history
    passive postnatal s.
    passive prenatal s.
smoking-induced angina
smooth
    s. coronary artery
    s. excimer laser coronary
      angioplasty (SELCA)
    s. lesion
    s. muscle actin (SMA)
    s. muscle cell (SMC)
    s. muscle relaxant
    s. muscle relaxation
    s. pseudo-Wigner-Ville distribution
      (SPWVD)
smoothing
    digital s.
    rate s.
smoothness index
SMVR
    supraanular mitral valve replacement
SMVT
    sustained monomorphic ventricular
      tachycardia
SMX/TMP
    sulfamethoxazole/trimethoprim
SN
    sinuatrial node
    sinus node
    suprasternal notch
SNA
    sella nasion point A
    sympathetic nerve activity
SNAC
    sodium N-[8-(2-
      hydroxybenzoyl)amino]caprylate
snack
    meat, eggs, dairy, invisible fat,
      condiments, s.'s (MEDICS)

snake
    s. graft
    s. venom
snake-tongue sign
SNAP
    sensory nerve action potential
    SNAP test
snap
    aortic second sound opening s.
      (A2-OS)
    closing s.
    mitral opening s. (MOS)
    opening s. (OS)
    tricuspid opening s.
snare
    s. catheter
    caval s.
    s. device
    endovascular s.
    EN Snare endovascular s.
    gooseneck s.
    Needle's Eye s.
    nitinol s.
    s. technique
    transvenous nitinol s.
snare-assisted
    s.-a. coil occlusion
    s.-a. coil occlusion of PDA
snare-drum effect
SNB
    sella nasion point B
SNCL
    sinus node cycle length
SNCV
    sensory nerve conduction velocity
SND
    sinus node dysfunction
SNE
    sinus node electrogram
Sneddon syndrome
sneeze
    s. reflex
    s. syncope
SNF
    sinus node formation
    skilled nursing facility
Snider match test
sniff
    s. nasal inspiratory pressure
    s. test
sniffing position
sniffling bronchophony
Sniper hydrophilic Nitinol guidewire
S-nitrosoglutathione (GSNO)
S-nitrosothiol
SNM
    Society of Nuclear Medicine
SNOAR open airway appliance

snooze-induced excitation of sympathetic triggered activity (SIESTA)
Snore-Ezzer oral appliance
Snorex mouthguard
snoring
  crescendo s.
  heroic s.
  s. rale
snowman
  s. abnormality
  s. configuration
  s. heart
  s. sign
snowplow effect
snowstorm
  cytokine s.
  s. shadow
SNP
  single-nucleotide polymorphism
  sinus node potential
SNRT
  sinus node recovery time
SNRTd
  sinus node recovery time, direct
    measuring
SNRTi
  sinus node recovery time, indirect
    measuring
SNS
  sympathetic nervous system
Snuggle Warm convective warming system
SNV
  Sin Nombre virus
SO$_2$
  oxygen saturation
  sulfur dioxide
^{82}So
  strontium-82
soap curd
SOB
  shortness of breath
SOBOE
  shortness of breath on exertion
sobria
  Aeromonas hydrophila biovar s.
society, pl. **societies**
  American Cancer S. (ACS)
  American Roentgen Ray S.
  American Thoracic S. (ATS)
  Associations of Professional Sleep
    Societies (APSS)
  British Cardiac S. (BCS)
  British Thoracic S. (BTS)
  Canadian Cardiovascular S. (CCS)
  Canadian Infectious Disease S.
  Canadian Thoracic S.
  S. for Cardiac Angiography and
    Interventions (SCAI)

S. of Cardiovascular and
  Interventional Radiology (SCVIR)
European Respiratory S. (ERS)
S. of Nuclear Medicine (SNM)
S. of Thoracic Surgeons (STS)
S. for Vascular Surgery (SVS)
sock array
sodium
  s. acetate
  s. aminosalicylate
  aminosalicylate s.
  ardeparin s.
  s. ascorbate
  beraprost s. (BPS)
  s. bicarbonate
  brequinar s.
  cefazolin s.
  cefmetazole s.
  cefonicid s.
  cefoperazone s.
  cefotaxime s.
  cefoxitin s.
  ceftizoxime s.
  ceftriaxone s.
  cephalothin s.
  cephapirin s.
  cerivastatin s.
  s. channel (I_{Na})
  s. channel blockade
  s. channel blocker
  s. channel gene
  s. chloride
  cloxacillin s.
  colistimethate s.
  s. content of food
  s. cromoglycate
  cromolyn s.
  s. current (I_{Na})
  dalteparin s.
  danaparoid s.
  dantrolene s.
  dextrothyroxine s.
  s. dichloroacetate
  dicloxacillin s.
  dietary s.
  s. dodecylsulfate polyacrylamide gel
    electrophoresis (SDS-PAGE)
  enoxaparin s.
  epoprostenol s.
  ertapenem s.
  s. excretion
  s. ferric gluconate complex
  fondaparinux s.
  fosinopril s.
  s. ion
  ioxaglate s.
  s. lactate
  Luminal S.
  meclofenamate s.

S

sodium *(continued)*
    s. meglumine diatrizoate
    s. meglumine ioxaglate
    mercaptomerin s.
    metam s.
    methicillin s.
    s. methylprednisolone
    mezlocillin s.
    montelukast s.
    morrhuate s.
    nafcillin s.
    nedocromil s.
    s. N-[8-(2-
      hydroxybenzoyl)amino]caprylate
      (SNAC)
    s. nitrite
    s. nitroprusside
    nitroprusside s.
    oxacillin s.
    s. oxybate
    pantoprazole s.
    paraaminosalicylate s.
    Pentothal S.
    pertechnetate s.
    s. pertechnetate technetium-99m
    s. phosphate
    piperacillin and tazobactam s.
    PMS-Levothyroxine S.
    s. polystyrene sulfonate
    s. polystyrene sulfonate enema
    pravastatin s.
    racemic warfarin s.
    s. reabsorption
    s. retention
    s. salicylate
    stibogluconate s.
    s. tetradecyl sulfate
    thiamylal s.
    thiopental s.
    thiopentone s.
    s. thiosulfate
    tinzaparin s.
    tosylchloramide s.
    treprostinil s.
    warfarin s.
sodium-potassium (Na+/K+)
    s.-p. exchange
    s.-p. pump (Na+/K+-ATPase)
Soemmerring
    arterial vein of S.
SOFA
    sepsis-related organ failure assessment
    sequential organ failure assessment
soft
    s. event
    s. phonation index
    s. pulse
    S. Thoracoport

    s. tissue calcification
    s. tissue sarcoma
Softclix lancet device
Softech endotracheal tube
Softgels
    Inflammation Defense S.
Softip
    S. catheter
    S. oxygen nasal cannula
Softouch diagnostic catheter
soft-tissue retractor
Soft-Vu Omni flush catheter
software
    CardIQ s.
    Clarity s.
    3-dimensional MSPECT s.
    Image-Measure morphometry s.
    ImageVue s.
    MedGraphics Breeze PF s.
    Solaris FLOW image analysis s.
    Stat View s.
    Tachyarrhythmia Detection S.
    TrakPro data analysis s.
    VISTA s.
SOH
    sympathetic orthostatic hypotension
Sokolow-Lyon
    S.-L. voltage
    S.-L. voltage criteria
SolAiris III, V oxygen concentrator
solani
    Fusarium s.
Solarcaine topical
Solaris FLOW image analysis software
Solcotrans autotransfusion unit
soldered bond
soldering
    s. flux
    s. fumes
soldier's
    s. heart
    s. patches
Solera thrombectomy catheter
solid
    s. angle concept
    s. organ transplantation
solitary
    s. coronary ostium
    s. fibrous tumor
    s. fibrous tumor of pleura (SFTP)
    s. pulmonary arteriovenous fistula
    s. pulmonary nodule (SPN)
solitus
    situs s.
    ventricular situs s.
    visceroatrial situs s.
solo
    S. balloon
    S. catheter

solubility
    lipid s.
soluble
    s. adhesion molecule
    s. dimeric TNF receptor
    s. intracellular adhesion molecule
      (sICAM)
    s. TREM-1 assay
    s. TREM-1 level
    s. tumor necrosis factor receptor
      (sTNFR)
Solu-Cortef Injection
Solu-Medrol injection
Solurex L.A.
Soluspan
    Celestone S.
solution
    agitated saline s.
    albuterol sulfate inhalation s.
    Atrovent Inhalation S.
    Belzer s.
    Bretschneider-HTK cardioplegic s.
    Brompton s.
    Burow s.
    Cafcit oral s.
    caffeine citrate oral s.
    cardioplegic s.
    cardioplegic perfusion s. (CPS)
    Carnoy s.
    Celsior s.
    Collins s.
    coronary perfusate s. (CPS)
    cromolyn sodium inhalation s.
    crystalloid cardioplegic s.
    Dakin s.
    Denhardt s.
    dextran s.
    Duration Nasal S.
    ECS cardioplegic s.
    Euro-Collins s.
    extracellular-like, calcium-free s.
      (ECS)
    Fowler s.
    Gey fixative s.
    hand agitated s.
    Hank's balanced salt s.
    Hartmann s.
    hypertonic saline s.
    iced saline s.
    ICS cardioplegic s.
    Intal Nebulizer S.
    intracellular-like, calcium-bearing
      crystalloid s. (ICS)
    iseganan HCl oral s.
    Isoetharine Inhalation S. USP 1%
    Krebs s.
    Krebs-Henseleit s.
    LET s.
    levalbuterol HCl inhalation s.

    low-chloride St. Thomas s.
    Lugol s.
    Massier s.
    Melrose s.
    Myers S.
    NasalCrom Nasal S.
    Neo-Synephrine 12 Hour Nasal S.
    Papanicolaou s.
    polyethylene glycol electrolyte
      lavage s. (PEG-LES)
    preservative-free s. (PFS)
    Resectisol Irrigation S.
    Ringer s.
    saturated s.
    Schlesinger s.
    Sepracoat coating s.
    Sporicidin sterilizing s.
    stroma-free hemoglobin s.
    St. Thomas s.
    TOBI Inhalation S.
    tobramycin s.
    Twice-A-Day Nasal S.
    Tyrode s.
    University of Wisconsin s.
    4-Way Long Acting Nasal S.
    Xopenex inhalation s.
    Xylocaine Topical S.
Solutrast contrast material
solvent vapor
SOM
    sustained outward movement
soman
SomaSensor
    S. device
    S. pad
somatic
    s. cell therapy
    s. nociceptive flexion reflex
    s. stem cell
somatization disorder
somatomedin
**Somatom Volume Zoom computed
  tomography system**
somatosensory
    s. evoked potential (SSEP)
    s. evoked potential test
somatostatin
somatotropic hormonal system
Somavert
somnambulism
somniloquism
somniloquy
Somnoplasty
    S. procedure
    S. system
Somnus Somnoplasty system
**So Much Improvement with a Little
  Exercise (SMILE)**
Sonazoid

S

Sondergaard procedure
Sones
    S. coronary catheter
    S. Hi-Flow catheter
    S. selective coronary arteriography
    S. technique
    S. woven Dacron catheter
sonicated
    s. albumin-dextrose contrast
    albumin microspheres s.
    s. contrast agent
    s. dextrose albumin
sonication technique
sonicator
Sonix 2000 ultrasonic nebulizer
sonogram
sonographic finding
sonography
    Acuson computed s.
    carotid B-mode s.
    contrast-enhanced transcranial color-coded real-time s. (CE-TCCS)
    2-dimensional transcranial color-coded s. (2D-TCCS)
    Doppler s. (DS)
    extracranial Doppler s. (ECD)
    functional transcranial Doppler s. (fTCD)
    TCD s.
    transcranial color-coded s. (TCCS)
SonoHeart
    S. Elite handheld ultrasound system
    S. Elite Ultrasound System
    S. hand-carried echocardiography
    S. handheld, all digital echocardiography system
    S. scanner
sonolucency
sonolucent
    s. distal imaging sheath
    s. zone
SonoLysis system
sonomicrometer piezoelectric crystal
sonomicrometry (SM)
    s. array localization
sonorous
    s. rale
    s. respiration
    s. rhonchus
Sonos
    S. 4500 echocardiography system
    S. 500 imaging system
    S. 1500, 2500 scanner
    S. 2000, 5500 ultrasound imager
    S. 5500 ultrasound system
SonoSite MicroMaxx ultrasound system
sonotherapy
    intravascular s. (IST)
    S. system

SonoVue ultrasound contrast media
soother
    SudaCare Shower S.'s
Sopha Medical gamma camera
Soprano
    S. bioprosthesis
    S. stented prosthesis
    S. valve
SOREM
    sleep-onset rapid eye movement
Sorin
    S. Bicarbon bileaflet aortic valve prosthesis
    S. Biomedica Cardio Solo stentless prosthesis
    S. Carbostent stent
    S. heart valve
    S. lead
    S. mitral valve prosthesis
    S. pacemaker
    S. prosthetic valve
Sorivudine
soroche
sorter
    cell s.
    fluorescence-activated cell s. (FACS)
SOS guidewire
Sotacor
sotalol
    s. HCl
    s. hydrochloride
Soucek
    Randall-Baker S.
souffle
    cardiac s.
    fetal s.
    funic s.
    mammary s.
soufflet
    bruit de s.
sound
    absent breath s.'s
    adventitious breath s.'s
    adventitious heart s.'s
    amphoric voice s.
    anodal closure s. (ACS)
    anodal opening s. (AOS)
    aortic s. (AS)
    aortic closure s.
    aortic ejection s. (AES)
    aortic first s. (A1)
    aortic second sound, pulmonary second s. (A2P2)
    aortic tunica adventitious breath s.'s
    atrial s.
    auscultatory s.
    bandbox s.

Beatty-Bright friction s.
bell s.
bellows s.
bottle s.
breath s.'s
bronchial breath s.'s
bronchovesicular breath s.'s
cannon s.
cardiac s.
coarse breath s.'s
coin s.
cracked-pot s.
crowing breath s.'s
crunching s.
decreased breath s.'s
distant breath s.'s
distant heart s.'s
double-shock s.
eddy s.
ejection s. (ES)
esophageal adventitious breath s.'s
FBPM spectral analysis of
  heart s.'s
fetal heart s. (FHS)
fifth Korotkoff s. (K5)
first heart s. (S_1)
flapping s.
fourth heart s. (S_4)
fourth Korotkoff s. (K4)
friction s.
gallop s.
heart s. (HS)
heart s.'s S_1, S_2, S_3, S_4
hippocratic s.
hippocratic succussion s.
s. intensity profile
Korotkoff s.
mammary souffle s.
metallic breath s.'s
mitral s.'s (MS)
mitral first s. (M_1)
mitral second s. (M_2)
muffled heart s.'s
pacemaker s.
paradoxically split S_2 s.
percussion s.
pericardial friction s.
physiologically split S_2 s.
physiologic third heart s.
pistol-shot s.
pistol-shot femoral s.
prosthetic valve s.
puffing s.
pulmonary component of second
  heart s.
pulmonic second heart s. (P2)
pulmonic valve closure s.
quiet breath s.'s
quiet heart s.'s

respiratory s.
sail s.
second heart s. (S_2)
second mitral s.
shaking s.
splitting of heart s.'s
squeaky-leather s.
succussion s.'s
tambour s.
third heart s. (S_3)
tic-tac s.
to-and-fro s.
tracheal breath s.'s
tricuspid first s. (T1)
tricuspid valve closure s. (T1)
tubular breath s.'s
tumor plop s.
tympanitic s.
vesicular breath s.'s
waterwheel s.
water-whistle s.
s. wave cycle
widely split second s.
xiphisternal crunching s.
source
  germanium-68 external s.
south
  S. Beach diet
  S. Carolina Organ Procurement
    Agency (SCOPA)
southern
  S. blot
  S. blot analysis
Souttar tube
soy
  s. isoflavone
  s. phytoestrogen
  s. protein
soybean lecithin asthma
SP
  shunt pressure
  shunt procedure
  spontaneous pneumothorax
  surfactant protein
  systolic pressure
    SP-A,-B,-C.-D
SP-10 spirometer
SP-A
  surfactant protein A
space
  air s.
  alveolar dead s.
  anatomic dead s.
  antecubital s.
  anterior clear s.
  Bogros s.
  Böttcher s.
  s. of Burns
  Cotunnius s.

S

space *(continued)*
    cystic s.
    dead s.
    echo-free s.
    extrapleural s.
    extravascular s.
    H s.
    Henke s.
    His perivascular s.
    Holzknecht s.
    intercostal s. (ICS)
    interelectrode s.
    interpleural s.
    interstitial s.
    intrapleural s.
    Larrey s.
    lateral pharyngeal s.
    mediastinal s.
    noncommunicating air s.
    parapneumonic s.
    peripharyngeal s.
    perivascular s.'s
    pharyngeal s.
    pharyngomaxillary s.
    physiologic dead s.
    pleural s.
    posterior airway s. (PAS)
    postpharyngeal s.
    prevertebral s.
    respiratory dead s.
    retrocardiac s.
    retropharyngeal s.
    retrosternal air s.
    retrotracheal s.
    subarachnoid s. (SAS)
    subphrenic s.
    Talairach s.
    Traube semilunar s.
    Virchow-Robin s.
    Westberg s.
    Zang s.
Spacehaler
Spacemaker balloon dissector
space-occupying
    s.-o. effect
    s.-o. lesion
spacer
    ACE MDI s.
    Ellipse compact s.
    MDI s.
spacing
spade-like configuration
SPAF
    spontaneous paroxysmal atrial fibrillation
SPAG
    small-particle aerosol generator
spalling effect

SPAMM
    spatial modulation of magnetization
      SPAMM technique
sPAP
    systolic pulmonary artery pressure
spare tire bulge
sparfloxacin
sparing
    myocardial s.
spark
    calcium s.
    s. erosion
Sparks mandrel technique
spasm
    arterial s.
    bronchial s.
    bronchopulmonary s.
    carpopedal s.
    catheter-induced s. (CIS)
    catheter-induced coronary artery s.
    catheter-related peripheral vessel s.
    catheter-tip s.
    coronary s.
    coronary artery s. (CAS)
    diffuse esophageal s. (DES)
    epicardial arterial s.
    ergonovine-induced s.
    esophageal s.
    post bypass s.
    vascular s.
    venous s.
    vessel s.
spasmodic
    s. asthma
    s. croup
spastica
    dysphagia s.
spasticity
SPAT
    slow paroxysmal atrial tachycardia
spatial
    s. average intensity (I_{sa})
    s. average pulse average (I_{sapa})
    s. average, temporal average
      intensity (I_{sata})
    s. modulation
    s. modulation of magnetization
      (SPAMM)
    s. modulation of magnetization
      technique
    s. peak intensity (I_{sp})
    s. peak pulse average intensity
      (I_{sppa})
    s. peak, temporal average intensity
      (I_{sapt})
    s. resolution
    s. tracking
    s. vector

s. vectorcardiogram (SVCG)
s. vectorcardiography
spatium, pl. **spatia**
s. intercostale
s. lateropharyngeum
s. parapharyngeum
s. pharyngeum laterale
s. retropharyngeum
s. suprasternale
Spatz-Lindenberg disease (SLD)
Spaulding classification system
SPCA
serum prothrombin conversion
accelerator
SPCG
spectral phonocardiography
SPE
septic pulmonary edema
sustained physical exercise
speaking valve
Spearman coefficient
Spears laser balloon
special
Lasix S.
specialized CC-chemokine secretion
species
reactive oxygen s. (ROS)
specific
s. bronchial challenge test
s. compliance
s. expiratory muscle training
(SEMT)
s. inhalation challenge test
s. inspiratory muscle training
(SIMT)
specificity
speckle
Doppler s.
speckling
SPECT
single-photon emission computed
tomography
adenosine ^{99m}Tc sestamibi SPECT
gated SPECT
SPECT imaging
MIBI SPECT
SPECT scintigraphy
sestamibi gated SPECT
stress perfusion and rest function
by sestamibi gated SPECT
technetium-99m sestamibi SPECT
technetium-sestamibi SPECT
spectacular shrinking deficit
spectography
magnetic resonance s.
Raman s.
spectra (*pl. of* spectrum)
Spectracef-TAP

spectral
s. analysis
s. Doppler
s. Doppler velocity measurement
s. envelope
s. leakage
s. peak velocity
s. phonocardiograph
s. phonocardiography (SPCG)
s. power
s. temporal mapping
s. turbulence mapping
s. waveform
Spectranetics
S. Extreme C laser catheter
S. laser
S. laser sheath (SLS)
S. Prima laser guidewire
spectrometer
Amis 2000 respiratory mass s.
Bruker Avance s.
InSpectra tissue s.
spectrometry
atomic absorption s.
gas chromatography-mass s. (GC-MS)
spectrophotometer
Cary 118C s.
Hitachi U-2000 s.
liquid scintillation s.
spectrophotometric oximetry
spectrophotometry
time of flight and absorbance s.
TOFA s.
spectroscope
argon plasma emission s.
spectroscopy
argon plasma emission s.
electron paramagnetic resonance s.
flame emission s. (FES)
fluorescence s.
graphite furnace atomic
absorption s.
magnetic resonance s. (MRS)
near-infrared s. (NIRS, NIS)
NMR s.
phosphorus-31 magnetic
resonance s. (^{31}P-MRS)
^{31}P nuclear magnetic resonance s.
proton s.
Raman s.
spectroscopy-directed laser
spectrum, pl. **spectra**
SpectRx test
specular echo
speculum, pl. **specula**
pharyngeal s.
Yankauer pharyngeal s.

S

speech
    alaryngeal s.
    esophageal s.
    s. mental stress test
    slurred s.
    speed reversal s.
speed
    s. of bronchoconstriction in response to methacholine (Sm)
    s. reversal speech
spell
    blackout s.
    breathholding s.
    grayout s.
    hypercyanotic s.
    hypoxic s.
    presyncopal s.
    syncopal s.
    Tet s.
    tetrad s.
    tetralogy of Fallot s.
Spembly cryoprobe
Spencer
    S. plication
    S. plication vena cava
Spens syndrome
spermine
SPET
    single-photon emission tomography
SPET imaging
SPF
    standard perfusion fluid
    systemic pulmonary fistula
SPGR
    spoiled gradient recalled
sphaericus
    Bacillus s.
Sphaerophorus necrophorus
sphenoidal fissure
sphere
    attraction s.
sphericalization
spherical pneumonia
sphericity index
spheroid left ventricular shape
spheroplast
sphincter
    cardioesophageal s.
    esophageal s.
    gastroesophageal s.
    hepatic s.
    inferior esophageal s.
    palatopharyngeal s.
    pharyngoesophageal s.
    precapillary s.
Sphingobacterium
sphingolipidosis

sphingomyelin
    s. hydrolysis
    s. phosphodiesterase
sphingomyelinase
    secretory s. (S-SMase)
sphingosine
Sphrintzen syndrome
sphygmic interval
sphygmocardiograph
sphygmocardioscope
sphygmochronograph
SphygmoCor
    S. non-invasive aortic blood pressure system
    S. Px Aortic BP Profile cardiovascular data collection device
sphygmogram
sphygmograph
sphygmographic
sphygmography
sphygmoid
sphygmomanometer, sphygmometer
    Ayers s.
    Baumanometer standard mercury s.
    Erlanger s.
    Faught s.
    Hawksley random zero mercury s.
    Janeway s.
    London School of Hygiene and Tropical medicine s.
    Mosso s.
    Physio-Control Lifestat s.
    random-zero s.
    Riva-Rocci s.
    Rogers s.
sphygmomanometry
sphygmometroscope
sphygmooscillometer
sphygmopalpation
sphygmophone
sphygmoscope
    Bishop s.
sphygmoscopy
sphygmosystole
sphygmotonograph
sphygmotonometer
sphygmoviscosimetry
spider
    s. angioma
    arterial s.
    s. burst
    S. embolic protection device
    S. filter
    s. projection
    vascular s.
    s. venom
    s. x-ray view
SpideRX embolic protection device

Spielberger Anger Expression scale
spigot
>   endobronchial Watanbe s. (EWS)
SPIH
>   superimposed pregnancy-induced
>   hypertension
spike
>   s. activity
>   atrial s.
>   H s.
>   pacemaker s.
>   pacing s.
>   sensing s.
>   wave s.
>   s. wave (SW, S/W)
spike-and-dome
>   s.-a.-d. configuration
>   s.-a.-d. potential
>   s.-a.-d. pulse
spike-wave stupor (SWS)
SPI-Lite sleep position indicator
spill
>   chylous s.
spillover
>   jugular venous catechol s.
spin
>   s. density
>   s. echo signal
>   s. tagging
spinal
>   s. cord stimulation (SCS)
>   s. embolism
>   s. muscle
>   s. muscle of thorax
>   s. nociceptive flexion reflex
spindle
>   aortic s.
>   s. cell carcinoma
>   s. cell sarcoma
>   s. fiber
>   His s.
>   sleep s.
spine
>   posterior nasal s. (PNS)
spin-echo (SE)
>   s.-e. imaging
>   s.-e. imaging sequence
>   s.-e. MRI
Spinhaler
spin-lattice time
spinnaker formation
spinocerebellar
>   s. ataxia
>   s. degeneration
spinothalamic tract
spin-spin time
spiral
>   s. computed tomography
>   s. CT scan

Curschmann s.
>   s. dissection
>   s. hypertrophic cardiomyopathy
>   s. reentrant wave
>   s. volumetric computed tomography
>   (SVCT)
spiral-embedded tube
spiralis
>   *Trichinella* s.
spiramycin
spirapril hydrochloride
Spiriva
spirochetal
>   s. disease
>   s. infection
>   s. myocarditis
spirochete
spirochetosis
>   bronchopulmonary s.
Spiroflex thrombectomy catheter
SpiroFlow children's peak flowmeter
spirogermanium
spirogram
>   forced expiratory s. (FES)
spirograph
spirography
spiro-index
Spirolite 201 spirometer
spirometer
>   Benedict-Roth s.
>   Calculair s.
>   chain-compensated s.
>   closed-circuit s.
>   Coach incentive s.
>   Collins Survey s.
>   Compact II desktop s.
>   Discovery handheld s.
>   Discovery portable s.
>   Eagle s.
>   Flash portable s.
>   flow-sensing s.
>   Gould Instrument Systems s.
>   Horizon PFT s.
>   incentive s.
>   Inspiron incentive s.
>   IQmark Digital S.
>   Krogh apparatus s.
>   MasterLab Pro pneumotachograph s.
>   MedicAIR Plus s.
>   Micro DiaryCard s.
>   MicroLab ML3500 desktop
>   diagnostic s.
>   MicroLoop II s.
>   MicroLoop pocket s.
>   Micro Plus s.
>   PiKo s.
>   Pneumotach s.
>   2120 Recording S.
>   Sensaire handheld s.

spirometer *(continued)*
 Simplicity S.
 SP-10 s.
 Spirolite 201 s.
 SpiroVision-3+ s.
 Stead-Wells water-seal type s.
 Tissot s.
 Vitalograph 2120 handheld
  recording s.
 Vitalor incentive s.
 volume-displacement s.
 water-sealed s.
 wedge s.
 Welch Allyn PneumoCheck s.
 Wright s.
spirometric
 s. evaluation
 s. screening
spirometry
 2170 S. Software system
 DX-Portable s.
 forced s.
 incentive s.
 MultiSPIRO Series SX/DX
  computerized s.
 stacked inspiratory s.
 SX/DX computerized s.
 Welch Allyn/Schiller SP-1
  budget s.
 Welch Allyn/Schiller SP-10
  diagnostic s.
spironolactone
 hydrochlorothiazide and s.
Spiros
 S. DPI
 S. dry powder inhaler
 S. inhalation system
spiroscope
SpiroSense
 S. flow sensor
 S. system
SpiroVision-3 spirometry system
SpiroVision-3+ spirometer
SpirOxCard
Spitzer theory
SPL
 superior parietal lobule
splanchnic
 s. bed perfusion
 s. blood flow
 s. circulation
 s. vessel
splanchnicotomy
splash
 succussion s.
splayed
 carina not s.
Splendore-Hoeppli phenomenon

splenic
 s. anemia
 s. flexure syndrome
 s. perfusion measurement
 s. portography
 s. venoconstriction
splenocyte
splenomegaly
splenopneumonia
splenoportal hypertension
splenoportography
splenorenal shunt
splenosis
 thoracic s.
splice
splint
 wrist positioning s.
splinter hemorrhage
splinting
split
 s. fused commissure
 paradoxical s.
 paradoxic s. of S_2
 physiological s. of S_2
split-function lung test
split-lung ventilation
split-sheath introducer
splitter
 beam s.
splitting
 commissural s.
 s. of heart sounds
SPN
 solitary pulmonary nodule
SpO$_2$
 oxygen saturation measured by pulse
 oximetry
spoiled gradient recalled (SPGR)
spondylitis
 ankylosing s.
spondyloarthropathy
 seronegative s.
sponge
 absorbable gelatin s.
 collagen s.
 Collostat hemostatic s.
 gelatin s.
 Gelfoam s.
 Ivalon s.
 laparotomy s.
 phantom s.
 porcine gelatin s.
spongy myocardium
spontaneous
 s. cervical artery dissection (sCAD)
 s. closure of fistula
 s. coronary artery disease (SCAD,
  sCAD)

s. coronary artery dissection (SCAD, sCAD)
s. echo contrast (SEC)
s. extrasystole
s. fibrillation (SF)
s. inspiratory flow rate
s. intracerebral hemorrhage (SICH)
s. lysis
s. paroxysmal atrial fibrillation (SPAF)
s. pneumomediastinum
s. pneumothorax (SP)
s. reentrant sustained ventricular tachycardia
s. resolution
s. respiration
s. ventilation

spontaneously hypertensive (SH)
Sporanox Oral
Sporicidin sterilizing solution
Sporothrix schenckii
sporotrichosis
sport
isometric s.
spot
Brushfield s.
café-au-lait s.
Campbell De Morgan s.
cold s.
cotton-wool s.
De Morgan s.'s
Horder s.'s
hot s.
Koplik s.
s. lesion
milk s.'s
rose s.
Roth s.
tendinous s.
ventricular milk s.'s
s. welding
white s.
spot-film fluorography
SPOT 3-shot Insight QE camera
spotty
s. coronary calcium
s. predicted stenosis
spray
Astelin nasal s.
Hurricaine s.
metered-dose s.
nicotine nasal s. (NNS)
Nicotrol NS nasal s.
Nitrolingual Translingual S.
Power Pulse s. (PPS)
spread
fomite-mediated s.
lymphangitic s.
venous s.

spreader
Bailey rib s.
Burford-Finochietto rib s.
DeBakey rib s.
Favaloro-Morse rib s.
Finochietto rib s.
Harken rib s.
Lilienthal-Sauerbruch rib s.
Medicon rib s.
Miltex rib s.
rib s.
Rienhoff-Finochietto rib s.
spreading depression (SD)
spring
S. catheter
s. coil
disc s.
spring-loaded
s.-l. resistor
s.-l. vascular stent
springwater cyst
sprint
S. Model 6942, 6943 tachyarrhythmia lead
S. Quattro quadripolar defibrillator lead
sprinting
SPT
skin prick test
SPTI
systolic pressure time index
spuria
angina s.
spurious aneurysm
spurium
septum s.
sputorum
Pandoraea s.
sputum, pl. sputa
s. aerogenosum
albuminoid s.
s. analysis
anchovy paste s.
blood-tinged s.
bloody s.
brown s.
chocolate sauce s.
s. coctum
copious s.
s. crudum
s. cruentum
currant jelly s.
s. cytology
egg-yolk s.
s. elastase
elastic fibers in s.
s. eosinophilia
s. expectoration
fetid s.

S

sputum *(continued)*
 frothy s.
 gelatinous s.
 globular s.
 green s.
 hemorrhagic s.
 icteric s.
 s. induction
 s. microscopy
 moss-agate s.
 mucoid s.
 mucopurulent s.
 nummular s.
 opalescent s.
 pink s.
 s. production
 productive s.
 prune juice s.
 purulent s.
 putrid s.
 red-streaked s.
 s. retention
 ropy s.
 rubbery s.
 rusty s.
 septicemia s.
 s. smear
 tenacious s.
 s. tenacity
 viscid s.
 s. viscoelasticity
 s. viscosity and elasticity
 s. volume
 white s.
 yellow s.
 yellowish-green s.
sputum-epithelium interface
SPV
 stentless porcine valve
SPWVD
 smooth pseudo-Wigner-Ville distribution
SPY
 SPY Intra-operative Imaging
  System
 SPY Paq
Spyglass angiography catheter
S$_1$Q$_3$ pattern
S-QRS interval
S$_1$Q$_3$T$_3$ pattern
squamous
 s. alveolar cell
 s. cell bronchogenic carcinoma
square
 s. root sign
 s. wave response
 s. wave stimulus
squared
 kilogram per meter s. (kg/m^2)

 liter per minute per meter s.
  (Lpm/m^2)
 meter per second s. (m/s^2)
square-shaped occluder
squeak
squeaky-leather sound
squeeze
 s. effect
 face s.
 reverse s.
 thoracic s.
 tussive s.
squeezer
SR
 sinus rhythm
 slew rate
 sustained release
  Aerolate JR, SR
  bupropion SR
  Calan SR
  SR calcium ATPase
  Cardene SR
  Deconamine SR
  Isoptin SR
  Procan SR
  Respaire-60 SR
  Respaire-120 SR
  Securon SR
SRA
 sewing ring area
 steroid-resistant asthma
Sramek formula
SRCBC
 serum reserve cholesterol binding
  capacity
Src kinase
SREBP
 sterol regulatory element-binding protein
SRMD
 stress-related mucosal disease
SRP
 synchronized retroperfusion
SRS-A
 slow-reacting substance of anaphylaxis
SRT
 segmented ring tripolar
 sinus node recovery time
  SRT lead
SRVT
 sustained reentrant ventricular
  tachyarrhythmia
SS
 selective shunt
 sidestream smoke
 subaortic stenosis
 systemic sclerosis
SSA
 senile systemic amyloidosis

SSAg
  Staphylococcus aureus superantigen
SSA/SSB
  Sjögren syndrome A and B antibody
SS-associated ILD
SSc
  systemic sclerosis
S-Scort New-Duet suction unit
S-segment airway conductance
SSEP
  somatosensory evoked potential
S-Series sleep system
SSI
  surgical site infection
S_1-S_2 **interval**
SSKI
  saturated solution of potassium iodide
S-sleep
  synchronized sleep
S-SMase
  secretory sphingomyelinase
SSP
  simultaneously stapled pneumonectomy
SSPS
  side-to-side portacaval shunt
SS-QOL
  stroke-specific quality of life
SSS
  sick sinus syndrome
  summed stress score
  superior sagittal sinus
SSSL
  secretin-stimulated serum lipase
S-Stent
S-sulfate
ST
  portion of segment between end of S
    wave and beginning of T wave
  sinus tachycardia
  stent thrombosis
  stress test
  systolic time
    ST alteration
    ST deviation
    ST elevation acute myocardial
      infarction (STEAMI)
    ST elevation myocardial infarction
    ST interval
    ST junction
    ST reelevation
    ST sag
    ST scooping
    ST segment
    ST wave
St.
  saint
    St. George Respiratory
      Questionnaire (SGRQ)
    St. Joseph Adult Chewable Aspirin

St. Joseph Cough Suppressant
St. Jude bileaflet prosthetic valve
St. Jude cardiac device
St. Jude composite prosthetic
St. Jude composite prosthetic valve
St. Jude heart valve prosthesis
St. Jude Medical (SJM)
St. Jude Medical bileaflet tilting-
  disc aortic valve
St. Jude Medical Biocor valve
St. Jude Medical Epic HF dual-
  chamber implantable
  cardioverter/defibrillator system
St. Jude Medical Port-Access
St. Jude Medical Port-Access
  mechanical heart valve
St. Jude Medical rigid saddle ring
St. Jude Medical valve prosthesis
St. Jude mitral valve
St. Jude prosthetic aortic valve
St. Jude sheath
St. Thomas Hospital cardioplegia
St. Thomas solution
St. Vitus dance
Stckert V142 series venous cannula
  with lighthouse tip
ST3 amplified stethoscope
STA
  serum thrombotic accelerator
stab
  s. electrode
  s. incision
  s. wound
stabilis
  Burkholderia s.
stability
  circulatory s.
  hemodynamic s.
  RR interval s.
stabilization
  internal pneumatic s.
  membrane s.
  plaque s.
  s. platform
  root s.
stabilizer
  Axius Vacuum 2 s.
  S. balanced performance guidewire
  Cohn cardiac s.
  S. marker wire
  S. marker wire steerable guidewire
  mast cell s.
  Octopus tissue s.
  S. Plus steerable guidewire
  S. XS steerable guidewire
stab-in epicardial electrode
stable
  s. angina (SA)
  s. angina pectoris (SAP)

S

staccato pain
Stachrom PAI chromogenic assay
Stachybotrys atra
stack
  S. autoperfusion balloon
  S. perfusion catheter
stacked inspiratory spirometry
stacking
  breath s.
Stadie-Riggs microtome
stadiometer
STAE
  subsegmental transcatheter arterial
    embolization
stage
  bacteria-free s.
  Scadding s. 0-IV
2-stage
  2-s. cannula
  ultrathin-walled 2-s. (UTTS)
staged
  s. angioplasty
  s. percutaneous coronary
    intervention
Stagesic
staging
  TNM s.
  videothoracoscopic operator s.
    (VOS)
stagnant
  s. anoxia
  s. hypoxia
stagnation
  contrast s.
STAI
  State-Trait Anxiety Inventory
stain, staining
  acetoorcein s.
  Alcian blue-PAS s.
  Azan-Mallory s.
  calcofluor s.
  Coomassie blue s.
  Dieterle s.
  Diff-Quik s.
  direct immunofluorescent s.
  endocardial s.
  Giemsa s.
  GMS s.
  Goldner trichrome s.
  Gomori methenamine silver s.
  Gram s.
  Grocott s.
  H&E s.
  hematoxylin and eosin s.
  immunoperoxidase s.
  Kinyoun s.
  Mallory s.
  Masson trichrome s.

May-Grünwald-Giemsa s.
methenamine silver s.
Miller elastic s.
Movat s.
mucicarmine s.
oil red O s.
Pappenheim s.
picrosirius red s.
Pizzolatto s.
propidium iodide s.
S100 s.
silver-methenamine s.
Sirius red s.
toluidine blue s.
TTC s.
TUNEL s.
van Gieson s.
Verhoeff elastica s.
Verhoeff tissue elastin s.
Weigert-van Gieson s.
Wright s.
Wright-Giemsa s.
Ziehl-Neelsen s.
staining
  growth factor-beta-1 s.
  histologic s.
  immunohistochemical s.
  nicotine s.
  Ponceau S s.
stainless
  s. steel balloon expandable stent
  s. steel guidewire
  s. steel mesh stent
staircase phenomenon
stair climbing
STALD
  Sheffield Screening Test for Acquired
    Language Disorders
Stamey test
stand-alone
  s.-a. balloon angioplasty
  s.-a. laser treatment
standard
  s. atmosphere
  Boehringer Mannheim s.
  s. Bruce protocol
  s. cardiopulmonary resuscitation
    (SCPR)
  s. deviation
  s. heparin (SH)
  hypertension s.
  s. Lehman catheter
  s. limb lead
  s. needle
  s. perfusion fluid (SPF)
  s. temperature and pressure, dry
  s. temperature and pulse (STP)
standardization wave

standby
 s. pacemaker
 s. pulse generator
Stand Displacement Amplification test
standing
 s. diastolic blood pressure (SDBP)
 s. venous pressure (SVP)
standstill
 atrial s.
 auricular s.
 cardiac s.
 persistent atrial s. (PAS)
 respiratory s.
 sinus s.
 ventricular s.
Stanford
 S. biopsy method
 S. bioptome
 S. classification
 S. treadmill exercise protocol
 S. type A, B aortic dissection
 S. type B AD
 S. type B anterior descending
stannic oxide
Stannius ligature
stannosis
stanol
 plant s.
stanozolol anabolic steroid
Stansel procedure
STAN S31 fetal heart monitor
staphyledema
staphylococcal
 s. bronchitis
 s. endocarditis
 s. infection
 s. pneumonia
Staphylococcus
 S. aureus
 S. aureus superantigen (SSAg)
 S. epidermidis
staphylokinase
staphylopharyngorrhaphy
stapled
 s. lung reduction
 s. wedge resection
stapler
 Androsov vascular s.
 CEEA s.
 Endo GIA s.
 Endopath EZ45 thoracic linear s.
 Ethicon Endopath EZ45 s.
stapling
 bleb s.
starch
 hydroxyethyl s.
StarClose
 S. ACD
 S. vascular closure system

STARFlex device
Starling
 S. curve
 S. curve of pancreas
 S. equation
 S. force
 S. law
 S. mechanism
Starr-Edwards
 S.-E. aortic valve prosthesis
 S.-E. ball-and-cage valve
 S.-E. ball valve prosthesis
 S.-E. cardiac valve prosthesis
 S.-E. disc valve prosthesis
 S.-E. heart valve prosthesis
 S.-E. mitral prosthesis
 S.-E. mitral valve
 S.-E. prosthetic valve
 S.-E. Silastic valve
Stary
 S. histology classification
 S. histology grading
 S. lesion classification system
stasis, pl. **stases**
 s. cirrhosis
 s. dermatitis
 s. edema
 pressure s.
 s. ulcer
 venous s.
Stat
 signal transducer and activator of
  transcription
stat
 alpha s.
 Stat 2 Pumpette
 Stat View software
STAT4 protein
STAT6 protein
state
 acute confusional s. (ACS)
 cardiovascular steady s.
 glycometabolic s.
 gradient recalled acquisition in a
  steady s. (GRASS)
 hypercoagulable s.
 hyperdynamic s.
 hyperinsulinemic euglycemic clamp
  metabolic s.
 hyperkinetic s.
 myocardial contraction s.
 nonfasting s.
 postabsorptive s.
 postictal s.
 prothrombotic s.
State-Trait Anxiety Inventory (STAI)
stathmokinesis
static
 s. dilation technique

S

static *(continued)*
    s. lung compliance
    s. lung volume
    s. obstruction
statin-fibrate therapy
statin therapy
station
    AJCC staging s.
    American Joint Committee on Cancer staging s.
    analog video acquisition s.
    DICOM acquisition s.
    s. pull-through
stationary
    s. arterial wave
    s. bicycle
StatLock Arterial Plus securement device
STAT protein family
status
    acute-on-chronic s.
    s. anginosus
    s. asthmaticus
    battery s.
    cardiac s.
    s. epilepticus
    functional s.
    IND s.
    investigational new drug s.
    mental s.
    neurologic s.
    OptiVol fluid s.
    pulmonary function s.
    work s.
staurosporine
stave cell
stavudine
stay
    length of s. (LOS)
Stayhealthy RT3 triaxial accelerometer
STD
    ST-segment depression
Stead-Wells water-seal type spirometer
steady Doppler
steady-state method
steal
    coronary s.
    s. effect
    endoperoxide s.
    iliac s.
    s. mechanism
    s. phenomenon
    pulmonary artery s.
    renal-splanchnic s.
    subclavian s.
    transmural s.
stealth angioplasty balloon
steam-fitter's asthma

STEAMI
    ST elevation acute myocardial infarction
steam tent
stearothermophilus
    Bacillus s.
steatorrhea
steatosis
    s. cardiaca
    s. cordis
    hepatic s.
Steell murmur
steel-winged butterfly needle
steep left anterior oblique projection
steeple sign
steepling
    s. of glottic airway
    s. of trachea
    tracheal s.
steerable
    s. angioplastic guidewire
    s. decapolar electrode catheter
    s. diagnostic catheter
    s. guidewire catheter
    s. over-the-wire angioplasty technique
    s. quadripolar catheter
Steerocath-Dx Spec. Procedure Octa Catheter
Steerocath-T temperature ablation catheter
Stegemann-Stalder method
Steidele complex
Steinberg thumb sign
Steinert
    S. disease
    S. myotonic dystrophy
Stelid II steroid eluting endocardial pacing lead
Stelix II steroid eluting endocardial pacing lead
stellate
    s. ganglion
    s. ganglion blockade
stem
    arterial s.
    s. bronchus
    s. cell factor (SCF)
    s. cell therapy
    left main s. (LMS)
    transposition of arterial s.'s
STEMI
    ST-segment elevation myocardial infarction
stenocardia
stenosal murmur
stenosed area
stenosis, pl. **stenoses**
    acute mitral s. (AMS)
    airway s.

aortic s.
aortic valve s. (AVS)
aqueductal s.
area of s. (AS)
atrial s. (AS)
benign airway s.
bottle neck s.
branch pulmonary artery s.
bronchial s.
buttonhole mitral s.
calcific aortic s. (CAS)
calcific mitral s.
calcific nodular aortic s.
caroticovertebral s.
carotid s.
carotid artery s. (CAS)
chronic aortic s.
cicatricial s.
congenital aortic s.
congenital mitral s.
congenital pulmonary s.
coronary artery s.
coronary luminal s.
coronary ostial s.
critical aortic s.
critical coronary s.
critical valvular s.
culprit s.
degenerative aortic s.
diameter s. (DS)
discrete subaortic s. (DSAS, DSS)
discrete subvalvular aortic s.
 (DSAS)
distal s.
Dittrich s.
double aortic s.
dynamic s.
eccentric s.
enucleation of subaortic s.
epicardial s.
fibrous subaortic s.
filiform s.
fish-mouth mitral s.
flow-limiting s.
focal eccentric s.
focal pulmonary vein s.
geometry of s.
granulation s.
hemodynamically significant s.
high-grade s.
hourglass s.
hypertrophic muscular subaortic s.
 (HMSAS)
hypertrophic subaortic s. (HSAS,
 HSS)
idiopathic hypertrophic subaortic s.
 (IHSS)
infundibular pulmonary s. (IPS)
in-segment s.

in-stent s.
left main coronary s.
linear s.
long axis-discrete subaortic s.
 (LAX-DSS)
low-gradient aortic s. (LGAS)
mitral s. (MS)
muscular subaortic s. (MSS)
myocardial infundibular s.
napkin-ring s.
nodular aortic s.
nonrheumatic valvular aortic s.
orificial s.
ostial s.
percent diameter s. (%DS)
peripheral pulmonary artery s.
 (PPAS)
peripheral pulmonic s. (PPS)
point of critical s.
postdiphtheritic s.
preinterventional high-grade s.
preventricular s.
prosthetic valve s. (PVS)
proximal s.
pulmonary s. (PS)
pulmonary arterial s. (PAS)
pulmonary artery s.
pulmonary branch s. (PBS)
pulmonary valve s.
pulmonary valvular s. (PVS)
pulmonic s. (PS)
pulmonic valve s.
radiotherapy-induced carotid s.
relative mitral s.
renal artery s. (RAS)
residual s.
s. resistance
rheumatic mitral s. (RMS)
rheumatic mitral valve s.
segmental s.
semilunar valve s.
senescent aortic s.
s. severity
silent mitral s.
single-vessel coronary s.
spotty predicted s.
subaortic s. (SAS, SS)
subglottic s.
subinfundibular s.
subpulmonary s.
subpulmonic s.
subvalvar aortic s.
subvalvar mitral s.
subvalvar pulmonary s.
supravalvar aortic s. (SAS, SVAS)
supravalvar pulmonary s.
supraventricular aortic s. (SVAS)
symptomatic aortic s.
tight s.

stenosis *(continued)*
    tracheobronchial s.
    tricuspid s. (TS)
    tunnel subaortic s.
    valvular aortic s.
    valvular pulmonic s.
    vascular s.
    Waterston anastomosis for
      congenital pulmonary s.
    X-linked aqueductal s. (XLAS)
stenothorax
stenotic
    s. flow reserve (SFR)
    s. jet
    s. lesion
    s. portion
    s. valvular heart disease
Stenotrophomonas maltophilia
stent
    Abbott TriMaxx drug-eluting s.
    Abbott ZoMaxx drug-eluting s.
    Absolute self-expanding s.
    access by radial artery multilink s.
      (ARMS)
    Acculink self-expanding s.
    ACS Multi-Link Duet coronary s.
    ACS Multi-Link RX Ultra s.
    ACS Multi-Link Tristar s.
    activated balloon expandable
      intravascular s.
    ACT-One s.
    Alveolus s.
    AneuRx s.
    angiopeptin-eluting s.
    antirestenotic s.
    s. apposition
    aSpire covered s.
    autologous vein graft-coated s.
      (AVGCS)
    AVE S540, S670 s.
    Axxion drug-eluting s.
    balloon-expandable flexible coil s.
    balloon-expandable intravascular s.
    Bard XT coronary s.
    bare metal s. (BMS)
    batimastat-coated BiodivYsio
      vascular s.
    BeStent 2 coronary s.
    BeStent Rival s.
    bifurcated s.
    biocompatible s.
    biodegradable s.
    BioDiamond F s.
    BioDiamond Micro s.
    BiodivYsio added support s.
    BiodivYsio AS PC-coated s.
    BiodivYsio OC over-the-wire s.
    BiodivYsio open cell s.
    BiodivYsio PC s.

BiodivYsio phosphorylcholine-coated
  coronary s.
BiodivYsio small vessel s.
BiodivYsio SV OTW s.
BiodivYsio SV PC-coated s.
BiodivYsio vascular s.
Biotronik Rithron-XR coronary s.
Biotronik Tenax s.
Biotronik Tensum s.
Bridge Assurant balloon-
  expandable s.
Bridge balloon-expandable s.
BxSonic coronary s.
Bx Velocity coronary artery s.
Bypass Speedy s.
Carbostent coronary s.
CardioCoil coronary s.
carotid s.
cell-coated s.
cell-seeded s.
cobalt alloy coronary s.
cobalt chromium s. (CoStar)
coil s.
Conor s.
Cook intracoronary s.
Cordis Bx Velocity s.
Cordis CrossFlex coronary s.
Cordis tantalum coil s.
Corinthian s.
coronary artery s.
CoStar s.
s. creep
CrossFlex coil s.
CrossFlex LC-stainless steel, laser-
  cut coronary s.
Crown s.
cutting balloon before s.
  (CBBEST)
Cypher sirolimus-eluting coronary s.
s. delivery system (SDS)
s. deployment
diaphragm of s.
DISA S-Flex coronary s.
DNA-coated s.
double-J s.
s. dressing
Driver coronary s.
drug-eluting s. (DES)
drug-loaded biodegradable
  polymer s.
Duet coronary s.
Dumon endobronchial silicone s.
Dumon tracheobronchial s.
Dumon Y s.
Dynamic Y s.
Elastalloy Ultraflex Strecker
  nitinol s.
Elgiloy s.
eluting s.

s. embolization
emergency bailout s.
Enforcer SDS coronary s.
Expander s.
s. expansion
Express balloon-expandable s.
flat wire coil s.
Flex s.
flexible coil s.
fork s.
Freitag s.
Genesis balloon-expandable s.
Genus s.
GFX Micro s. III
GFX over-the-wire coronary s.
Gianturco expandable wire s.
  (GEWS)
Gianturco-Roubin Flex II s.
Gianturco-Roubin Flex-Stent
  coronary s.
Gianturco Z s.
Global Therapeutics V-Flex s.
gold-coated Inflow coronary s.
gold-coated NIR s.
s. graft (SG)
Guidant Vision Multi-Link S.
heat-activated recoverable
  temporary s. (HARTS)
helical coil s.
HepaCoat coronary s.
Hepamed-coated s.
Herculink balloon-expandable s.
Hood stoma s.
hybrid s.
Igaki-Tamai s.
s. implantation
Infinnium Paclitaxel system drug-
  eluting s.
InStent VascuCoil s.
IntraCoil self-expanding nitinol s.
IntraCoil self-expanding
  peripheral s.
IntraStent DoubleStrut s.
intravascular s.
INX s.
Iris coronary s.
Iris II s.
s. jail
J & J s.
Johnson & Johnson coronary s.
Johnson & Johnson Interventional
  Systems s.
Jostent coronary s.
kissing s.'s
laser-cut, self-expanding nitinol s.
Liberté s.
LifeStent self-expanding s.
Logic coronary s.
Logic drug-eluting s.

low-profile, balloon-expandable s.
LP s.
Luminexx self-expanding s.
Mac s.
Magic Wallstent s.
Medex coronary C1 s.
Medinol NIR s.
Medivent self-expanding coronary s.
Medivent vascular s.
Medtronic 57 s.
Medtronic AVE S660 coronary s.
Medtronic BeStent s.
Medtronic Driver s.
Medtronic interventional vascular s.
Medtronic MicroDriver coronary s.
Memotherm s.
mesh s.
metallic s.
MicroDriver coronary s.
s. migration
Mini Crown s.
multicellular s.
Multi-Link Ascent s.
Multi-Link Duet coronary s.
Multi-Link Penta coronary s.
Multi-Link Pixel coronary s.
Multi-Link Solo s.
Multi-Link Tetra coronary s.
Multi-Link Ultra coronary s.
Neville s.
NexStent carotid s.
Nexus coronary s.
NIR s.
NIRflex coronary s.
nitinol mesh s.
nitinol self-expandable s.
nitinol self-expanding coil s.
nitinol thermal memory s.
nonarticulated s.
nonpolymer-based paclitaxel-
  eluting s.
nonpolymer-based rapamycin-
  eluting s.
nuclear s.
Omega s.
Omnilink balloon-expandable s.
ostial s.
s. overlap
paclitaxel-coated coronary s.
paclitaxel-eluting s. (PES)
Palmaz Genesis s.
Palmaz-Schatz s. (PSS)
Palmaz-Schatz balloon-expandable s.
Palmaz-Schatz coronary s.
Palmaz-Schatz Crown s.
Palmaz-Schatz PS-204 s.
Palmaz vascular s.
Paragon coronary s.
Paragon nitinol s.

S

stent *(continued)*

Paragon PAS s.
s. patency
PC-coated s.
Penta s.
Phytis s.
s. placement
Polyflex s.
poly-L-lactic acid s.
polymeric endoluminal paving s.
polyorganophosphazene-coated s.
polypropylene s.
polytetrafluoroethylene covered s.
Power Grip s.
^{32}P radioactive s.
Precise self-expanding s.
predilated polytetrafluoroethylene s.
premounted s.
Protg GPS nitinol self-expanding
long s.
PS 153 s.
PTFE-covered s.
Pura-Vario s.
QuaDDS s.
Quanam QP2 coronary s.
Quanam QuaDDS s.
Racer balloon-expandable s.
radioactive s.
radiopaque tantalum s.
Radius self-expanding s.
s. reconstruction
restenosed s.
Rithron-XR coronary s.
R-Stent s.
s. sandwich
Schatz-Palmaz intravascular s.
Schneider Speedy s.
Scimed s.
S7 coronary s.
S670 coronary s.
screw-thread s.
self-expandable metallic s.
self-expanding s. (SES)
self-expanding microporous s.
(SEMS)
self-expanding nitinol s.
self-expanding wire mesh s.
Sentinel self-expanding s.
short s.
silicone s.
simultaneous kissing s. (SKS)
sirolimus-coated s.
sirolimus-eluting s. (SES)
slotted tube articulated s.
Smart Control self-expanding s.
Sorin Carbostent s.
spring-loaded vascular s.
S660 small vessel coronary s.

stainless steel balloon
expandable s.
stainless steel mesh s.
Strecker balloon-expandable s.
Strecker tantalum s.
s. strut
STS s.
Supra G coronary s.
s. or surgery
Symbiot covered s.
Symbiot PTFE-covered s.
Symphony nitinol s.
T s.
tantalum s.
Taxus coronary s.
Taxus drug-eluting s.
Taxus Express s.
Taxus Libèrtè s.
Terumo s.
Tetra coronary s.
thermal memory s.
thermoexpandable s.
s. thrombosis (ST)
Tristar coronary s.
T-shaped s.
tubular slotted s.
T-Y s.
Ultra s.
Ultraflex nitinol s.
Ultraflex self-expanding s.
Ultraflex tracheobronchial s.
VascuCoil peripheral vascular s.
Velocity s.
Veriflex s.
V-Flex FMJ s.
V-Flex Plus s.
Viabahn covered s.
Vision bare-metal s.
Wallgraft s.
Wallstent flexible, self-expanding
wire-mesh s.
Wallstent Magic s.
Wallstent Monorail carotid s.
Wallstent spring-loaded s.
Westaby tracheobronchial silicone s.
Wiktor balloon expandable
coronary s.
Wiktor GX coronary s.
Wiktor-I implantable s.
wire mesh self-expandable s.
Xact carotid s.
Xceed self-expanding s.
Xience V everolimus eluting
coronary s.
XT radiopaque coronary s.
X-Trode s.
Y s.
Z s.
Zeta s.

zigzag s.
Zilver self-expanding s.
Zilver vascular s.
ZoMaxx drug-eluting s.
stent-anchoring device
stent-assisted coiling of basilar fusiform aneurysm
stented bioprosthetic valve
stent-graft
Ancure s.-g.
Hemobahn s.-g.
Inoue endovascular s.-g.
Lifepath s.-g.
s.-g. placement
transluminally placed Inoue endovascular s.-g.
Viabahn endoprosthesis s.-g.
stenting
airway s.
bailout s.
Brockenbrough atrial s.
carotid angioplasty and s. (CAS)
carotid artery s.
conduit s.
coronary s.
direct s.
drug-delivery s.
endoluminal s.
femoropopliteal s.
high-pressure balloon s.
intracoronary s.
kissing s.
provisional side-branch s.
provisional spot s.
side-branch s.
s. in small arteries (SISA)
transradial primary s.
Y s.
stent-jail orifice
stentless
s. porcine aortic valve
s. porcine aortic valve prosthesis
s. porcine bioprosthesis
s. porcine valve (SPV)
s. porcine xenograft
s. tissue valve
stent-mounted
s.-m. allograft valve
s.-m. heterograft valve
stent/system
stent-to-artery (S/A)
STEP
short transitional edge protection
step
Krönig s.'s
s. treadmill protocol
2-step
2-s. dilation
2-s. exercise test

step-down therapy
Step-One Diet
stepped bur approach
stepped-care antihypertensive regimen
Step-Two Diet
step-up in oxygen saturation
stepwise
Sterapred Oral
stercoralis
Strongyloides s.
stereoauscultation
stereolithography
stereoscopic interrogation
Steri-Cath catheter
sterilant
sterile saline aerosol
Steri-Neb
Sterles sign
Sterling Edwards procedure
sternad
sternal
s. border
s. compression
s. dehiscence
s. extremity of clavicle
s. fracture
s. notch
s. part of diaphragm
s. plane
s. synchondrosis
s. wiring
sternalgia
sternal-splitting incision
Sternberg
S. myocardial insufficiency
S. pericarditis
S. sign
Sterneedle tuberculin test
sternochondral junction
sternoclavicular angle
sternocleidomastoid artery
sternocostal triangle
sternodynia
sternomastoid
sternotomy
median s.
sternotracheal
sternoxiphoid plane
Stern posture
sternum
s. saw
wiring of s.
steroid
s. aerosol
anabolic s.
s. elution
high-dose s.
nasal s. (NS)

S

steroid *(continued)*
    sex s.
    stanozolol anabolic s.
steroid-dependent
    s.-d. asthma
    s.-d. asthmatic
steroid-eluting
    s.-e. electrode
    s.-e. pacemaker lead
steroidogenesis
steroid-resistant
    s.-r. asthma (SRA)
    s.-r. BOOP
    s.-r. bronchiolitis obliterans organizing pneumonia
steroids
    stress-dose s.
steroid-sparing agent
sterol
    plant s.
    s. regulatory element-binding protein (SREBP)
stertor
    hen-cluck s.
stertorous respiration
Stertzer
    S. brachial catheter
    S. guiding catheter
STET
    submaximal treadmill exercise test
stethoscope
    Acoustascope esophageal s.
    bell s.
    Cardiology II s.
    Classic II s.
    differential s.
    Doppler fetal s.
    double-headed s.
    E-Scope II electronic s.
    Harvey Elite s.
    Labtron s.
    Littman class II pediatric s.
    Rappaport-Sprague s.
    ST3 amplified s.
stethoscopic phonocardiograph
Stevens-Johnson syndrome
Stewart-Hamilton cardiac output technique
STG
    superior temporal gyrus
sthenic fever
ST/HR
    ST-segment divided by heart rate
    ST/HR index
    ST/HR slope
STI
    systolic time interval
stibogluconate sodium

stick
    arterial s.
    Vaxcel mini s.
Stifcore
    S. aspiration needle
    S. biopsy injection needle
stiff
    s. heart
    s. heart syndrome
    s. left atrium syndrome
    s. lung
stiffness
    active dynamic s.
    arterial s.
    chamber s.
    diastolic s.
    dynamic s.
    elastic s.
    end-diastolic chamber s. (EDCS)
    s. index
    muscle s.
    myocardial s.
    systolic s.
    vascular s.
    ventricular systolic s.
    volume s.
stigma, pl. **stigmata**
    peripheral stigmata
Still
    S. disease
    S. murmur
Stilphostrol
stimulant
    adrenergic s.
stimulated acoustic emission
stimulation
    alpha-adrenergic s.
    atrial s.
    beta-adrenergic s. (BAS)
    beta-1 adrenergic s.
    beta-2 adrenergic s.
    beta adrenoceptor s.
    beta-2 adrenoreceptor s.
    biventricular pacing s.
    blood monocyte s.
    carotid sinus s.
    s. catheter
    chest wall s. (CWS)
    direct s.
    functional magnetic s.
    intracardiac s.
    muscarinic s.
    neurohormonal s.
    noninvasive programmed s. (NIPS)
    paired electrical s.
    postganglionic vagal s. (PGVS)
    programmed electrical s. (PES)
    programmed ventricular s. (PVS)
    rapid atrial s. (RAS)

reflex s.
slaved programmed electrical s.
spinal cord s. (SCS)
subthreshold s.
supramaximal tetanic s.
synchronous atrial s. (SAS)
s. threshold
transcutaneous electrical s. (TES)
transesophageal atrial s. (TRAS)
ultrarapid subthreshold s.
vagal s.
vagus nerve s.
ventricular-programmed s.
stimulator
Atrostim phrenic nerve s.
Bloom programmable s.
Grass S88 muscle s.
InSync multisite cardiac s.
stimulus, pl. **stimuli**
chemical s.
chemoattracting stimuli
heterotopic s.
hypercapnic s.
hyperemic s.
ischemic-type preconditioning s.
neurohumoral s.
pacing s.
paired s.
physical s.
preconditioning s.
premature atrial s. (PAS)
psychological s.
square wave s.
thrombogenic s.
train-of-4 s.
triple s.
stimulus-T interval
Stinger S ablation catheter
stippled calcification
stippling of lung field
sTNFR
soluble tumor necrosis factor receptor
stochastic
s. effect
s. risk
Stockert 70 RF generator
stocking-glove distribution
stockings
Bellavar medical support s.
Carolon life support
antiembolism s.
compression s.
elastic s.
Fast-Fit vascular s.
Florex medical compression s.
graduated compression s. (GCS)
Jobst Vairox gradient compression
vascular s.
Juzo s.

pneumatic compression s.
Sigvaris compression s.
TED antiembolism s.
thigh-high antiembolic s.
Vairox high compression
vascular s.
venous pressure gradient support s.
(VPGSS)
Zimmer antiembolism support s.
stocking-seam incision
stoichiometric fashion
Stokes
collar of S.
Stokes-Adams
S.-A. attack
S.-A. disease
S.-A. syndrome
Stokvis-Talma syndrome
Stoll pneumonia
stoma, pl. **stomas, stomata**
tracheostomy s.
stomach
s. cough
left coronary artery of s.
Stomatococcus
stone
cholesterol s. (CS)
s. cutter's phthisis
s. heart
lung s.
s. stripper's asthma
stone-like myxoma
stool
melenic s.
stopcock
3-way s.
stopped flow pressure (SFP)
stop-valve airway obstruction
storage
s. cardiomyopathy
continuous electrogram s.
electrogram s.
tracer s.
store
myocyte magnesium s.
stored electrocardiogram
storm
electric s.
thyroid s.
Stormer OTW balloon dilation catheter
Storz bronchoscope
Storz-Hopkins laryngoscope
STP
standard temperature and pulse
straddling
s. aorta
s. atrioventricular valve
s. embolism
s. thrombus

S

straddling *(continued)*
  s. tricuspid valve
  s. of valve
straight
  s. back syndrome
  s. blade
  s. flush percutaneous catheter
  s. hemostat
  s. sinus thrombosis
  s. stylet
  s. tipped catheter
  s. tube graft
straight-line ECG
StraightShot arterial cannula
straight-tined pacing lead
strain
  avian influenza virus s. H5N1
    (AIV H5N1, AIV H5N1, H5N1)
  carer s.
  cell s.
  Eulerian s.
  0157-H7 s.
  Lagrangian s.
  left heart s. (LHS)
  left ventricular s. (LVS)
  natural s.
strain-gauge plethysmography
stramonium
strand
  iridium s.
stranding effusion
strandy infiltrate
strap
  hook-and-loop fastener s.
  s. muscle
  Pepper Medical Antidisconnect
    Device s.
Strasburger cell plate
strategy, pl. **strategies**
  lung volume s.
  protective ventilator s.
  treatment s.
  ventilatory s.
stratification
  postinfarction risk s. (PIRS)
  risk s.
stratified thrombus
stratify
  risk s.
stratigraphy
stratum segmentorum
Stratus cardiac troponin I test
Straub Aspirex pulmonary embolectomy catheter
Strauss method
strawberry tongue
streak
  fatty s.

streaking
  basophilic vascular s.
streaky infiltrate
Strecker
  S. balloon-expandable stent
  S. tantalum stent
strength
  Allerest Maximum S.
  Bayer Low Adult S.
  double s. (DS)
  peripheral muscle s.
  s. training
strenuous exercise
Streptase
streptavidin
Streptobacillus moniliformis
streptococcal
  s. antibody
  s. bacteremia
  s. bronchitis
  s. carditis
  s. empyema
  s. endocarditis
  s. infection
  s. pneumonia
Streptococcus
  S. *acidominimus*
  S. *agalactiae*
  S. *anginosus*
  S. *anginosus-constellatus*
  S. *faecalis*
  group A S. (GAS)
  S. *milleri*
  S. *mitis*
  S. *pneumoniae*
  S. *pneumoniae*
  S. *pyogenes*
  S. *pyogenes* infection
  S. *salivarius*
  S. *viridans*
streptodornase
streptogramin antibiotic
streptokinase (SK)
  s. antibody
  intracoronary s. (ICSK)
streptokinase-plasminogen complex
streptokinase-streptodornase
streptokinase-urokinase myocardial infarct test (SUMIT)
streptolysin O
Streptomyces tsukubaensis
streptomycin sulfate
streptozocin
STRESS
  subject's treatment-emergent symptom
    scale
stress
  adenosine s.

circumferential end-systolic s.
(cESS)
circumferential wall s. (CWS)
dipyridamole s.
S. Echo bed
s. echocardiography
s. electrocardiography (SECG)
emotional s.
end-diastolic circumferential s.
(EDCS)
end-systolic s. (ESS)
end-systolic circumferential wall s.
end-systolic left ventricular s.
end-systolic wall s. (ESWS)
handgrip s.
left ventricular end-systolic
circumferential wall s.
left ventricular end-systolic wall s.
(LVESWS)
left ventricular wall s.
mental s.
meridional wall s.
s. MUGA electrocardiogram
nitrosative s.
oxidant s.
oxidative s.
s. perfusion and rest function
s. perfusion and rest function by
sestamibi gated SPECT
s. perfusion scintigraphy
pharmacologic s.
physiological s.
s. relaxation
shear s.
s. signaling pathway
s. SPECT perfusion imaging
tend-and-befriend response to s.
tensile s.
s. test (ST)
s. thallium-201 myocardial
perfusion imaging
s. thallium scintigraphy
ventricular end-systolic wall s.
wall s.
s. washout myocardial perfusion
image
stress-activated protein kinase (SAPK)
stress-dose steroids
**stress-injected sestamibi-gated SPECT
with echocardiography**
stressor
remedial psychological s.
**stress-redistribution-reinjection thallium-
201 imaging**
stress-related
s.-r. arrhythmia
s.-r. hypertension
s.-r. mucosal disease (SRMD)
stress-shortening relationship

stretch
atrial s.
s. receptor
stretched
s. bronchus sign
s. diameter
**stretch-induced cardiomyocyte
hypertrophy**
stretching
side s.
s. syncope
stria, pl. **striae**
striae cutis distensae
lipidic s.
striation
tabby cat s.
tigroid s.
striatocapsular infarction
stricture
anastomotic s.
esophageal s.
Wickwitz esophageal s.
strident
stridor
biphasic s.
congenital laryngeal s.
inspiratory s.
laryngeal s.
Münchausen s.
psychogenic s.
respiratory s.
s. serraticus
stridulosa
laryngitis s.
stridulous respiration
stridulus
laryngismus s.
strike
heel s.
string
s. of pearls
s. sign
strip
bovine pericardium s.
Breathe Right nasal s.
cardiac monitor s.
Cover-Strip wound closure s.'s
ECG monitor s.
felt s.
nasal s.
s. percussion
rhythm s.
stripchart tracing
stripe
s. sign
subepicardial fat s.
stripper
Alexander rib s.
Dorian rib s.

S

stripper *(continued)*
   hydraulic vein s.
   Kurten vein s.
   Linton vein s.
   Matson-Alexander rib s.
   rib s.
   thrombus s.
   Zollinger-Gilmore intraluminal
      vein s.
stroke
   acute caudate s.
   acute hemispheric s.
   acute ischemic s. (AIS)
   atheroembolic s.
   atherothrombotic s.
   s. belt
   brain stem s.
   bulbar s.
   cardioembolic s. (CES)
   cardiogenic s.
   caudate hemorrhagic s.
   caudate ischemic s.
   cortical s.
   crude s.
   cryptogenic s.
   early progressing s. (EPS)
   effective s.
   s. ejection rate
   embolic s.
   s. guidance system (SGS)
   heart s.
   heat s.
   hemorrhagic s.
   S. Impact Scale (SIS)
   s. index (SI)
   ipsilateral s.
   ischemic s.
   lacunar s.
   late progressing s. (LPS)
   left hemisphere s. (LCVA)
   light s.
   migraine s.
   mini s.
   MRI-identified s.
   National Institutes of Neurological
      Disorders and S. (NINDS)
   s. output
   pure motor s.
   pure sensorimotor s.
   pure sensory s.
   right hemisphere s.
   sensorimotor s.
   silent s.
   subcortical s.
   thromboembolic s.
   undetermined pathological-type s.
   s. unit (SU)
   s. volume (SV)
   s. volume index (SVI)

   s. work (SW, S/W)
   s. work index (SWI)
stroke-specific quality of life (SS-QOL)
stroma-free
   s.-f. hemoglobin pyridoxalated
      (SFHb)
   s.-f. hemoglobin solution
strong
   Thyroid S.
   S. unbridling of celiac artery axis
Strongyloides stercoralis
strongyloidiasis
strontium-82 (^{82}So)
Stroop
   S. color word conflict test
   S. color word interference test
Strophanthus gratus
Strouhal number
structural
   s. heart disease (SHD)
   s. valve deterioration (SVD)
structure
   chordal s.
   echodense s.
   tubuloreticular s.
   vestigial s.
   wall s.
structured interview
struma, pl. **strumae**
   Riedel s.
strut
   central bridging s.
   George Washington s.
   outlet s.
   stent s.
   s. thickness
   tricuspid valve s.
   variable thickness s. (VTS)
strutting
   plaque s.
Stryker saw
STS
   Society of Thoracic Surgeons
   STS stent
ST-segment
   ST-s. alternans
   ST-s. changes
   ST-s. coving
   ST-s. depression (STD)
   ST-s. displacement
   ST-s. divided by heart rate
      (ST/HR)
   ST-s. elevation
   ST-s. elevation myocardial
      infarction (STEMI)
   ST-s. reelevation
   ST-s. resolution
ST-T
   ST-T. deviation

ST-T. segment changes
ST-T. vector
ST-T. wave
ST-T. wave changes

STT
    serial thrombin time
Stuart-Prower factor
study, pl. **studies** (*See also* trial, program, protocol)
    bubble s.
    case-control s.
    electrophysiologic s.
    elegant s.
    flow-volume loop studies
    Persantine myocardial perfusion s.
    postoperative pacing s. (POPS)
    segmental arterial Doppler s.
stuffer
stump
    bronchial s.
    cardiac s.
    s. pressure
stunned
    s. atrium
    s. myocardium
stunning
    atrial s.
    left atrial appendage s.
    myocardial s.
    repetitive s.
stupor
    spike-wave s. (SWS)
Sturge-Weber syndrome
stuttering
    s. myocardial infarction
    s. of perfusion
stutzeri
    Pseudallescheria s.
    Pseudomonas s.
stylet
    Bing s.
    Cook locking s.
    K s.
    Liberator locking s.
    lighted s.
    locking s.
    straight s.
    transmyocardial pacing s.
    transthoracic pacing s.
    wire s.
styrene asthma
SU
    stroke unit
Sub-4 small vessel balloon dilation catheter
subacute
    s. bacterial endocarditis (SBE)
    s. bronchopneumonia
    s. care

s. coronary disease (SCD)
s. infective endocarditis
s. myocardial infarction
s. pericarditis
s. suppurative infection
s. tamponade
s. thrombosis (SAT)
s. unit
s. ventricular free wall
subantihypertensive dose
subanular mattress suture
subaortic
    s. lymph node
    s. obstruction
    s. stenosis (SAS, SS)
subapicale
    segmentum s.
subapical segment
subarachnoid
    s. hemorrhage (SAH)
    s. space (SAS)
subcarinal node
subcellular mechanism
subclavian
    s. approach for cardiac catheterization
    s. arteriovenous fistula
    s. artery
    s. artery bypass graft
    s. flap
    s. flap aortoplasty (SFA)
    s. lymphatic
    s. murmur
    s. peel-away sheath
    s. steal
    s. steal syndrome
    s. triangle
    s. vein
    s. vein catheterization (SVC)
    s. vein thrombosis (SVT)
    s. vessel
subclavian-carotid bypass
subclavian-subclavian bypass
subclavicular murmur
subclinical
    s. asthma
    s. atherosclerotic disease
    s. hypothyroidism
subcoronary aortic valve implantation
subcortical
    s. junctional infarct
    s. stroke
    s. vascular encephalopathy (SVE)
subcostal
    s. outflow
    s. right ventricle view
    s. zone
subcrepitant rale

S

subcutanea
  bursa s.
subcutaneous
  s. bursa
  s. bursa of laryngeal prominence
  s. emphysema
  s. nodule
  s. patch
  s. patch electrode
  s. suture
  s. tunneling device
subcuticular suture
subdiaphragmatic abscess
subdural hematoma (SDH)
subendocardial
  s. to epicardial resting perfusion ratio
  s. fibrosis
  s. infarction (SEI)
  s. ischemia
  s. layer
  s. myocardial infarction (SEMI)
  s. sclerosis
  s. zone
subendocardium
subendothelial matrix
subendothelium
subepicardial
  s. fat stripe
  s. fatty infiltration
  s. ventricular tachycardia
subepithelial fibrosis
suberosis
subeustachian isthmus
subfascial endoscopic perforator surgery (SEPS)
subgaleal emphysema
subglottic
  s. laryngitis
  s. secretion
  s. stenosis
subinfundibular stenosis
subjective fremitus
subject's treatment-emergent symptom scale (STRESS)
subjunctional heart block
sublethal
Sublimaze Injection
sublingual
  s. artery
  s. bursa
  s. carbon dioxide level
  s. caruncula
  s. CO_2
  s. crescent
  s. gland
  Nitrostat s.
  s. vein

sublingualis
  bursa s.
  caruncula s.
  glandula s.
  vena s.
submassive pulmonary embolism
submaximal
  s. effort tourniquet test
  s. heart rate
  s. maneuver
  s. treadmill exercise test (STET)
submaximum heart rate
submucosa
  airway s.
submucosal
  s. gland
  s. gland hypertrophy
  s. plaque
submucous
suboptimally visualized
suboptimal visualization
subpectoral
  s. implantation of cardioverter-defibrillator
  s. implantation of pulse generator
subpharyngeal
subphrenic
  s. abscess
  s. recess
  s. space
subphysiological
  s. volume
  s. volumes of gas
subpleural
  s. caseous focus
  s. edema
  s. honeycombing
subpulmonary
  s. obstruction
  s. stenosis
  s. ventricle
  s. VSD
subpulmonic
  s. effusion
  s. stenosis
Sub-Q-Set subcutaneous continuous infusion device
Subramanian clamp
subsalicylate
  bismuth s.
subsarcolemmal cisterna
subsartorial tunnel
subscript
subsegment
subsegmental
  s. atelectasis
  s. bronchus
  s. transcatheter arterial embolization (STAE)

subselection catheter
subset
 T-cell s.
subsidiary atrial pacemaker
substance
 digoxin-like immunoreactive s. (DLIS)
 myocardial depressant s. (MDS)
 neurotransmitter s.
 s. P
 paramagnetic s.
 proinflammatory s.
 rabbit aorta-contracting s. (RCS)
 thiobarbituric acid-reactive s. (TBARS)
 vasoactive s.
 vasoconstrictor s. (VCS)
 vasodepressor s.
 vasodilator s. (VDS)
substernal thyroid
substitute
 blood s.
 fat s.
 hemoglobin product s.
 Hemolink investigational hemoglobin product or blood s.
 Nu-Trim dietary fat s.
 PolyHeme blood s.
substitutional cardiac surgery
substrate
 arrhythmogenic s.
 enzyme s.
 exogenous s.
 fluorogenic s.
 s. gel zymography
 s. metabolism
 neural s.
 tachyarrhythmic s.
subsuperior segment
subsuperius
 segmentum s.
subthreshold
 s. pacing
 s. stimulation
subtilis
 Bacillus s.
subtilisin
subtraction
 s. angiography
 digital s.
 functional s.
 intraoperative digital s. (IDIS)
 mask-mode s.
subtype
 Sudan s.
 Zaire s.
subvalvar, subvalvular
 s. aortic obstruction (SAO)
 s. aortic stenosis

 s. apparatus
 s. mitral stenosis
 s. obstruction
 s. pulmonary stenosis
 s. thickening (SVTh)
subventricular (SV)
subxiphoid
 s. area
 s. limited pericardiotomy
 s. window
succession of losses
succinate
 cifenline s.
 hydrocortisone hydrogen s.
 hydrocortisone sodium s.
 methylprednisolone s.
 metoprolol s.
succinylcholine chloride
succussion
 hippocratic s.
 s. sounds
 s. splash
sucker
 intracardiac s.
sucking chest wound
suck reflex
Sucquet anastomosis
Sucquet-Hoyer anastomosis
suction
 diastolic s.
 s. feeling
 hydrostatic s.
 nasotracheal s.
 pleural s.
 Pleur-evac s.
suctioning
 cuff s.
SudaCare Shower Soothers
Sudafed
 S. Cold & Cough Liquid cap
 S. Severe Cold
Sudan subtype
sudden
 s. arrhythmic death syndrome (SADS)
 s. cardiac arrest (SCA)
 s. cardiac death (SCD)
 s. coronary death (SCD)
 s. death heart disease (SDHD)
 s. death ischemic heart disease (SDIHD)
 s. heart death (SHD)
 s. infant death syndrome (SIDS)
 s. rate onset
 s. unexplained death
 s. unexplained death syndrome (SUDS)
 s. unexplained nocturnal death (SUND)

S

sudden *(continued)*
>s. unexplained nocturnal death syndrome

SUDS
>sudden unexplained death syndrome

sufentanil citrate
suffocate
suffocating gas
suffocation
suffocative
>s. bronchitis
>s. catarrh
>s. goiter

sugar
>blood s.
>capillary blood s. (CBS)
>S. clip
>fasting blood s.
>postprandial blood s.
>s. tumor

Sugarbaker staging system
Sugita clip
Sugiura procedure
suicide ventricle
suis
>*Actinobacillus s.*
>bronchus s.

suit
>antigravity s., anti-G s.
>Life S.
>MAST s.

Sular
sulbactam
>ampicillin and s.

sulcus, pl. **sulci**
>atrioventricular s.
>bulboventricular s.
>coronary s.
>costophrenic s.
>interventricular s.
>intraparietal s. (IPS)
>s. pulmonalis
>pulmonary s.
>s. terminalis

sulfadiazine
>silver s.
>s., sulfamethazine, sulfamerazine

sulfadoxine and pyrimethamine
sulfamerazine
>sulfadiazine, sulfamethazine, s.

sulfamethoxazole/trimethoprim (SMX/TMP)
sulfasalazine
sulfate
>amikacin s.
>amphetamine s.
>atropine s.
>bleomycin s.
>Capastat S.

capreomycin s.
cholesterol s. (CS)
chondroitin s.
codeine s.
debrisoquine s.
dermatan s.
dextran s.
dextroamphetamine s.
dimethyl s.
ephedrine s.
ferrous s.
gentamicin s.
guanadrel s.
guanethidine s.
hydroxychloroquine s.
isoprenaline s.
isoproterenol s.
lobeline s.
magnesium s.
metaproterenol s.
neomycin s.
netilmicin s.
orciprenaline s.
paromomycin s.
penbutolol s.
protamine s.
quinidine s.
quinine s.
sodium tetradecyl s.
streptomycin s.
terbutaline s.
trimethoprim s.
trospectomycin s.
vinblastine s.
vincristine s.
Wyamine S.

Sulfatrim DS
sulfhemoglobin level
sulfhydryl depletion hypothesis
sulfide
>hydrogen s.
>selenium s.

sulfinpyrazone
sulfisoxazole
>erythromycin and s.
>s. and phenazopyridine

sulfonamide sensitivity
sulfonate
>sodium polystyrene s.

sulfonylurea
sulfosalicylic acid
sulfotepp
sulfoxide
>albendazole s.
>dimethyl s.

sulfur
>s. dioxide (SO_2)
>s. hexafluoride (SF_6)

sulindac

Sullivan
    S. bubble cushion
    S. HumidAire heated humidifier
    S. III CPAP
    S. Mirage nasal mask
    S. nasal variable positive airway
    pressure unit
    S. V Elite Real Time Clock
    CPAP machine
    S. VPAP II
sulmazole
Sulphan Blue
sum
    ray s.
sumatriptan
SUMIT
    streptokinase-urokinase myocardial
    infarct test
summation
    s. beat
    s. gallop (S_7)
    impulse s.
    s. shadow
summed stress score (SSS)
sump pump
Sumycin Oral
SunBox light box
SUND
    sudden unexplained nocturnal death
    SUND syndrome
sundowning
Sundt carotid endarterectomy shunt
sunflower asthma
**Sunshine Heart C-Pulse implantable
mechanical heart assist device**
super
    S. ArrowFlex catheterization sheath
    s. stress test
    S. Torque Plus catheter
Super-4 catheter ablation system
superantigen
    Staphylococcus aureus s. (SSAg)
superdicrotic
superDimension bronchus system
superdominant artery
superficial
    s. circumflex iliac vein
    s. external pudendal artery
    s. femoral artery (SFA)
    s. medial artery of foot
    s. phlebitis
    s. pneumonia
superficialis
    esophagitis dissecans s.
    vena circumflexa iliaca s.
superimposed
    s. echodensity

    s. pregnancy-induced hypertension
    (SPIH)
    s. thrombosis
superimposition
superinfection
    bacterial s.
superior
    arteria glutealis s.
    arteria laryngea s.
    s. articular facet of atlas
    s. carotid artery
    s. cerebellar artery (SCA)
    s. costal facet
    s. femoral artery (SFA)
    fovea costalis s.
    s. laryngeal artery
    s. laryngeal cavity
    s. laryngeal nerve
    s. laryngeal vein
    s. lobe
    s. lobe of right/left lung
    s. mesenteric artery (SMA)
    s. mesenteric artery bypass
    s. mesenteric artery filling
    s. mesenteric artery syndrome
    s. mesenteric vascular occlusion
    s. mesenteric vein
    s. omental recess
    s. parietal lobule (SPL)
    s. phrenic lymph node
    posterior branch of right s.
    s. pulmonary sulcus tumor
    s. pulmonary vein
    s. pulmonary vein ablation
    s. QRS axis
    s. sagittal sinus (SSS)
    s. temporal gyrus (STG)
    s. thalamostriate vein
    s. thyroid artery
    s. tracheobronchial lymph node
    s. triangle sign
    s. vascular mediastinum
    s. vascular plexus (SVP)
    s. vena cava (SVC)
    s. vena cava compression syndrome
    (SVCCS)
    s. vena cava obstruction (SVCO)
    s. vena cava syndrome (SVCS)
    s. vena cava thrombosis
    vena laryngea s.
superiores
    nodi lymphoidei phrenici s.
    nodi lymphoidei
    tracheobronchiales s.
superioris
    ramus internus nervi laryngei s.
    ramus posterior venae pulmonalis
    dextrae s.

S

superius
>   segmentum bronchopulmonale
>   lingulare s.
>   tuberculum thyroideum s.

supernatant

supernormal
>   s. conduction
>   s. recovery phase

supernumerary bronchus

superoinferior
>   s. dimension
>   s. heart

superoxide
>   s. anion
>   s. catalase
>   s. dismutase
>   s. dismutase gene

supersaturation
>   tissue s.

supersensitivity
>   denervation s.

SuperStitch suture-mediated device

**supersystemic pulmonary artery
   pressure**

supertension

superwarfarin ingestion

supine
>   s. bicycle ergometry
>   s. bicycle stress echocardiography
>   (SBSE)
>   s. diastolic blood pressure (SDBP)
>   s. exercise
>   s. hypotension syndrome
>   s. rest gated equilibrium image

suplatast tosilate

supplement
>   Airozin nutritional s.
>   high cholesterol and tocopherol s.
>   (HCTS)
>   Vivonex Plus nutritional s.

supplemental
>   s. air
>   s. motor area (SMA)
>   s. oxygen

supplementary respiration

supplementation
>   magnesium s.

supply, pl. **supplies**
>   adequate blood s.
>   blood s.
>   energy s.
>   gas s.
>   high-pressure gas s.
>   myocardial oxygen s.
>   oxygen s.

support
>   Abee s.
>   added s. (AS)
>   advanced cardiac life s. (ACLS)
>   advanced life s. (ALS)
>   advanced trauma life s. (ATLS)
>   basic cardiac life s. (BCLS)
>   basic life s. (BLS)
>   biventricular s. (BVS)
>   bradycardia pacing s.
>   cardiopulmonary s. (CPS)
>   esophageal-directed pressure s.
>   (EDPS)
>   extracorporeal life s. (ECLS)
>   inotropic s.
>   intravenous inotropic s.
>   life s.
>   mechanical ventilatory s.
>   noninvasive positive pressure
>   ventilatory s.
>   noninvasive ventilatory s. (NIVS)
>   pediatric life s. (PALS)
>   percutaneous cardiopulmonary s.
>   (PCPS)
>   percutaneous cardiopulmonary
>   bypass s. (PCBS)
>   respiratory s.
>   vasopressor s.
>   ventilatory s.
>   volume-assured pressure s. (VAPS)

support-defibrillation
>   basic life s.-d. (BLS-D)

supported angioplasty

suppressant
>   cough s.
>   St. Joseph Cough S.

suppressed respiration

suppressible ventricular tachycardia

suppression
>   s. of arrhythmia
>   overdrive s.

suppressor
>   gastric acid s.

suppuration

suppurative
>   s. bronchiectasis
>   s. necrotizing aspergillosis
>   s. pericarditis
>   s. pleurisy
>   s. pneumonia

Supra
>   S. G coronary stent
>   Lipidil S.

supraanular, supraannular
>   s. constriction
>   s. implant
>   s. mitral valve replacement
>   (SMVR)
>   s. prosthesis
>   s. suture ring

supraaortic
>   s. ridge (SAR)
>   s. ring (SAR)

suprabulbar palsy
suprachiasmatic nucleus
supraclavicular
    s. examination
    s. fossa
    s. lymph node
    s. lymph node biopsy
supracoronary
supracristal ventricular septal defect
supradiaphragmatic
supraglottoplasty
suprahepatic caval clamp
suprahisian block
supramarginal gyrus (SMG)
supramaximal tetanic stimulation
Suprane
supranormal
    s. excitability
    s. excitation
suprapleural membrane
suprasellar aneurysm
suprasternal
    s. examination
    s. notch (SN)
    s. pulsation
    s. view
suprasternale
    spatium s.
suprastomal ring fracture
suprasystolic
supratentorial
    s. ICH
    s. intracerebral hemorrhage
suprathreshold pacing
supratonsillar recess
supratrochleares
    venae s.
supravalvar, supravalvular
    s. aortic stenosis (SAS, SVAS)
    s. aortic stenosis-infantile
      hypercalcemia syndrome
    s. aortic stenosis syndrome
    s. aortography
    s. pulmonary stenosis
supraventricular
    s. aortic stenosis (SVAS)
    s. arrhythmia
    s. crest
    s. ectopy
    s. extrasystole (SVE)
    s. premature beat (SVPB)
    s. premature complex (SVPC)
    s. premature contraction
    s. tachyarrhythmia (SVT)
    s. tachycardia (SVT)
supraventricularis
    crista s.
Suprax
Supreme electrophysiology catheter

surcingle
surdocardiac syndrome
SureGrip breathing bag
SureStepPro professional blood glucose
    management system
SureTemp electronic thermometer
surface
    s. adherent monocyte (SAM)
    articular s.
    Carmeda BioActive S.
    costal s.
    diaphragmatic s.
    high-density lipoprotein-cell s.
      (HDL-c)
    interlobar s.
    isovelocity s.
    medial s.
    s. modification technique
    pleural s.
surfactant
    aerosolized s.
    s. apoprotein B
    bovine lavage extract s. (BLES)
    s. deficiency
    heterologous s.
    hydrolysis of s.
    s. phospholipid
    s. protein (SP)
    s. protein A (SP-A)
    s. protein A, B, C
    pulmonary s.
    s. replacement therapy
surfactant-specific protein
Surfaxin
surf test
surgeon
    Society of Thoracic S.'s (STS)
    thoracic s.
surgery, pl. **surgeries**
    ablative cardiac s.
    antiarrhythmic s.
    beating heart s.
    bench s.
    bypass s.
    cardiac s.
    cardiopulmonary bypass s.
    cardiothoracic s. (CTS)
    cardiovascular s. (CVS)
    cervical plexus block for carotid
      endarterectomy s.
    closed heart s.
    computer-assisted pericardial s.
      (CASPER)
    conduit s.
    conservative s. (CS)
    coronary artery bypass s. (CABS)
    coronary artery bypass graft s.
      (CABGS)
    coronary artery bypass grafting s.

S

surgery *(continued)*
    endoscopic beating heart s.
    endoscopic vascular s. (ESVS)
    excisional cardiac s.
    extracranial/intracranial bypass s.
    heart valve replacement s.
    keyhole s.
    left ventricular reduction s.
    lung reduction s.
    lung volume reduction s. (LVRS)
    maze III s.
    MICAB s.
    MIDCAB s.
    mitral redo s.
    noncardiac s.
    off-pump beating heart s.
    off-pump vascular s.
    open s. (OS)
    open chest s.
    open heart s. (OHS)
    palatal s.
    palliative s.
    Port-Access minimally invasive
      cardiac s.
    postoperative atrial fibrillation in
      cardiac s. (PACS)
    reparative cardiac s.
    robotic heart s.
    site-specific s.
    Society for Vascular S. (SVS)
    stent or s.
    subfascial endoscopic perforator s.
      (SEPS)
    substitutional cardiac s.
    untouched aortic off-pump
      coronary s.
    valve-preserving s.
    ventricular reduction s.
    ventricular restoration s.
    video-assisted thoracic s. (VATS)
    video-assisted thoracoscopic s.
      (VATS)
surgical
    s. ablation
    s. ablation of pathway
    s. ablation probe
    s. ablation system
    s. anterior ventricular endocardial
      restoration (SAVER)
    s. anterior ventricular restoration
      (SAVR)
    s. closure device
    s. embolectomy
    s. emphysema
    s. intensive care unit (SICU)
    s. lung biopsy (SLB)
    s. osteosynthesis
    s. reexploration
    s. revascularization

    s. risk
    s. site infection (SSI)
    s. tuberculosis
    s. ventricular restoration (SVR)
Surgicel gauze
Surgiclip
    Auto Suture S.
Surgilase 150 laser
Surgilon suture
Surg-I-Loop
Surgitool prosthetic valve
Surgitron unit
Surmontil
Surpasse Superfusion perfusion catheter
surrogate endpoint biomarker (SEB)
Survanta
surveillance
    s. angiography
    s. bronchoscopy
    imaging s.
    National Nosocomial Infection s.
survey
    environmental s.
    European Heart S.
    Jenkins Activity S.
    National Health Interview S.
      (NHIS)
    National Health and Nutrition
      Examination S. (NHANES)
    National Health and Nutrition
      Examination S. I
    SF-36 Health S.
    Short-Form 36 Health S.
Surveyor recording device
survival
    posttransplantation s.
    s. time
survivor
susceptibility
    s. artifact
    R-on-T arrhythmia s.
susceptible
    high-altitude pulmonary edema s.
      (HAPE-s)
suspected coronary artery disease
suspended
    s. heart
    s. heart syndrome
suspension
    Aristocort Intralesional S.
    budesonide inhalation s.
    calfactant intratracheal s.
    CellCept oral s.
    Children's Motrin S.
    Curosurf intratracheal s.
    hyoid s.
    s. laryngoscopy
    mycophenolate mofetil oral s.

Optison injectable s.
Rynatuss Pediatric S.

suspensory
s. ligament
s. ligament of esophagus

suspicion
index of s.

sustained
s. maximal inspiration (SMI)
s. monomorphic ventricular
  tachycardia (SMVT)
s. outward movement (SOM)
s. physical exercise (SPE)
s. pulse
s. rate duration
s. reentrant ventricular
  tachyarrhythmia (SRVT)
s. release (SR)
s. tachycardia
s. ventricular tachycardia (SVT)

Sustiva
susurrus
Sutterella wadsworthensis
Sutton law
suture
absorbable s.
Cardioflon s.
chromic catgut s.
Deklene II cardiovascular s.
Dermalon s.
Dexon Plus s.
Endoknot s.
end-to-side s.
ePTFE vascular s.
Ethibond s.
everting mattress s.
figure-of-8 s.
Gabbay-Frater valve s.
s. hole
interrupted pledgeted s.
mattress s.
Mersilene braided nonabsorbable s.
Mersilk black silk s.
Micrins microsurgical s.
monofilament absorbable s.
monofilament polypropylene s.
NextStitch cardiovascular valve s.
Nurolon s.
pericostal s.
pledgeted mattress s.
Pronova s.
pursestring s.
reabsorbable s.
Serralnyl s.
Serralsilk s.
subanular mattress s.
subcutaneous s.
subcuticular s.

Surgilon s.
Techstar percutaneous s.
through-and-through continuous s.
through-the-wall mattress s.
Ti-Cron s.
traction s.
transfixion s.
U s.'s

sutured plaque electrode
sutureless anastomosis
suturing
coupled s.
suxamethonium
SV
saphenous vein
small vessel
stroke volume
subventricular
  SV OTW
SV40
simian virus 40
Sv
sievert
SVA
sequential ventriculoatrial
  SVA pacing
SVAS
supravalvar aortic stenosis
supraventricular aortic stenosis
SVB
saphenous vein bypass
SVBG
saphenous vein bypass grafting
SVC
saphenous vein cutdown
segmental venous capacitance
selective venous catheterization
slow vital capacity
subclavian vein catheterization
superior vena cava
  SVC lead
  SVC syndrome
SVCCS
superior vena cava compression
  syndrome
SVCG
spatial vectorcardiogram
SVCO
superior vena cava obstruction
SVCR
segmental venous capacitance ratio
SVCS
superior vena cava syndrome
SVCT
spiral volumetric computed tomography
SVD
single-vessel disease
structural valve deterioration

S

SVE
subcortical vascular encephalopathy
supraventricular extrasystole
Svedberg flotation rate
SVG
saphenous vein graft
SVH
saphenous vein harvesting
SVI
small vessel infarction
stroke volume index
systolic velocity integral
SVN
small-volume nebulizer
SvO$_2$
mixed venous oxygen saturation
continuous cardiac output with SvO$_2$
SVP
standing venous pressure
superior vascular plexus
SVPB
supraventricular premature beat
SVPC
supraventricular premature complex
SVR
sequential vascular response
surgical ventricular restoration
systemic vascular resistance
SVRI
systemic vascular resistance index
SVS
slit ventricle syndrome
Society for Vascular Surgery
SVT
sinoventricular tachycardia
subclavian vein thrombosis
supraventricular tachyarrhythmia
supraventricular tachycardia
sustained ventricular tachycardia
SVTh
subvalvar thickening
SW
spike wave
stroke work
S/W
spike wave
stroke work
swallow
barium s.
s. syncope
wet s.
swallowing
fiberoptic endoscopic evaluation of s. (FEES)
Swan-Ganz
S.-G. balloon flotation catheter
S.-G. bipolar pacing catheter
S.-G. flow-directed catheter
S.-G. Pacing TD catheter
S.-G. syndrome
S-warfarin
S′ wave
sweat
s. chloride test
night s.'s
s. testing
sweating
sweep
Sweet Tip bipolar lead
swelling
ventricular mural s.
SWI
stroke work index
swimmer's view
swimming
hypoxic lap s.
s. pool granuloma
swing
respiratory s.
s. test
swinging heart
Swiss
S. cheese defect
S. cheese interventricular septum
switch
atrial s.
DNA s.
internal reed s.
isoactin s.
isomyosin s.
late arterial s.
mode s.
s. operation
s. procedure
switch-conversion of transposition
switching
automatic mode s. (AMS)
mode s.
SWM
segmental wall motion
SWMA
segmental wall motion analysis
SWOP
second window of protection
SWS
slow-wave sleep
spike-wave stupor
Swyer-James syndrome
SX/DX computerized spirometry
Sydenham
S. chorea
S. cough
sydowi
Aspergillus s.
Sylvest disease
Sylvian fissure

Sylvius
    valve of S.
Symbicort
    S. 100/6 Turbuhaler
    S. 200/6 Turbuhaler
Symbion
    S. cardiac device
    S. total artificial heart
Symbios 7006 pacemaker
Symbiot
    S. covered stent
    S. PTFE-covered stent
Symmetrel
symmetric
    s. asphyxia
    s. dimethylarginine
symmetrical
    bilateral s. (BS)
    s. phased array
Symmetry bypass system aortic connector
sympathectomy, sympathetectomy
    cervicothoracic s.
    lumbar s.
sympathetic
    s. effusion
    s. fiber
    s. nerve
    s. nerve activity (SNA)
    s. nervous system (SNS)
    s. nervous system activity
    s. neurotransmission
    s. orthostatic hypotension (SOH)
sympathoadrenal system
sympathoexcitation
    reflex s.
sympathoexcitatory response
sympathoinhibition
sympathoinhibitory response
sympatholytic
sympathomimetic
    s. amine
    s. drug
sympathovagal
    s. balance
    s. imbalance
    s. transition
symphony
    S. nitinol stent
    S. patient monitoring system
symphysis, pl. **symphyses**
    cardiac s.
    pericardial s.
symptom
    Baumès s.
    Burghart s.
    cardinal s.
    Duroziez s.
    Fischer s.

Kussmaul s.
    NYHA class I-IV s.'s
    Oehler s.'s
    prodromal s.
    Trunecek s.
symptomatic
    s. airway obstruction
    s. aortic stenosis
    s. asthma
    s. hemorrhage
    s. ischemic heart disease
    s. peripheral arterial disease
    s. therapy
symptomaticity
symptom-free interval
symptom-limited
    s.-l. graded exercise test (SL-GXT)
    s.-l. maximal treadmill test
    s.-l. treadmill exercise test
Synacol CF
Synagis
synaptene
synaptic
synaptophysin
synchondrosis
    sternal s.
Synchrocor pacemaker
SynchroMed programmable pump
synchronicity
    cardiac s.
synchronization
synchronized
    s. DC cardioversion
    s. direct current cardioversion
    s. intermittent mandatory
    s. intermittent mandatory ventilation (SIMV)
    s. retroperfusion (SRP)
    s. shock
    s. sleep (S-sleep)
synchronizer
    CardioSync cardiac s.
synchronous
    s. airway lesions
    s. atrial contraction
    s. atrial stimulation (SAS)
    s. biatrial pacing therapy
    s. endobronchial disease
synchrony
    atrial s.
    atrioventricular s.
    A-V s.
    S. II, III DDDR pulse generator
    ventricular contractile s.
synchrotron-based transvenous angiography
syncopal
    s. migraine

S

syncopal *(continued)*
    s. migraine headache
    s. spell
syncope
    Adams-Stokes s.
    s. anginosa
    cardiac s.
    cardiogenic s.
    cardioinhibitory vasovagal s.
    cardioneurogenic s.
    carotid sinus s.
    cerebrovascular s.
    cough s.
    defecation s.
    deglutition s.
    diver's s.
    exertional s.
    factitious s.
    head-up, tilt-induced s.
    high-altitude s.
    hypoglycemic s.
    hypoxic s.
    hysterical s.
    isoproterenol-induced vasovagal s.
    laryngeal s.
    local s.
    metabolic s.
    micturition s.
    migraine s.
    mixed neurally mediated s.
    Morgagni-Adams-Stokes s.
    near s.
    neurally mediated s. (NMS)
    neurally mediated vasovagal s.
     (NMVS)
    neurocardiac s.
    neurocardiogenic s.
    neurologic s.
    neuromediated s.
    noncardiac s.
    orthostatic s.
    postmicturition s.
    posttussive s.
    postural s.
    psychogenic s.
    refractory neurocardiogenic s.
    severe refractory
     neurocardiogenic s.
    sexual s.
    situational s.
    sneeze s.
    stretching s.
    swallow s.
    toilet-seat s.
    transient s.
    tussive s.
    vasodepressor s.
    vasodepressor-cardioinhibitory s.
    vasomotor s.
    vasovagal s. (VVS)
    visceral s.
Syncrus internal cardioversion system
syncytia (*pl. of* syncytium)
syncytial virus
syncytiovascular membrane
syncytium, pl. **syncytia**
    s. formation
    myocardial s.
syndactyly
Syn-Diltiazem
syndrome
    abdominal compartment s. (ACS)
    acquired immunodeficiency s.
     (AIDS)
    acquired valvular heart s. (AVHS)
    acute brain s.
    acute chest s. (ACS)
    acute coronary s. (ACS)
    acute ischemic coronary s. (AICS)
    acute respiratory distress s.
     (ARDS)
    acute retroviral s.
    acute right heart s. (ARHS)
    acute sickle cell chest s.
    acute sickle chest s. (ASCS)
    Adams-Stokes s.
    adrenogenital s.
    adult respiratory distress s. (ARDS)
    advanced sleep phase s.
    AFA s.
    agitation s.
    Alagille s.
    Albright s.
    ALCAPA s.
    Alport s.
    ALPS s.
    Alstrom s.
    amniotic fluid s.
    anaphylactoid s.
    Andersen s.
    angioosteohypertrophy s.
    anomalous first rib thoracic s.
    anomalous origin of left coronary
     artery from pulmonary artery s.
    antiphospholipid s.
    aortic arch s. (AAS)
    aortic arteritis s.
    aortocaval compression s.
    apallic s.
    Apert s.
    Ardystil s.
    arterial thoracic outlet s.
    arteriohepatic dysplasia s.
    Asherson s.
    Ask-Upmark s.
    ataxia telangiectasia s.
    Austrian s.
    Ayerza s.

Babinski s.
ballooning mitral cusp s.
ballooning mitral valve s.
ballooning posterior leaflet s.
Bamberger-Marie s.
bangungot s.
Bannwarth s.
Barlow s.
Barsony-Polgar s.
Barth s.
Bartter s.
Bauer s.
Beau s.
beer and cobalt s.
Behçet s.
Bernheim s.
Besnier-Boeck-Schaumann s.
Beuren s.
billowing mitral leaflet s. (BMLS)
billowing mitral valve s.
Blackfan-Diamond s.
Bland-Garland-White s.
Bland-White-Garland s.
Bloom s.
blue digit s.
blue finger s.
blue toe s.
blue velvet s.
Boerhaave s.
brachial s.
Bradbury-Eggleston s.
bradycardia-tachycardia s. (BTS)
bradytachycardia s.
Brett s.
Brock s.
broken heart s.
bronchiolitis obliterans s. (BOS)
Brugada s.
bubbly lung s.
Budd-Chiari s.
Bürger-Grütz s.
busulfan lung s.
Cantrell s.
capillary leak s. (CLS)
Caplan s.
carcinoid s.
cardiac destabilization s.
cardiac disturbance s.
cardiac s. X
cardioauditory s.
cardiofacial s.
cardiofaciocutaneous s.
carotid sinus s.
carotid sinus hypersensitivity s.
carotid steal s.
Carpenter s.
CATCH-22 s.
cat cry s.
cat's eye s.

cauda equina s.
Ceelen-Gellerstedt s.
central sleep apnea s. (CSAS)
Cepacia s.
cervical rib s.
CFC s.
Char s.
Charcot s.
Charcot-Weiss-Baker s.
CHARGE s.
Chédiak-Higashi s.
chemoreceptor s.
chest pain s. (CPS)
Chiari s.
Chiari-Budd s.
Chinese restaurant asthma s.
cholesterol emboli s.
chronic fatigue s. (CFS)
chronic hyperventilation s.
Churg-Strauss s. (CSS)
chylomicronemia s.
Clarke-Hadfield s.
CLH s.
click s.
click-murmur s.
Cockayne s.
Cogan s.
combination s.
compartment s.
compensatory antiinflammatory
  response s. (CARS)
complete form of DiGeorge s.
  (cDGS)
congenital central hypoventilation s.
congenital long QT interval s.
Conn s.
Conradi-Hünermann s.
Cornelia de Lange s.
coronary slow flow s. (CSFS)
coronary-subclavian steal s. (CSSS)
costochondral s.
costoclavicular rib s.
costosternal s.
craniocerebellocardiac s.
CREST s.
cricopharyngeal achalasia s.
cri du chat s.
critical malperfusion s.
Crow-Fukase s.
cryptophthalmos s.
Cushing s.
cutis laxa s.
Cyriax s.
cytokine release s.
DaCosta s.
4-day s.
deadly quartet s.
declamping shock s.
defects s.

S

syndrome *(continued)*
    de Lange s.
    delayed pulmonary toxicity s.
      (DPTS)
    Desert Storm s.
    Determann s.
    DG/VCF s.
    diffuse obstructive pulmonary s.
      (DOPS)
    DiGeorge s. (DGS)
    distal intestinal obstruction s.
    distal intestinal obstructive s.
    disturbance of function occlusion s.
      (DOFOS)
    Down s. (DS)
    Dressler s.
    drowned newborn s.
    drug-induced lupus s.
    Duncan s.
    dysarthria-clumsy hand s. (DCHS)
    dyskinesia s.
    dyslipidemic hypertension s.
    early repolarization s.
    early ventricular repolarization s.
      (EVRS)
    Eaton-Lambert s.
    economy class s.
    effort s.
    Ehlers-Danlos s. (EDS)
    Eisenmenger s.
    elfin facies s.
    Ellis-van Creveld s.
    engraftment s. (ES)
    eosinophilia-myalgia s. (EMS)
    eosinophilic lung s.
    eosinophilic pulmonary s.
    epibronchial right pulmonary
      artery s.
    euthyroid sick s.
    familial aortic ectasia s.
    familial atrial myxoma s.
    familial cholestasis s.
    familial chylomicronemia s.
    fat embolism s. (FES)
    fear of food s.
    Fechtner s.
    fetal alcohol s. (FAS)
    fetal aspiration s.
    fibrinogen-fibrin conversion s.
    flapping valve s.
    Fleischner s.
    floppy valve s.
    Foix-Cavany-Marie s.
    folded lung s.
    Forney s.
    Forrester s.
    FRAX-MR s.
    Gaisböck s.
    gastrocardiac s.

    Gerhardt s.
    Goldenhar s.
    Goodpasture s.
    Gorlin s.
    Gowers s.
    Grönblad-Strandberg s.
    Guillain-Barré s.
    Gulf War s.
    Halbrecht s.
    Hamman s.
    Hamman-Rich s. (HRS)
    Hantavirus pulmonary s.
    Hare s.
    heart-hand s.
    Hegglin s.
    Heiner s.
    HELLP s.
    hemangioma-thrombocytopenia s.
    hemolysis, elevated liver function
      tests, low platelets s.
    Henoch-Schönlein s.
    heparin-induced thrombosis-
      thrombocytopenia s. (HITTS)
    hepatopulmonary s. (HPS)
    Hermansky-Pudlak s.
    Herner s.
    heterotaxy s.
    high-altitude hypertrophic
      cardiomyopathy s. (HHCS)
    high-pressure neurologic s. (HPNS)
    HO s.
    holiday heart s.
    Holt-Oram s. (HOS)
    homocystinuria s.
    Horner s.
    Howel-Evans s.
    Hughes-Stovin s.
    Hunter s.
    Hunter-Hurler s.
    Hurler s.
    hyaline membrane s.
    hyperabduction s.
    hyperapolipoprotein B s.
    hypercalcemia s.
    hypereosinophilia s.
    hypereosinophilic s.
    hyperimmunoglobulin E s.
    hyperkinetic heart s. (HHS)
    hyperlucent lung s.
    hyperperfusion s.
    hypersensitive carotid sinus s.
    hypersensitive xiphoid s.
    hyperventilation s. (HVS)
    hyperviscosity s.
    hyponatremic-hypertensive s.
    hypoplastic left heart s. (HLHS)
    hypoplastic left ventricle s. (HLVS)
    idiopathic hypereosinophilic s.
      (IHES, IHS)

idiopathic hyperkinetic heart s.
(IHHS)
idiopathic long QT interval s.
idiopathic pneumonia s. (IPS)
immotile cilia s.
immune reconstitution s.
s. of inappropriate antidiuresis
(SIAD)
s. of inappropriate antidiuretic
hormone (SIADH)
s. of inappropriate antidiuretic
hormone secretion (SIADH)
incontinentia pigmenti s.
infant respiratory distress s. (IRDS)
insulin resistance s.
intermediate coronary s.
irritable larynx s.
ischemic steel s.
Ivemark s.
Jackson s.
Janus s.
Jervell and Lange-Nielsen s.
Jeune s.
Job s.
Kallmann s.
Kartagener s.
Kasabach-Merritt s.
Kawasaki s.
Kearns-Sayre s.
Kimmelstiel-Wilson s.
Klein-Waardenburg s.
Klinefelter s.
Klippel-Feil s.
Klippel-Trenaunay-Weber s.
Kohlmeier-Degos s.
Kostmann s.
Kugelberg-Welander s.
Kussmaul s.
Labbe neurocirculatory s.
lacunar s. (LACS)
Lady Windermere s.
LAMB s.
Lambert-Eaton myasthenic s.
Landouzy-Dejerine s.
Landry-Guillain-Barré s.
Laron s. (LS)
Laubry-Soulle s.
Laurence-Moon-Bardet-Biedl s.
Laurence-Moon-Biedl s.
Leitner s.
Lemierre s.
Lenègre s.
Lenz s.
LEOPARD s.
Leredde s.
Leriche s.
Lev s.
Libman-Sacks s.
Liddle s.

Löffler s.
Löfgren s.
long QT s. (LQTS)
long QTU s.
low cardiac output s. (LCOS,
LOS)
Lown-Ganong-Levine s.
low salt s.
low sodium s.
LQT s.
lupus-like s.
Lutembacher s.
Macleod s.
malignant carcinoid s.
malignant superior vena caval s.
malignant SVC s.
malignant vasovagal s.
Mallory-Weiss s.
Marfan s.
Marie s.
Marie-Bamberger s.
Maroteaux-Lamy s.
Martorell s.
mastocytosis s.
McArdle s.
Meadows s.
meconium aspiration s. (MAS)
Meigs s.
MEN 2 s.
Mendelson s.
Ménière s.
metabolic s.
metastatic carcinoid s.
middle lobe s.
midsystolic click s.
milk-alkali s.
Miller Fisher variant of Guillain-
Barré s.
mirror-image lung s.
mitral valve prolapse s. (MVPS)
Mönckeberg s.
Mondor s.
Morestin s.
Morgagni-Adams-Stokes s.
Morquio s.
Mounier-Kuhn s.
Moynahan s.
mucocutaneous lymph node s.
multiple cholesterol emboli s.
(MCES)
multiple lentigines s.
multiple-organ dysfunction s.
(MODS)
myocardial ischemic s.
NAME s.
neonatal respiratory distress s.
(NRDS)
nephrotic s.
Netherton s.

S

723

syndrome *(continued)*

neurally mediated syncopal s.
nonpyramidal hemimotor s.
Noonan s.
no-reflow s.
obesity hypoventilation s. (OHS)
obstructive sleep apnea s. (OSAS)
obstructive sleep apnea-hypopnea s.
  (OSAHS)
oculomucocutaneous s.
Opitz s.
organic dust toxic s. (ODTS)
Ortner s.
Osler-Weber-Rendu s.
osmotic demyelination s.
overlap s.
PAC s.
pacemaker s. (PS)
Paget-von Schrötter s.
PAGOD s.
Pancoast s.
papillary muscle s.
paraneoplastic s.
partial anterior circulation s.
  (PACS)
pericarditis-myocarditis s.
Perthes s.
pharyngeal pouch s.
PHAVER s.
Pick s.
pickwickian s.
PIE s.
Pierre Robin s.
Pins s.
platypnea-orthodeoxia s.
Plummer-Vinson s.
POEMS s.
pokkuri sudden arrhythmia-death s.
Polhemus-Schafer-Ivemark s.
polyglandular autoimmune s. type
  II
polymetabolic s.
polymyalgia rheumatica s.
polysplenia s.
positional obstructive sleep
  apnea s.
postcardiac injury s. (PCIS)
postcardiotomy s. (PCS)
postcardiotomy psychosis s.
postcommissurotomy s.
posterior circulation s. (POCS)
postinfarction s.
postmyocardial infarction s. (PMIS)
postnasal drainage s. (PNDS)
postnasal drip s. (PNDS)
postparalytic s.
postperfusion s.
postpericardiotomy s. (PPS)
postphlebitic s.
postpump s.
posttransfusion s.
postural orthostatic tachycardia s.
  (POTS)
P pulmonale s.
precordial catch s.
preexcitation s. (PES)
preinfarction s. (PIS)
premonitory s.
prolapsed mitral valve s.
prolonged QT interval s.
Proteus s.
pseudoxanthoma elasticum s.
pulmonary acid aspiration s.
pulmonary disease anemia s.
pulmonary dysmaturity s.
pulmonary fat embolism s.
pulmonary hyperinfection s.
pulmonary infarction s.
pulmonary infiltrates with
  eosinophilia s.
pulmonary sling s.
pure sensory s. (PSS)
QT s.
quinidine syncope s.
radiologic scimitar s.
Raeder-Harbitz s.
Rasmussen s.
Raynaud s.
reactive airways disease s. (RADS)
reactive airways dysfunction s.
  (RADS)
reactive upper airways
  dysfunction s. (RUDS)
Reaven s.
redundant cusp s.
Reel s.
refeeding s.
Refsum s.
Reiter s.
Rendu-Osler-Weber s.
respiratory distress s. (RDS)
Reye s.
Riley-Day s.
Romano-Ward s.
Rosenbach s.
Rosenberg s.
Roussy-Lévy s.
rubella s.
Rubinstein-Taybi s.
salt depletion s.
Sanchez-Cascos cardioauditory s.
Sandifer s.
Sanfilippo s.
scalenus anterior s.
scalenus anticus s.
Schaumann s.
Scheie s.
Schmidt s.

scimitar s.
Sebastiani s.
senile cardiac calcification s.
severe acute respiratory s. (SARS)
shallow-water blackout s.
Shone s.
shoulder-hand s.
Shprintzen s.
shrinking lung s. (SLS)
Shwachman s.
Shy-Drager s.
sicca s.
sick building s. (SBS)
sick sinus s. (SSS)
silicone embolism s.
Silver s.
Simpson-Golabi-Behmel s.
single papillary muscle s.
Singleton-Merten s.
sinobronchial s.
sinuatrial node weakness s.
 (SANWS)
Sjögren s.
sleep apnea/hypopnea s. (SAHS)
slipping rib s.
slit ventricle s. (SVS)
small aorta s. (SAS)
Smith-Lemli-Opitz s.
Sneddon s.
Spens s.
Sphrintzen s.
splenic flexure s.
Stevens-Johnson s.
stiff heart s.
stiff left atrium s.
Stokes-Adams s.
Stokvis-Talma s.
straight back s.
Sturge-Weber s.
subclavian steal s.
sudden arrhythmic death s. (SADS)
sudden infant death s. (SIDS)
sudden unexplained death s.
 (SUDS)
sudden unexplained nocturnal
 death s.
SUND s.
superior mesenteric artery s.
superior vena cava s. (SVCS)
superior vena cava compression s.
 (SVCCS)
supine hypotension s.
supravalvar aortic stenosis s.
supravalvar aortic stenosis-infantile
 hypercalcemia s.
surdocardiac s.
suspended heart s.
SVC s.
Swan-Ganz s.

Swyer-James s.
systemic inflammatory response s.
 (SIRS)
systolic click s. (SCS)
systolic click-late systolic
 murmur s.
systolic click-murmur s.
tachybrady s.
tachybradycardia s.
tachycardia-bradycardia s.
tachycardia-polyuria s.
Takayasu s.
takotsubo s.
TAR s.
Taussig-Bing s.
Taybi s.
telangiectasia s.
thoracic compressive s.
thoracic endometriosis s. (TES)
thoracic outlet s. (TOS)
thoracic outlet compression s.
thrombocytopenia-absent radius s.
thromboembolic s.
Tietze s.
total anterior circulation s. (TACS)
Townes-Brocks s.
toxic oil s. (TOS)
Treacher Collins s.
Trousseau s.
Turner s.
twiddler's s.
TWISTED s.
Uhl s.
Ulick s.
Ullmann s.
unroofed coronary sinus s.
upper airway cough s. (UACS)
upper airway resistance s. (UARS)
Urbach-Wiethe s.
V_1-like ambulatory lead s.
V_5-like ambulatory lead s.
VACTERL s.
vascular leak s. (VLS)
vasovagal s.
VATER association s.
VCF s.
velocardiofacial s. (VCFS)
vena cava s.
venolobar s.
venous insufficiency s. (VIS)
Vernet s.
Villaret s.
Vogt-Koyanagi-Harada s.
von Recklinghausen s.
Waardenburg s.
Wallenberg s.
Ward-Romano s.
wasting s.
Watson s.

S

syndrome *(continued)*
    Weber-Osler-Rendu s.
    Werner s.
    West s.
    white clot s.
    Willebrand-Jürgens s.
    Williams s.
    Williams-Campbell s.
    Wilson-Mikity s.
    Wiskott-Aldrich s.
    Wolff-Parkinson-White s.
    WPW s.
    Wright s.
    s. X
    XO s.
    XXXX s.
    XXXY s.
    yellow nail s. (YNS)
    Yentl s.
    Young s.
synechia, pl. **synechiae**
    bronchial s.
    pericardial s.
    s. pericardii
Synercid
synergism
synergistic
SynerGraft
    S. implant
    S. pulmonary heart valve
    S. tissue-engineered heart valve
Synergy model 700 pulmonary heart valve
Synergyst
    S. DDD pacemaker
    S. II pacemaker
Syngamus laryngeus
syngenesioplastic transplant
Syn-Nadolol
synovial sarcoma
Synox fractal pacemaker lead
synpneumonic empyema
Syntel
    S. graft cleaning catheter
    S. latex-free embolectomy catheter
synthase
    aldosterone s.
    constitutive nitric oxide s. (cNOS)
    endothelial constitutive nitric
      oxide s. (ecNOS, eNOS)
    endothelial nitric oxide s. (eNOS)
    endothelial oxide s. (eNOS)
    glycogen s.
    inducible nitric oxide s. (iNOS)
    nitric oxide s. (NOS)
    nitric oxide s. 1 (NOSI)
    promotor region of endothelial
      oxide s.
synthesis, pl. **syntheses**

    cytokine-induced endothelial s.
    leukotriene s.
    matrix s.
    s. polyneuropathy
    thromboxane s.
synthetase
    alanyl-tRNA s.
    aminoacyl-tRNA s.
    histidyl-tRNA s.
    inducible nitric oxide s. (iNOS)
    isoleucyl-tRNA s.
    pantothenate s.
    purified histidyl-tRNA s.
Synthroid
synvinolin
syphilis
    cardiovascular s.
    nonvenereal s.
    tertiary s.
syphilitic
    s. aortic aneurysm
    s. aortic valvulitis
    s. aortitis
    s. arteritis
    s. endarteritis
    s. endocarditis
    s. laryngitis
    s. myocarditis
Syracol-CF
syringe
    anaerobic Pulsator s.
    Angioject s.
    flow-volume s.
    Gas-Lyte ABG s.
    Lyo-Ject s.
    Namic angiographic s.
    Osciflator balloon inflation s.
    Pulsator s.
    Raulerson s.
    s. technique
    Ultraject prefilled s.
syringomyelobulbia
syrup
    albuterol sulfate s.
    Allerphed S.
    Ambenyl Cough S.
    Amgenal Cough S.
    Aprodine S.
    Bromanyl Cough S.
    Bromotuss w/Codeine Cough S.
    Cardec-S S.
    Decofed S.
    Deconamine S.
    Histalet S.
    Phanatuss Cough S.
    Rondec S.
    Silafed S.
    Tusstat S.

SYS-BP
   systolic blood pressure
system
   Abiomed biventricular support s.
   ABI Vest Airway Clearance s.
   ABL 625 s.
   ABL 520 blood gas
     measurement s.
   ABO blood group s.
   Access MV s.
   Accunet embolic protection s.
   Achieve Off-Pump s.
   ACIST contrast delivery s.
   ACIST contrast injection s.
   ACS Concorde over-the-wire
     catheter s.
   ACS Multi-Link RX Ultra
     coronary stent s.
   ACS Multi-Link Tristar coronary
     stent s.
   Active Can defibrillator lead s.
   ACT MicroCoil delivery s.
   Acuson cardiovascular s.
   adrenergic nervous s.
   Advanced Cardiovascular S.'s
     (ACS)
   Advantx LC+ cardiovascular
     imaging s.
   Aegis ICD s.
   AeroNOx nitric oxide delivery and
     analysis s.
   AeroNOx nitric oxide transport s.
   AeroView optical intubation s.
   AirSep OxiScan Oximetry
     recording, reporting, and
     archiving s.
   Aladdin Infant Flow s.
   Aladdin nasal CPAP s.
   Albert Grass Heritage EEG s.
   Albert Grass Heritage PSG s.
   Alcon Closure S.
   AlereNet s.
   Alice 3, 5 diagnostic sleep s.
   Alliance catheter delivery s.
   Alveolus stent technology s.
   Anaconda device and delivery s.
   Ancor imaging s.
   Ancure abdominal aortic
     aneurysm s.
   Androderm Transdermal s.
   AneuRx DTA stent graft s.
   AneuRx fully supported modular s.
   AneuRx IDS delivery s.
   AngioJet rapid thrombectomy s.
   AngioJet rheolytic thrombectomy s.
   Angiomat Illumena contrast
     delivery s.
   AngioRad Afterloader s.
   AngioRad radiation s.

AnnuloFlo annuloplasty ring s.
anular phased array s. (APAS)
Aortic Connector s.
Apollo Light S.'s
Aptaer heliox delivery s.
Aria LX CPAP s.
arrhythmia mapping s.
artificial heart energy s. (AHES)
aSpire controlled expansion
  delivery s.
aSpire covered stent and Controlled
  Release delivery s.
Atakr II RF ablation s.
ATL Ultramark 9 ultrasound s.
atrial septal defect occlusion s.
  (ASDOS)
atrial septum defect occluder s.
  (ASDOS)
atrioventricular conduction s.
  (AVCS)
AutoCapture pacing s.
autologous blood management s.
automated cervical cell screening s.
automatic exposure s.
automatic titration s.
autonomic nervous s. (ANS)
AutoPulse resuscitation s.
AutoSet T titration s.
Autotrans s.
autotransfusion s. (ATS)
Autovac LF autotransfusion s.
Axcis PMR s.
BACTEC MGIT 960 S.
balloon-delivery s.
balloon-on-a-wire dilation s.
Bard percutaneous cardiopulmonary
  support s.
Baylor autologous transfusion s.
BD ProbeTec Direct TB S.
Beckman ICS Nephelometer s.
Bedbugg s.
BeStent Rival coronary stent s.
BeStent 2 with Discrete
  Technology Over-The-Wire and
  Rapid Exchange coronary stent
  delivery s.
Beta-Cath s.
bias flow s.
BiliBlanket phototherapy s.
Biodex S.
bionic baroreflex s.
Biosound Genesis II scanning s.
biotin/streptavidin s.
Biotronik Home Monitoring S.
BioZ hemodynamic monitoring s.
BioZ noninvasive cardiac function
  monitoring s.
BioZ.pc s.
BiPAP duet s.

S

system *(continued)*
  BiPAP S/T-D 30 s.
  BiPAP S/T-D ventilatory support s.
  BiPAP Vision s.
  blood-vascular s.
  Boomerang ClosureWire vascular
    closure s.
  2-bottle thoracic drainage s.
  brachiocephalic s.
  brachytherapy s.
  BRAT s.
  Breeze E150 ventilation s.
  Bridge extra support over-the-wire
    renal stent s.
  Bridge X3 renal stent s.
  Burette multiple patient delivery s.
  BVS 5000 biventricular support s.
  Bx Velocity stent with Raptor
    OTW delivery s.
  Bx Velocity with Hepacoat on
    Raptor stent s.
  Cadence tiered therapy
    defibrillator s.
  CAESAR analysis s.
  Cambridge Heart CH2000 stress
    test s.
  Cancion cardiac recovery s.
  CapnoProbe model 2000 s.
  CapnoProbe SL s.
  CapnoProbe sublingual CO_2 s.
  cardiac assist s.
  cardiac conduction s. (CCS)
  cardiac recovery s. (CRS)
  cardiac surgery reporting s. (CSRS)
  Cardia Horizon Legacy cannulated
    implant s.
  Cardima surgical ablation s.
  Cardioblate BP, RF surgical
    ablation s.
  Cardioblate BP2 surgical
    ablation s.
  Cardioblate RF surgical ablation s.
  CardioGenesis TMR s.
  CardioLab 2000 single monitor
    EP s.
  CardioSEAL septal occlusion s.
  CardioTek electrophysiologic
    tracer s.
  cardiovascular s. (CVS)
  Cardiovascular Angiography
    Analysis S. (CAAS)
  cardiovascular imaging s. (CVIS)
  cardiovascular measurement s.
    (CMS)
  cardiovascular reflex conditioning s.
    (CRCS)
  Carto EP navigation s.
  Carto XP s.
  CASE exercise testing s.

  Cathcor LX hemodynamic
    recording s.
  catheter delivery s.
  catheter-snare s.
  catheter-tip micromanometer s.
  Cath-Finder catheter tracking s.
  CCT.2 CryoConsole s.
  CDI 2000 blood gas monitoring s.
  Cell Saver autologous blood
    recovery s.
  Cell Saver Haemonetics
    Autotransfusion s.
  central nervous s. (CNS)
  CFC-free delivery s.
  CGR biplane angiographic s.
  CH 2000 cardiac diagnostic s.
  Checkmate gamma brachytherapy s.
  Checkmate intravascular
    brachytherapy s.
  Chilli cooled ablation s.
  Cholestech LDX s.
  cholesterol monitoring s.
  cineangiographic s.
  cineless recording s.
  cine-pulse s.
  CineView Plus Freeland s.
  Circulaire aerosol drug delivery s.
  circulatory support s.
  Clarity multiparameter monitoring s.
  Clearglide endoscopic vessel
    harvesting s.
  CLeaRS cardiac lead removal s.
  CMS AccuProbe 450 s.
  CoaguChek aPTT testing s.
  codominant s.
  COER-24 delivery s.
  ColorZone Management s.
  CompAir Elite compressor
    nebulizer s.
  complement s.
  complete pacemaker patient
    testing s. (CPPTS)
  computerized sleep analysis s.
  Concentric retriever s.
  conduction s.
  conductive s.
  Cook-Swartz Doppler flow
    monitoring s.
  coordinate s.
  coordinate reduction time
    encoding s. (CORTES)
  Cordis Checkmate s.
  Cordis LC Multipurpose stent s.
  Cordis Mini stent s.
  coronary implant s. (CIS)
  CorRestore s.
  Cosgrove-Edwards annuloplasty s.
  CoStar cobalt chromium paclitaxel-
    eluting coronary stent s.

CoumaCare Coumadin management s.
CoumaCare patient management s.
CPS s.
CryCor cardiac cryoablation s.
Cryocare cardiac surgical s.
CryoCor cryoablation s.
CryoHit s.
C-Vest radiation detector s.
CVProfilor DO-2020 s.
CVX-300 excimer laser s.
cytochrome P450 s.
Dallas Classification S.
DAR breathing s.
Datex-Ohmeda S/5 telemetry s.
da Vinci robotic surgical s.
DCI-S automated coronary analysis s.
demand oxygen delivery s. (DODS)
Desai VectorCath mapping s.
Diameter Index Safety S. (DISS)
Digital Cardiac Imaging s.
digital vascular imaging s. (DVIS)
dilator-sheath s.
Dinamap s.
Discrete Technology coronary stent s.
distal perfusion s. (DPS)
2D TEE s. Ultra-Neb 99
dual-chamber defibrillation s.
Duct-Occlud s.
Dupel drug delivery s.
Dymer excimer delivery s.
Dynalink biliary self-expanding stent s.
Dynasty delivery s.
Eagle portable ventilation s.
EasyOne spirometry s.
echocardiographic automated boundary detection s.
echocardiographic scoring s.
EchoFlow blood velocity meter s.
Echovar Doppler s.
Eclipse PTMR s.
EdenTrace II multichannel polysomnographic s.
edge-detection s.
Elecsys troponin T immunoassay s.
electroanatomical mapping s.
electrode s.
electromagnetic navigation s.
Electronic HouseCall s.
emboli containment s.
Embol-X arterial cannula and filter s.
endocannabinoid s. (ECS)
endocrine s.
Endologix PowerLink s.

Endosaph vein harvest s.
Endotak lead s.
EnSite 3000 s.
EnSite NavX intracardiac nonfluoroscopic navigation s.
Entrata aortic valve s.
EPT-1000 XP cardiac ablation s.
Equinox digital EEG s.
Equinox occlusion balloon s.
Erie S.
ES 300-Cardiac T ELISA troponin T immunoassay s.
Estes point s.
Estes-Romhilt ECG point-score s.
European Antimicrobial Resistance Surveillance S. (EARSS)
eVent Inspiration ventilator s.
event-link data s.
EVS vascular closure s.
Express2 coronary stent s.
factor XII-kallikrein-kinin s.
FemoStop femoral compression s.
fiberoptic catheter delivery s.
fibrinolytic s.
FilterWire EX embolic protection s.
Finger Phantom pulse oximeter testing s.
fixed-wire balloon dilation s.
Flowtron DVT pump s.
Frank ECG lead placement s.
Frank XYZ orthogonal lead s.
Freezor CryoAblation s.
3.2-French Monorail s.
Frostline linear cryoablation s.
Galaxy IVUS imaging s.
Galileo intravascular radiotherapy s.
gamma radiation therapy s.
gated s.
GE Advantx s.
GE CT Advantage high-speed CT s.
Gem SensiCath blood gas monitoring s.
GenBank information s.
General Electric Vivid 3, 4, and 7 echocardiology s.
GenESA closed-loop delivery s.
Genesis s.
Genic coronary stent delivery s.
GE Signa 1.5-T MRI s.
GFX 2 coronary stent s.
GOLD staging s.
GoodKnight 418A, 418G, 418P CPAP s.
GoodKnight home care s.
GS Modular pulmonary testing s.
GuardDOG Embolic Protection S.
GuardWire Plus s.

S

system *(continued)*

Guidant cardiac resynchronization therapy defibrillator s.

Guidant Heart Rhythm Technologies Linear Ablation s.

Guidant Multi-Link Tetra coronary stent s.

Günther Tulip Vena Cava MReye filter and retrieval s.

Gyroscan HP Philips 15S whole-body s.

Haemolite autologous blood recovery s.

Haemonetics Cell Saver s.

HaloLite AAD s.

Healthy Early Alarm Recognition and Telemonitoring S. (HEARTS)

Heart Laser s.

HeartMate implantable pneumatic left ventricular assist s.

HeartMate vented electric left ventricular assist s.

Heartport Port-Access s.

Heartstring Proximal Seal S.

HearTwave s.

HELiOS oxygen delivery s.

hematopoietic s.

hemoglobin-based therapeutic s.

Hemopump cardiac assist s.

hemostatic splittable valved sheath s.

HEPAtech air purification s.

Hewlett-Packard Sonos 1000, 1500, 2500 ultrasound s.

hexaxial reference s.

Hi-Care closed suction and pulmonary hygiene s.

HICOR s.

His-Purkinje s.

Hitachi PCT-3600W PET s.

HomMed monitoring s.

Horizon AutoAdjust CPAP s.

Horizon LT CPAP s.

Horizon nasal CPAP s.

Housecall transtelephonic monitoring s.

HP Sonos 2000 ultrasound s.

hub and spoke referral s.

Hunt and Hess grades I through V aneurysm grading s.

HydroCoil embolization s. (HES)

HydroDot neuromonitoring s.

HyperQ s.

hypoxia warning s.

IBI Therapy cardiac ablation s.

iliofemoral venous s.

ImageView s.

Immedia PT s.

implantable left ventricular assist s. (IPLVAS)

INCA s.

Incardia valve s.

indirect blood pressure measuring s. (IBPMS)

Infant Flow noninvasive nasal CPAP s.

Infant Resuscitation s.

Infinix DP-i dual C-arm s.

infrahisian conduction s.

Inhale deep lung delivery s.

Innervasc expandable vascular access s.

INOvent delivery s.

INR home anticoagulation blood monitoring s.

InSync Biventricular Cardiac Pacing S.

InSync cardiac resynchronization s.

integrated lead s.

Integris cardiac imaging s.

Integris H5000 digital x-ray imaging s.

Integrity AFx AutoCapture pacing s.

Integrity Micro AutoCapture pacing s.

Interceptor Plus filter s.

intravascular brachytherapy s.

Invacare Venture HomeFill complete home oxygen s.

iQ200 analysis s.

IRMA blood gas analysis s.

Irri-Cath suction s.

isocenter s.

Jinotti closed suctioning s.

Johnson & Johnson Interventional S.'s

kallikrein-bradykinin s.

Karl Storz D-LIGHT AF autofluorescence s.

Kerberos Rinspiration s.

King double umbrella closure s.

KK s.

KnightStar 335 respiratory-support s.

lead extraction s.

left ventricle assist s.

left ventricular assist s. (LVAS)

Leocor hemoperfusion s.

lesion marking s.

Leukotrap red cell storage s.

LIFE-Lung S.

Lifepath AAA endovascular graft s.

LifeShirt noninvasive ambulatory s.

LifeSync s.

LionHeart left ventricular assist s.

Liposorber LA-15 s.

Lown grading s.
Luxtec fiberoptic s.
lymphohematogenous drainage s.
Lyra laser s.
Mallinckrodt Hi-Care Pulmonary
  Hygiene s.
Mark V ProVis injection s.
Marquette Case-12
  electrocardiographic s.
Marquette Case-12 exercise s.
Mason-Likar 12-lead ECG s.
Matrix VSG s.
M/D 4 defibrillator s.
MDS s.
MedGraphics Cardio O2 s.
Medical Graphics Cardiopulmonary
  Exercise S. 2001
medication monitoring event s.
  (MEMS)
Medi-Facts s.
Medi-Tech catheter s.
MedNova NeuroShield cerebral
  protection s.
Medos mechanical circulatory
  support s.
Medtronic CardioRhythm Atakr II
  RF ablation s.
Medtronic Hemopump s.
Medtronic Interactive Tachycardia
  Terminating s.
Medtronic Interceptor Plus filter s.
Medtronic Octopus 2+ tissue
  stabilizing s.
Meier-Magnum s.
Metrix atrial defibrillation s.
MicroAir ultrasonic nebulizer s.
Micro Delta/Max Delta s.
MicroGas 7650 transcutaneous
  monitoring s.
MicroLysUS s.
micromanometer catheter s.
Microny II SR+ AutoCapture
  pacing s.
microsurgical dilation catheter s.
Microvascular Anastomotic
  Coupler S.
MicroVein Vascular s.
microwave cardiac ablation s.
MIDCAB s.
minimum data set s.
mobile artery and vein imaging s.
  (MAVIS)
Mobin-Uddin filter s.
modular electrocardiogram
  analysis s. (MEANS)
Monaldi drainage s.
Monorail delivery s.
Monovial drug delivery s.
MPatch vascular closure s.

MT-100 ECG Holter s.
mucociliary s.
Mullins sheath s.
MULTIFIT computer-based chronic
  illness management s.
Multi-Link Frontier coronary
  stent s.
Multi-Link Penta coronary stent s.
Multi-Link Pixel stent s.
Multi-Link Tetra coronary stent s.
Multi-Link Tristar stent s.
Multi-Link Vision RX and OTW
  coronary stent s.
Multi-Link Zeta coronary stent s.
Multitest cell-mediated immunity s.
Myocardial Infarction Data
  Acquisition S.
myocardial protection s. (MPS)
MyoSIGHT dedicated nuclear
  cardiology camera s.
MYOtherm XP cardioplegia
  delivery s.
nasal CPAP s.
Nellcor Puritan Bennett 840
  ventilator s.
Neotrend s.
nervous s.
Neuroform microdelivery stent
  delivery s.
Neurostar angiography s.
Nihon Kohden polygraph s.
NIOX nitric oxide breath test s.
NIRflex stent s.
NIRoyal Elite Monorail coronary
  stent s.
nitric oxide s.
NNMT Medical CardioSEAL septal
  occlusion s.
node-His-Purkinje s.
NOGA cardiac navigation s.
nonimplantable s.
nonthoracotomy defibrillation
  lead s.
Novacor left ventricular assist s.
Novacor mechanical circulatory
  support s.
Novametrix NICO cardiopulmonary
  management s.
Novoste Beta-Cath s.
NOxBOX mobile nitric oxide
  delivery and monitoring s.
Nuvolase 660 laser s.
Oasis thrombectomy s.
Octopus 2+, 3 tissue
  stabilization s.
Omnicell supply s.
Omni-Tract s.
ON-Q PainBuster postoperative pain
  relief s.

S

system *(continued)*

Onyx liquid embolic s.
Optical Sensors stand-alone arterial blood gas monitoring s.
OptiCor digital cardiac communication and storage s.
OptiHaler drug delivery s.
oral L-arginine s.
organ transplantation s.
orthogonal lead s.
over-the-wire balloon dilation catheter s.
OxiFirst fetal oxygen saturation monitoring s.
Oximetrix 3 S.
OxiScan oximetry recording and reporting s.
Oxyfill oxygen refilling s.
Oxylator-EM 100 automatic resuscitation and inhalation s.
Oxylite ambulatory oxygen s.
Oxy-Ultra-Lite ambulatory oxygen s.
Paceart complete pacemaker patient testing s.
pacemaker code s.
PARAFlow circulatory support s.
parasympathetic nervous s.
Parodi Anti-Embolism S.
patch-coil s.
Patil stereotactic s.
PCA s.
PCD Transvene implantable cardioverter-defibrillator s.
PDB preperitoneal distention balloon s.
p53-dependent signaling s.
PediaFlow s.
Pediatric LifeShirt s.
Pelorus stereotactic s.
PenChant coronary stent delivery s.
Perclose vascular surgical closure s.
PercuSurge Guardwire Plus distal protection s.
percutaneous mechanical thrombectomy s.
Percutaneous Mitral Annuloplasty S.
Performer cardiopulmonary bypass s.
peripheral access s. (PAS)
Peripheral AngioJet s.
peripheral atherectomy s.
phased array s.
Physios CTM 01 noninvasive cardiac transplant monitoring s.
Picker Voxel image analysis s.
Pie Medical CAAS II analysis s.
Pittman IMA retractor s.

plasma coagulation s.
Pleur-evac autotransfusion s.
2010 Plus Holter s.
PneuView ventilator testing and training s.
polarcardiography computing s.
PolarCath Peripheral Dilation S.
PolarCath peripheral transluminal angioplasty s.
Polaris CPAP s.
Port-A-Cath implantable catheter s.
Portex Soft-Seal cuff s.
Power Grip Over the Wire Stent Delivery s.
Powerlink s.
Presto-Flash spirometry s.
Presto spirometry s.
PreVue III digitizing s.
Prima total occlusion s.
Prime ECG electrocardiac mapping s.
Primo noninvasive blood pressure measurement s.
Prodose AAD s.
programmable implantable medication s. (PIMS)
Progreat coaxial microcatheter s.
Prostar 9F, 11F percutaneous vascular surgery s.
Prostar XL 8, 10 suture mediated closure s.
Proxis Embolic Protection S.
P-Series sleep monitoring s.
pulmonary arterial s.
Pulsar Max II pacemaker s.
PulseDose portable compressed oxygen s.
PulseSpray infusion s.
PulStar pneumatic wrap s.
Puritan Bennett 840 ventilator s.
Purkinje s.
Q-cath catheterization recording s.
Quanam QuaDS-QP2 stent s.
Quartet s.
Quest Medical microplegia s.
Quest MPS microplegia s.
Quest MPS myocardial protection s.
QuickFlow DPS distal perfusion s.
QuickSeal femoral arterial closure s.
Quinton Synergy cardiac information management s.
RadiStop radial compression s.
Rapidlab 800 Critical Care s.
Rasor blood pumping s. (RBPS)
RDC classification s.
RDX coronary radiation catheter delivery s.

real-time position management tracking s.
Red s.
regeneration heat exchanger cycle s.
Remac s.
Remedy sleep therapy s.
REMstar CPAP s.
Renaissance spirometry s.
renal kallikrein-kinin s.
renin-angiotensin s. (RAS)
renin-angiotensin-aldosterone s. (RAAS)
Rescue thrombus management s.
respiratory s.
Response CV catheter s.
reticuloendothelial s.
revascularization s.
Rithron-XR coronary stent s.
Robert David Cerfolio classification s.
Roda Patient Monitoring S.
Romhilt-Estes point scoring s.
rotational angioplasty catheter s. (ROTACS)
rotational atherectomy s. (RAS)
RPM tracking s.
Rubicon filter s.
Safe-Steer Total Occlusion Crossing S.
Sahara S1100a Pleur-evac Chest Drainage S.
SAM s.
Sandman s.
saphenofemoral s.
sarcotubular s.
Schneider-Meier-Magnum s.
ScleroPLUS HP laser s.
secondary anticoagulation s. (SACS)
SenDx 100 blood gas and electrolyte analysis s.
Septi-Check mycobacteria culture s.
Sequel compression s.
Sequestra 1000 s.
800 series blood gas and critical analyte s.
SetPoint endovascular temperature cooling s.
sheath and dilator s.
SICOR recording s.
Siemens biplane Neurostar digital subtraction angiography s.
Sigma II Dualplace hyperbaric oxygen therapy s.
Sigma I monoplace hyperbaric therapy s.
Sigma Plus monoplace hyperbaric oxygen therapy s.
Signa EXCITE 3.0T MRI s.

SilverHawk plaque excision s.
Simpson AtheroCath s.
Simpson-Robert vascular dilation s.
single-chamber cardiac pacing s.
SinuScope s.
SJM Genesis s.
Sleepscan Traveler ambulatory polysomnography s.
Sleepscan Traveler home monitoring s.
SLK-View stent and delivery s.
Smart MAC-Line capnography s.
SmartMist asthma management s.
SmartMist respiratory management s.
Snuggle Warm convective warming s.
Somatom Volume Zoom computed tomography s.
somatotropic hormonal s.
Somnoplasty s.
Somnus Somnoplasty s.
SonoHeart Elite handheld ultrasound s.
SonoHeart Elite Ultrasound S.
SonoHeart handheld, all digital echocardiography s.
SonoLysis s.
Sonos 4500 echocardiography s.
Sonos 500 imaging s.
SonoSite MicroMaxx ultrasound s.
Sonos 5500 ultrasound s.
Sonotherapy s.
Spaulding classification s.
SphygmoCor non-invasive aortic blood pressure s.
2170 Spirometry Software s.
SpiroSense s.
Spiros inhalation s.
SpiroVision-3 spirometry s.
SPY Intra-operative Imaging S.
S-Series sleep s.
StarClose vascular closure s.
Stary lesion classification s.
stent delivery s. (SDS)
St. Jude Medical Epic HF dual-chamber implantable cardioverter/defibrillator s.
stroke guidance s. (SGS)
Sugarbaker staging s.
Super-4 catheter ablation s.
superDimension bronchus s.
SureStepPro professional blood glucose management s.
surgical ablation s.
S660 with Discrete Technology coronary stent s.
S670 with Discrete Technology coronary stent s.

S

system *(continued)*

sympathetic nervous s. (SNS)
sympathoadrenal s.
Symphony patient monitoring s.
Syncrus internal cardioversion s.
T s.
Talent LPS endoluminal stent-graft s.
TAM s.
TBird ventilator s.
TCD100M digital transcranial Doppler s.
TCI HeartMate mechanical circulatory support s.
TEC atherectomy s.
Technos ultrasound s.
Techstar XL 6F percutaneous vascular surgical s.
Techstar XL 6F PVS s.
Telectronics Pacing S.'s
ThAIRapy vest airway clearance s.
The Closer suture-mediated closure s.
TheraPEP PEP therapy s.
Therapeutic Intervention Scoring S. (TISS)
ThermoChem-HT s.
ThermoFlo s.
TherOx Aqueous Oxygen s.
Thora-Klex chest drainage s.
Thora-Seal III 3-chamber s.
Thoratec VAD s.
Thrombex PMT s.
Thrombolytic Assessment S. (TAS)
Thumper 1007 CPR s.
TMS 1000 tachyarrhythmia monitoring s.
TomTec Imaging S.'s
tonsillar Somnoplasty s.
Total O_2 delivery s.
Total O_2 supplementary oxygen s.
Total Synchrony S.
TRAKE-fit s.
Tranquility Quest CPAP S.
transesophageal pacing s.
transluminal lysing s.
transtelephonic ambulatory monitoring s.
Trap cardiovascular filtration s.
Trap neurovascular filtration s.
Trap vascular filtration s.
Traveler portable oxygen s.
Trellis-8 infusion s.
TriActiv balloon-protected flush extraction s.
Triad defibrillator s.
Triage cardiac rapid diagnostic test s.
triaxial reference s.

TriVex s.
TrueMax 2400 metabolic measuring s.
Trufill n-BCA liquid embolic s.
TruTrak data sampling s.
turbine-powered ICU ventilator s.
Ultraflex esophageal stent s.
Unified Medical Language s. (UMLS)
Uni-Lead ECG electrode s.
Unilink s.
Unistep catheter delivery s.
Unistep Plus delivery s.
Uni-Vent Eagle ventilation s.
Univision echocardiographic s.
URx intravascular Sonotherapy s.
USCI Probe balloon-on-a-wire dilation s.
vacuum-assisted venous return s.
Vanguard modular endograft s.
Vapor-Phase heated humidification s.
Vapotherm 2000i oxygen delivery s.
Vario s.
vascular s.
Vascular Solutions Acolysis ultrasound thrombolysis s.
Vasotrac blood pressure monitoring s.
VasoView 6 endoscopic vessel harvesting s.
VasoView Uniport endoscopic saphenous vein harvesting s.
VDD pacing s.
VeinViewer imaging s.
VenaFlow compression s.
VenaFlow DVT prophylaxis s.
Venodyne EPS-410 external pneumatic compression s.
venous s.
venous arterial blood management protection s. (VAMP)
Ventak Prizm 2 s.
Ventak Prizm HE s.
Ventak PRx defibrillation s.
Ventak PRx III/Endotak s.
840 ventilator s.
ventricular resynchronization s.
Ventritex TVL s.
VersaStep laparoscopy s.
vessel occlusion s.
Veterans Affairs Medical Center scoring s.
Viagraph ECG s.
video s.
videodensitometric analysis s.
Vigilance monitoring s.

Vingmed CFM 800 echocardiographic s.
Virtuoso LX Smart CPAP s.
Visa Iris s.
Vision blood cardioplegia s.
Vitatron pacing s.
VNUS Closure s.
VPAP II ST ventilatory support s.
Wallstent endoprosthesis with Unistep Plus delivery s.
wall tracking s.
WaveMap intracoronary blood pressure measurement s.
WaveWire intracoronary blood pressure measurement s.
WCD 2000 S.
Welch Allyn/Schiller AT-10 Exercise Testing s.
White s.
Wiktor GX Hepamed coated coronary stent s.
Wiktor Prime coronary stent s.
Wingspan stent s.
Xact carotid stent s.
Xcelerant delivery s.
Xillix LIFE-Lung s.
X-Press vascular closure s.
X-Scribe stress testing s.
X-Sizer single-use catheter s.
XYZ lead s.
Yellow IRIS s.
Zenith AAA endovascular graft s.
Zeus s.

systema
s. cardiovasculare
s. conducens cordis
s. respiratorium

system/catheter
RPM tracking s./c.

systemic
s. arterial air embolism
s. arterial catheter
s. arterial pressure (SAP)
s. arterial resistance (Rsa)
s. betamethasone
s. blood flow (Qs, SBF)
s. blood pressure (Psa)
s. circulation
s. collateral
s. corticosteroid
dexamethasone s.
s. erythromycin
s. granulomatous vasculitis
s. heart
s. hemodynamic parameters
s. hemodynamics
s. hydration
s. hydrocortisone
s. infection

s. inflammatory response syndrome (SIRS)
s. ischemic branch vessel involvement (SIBVI)
s. lupus erythematosus (SLE)
s. mean arterial pressure (SMAP)
s. necrotizing vasculitis
s. prednisolone
s. prothrombosis
s. to pulmonary artery anastomosis
s. to pulmonary connection
s. pulmonary fistula (SPF)
s. to pulmonary shunt
s. sclerosis (SS, SSc)
s. thromboembolism
s. thrombotic propensity
triamcinolone (s.)
s. vascular hypertension
s. vascular resistance (SVR)
s. vascular resistance index (SVRI)
s. vasoconstriction
s. venous atrium
s. venous hypertension
s. venous return

systodiastolic flow
systogram
systole (S)
aborted s.
s. alternans
anticipated s.
atrial s.
auricular s.
cardiac s.
duration of s. (DS)
electrical s.
electromechanical s.
frustrate s.
hemic s.
isovolumic s.
late s.
premature s.
premature ventricular s. (PVS)
total electromechanical s. (QS₂)
ventricular s.
ventricular ectopic s.

systolic
s. acceleration time (SAT)
s. anterior motion (SAM)
s. apical impulse
s. apical murmur
s. arterial blood pressure (SABP)
s. atrial pressure (SAP)
basal s.
s. blood pressure (BPS, SBP, SYS-BP)
s. bruit
s. bulging
s. click (SC)

systolic *(continued)*
  s. click-late systolic murmur syndrome
  s. click-murmur syndrome
  s. click syndrome (SCS)
  s. coronary artery narrowing (SCAN)
  s. current
  s. current of injury
  s. discharge (SD)
  s. doming
  s. dysfunction
  s. ejection murmur (SEM)
  s. ejection period (SEP)
  s. ejection rate (SER)
  s. function
  s. gallop
  s. gallop rhythm
  s. gradient
  s. heart failure (SHF)
  s. honk
  s. hypertension
  s. left ventricular pressure
  s. motion (SM)
  s. murmur (SM)
  s. pressure (Ps, SP)
  s. pressure time index (SPTI)
pulmonary artery s. (PAS)
  s. pulmonary artery pressure (sPAP)

pulmonary venous s. (PVs)
  s. pulmonary venous velocity
  s. recoil
  s. reflection wave
  s. regurgitant murmur
  s. reserve
  s. reversal
segment length, s. (SLS)
  s. shock
  s. stiffness
  s. S wave
  s. thrill
  s. time (ST)
  s. time interval (STI)
  s. trough
  s. true lumen collapse
  s. twist
  s. upstroke time
  s. velocity integral (SVI)
  s. velocity ratio
  s. wall motion velocity (Vsys)
  s. whipping
  s. whoop
systolic/diastolic (S/D)
systolometer
SyvekPatch topical hemostasis patch
szulgai
  Mycobacterium s.

T
 electrocardiographic wave corresponding
  to repolarization of ventricles
 temperature
 thrombus
  T artifact
  T axis
  T cell
  T cell defect
  T $_H$2-cell dominance
  T graft
  T loop
  T lymphocyte
  nonspecific ST and T (NSSTT)
  T sign
  T stent
  T system
  T technique
  T tube
  T tubule
  T wave
T1
 tricuspid first sound
 tricuspid valve closure sound
T$_4$
 thyroxine
T$_E$
 duration of expiration
 expiratory time
T$_I$
 duration of inspiration
 inspiratory time
T$_b$
 buildup time
T1-weighted image
T2 relaxation time
T2-weighted MRI
TA
 arterial tension
 tantalum
 transposition of aorta
 tricuspid atresia
 truncus arteriosus
T + A
 ticlopidine plus aspirin
^{178}TA
 tantalum-178
Ta
  Ta segment
  Ta wave
TAA
 thoracic aortic aneurysm
 transcoronary alcohol ablation
 transverse aortic arch
 triamcinolone acetonide

TAB
 total atrial blanking
  TAB period
tabacosis
tabby
  t. cat heart
  t. cat striation
tabetic cuirass
table
  Akron tilt t.
  anterior t.
  t. binding
  decompression t.
  Diamond-Forrester t.
  Siemens open heart t.
  tilt t.
tablet
  Afrin T.
  Aprodine T.
  Aristocort T.
  Atacand Plus t.
  Avelox t.
  Betapace AF t.
  Cardizem T.
  CellCept t.
  Cenafed Plus T.
  cerivastatin sodium t.
  Deconamine T.
  diltiazem HCl extended-release t.
  Genac T.
  Mevacor lovastatin t.
  mycophenolate mofetil t.
  NitroQuick sublingual t.
  Nolvadex t.
  Pacerone t.
  Taztia XT extended-release t.
  Triposed T.
  Wobenzym t.
tabourka
  bruit de t.
tabun
TAC
 truncus arteriosus communis
Tac-3 injection
tache
  t. blanche
  t. laiteuse
tachogram
tachometer
tachyarrhythmia
  atrial t.
  T. Detection Software
  double ectopic t.
  malignant ventricular t.
  multifocal supraventricular t.

tachyarrhythmia *(continued)*
- reentrant ventricular t.
- supraventricular t. (SVT)
- sustained reentrant ventricular t. (SRVT)
- triple ectopic t.
- ventricular t. (VTA)

tachyarrhythmic substrate

tachybrady
- t. arrhythmia
- t. syndrome

tachybradycardia syndrome

tachycardia
- accelerated idioventricular t.
- accessory pathway mediated t.
- alternating bidirectional t.
- antidromic circus movement t.
- antidromic reciprocating t.
- artificial circus movement t. (ACMT)
- atrial t. (AT)
- atrial chaotic t.
- atrial ectopic t. (AET)
- atrial paroxysmal t.
- atrial ventricular nodal reentry t.
- atrial ventricular reciprocating t. (AVRT)
- atriofascicular Mahaim reentrant t.
- atrioventricular junctional reciprocating t.
- atrioventricular nodal t. (AVNT)
- atrioventricular nodal reentrant t. (AVNRT)
- atrioventricular nodal reentry t. (AVNRT)
- atrioventricular reciprocating t. (AVRT)
- atrioventricular reentrant t. (AVRT)
- atypical atrioventricular nodal reentrant t. (AAVNRT)
- auricular t.
- automatic atrial t. (AAT)
- automatic ectopic t.
- A-V junctional t.
- A-V nodal reentry t.
- A-V node reentrant t.
- A-V reciprocating t.
- Belhassen t.
- bidirectional ventricular t.
- bundle branch reentrant t.
- burst of ventricular t.
- catecholaminergic polymorphic ventricular t. (CPVT)
- chaotic atrial t.
- chronic ectopic atrial t. (CEAT)
- circus movement t. (CMT)
- Coumel t.
- t. cycle length
- double t. (DT)
- drug-refractory t.
- ectopic atrial t. (EAT)
- ectopic junctional t.
- endless loop t. (ELT)
- endocardial mapping of ventricular t.
- t. en salves
- entrainment of t.
- essential t.
- exercise-induced ventricular t.
- t. exophthalmica
- familial t.
- familial polymorphic ventricular t. (FPVT)
- fascicular t.
- fetal t.
- idiopathic left bundle branch block-shaped ventricular t.
- idiopathic ventricular t. (IVT)
- idioventricular t.
- inappropriate sinus t. (IST)
- incessant atrial t.
- incessant ventricular t.
- inducible polymorphic ventricular t.
- intraatrial reentrant t.
- intraatrial reentry t. (IART)
- junctional t. (JT)
- junctional ectopic t. (JET)
- junctional reciprocating t.
- left ventricular outflow tract t.
- macroreentrant atrial t.
- Mahaim-type t.
- malignant ventricular t.
- monoform t.
- monomorphic ventricular t. (MVT)
- multifocal atrial t. (MAT, MFAT, MFT)
- multiform t.
- narrow-complex t.
- nodal paroxysmal t.
- nodal reentrant t.
- nonparoxysmal atrioventricular junctional t. (NPJT)
- nonsuppressible ventricular t.
- nonsustained ventricular t. (NSVT)
- orthodromic atrioventricular reciprocating t.
- orthodromic A-V reentrant t.
- orthodromic circus movement t.
- orthodromic reciprocating t. (ORT)
- orthostatic t.
- pacemaker circus movement t. (PCMT)
- pacemaker-mediated t. (PMT)
- pacing-induced t. (PIT)
- parasystolic ventricular t.
- paroxysmal t. (PT)
- paroxysmal atrial t. (PAT)

paroxysmal atrioventricular nodal
  reciprocal t. (PAVNRT)
paroxysmal junctional t. (PJT)
paroxysmal nodal t.
paroxysmal reentrant
  supraventricular t.
paroxysmal sinus t.
paroxysmal supraventricular t. (PST,
  PSVT)
paroxysmal ventricular t. (PVT)
t. pathway mapping
permanent atrial t.
permanent junctional reciprocating t.
  (PJRT)
pleomorphic t.
polymorphic ventricular t.
polymorphous ventricular t.
primary ventricular t. (PVT)
rapid nonsustained ventricular t.
reciprocating t. (RT)
reciprocating macroreentry
  orthodromic t.
reentrant t. (RT)
reentrant atrial t.
reentrant supraventricular t.
reflex t.
refractory t.
repetitive monomorphic
  ventricular t.
repetitive paroxysmal ventricular t.
resting sinus t.
right ventricular outflow tract t.
salvo of ventricular t.
S-A nodal reentrant t.
scar-related ventricular t.
self-terminating t.
sinoventricular t. (SVT)
sinus t. (ST)
sinus nodal reentrant t.
sleeping t.
slow-fast t.
slow paroxysmal atrial t. (SPAT)
spontaneous reentrant sustained
  ventricular t.
subepicardial ventricular t.
suppressible ventricular t.
supraventricular t. (SVT)
sustained t.
sustained monomorphic
  ventricular t. (SMVT)
sustained ventricular t. (SVT)
torsade de pointes ventricular t.
ventricular t. (VT)
ventricular fibrillation/ventricular t.
  (VF/VT)
wide QRS t.
t. window
Wolff-Parkinson-White reentrant t.
tachycardia-bradycardia syndrome

tachycardiac
tachycardia-dependent aberrancy
tachycardia-induced
  t.-i. cardiomyopathy
  t.-i. heart failure
  t.-i. myopathy
tachycardia-polyuria syndrome
tachycardic
tachycrotic
tachydysrhythmia
tachykinin
  t. receptor
  t. receptor antagonist
tachypacing
tachyphylactic
tachyphylaxis
tachypnea
  happy t.
  nervous t.
tachyrhythmia
tachysystole
TACI
  total anterior circulation infarct
tacrolimus
TACS
  total anterior circulation syndrome
tactile fremitus
tadalafil
TAE
  transcatheter arterial embolization
Taema ventilator
tag
  2-dimensional t.
  emergency medical t. (EMT)
  epicardial fat t.
  pleural t.
Tagarno 3SD cineangiography projector
tagged
  t. acquisition
  expression sequence t. (EST)
  t. magnetic resonance imaging
tagging
  spin t.
Tag-It cystic fibrosis kit
TAH
  total artificial heart
    Berlin TAH
    CardioWest TAH
    Penn State TAH
    University of Akron TAH
    Utah TAH
    Vienna TAH
TAH-t
  temporary total artificial heart
tailoring
  apical t.
  root t.
tail sign
Taiwan acute respiratory (TWAR)

T

Takayasu
- T. aortitis
- T. arteritis
- T. disease
- idiopathic arteritis of T.
- T. syndrome

Takayasu-Onishi disease

Take Control

takotsubo, tako tsubo
- t. cardiomyopathy (TTC)
- t. heart
- t. syndrome

Talairach space

talc
- t. granulomatosis
- t. operation
- t. pleurodesis
- t. pneumoconiosis
- t. poudrage
- t. slurry

talcosis

talent
- T. bifurcated endograft
- T. graft
- T. LPS endoluminal stent-graft system

tall
- t. oil asthma
- t. T wave

Talon balloon dilation catheter

TAM
- transtelephonic ambulatory monitoring
- tricuspid anular motion
- TAM system

Tambocor

tambour
- bruit de t.
- t. sound

TAMI
- transmural anterior myocardial infarction
- TAMI protocol

Tamiflu

Tamm-Horsfall protein

Tamofen

Tamone

tamoxifen

tamponade, tamponage
- acute t.
- atypical t.
- balloon t.
- cardiac t. (CT)
- chronic t.
- endobronchial t.
- esophageal t.
- esophagogastric t.
- heart t.
- left ventricular cardiac t. (LVCT)
- low-pressure t.
- pericardial t. (PT)

- Rose t.
- subacute t.
- traumatic t.

TAN
- total adenine nucleotide

Tanatril

tandem
- T. cardiac device
- t. lesion
- t. needle approach

TandemHeart
- T. centrifugal pump/ventricular assist device
- T. pVAD

tangential
- t. flow filtration (TFF)
- t. percussion

Tangier disease

TANI
- total axial node irradiation

tank respirator

tannate
- methyclothiazide and cryptenamine t.

Tanner operation

tantalum (TA)
- t. bronchogram
- t. mesh
- t. myocardial marker
- t. plate
- powdered t.
- radioactive t.
- t. ring
- t. stent
- t. wire

tantalum-178 (^{178}TA)
- t.-178 generator

TAO
- troleandomycin

TAP
- Thornton anterior positioner
- transesophageal atrial pacing
- transluminal angioplasty

tap
- bloody t.
- mitral t.
- pericardial t.
- pleural t.

TAPE
- temporary atrial pacemaker electrode

tape
- B101 ET Tape II adhesive t.
- ColorZone t.
- Hy-Tape waterproof adhesive t.
- Original Pink Tape waterproof adhesive t.
- Silastic t.
- twill t.
- umbilical t.

vascular t.
waterproof t.

TapeMeasure computerized planimetry

taper

short T.

tapered movable core curved wire guide

tapering

airway t.

tapotage

taprostene

TAPSE

transesophageal atrial pacing stress echocardiography

TAPVC

total anomalous pulmonary venous connection

TAPVD

total anomalous pulmonary venous drainage

TAPVR

total anomalous pulmonary venous return

Taq

T. DNA polymerase
T. extender

TAQW

transient abnormal Q wave

TAR

thoracic aortic rupture
thrombocytopenia-absent radius
TAR syndrome

tar

coal t.

tardive

cyanose t.
t. cyanosis
t. muscular dystrophy

tardokinesis

tardus

pulsus t.
pulsus parvus et t.

target

dyspnea t.
t. heart rate (THR)
t. INR
t. lesion
t. lesion revascularization (TLR)
t. organ disease/clinical cardiovascular disease (TOD/CCD)
plateau-pressure t.
t. site
T. Therapeutics Stealth angioplasty balloon
T. Tip lead
t. vessel
t. vessel failure
t. vessel revascularization (TVR)

target-6

early secretory antigenic t.-6 (ESAT-6)

targeted area

Tarka

Taro-Ampicillin

Taro-Atenol

Taro-Cloxacillin

TARP

total atrial refractory period

TARTI

total apexcardiographic relaxation time index

tartrate

antimony potassium t.
metoprolol t.
phenindamine t.
vinorelbine t.
zolpidem t.

tartrazine asthma

TAS

Thrombolytic Assessment System

TASH

transcoronary ablation of septal hypertrophy

task

bean-spooning t.
metabolic equivalent of t. (MET)

tasosartan

TAT

thrombin-antithrombin
turnaround time

Tatlockia micdadei

taurinum

cor t.

Taussig-Bing

T.-B. anomaly
T.-B. complex
T.-B. disease
T.-B. heart
T.-B. malformation
T.-B. syndrome

TAV

transvenous aortovelography

TAVB

total atrioventricular block

Tawara atrioventricular node

taxane

Taxol

taxonomic

taxonomy

Taxotere

Taxus

T. coronary stent
T. drug-eluting stent
T. Express stent
T. Libèrtè stent

Taybi syndrome

Taylor dispersion

Tay-Sachs disease
Tazicef
Tazidime
tazobactam
Taztia XT extended-release tablet
TB
    tuberculosis
        TB tine test
TBARS
    thiobarbituric acid-reactive substance
TBB, TBBX, TBBx
    transbronchial biopsy
TBFV
    tidal breathing flow volume
TBI
    thrombotic brain infarction
    total body irradiation
TBird ventilator system
TBLB
    transbronchial lung biopsy
TBNA
    transbronchial needle aspiration
TBP
    total bypass
TBV
    total blood volume
TC
    total cholesterol
3TC
    lamivudine
Tc
    tricuspid closure
^{99m}Tc, Tc-99^m
    technetium-99m
        ^{99m}Tc MIBI-SPECT
        ^{99m}Tc sestamibi
        ^{99m}Tc sestamibi imaging
        ^{99m}Tc sestamibi scintigraphy
        ^{99m}Tc tetrofosmin imaging
TCA
    total circulatory arrest
TCABG
    triple coronary artery bypass graft
TCAD
    transplant coronary artery disease
TCAG
    triple coronary artery graft
TCB
    total cardiopulmonary bypass
    transcatheter biopsy
TCC
    transcatheter closure
TCCS
    transcranial color-coded sonography
TCD
    transverse cardiac diameter
        TCD sonography
        TCD ultrasonography
        TCD ultrasound

TCD100M digital transcranial Doppler system
Tc-diethylenetriamine pentaacetic acid
T-cell
    T-c. expansion
    T-c. repertoire
    T-c. subset
TCF
    total coronary flow
TCG
    time compensation gain
T-channel
TC/HDL
    total cholesterol/high-density lipoproteins
        TC/HDL ratio
TCI HeartMate mechanical circulatory support system
TCM30 transcutaneous oxygen monitor
TCN-P
    triciribine phosphate
TCOM
    transcutaneous oxygen monitor
T-composite arterial graft
TCP
    transcutaneous pacemaker
    transcutaneous pacing
TCPC
    total cavopulmonary connection
TCPS
    total cavopulmonary shunt
TCS
    total coronary score
TCT
    thoracic computed tomography
    thrombin clotting time
    transcardial catheter therapy
    transcatheter therapy
    trunk control test
        TCT scan
tcu-PA
    2-chain urokinase plasminogen activator
TDCO
    thermodilution cardiac output
        TDCO measurement
TDD
    thermal-dye dilution
    thoracic duct drainage
TDI
    tissue Doppler imaging
    toluene diisocyanate
        TDI M-mode echocardiography
TDI-induced asthma
TDI-Tei index
TDP
    therapist-driven protocol
    torsade de pointes

TdP
torsade de pointes
TdT-mediated dUTP nick-end labeling (TUNEL)
TE
echo delay time
thromboembolism
tracheoesophageal
treadmill exercise
TE fistula
TEA
thromboendarterectomy
transluminal extraction atherectomy
tea
black t.
pectoral t.
t. taster's cough
teacher's node
team
Bimodality Lung Oncology T. (BLOT)
cardiac resuscitation T. (CRT)
code blue T. (CBT)
code response T. (CRT)
Public Health Response T. (PHRT)
TEAP
transesophageal atrial pacing
tear
Boerhaave t.
distal reentry t.
t. gas, teargas
great vessel t.
intimal t.
Mallory-Weiss t.
medial t.
neointimal t.
proximal entry t.
teardrop heart
teargas (*var. of* tear gas)
TEB
thoracic electrical bioimpedance
teboroxime
t. imaging
t. scan
technetium-99m t.
Tebrazid
TEC
thromboembolic complication
transluminal endarterectomy catheter
transluminal extraction catheter
TEC atherectomy device
TEC atherectomy system
TEC extraction catheter
TEC guide catheter
TECAB
totally endoscopic coronary artery bypass
tecadenoson
technetium
t. depreotide

t. glucarate
t. pyrophosphate
technetium-99m-sestamibi single-photon emission computed tomography
technetium-99m (^{99m}Tc, Tc-99^{m})
t.-99m hexakis 2-methoxyisobutyl isonitrile
t.-99m hexamibi scan
t.-99m 2-methoxyisobutyl isonitrile
t.-99m methylene diphosphonate
t.-99m MIBI
t.-99m MIBI imaging
t.-99m pyrophosphate
t.-99m sestamibi SPECT
t.-99m sestamibi stress test
t.-99m sestamibi tomographic imaging
sodium pertechnetate t.-99m
t.-99m stannous pyrophosphate scintiscan
t.-99m teboroxime
t.-99m tetrofosmin
t.-99m tetrofosmin imaging
technetium-99m-labeled annexin V
technetium-99m mercaptoacetyltriglycine
technetium-sestamibi
t.-s. SPECT
t.-s. stress test
technetium-teboroxime
Technicare Omega 500 CT
technique
ablative t.
airway occlusion t.
Amplatz t.
Angus t.
antegrade double balloon/double wire t.
antegrade/retrograde cardioplegia t.
anterior sandwich patch t.
anterograde transseptal t.
antialiasing t.
arch-first t.
atrial-well t.
background subtraction t.
ballpoint pen t.
beating heart edge-to-edge t.
Bentall inclusion t.
Bergstrom needle biopsy t.
black-white interface t. (BWIT)
Bland-Altman t.
blood oxygenation level-dependent t.
BOLD t.
bootstrap 2-vessel t.
breathing t.
Brecher and Cronkite t.
Brockenbrough t.
Brompton t.
button t.

technique *(continued)*

Carpentier t.
Carrie coronary stent placement t.
catheterization t.
chloramine-T t.
Ciaglia serial dilation t.
cine t.
clearance t.
clonogenic t.
Collins chain compensated
  gasometer t.
Colombo inverted Y t.
combo t.
Copeland t.
coronary flow reserve t.
cough CPR t.
crash t.
Crawford graft inclusion t.
Creech t.
crush stent t.
cryosurgical t.
CT-guided stereotaxic t.
culotte coronary stenting t.
culotte stent t.
cutdown t.
Davies t.
DCA debulking t.
digital subtraction t.
dilator and sheath t.
direct insertion t.
directional atherectomy debulking t.
Doppler auto-correlation t.
Dotter t.
Dotter-Judkins t.
double-balloon (9-11) t.
double-dummy t.
double-syringe t.
double-wire t.
Douglas bag t.
drawback stent deployment t.
dye-dilution t.
ECG signal-averaging t.
elephant trunk t.
en bloc no-touch t.
endocardial mapping t. (EMT)
endovascular edge-to-edge t.
entangling t.
exchange t.
Exorcist t.
Fantoni translaryngeal
  tracheostomy t.
Fick t.
Finapres t.
first-pass t.
flotation catheter t.
flow mapping t.
flush and bathe t.
forced expiratory t.
forced oscillation t. (FOT)

fork stenting t.
Forssmann t.
forward triangle t.
Fourier-acquired steady-state t.
  (FAST)
frozen elephant trunk t.
gated t.
George-Lewis t.
gloved fist t.
Goris background subtraction t.
grabbing t.
Grüntzig t.
guidewire t.
harmonic imaging ultrasound t.
Heartport t.
high-pressure inflation t.
hydrogen inhalation t.
immunofluorescent t.
immunostaining t.
5-in-6 t.
indicator dilution t.
indocyanine green indicator
  dilution t.
inhaled radioaerosol t.
Inoue balloon t.
Inoue single-balloon t.
inverted crush t.
inverted V, Y t.
Jatene t.
J-loop t.
Judkins t.
Judkins-Sones t.
Kern t.
kissing balloon t.
laser-assisted internal fabrication t.
  (LIFT)
LocaLisa t.
long-leg venography t.
Lown t.
magnetization t.
Marbach-Weil t.
Mason Sones transbrachial t.
McGoon t.
Merendino t.
minimal leak t.
modified brachial t.
modified Seldinger t.
Mullins blade t.
multibreath nitrogen washout t.
multiplanar reconstruction t.
multiple-dilator t.
multislab t.
nasal pool t.
Nikaidoh-Bex t.
nitrogen washout t.
no-clamp t.
noise-canceling t.
no-leak t.
no-touch t.

occluder balloon wash-out t.
open t.
oscillation t.
Oxford t.
2-patch t.
percutaneous t.
percutaneous edge-to-edge t.
PI MRI t.
Porstmann t.
port access t.
posture t.
pranayama breathing t.
pressure-controlled ventilation t.
pressure half-time t.
pressure-volume curve measurement
  using syringe t.
pullback t.
Rabinov venography t.
radiographic t.
radionuclide t.
raised-volume rapid
  thoracoabdominal compression t.
Rashkind balloon t.
rebreathing t.
relaxation t.
Ricketts-Abrams t.
Robicsek t.
Rosalki t.
scatterplot smoothing t.
Schonander t.
Schoonmaker-King single catheter t.
Sealy-Laragh t.
second harmonic imaging
  ultrasound t.
Seldinger percutaneous t.
Semple t.
Sewall t.
shaping behavioral t.
Sheehan and Dodge t.
SHI ultrasound t.
single-dilator t.
skewer t.
skirt t.
snare t.
Sones t.
sonication t.
SPAMM t.
Sparks mandrel t.
spatial modulation of
  magnetization t.
static dilation t.
steerable over-the-wire
  angioplasty t.
Stewart-Hamilton cardiac output t.
surface modification t.
syringe t.
T t.
telescoping anastomotic t.
T-graft configuration t.

thermal dilution t.
thermodilution t.
track-ball t.
translaryngeal tracheostomy t.
trouser legs and seat t.
Trusler aortic valve t.
TurboFLASH t.
upgated t.
velocity catheter t.
ventilatory t.
video-assisted diagnostic
  thoracoscopic t.
Waldhausen subclavian flap t.
wax-matrix t.
xenon washout t.
Y t.
Zavala t.

technologist
cardiovascular t. (CVT)
National Alliance of
  Cardiovascular T.'s (NACT)
National Society of
  Cardiovascular T.'s (NSCT)

technology
acquisition zoom t.
Alkermes AIR pulmonary drug
  delivery t.
American Society of Extra-
  Corporeal T. (AmSECT)
angiographic contrast injection
  system t. (ACIST)
AZ t.
BioZ impedance cardiography t.
biventricular resynchronization t.
CardioFix pericardium with
  PhotoFix t.
Coblation t.
demineralization t.
Extracorporeal Circulation T. (ECT)
FilterLine sampling t.
Focus t.
Focus Angioplasty Catheter T.
  (FACT, FACT-22)
2H T. Breathing Circuit Filter
  (2HBCF)
Lingraphica system treatment t.
Oxismart advanced signal
  processing and alarm t.
perfusion t.
phased array t.
PORxin t.
PulseDose oxygen delivery t.
SAC data acquisition t.
serial autocorrelation data
  acquisition t.
vein-to-vein t.
VTS t.
Vueport balloon t.
Technos ultrasound system

Techstar
> T. device
> T. percutaneous suture
> T. XL 6F percutaneous vascular surgical system
> T. XL 6F PVS system

TECSAC
> telecollaboration for signal analysis in cardiology

TED
> thromboembolic disease
> TED antiembolism stockings
> TED hose

TEDD
> total end-diastolic diameter

tedisamil

Tedlar bag

TEE
> transesophageal echocardiography
> 3D TEE
> TEE transducer

TEE-DSE
> transesophageal echocardiography-dobutamine stress echocardiography

Teejel

TEEP
> transesophageal echocardiography with pacing

TEF
> tracheoesophageal fistula

TEF$_{25}$
> tidal expiratory flow at 25% of tidal volume

TEF$_{25}$/PTEF
> ratio of tidal expiratory flow at 25% of tidal volume and peak tidal expiratory flow

TEF$_{50}$
> tidal expiratory flow at 50% of tidal volume

TEF$_{50}$/TIF$_{50}$
> ratio of tidal expiratory and inspiratory flow at 50% of tidal volume

TEF$_{75}$
> tidal expiratory flow at 75% of tidal volume

Tefcor movable core straight wire guide

Teflon
> T. Bardic plug
> T. catheter
> T. coating
> T. felt bolster
> T. felt patch
> T. graft
> T. intracardiac patch
> T. pledget
> T. pledget suture buttress
> T. sheath

> T. trileaflet prosthesis
> woven T.
> T. woven prosthesis

Teflon-coated
> T.-c. guidewire
> T.-c. wire skeleton

TEG
> thromboelastogram
> thromboelastography

tegafur
> uracil and t. (UFT)

TEH
> theophylline, ephedrine, hydroxyzine

Tei
> T. index
> T. index of myocardial performance

Teichholz
> T. correction
> T. ejection fraction
> T. equation
> T. formula

teichoic acid antibody

teicoplanin
> glycopeptide t.

telangiectasia
> ataxia t.
> calcinosis, Raynaud phenomenon, esophageal involvement, sclerodactyly, t. (CREST)
> hemorrhagic hereditary t.
> hereditary hemorrhagic t. (HHT)
> t. syndrome

teleauscultation

telecardiogram

telecardiophone

telecollaboration for signal analysis in cardiology (TECSAC)

Telectronics
> T. Accufix pacing lead
> T. ATP implantable cardioverter-defibrillator
> T. Guardian ATP 4210 device
> T. Guardian ATP II ICD
> T. pacemaker
> T. Pacing Systems

telecurietherapy

telediastolic

telelectrocardiogram

telemetry
> cardiac t.
> Conexus wireless t.
> multiple-parameter t. (MPT)
> pacemaker t.
> real-time t.

telemonitor

telemonitored polysomnography

teleradiology

telescope

telescoping anastomotic technique
telesystolic
telethermometer
    YSI 4000 t.
telithromycin
telmisartan
telomere
telomeric shortening
telopeptide
    type I collagen t. (ICTP)
TEM
    transmission electron microscopy
    transtelephonic exercise monitor
temafloxacin
temazepam
temozolomide
tempeh
temperature (T)
    central venous t. (CVT)
    core t.
    esophageal t.
    t. and pulse (T&P, T+P)
    t., pulse, respiration (TPR)
temperature-sensing pacemaker
TempLink extension cable
Tempo diagnostic catheter
temporal
    t. arteritis
    t. average intensity (I_{ta})
    t. dispersion
    t. peak intensity (I_{tp})
    t. resolution
temporary
    t. atrial pacemaker electrode (TAPE)
    t. filter
    t. pacemaker (TPM)
    t. pacemaker placement
    t. pacing
    t. pervenous lead
    t. total artificial heart (TAH-t)
    t. unilateral pulmonary artery occlusion
tenacious
    t. mucus
    t. sputum
tenacity
    sputum t.
tenascin-C
tenase complex
tend-and-befriend
    t.-a.-b. response
    t.-a.-b. response to stress
tenderness
    point t.
tendinea
    macula t.
tendineae
    chordae t.

tendinosum
    xanthoma t.
tendinous
    t. spot
    t. xanthoma
    t. zone
    t. zones of heart
tendo
    t. cricoesophageus
    t. infundibuli
tendon
    t. of conus
    coronary t.
    cricoesophageal t.
    false t.
    t. of infundibulum
    t. of Todaro
    trefoil t.
tendophony
tendril
    T. DX implantable pacing lead
    T. DX steroid-eluting active-fixation pacing lead
    T. SDX model 1688 active-fixation pacing lead
tenecteplase (TNKase, TNK-tPA)
Tenex
Tenif
teniposide
tennis racket peripheral angiographic catheter
tenonometer
tenophony
Tenoretic
Tenormin
Tenox
tense
    t. edema
    t. pulse
tensile stress
Tensilon injection
tension
    alveolar-arterial oxygen t. ($A-aO_2$)
    alveolar carbon dioxide t.
    alveolar oxygen t.
    arterial t. (TA)
    arterial carbon dioxide t. ($PaCO_2$)
    arterial oxygen t. (PaO_2)
    carbon dioxide t.
    isometric systolic t. (IST)
    left ventricular t. (LVT)
    myocardial t.
    oxygen t.
    t. pneumopericardium
    t. pneumothorax
    wall t.
tension-length relation
tension-time index
tensor palatini

T

Tensys T-line blood pressure monitor
tent
>croup t.
>Croupette child t.
>mist t.
>oxygen t.
>pleural t.
>steam t.

tenting
>t. of hemidiaphragm
>t. sign
>t. of skin

tenuis
>*Alternaria* t.

TEP
>transesophageal pacing

Teq-Paq
>Tequin T.-P.

Tequin Teq-Paq
teratogenicity
teratoma
>benign t.
>pericardial t.
>t. tumor

terazosin hydrochloride
terbutaline sulfate
terconazole
terephthalate
>polyethylene t. (PET)

terfenadine
terikalant
terminal
>t. aorta
>t. bronchiole
>t. cisterna
>t. edema
>t. endocarditis
>t. filtered QRS signal
>t. groove
>t. internal carotid artery (TICA)
>t. phase
>t. pneumonia
>t. Purkinje fibers
>t. respiratory unit (TRU)
>t. weaning
>Wilson central t.

Terminalia arjuna
terminalis
>bronchiolus t.
>crista t.
>sulcus t.

termination
>exercise t.
>underdrive t.

terminus
terodiline
terrae
>*Mycobacterium* t.

Terramycin IM injection

terreus
>*Aspergillus* t.

terror
>night t.'s

tertiary
>t. bronchus
>t. contraction
>t. syphilis

tertile
Terumo
>T. Crosswire guidewire
>T. Crosswire NT guidewire
>T. Pinnacle sheath
>T. Radifocus Glidewire
>T. SP coaxial catheter
>T. stent

TES
>thoracic endometriosis syndrome
>transcutaneous electrical stimulation

TESD
>total end-systolic diameter

tesla
Teslac
Tessalon Perles
test
>Aachen Aphasia T. (AAT)
>abdominal jugular t.
>ABG point-of-care t.
>Acarex-t.
>ACB t.
>Access AccuTnI troponin I t.
>AccuMeter theophylline t.
>AccuTnI troponin I t.
>acetylcholine t.
>acid infusion t.
>Action Research Arm T.
>adenosine thallium t.
>Adson t.
>Advanced Care cholesterol t.
>aerobic exercise stress t.
>aerosol challenge t.
>ajmaline t.
>AlaSTAT latex allergy t.
>albumin cobalt binding t.
>alertness t.
>Allen t.
>alternans t.
>Amplicor *Mycobacterium tuberculosis* t.
>amplified *Mycobacterium tuberculosis* direct t. (AMTDT)
>Anderson t.
>angiotensin sensitivity t. (AST)
>ankle-brachial index t.
>anoxemia t.
>antistreptozyme t.
>apoE t.
>Apt t.
>arginine tolerance t. (ATT)

Arloing-Courmont t.
arm exercise stress t.
arm-tongue time t.
arterial blood gas point-of-care t.
  (ABG PCT)
Aspergillus skin prick t.
Astrand bicycle exercise stress t.
atrial pacing stress t.
atropine t.
Balke exercise stress t.
Balke-Ware t.
balloon distention t.
Benton Lines T.
Bernstein t.
beryllium lymphocyte
  proliferation t. (BeLPT)
beta-D-glucan t.
bicycle ergometer exercise stress t.
bile solubility t.
Biosafe Hemo-Quant rapid
  anemia t.
Blake exercise stress t.
blanch t.
blot t.
Blumenau t.
Bordet-Gengou t.
brachial plexus tension t.
breath excretion t.
breathholding t.
breath pentane t.
Breslow-Day t.
Brodie-Trendelenburg tourniquet t.
bronchial challenge t.
bronchial provocation t.
bronchoprovocation t.
broth t.
Bruce exercise stress t.
Bruce maximum stress t. (BMST)
Brunnstrom-Fugl-Meyer Scale for
  motor t.
CAMP t.
carbachol provocation t.
carbohydrate utilization t.
Cardiac STATus CK-MB t.
Cardiac STATus CK-MB/myoglobin
  panel t.
Cardiac STATus rapid format
  troponin I panel t.
cardiac stress t. (CST)
cardiolipin flocculation t. (CFT)
cardiolipin microflocculation t.
  (CMFT)
Cardiolite stress t.
Caregiver Strain T.
carotid sinus t.
Casoni t.
ChemTrak AccuMeter
  theophylline t.
Cholesterol 1,2,3 t.

CLA for infusion of catecholamine
  in heart stress t.
Clearview Troponin I t.
coccidioidin t.
coin t.
cold pressor t.
complement-fixation t.
Coombs t.
CPX t.
Crampton t.
^{14}C-triolein breath t.
^{13}C-triolein breath t.
cuff t.
cuff-leak t.
cystatin C t.
Davidson protocol exercise t.
D-dimer t.
Dehio t.
dexamethasone suppression t.
digit span memory t.
dipalmitoyl phosphatidylcholine t.
dipyridamole echocardiography t.
  (DET)
dipyridamole handgrip t.
dipyridamole thallium stress t.
direct amplification t. (DAT)
dobutamine stress t.
double simultaneous stimulation t.
DPPC t.
DR-70 tumor marker t.
duodenal string t.
electrophysiologic t.
ELISPOT t.
Ellestad exercise stress t.
ergonovine provocation t.
Escherich t.
ether t.
euglobin clot t.
euglobulin clot t. (ECT)
euglycemic hyperinsulinemic glucose
  clamp t.
exercise t. (ET)
exercise stress t. (EST)
exercise tolerance t. (ETT)
exercise treadmill t. (ETT)
extrastimulus t.
Farr t.
fetal heart rate nonstress t.
  (FHRNST)
flashing checkerboard t.
fluorescent treponemal antibody
  absorption t.
foam stability t.
Fowler single-breath t.
Frenchay Aphasia Screening T.
  (FAST)
FTA-ABS t.
galactomannan antigen t.

T

test *(continued)*

GenESA system for radionuclide imaging stress t.
Gibbon-Landis t.
Goethlin t.
goodness-of-fit t.
gradational step exercise stress t.
graded exercise t. (GXT)
Griess t.
guidewire traversal t.
Hallion t.
Ham t.
Hamburger t.
handgrip apexcardiographic t. (HAT)
head-down tilt t.
head-up tilt t.
head-up tilt-table t. (HUTTT)
Heaf t.
Heart Failure Knowledge T.
heart rate variability t.
Heartscan heart attack prediction t.
Henle-Coenen t.
hepatojugular reflux t.
Hess capillary t.
high-altitude simulation t. (HAST)
Hines-Brown t.
Hitzenberg t.
HIVAGEN t.
Hosmer-Lemeshow Goodness-of-Fit t.
Hotelling T2 t.
Howell t.
HRV t.
hyperventilation challenge t.
hypoxemia t.
IgG avidity t.
implantation t. (IT)
incremental shuttle walking t. (ISWT)
inhalation challenge t.
intravenous glucose tolerance t. (IVGTT)
isometric handgrip t.
isoproterenol stress t.
isoproterenol tilt-table t.
Jaeger body t.
Jebsen Hand Function T.
Kattus exercise stress t.
Kleihauer t.
Kleihauer-Betke t.
Korotkoff t.
Kveim antigen skin t.
Kveim-Siltzbach t.
laryngeal cough reflex t.
LDL direct blood t.
left atrial transesophageal pacing t. (LATPT)
lepromin t.

Levy Chimeric Faces T.
Lewis-Pickering t.
Liebermann-Burchard t.
Lignieres t.
limited treadmill t. (LTT)
liver function t. (LFT)
Livierato t.
loaded breathing t. (LBT)
low-range heparin management t. (LHMT)
LungAlert t.
lymphocyte transformation t.
Machado-Guerreiro t.
maintenance of wakefulness t. (MWT)
Mantoux t.
Master exercise stress t.
Master 2-step exercise t.
Matas t.
maximal exercise t. (MET)
maximal treadmill stress t. (MTST)
maximum exercise tolerance t. (METT)
methacholine challenge t.
MHA-TP t.
MIBI stress t.
microneutralization t.
6-minute corridor walk t.
10-minute supine/30-minute tilt t.
6-minute walking t. (6MWT, 6-MWT)
modified shuttle t.
modified treadmill exercise t. (MTET)
Moschcowitz t.
MTD t.
MUGA exercise stress t.
Müller t.
multiple sleep latency t. (MSLT)
multistage exercise t. (MET)
multistage maximal effort exercise stress t.
MycoAKT latex bead agglutination t.
Mycobacterium Tuberculosis Direct T.
myoglobulin cardiac diagnostic t.
Nagle exercise stress t.
Nathan t.
Naughton cardiac exercise treadmill t.
Naughton graded exercise stress t.
near patient t. (NPT)
N-geneous automated HDL cholesterol t.
Nickerson-Kveim t.
noninvasive t.
nonspecific challenge t.
Norris t.

Nottingham Sensory Assessment t.
nucleic acid direct amplification t.
Ochsner-Mahorner t.
Optochin disc t.
oral glucose tolerance t. (OGTT)
Osteomark t.
oxygen challenge t.
Pachon t.
p24 antigen t.
paracoccidioidin skin t.
PCR t.
pendulum t.
peppermint t.
Persantine-isonitrile stress t.
Persantine thallium stress t.
Perthes t.
Phalen stress t.
Physical Work Capacity exercise
  stress t.
pilocarpine iontophoresis t.
planar thallium t.
plantar ischemia t.
Plesch t.
POC blood gas t.
point of care t.
postdischarge graded-exercise t.
  (PD-GXT)
PPD skin t.
PPL skin t.
prediscarge t.
PREVU(x) skin sterol t.
primed lymphocyte t.
proBNP t.
progressive exercise t. (PET)
provocation t.
pulmonary function t. (PFT)
purified protein derivative t.
Q-Stress treadmill stress t.
QuantiFeron-TB t.
Quick intravenous liver function t.
radioactive xenon t.
radioallergosorbent t. (RAST)
Ramp cardiac marker t.
Ramp Reader and Ramp
  Myoglobin T.
rapid antigen-detection t.
rapid plasma t.
Read t.
Recurring Figures T. (for short-
  term memory)
Recurring Words T. (for short-term
  memory)
reflex cough t.
Reflotron bedside theophylline t.
t. result
reverse transcriptase polymerase
  chain reaction t.
Rey figure copying t.
Rivermead Behavioral Memory T.

Roos t.
Rumpel-Leede t.
Sabin-Feldman dye t.
Salkowski t.
Sandrock t.
Schapiro-Wilks t.
Schellong t.
Schiff t.
Schlichter t.
Schultze t.
selective arterial secretin
  injection t. (SAST)
serological t.
sestamibi technetium-99m SPECT
  with dipyridamole stress t.
shake t.
Sheffield exercise stress t.
shuttle t.
Sickledex t.
single-breath carbon monoxide t.
single-breath nitrogen washout t.
single-stage exercise stress t.
skin prick t. (SPT)
SNAP t.
Snider match t.
sniff t.
somatosensory evoked potential t.
specific bronchial challenge t.
specific inhalation challenge t.
SpectRx t.
speech mental stress t.
split-function lung t.
Stamey t.
Stand Displacement Amplification t.
2-step exercise t.
Sterneedle tuberculin t.
Stratus cardiac troponin I t.
streptokinase-urokinase myocardial
  infarct t. (SUMIT)
stress t. (ST)
Stroop color word conflict t.
Stroop color word interference t.
submaximal effort tourniquet t.
submaximal treadmill exercise t.
  (STET)
super stress t.
surf t.
sweat chloride t.
swing t.
symptom-limited graded exercise t.
  (SL-GXT)
symptom-limited maximal
  treadmill t.
symptom-limited treadmill
  exercise t.
TB tine t.
technetium-99m sestamibi stress t.
technetium-sestamibi stress t.
thallium-201 exercise stress t.

test *(continued)*
   thallium stress t.
   The Cambridge Heart T-Wave
      Alternans T.
   thermodilution t.
   thyroid function t.
   tilt t.
   tilt-table t. (TTT)
   tine t.
   tiptoe t.
   tolazoline t.
   treadmill t. (TT)
   treadmill exercise t. (TET, TMET)
   treadmill exercise stress t.
   treadmill performance t. (TPT)
   treadmill stress t. (TMST, TST)
   Trendelenburg t.
   treponemal t.
   Triage BNP blood t.
   Tris-buffer infusion t.
   true-positive stress t. (TPST)
   trunk control t. (TCT)
   tuberculin skin t.
   tuberculin tine t.
   Tuffier t.
   Tzanck t.
   Valsalva t.
   vasodilator plus exercise
      treadmill t.
   VDRL t.
   venous occlusion t.
   ventricular accommodation t. (VAT)
   VerifyNow t.
   VEX treadmill t.
   Visov t.
   Vitalometer t.
   Vitalor screening pulmonary
      function t.
   in vitro allergy t.
   Vollmer t.
   volume-challenge t.
   von Recklinghausen t.
   Wada t.
   walk distance t.
   walking ventilation t.
   water-gurgle t.
   Weinberg t.
   whiff t.
   Widal t.
   Wideroe t.
   Wilks-Schapiro t.
   William t.
   Winslow t.
   Wolf Motor Function T. (WMFT)
   word association t. (WAT)
   worksite challenge t.
   X-Scribe stress t.
   Youman-Parlett t.
   Zwenger t.

tester
   IRMA SL blood glucose strip t.
   Polar Electro sport t.
   Quik-Chek external pacer t.
testing *(See also* test)
   cardiopulmonary exercise t. (CPET)
   exercise stress t.
   genetic t.
   histamine challenge t.
   immediate exercise treadmill t.
      (IETT)
   maximal treadmill t. (MTT)
   t. method
   methylcholine challenge t. (MCT)
   mycobacteria t.
   point-of-care t. (POCT)
   serum precipitin t.
   skeletal muscle strength t.
   sweat t.
testolactone
testosterone
Testred
TET
   total ejection time
   treadmill exercise test
Tet, tet
   tetralogy of Fallot
      Tet spell
tetani
      Clostridium t.
tetanus
   anodal closure t. (ACTe)
   anodal duration t. (ADTe, AnDTe)
   anodal opening t. (AOT, AOTe)
   cathodal closure t. (CCTe)
   cathodal duration t. (CDTe)
   cathodal opening t. (COTe)
tethered leaflet
tethering
tetracaine
   t. hydrochloride
   lidocaine, epinephrine, t. (LET)
tetrachloride
   zirconium t.
Tetra coronary stent
tetracrotic
tetracycline
tetrad
   Fallot t.
   t. spell
tetraethylammonium chloride
tetrahedron chest
tetrahydrobiopterin (BH$_4$)
tetrahydrochloride
   diaminobenzidine t.
tetralogy
   Eisenmenger t.
   Fallot t. (FT)

t. of Fallot (Tet, tet, TF, TOF)
t. of Fallot spell

tetranitrate
erythrityl t.
pentaerythritol t. (PETN)

tetrapolar esophageal catheter

tetrazolium
nitroblue t.

tetrodotoxin

tetrofosmin
technetium-99m t.

tE/tTOT
ratio of expiration time and total time of
breathing cycle

Teutleben ligament

Teveten

texaphyrin
lutetium t.

Texas
T. Heart Institute (THI)
T. influenza

textbook
Sleep Multimedia 2.6
computerized t.

tezosentan

TF
tetralogy of Fallot
Thomsen-Friedenreich
tissue factor
TF antigen

TFA
trans fatty acid

TFB
tracheobronchial foreign body

TFCI
transient focal cerebral ischemia

TFE
turbo field echo

TFF
tangential flow filtration

TFF-domain peptide

TFPI
tissue factor pathway inhibitor

TFT
thrombus formation time

TFVL
tidal flow volume loop

TFX Medical
TFX M. catheter stylet
TFX M. safety needle with
introducer

TG
thrombin generation
triglyceride

TGA
transposition of great arteries

TGC
time-gain compensation

time-gain control
time-varied gain control

T-Gesic

TGF
transforming growth factor

TGFA
triglyceride fatty acid

TGI
tracheal gas insufflation

TGL
triglyceride

T-graft configuration technique

TGV
thoracic gas volume
transposition of great vessels

ThA
thoracic aorta

ThAIRapy
T. vest
T. vest airway clearance system

thalamic dementia

thalassemia
sickle cell t.

thalidomide

Thalitone

thallium (Tl)
t. electrocardiogram
t. myocardial scintigraphy (TMS)
t. perfusion imaging
t. rest-redistribution scintigraphy
t. scan
t. scanning
t. SPECT imaging
t. stress test
t. tomography
t. uptake
t. uptake defect
t. washout

thallium-201 (^{201}Tl)
t.-201 exercise stress test
t.-201 perfusion scintigraphy
t.-201 planar scintigraphy
t.-201 sestamibi
t.-201 SPECT scintigraphy

thallous chloride (^{201}Tl)

Thal procedure

Tham

THB
Todd-Hewitt broth
total heart beats

tHcy
total homocysteine

THC:YAG laser

THD
transverse heart diameter

the
T. Cambridge Heart T-Wave
Alternans Test

the *(continued)*
    T. Closer suture-mediated closure system
    T. Global Initiative for Chronic Obstructive Pulmonary Disease (GOLD)
    T. Sports Breather
thebesian
    t. circulation
    t. foramina
    t. valve
    t. vein
Thebesius
    vein of T.
theca cordis
Theden method
Theis rib retractor
Thelin
T-helper 1-type cytokine production
Theo-24
theobromine
Theochron
Theolair
Theolate
theophyllinate
    choline t.
theophylline
    t., ephedrine, hydroxyzine (TEH)
    t., ephedrine, phenobarbital
    t. ethylenediamine
    t. and guaifenesin
    t. sodium glycinate
theorem
    Bayes t.
    Bernoulli t.
theory, pl. **theories**
    Bayliss t.
    Cannon t.
    chaos t.
    crosslinkage t.
    dipole t.
    immunological t.
    Melzack-Wall gate t.
    myogenic t.
    neuroendocrine t.
    neurogenic t.
    Ornish t.
    reentry t.
    response-to-injury t.
    sliding filament t.
    Spitzer t.
TheraCys
TheraKair mattress
TheraPEP PEP therapy system
therapeutic
    t. angiogenesis
    t. bronchoscopy
    t. dissection
    t. efficacy

    t. endpoint
    t. exercise
    t. hypothermia
    T. Intervention Scoring System (TISS)
    t. modality
    t. pneumothorax
therapist-driven protocol (TDP)
therapy, pl. **therapies**
    AAV-CF t.
    ACE antisense gene t.
    adjunctive medical t.
    amiodarone t.
    angina-guided t.
    angiotensin-converting enzyme antisense gene t.
    anitplatelet t.
    antiaggregant t.
    antialdosterone t.
    antiarrhythmic t.
    anticlot t.
    anticoagulant t. (ACT)
    anticytokine t.
    antiendotoxin t.
    antihypertensive diuretic t.
    antiischemic t.
    antimicrobial t.
    antiplatelet t.
    antireflux t.
    antiretroviral t.
    antitachycardia pacing t.
    antituberculous t.
    atrial low energy reversion t. (ALERT)
    augmentation t.
    behavioral t.
    beta-blocker t.
    bone marrow toxic t.
    bretylium t.
    bronchodilator t.
    cardiac resynchronization t. (CRT)
    cardiac shock wave t. (CSWT)
    cell t.
    cell-based myocardial regenerative t.
    cerebral protective t.
    chest physical t. (CPT)
    chimeric-7E3 antiplatelet t.
    CI t.
    Circulator Boot t.
    Clinitron air-fluidized t.
    CO2 heart laser angina relief t.
    collapse t.
    constraint-induced movement t.
    Contak Renewal 3 system cardiac resynchronization t.
    continuous nebulization t. (CNT)
    coronary radiation t.
    corrective t. (CT)
    corticosteroid t.

CryoPlasty t.
cytotoxic gene t.
deep chest t.
device t.
directly observed t. (DOT)
diuretic t.
drug t.
ECMO t.
EECP t.
efficacy of drug t.
electroconvulsive t.
embolization t.
empiric t.
endobronchial laser t.
endolaser venous t. (ELVT)
endovascular radiation t.
enoxaparin bridge t.
estrogen replacement t. (ERT)
extracorporeal cardiac shock
  wave t.
extracorporeal membrane
  oxygenation t.
fibrinolytic t.
first-line t.
fluid t.
gene t.
Generx gene t.
HBO t.
highly active antiretroviral t.
  (HAART)
high-output extended aerosol
  respiratory t.
Holter-guided antiarrhythmic drug t.
hormone replacement t. (HRT)
12-hour antiplatelet t.
hyperbaric oxygen t. (HBOT)
hypertensive hypervolemic t. (HHT)
immunosuppression t.
inhalation t.
inodilator t.
interventional t.
intracoronary radiation t. (ICRT,
  IRT)
intraoperative intraarterial
  fibrinolytic t. (IIFT)
intravascular red light t. (IRLT)
intravenous immunoglobulin t.
ischemia-guided medical t.
ISS t.
kinetic t.
lipid-lowering t.
long-term oxygen t. (LTOT)
Lymphapress compression t.
malignancy and low molecular
  weight heparin t. (MALT)
maximum medical t.
medical t.
monophasic shock t.

mucoactive t.
NCPAP t.
nebulized Ig t.
nicotine replacement t. (NRT)
nitric oxide synthase gene t.
nonballoon t.
noncommitted biphasic shock t.
nonsurgical septal reduction t.
  (NSRT)
open-label ACE-inhibitor t.
oral anticoagulant t.
oral flecainide t.
oxygen t.
percutaneous intrapericardial fibrin-
  glue infusion t.
photodynamic t. (PDT)
physical t.
plaque stabilization t.
postthrombolytic t.
prophylactic t.
prostaglandin t.
radiation t.
rapid empiric t.
red light t. (RLT)
refractory to medical t.
Remedy sleep t.
reperfusion t.
respiratory t.
rheologic t.
shock t.
somatic cell t.
statin t.
statin-fibrate t.
stem cell t.
step-down t.
surfactant replacement t.
symptomatic t.
synchronous biatrial pacing t.
thoracic radiation t. (TRT)
thrombolytic t. (TT)
transcardial catheter t. (TCT)
transcatheter t. (TCT)
transtracheal oxygen t. (TTOT)
TriaDyne II kinetic t.
TTO t.
ultrasound t.
VEGF gene t.
ventricular resynchronization t.
warfarin t.
zone t.
TheraSnore oral appliance
thermal
  t. angiography
  t. dilution curve
  t. dilution technique
  t. dysregulation
  t. epiglottitis
  t. inhalation injury

755

thermal *(continued)*
    t. memory stent
    t. sensation
thermal-dye dilution (TDD)
Thermedics cardiac device
thermic fever
thermistor plethysmography
thermoacoustic refrigeration
Thermoactinomyces
    T. candidus
    T. sacchari
    T. viridis
    T. vulgaris
Thermocardiosystems left ventricular assist device
ThermoChem-HT system
thermocouple, thermocoupler
thermodilution
    t. balloon catheter
    cardiac output by t. (COTD)
    t. cardiac output (TDCO)
    coronary sinus t.
    t. curve
    t.-derived
    Kim-Ray t.
    t. measurement
    t. method
    t. Swan-Ganz catheter
    t. technique
    t. test
thermoexpandable stent
ThermoFlo system
thermography
    infrared t.
thermometer
    infrared t.
    SureTemp electronic t.
    Thermoscan Pro-1-Instant t.
thermophilic actinomycetes
thermoplastic head mask
thermoresistibile
    Mycobacterium t.
Thermoscan Pro-1-Instant thermometer
thermosetting resin
ThermoVent heat and moisture exchanger
TherOx Aqueous Oxygen system
thesaurosis
    hairspray t.
THI
    Texas Heart Institute
    THI needle
thiabendazole
thiacetazone
thiamine deficiency
thiamylal sodium
thiazide diuretic
thiazolidinedione derivative
thick and sticky mucus

thickened pericardium
thickening
    apical pleural t.
    basal pleural t.
    cardiac wall t.
    diffuse intimal t.
    endocardial t.
    intimal t.
    intimal-medial t.
    leaflet t.
    mediastinal t.
    neointimal t.
    nodular interlobular septal t.
    peribronchovascular t.
    pleural t.
    pressure overload-induced aortic valve calcific t.
    residual pleural t.
    reticular basement membrane t.
    septal t.
    subvalvar t. (SVTh)
    valve t.
    valvular t.
    wall t.
thickness
    cap t.
    carotid intima-medial t. (CIMT)
    common carotid artery intima-media t. (CCA-IMT)
    end-diastolic t. (EDT)
    end-diastolic wall t. (EDWTH)
    interventricular septal t. (IVS)
    intimal-medial t. (IMT)
    left ventricular wall t. (LVWT)
    media t.
    myocardial wall t. (MWT)
    posterior wall t.
    relative wall t. (RWT)
    right ventricular wall t. (RVWT)
    skin-fold t.
    strut t.
    wall t. (WT)
thienopyridine
thigh-high antiembolic stockings
thimble valvotomy
ThinLine
    T. EZ bipolar pacemaker lead
    T. EZ pacing lead
thinning
    infarct t.
    shear t.
    ventricular wall t.
thin-section CT
thin-slice CT scan
thin-walled
    t.-w. catheter
    t.-w. needle
thioamide

thiobarbituric
    t. acid-reactive
    t. acid-reactive substance (TBARS)
thiocarlide
thiocyanate
thiolprotease
thionamide
thiopental sodium
thiopentone sodium
thiophosphate
    organic t.
thioridazine hydrochloride
thiosemicarbazide
thiosemicarbazone
thiosulfate
    sodium t.
thiotepa
thioxanthene
third
    t. heart sound (S_3)
    t. sound rumble
third-degree
    t.-d. atrioventricular block
    t.-d. A-V block
    t.-d. heart block
third-generation cephalosporin
third-order Butterworth filter
thixotropy
Thoma ampulla
Thomas
    T. LT endotracheal tube holder
    T. Quick Block endotracheal tube holder
    T. shunt
Thom flap laryngeal reconstruction method
Thompson-Hatina method
Thomsen disease
Thomsen-Friedenreich (TF)
    T.-F. antigen
thoracalgia
thoracalis
    aorta t.
thoracentesis
    Argyle-Turkel t.
    blind t.
    t. needle
thoraces (*pl. of* thorax)
thoracic
    t. actinomycosis
    t. aorta (ThA)
    t. aortic aneurysm (TAA)
    t. aortic atherosclerotic plaque
    t. aortic dissection
    t. aortic knob
    t. aortic rupture (TAR)
    t. arch aortography
    t. asphyxiant dystrophy
    t. axis

    t. cage
    t. compliance
    t. compressive syndrome
    t. computed tomography (TCT)
    t. crisis
    t. crush injury
    t. duct
    t. duct drainage (TDD)
    t. duct ligation
    t. electrical bioimpedance (TEB)
    t. empyema
    t. endometriosis syndrome (TES)
    t. expanding action
    t. gas
    t. gas volume (TGV, V_{TG})
    t. impedance
    t. inferior vena cava (TIVC)
    t. injury
    t. inlet
    t. irradiation
    t. limb
    t. nerve
    t. outlet compression syndrome
    t. outlet syndrome (TCS)
    t. paracentesis
    t. part
    t. part of esophagus
    t. percutaneous needle aspiration (TPNA)
    t. radiation therapy (TRT)
    t. radiologist
    t. respiration
    t. splenosis
    t. squeeze
    t. stent graft
    t. surgeon
    t. trauma
    t. vertebral body
    t. vessel
    t. volume
thoracica, pl. thoracicae
    aorta t.
    rami esophageales aortae thoracicae
thoracic-pelvic-phalangeal dystrophy
thoracicus
    ductus t.
thoracis
    paracentesis t.
thoracoabdominal
    t. aortic aneurysm
    t. dyssynchrony
    t. excursion
    t. paradox
    t. wall motion
thoracocardiography
thoracocentesis
    repeated ultrasound-guided needle t.
thoracodorsal artery
thoracodynia

T

thoracolaparotomy
thoracolumbar
thoracopagus twin
thoracophrenolaparotomy
thoracoplasty
    apical tailoring t.
    costoversion t.
    Delorme t.
    Fowler t.
    Schede t.
    Wilms t.
Thoracoport
    T. placement
    Soft T.
    T. trocar
thoracopulmonary morphology and mechanics
thoracoschisis
thoracoscope
    rigid t.
thoracoscopic
    t. apical pleurectomy
    t. talc insufflation
    t. talc pleurodesis
thoracoscopy
    medical t. (MT)
    video-assisted t. (VAT, VATS)
thoracosternotomy
    transverse t.
thoracostomy
    closed chest t.
    closed-tube t.
    needle t.
    prophylactic t.
    tube t.
    t. tube
thoracotome
    Bettman-Fovash t.
thoracotomy
    anterior t.
    emergent t.
    t. incision
    Lewis t.
    muscle-sparing t.
    posterolateral t.
    video t.
Thora-Klex chest drainage system
Thora-Port
    T.-P. cannula
    T.-P. obturator
thorascopic
    t. biopsy
    t. talc pleurodesis
Thora-Seal
    T.-S. III 3-chamber system
    T.-S. III chest drainage unit
Thoratec
    T. biventricular assist device
    T. cardiac device

    T. HeartMate implant
    T. IVAD
    T. pump
    T. right ventricular assist device
    T. VAD system
thorax, pl. **thoraces**
    amazon t.
    t. asthenicus
    barrel-shaped t.
    cholesterol t.
    compages t.
    empyema t.
    frozen t.
    muscle of t.
    t. paralyticus
    Peyrot t.
    piriform t.
    semispinal muscle of t.
    spinal muscle of t.
    transverse muscle of t.
Thorel
    T. bundle
    T. pathway
Thornell microlaryngoscopy
Thornton anterior positioner (TAP)
Thorotrast
Thorpe flowmeter
THP
    transthoracic portography
THR
    target heart rate
thread
    mucous t.
thready pulse
threatened
    t. abrupt closure
    t. closure of arteries
    t. myocardial infarction (TMI)
threonine protein kinase
thresher's lung
threshing fever
threshold
    aerobic t.
    anaerobic t. (AT)
    anginal perceptual t.
    atrial capture t.
    atrial defibrillation t.
    atrial fibrillation t.
    backscatter t.
    capture t.
    cardioversion t.
    cough t.
    defibrillation t. (DFT, DT)
    t. dose
    fibrillation t.
    flicker fusion t.
    ischemic t.
    lactate t.
    lead t.

t. limit value
nociceptive t.
pacemaker t.
pacing t.
t. pacing
T. PEP device
t. percussion
t. resistor
risk t.
stimulation t.
t. trend
unipolar pacing t.
ventilation t.
ventilatory anaerobic t. (VAT)
ventricular capture t.
ventricular premature contraction t. (VPCT)
work t.

threw an embolus
thrill
aneurysmal t.
aortic t.
arterial t.
coarse t.
dense t.
diastolic t.
parasternal systolic t.
precordial t.
presystolic t.
purring t.
systolic t.

throb
thrombasthenia
Glanzmann t.
Thrombate III
thrombectomize
thrombectomy
catheter t.
intracoronary aspiration t. (ICAT)
mechanical t.
percutaneous mechanical t. (PMT)
percutaneous rotational t. (PRT)
rheolytic coronary t.
shredding embolectomy t. (SET)
Thrombex
T. PMT
T. PMT system
thrombi (*pl. of* thrombus)
thrombin
clot-bound t.
t. clotting time (TCT)
t. generation (TG)
t. receptor activating peptide (TRAP)
t. time (TT)
topical t.
thrombin-antithrombin (TAT)
t.-a. III complex
thrombin-soaked Gelfoam

thromboangiitis obliterans
thromboaortopathy
occlusive t.
thromboarteritis
thromboaspiration
thromboclasis
thromboclastic
thrombocystis
thrombocytapheresis
thrombocythemia
thrombocytopenia
drug-induced t.
essential t.
heparin-associated t. (HAT)
heparin-induced t. (HIT)
idiopathic t.
immune t.
lipopolysaccharide-induced t.
malignant t.
thrombocytopenia-absent
t.-a. radius (TAR)
t.-a. radius syndrome
thrombocytosis
thromboelastogram (TEG)
thromboelastograph
thromboelastography (TEG)
thromboembolectomy
thromboembolic
t. complication (TEC)
t. disease (TED)
t. pulmonary hypertension
t. stroke
t. syndrome
thromboembolism (TE)
pulmonary t.
pulmonary artery t. (PATE)
recurring venous t. (RVTE)
septic t.
systemic t.
venous t. (VTE)
thromboendarterectomy (TEA)
thromboendarteritis
thromboendocarditis
Thrombogen
thrombogenic
t. component
t. factor
t. stimulus
thrombogenicity
coil t.
thromboglobulin
beta t.
thromboid
thrombolic
thrombolizer
Angiocor rotational t.
T. catheter
thrombolus

thrombolysis
    catheter-based t.
    coronary t.
    t. in myocardial infarction (TIMI)
    t. in myocardial infarction flow
    t. in myocardial infarction frame
     count
    t. in myocardial infarction risk
     score
    pharmacomechanical t.
    rescue t.
    selective intracoronary t. (SICT)
thrombolysis-related intracranial hemorrhage (TICH)
thrombolytic
    t. agent
    T. Assessment System (TAS)
    t. predictive instrument (TPI)
    t. therapy (TT)
thrombomodulin (TM)
thrombophilia
thrombophilic factor V Leiden mutation
thrombophlebitis (TP)
    t. migrans (TPM)
    t. saltans
thromboplastin time (TT)
thrombopoietin (TPO)
thromboresistant turbostratic carbon
thrombosed
thrombosis, pl. **thromboses**
    abacterial t.
    t. activation
    acute t. (AT)
    acute occlusive t. (AOT)
    agonal t.
    aortic t.
    aortoiliac t.
    arterial t.
    atrophic t.
    baffle t.
    brachial artery t.
    calf-vein t.
    cardiac t.
    catheter-induced t.
    cavernous sinus t.
    central splanchnic venous t. (CSVT)
    cerebral t.
    cerebral venous t. (CVT)
    cerebrovascular t.
    coagulation t.
    compression t.
    coronary t. (CT)
    coronary artery t.
    cortical vein t.
    creeping t.
    deep vein t. (DVT)
    deep venous t. (DVT)
    dilation t.

    effort-induced t.
    embolic t.
    femoral artery t.
    femoral venous t.
    heparin-associated thrombocytopenia and t. (HATT)
    heparin-induced thrombocytopenia and t. (HITT)
    iliac vein t.
    incomplete t.
    infective t.
    inferior vena cava t. (IVCT)
    in situ t.
    in-stent t.
    intraarterial t.
    intramural t.
    intraprocedural stent t. (IPST)
    IVC t.
    t. of jugular bulb
    jumping t.
    laser-induced t.
    marantic t.
    marasmic t.
    mural t. (MT)
    nonobstructive valve t.
    obstructive valve t.
    occlusive t.
    Paget-von Schrötter venous t.
    panvascular t.
    partial confluens sinuum t.
    perigraft t.
    plate t.
    platelet t.
    platelet-mediated t.
    portal vein t. (PVT)
    t. prevention trial (TPT)
    propagating t.
    prosthetic mitral valve t.
    puerperal t.
    pulmonary t. (PT)
    residual deep vein t.
    Ribbert t.
    sinus t.
    stent t. (ST)
    straight sinus t.
    subacute t. (SAT)
    subclavian vein t. (SVT)
    superimposed t.
    superior vena cava t.
    traumatic t.
    upper extremity deep venous t. (UEDVT)
    venous t.
thrombospondin-1
thrombospondin-2
thrombostasis
Thrombotest
thrombotic
    t. brain infarction (TBI)

t. endocarditis
t. microangiopathy (TMA)
t. occlusion (TO)
t. thrombocytopenic purpura (TTP)
Thrombo-Wellcotest method
thromboxane
t. A$_2$
t. receptor antagonist
serum t.
t. synthesis
t. synthetase inhibitor
thrombus, pl. thrombi (T)
acute occlusive t. (AOT)
adherent mobile t.
adherent mural t.
agglutinative t.
agonal t.
antemortem t.
anular t.
atrial t.
ball t.
ball-valve t.
bland t.
blood platelet t.
t. burden
calcified t.
capillary thrombi
coral t.
currant jelly t.
fibrin t.
t. formation time (TFT)
free-floating t. (FFT)
free-floating vena caval t.
globular t.
t. grade
hyaline t.
infective t.
intracardiac t. (ICT)
intragraft t.
intraluminal t.
intramural t.
intravascular t.
juxtaluminal t.
LAA thrombi
laminated t.
lateral t.
left atrial t. (LAT)
marantic t.
marasmic t.
massive t.
migratory t.
mixed t.
mobile t.
mural t. (MT)
obstructive t.
occluding t.
occlusive t.
organized t.
organizing t.

pale t.
parietal t.
pedunculated t.
plate t.
platelet t.
postmortem t.
t. precursor protein (TpP)
T. Precursor Protein immunoassay
primary t.
progressive t
propagated t.
propagation of t.
red coronary t.
right atrial t.
right atrial mobile t. (RAMT)
saddle t.
secondary t.
straddling t.
stratified t.
t. stripper
traumatic t.
valvular t.
ventricular t.
white t.
white coronary t.
thrombus-filled cavity
ThromCat thrombectomy catheter
through-and-through
t.-a.-t. continuous suture
t.-a.-t. myocardial infarction
through-the-balloon ultrasound
through-the-needle catheter
through-the-wall mattress suture
throw an embolus
thrush
t. breast
t. breast heart
thrust
cardiac t.
thulium
thulium-holmium-chromium:yttrium-
aluminum-garnet laser
thulium-holmium:YAG laser
thulium:YAG laser angioplasty
thumbprint bronchus sign
thump
chest t.
precordial t.
Thumper 1007 CPR system
thumpversion
precordial t.
thymectomy
video-assisted thoracoscopic t.
thymic
t. asthma
t. carcinoid tumor
t. carcinoma
t. cyst
t. hyperplasia

thymidine phosphorylase
thymoglobulin
thymolipoma
thymoma
    malignant t.
thymopentin
thymostimuline
thymusectomy
Thyro-Block
thyrocardiac disease
thyrocervicalis
    truncus t.
thyroid
    aberrant t.
    accessory t.
    t. antibody
    Armour T.
    t. bruit
    t. cachexia
    t. disease
    t. extract
    t. function test
    t. gland
    intrathoracic t.
    t. isthmus
    lingual t.
    t. notch
    t. panel
    retrosternal t.
    t. storm
    T. Strong
    substernal t.
    t. tumor
thyroideae
    musculus levator glandulae t.
thyroidectomy
thyroiditis
    chronic lymphocytic t.
    de Quervain t.
    Hashimoto t.
    Riedel t.
    woody t.
thyroid-stimulating hormone (TSH)
thyrointoxication
Thyrolar
thyrolaryngeal
thyrolingual duct
thyromegaly
thyropalatine
thyropharyngeal
thyroprival
thyrotoxic heart disease
thyrotoxicosis
thyrotoxin radioisotope assay
thyrotropin
thyrotropin-releasing hormone response
thyroxine, thyroxin (T$_4$)
D-thyroxine
L-thyroxine

TI
    tricuspid incompetence
    tricuspid insufficiency
TIA
    transient ischemic attack
        crescendo TIA
        vertebrobasilar TIA
TIAH
    total implantation of artificial heart
tiamenidine
tiapamil
Tiazac extended-release capsule
TIB
    time in bed
Tibbs arterial cannula
tibial
    t. artery
    t. pulse
tibioperoneal vessel angioplasty
TICA
    terminal internal carotid artery
Ticar
ticarcillin
    t. and clavulanate potassium
    t. and clavulanic acid
    t. disodium
TICH
    thrombolysis-related intracranial
    hemorrhage
tick
    t. anticoagulant peptide
    t. paralysis
Ticlid
ticlopidine
    t. hydrochloride
    t. plus aspirin (T + A)
Ti-Cron suture
tic-tac
    t.-t. rhythm
    t.-t. sound
TICU
    trauma intensive care unit
TID
    transient ischemic dilation
tidal
    t. air
    T. balloon catheter
    t. breathing
    t. breathing flow volume (TBFV)
    t. expiratory flow at 25% of tidal
    volume (TEF$_{25}$)
    t. expiratory flow at 50% of tidal
    volume (TEF$_{50}$)
    t. expiratory flow at 75% of tidal
    volume (TEF$_{75}$)
    t. expiratory volume (TV$_E$)
    t. flow
    t. flow volume loop (TFVL)

t. inspiratory flow at 50% of tidal
volume (TIF$_{50}$)
t. inspiratory volume (TV$_I$)
t. loop
t. ventilation
t. volume (TV, V$_T$, Vt)
t. wave
T. Wave handheld capnograph
t. wave pulse
T. Wave Sp capnometer/pulse
oximeter

TIE
transient ischemic episode
transient ischemic event

tiered-therapy
t.-t. antiarrhythmic device
t.-t. implantable cardioverter-
defibrillator
t.-t. programmable cardioverter-
defibrillator

Tietze syndrome
TIF$_{50}$
tidal inspiratory flow at 50% of tidal
volume

tifacogin
tiger lily heart
tight
t. asthmatic
t. junction
t. stenosis

tightness
chest t.

tigroid striation
TIJ lead
Tikosyn
Tilade Inhalation Aerosol
Tildiem
tilt
first-phase t.
head-up t. (HUT)
second-phase t.
t. table
t. test
t. vital signs

tilting
t. disc aortic valve prosthesis
t. disc heart valve
t. disc occluder
t. disc prosthetic valve
passive t.

tilt-table test (TTT)
TIM
tissue-infiltrating macrophage
transthoracic intracardiac monitoring

Tim-AK
time
acceleration t.
acquisition t.
activated clotting t. (ACT)

activated coagulation t. (ACT)
activated partial thromboplastin t.
(APTT, aPTT)
AH conduction t.
arm-tongue t.
arteriovenous passage t. (AVP)
aspirin tolerance t. (ATT)
atrioventricular t.
t. in bed (TIB)
t. between P wave and beginning
of QRS complex (PR)
bleeding t. (BLT, BT)
blood clot lysis t.
buildup t. (T$_b$)
bypass t.
capacitor forming t.
carotid ejection t.
central motor conduction t.
(CMCT)
cerebral transit t. (cTT)
charge t.
circulation t.
clot lysis t. (CLT)
clot retraction t.
clotting t. (CLT, CT)
coagulation t. (CT)
cold ischemic t. (CIT)
t. compensation gain (TCG)
conduction t.
corrected ejection t. (ETc)
corrected sinus node recovery t.
(CSNRT)
cross-clamp t.
dead t.
deceleration t. (DT)
detect t.
direct sinuatrial conduction t.
(DSACT, D-SACT)
t. domain
t. domain signal-averaged
electrocardiogram
t. domain signal-averaged
electrocardiography
donor organ ischemic t.
door-to-balloon t.
door-to-needle t.
Doppler deceleration t.
doubling t.
Duke bleeding t.
echo delay t. (TE)
ejection t. (ET)
esophageal transit t.
euglobulin clot lysis t.
expiratory t. (T$_E$)
extubation t.
t. of flight (TOF)
t. of flight and absorbance
(TOFA)

time *(continued)*
    t. of flight and absorbance spectrophotometry
    flushing t.
    forced expiratory t. (FET)
    t. forced expiratory rate
    His-ventricle conduction t.
    HR conduction t.
    HV conduction t.
    hydrogen appearance t.
    inspiratory t. (T_I)
    interatrial conduction t.
    intraatrial conduction t.
    intubation t.
    isovolumetric t. (IVT)
    isovolumetric relaxation t. (IVRT)
    isovolumic relaxation t. (IVRT)
    Ivy bleeding t.
    junctional recovery t. (JRT)
    kaolin-cephalin clotting t. (KCCT)
    kaolin partial thromboplastin t. (KPTT)
    lag t. (LT)
    left ventricular ejection t. (LVEJT, LVET)
    longitudinal relaxation t.
    lung-to-finger circulation t. (LFCT)
    lysis t.
    magnetic relaxation t.
    maximum walking t.
    median survival t. (MST)
    PA conduction t.
    partial thromboplastin t. (PTT)
    t. to peak (TTP)
    peak ejection t. (PET)
    t. to peak expiratory flow (tPTEF)
    t. to peak expiratory flow and total expiration t. (tPTEF/tE)
    t. to peak inspiratory flow (tPTIF)
    pH conduction t.
    prothrombin t. (PTT)
    prothrombin time/partial thromboplastin t. (PT/PTT)
    pulse transmission t. (PTT)
    quick prothrombin t.
    ratio of inspiratory time to total breathing cycle t. (T_I/T_{TOT})
    relaxation t.
    repetition t. (TR)
    right ventricular ejection t. (RVET)
    right ventricular isovolumic relaxation t. (RV-IVRT)
    rise t.
    saturation t.
    serial thrombin t. (STT)
    Simplate bleeding t.
    sinuatrial conduction t. (SACT)
    sinuatrial recovery t. (SART)
    sinus node recovery t. (SNRT, SRT)
    spin-lattice t.
    spin-spin t.
    survival t.
    systolic t. (ST)
    systolic acceleration t. (SAT)
    systolic upstroke t.
    thrombin t. (TT)
    thrombin clotting t. (TCT)
    thromboplastin t. (TT)
    thrombus formation t. (TFT)
    total ejection t. (TET)
    total sleep t. (TST)
    transmitral E-wave deceleration t.
    T2 relaxation t.
    turnaround t. (TAT)
    venous clotting t. (VCT)
    ventilator t.
    ventricular activation t. (VAT)
    ventricular ejection t. (VET)
    wake after sleep onset t. (WASO)

time-activity curve
time-averaged peak velocity
time-based
    t.-b. counter
    t.-b. event recording
time-compensated gain
time-cycled ventilation
time-cycling
timed
    t. forced expiratory volume
    t. vital capacity
time-domain analysis
time-gain
    t.-g. compensation (TGC)
    t.-g. compensationtime-varied gain control
    t.-g. control (TGC)
Timentin
time-of-flight
    3-dimensional t.-o.-f. (3DTF)
    t.-o.-f. effect
    t.-o.-f. magnetic resonance angiography
time-resolved imaging by automatic data segmentation (TRIADS)
time-to-peak
    t.-t.-p. contrast
    t.-t.-p. filling rate
time-triggered
time-varied
    t.-v. gain (TVG)
    t.-v. gain control (TGC, TVGC)
time-weighted average
TIMI
    thrombolysis in myocardial infarction
    transmural inferior myocardial infarction
    TIMI blush score

TIMI classification
TIMI criteria
TIMI flow
TIMI flow grade 0–3
TIMI frame count
TIMI frame count index
TIMI myocardial perfusion grade
TIMI patency
TIMI risk score

timing
aortic cross-sectional area/height ratio t.
t. circuit

Timolide
timolol maleate
timori
Brugia t.
TIMP
tissue inhibitor of metalloproteinase
TIMP-3
tissue inhibitor of metalloproteinase-3
TIMP-3 overexpression
Tina-quant immunoturbidimetric assay
tined
t. lead pacemaker
t. ventricular electrode
tine test
tinidazole
tinkle
Bouillaud t.
metallic t.
tin oxide
TintElize PAI-1 ELISA kit
tinzaparin
t. sodium
t. sodium injection
tiotropium bromide
tip
t. extrasystole
lighthouse t.
Luer-Lok needle t.
Medtronic t.
mitral leaflet t.
t. occluder
papillary muscle t.
Sensor PTFE-nitinol guidewire with hydrophilic t.
Skimmer laryngeal blade t.
Stckert V142 series venous cannula with lighthouse t.
tip-deflecting wire
TIPP
transilluminated powered phlebectomy
tiprenolol hydrochloride
TIPS
transjugular intrahepatic portosystemic shunt
tiptoe test
tirilazad mesylate

tirofiban
TISS
Therapeutic Intervention Scoring System
Tissomat application device and spray set
Tissot spirometer
tissue
t. ablation
adipose t.
atrioventricular conduction t.
autodigestion of connective t.
t. bank
bovine pericardial t.
bronchopulmonary t.
bronchus-associated lymphoid t. (BALT)
bullous lung t.
caseated t.
connective t.
dissected t.
t. Doppler imaging (TDI)
t. engineering
extrathoracic soft t.
exuberant granulation t. (EGT)
t. factor (TF)
t. factor pathway inhibitor (TFPI)
fast t.
fibromyxoid connective t.
t. fissure
granulation t.
gut-associated lymphoid t. (GALT)
His-Purkinje t.
t. hypoperfusion
t. hypoxia
t. inhibitor of metalloproteinase (TIMP)
t. inhibitor of metalloproteinase-3 (TIMP-3)
t. inhibitor of metalloproteinase-3 overexpression
interfascicular fibrous t.
laminated connective t.
loose connective t.
myocardial t.
myocardial scar t.
myxoid fibroblastic t.
t. necrosis
neointimal t.
nodal t.
nonmalignant t.
perinodal t.
t. plasminogen activator (t-PA, tPA)
t. plasminogen activator inhibitor (tPAI)
t. plasminogen activator release deficiency
t. preservation
proteoglycan-rich t.

T

tissue *(continued)*
>>resistance to movement of lung t. (Rti)
>>t. septa
>>skeletal muscle t.
>>slow t.
>>t. supersaturation
>>t. valve

tissue-infiltrating macrophage (TIM)
tissue-specific antibody
tissue-type plasminogen activator
titanium
>>t. cage
>>t. Greenfield IVC filter
>>t. port

Titan Mega XL PTCA dilation catheter
titer
>>antiheart antibody t.
>>anti-Rho(D) t.
>>bactericidal t.
>>Lyme t.
>>serum bactericidal t. (SBT)

titin isoform
titration regimen
titrator
tI/tTOT
>>ratio of inspiration time and total time of breathing cycle

TIVC
>>thoracic inferior vena cava

tizanidine hydrochloride
Tl
>>thallium

²⁰¹Tl
>>thallium-201
>>thallous chloride
>>²⁰¹Tl perfusion tracer
>>²⁰¹Tl sestamibi

TLA
>>translumbar aortogram
>>transluminal angioplasty

TLC
>>total lung capacity

TLC-II portable VAD driver
TLCO, TLco
>>carbon monoxide transfer factor

TLI
>>total lymphoid irradiation

TLR
>>target lesion revascularization
>>toll-like receptor

TM
>>thrombomodulin
>>transatrial membranotomy

TMA
>>thrombotic microangiopathy

TMC
>>Tokyo Medical College

transmyocardial mechanical channeling
>>TMC needle

TMET
>>treadmill exercise test

TMI
>>threatened myocardial infarction
>>transmural myocardial infarction

TMLR
>>transmyocardial laser revascularization

TMP-SMX
>>trimethoprim-sulfamethoxazole

TMR
>>transmyocardial revascularization
>>Heart Laser for TMR

TMS
>>thallium myocardial scintigraphy
>>TMS 1000 tachyarrhythmia monitoring system

TMST
>>treadmill stress test

TMZ
>>trimetazidine 1

TNB
>>transthoracic needle biopsy

TNF
>>tumor necrosis factor

TNF2
>>tumor necrosis factor-2
>>TNF2 allele

TNF-alpha
>>tumor necrosis factor-alpha
>>TNF-alpha antagonist
>>TNF-alpha promotor polymorphism

TNFR
>>tumor necrosis factor receptor

TNKase, TNK-tPA
>>tenecteplase

TNM
>>tumor, node, metastasis
>>TNM classification
>>TNM staging

TnT
>>troponin T

TO
>>thrombotic occlusion
>>total obstruction

To
>>tricuspid opening

to-and-fro
>>t.-a.-f. murmur
>>t.-a.-f. sound

tobacco heart
TOBI Inhalation Solution
toborinone
tobramycin
>>nebulized t.
>>t. solution
>>t. solution for inhalation

tocainide hydrochloride

tocolytic pulmonary edema
Todaro
    tendon of T.
    T. triangle
TOD/CCD
    target organ disease/clinical
    cardiovascular disease
Todd-Hewitt broth (THB)
Todd unit
toe
    clubbing of t.'s
TOF
    tetralogy of Fallot
    time of flight
    TOF MRA
TOFA
    time of flight and absorbance
    TOFA spectrophotometry
Tofranil
tofu
Togaviridae virus
toilet, toilette
    bronchial t.
    pleural t.
    pulmonary t.
    respiratory t.
    tracheobronchial t.
toilet-seat
    t.-s. angina
    t.-s. syncope
Tokyo Medical College (TMC)
tolazamide
tolazoline
    t. hydrochloride
    t. test
tolbutamide
tolerance
    exercise t.
    hemodynamic t.
    impaired glucose t. (IGT)
    ischemic t.
    poor exercise t. (PET)
Tolinase
toll-like receptor (TLR)
toluene
    t. diisocyanate (TDI)
    t. diisocyanate-induced asthma
toluidine blue stain
Tolu-Sed DM
tolvaptan
Tolypocladium inflatum
tombstoning ST-segment elevation
Tomcat PTCA guidewire
tomogram
    horizontal long-axis t.
    short-axis t.
    vertical long-axis t.
tomograph
    ECAT III positron t.

tomographic
    high-resolution thin section
    computed t.
    t. radionuclide imaging
    t. radionuclide ventriculography
tomography
    adaptive current t. (ACT)
    adenosine triphosphate single-photon
    emission computed t. (ATP-
    SPECT)
    atrial bolus dynamic computer t.
    axial computed t. (ACT)
    biplanar t.
    Cardiac Protect t.
    cardiovascular computed t. (CVCT)
    cine computed t.
    computed t. (CT)
    computerized axial t. (CAT)
    3-dimensional helical computed t.
    dual-isotope simultaneous acquisition
    single-photon emission
    computed t. (DISA-SPECT)
    electrical impedance t. (EIT)
    electron beam computed t. (EBCT)
    electronic beam t. (EBT)
    fluorodeoxyglucose-positron
    emission t. (FDG-PET)
    gated computed t.
    HeartCam electronic beam t.
    high-resolution computed t. (HRCT)
    intravenously enhanced computed t.
    (IVCT)
    2-methoxyisobutyl isonitrile single-
    photon emission computed t.
    (MIBI-SPECT)
    multidetector computed t. (MDCT)
    multidetector row helical
    computed t.
    multislice spiral computed t.
    (MSCT)
    myocardial single photon
    emission t. (MSPECT)
    N-13 ammonia positron emission t.
    optical coherence t. (OCT)
    7-pinhole t.
    positron emission t. (PET)
    quantitative computed t. (QCT)
    rapid acquisition computed axial t.
    (RACAT)
    rest-reinjection thallium t.
    rubidium-82 positron emission t.
    single-photon emission t. (SPET)
    single-photon emission computed t.
    (SPECT)
    slant-hole t.
    16-slice spiral computed t.
    spiral computed t.
    spiral volumetric computed t.
    (SVCT)

T

tomography *(continued)*
  technetium-99m-sestamibi single-photon emission computed t.
  thallium t.
  thoracic computed t. (TCT)
  ultrafast computed t. (UFCT)
  ultrafast contrast-enhanced chest computed t.
  xenon-enhanced computed t. (XECT)
  x-ray cine computed t.
TomTec
  T. echo platform
  T. Imaging Systems
tone
  bronchial smooth muscle t.
  cardiac vagal t.
  cholinergic t.
  depression-induced altered autonomic t.
  fetal heart t. (FHT)
  heart t. (HT, Ht, ht)
  peripheral arterial t. (PAT)
  resting vascular t.
  Traube double t.
  vagal t.
  vasomotor t.
  Williams tracheal t.
tongs
  Trippi-Wells t.
tongue
  smoker's t.
  strawberry t.
  t. traction
tongue-jaw lift
tongue-retaining device (TRD)
tongue-rolling effect
tonometer
  air-puff t.
  Gärtner t.
  Linear KGT t.
tonometered whole blood
tonometry
  applanation t.
  peripheral artery t.
tonoscillograph
tonsil
  Gerlach t.
  kissing t.'s
  laryngeal t.
  lingual t.
  Luschka t.
  palatine t.
  pharyngeal t.
tonsilla
  t. lingualis
  t. palatina
  t. pharyngealis

tonsillar
  t. pillar
  t. ring
  t. Somnoplasty procedure
  t. Somnoplasty system
tonsillaris
  angina t.
tonsillitis
  caseous t.
  chronic catarrhal t.
  diphtherial t.
tonsilloadenoidectomy
tonus
  vasomotor t. (VMT)
tool
  cardiovascular self-assessment t. (CST)
  congestive heart failure data t. (CHFDT)
  LIMA-Lift t.
  LIMA-Loop t.
  vascular anatomy teaching t. (VATT)
Top-Hat supraannular aortic valve
topical
  t. anesthesia
  Aquacare t.
  Bactroban T.
  Benadryl T.
  Carmol t.
  t. cooling
  Efudex T.
  Fluoroplex T.
  Gelfoam T.
  t. hypothermia
  Lanaphilic t.
  Mycostatin T.
  Nutraplus t.
  Oxsoralen T.
  Rogaine t.
  Solarcaine t.
  t. thrombin
  Ultra Mide t.
topiramate
topography
  NMR t.
Toposar injection
topotecan
Toprol XL
torcetrapib
Torcon
  T. NB Advantage coronary angiographic catheter
  T. NB selective angiographic catheter
Torek resection of thoracic esophagus
toremifene
Tornado embolization coil
Tornwaldt cyst

toroidal valve
Toronto
    T. Alexithymia Scale
    T. SPV aortic valve
    T. SPV bioprosthesis
    T. SPV stentless porcine heart
      valve
torpedo-shaped pattern
Torq-Flex wire guide
torque
    clockwise t.
    t. control
    t. control balloon catheter
    t. tube catheter
    t. vise
torquer
    Clip On t.
torquing ability
torr
    t. pressure
    t. unit
Torricelli
    T. law
    T. model
    T. orifice equation
torsade
    t. de pointes (TDP, TdP)
    t. de pointes ventricular tachycardia
torsemide
torsion
    lobar t.
tortuosity
tortuous
    t. right coronary artery
    t. veins
    t. vessel
Torula histolytica
Torulopsis glabrata
torulosis
torus aorticus
TOS
    thoracic outlet syndrome
    toxic oil syndrome
Toshiba
    T. biplane transesophageal
      transducer
    T. electrocardiography machine
    T. MRT 200 MRI
    T. scanner
    T. Sonolayer SSH-140A ultrasound
tosilate
    suplatast t.
tosylate
    bretylium t.
tosylchloramide sodium
total
    t. absence of circulation on 4-
      vessel angiography
    t. acidity

t. adenine nucleotide (TAN)
t. airway resistance (Rtot)
t. alternans
t. anomalous pulmonary venous connection (TAPVC)
t. anomalous pulmonary venous drainage (TAPVD)
t. anomalous pulmonary venous return (TAPVR)
t. anterior circulation infarct (TACI)
t. anterior circulation syndrome (TACS)
t. apexcardiographic relaxation time index (TARTI)
t. arterial off-pump coronary artery bypass
t. artificial heart (TAH)
t. atrial blanking (TAB)
t. atrial blanking period
t. atrial refractory period (TARP)
t. atrioventricular block (TAVB)
t. axial node irradiation (TANI)
t. blood volume (TBV)
t. body irradiation (TBI)
t. bypass (TBP)
t. cardiopulmonary bypass (TCB)
t. cavopulmonary anastomosis
t. cavopulmonary connection (TCPC)
t. cavopulmonary shunt (TCPS)
t. cholesterol (TC)
t. cholesterol/high-density lipoproteins (TC/HDL)
t. chordal-sparing mitral valve replacement
t. circulatory arrest (TCA)
t. coronary flow (TCF)
t. coronary score (TCS)
t. ejection time (TET)
t. electromechanical systole (QS_2)
t. end-diastolic diameter (TEDD)
t. end-systolic diameter (TESD)
t. exhaled nitric oxide (FENO)
t. heart beats (THB)
t. hemoglobin
t. homocysteine (tHcy)
t. homocysteine level
t. implantation
t. implantation of artificial heart (TIAH)
t. lung capacity (TLC)
t. lung compliance
t. lymphoid irradiation (TLI)
t. obstruction (TO)
T. O_2 delivery system
T. O_2 supplementary oxygen system
t. patient shock count

total *(continued)*
    t. peripheral resistance (TPR)
    t. peripheral resistance index (TPRI)
    t. peripheral vascular resistance (TPVR)
    t. peroxyl radical-trapping antioxidant potential (TRAP)
    t. plasma cholesterol (TPC)
    positive symptom t. (PST)
    t. pressure (P_T)
    t. pulmonary blood flow (TPBF)
    t. pulmonary resistance
    t. pulmonary vascular resistance (TPVR)
    t. repair of tetralogy of Fallot
    t. right ventricular volume (TRVV)
    t. sleep time (TST)
    T. Synchrony System
    t. systemic vascular resistance (TSVR)
    t. vascular resistance (TVR)
    t. ventilator days

totalis
    situs inversus t.

totally endoscopic coronary artery bypass (TECAB)
touch shock count
Toupet hemifundoplication
Tourguide guiding catheter
tourniquet
    Esmarch t.
    pneumatic t.
    Rumel t.
    Shenstone t.
Touro
    T. CC
    T. DM
TOVA
    trigger of ventricular arrhythmia
Tovell tube
Towbin
    method of T.
Townes-Brocks syndrome
ToxCO+ breath carbon monoxide monitor
toxemia
toxemic pneumonia
toxic
    t. agent
    t. delirium
    t. epidermal necrolysis
    t. fume inhalation
    t. fumes
    t. level
    t. myocarditis
    t. oil syndrome (TOS)
    t. shock

toxicant
    urban t.
toxicity, pl. toxicities
    amphetamine t.
    anthracycline t.
    antimony t.
    cobalt t.
    dextroamphetamine t.
    digitalis t.
    digoxin t.
    doxorubicin-induced cardiac t.
    emetine t.
    fluoride t.
    hydrocarbon t.
    oxygen t.
    phenylpropanolamine t.
    plant t.
toxicosis
    Aspergillus t.
toxin
    adenylate cyclase t.
    botulinum t. type A
    t. exposure
    pertussis t.
    RNA glycosidase t.
toxin-insensitive current
Toxocara canis
toxoid
    diphtheria and tetanus t.
Toxoplasma gondii
toxoplasmosis
ToxR protein
TP
    thrombophlebitis
    TP baseline
    TP interval
    TP segment
T&P, T+P
    temperature and pulse
TPA
    alteplase
t-PA, tPA
    tissue plasminogen activator
tPAI
    tissue plasminogen activator inhibitor
TPBF
    total pulmonary blood flow
TPC
    total plasma cholesterol
TPE
    tropical pulmonary eosinophilia
TPG
    transpulmonary gradient
    transvalvular pressure gradient
T-Phyl
TPI
    thrombolytic predictive instrument

T-piece
    T-p. oxygen
    T-p. weaning
TPM
    temporary pacemaker
    thrombophlebitis migrans
TPNA
    thoracic percutaneous needle aspiration
TPO
    thrombopoietin
TpP
    thrombus precursor protein
T-P-Q segment
TPR
    temperature, pulse, respiration
    total peripheral resistance
TPRI
    total peripheral resistance index
TPST
    true-positive stress test
TPT
    thrombosis prevention trial
    treadmill performance test
tPTEF
    time to peak expiratory flow
tPTEF/tE
    time to peak expiratory flow and total
      expiration time
tPTIF
    time to peak inspiratory flow
TPVL
    transient pulmonary vascular lability
TPVR
    total peripheral vascular resistance
    total pulmonary vascular resistance
TQa
    transcutaneous access flow
      TQa device
TQ segment
TR
    repetition time
    tricuspid regurgitation
trabeculae carneae
trabecular
    t. hypertrophy
    t. VSD
trabecula septomarginalis
trabeculation
    muscle t.
trace metal
tracer
    carbon-11 palmitic acid
      radioactive t.
    CardioTek electrophysiologic t.
    t. distribution
    frequency t.
    t. homogeneity
    iodine-123 heptadecanoic acid
      radioactive t.

    T. over-the-wire mapping
      microcatheter
    t. retention
    t. storage
    ^{201}Tl perfusion t.
    t. uptake
TrachCare
    neonatal Y T.
trachea, pl. tracheae
    anular ligament of t.
    bifurcatio tracheae
    bifurcation of t.
    carina of t.
    carina tracheae
    membranous wall of t.
    muscular coat of t.
    paries membranaceus tracheae
    saber-sheath t.
    scabbard t.
    steepling of t.
    tunica mucosa tracheae
    tunica muscularis tracheae
tracheal
    t. aspirate
    t. bifurcation
    t. branch
    t. breath sounds
    t. bronchus
    t. button
    t. cartilage
    t. deviation
    t. diverticuli
    t. gas insufflation (TGI)
    t. gland
    t. intubation
    t. lymph node
    t. mucosa
    t. mucus velocity
    t. rale
    t. ring
    t. steepling
    t. triangle
    t. tube
    t. tug
    t. vein
    t. wall cave-in
    t. wall injury with intermittent
      stoppage of tracheostomy and
      episodes of dyspnea (TWISTED)
tracheales
    cartilagines t.
    glandulae t.
    venae t.
trachealia
    ligamenta anularia t.
trachealis
    angina t.
    t. muscle
tracheitis

tracheobiliary
tracheobronchial
- t. amyloidosis
- t. angle
- t. aspergillosis
- t. aspirate
- t. clearance
- t. collapse
- t. diverticulum
- t. dyskinesia
- t. flora
- t. foreign body (TFB)
- t. lavage
- t. stenosis
- t. toilet
- t. tree
- t. tuberculosis

tracheobronchitis
- *Aspergillus* t.
- influenza t.
- lymphocytic t.
- pseudomembranous *Aspergillus* t.

tracheobronchomalacia
tracheobronchomegaly
tracheobronchopathia osteoplastica
tracheobronchoscopy
tracheoesophageal (TE)
- t. fistula (TEF)
- t. junction
- t. puncture

tracheolaryngeal
Tracheolife HME
tracheomalacia
tracheopathia osteoplastica
tracheopharyngeal
tracheophonesis
tracheophony
tracheoscope
tracheostenosis
tracheostomized
tracheostomy
- balloon-facilitated percutaneous t.
- t. button
- Ciaglia Blue Dolphin t.
- Ciaglia percutaneous t.
- t. cuff
- early t.
- epithelized t.
- Fantoni translaryngeal t.
- flap t.
- Great Ormond Street t.
- Griggs t.
- late t.
- Montgomery t.
- percutaneous t. (PCT)
- percutaneous dilational t. (PDT)
- PercuTwist t.
- t. plate
- t. stoma

T. TOM anatomical model
- t. tube

tracheotome
tracheotomy
- percutaneous t.

trachomatis
- *Chlamydia* t.

trach plate
Trach-Talk tracheostomy tube
trachyphonia
tracing
- carotid pulse t.
- diamond-shaped t.
- fetal heart monitor t.
- jugular venous pulse t. (JVPT)
- pressure t.
- pulmonary capillary wedge pressure t.
- pulse t.
- serial ECG t.
- serial electrocardiogram t.
- stripchart t.
- venous pressure t.
- venous pulse t.

track
- tram t.

trackability
track-ball technique
tracker
- T. microcatheter
- Purkinje image t.

tracking
- bolus t.
- spatial t.
- wall t.

Tracleer
Tracrium
tract
- aneurysm of right ventricle or right ventricular outflow t.
- anterior internodal t.
- atriodextrofascicular t.
- atriofascicular t.
- atrio-His bypass t.
- atrionodal bypass t.
- bronchopulmonary t.
- bypass t.
- concealed bypass t.
- corticobulbar t.
- inflow t.
- internodal t.
- James accessory t.'s
- left ventricular outflow t. (LVOT)
- lower respiratory t.
- nodohisian bypass t.
- nodoventricular t.
- outflow t.
- pulmonary outflow t.
- respiratory t.

right ventricular inflow t. (RVIT)
right ventricular outflow t. (RVOT)
spinothalamic t.
upper aerodigestive t.
venous outflow t.
Wolff-Parkinson-White bypass t.

traction
t. aneurysm
bilateral carotid artery t. (BiCAT)
t. bronchiectasis
t. bronchiolectasis
Crego t.
t. endarterectomy
papillary muscle t.
t. suture
tongue t.

trafficking
intracellular t.

tragacanth asthma
trailing edge
train
drive t.
t.'s of ventricular pacing

trainer
CardioGrip cardiovascular t.

training
CDBR respiratory muscle t.
t. effect
expiratory muscle t.
inspiratory muscle t. (IMT)
relaxation t.
resistance t. (RT)
specific expiratory muscle t.
(SEMT)
specific inspiratory muscle t.
(SIMT)
strength t.

train-of-4
t.-o.-4 monitoring
t.-o.-4 stimulus

trainwheel rhythm
trait
sickle cell t.

Trak Back pullback device
TRAKE-fit system
TrakPro data analysis software
TRALI
transfusion-related acute lung injury

tram
t. line
t. tracks

Trandate
T. injection
T. Oral

trandolapril and verapamil
tranexamic acid
tranilast

tranquility
T. Bilevel airway patency
maintenance device
T. Bilevel CPAP unit
T. Bilevel positive airway pressure
therapy device
T. Quest CPAP device
T. Quest CPAP System

tranquilizer
trans
t. fat
t. fatty acid (TFA)

TransAccess catheter
TransAct intraaortic balloon pump
transaminase
glutamic-oxaloacetic t. (GOT)
serum glutamic-oxaloacetic t.
(SGOT)
serum glutamic-pyruvic t. (SGPT)

transaminitis
transanular, transannular
t. patch

transaortic valve gradient
transatrial
t. membranotomy (TM)
t. pacing

transaxial
t. plane
t. slice

transaxillary apical bullectomy
transbrachial aortography
transbronchial
t. biopsy (TBB, TBBX, TBBx)
t. lung biopsy (TBLB)
t. needle
t. needle aspiration (TBNA)

transcapillary refill
transcardiac
t. gradient
t. monocyte
t. vein perfusion

transcardial catheter therapy (TCT)
transcarotid balloon valvoplasty
transcatheter
t. ablation
t. arterial embolization (TAE)
t. biopsy (TCB)
t. closure (TCC)
t. closure of atrial defect
t. closure of atrial septal defect
operation
t. coil occlusion
t. device
t. embolization
t. embolotherapy
t. occlusion of atrial septal defect
t. patch
t. therapy (TCT)
t. umbrella

T

transcatheter *(continued)*
    t. valve implantation
    t. valvotomy
transcoronary
    t. ablation of septal hypertrophy
    (TASH)
    t. alcohol ablation (TAA)
    t. chemical ablation
transcranial color-coded sonography
    (TCCS)
transcricothyroid puncture
transcription
    t. factor
    gene t.
    Janus kinase/signal transducer and
    activator of t.
    signal transducer and activator
    of t. (Stat)
transcutaneous
    t. access flow (TQa)
    t. echo
    t. electrical stimulation (TES)
    t. extraction catheter
    t. lead
    t. oxygen monitor (TCOM)
    t. pacemaker (TCP)
    t. pacing (TCP)
    t. pCO_2 monitoring
transdermal
    t. 17-beta-estradiol
    Catapres-TTS T.
    Duragesic T.
Transderm-Nitro Patch
transdiaphragmatic pressure
transducer
    Acuson V5M multiplane
    transesophageal
    echocardiographic t.
    Aloka model SSD-830 2.5- and
    3.5-MHz t.
    anular array t.
    t. aperture
    arterial line t.
    Bentley t.
    charge-coupled device t.
    Deltran disposable t.
    diaphragm t.
    Diasonics t.
    differential pressure t.
    Doppler t.
    echocardiographic t.
    footprint of t.
    Gould Statham pressure t.
    HP SONOS 2500 t.
    Medex t.
    2-MHz pulsed-wave Doppler t.
    Mikro-Tip t.
    Millar Mikro-Tip catheter
    pressure t.

    Millar TCB-500 t.
    M-mode t.
    Pedoff continuous wave t.
    phased array sector t.
    phonocardiographic t.
    piezoelectric ultrasound t.
    pressure t.
    quartz t.
    range-gated t.
    sector t.
    Sleepscan Airflow Pressure T.
    TEE t.
    Toshiba biplane transesophageal t.
    ultrasound t.
    V510B biplane TEE t.
    Vingmed CFM 750 t.
    V5M multiplane TEE t.
transducer-tipped catheter
transendothelial
transesophageal
    t. atrial pacing (TAP, TEAP)
    t. atrial pacing stress
    echocardiography (TAPSE)
    t. atrial stimulation (TRAS)
    t. contrast echocardiography
    t. dobutamine stress
    echocardiography
    t. echo
    t. echocardiography (TEE)
    t. echocardiography-dobutamine
    stress echocardiography (TEE-
    DSE)
    t. echocardiography with pacing
    (TEEP)
    t. echo probe
    t. pacing (TEP)
    t. pacing system
    t. pressure
transfection
    gene t.
transfemoral endoaortic occlusion
    catheter
transfer
    adenovirus-mediated gene t.
    Akt gene t.
    cholesterol ester t. (CET)
    chordal t.
    ex vivo gene t.
    intraarterial gene t.
    intravascular gene t.
    in vivo gene t.
    vascular gene t.
transferase
    chloramphenicol t.
transfixion suture
transform
    3-dimensional Fourier t. (3DFT)
    fast Fourier t. (FFT)
    Fourier t.

gradient field t. (GFT)
Karhunen-Loéve t. (KLT)

transformation
epicardial-mesenchymal t.
Haldane t.
hemorrhagic t. (HT)
Richter t.

transformer
vesicular monoamine t. (VMAT)

transforming
t. growth factor (TGF)
t. growth factor-beta

transfusion
allogenic-blood t.
autologous t.
Baylor rapid autologous t. (BRAT)
donor-specific t.
exchange t.
t. factor
perioperative blood t.
perioperative platelet t.

transfusional hemosiderosis
transfusion-related acute lung injury
  (TRALI)
transgenesis
transient
t. abnormal Q wave (TAQW)
t. asystole
calcium t.
t. depolarization
t. early wheezing
t. entrainment
t. focal cerebral ischemia (TFCI)
t. heart block
t. hiccups
t. inward current
t. ischemic attack (TIA)
t. ischemic attack plus carotid
  endarterectomy
t. ischemic dilation (TID)
t. ischemic episode (TIE)
t. ischemic event (TIE)
t. leukocytosis
t. mesenteric ischemia
t. pericarditis
t. pulmonary vascular lability
  (TPVL)
t. receptor potential vanilloid-1
  (TRPV-1)
t. response imaging (TRI)
t. spastic occlusion (TSO)
t. spontaneous circulation (TSC)
t. ST-segment elevation
t. syncope
t. tachypnea of newborn (TTNB)
t. wall motion abnormality

transilluminated powered phlebectomy
  (TIPP)

transition
t. dyspnea index focal score
forced ischemia-reperfusion t.
sympathovagal t.

transitional
t. cell
t. cell carcinoma
t. cell zone
t. respiration

transjugular
t. balloon valvoplasty procedure
t. catheter
t. intrahepatic portosystemic shunt
  (TIPS)

translaryngeal tracheostomy technique
translesional spectral flow velocity
translocation
Nikaidoh t.

translocator
adenine nucleotide t. (ANT)

translumbar
t. aortogram (TLA)
t. aortography

transluminal
t. angioplasty (TAP, TLA)
t. angioplasty catheter
t. coronary angioplasty
t. endarterectomy
t. endarterectomy catheter (TEC)
t. extraction atherectomy (TEA)
t. extraction catheter (TEC)
t. extraction coronary atherectomy
t. lysing system
percutaneous t.

transluminally
t. placed endovascular branched
  stent graft
t. placed Inoue endovascular stent-
  graft

transmembrane
t. calcium flux
t. potential
t. signaling
t. voltage

transmission
airborne t.
t. electron microscopy (TEM)
electrotonic t.
genetic t.
t. imaging
mitral E-wave t.
t. scan
transtelephonic t.

transmitral
t. Doppler E:A ratio
t. E:A ratio
t. E-wave deceleration time
t. flow velocity
t. gradient

transmitted murmur
transmucosal
    Actiq Oral T.
transmural
    t. anterior myocardial infarction
      (TAMI)
    t. antitachycardia pacemaker
    t. channel
    t. inferior myocardial infarction
      (TIMI)
    t. myocardial infarction (TMI)
    t. myocardial ischemia
    t. pressure
    t. pressure of collapsible segment
      (Ptm)
    t. steal
transmyocardial
    t. laser channel
    t. laser revascularization (TMLR)
    t. mechanical channeling (TMC)
    t. pacing stylet
    t. perfusion pressure
    t. revascularization (TMR)
    t. revascularization with laser
transnexus channel
Transonic flowmeter
transPAC ventilator
transpiration
    pulmonary t.
transplant (Tx) (*See also* transplantation)
    allogeneic t.
    bilateral lung t. (BLT)
    bilateral sequential single lung t.
    bone marrow t.
    cardiac t.
    t. coronary artery disease (TCAD,
      TxCAD)
    double lung t. (DLT)
    en bloc bilateral lung t.
    heart t. (HT)
    heart-lung t. (HLT, HLTx)
    heterologous cardiac t.
    heterotopic cardiac t.
    heterotopic heart t. (HHT)
    homologous cardiac t.
    living related t. (LRT)
    Lower-Shumway cardiac t.
    lung t. (LT, LTx)
    natural heart t.
    orthotopic cardiac t.
    orthotopic heart t. (OHT)
    t. pneumonia
    rejection cardiomyopathy t.
    right single lung t. (RSLTx)
    single-lung t. (SLT)
    syngenesioplastic t.
transplantation (TX, Tx) (*See also*
  transplant)
    cardiac t. (CTx)

hBMSC t.
heart t. (HT)
heart-lung t. (HLT)
heterotopic heart t. (HHT)
International Society for Heart T.
  (ISHT)
International Society for Heart and
  Lung T. (ISHLT)
orthotopic cardiac t. (OCT)
solid organ t.
transplanted heart
transplant-related angiogenesis
transpleural
transport
    active t.
    T. dilation balloon catheter
    T. drug delivery catheter
    lactic acid t.
    mucociliary t.
    mucus t.
    oxygen t.
    sarcolemmal reticular t.
    sarcoplasmic reticular t.
transportability
    cough t.
transportation
    air medical t. (AMT)
transporter
    monocarboxylate t.
transposition
    t. of aorta (TA)
    t. of arterial stems
    t. assessment
    t. complex
    corrected t. (CT)
    t. of great arteries (TGA)
    t. of great vessels (TGV)
    portacaval t. (PCT)
    switch-conversion of t.
transprosthetic
    t. flow velocity
    t. gradient
transpulmonary
    t. gradient (TPG)
    t. pressure (Ptp)
    t. thermal-dye dilution
transradial
    t. approach
    t. cardiac catheterization
    t. coronary angioplasty
    t. primary stenting
transsarcolemmal
    t. calcium current
    t. calcium entry
    t. calcium influx
transseptal
    t. angiocardiography
    t. approach
    t. catheter

t. conduction
t. left heart catheterization
t. needle
t. puncture
t. sheath
transstenotic
t. pressure gradient
t. pressure gradient measurement
transtelephonic
t. ambulatory monitoring (TAM)
t. ambulatory monitoring system
t. arrhythmia monitoring
t. cardiac event monitoring
t. exercise monitor (TEM)
t. monitoring (TTM)
t. recording
t. transmission
transthoracic
t. acoustic window
t. color Doppler echocardiography
t. contrast echocardiography
t. direct current electrical cardioversion
t. Doppler harmonic echocardiography
t. echocardiogram (TTE)
t. echocardiographic Doppler assessment
t. echocardiography (TTE)
t. impedance
t. implantable cardioverter-defibrillator
t. intracardiac monitoring (TIM)
t. needle aspiration (TTNA)
t. needle aspiration biopsy
t. needle biopsy (TNB)
t. pacemaker
t. pacing stylet
t. portography (THP)
t. pressure
t. shock
transthoracically implanted ICD
transthyretin (TTR)
amyloidogenic t. (ATTR)
t. monomer
transtracheal
t. aspiration
t. oxygen (TTO)
t. oxygen catheter
t. oxygen therapy (TTOT)
transudate
transudation
transudative pleural effusion
transvalensis
Nocardia t.
transvalvular
t. aortic gradient
t. E velocity
t. flow

t. flow rate
t. hemodynamics
t. pressure gradient (TPG)
t. reflux
Transvene
T. lead
T. nonthoracotomy implantable cardioverter-defibrillator
T. tripolar electrode
transvenous (TV)
t. ablation
t. aortovelography (TAV)
t. biopsy
t. cardioversion (TVCV)
t. catheter extraction
t. defibrillator lead
t. device
t. electrode
t. implantable defibrillator
t. internal cardioversion
t. nitinol snare
t. pacemaker (TVP)
transventricular
t. closed valvotomy
t. mitral valve commissurotomy
transverse
t. aortic arch (TAA)
t. artery of face
t. artery of neck
t. cardiac diameter (TCD)
t. cervical artery
t. costal facet
t. fissure
t. fissure of right lung
t. heart diameter (THD)
t. incision
t. muscle
t. muscle of nape
t. muscle of thorax
t. section of heart
t. sinus (TS)
t. thoracosternotomy
t. tubule
transverse/sigmoid sinus (TS/SS)
transversi
fovea costalis processus t.
transversus
t. nuchae muscle
situs t.
transxiphoid approach
tranylcypromine
TRAP
thrombin receptor activating peptide
total peroxyl radical-trapping antioxidant potential
TRAP assay
trap
T. cardiovascular filtration system
T. neurovascular filtration system

trap (*continued*)
    T. vascular filtration system
    VEGF T.'s
trapdoor approach
TrapEase permanent vena cava filter
trapezius ridge sign
trapezoidal rule
trapidil
trapped
    t. gas
    t. gas volume
    t. lung
Trapper catheter exchange device
trapping
    air t.
    gas t.
TRAS
    transesophageal atrial stimulation
trash foot
Trasicor
trastuzumab
Trasylol
Traube
    T. bruit
    T. curve
    T. double tone
    T. dyspnea
    T. heart
    T. murmur
    T. plug
    T. semilunar space
    T. sign
trauma
    American Association for the
      Surgery of T. (AAST)
    blunt chest t. (BCT)
    blunt thoracic t.
    iatrogenic t.
    t. intensive care unit (TICU)
    isolated chest t.
    mechanical t.
    t. patient
    penetrating thoracic t.
    thoracic t.
    truncal t.
    vessel t.
traumatic
    t. aortic aneurysm
    t. aortic disruption
    t. aortography
    t. apnea
    t. asphyxia
    t. chylothorax
    t. emphysema
    t. fistula
    t. heart disease
    t. hemopericardium
    t. hemorrhage
    t. pericarditis

    t. pneumonia
    t. pneumothorax
    t. rupture
    t. tamponade
    t. thrombosis
    t. thrombus
traveler
    T. portable oxygen system
    Pulmo-Aide T.
Travenol infusion pump
tray
    lock pericardiocentesis set and t.
trazodone hydrochloride
TRD
    tongue-retaining device
Treacher Collins syndrome
treadmill
    arm ergometry t.
    t. echocardiography
    t. electrocardiogram
    t. ergometer
    exercise t. (ET)
    t. exercise (TE)
    t. exercise stress test
    t. exercise test (TET, TMET)
    t. incline
    Marquette t.
    t. performance test (TPT)
    Q-Stress t.
    t. score (TS)
    self-powered t.
    t. stress test (TMST, TST)
    t. test (TT)
treadmill-induced angina
treat
    number needed to t. (NNT)
treatment
    ablation t.
    Albertini t.
    antianginal t.
    arrest-and-reversal t.
    atherosclerosis prevention and t.
    Brehmer t.
    Coapsys surgical t.
    coronary artery risk assessment
      and t.
    Cosgrove-Edwards annuloplasty
      system with Duraflo t.
    Debove t.
    directly observed t. (DOT)
    efficacy of t.
    emergency medical t. (EMT)
    endovascular t.
    Forlanini t.
    Frankel t.
    HELP-apheresis t.
    Karell t.
    Lingraphica aphasic t.
    McPheeters t.

Nauheim t.
nonpharmacologic measure of t.
Nordach t.
Oertel t.
PICVA t.
pigmented t.
preventive allergy t.
rapid early action in coronary t.
  (REACT)
SAVR surgical t.
Schott t.
stand-alone laser t.
t. strategy
Tuffnell t.
vascular t.
VenaCure laser vein t.

Trecator-SC
Tredex powered bicycle
tree
bronchial t.
coronary t.
endobronchial t.
tracheobronchial t.
tree-in-winter appearance
trefoil
t. balloon catheter
t. Schneider balloon
t. tendon
Trellis-8 infusion system
tremolite
tremor
flapping t.
tremulus
pulsus t.
trench lung
trend
threshold t.
Trendelenburg
T. operation
T. position
T. test
Trental
trepidatio cordis
treponemal
t. antibody
t. test
Treponema pallidum
trepopnea
treppe
negative t.
t. phenomenon
positive t.
treprostinil sodium
TRI
transient response imaging
TriActiv balloon-protected flush
  extraction system
triad
acute compression t.

adrenomedullary t.
Andersen t.
t. asthma
atherogenic metabolic t.
Beck t.
Carney t.
Cushing t.
T. defibrillator system
Fallot t.
Grancher t.
Hull t.
Kartagener t.
lipid t.
Osler t.
Virchow t.
Widal-Abrami-Lermoyez t.

triadic junction
TRIADS
time-resolved imaging by automatic data
  segmentation
TriaDyne II kinetic therapy
triage
T. BNP blood test
T. cardiac rapid diagnostic test
  system
T. Cardio ProfilER panel
trial (*See also* study, program, protocol)
controlled clinical t. (CCT)
Philadelphia Association of
  Clinical T.'s (PACT)
randomized t.
randomized clinical t. (RCT)
randomized, controlled t. (RCT)
thrombosis prevention t. (TPT)
Zwolle t. (ZT)
Triam-A Injection
triamcinolone
t. acetonide (TAA)
t. diacetate
t. inhalation, nasal
t. (systemic)
Triam Forte Injection
Triaminic
T. AM Decongestant Formula
T. DM
Triamonide injection
triamterene
hydrochlorothiazide and t.
triangle
aortic t.
ausculatory t.
axillary t.
Burger scalene t.
Calot t.
cardiohepatic t.
carotid t.
clavipectoral t.
t. of dysplasia
Einthoven t.

triangle *(continued)*
    endocardial t.
    Gerhardt t.
    infraclavicular t.
    Jackson safety t.
    Koch t.
    t. of Koch
    Rauchfuss t.
    sternocostal t.
    subclavian t.
    Todaro t.
    tracheal t.
triangular
    t. resection
    t. resection of leaflet operation
Triatoma infestans
triatrial heart
triatriatum
    cor t.
triaxial
    t. accelerometer
    t. accelerometry
    t. reference system
triazolam
tribromide
    phosphorus t.
tribromide
tributyltin oxide
Trichinella spiralis
trichinosis
trichinous embolism
trichiura
    Trichuris t.
trichloramine
trichloride
    antimony t.
trichlormethiazide
Trichosporon
    T. asahii
    T. beigelii
    T. beigelii pneumonia
trichosporonosis
Trichosporum cutaneum
Trichuris trichiura
triciribine phosphate (TCN-P)
TriCor capsule
tricrotic, tricrotous
tricrotism
tricrotous
tricuspid
    t. anular motion (TAM)
    t. aortic valve
    t. atelectasis
    t. atresia (TA)
    t. closure (Tc)
    t. commissurotomy
    t. first sound (T1)
    t. incompetence (TI)
    t. insufficiency (TI)

    t. murmur
    t. opening (To)
    t. opening snap
    t. orifice
    t. position
    pulmonic t.
    t. regurgitant jet
    t. regurgitation (TR)
    t. restenosis
    t. stenosis (TS)
    t. valve (TV)
    t. valve annuloplasty
    t. valve anulus
    t. valve area
    t. valve closure
    t. valve closure sound (T1)
    t. valve disease
    t. valve doming
    t. valve dysplasia
    t. valve endocarditis
    t. valve flow
    t. valve prolapse (TVP)
    t. valve regurgitation (TVR)
    t. valve replacement (TVR)
    t. valve strut
    t. valve vegetation
    t. valvoplasty
    t. valvular leaflet
tricuspidalis
    cuspis anterior valvae t.
tricuspid-inferior vena cava isthmus
tricyclic antidepressant
triethanolamine
triethiodide
    gallamine t.
trifascicular block
triflupromazine
trigeminal
    t. cough
    t. nerve
    t. pulse
    t. rhythm
trigeminus
    pulsus t.
trigeminy
trigger
    asthma t.
    EKG t.
    pathologic t.
    rupture t.
    Smart T.
    t. of ventricular arrhythmia (TOVA)
triggered
    t. activity
    atrial t.
    atrial demand t. (AAT)
    t. harmonic power Doppler imaging
    t. mode

t. pacing
ventricular t. (VVT)
triggering
t. mechanism
respiratory t.
triglyceride (TG, TGL)
t. fatty acid (TGFA)
t. level
medium chain t.'s
remnant lipoprotein t.
serum t.
triglyceridemia
normal t. (NTG)
triglyceride-rich lipoprotein (TRL, TRLP)
trigone
anterior fibrous t.
vertebrocostal t.
trigonum omotracheale
Tri-Hydroserpine
triiodothyronine
trileaflet
trilinear cylindric interpolation algorithm
triloculare
cor t.
trilocular heart
trilogy
T. DC, DR, SR pulse generator
Fallot t.
t. of Fallot
Trimadeau sign
trimazosin
trimellitic
t. anhydride
t. anhydride asthma
trimetazidine 1 (TMZ)
trimethaphan camsylate
trimethoprim-sulfamethoxazole (TMP-SMX)
trimethoprim sulfate
trimetrexate glucoronate
trimipramine maleate
Trimox
trinitrate
glyceryl t.
trinucleotide
cytosine-thymine-guanine T.
triolet
bruit de t.
Triostat injection
trioxide
antimony t.
arsenic t.
Tripedia
tripelennamine
tripe palm
triphammer pulse

triphenyl
t. tetrazolium chloride
t. tetrazolium staining method
triphosphatase
adenosine t. (ATPase)
triphosphate
adenosine t. (ATP)
guanosine t. (GTP)
inositol t.
purine nucleotides adenosine t.
uridine t. (UTP)
triphosphate-dependent potassium channel
triple
t. coronary artery bypass graft (TCABG)
t. coronary artery graft (TCAG)
t. ectopic tachyarrhythmia
t. extrastimulus
t. rhythm
t. stimulus
triple-balloon valvoplasty
triple-bandpass filter
triple-drug maintenance regimen
triple-humped pressure pulse
triplet
tripoding
tripod sign
tripolar
t. defibrillation coil electrode
t. lead
segmented ring t. (SRT)
t. with Damato curve catheter
triport cannula
TriPort hemostasis introducer sheath kit
Triposed Tablet
Trippi-Wells tongs
triprolidine
t. and pseudoephedrine
t., pseudoephedrine, codeine
trisalicylate
choline magnesium t.
Tris-buffer infusion test
trisection
pulse t.
tris(hydroxymethyl)aminomethane
trisomy 13, 18, 21
Tristar coronary stent
Tritace
TriTrac-R3D accelerometer
Triumph VTX port
TriVex system
TRL, TRLP
triglyceride-rich lipoprotein
trocar
Axiom thoracic t.
B-D Potain thoracic t.
Davidson thoracic t.

T

trocar *(continued)*
    Entree thoracoscopy t.
    Flexipath surgical thoracic t.
    Hunt angiographic t.
    large-bore t.
    Thoracoport t.
trochleae
    vagina synovialis t.
trochocardia
trochorizocardia
troglitazone
Troisier sign
troleandomycin (TAO)
trolley
tromethamine
Trooper extra support guidewire
Tropheryma whippleii
trophic changes
trophoblastic tumor
tropical
    t. endomyocardial fibrosis
    t. pulmonary eosinophilia (TPE)
tropicalis
    Xenopus t.
tropomyosin
troponin
    t. C
    cardiac t. I (CTI, cTnI, cTn-I)
    cardiac t. T (cTnT)
    t. I
    t. T (TnT)
trospectomycin sulfate
trough
    t. dosing
    peak and t.
    t. and peak levels
    systolic t.
    X-descent t.
    Y-descent t.
trough-to-peak ratio
trouser
    t. legs and seat technique
    military antishock t.'s (MAST)
    pneumatic t.'s
Trousseau syndrome
trovafloxacin
TRPV-1
    transient receptor potential vanilloid-1
TRT
    thoracic radiation therapy
TRU
    terminal respiratory unit
Tru-Cut biopsy needle
true
    t. aortic aneurysm
    t. asthma
    t. cyst
    t. lumen

    T. Sheathless intraaortic balloon catheter
    t. versus false aneurysm aortography
    t. vocal cord
TrueMax 2400 metabolic measuring system
true-negative test result
true-positive
    t.-p. stress test (TPST)
    t.-p. test result
Trufill n-BCA liquid embolic system
TruFisp cine
trumpet
    angel's t.
    nasal t.
truncal
    t. distribution of body fat
    t. trauma
truncoconal area
truncus, pl. **trunci**
    t. arteriosus (TA)
    t. arteriosus communis (TAC)
    bifurcatio trunci
    t. brachiocephalicus
    t. celiacus
    t. costocervicalis
    t. fascicularis atrioventricularis
    t. linguofacialis
    t. lymphaticus bronchiomediastinalis
    t. pulmonalis
    t. thyrocervicalis
Trunecek
    T. sign
    T. symptom
trunk
    bifurcation of pulmonary t.
    brachiocephalic t.
    bronchomediastinal lymphatic t.
    t. control test (TCT)
    t. forward flexion
    left-sided innominate t.
    loose elephant t.
    orifice of pulmonary t.
    pulmonary t.
    valve of pulmonary t.
Trusler
    T. aortic valve technique
    T. rule for pulmonary artery banding
    T. technique of aortic valvoplasty
TruTrak data sampling system
TruZone
    T. asthma action plan wallet card
    T. peak flowmeter
    T. PFM
TRVV
    total right ventricular volume

Trypanosoma
    T. brucei
    T. cruzi
    T. gambiense
    T. rhodesiense
trypanosomiasis
    American t.
trypsin, balsam peru, castor oil
trypsinogen
    serum immunoreactive t.
TS
    transverse sinus
    treadmill score
    tricuspid stenosis
        forme fruste of TS
TSC
    transient spontaneous circulation
TSC2 gene
TSH
    thyroid-stimulating hormone
T-shaped stent
TSO
    transient spastic occlusion
TS/SS
    transverse/sigmoid sinus
TST
    total sleep time
    treadmill stress test
tsukubaensis
    Streptomyces t.
TSVR
    total systemic vascular resistance
TT
    thrombin time
    thrombolytic therapy
    thromboplastin time
    treadmill test
        TT form of MTP gene
T_I/T_{TOT}
    ratio of inspiratory time to total breathing
        cycle time
TTC
    takotsubo cardiomyopathy
        TTC stain
TTE
    transthoracic echocardiogram
    transthoracic echocardiography
TTM
    transtelephonic monitoring
TTNA
    transthoracic needle aspiration
TTNB
    transient tachypnea of newborn
TTO
    transtracheal oxygen
        TTO therapy
TTOT
    transtracheal oxygen therapy

TTP
    thrombotic thrombocytopenic purpura
    time to peak
TTR
    transthyretin
TTT
    tilt-table test
T-type calcium channels
Tubasal
Tubbs dilator
tube, tubing
    AccuMark calibrated infant
        feeding t.
    air t.
    Aire-Cuf tracheostomy t.
    American tracheotomy t.
    Andrews-Pynchon t.
    Arm-a-Med endotracheal t.
    Atkins-Cannard tracheal t.
    Bivona Fome-Cuff t.
    Bivona TTS tracheostomy t.
    Blue Line cuffed endotracheal t.
    bronchial t.
    Broncho-Cath double-lumen
        endotracheal t.
    bulboventricular t.
    Caluso PEG t.
    Carabelli t.
    Carlen double-lumen endotracheal t.
    Celestin esophageal t.
    Chaussier t.
    chest t. (CT)
    Cooley sump t.
    cuffed endotracheal t.
    cuffed tracheostomy t.
    Dacron t.
    Dale-Schwartz t.
    decompressive chest t
    double-lumen endobronchial t.
    Dow Corning t.
    dual-lumen endotracheal t.
    Durham t.
    endobronchial t.
    endocardial t.
    Endoflex endotracheal t.
    endotracheal t. (ETT)
    Endotrol endotracheal t.
    Endotrol tracheal t.
    esophageal combination t. (ECT)
    ETView endotracheal t.
    Ewald t.
    fenestrated tracheostomy t.
    Flex DIC tracheostomy t.
    fluffy-cuffed t.
    Fome-Cuf tracheostomy t.
    glutaraldehyde-tanned bovine
        collagen t.
    Gore-Tex t.
    Haldane-Priestley t.

T

tube *(continued)*
   high pressure connecting t.
   high-volume cuffed endotracheal t.
   Hi-Lo Evac endotracheal t.
   Hi-Lo Jet tracheal t.
   Holter t.
   Hyperflex tracheostomy t.
   inner t.
   interposition of Dacron t.
   intratracheal t.
   J-shaped t.
   Kuhn t.
   Lanz low-pressure cuff
    endotracheal t.
   large-bore chest t.
   large-caliber chest t.
   Laryngoflex reinforced
    endotracheal t.
   laser t.
   lidocaine, atropine, naloxone,
    epinephrine [drugs that may be
    administered via endotracheal t.]
    (LANE)
   Lindholm tracheal t.
   Lo-Pro tracheal t.
   Lore-Lawrence trachea t.
   Luer tracheal t.
   Mackler t.
   Magill Safety Clear Plus
    endotracheal t.
   Mallinckrodt cuffed endotracheal t.
   Montgomery Safe-T T.
   Mosher life-saving tracheal t.
   mycobacterial growth indicator t.
    (MGIT)
   Nachlas t.
   nasogastric t.
   nasotracheal t.
   NG t.
   Olympus One-Step Button t.
   oroendotracheal t.
   orotracheal t.
   otopharyngeal t.
   PEG t.
   PEJ t.
   pleural t.
   polyvinyl chloride t.
   Portex Per-fit tracheostomy t.
   primordial catheter t.
   RAE endotracheal t.
   right-angle chest t.
   Robertshaw t.
   Ruschelit polyvinyl chloride
    endotracheal t.
   Safe-T T.
   Sarns intracardiac suction t.
   scavenging t.
   Shiley tracheostomy t.
   Softech endotracheal t.

   Souttar t.
   spiral-embedded t.
   T t.
   thoracostomy t.
   t. thoracostomy
   Tovell t.
   tracheal t.
   tracheostomy t.
   Trach-Talk tracheostomy t.
   Univent t.
   UTTS endotracheal t.
   Vacutainer t.
   Venturi t.
   Vivonex Moss t.
   water-seal chest t.
   wire-wound endotracheal t.
   x-ray t.
**TubeChek esophageal intubation
  detector**
tubercle
   corniculate t.
   cuneiform t.
   Ghon t.
tuberculin
   Koch old t.
   purified protein derivative of t.
   t. skin test
   t. tine test
tuberculocidal
tuberculoid myocarditis
tuberculoma
tuberculosilicosis
tuberculosis (TB)
   active t.
   acute miliary t.
   adult t.
   aerogenic t.
   Amplicor assay for
    Mycobacterium t.
   anthracotic t.
   arrested t.
   atypical t.
   avian t.
   basal t.
   t. of bones and joints
   cerebral t.
   cestodic t.
   childhood t.
   childhood-type t.
   disseminated t.
   endobronchial t.
   ESAT-6 protein *mycobacterium t.*
   extrapulmonary t.
   exudative t.
   generalized t.
   healed t.
   hematogenous t.
   hilum t.
   inactive t.

inhalation t.
t. of larynx
t. lichenoides
t. of lung
miliary t.
multidrug-resistant t. (MDR-TB)
mycobacteria other than t. (MOTT)
Mycobacterium t. (MTB)
open t.
oral t.
orificial t.
papulonecrotic t.
paradoxical worsening of t.
postprimary t.
primary t.
productive t.
pulmonary t. (PTB)
pulmonary parenchymal t.
reactivation t.
reinfection t.
renal t.
secondary t.
smear-negative t.
smear-positive t.
surgical t.
tracheobronchial t.
t. vaccine
W-strain t.
tuberculostat
tuberculostatic
tuberculous
t. arteritis
t. bronchopneumonia
t. caseation
t. chemotherapy
t. empyema
t. empyesis
t. endocarditis
t. laryngitis
t. lymphadenitis
t. mycotic aneurysm
t. mycotic aneurysm of aorta
t. nephritis
t. pericarditis
t. pleurisy
t. pleuritis
t. pneumonia
t. rheumatism
tuberculum
t. thyroideum inferius
t. thyroideum superius
tuberoeruptive xanthoma
tuberous
t. sclerosis
t. xanthoma
Tubersol
tubing (*var. of* tube)
tubular
t. breath sounds

t. necrosis
t. respiration
t. shadow
t. slotted stent
tubule
distal convoluted t.
lower t.
proximal convoluted t.
T t.
transverse t.
tubuloreticular structure
Tuffier test
Tuffnell treatment
tug, tugging
tracheal t.
Tukey-Kramer posttest
tularemia
oropharyngeal t.
tularemic pneumonia
tularensis
Francisella t.
tumefaciens
Agrobacterium t.
tumor
adenomatoid t.
anaplastic t.
Askin t.
t. blush
bronchopulmonary carcinoid t.
carcinoid t.
cardiac t.
carotid body t.
chromaffin cell t.
clear cell t.
congenital peribronchial
  myofibroblastic t.
craniopharyngeal duct t.
desmoplastic small round cell t.
t. embolism
endodermal sinus t.
extrathoracic t.
fibrous t.
t. fixation
germ cell t.
glomus t.
Godwin t.
granular cell t.
Hürthle cell t.
iceberg t.
inflammatory myofibroblastic t.
intracardiac t.
intravascular bronchoalveolar t.
t. marker
mesenchymal-derived t.
mesodermal t.
mesothelial t.
migrated t.
mixed germ cell t.
myxoma t.

T

tumor *(continued)*
    t. necrosis factor (TNF)
    t. necrosis factor-2 (TNF2)
    t. necrosis factor-2 allele
    t. necrosis factor-alpha (TNF-alpha)
    t. necrosis factor-alpha promotor
      polymorphism
    t. necrosis factor receptor (TNFR)
    nerve sheath t.
    neuroectodermal t.
    neuroendocrine t.
    neurogenic t.
    t., node, metastasis (TNM)
    nonseminomatous germ cell t.
    Pancoast t.
    papillary t.
    paraganglioma t.
    pericardiac t.
    phantom t.
    t. plop
    t. plop sound
    polycystic t.
    preganglionic t.
    primitive neuroectodermal t.
      (PNET)
    Purkinje t.
    Rathke pouch t.
    sarcomatous t.
    solitary fibrous t.
    sugar t.
    superior pulmonary sulcus t.
    t. suppressor gene inactivation
    teratoma t.
    thymic carcinoid t.
    thyroid t.
    trophoblastic t.
    vanishing t.
tumorigenic
tumorlet
tumultus cordis
tunable pulsed dye laser
TUNEL
    TdT-mediated dUTP nick-end labeling
    TUNEL assay
    TUNEL method
    TUNEL stain
tungsten
    t. carbide pneumoconiosis
    t. microelectrode
tunic
    Bichat t.
    vascular t.
tunica
    t. mucosa
    t. mucosa bronchi
    t. mucosa esophagi
    t. mucosa laryngis
    t. mucosa linguae
    t. mucosa pharyngis

    t. mucosa tracheae
    t. muscularis bronchiorum
    t. muscularis esophagi
    t. muscularis pharyngis
    t. muscularis tracheae
tunnel
    aortic and left ventricular t.
      (ALVT)
    Kawashima intraventricular t.
    percutaneous t.
    t. subaortic stenosis
    subsartorial t.
tunneled segment
tunneler
Tunturi EL400 bicycle ergometer
Tuohy-Borst
    T.-B. adapter
    T.-B. introducer
Tuohy needle
TUPLE-1 gene
turbinate
turbine-powered ICU ventilator system
Turboaire Challenger cold-air bronchial
    provocation device
turbo field echo (TFE)
TurboFLASH technique
Turbuhaler
    Bricanyl T.
    Oxis T.
    Pulmicort T.
    Symbicort 100/6 T.
    Symbicort 200/6 T.
turbulence
    heart rate t.
turbulent
    t. diastolic mitral inflow
    t. jet
turgor
    coronary vascular t.
    skin t.
turn
    2-t. epicardial lead
    3-t. epicardial lead
turnaround time (TAT)
Turner syndrome
Tussafed drops
Tussigon
Tussin
    Safe T. 30
Tussionex
Tussi-Organidin DM NR
tussive
    t. fremitus
    t. squeeze
    t. syncope
Tusstat Syrup
Tuttle thoracic forceps
TV
    tidal volume

transvenous
tricuspid valve

TV$_I$
tidal inspiratory volume

TV$_E$
tidal expiratory volume

TVCV
transvenous cardioversion

TVG
time-varied gain

TVGC
time-varied gain control

TVP
transvenous pacemaker
tricuspid valve prolapse

TVR
target vessel revascularization
total vascular resistance
tricuspid valve regurgitation
tricuspid valve replacement

TWA
T-wave alternans

TWAR
Taiwan acute respiratory
TWAR agent
TWAR disease
TWAR pneumonia

T-wave
T-w. alternans (TWA)
T-w. change
T-w. flattening
T-w. inversion
T-w. loop
T-w. pseudonormalization
T-w. shock

Tween 80
tweezers
optic t.

Twice-A-Day Nasal Solution
twiddler's syndrome
twill tape
twin
Bennett t.
T. Jet nebulizer
thoracopagus t.
VersaLab APM2 for t.'s

Twin-Pass dual access catheter
twist
systolic t.

TWISTED
tracheal wall injury with intermittent
stoppage of tracheostomy and episodes
of dyspnea
TWISTED syndrome

Twisthaler
Asmanex T.

TwistLock
T. Cath-Gard

Hands-Off infusion port heparin-
coated thermodilution catheter
with T.

twitch
t. esophageal pressure
t. force
t. gastric pressure
t. potentiation
t. transdiaphragmatic pressure

TX
transplantation

Tx
transplant
transplantation

TxCAD
transplant coronary artery disease

Tylenol Cold No Drowsiness
tylophorine
alkaloid t.

tylosin tartrate asthma
tyloxapol
tympanitic
t. resonance
t. sound

tympany
bell t.

type
t. A, B behavior
Ambrose plaque t.
cardioinhibitory t.
cell t.
t. 1-4 dextrocardia
t. I collagen telopeptide (ICTP)
t. I, Ia, Ib, Ic, II, III lesion
t. II cell hyperplasia
t. III antiarrhythmic agent
t. I, II dip
t. I, III procollagen
t. II pneumocyte
t. Va, Vb, Vc lesion

typhoid
t. fever
t. pleurisy
t. pneumonia

typhus
African tick t.
Queensland tick t.
scrub t.

typical small cell
typing
human lymphocyte antigen t.

tyramine
Tyrode solution
tyrosine
t. hydroxylase
t. phosphorylated protein

Tyshak
T. balloon
T. balloon valvoplasty catheter

T-Y · Tzanck

T-Y stent   Tzanck test

U

U loop
U suture
U virus
U wave

UA

ultrasonic arteriography
unstable angina

UACP

upper airway closing pressure

UACS

upper airway cough syndrome

UAE

unsupported arm exercise

UA/NQMI

unstable angina/non-Q-wave myocardial
infarction

UAO

upper airway obstruction

UAOP

upper airway opening pressure

UAP

unstable angina pectoris

UAPA

unilateral absence of pulmonary artery

UARS

upper airway resistance syndrome

ubiquinol

ubiquinone

ubiquitin

ubiquitin-conjugated protein

ubonensis

Burkholderia u.

UCA

ultrasound contrast agent

UCAD

unstable coronary artery disease

UCG

ultrasonic cardiography

UCI-Barnard aortic valve

UCO

ultrasonic cardiac output

UEDVT

upper extremity deep venous thrombosis

UFA

unesterified fatty acid

UFCT

ultrafast computed tomography

UFH

unfractionated heparin

UFT

uracil and tegafur

UGNB

ultrasonically guided needle biopsy

UHFV

ultra high frequency ventilation

Uhl

U. anomaly
U. disease
U. malformation
U. syndrome

UHR

underlying heart rhythm

UIP

usual interstitial pneumonia
usual interstitial pneumonitis

UK

urokinase

ulcer

Bairnsdale u.
decubitus u.
diabetic u.
foot u.
penetrating aortic u. (PAU)
penetrating atherosclerotic u. (PAU)
peptic u.
stasis u.
venous u.

ulcerans

Mycobacterium u.

ulcerated

u. lesion
u. plaque

ulcerative endocarditis

ulcerogangrenous

ulceromembranous

ulcerosa

angina u.
pharyngitis u.

Uldall subclavian hemodialysis catheter

Ulick syndrome

Ullmann syndrome

ULM

unprotected left main

ulnar

u. nerve
u. pulse

ULP

ultra low profile
ULP catheter

ULPE

upper lobe pulmonary edema

Ultegra

U. rapid platelet function assay
U. RPFA-TRAP

ultimate

U. nasal mask
U. Seal CPAP mask seal
U. Seal gel interface

U

ultimum
U. hemostasis introducer
u. moriens

ultra
U. 8 balloon catheter
u. high frequency ventilation
(UHFV)
U. ICE catheter
u. low profile (ULP)
u. low profile fixed-wire balloon
dilation catheter
U. low resistance voice prosthesis
U. Mide topical
U. pacemaker
U. stent

Ultracef

ultracentrifugation

UltraCision ultrasonic knife

UltraCross profile imaging catheter

ultrafast
u. computed tomographic scanner
u. computed tomography (UFCT)
u. computed tomography scan
u. contrast-enhanced chest computed
tomography
u. CT scan
u. CT scanner

ultrafiltration
continuous arteriovenous u.
(CAVU)
modified u. (MUF)

Ultraflex
U. esophageal stent system
U. nitinol stent
U. self-expanding stent
U. tracheobronchial stent

UltraFuse infusion catheter

Ultraject prefilled syringe

Ultra-Lite portable aspirator

Ultramark 9 echocardiograph

Ultramax woven velour vascular graft

ultrarapid subthreshold stimulation

Ultra-Select nitinol PTCA guidewire

UltraSom computerized sleep analyzer

ultrasonic
u. arteriography (UA)
u. cardiac output (UCO)
u. cardiac output monitoring
(USCOM)
u. cardiography (UCG, USCG)
u. integrated backscatter imaging
u. nebulizer (USN)
u. tissue characterization relation

ultrasonically guided needle biopsy
(UGNB)

ultrasonographer

ultrasonography
B-mode u.
compression u.

Doppler u.
duplex pulsed-Doppler u.
endobronchial u. (EBUS)
high-resolution B-mode u.
intracaval endovascular u. (ICEUS)
intracoronary u.
TCD u.

ultrasonoscope
Acuson XP-5 u.
Acuson XP-10 u.
Acuson XP-128 u.

ultrasound
u. ablation catheter
Aloka u.
u. angiography
ATL UltraMark 4 u.
ATL UltraMark 7 colorflow u.
B-mode u.
bronchoscopic u.
cardiac u.
u. cardiography
continuous-wave Doppler u.
u. contrast agent (UCA)
contrast-enhanced u. (CEU)
U. Contrast Microsphere
coronary intravascular u.
3-dimensional intravascular u.
Doppler u.
duplex u.
echo-guided u.
endobronchial u. (EBUS)
gray-scale u.
Hewlett-Packard 2500 Sonos u.
high-resolution deep penetration 2D
intracardiac u.
u. holography
u. instrument
InterTherapy intravascular u.
intracoronary u. (ICUS)
intracoronary vascular u. (IVUS)
intraluminal u. (ILUS)
intravascular u. (IVUS)
Irex Exemplar u.
u. machine
matrix-array u.
negative-contrast intravascular u.
power Doppler u.
qualitative coronary u. (QCU)
real-time u.
Shimadzu cardiac u.
Siemens SI 400 u.
TCD u.
u. therapy
through-the-balloon u.
Toshiba Sonolayer SSH-140A u.
u. transducer

ultrasound-guided bronchoscopy

ultrasound-tipped catheter

UltraStethoscope

ultrastructure
Ultra-Thin balloon catheter
ultrathin-walled 2-stage (UTTS)
ultraviolet laser
Ultravist
    U. contrast
    U. injection
umbilical
    u. artery
    u. tape
    u. vein
umbilicalis
    arteritis u.
umbrella
    ASDOS u.
    atrial septal defect u.
    Bard Clamshell septal u.
    Clamshell septal u.
    u. closure
    double u.
    u. filter
    patent ductus arteriosus u.
    PDA u.
    transcatheter u.
UMI
    UMI catheter
    UMI transseptal Cath-Seal catheter
    introducer
U-Mid-O$_2$ Jet Set
UMLS
    Unified Medical Language system
unassisted spontaneous ventilation
Unasyn
unattended polysomnography
unbalanced A-V canal
uncoupling
    eNOS u.
uncrossable
underdrive
    u. pacing
    u. termination
underexpressed protein
underinflation
underlying heart rhythm (UHR)
underperfused myocardium
underperfusion
undersedation
undersensing
    atrial u.
    functional u.
    pacemaker u.
undertreatment
underventilation
underwater
    u. seal drainage
    u. seal resistor
undetermined pathological-type stroke
undifferentiated small-cell carcinoma
undilatable

undulating
    u. deflection
    u. deflection that follows T wave
    u. pulse
unequal pulse
unesterified
    u. cholesterol
    u. fatty acid (UFA)
unfractionated heparin (UFH)
uniaxial accelerometer
unicommissural
unicuspid aortic valve
unidirectional block
unifascicular block
Unified Medical Language system
    (UMLS)
unifocalization
unifocal ventricular ectopic beat
    (UVEB)
UniHeart IV universal nebulizer
unilateral
    u. absence of pulmonary artery
    (UAPA)
    u. hyperlucency
    u. hyperlucency of lung
    u. hyperlucent lung
    u. lobar emphysema
    u. nonfunctioning lung
    u. pneumonia
    u. pneumothorax
    u. spatial neglect (USN)
Uni-Lead ECG electrode system
unileaflet prolapse
Unilink
    U. anastomotic device
    U. system
unilocular
    u. cyst
    u. hydatid disease
unintended positive end-expiratory
    pressure (autoPEEP, intrinsic PEEP)
unintubated
Uniphyl
unipolar
    u. atrial pacemaker
    u. connector
    u. defibrillation coil electrode
    u. electrocardiogram
    u. limb lead
    u. limb lead on left leg in
    electrocardiography (aVF, aVL)
    u. limb lead on right arm in
    electrocardiography (aVR)
    u. pacing threshold
    u. Pisces Sigma
    u. precordial lead
    u. sequential pacemaker
Uniretic
Uni-Silicone lead

U

Unisom
Unisperse blue dye
Unistasis valve
Unistep
 U. catheter delivery system
 U. Plus delivery system
 Wallstent venous endoprosthesis
  with U.
 Wallstent with U.
unit (*See also* device)
 Acrodisc u.
 acute coronary care u.
 Aqua-Seal chest drainage u.
 arbitrary densitometric u. (ADU)
 ATA u.
 BCD Plus cardioplegic u.
 BICAP u.
 Biosound 2000 II ultrasound u.
 Biosound 3000 ultrasound u.
 BiPAP u.
 cardiac u. (CU)
 cardiac care u. (CCU)
 cardiac diagnostic u. (CDU)
 cardiac intensive care u. (CICU)
 cardiac observation u. (COU)
 cardiac rehabilitation u. (CRU)
 cardiac surgical intensive care u.
  (CSICU)
 cardiothoracic u. (CTU)
 cardiothoracic intensive care u.
  (CTICU)
 cardiovascular intensive care u.
  (CVICU)
 chest pain observation u. (CPOU)
 clinical research u. (CRU)
 comprehensive cardiac care u.
  (CCCU)
 coronary care u. (CCU)
 critical care u.
 defibrillator u.
 digital fluoroscopic u.
 ECG triggering u.
 electromyography u.
 enhanced external
  counterpulsation u.
 FreeDop portable Doppler u.
 high-dependency u. (HDU)
 Hounsfield u. (HU)
 hybrid u.
 intensive coronary care u. (ICCU)
 intrapleural sealed drainage u.
 kallidinogenase inactivator u.
 kallikrein inactivating u. (KIU)
 Karmen u.'s
 Kreiselman u.
 life change u.
 lung u.
 medical coronary intensive care u.
  (MCICU)

 medical intensive care u. (MICU)
 million international u.'s (MIU)
 mobile coronary care u. (MCCU)
 myocardial infarction research u.
  (MIRU)
 Myotrace Plus electromyography u.
 peripheral resistance u. (PRU)
 postanesthesia care u. (PACU)
 postcoronary care u. (PCCU)
 Q-Plex metabolic cart and
  pulmonary function u.
 R u.
 respiratory special care u. (ReSCU)
 RinoFlow ENT wash u.
 Sentinal seal pleural drainage u.
 Solcotrans autotransfusion u.
 S-Scort New-Duet suction u.
 stroke u. (SU)
 subacute u.
 Sullivan nasal variable positive
  airway pressure u.
 surgical intensive care u. (SICU)
 Surgitron u.
 terminal respiratory u. (TRU)
 Thora-Seal III chest drainage u.
 Todd u.
 torr u.
 Tranquility Bilevel CPAP u.
 trauma intensive care u. (TICU)
 Wood u.
united
 U. Network for Organ Sharing
  (UNOS)
 U. States Air Force School of
  Aerospace Medicine
 U. States Catheter and Instrument,
  Inc.
 U. States Pharmacopeia (USP)
univariate
 u. analysis
 u. predictor
Univasc
Univent
 U. tube
 U. ventilator
Uni-Vent Eagle ventilation system
univentricular
 u. atrioventricular connection
 u. heart
 u. pacing
universal
 u. ACE
 u. aerosol cloud enhancer
 A-V u. (DDD)
 u. pacemaker
universalis
 adiposis u.

university
> U. of Akron TAH
> U. of Wisconsin solution

Univision echocardiographic system
unlabored respiration
unloading
> left ventricular u.

unmyelinated C-fiber
UNOS
> United Network for Organ Sharing

unpotentiated twitch force
unprotected
> u. artery
> u. left main (ULM)

unrelated donor (URD)
unresolved pneumonia
unrestricted somatic stem cell (USSC)
unroofed
> u. coronary sinus
> u. coronary sinus syndrome

unsaturated pyrrolizidine alkaloid (UPA)
Unschuld sign
unstable
> u. angina (UA)
> u. angina/non-Q-wave myocardial
>   infarction (UA/NQMI)
> u. angina pectoris (UAP)
> u. coronary artery disease (UCAD)
> u. plaque

unstented xenograft valve
unsupported arm exercise (UAE)
untouched aortic off-pump coronary
  surgery
untwist
untwisting
up
> pinked u.

UPA
> unsaturated pyrrolizidine alkaloid

uPA
> urokinase plasminogen activator

updraft
> albuterol nebulizer u.
> U. handheld nebulizer
> Ventolin u.

upgated technique
upgoing Babinski
UPP
> uvulopalatoplasty

upper
> u. aerodigestive tract
> u. airway
> u. airway closing pressure (UACP)
> u. airway cough syndrome (UACS)
> u. airway obstruction (UAO)
> u. airway opening pressure
>   (UAOP)
> u. airway resistance syndrome
>   (UARS)

> u. chamber
> u. extremity deep venous
>   thrombosis (UEDVT)
> u. infection point
> u. lobe
> u. lobe bronchus
> u. lobe of lung
> u. lobe pulmonary edema (ULPE)
> u. lung zone
> u. nodal extrasystole
> u. respiratory infection (URI)
> u. ribs

UPPGP
> uvulopalatopharyngoglossoplasty

UPPP
> uvulopalatopharyngoplasty

up-regulated tissue factor
up-regulation
upright
> u. exercise
> u. T wave

upsloping
> u. ST elevation
> u. ST segment
> u. ST-segment depression

upstairs-downstairs heart
upstream
> u. airway conductance
> u. airways
> u. segment

upstroke
> carotid u.
> diastolic u.
> u. and falloff
> u. pattern
> u. phase
> R-wave u.
> u. velocity

uptake
> cardiac antimyosin antibody u.
> glucose u.
> I-123 MIBG u.
> insulin-mediated glucose u. (IMGU)
> iodine-123
>   metaiodobenzylguanidine u.
> lung u.
> maximum oxygen u.
> myocardial oxygen u.
> myocardial substrate u. (MSU)
> N-13 ammonia u.
> norepinephrine u. 1
> oxygen u. (oxygen uptake peak VO_2)
> peak oxygen u.
> thallium u.
> tracer u.

uptake-mismatch pattern
uracil and tegafur (UFT)
urapidil
urate

U

Urbach-Wiethe syndrome
urban
- u. allergen
- u. asthma
- u. toxicant

URD
unrelated donor

ureae
- *Actinobacillus u.*

urea-formaldehyde resin
urealyticum
- *Ureaplasma u.*

urea nitrogen
Ureaphil Injection
Ureaplasma urealyticum
Urecholine
ureidopenicillin
uremia
uremic
- u. lung
- u. pericarditis
- u. pneumonia
- u. pneumonitis

Uremol
Uresil
- U. radiopaque silicone band vessel loops
- U. Vascu-Flo carotid shunt

urethane
- polycarbonate u.

urethralis
- *Oligella u.*

urgency
- hypertensive u.

URI
upper respiratory infection

uric acid
uridine triphosphate (UTP)
Uridon
urinary
- u. catheter
- u. equol excretion

urine
- brown u.
- u. volume

urinothorax
Urisec
Uritol
urocanic acid
urodiolenone
Urografin-76 contrast medium
urokinase (UK)
- u. plasminogen activator (uPA)
- recombinant u. (r-UK)

Uro-Mag
urorosein
Urozide

urticaria
- aquagenic u.
- pressure u.

URx
- URx intravascular Sonotherapy catheter
- URx intravascular Sonotherapy system
- URx Sonotherapy instrument

USAFSAM treadmill exercise protocol
USCG
ultrasonic cardiography

USCI
- USCI catheter
- USCI Goetz bipolar electrode
- USCI introducer
- USCI NBIH bipolar electrode
- USCI Probe balloon-on-a-wire dilation system
- USCI shunt

USCOM
ultrasonic cardiac output monitoring

use
- amount of u. (AOU)
- u. dependence

U-shaped catheter loop
USN
- ultrasonic nebulizer
- unilateral spatial neglect

USP
United States Pharmacopeia

USSC
unrestricted somatic stem cell

ustus
- *Aspergillus u.*

usual
- u. interstitial pneumonia (UIP)
- u. interstitial pneumonia of Liebow
- u. interstitial pneumonitis (UIP)

usurpation
Utah
- U. TAH
- U. total artificial heart

utilization
- MO2 u.

UTP
uridine triphosphate

UTTS
- ultrathin-walled 2-stage
- UTTS endotracheal tube

UVEB
unifocal ventricular ectopic beat

uvulopalatopharyngoglossoplasty (UPPGP)
uvulopalatopharyngoplasty (UPPP)
- laser-assisted u. (LAUPPP)

uvulopalatoplasty (UPP)
- laser-assisted u. (LAUP)

U-wave
    U-w. alternans

U-w. inversion

U

V
    ventricular
    volt
    volume
        V lead
        V peak of jugular venous pulse
        V wave
V$_O$
    oral airflow in liters per second
V$_{TG}$
    thoracic gas volume
V$_{pe}$
    peak ejection velocity
V$_E$
    minute ventilation
    peak exercise ventilation
V$_T$
    tidal volume
V$_{MAX}$, Vmax
    maximal velocity
    maximum velocity
V510B biplane TEE transducer
V5M multiplane TEE transducer
VA
    alveolar volume
    variant angina
    vasodilator agent
    ventricular aneurysm
    ventricular arrhythmia
    ventriculoatrial
    ventroanterior
    vertebral artery
    Veterans Administration
        VA conduction
        VA interval
V$_A$
    alveolar ventilation per minute
VABP
    venoarterial bypass pumping
VAC
    vacuum-assisted closure
    ventriculoatrial conduction
        Wound VAC
vaccae
    Mycobacterium v.
vaccine
        ActHIB v.
        BCG v.
        diphtheria, tetanus toxoids, acellular
            pertussis v.
        diphtheria, tetanus toxoids, whole-
            cell pertussis v.
        diphtheria, tetanus toxoids, whole-
            cell pertussis vaccine,
        Haemophilus type b conjugate v.

Haemophilus type b conjugate v.
HbOC v.
Imovax v.
inactivated poliovirus v.
influenza virus v.
lipopolysaccharide v.
meningococcal v.
pneumococcal v.
PRP-D v.
PRP-OMPC v.
tuberculosis v.
14-valent v.
23-valent polysaccharide v.
vaccinia
Vaccinium myrtillus
Vac-Pak-II ultra-lite portable aspirator
VACTERL
    vertebral, vascular, anal, cardiac,
        tracheoesophageal, renal, limb
        anomalies
        VACTERL association
        VACTERL Association Support
            Group
        VACTERL syndrome
Vacu-Aide home-use aspirator
vacuolated cell
Vacutainer tube
vacuum
        v. controller
        high v. (HV)
vacuum-assisted
        v.-a. closure (VAC)
        v.-a. closure treated mediastinitis
        v.-a. venous return system
vacuus
        pulsus v.
VAD
    venous access device
    ventricular assist device
        DeBakey VAD
        HeartSaver VAD
VAE
    venous air embolism
VA-ECMO
    venoarterial extracorporeal membrane
        oxygenation
VAG
    vascular access graft
        Vectra VAG
vagal
        v. atrial fibrillation
        v. attack
        v. block
        v. body
        v. bradycardia

V

vagal *(continued)*
    v. escape
    v. neural crest
    v. reaction
    v. reflex
    v. response
    v. stimulation
    v. tone
vagectomy
vagi (*pl. of* vagus)
vagina synovialis trochleae
vagolytic
    v. agent
    v. property
vagomimetic intervention
vagotonic baroreceptor response
vagus, pl. **vagi**
    v. arrhythmia
    ganglion inferius nervi vagi
    v. nerve
    v. nerve stimulation
    v. pneumonia
    v. pulse
    rami esophagei nervi vagi
Vairox high compression vascular stockings
Vak
    atrial volume constant
valacyclovir
valdecoxib
valent
    23-v. polysaccharide vaccine
    14-v. vaccine
valgus
    cubitus v.
VALI
    ventilator-associated lung injury
validity
    face v.
vallecula, pl. **valleculae**
vallecular dysphagia
valley fever
Valleylab Force 2 electrosurgical device
Valpha
    alpha variable
valproic acid
valrubicin
Valsalva
    aneurysm of sinus of V.
    aortic sinus of V. (ASOV)
    Gelweave V.
    V. maneuver (VM)
    ruptured sinus of V.
    sinus of V.
    V. sinus
    V. test
valsalviana
    dysphagia v.
valsartan and hydrochlorothiazide

value
    Astrup blood gas v.
    index v.
    negative predictive v. (NPV)
    positive predictive v. (PPV)
    predictive v.
    QRS-T v.
    reference v.
    resting v.
    threshold limit v.
valva trunci pulmonalis
valve
    abnormal cleavage of cardiac v.
    Abrams-Lucas flap heart v.
    absent pulmonary v.
    Access-9 large-bore hemostasis v.
    Allcarbon monodisc v.
    Angell-Shiley bioprosthetic v.
    Angell-Shiley xenograft prosthetic v.
    anterior cusp of mitral v.
    anterior cusp of right atrioventricular v.
    anterior cusp of tricuspid v.
    anterior leaflet of mitral v. (ALMV)
    aortic v. (AOV, AoV, AV)
    aortic bioprosthetic v.
    artificial cardiac v.
    atretic pulmonary v.
    atrial v.
    atrioventricular v. (AVV)
    ATS Open Pivot bileaflet heart v.
    ATS standard aortic v.
    ATS standard mitral v.
    ball-and-cage prosthetic v.
    ball heart v.
    ball-occluder v.
    Beall prosthetic v.
    Beall-Surgitool ball-cage prosthetic v.
    Bianchi v.
    Bicarbon Sorin v.
    bicommissural aortic v. (BAV)
    bicuspid aortic v.
    bileaflet tilting disc prosthetic v.
    Biocor porcine v.
    biological aortic v.
    bioprosthetic v. (BPV)
    bioprosthetic porcine heart v.
    Bio-Vascular prosthetic v.
    Björk-Shiley convexoconcave disc prosthetic v.
    Björk-Shiley mitral v.
    Björk-Shiley monostrut v.
    Blom-Singer v.
    Bonhoeffer v.
    bovine heart v.
    bovine pericardial v.

B-S v.
BSCC heart v.
butterfly heart v.
caged ball v.
calcification of tips of mitral v.
calcified aortic v.
Capetown prosthetic v.
Carbomedics bileaflet prosthetic
  heart v.
Carbomedics top-hat supra-anular v.
cardiac v.
Carpentier-Edwards mitral
  annuloplasty v.
Carpentier-Edwards pericardial v.
Carpentier-Edwards Perimount
  mitral v.
Carpentier-Edwards porcine
  prosthetic v.
Carpentier-Edwards porcine
  supraannular v.
Carpentier pericardial v.
caval v.
C-C heart v.
C-E Perimount stented v.
CirKuit-Guard pressure relief v.
cleft A-V v.
cleft mitral v.
v. commissure
congenital anomaly of mitral v.
Cooley-Bloodwell-Cutter v.
Cooley-Cutter disc prosthetic v.
CPHV OptiForm mitral v.
Cribier v.
Cribier-Edwards percutaneous v.
crisscross atrioventricular v.
Cross-Jones disc prosthetic v.
Cross-Jones mitral v.
Cryolife-O'Brien stentless aortic
  porcine v.
cryopreserved homograft v.
Cutter-Smeloff disc v.
Cutter-Smeloff mitral v.
DeBakey-Surgitool prosthetic v.
v. debris
Delrin heart v.
diastolic fluttering aortic v.
disc-cage v.
diseased heart v.
Double Play large-bore double Y
  hemostasis v.
Duostat rotating hemostatic v.
Duromedics mitral v.
dysplastic v.
early opening v.
Ebstein malformed v.
echodense v.
Edmark mitral v.
Edwards-Duromedics bileaflet
  heart v.

Edwards heart v.
Edwards Prima Plus v.
Edwards Prima Plus porcine
  tissue v.
Emphasys endobronchial v.
Enable aortic hear v.
eustachian v.
v. excursion
flail mitral v.
floppy aortic v. (FAV)
floppy mitral v. (FMV)
Freestyle bioprosthetic heart v.
Freestyle stentless aortic heart v.
glutaraldehyde-tanned bovine
  heart v.
glutaraldehyde-tanned porcine
  heart v.
Gott butterfly heart v.
Guangzhou GD-1 prosthetic v.
Hall-Kaster prosthetic v.
Hall prosthetic heart v.
Hancock II tissue v.
Hancock modified orifice v.
Hancock M.O. II bioprosthesis
  porcine v.
Hans Rudolph nonbreathing v.
Harken ball v.
heart v.
Heimlich chest drainage v.
Heimlich heart v.
hemostasis v.
hockey-stick tricuspid v.
Hufnagel prosthetic v.
impedance threshold v. (ITV)
Inspector large-bore in-line
  hemostasis v.
intact v.
Ionescu-Shiley pericardial v.
Ionescu trileaflet v.
Kay-Shiley caged-disc v.
Labcor Synergy v.
left atrial ball v. (LABV)
4-legged cage v.
LeVeen v. (LVV)
Lillehei-Kaster pivoting-disc
  prosthetic v.
Lillehei-Nakib toroidal v.
Liotta-BioImplant low-profile
  bioprosthesis prosthetic v.
Malteno v.
v. mapper Steerocath-Dx mapping
  catheter
MBA hemostasis v.
mechanical heart v.
Medtronic-Hall monocuspid tilting
  disc v.
Medtronic-Hall prosthetic heart v.
Medtronic Hancock II tissue v.
Medtronic Intact bioprosthetic v.

V

valve *(continued)*
    Medtronic Mosaic bioprosthetic v.
    midsystolic buckling of mitral v.
    midsystolic closure of aortic v.
    Mitroflow Synergy PC stented
      pericardial v.
    Montgomery speaking v.
    Mosaic porcine bioprosthetic
      heart v.
    native v.
    noncalcified v.
    nonrebreathing v.
    nonrheumatic stenotic aortic v.
    O'Brien stentless porcine heart v.
    Omnicarbon prosthetic heart v.
    On-X aortic v.
    On-X mechanical bi-leaflet
      prosthetic heart v.
    Open Pivot heart v.
    Optiform mitral v.
    v. orifice area
    overriding v.
    parachute mitral v.
    Passage hemostasis v.
    Passy-Muir tracheostomy
      speaking v.
    PEEP v.
    Pericarbon More v.
    pericardial v.
    Phonate speaking v.
    Plegiaguard pressure relief v.
    PMV 2000 series speaking V.
    pop-off v.
    porcine aortic v.
    porcine prosthetic v.
    posterior leaf mitral v. (PLMV)
    Prima Plus porcine tissue v.
    Prima Plus stentless v.
    prolapse of mitral v. (PMV)
    v. prosthesis
    prosthetic aortic v.
    prosthetic ball v.
    prosthetic cardiac v.
    prosthetic heart v.
    Provox speaking v.
    pulmonary v. (PV)
    pulmonary autograft v.
    v. of pulmonary trunk
    pulmonic v.
    pyrolytic carbon aortic v.
    quadricuspid aortic v. (QAV)
    reducing v.
    v. regurgitation
    v. replacement (VR)
    v. resistance
    v. rupture
    semilunar v.
    Shiley convexoconcave heart v.
    Shiley Phonate speaking v.

    short-axis mitral v. (SAX-MV)
    short-axis plane mitral v.
    v. sizer
    SJM Biocor supra v.
    SJM Masters Series heart v.
    SJM mechanical heart v.
    SJM Quattro mitral v.
    SJM Regent mechanical aortic
      heart v.
    Smeloff-Cutter ball-and-cage
      prosthetic v.
    Smeloff heart v.
    Soprano v.
    Sorin heart v.
    Sorin prosthetic v.
    speaking v.
    Starr-Edwards ball-and-cage v.
    Starr-Edwards mitral v.
    Starr-Edwards prosthetic v.
    Starr-Edwards Silastic v.
    stented bioprosthetic v.
    stentless porcine v. (SPV)
    stentless porcine aortic v.
    stentless tissue v.
    stent-mounted allograft v.
    stent-mounted heterograft v.
    St. Jude V. (SJM)
    St. Jude bileaflet prosthetic v.
    St. Jude composite prosthetic v.
    St. Jude Medical bileaflet tilting-
      disc aortic v.
    St. Jude Medical Biocor v.
    St. Jude Medical Port-Access
      mechanical heart v.
    St. Jude mitral v.
    St. Jude prosthetic aortic v.
    straddling of v.
    straddling atrioventricular v.
    straddling tricuspid v.
    Surgitool prosthetic v.
    v. of Sylvius
    SynerGraft pulmonary heart v.
    SynerGraft tissue-engineered
      heart v.
    Synergy model 700 pulmonary
      heart v.
    thebesian v.
    v. thickening
    tilting disc heart v.
    tilting disc prosthetic v.
    tissue v.
    Top-Hat supraannular aortic v.
    toroidal v.
    Toronto SPV aortic v.
    Toronto SPV stentless porcine
      heart v.
    tricuspid v. (TV)
    tricuspid aortic v.
    UCI-Barnard aortic v.

unicuspid aortic v.
Unistasis v.
unstented xenograft v.
Vascor porcine prosthetic v.
v. vegetation
ventilator speaking v.
Vieussens v.
v. of Vieussens
Wessex prosthetic v.
Xenotech prosthetic v.
valve-conserving operation
valvectomy
valved holding chamber (VHC)
valve-preserving surgery
valve-sparing aortic root replacement
valvopathy, valvulopathy
valvoplasty, valvuloplasty
  aortic v.
  bailout v.
  balloon v. (BV)
  balloon aortic v. (BAV)
  balloon mitral v. (BMV)
  balloon pulmonary v. (BPV)
  Carpentier tricuspid v.
  catheter balloon v. (CBV)
  double-balloon v.
  intracoronary thrombolysis
    balloon v.
  mitral v.
  multiple-balloon v.
  percutaneous aortic v. (PAV)
  percutaneous aortic balloon v.
    (PABV)
  percutaneous balloon v. (PBV)
  percutaneous balloon aortic v.
  percutaneous balloon mitral v.
  percutaneous balloon pulmonary v.
    (PBPV)
  percutaneous balloon pulmonic v.
  percutaneous mitral v. (PMV)
  percutaneous mitral balloon v.
    (PMBV)
  percutaneous transluminal balloon v.
  pulmonary v.
  pulmonary balloon v. (PBV)
  single-balloon v.
  transcarotid balloon v.
  tricuspid v.
  triple-balloon v.
  Trusler technique of aortic v.
valvotomy, valvulotomy
  aortic v.
  balloon aortic v. (BAV)
  balloon pulmonary v.
  balloon tricuspid v.
  double-balloon v.
  Inoue balloon mitral v.
  v. knife
  Longmire v.

mitral balloon v. (MBV)
mitral valve v.
open surgical v.
percutaneous mitral v. (PMV)
percutaneous mitral balloon v.
  (PMBV)
pulmonary v.
radiofrequency-assisted v.
repeat balloon mitral v.
single-balloon v.
thimble v.
transcatheter v.
transventricular closed v.
valvula, pl. **valvulae**
  v. coronaria dextra valvae aortae
  v. semilunaris dextra
valvular
  v. aortic stenosis
  v. calcification
  v. cardiomyopathy
  v. disease of heart (VDH)
  v. dysfunction
  v. endocarditis
  v. function
  v. heart disease (VHD)
  v. incompetence
  v. insufficiency
  v. leaflet
  v. morphology
  v. orifice
  v. pneumothorax
  v. prolapse
  v. pulmonic stenosis
  v. reflux
  v. regurgitation
  v. sclerosis
  v. thickening
  v. thrombus
  v. vegetation
valvulitis
  aortic v.
  chronic v.
  mitral v.
  rheumatic v.
  syphilitic aortic v.
valvulopathy (*var. of* valvopathy)
valvuloplasty (*var. of* valvoplasty)
valvulotome
  angioscopic v.
  Hall v.
valvulotomy (*var. of* valvotomy)
VAM
  ventricular arrhythmia monitor
VAMC prognostic score
VAMP
  venous arterial blood management
    protection system
**vampire bat salivary plasminogen
  activator (DSPA)**

V

van
 v. Aman pulmonary pigtail catheter
 v. Andel catheter
 v. den Bergh disease
 v. Gieson stain
 v. Helmont mirror
 v. Horne canal
vanadium
vanadiumism
Vancocin
 V. CP
 V. Oral
Vancoled injection
vancomycin hydrochloride
vancomycin-resistant enterococcus
Vanguard
 V. device
 V. endograft
 V. III endovascular aortic graft
 V. modular endograft system
vanilloid-1
 transient receptor potential v.-1 (TRPV-1)
vanishing
 v. lung
 v. tumor
Van Slyke method
Vantex central venous catheter
Vantin
VAP
 variant angina pectoris
 ventilator-acquired pneumonia
 ventilator-associated pneumonia
vapor
 body temperature, ambient pressure, saturated with water v. (BTPS)
 inorganic acid v.
 v. massage
 mercury v.
 solvent v.
vaporize
vaporizer
 Fluotec v.
 Maxi-Myst v.
Vapor-Phase heated humidification system
vapotherapy
Vapotherm 2000i oxygen delivery system
VAPS
 volume-assured pressure support
vaptan
Va/Q
 alveolar ventilation/perfusion
Vaquez disease
Varco thoracic forceps
vardenafil
varenicline

variability
 baseline v.
 beat-to-beat v. (BTBV)
 cardiac v.
 diurnal peak flow v.
 heart rate v. (HRV)
 interlead QT v.
 interobserver v.
 intraobserver v.
 peak flow v.
 relative heart rate v. (RHRV)
variable
 alpha v. (Valpha)
 v. angle slant-hole collimator
 beta v. (Vbeta, Vbeta3)
 v. coupling
 v. deceleration
 v. extrathoracic obstruction
 impedance v.
 v. intrathoracic obstruction
 v. positive airway pressure (VPAP)
 scintigraphic v.
 v. stiffness wire guide
 v. thickness strut (VTS)
 v. threshold angina
variance
 ball v.
 v. cardiography (VC)
variant
 v. angina (VA)
 v. angina pectoris (VAP)
 Miller Fisher v.
variation
 circadian v.
 diurnal v.
 respiratory waveform v.
variceal
 v. ligation
 v. sclerosing
 v. sclerotherapy
varicella
 v. pneumonia
 v. pneumonitis
varicella-zoster (VZ)
 v.-z. immunoglobulin (VZIG)
 v.-z. infection
 v.-z. virus (VZV, VZ)
varices (*pl. of* varix)
varicose
 v. bronchiectasis
 v. vein
 v. vein stripping and ligation
varicosity
 saphenous vein v.
Vari-Lase endovenous laser procedure kit
Vario system

variotii
    Paecilomyces v.
varix, pl. **varices**
    aneurysmal v.
    cirsoid v.
    downhill esophageal v.
    esophageal varices
VAS
    vascular access service
    vasculotropin
    ventriculoatrial shunt
    visual analog scale
        horizontal VAS
        mechanical VAS
        vertical VAS
vas, pl. **vasa**
    v. afferentia
    v. nervorum
    v. vasorum
Vascoray
Vascor porcine prosthetic valve
VascuClamp vascular clamp
VascuCoil peripheral vascular stent
Vascu-Flo carotid shunt
Vascugel device
vascular
    v. access catheter
    v. access graft (VAG)
    v. access service (VAS)
    v. acoustic emission
    v. anatomy teaching tool (VATT)
    v. attenuation
    v. bed
    v. blush
    v. brachytherapy
    v. bundle
    v. cadherin
    v. cell adhesion molecule-1
      (VCAM-1)
    v. change (VC)
    v. choir
    v. clamp
    v. clip
    v. collapse
    v. compromise
    v. death
    v. dementia
    v. depression
    v. disease (VD)
    v. ectasia
    v. endothelial dysfunction
    v. endothelial growth factor
      (VEGF)
    v. funnel
    v. gene transfer
    v. graft prosthesis
    v. groove
    v. hemostatic device (VHD)
    v. impedance

    v. incident
    v. injury
    v. insult
    v. leak syndrome (VLS)
    v. marking
    v. matrix
    v. murmur
    v. Parkinson disease
    v. pattern
    v. peripheral resistance
    v. permeability factor (VPF)
    v. profiling (VP)
    v. puncture site
    v. reactivity
    v. reconstruction
    v. redistribution
    v. reflex
    v. remodeling
    v. resistance (VR)
    v. resistance index
    v. ring
    v. ring division
    v. sclerosis
    v. sealing device
    v. sheath
    v. sling
    v. smooth muscle cell (VSMC)
    V. Solutions Acolysis ultrasound
      thrombolysis system
    v. spasm
    v. spider
    v. stenosis
    v. stiffness
    v. system
    v. tape
    v. treatment
    v. tunic
    v. wall (VW)
    v. zone
vascularity
vascularization
vasculature
    coronary v.
    pulmonary v.
VascuLink vascular access graft
vasculitic neuropathy
vasculitis, pl. **vasculitides**
    allergic v.
    cardiac v.
    Churg-Strauss v.
    consecutive v.
    Henoch-Schönlein v.
    hypersensitivity v.
    immune-mediated v.
    leukocytoblastic v.
    livedo v.
    lymphoreticular granulomatous v.
    necrotizing granulomatous v.
    nodular v.

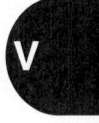

vasculitis *(continued)*
    overlap v.
    primary systemic v.
    pulmonary v.
    secondary v.
    segmented hyalinizing v.
    systemic granulomatous v.
    systemic necrotizing v.
vasculocardiac syndrome of hyperserotonemia
vasculogenesis
vasculogenic impotence
vasculopathy
    allograft v.
    cardiac allograft v. (CAV)
    cerebral v.
    cutaneous v.
    graft v.
    hypertensive v.
    primary fibroproliferative
      pulmonary v.
vasculotropin (VAS)
Vascutek
    V. Gelseal vascular graft
    V. knitted vascular graft
    V. woven vascular graft
Vaseretic
vasinfectum
    Fasarium v.
vasoactive
    v. drug
    v. intestinal peptide (VIP)
    v. mediator
    v. substance
vasoactivity
vasoconstriction (VC)
    coronary microcirculatory v.
    delayed cerebral v. (DCV)
    hypoxic v.
    hypoxic pulmonary v. (HPV)
    microcirculatory v.
    paradoxical v.
    peripheral v.
    pulmonary v.
    v. rate (VCR)
    reflex v.
    reflex pulmonary arterial v.
    systemic v.
vasoconstrictive reflex
vasoconstrictor
    v. center (VCC)
    v. peptide
    pulmonary alveolar hypoxic v. (PAHVC)
    v. substance (VCS)
vasodepression
vasodepressor
    v. lipid (VDL)
    v. material (VDEM, VDM)

    v. substance
    v. syncope
vasodepressor-cardioinhibitory syncope
vasodepressor-prone
vasodilatation
vasodilation (VD)
    cholinergic v.
    coronary v.
    endothelium-dependent v.
    flow-mediated v.
    myocardial v. (MVD)
    peripheral v.
    profound systemic v.
    pulmonary v.
    reflex v.
    regional v.
vasodilator (VD)
    v. agent (VA)
    balanced v.
    v. center (VDC)
    v. effect
    parenteral v.
    v. plus exercise treadmill test
    v. reserve
    v. substance (VDS)
vasodilatory
    v. hypotension
    v. response
    v. shock
vasoexcitor material (VEM)
vasofactive cell
vasogenic
    v. edema
    v. shock
vasogram
vasoinhibitor
vasoinhibitory
    v. center
    v. peptide (VIP)
vasomodulator
vasomotion
    coronary v.
vasomotor (VM)
    v. angina
    v. center (VMC)
    v. flushing (VMF)
    v. paralysis
    v. response (VMR)
    v. rhinitis
    v. syncope
    v. tone
    v. tonus (VMT)
vasomotoria
    angina pectoris v.
vasoneuronal coupling
vasoocclusive pain (VOP)
vasopeptidase inhibitor (VPI)
vasopressin (VP)
    abnormal v. (AVP)

aqueous v. (AVP)
arginine v. (ARVP, AVP)
v. blocker
deamino-8-D-arginine v. (DDAVP, dDAVP)
1-deamino-4-valine-D-arginine v. (dVDAVP)
immunoreactive arginine v. (IAVP, irAVP)
intraarterial v. (IAV)
intravenous v. (IVV)
plasma arginine v. (pAVP)

vasopressor
v. deficiency
v. reflex
v. support

vasoreactivity

vasoregulatory asthenia

vasorelaxant peptide

vasorelaxation

vasoresponse

vasorum
adventitial vasa v.
aortic vasa v.
vasa v.

VasoSeal
V. vascular hemostasis device
V. VHD

vasospasm
cerebral v. (CVS)
coronary v.
diffuse v.
ergonovine-induced coronary v.
focal v.

vasospastic
v. angina (VSA)
v. angina pectoris
v. disease

Vasotec
V. IV
V. Oral

vasotocin
arginine v. (AVT)

vasotonic angina

Vasotrac
V. blood pressure monitor
V. blood pressure monitoring system

Vasotrax handheld monitor

vasovagal
v. attack
v. episode
v. hypotension
v. orthostatism
v. reaction
v. syncope (VVS)
v. syndrome

VasoView
V. balloon dissection device

V. 6 endoscopic vessel harvesting system
V. Uniport endoscopic saphenous vein harvesting system

vastus lateralis

VAT
ventilatory anaerobic threshold
ventricular accommodation test
ventricular activation time
video-assisted thoracoscopy
VAT pacemaker
VAT pacing

VATER
vertebral defects, imperforate anus, transesophageal fistula, radial and renal dysplasia
VATER association syndrome
VATER complex

VATS
video-assisted thoracic surgery
video-assisted thoracoscopic surgery
video-assisted thoracoscopy

VATT
vascular anatomy teaching tool

Vaughan-Williams
V.-W. antiarrhythmic drug classification
V.-W. class effect

Vaxcel
V. catheter
V. mini stick
V. Mini Stick vascular entry kit

VB
venous blood
virtual bronchoscopy

Vbeam pulsed dye laser

Vbeta
beta variable

Vbeta3
beta variable

VBG
venous bypass graft

VBI
vertebrobasilar territory ischemia

VBP
venous blood pressure

VC
variance cardiography
vascular change
vasoconstriction
vena cava
venous capacitance
ventricular contraction
vital capacity
volume control

V/C
ventilation-to-circulation
V/C ratio

V

Vc
pulmonary capillary blood volume
VCA
viral capsid antigen
VCAM-1
vascular cell adhesion molecule-1
VCC
vasoconstrictor center
VCD
vocal cord dysfunction
VCDF
volume-cycled decelerating-flow
ventilation
VCF
velocardiofacial
velocity of circumferential fiber
shortening
VCF syndrome
V$_{cf}$
fiber shortening velocity
VCFS
velocardiofacial syndrome
VCG
vectorcardiogram
vectorcardiography
VCO$_2$
venous carbon dioxide production
VCPC
vindesine, cisplatin, lomustine,
cyclophosphamide
VCR
vasoconstriction rate
VCS
vasoconstrictor substance
VCT
venous clotting time
VCV
ventricular conduction velocity
volume-controlled ventilation
VD
vascular disease
vasodilation
vasodilator
ventricular dilator
V$_D$
physiological dead space ventilation per
minute
VDC
vasodilator center
VDD
atrial synchronous ventricular inhibited
VDD mode
VDD pacemaker
VDD pacing
VDD pacing system
V-Dec-M
VDEM
vasodepressor material

VDF
ventricular diastolic fragmentation
VDH
valvular disease of heart
VDI
both ventricles inhibited
venous distensibility index
VDI pacing
VDI pacing mode
VDL
vasodepressor lipid
VDM
vasodepressor material
VDR
venous diameter ratio
volumetric diffusive respirator
VDRL
Venereal Disease Research Laboratory
VDRL test
VDS
vasodilator substance
venous duplex scanning
V$_{DS}$/V$_T$
dead space gas volume to tidal gas
volume ratio
VDV
ventricular end-diastolic volume
V$_D$/V$_T$
physiologic dead space/tidal volume ratio
physiologic dead space ventilation
VE
venous extension
ventricular elasticity
ventricular extrasystole
VEA
ventricular ectopic activity
VEB
ventricular ectopic beat
VECG
vector electrocardiogram
VE-cMRI
velocity-encoded cine-magnetic
resonance imaging
vector
adeno-associated viral v.
adenoviral v.
angle between QRS and T v.'s
v. cardiography
electric heart v. (EHV)
v. electrocardiogram (VECG)
instantaneous v.
v. loop
magnetic heart v. (MHV)
v. magnetocardiogram (VMCG)
manifest v.
mean manifest v.
P v.
v. phased-array ultrasound tipped
catheter

QRS v.
retroviral v.
spatial v.
ST-T v.
viral v.
vectorcardiogram (VCG)
spatial v. (SVCG)
vectorcardiography (VCG)
left foot electrode in v.
spatial v.
VectorCath
Desai V.
Vector-X coronary guiding catheter
Vectra
V. VAG
V. vascular access graft
vecuronium
VED
ventricular ectopic depolarization
Veetids Oral
VEF
ventricular ejection fraction
VEFR
visually evoked flow response
vegetal bronchitis
vegetarian diet
vegetation
aortic valve v.
bacterial v.
endocardial v.
leaflet v.
mobile v.
prosthetic valve v.
pulmonary valve v.
tricuspid valve v.
valve v.
valvular v.
ventricular septal defect v.
verrucous v.
vegetative
v. endocarditis
v. lesion
VEGF
vascular endothelial growth factor
VEGF gene therapy
VEGF TRAP
veiled puff
veiling glare
Veillonella parvula
vein
accessory saphenous v.
allantoic v.
anastomotic v.
angular v.
anomalous pulmonary v.
antecubital v.
aortocoronary saphenous v. (ACSV)
arrhythmogenic pulmonary v.
autogenous v.

autogenous saphenous v. (ASV)
autologous saphenous v. (ASV)
axillary v.
azygos v.
basilic v.
Boyd perforating v.
brachial v.
brachiocephalic v.
bronchial v.
Burow v.
cardiac v.
cardinal v.
v. of caudate nucleus
cavernous v.
central v.
cephalic v.
common femoral v.
coronary v.
cryopreserved v.
deep lingual v.
Dodd perforating v.
electrical isolation of v.
esophageal v.
external jugular v.
external pudendal v.
facial v.
femoral v.
v. graft
v. graft cannula
v. graft patency
v. graft ring marker
great cardiac v. (GCV)
hemiazygos v.
hepatic v.
human umbilical v. (HUV)
iliac v.
inferior laryngeal v.
inferior thyroid v.
infrasegmental v.
innominate v.
internal cerebral v. (ICV)
internal jugular v.
internal pudendal v.
internal thoracic v.
intersegmental part of pulmonary v.
interventricular v.
intrapulmonary v. (IPV)
jugular v. (JV)
Kohlrausch v.
Krukenberg v.
Kuhnt postcentral v.
laryngeal v.
left inferior pulmonary v.
left internal jugular v.
left lower pulmonary v. (LLPV)
left median v.
left pulmonary v. (LPV)
left superior pulmonary v.
left upper pulmonary v. (LUPV)

V

vein *(continued)*
    levoatriocardinal v.
    lingual v.
    main portal v. (MPV)
    main renal v.
    Marshall oblique v.
    nest of v.'s
    partial anomalous pulmonary v.'s
    percutaneous isolation of multiple
      pulmonary v.'s
    pharyngeal v.
    portal v. (PV)
    profunda femoris v.
    prominent pulmonary v.
    pulmonary v. (PV)
    renal v.
    Retzius v.'s
    reverse saphenous v.
    right brachial v. (RBV)
    right inferior pulmonary v.
    right lower pulmonary v. (RLPV)
    right portal v. (RPV)
    right pulmonary v. (RPV)
    right superior pulmonary v.
    right upper pulmonary v. (RUPV)
    saphenous v. (SV)
    sausaging of v.
    scimitar v.
    subclavian v.
    sublingual v.
    superficial circumflex iliac v.
    superior laryngeal v.
    superior mesenteric v.
    superior pulmonary v.
    superior thalamostriate v.
    thebesian v.
    v. of Thebesius
    tortuous v.'s
    tracheal v.
    umbilical v.
    varicose v.
    ventricular v.
vein-to-vein technology
VeinViewer imaging system
Velban
Velbe
Velcro
    V. crackle
    V. rale
Veletri
velocardiofacial (VCF)
    v. syndrome (VCFS)
Velocimed Proxis catheter
velocimeter
    FloMap v.
velocimetry
    Doppler v.
velocity
    airflow v.

aortic flow v. (AFV)
aortic jet v.
aortic pulse-wave v.
A-peak v.
average peak v. (APV)
basal average peak v. (BAPV)
baseline average peak v. (BAPV)
blood flow v. (BFV)
blunted systolic v.
v. catheter technique
cerebral blood flow v. (CBFV)
v. of circumferential fiber
  shortening (VCF)
conduction v.
coronary blood flow v. (CBFV)
coronary flow v.
detachment v.
diastolic closing v.
diastolic pulmonic regurgitation v.
Doppler peak flow v. (Vmax)
ejection v.
v. encoding
end-diastolic pulmonic
  regurgitation v.
E-peak v.
E-wave v.
fiber shortening v. (V_{cf})
field flow v.
flow v.
forward flow of v.
high regional wall motion v.
  (Vhigh)
hyperemic v.
inflow propagation v.
instantaneous spectral peak v.
jet v.
left atrial appendage flow v.
left ventricular outflow tract v.
long-axis shortening v.
maximal v. (V_{MAX}, Vmax)
maximum v. (V_{MAX}, Vmax)
mitral v.
myocardial Doppler v. (MDV)
nerve conduction v. (NCV)
v. parameter
peak A, E v.
peak diastolic v. (PDV)
peak ejection v. (V_{pe})
peak systolic v. (PSV)
peak transaortic flow v.
phasic intragraft flow v.
pulse wave v. (PWV)
v. ratio (VR)
sensory nerve conduction v.
  (SNCV)
shortening v.
spectral peak v.
V. stent
systolic pulmonary venous v.

systolic wall motion v. (Vsys)
time-averaged peak v.
v. time integral
tracheal mucus v.
translesional spectral flow v.
transmitral flow v.
transprosthetic flow v.
transvalvular E v.
upstroke v.
ventricular conduction v. (VCV)
wall motion v.
velocity-encoded cine-magnetic resonance imaging (VE-cMRI)
Velogene rapid TB assay
velopharyngeal
v. endoscope
v. insufficiency
velopharynx
Velosef
Velosulin Human
velour collar graft
Velpeau hernia
VEM
vasoexcitor material
vena, pl. **venae**
agger valvae venae
venae bronchiales
venae cardiacae anteriores
venae cardiacae minimae
v. cava (VC)
v. cava cannula
v. cava clip
venae cavae
v. cava filter
v. caval foramen
v. caval obstruction
v. cava obstruction
v. cava syndrome
venae circumflexae femoris laterales
v. circumflexa humeri anterior
v. circumflexa iliaca profunda
v. circumflexa iliaca superficialis
v. contracta
venae cordis
venae cordis minimae
venae dorsales linguae
venae esophageales
v. laryngea inferior
v. laryngea superior
v. lingularis
v. obliqua atrii sinistra
venae pharyngeae
v. profunda linguae
venae pulmonales
v. pulmonalis inferior dextra
v. pulmonalis inferior sinistra
v. pulmonalis superior dextra
v. pulmonalis superior sinistra
v. sublingualis

venae supratrochleares
V. Tech IVC filter
V. Tech LGM filter
venae tracheales
venacavogram
venacavography
inferior v. (IVCV)
VenaCure laser vein treatment
venae (*pl. of* vena)
VenaFlow
V. compression system
V. DVT prophylaxis system
Venaport
V. coronary sinus access catheter
V. coronary sinus guiding catheter
Vena Tech
Vena Tech IVC filter
Vena Tech LGM filter
venectasia
Venereal Disease Research Laboratory (VDRL)
venereum
lymphogranuloma v. (LGV)
venesection (VS, Vs)
Venflon needle
venipuncture
antecubital v.
contrast-guided v.
venoarterial
v. bypass pumping (VABP)
v. extracorporeal membrane oxygenation (VA-ECMO)
v. shunting
venoatrial junction
venoconstriction
splenic v.
venodilation
Venodyne EPS-410 external pneumatic compression system
Venoglobulin-S
venogram
venography
balloon v.
contrast v.
helical CT v.
magnetic resonance v. (MRV)
radionuclide v. (RNV)
renal v.
venolobar syndrome
venom
arthropod v.
bee v.
black widow spider v.
scorpion v.
snake v.
spider v.
venoocclusive disease (VOD)
venopathy
pulmonary occlusive v. (POV)

venopressor
venorespiratory reflex
Venoscope
venosinal
venosity
venostasis
venosus
    ductus v.
    pulsus v.
    sinus v.
venous
    v. access
    v. access device (VAD)
    v. admixture
    v. air embolism (VAE)
    v. arterial blood management
      protection system (VAMP)
    v. blood (VB)
    v. blood pressure (VBP)
    v. bypass graft (VBG)
    v. cannula
    v. capacitance (VC)
    v. capacitance bed
    v. carbon dioxide production
      (VCO_2)
    central v. (CV)
    v. clotting time (VCT)
    v. collateral
    v. congestion
    v. coronary graft patency
    v. Corrigan wave
    v. cutdown
    v. diameter ratio (VDR)
    v. digital angiogram
    v. dilation
    v. distensibility index (VDI)
    v. duplex scanning (VDS)
    v. embolism
    v. engorgement
    v. extension (VE)
    v. filling index (VFI)
    v. flow controller (VFC)
    v. flow measurement
    v. flow reversal
    v. graft myringoplasty (VGM)
    v. groove
    v. heart
    v. hum
    v. hyperemia
    v. hypertension
    v. impedance plethysmography
      (VIP)
    v. insufficiency syndrome (VIS)
    v. intravasation
    v. lakes
    v. mesenteric vascular occlusion
    v. murmur
    v. occlusion plethysmography
      (VOP)

    v. occlusion test
    v. ostium
    v. outflow tract
    v. phase
    v. plasma norepinephrine
      concentration
    v. pressure (VP)
    v. pressure gradient support
      stockings (VPGSS)
    v. pressure tracing
    v. pulse
    v. pulse tracing
    v. puncture
    v. reflux (VR)
    v. reservoir
    v. return (VR)
    v. return curve
    v. runoff
    v. saturation
    v. sclerosis
    v. sheath
    v. smooth muscle
    v. spasm
    v. spread
    v. stasis
    v. stop flow pressure (VSFP)
    v. system
    v. thromboembolism (VTE)
    v. thrombosis
    v. ulcer
    v. valvular insufficiency
    v. volume (VV)
    v. web
venovenostomy
venovenous (VV)
    v. access
    v. double-lumen (VVDL)
    v. dye dilution curve
vent
    ventricle
    ventricular
Ventak
    V. AICD
    V. AICD pacemaker
    V. A-V III DR automatic
      implantable cardioverter-
      defibrillator
    V. ECD
    V. Mini II and III automatic
      implantable cardioverter-defibrillator
    V. Prizm 2 automatic implantable
      cardioverter-defibrillator
    V. Prizm AVT pulse
      generator/defibrillator
    V. Prizm dual-chamber implantable
      defibrillator
    V. Prizm HE system
    V. Prizm 2 system
    V. PRx cardioverter-defibrillator

V. PRx defibrillation system
V. PRx III/Endotak system
V. PRx pacemaker
Ventavis
VentCheck handheld respiratory monitor
vented-electric HeartMate LVAD
ventilate
ventilated alveoli
ventilation
    adaptive support v. (ASV)
    airway pressure release v. (APRV)
    alveolar v.
    artificial v.
    assist-control v. (ACV)
    assist-control mode v.
    assisted mechanical v. (AMV)
    backup v. (BUV)
    bag v.
    bag-mask v.
    bag-valve-mask v.
    v. bronchoscope
    BVM v.
    v. collateralization
    continuous-flow v.
    continuous mandatory v.
    continuous positive pressure v.
    controlled mechanical v.
    control-mode v.
    conventional v. (CV)
    conventional mechanical v. (CMV)
    cuirass v.
    dead space v.
    v. episode
    v. equivalent
    forced mandatory intermittent v. (FMIV)
    high-frequency v. (HFV)
    high-frequency jet v. (HFJV)
    high-frequency percussive v. (HFPV)
    high-frequency positive pressure v. (HFPPV)
    intermittent demand v. (IDV)
    intermittent mandatory v. (IMV)
    intermittent mechanical v. (IMV)
    intermittent percussive v. (IPV)
    intermittent positive pressure v. (IPPV)
    intrapulmonary percussive v. (IPV)
    invasive mechanical v.
    invasive positive pressure mechanical v.
    inverse-ratio v. (IRV)
    jet v.
    liquid v.
    mandatory minute v.
    manual v.
    v. mask

    maximal v. (MV)
    maximum voluntary v. (MVV)
    mechanical v. (MV)
    v. meter
    minute v. (V_E)
    mouth-to-face shield v.
    mouth-to-mask v.
    mouth-to-mouth v.
    mouth-to-nose v.
    mouth-to-stoma v.
    nasal nocturnal v. (NNV)
    nasal positive pressure v. (NPPV)
    negative pressure v. (NPV)
    nocturnal v.
    noninvasive v. (NIV)
    noninvasive face mask v.
    noninvasive mechanical v.
    noninvasive positive pressure v. (NIPPV, NPPV)
    partial liquid v. (PLV)
    patient-triggered v.
    peak exercise v. (V_E)
    percutaneous transtracheal jet v. (PTJV)
    percutaneous transtracheal needle v.
    permissive hypercapnic v.
    physiologic dead space v. (V_D/V_T)
    positive airway pressure v.
    positive pressure v. (PPV)
    positive pressure mechanical v.
    pressure control v.
    pressure-controlled v. (PCV)
    pressure-controlled inverse ratio v. (PCIRV)
    pressure-cycled v.
    pressure-regulated volume control v.
    pressure support v. (PSV)
    proportional assist v. (PAV)
    protective v.
    PRVC v.
    pulmonary v.
    QT v.
    v. scintigraphy
    split-lung v.
    spontaneous v.
    synchronized intermittent mandatory v. (SIMV)
    v. threshold
    tidal v.
    time-cycled v.
    ultra high frequency v. (UHFV)
    unassisted spontaneous v.
    volume-controlled v. (VCV)
    volume-cycled decelerating-flow v. (VCDF)
    wasted v.
ventilation/carbon dioxide production (VE/VCO$_2$)
ventilation/perfusion (V/Q)

V

ventilation/perfusion *(continued)*
    alveolar v. (Va/Q)
    v. defect
    v. imaging
    v. lung scan
    v. matching
    v. mismatch
    v. ratio
    v. relation
    v. relationship
ventilation-to-circulation (V̊/C̊)
ventilator
    740 V.
    Acutronic Mistral v.
    Acutronic Monsoon v.
    Adult Star 2000 v.
    Aequitron Medical LP-6 v.
    AirMed v.
    Airox Home 1, 2 v.
    Avian transport v.
    babyPac v.
    Bear 1000 v.
    Bear 1, 2 adult volume v.
    Bear Cub infant v.
    Bennett MA-1, PR-2 v.
    3100B high-frequency oscillatory v.
    Bio-Med MVP-10 pediatric v.
    Bird Ascension v.
    Bird VDR v.
    blow-by v.
    Bourns-Bear v.
    Bourns infant v.
    Breas v.
    Bunnell Life Pulse high frequency
     jet v.
    compPAC v.
    Critical Care V.
    cuirass v.
    Datex-Ohmeda v.
    v. dependency
    Dräger v.
    E-150 Breeze v.
    Emerson postoperative v.
    Esprit v.
    Galileo v.
    Hamilton v.
    Healthdyne Quantum PSV v.
    high-frequency chest wall v.
    high-frequency jet v.
    high-frequency oscillation v.
    Impact Uni-Vent v.
    Infant Star 100, 200 v.
    Infant Star v. 500/950
    Inter 3 v.
    Intermed Inter 3 v.
    KnightStar 330 v.
    Lifecare PLV-100 portable v.
    v. management
    Maquet Servoi v.

    mechanical v.
    MicroVent v.
    Monaghan 300 v.
    Nellcor Puritan-Bennett v.
    Neumovent Bebé infant v.
    Newport E100M v.
    Newport Wave V200 v.
    noninvasive extrathoracic v. (NEV)
    paraPAC v.
    pneuPAC v.
    portable volume v.
    positive support v. (PSV)
    pressure cycled v.
    pressure support v. (PSV)
    Puritan Bennett v.
    v. rate
    rescuPAC v.
    respiratory v.
    Respironics BIPAP bilevel v.
    responder v.
    Sechrist 500A hyperbaric v.
    Sechrist IV-100 infant v.
    SensorMedics v.
    Servo V. 300
    Siemens v.
    SLE 2000 neonatal, infant, and
     pediatric v.
    Smart Trigger Bear 1000 v.
    v. speaking valve
    840 v. system
    Taema v.
    v. time
    transPAC v.
    Univent v.
    ventiPAC v.
    Venturi v.
    volume v.
    volume-cycled v.
    Wave VM200 v.
    v. weaning
ventilator-acquired pneumonia (VAP)
ventilator-associated
    v.-a. lung injury (VALI)
    v.-a. pneumonia (VAP)
ventilator-induced
    v.-i. lung injury (VILI)
    v.-i. pneumopericardium
    v.-i. pneumothorax
ventilatory
    v. anaerobic threshold (VAT)
    v. assistance
    v. capacity
    v. compliance
    v. effort
    v. equivalent
    v. failure
    v. function
    v. objective
    v. problem

v. response
v. strategy
v. support
v. technique
VentiMask
venting
ventiPAC ventilator
Ventolin
    V. HFA
    V. Nebules
    V. Rotacaps
    V. updraft
VenTrak respiratory mechanics monitor
ventral lead 1–6 (V1-V6)
VentrAssist
    V. device
    V. heart pump
ventricle (vent)
    AIS model of a beating v.
    anterior papillary muscle of left v.
    anterior right v. (ARV)
    anteroventral third v. (Av3V)
    atrialized v.
    banana-shaped left v.
    calcified papillary muscle in
      right v.
    double-inlet left v. (DILV)
    double-outlet left v. (DOLV)
    double-outlet right v. (DORV)
    effective refractory period of
      left v. (ERPLV)
    electrocardiographic wave
      corresponding to repolarization
      of v.'s (T)
    1-v. heart
    hypoplasia of right v.
    hypoplastic left v. (HLV)
    indeterminate single v.
    ischemic contracture of left v.
    laryngeal v.
    left v. (LV)
    L-looping of v.
    Mary Allen Engle v.
    noncompliant v.
    over-and-under v.'s
    parchment right v.
    posterior left v. (PLV)
    posterior wall of left v. (PWLV)
    right v. (RV)
    right atrium to right v. (RA-RV)
    single v.
    subpulmonary v.
    suicide v.
    volume-overloaded left v.
Ventricor pacemaker
ventricular (V, vent)
    v. aberration
    v. accommodation test (VAT)
    v. activation time (VAT)

v. afterload
v. aneurysm (VA)
v. angiography
v. apex
v. architecture
v. arrhythmia (VA)
v. arrhythmia monitor (VAM)
v. assist device (VAD)
v. asynchronous (VOO)
v. asynchronous pacemaker
v. atresia
atrial carotid v. (ACV)
v. autocapture
v. band of larynx
bidirectional v.
v. bigeminy
v. biopsy
v. block
v. bradycardia
v. canal
v. capture
v. capture beat
v. capture threshold
v. cavity
v. chamber
v. complex
v. conduction
v. conduction velocity (VCV)
v. containment device
v. contour
v. contractile synchrony
v. contraction (VC)
v. contraction pattern
v. couplet
v. demand-inhibited pacemaker
v. demand-triggered (VVD)
v. demand-triggered pacemaker
v. depolarization abnormality
v. diastole
v. diastolic fragmentation (VDF)
v. diastolic pressure
v. dilation
v. dilator (VD)
v. distensibility
v. drive
v. dysfunction
v. dyssynchrony
v. dyssynergy
v. echo
v. ectopic activity (VEA)
v. ectopic beat (VEB)
v. ectopic depolarization (VED)
v. ectopic systole
v. ectopy
v. effective refractory period
  (VERP)
v. ejection fraction (VEF)
v. ejection time (VET)
v. elasticity (VE)

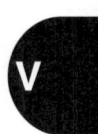

ventricular *(continued)*
v. end-diastolic volume (VDV)
v. endoaneurysmorrhaphy
v. endocardial border
v. end-systolic pressure-volume relation
v. end-systolic wall stress
v. escape
v. escape beat
v. escape rate
v. extension branch
v. extrasystole (VE)
v. failure
v. far-field signal
v. fibrillation (VF)
v. fibrillation arrest
v. fibrillation/ventricular tachycardia (VF/VT)
v. filling
v. filling pressure
v. fluid (VF)
v. flutter (VF)
v. function (VF)
v. function curve (VFC)
v. fusion beat
v. gallop (VG)
v. geometry
v. geometry change
v. gradient
v. heart rate (VHR)
v. hypertrophy (VH)
v. imbalance
v. impedance
v. implantable cardioverter-defibrillator (VICD, V-ICD)
v. inflow anomaly
v. inflow tract obstruction
v. inhibited (VVI)
v. inhibited pulse generator
v. injury
v. inlet
v. inotropic parameter (VIP)
v. interdependence
v. inversion
v. late potential (VLP)
v. lead
left v. (LV)
v. ligament
v. mapping
v. mass
v. milk spots
v. mural swelling
v. myocyte
v. myxoma
v. outflow tract obstruction
v. paced rhythm (VPR)
v. pacing (VP)
v. parasystole
v. pause

v. perforation
v. performance
v. perfusion index (VQI)
v. pericardium (VP)
v. plateau
v. ponderance
v. power
v. preexcitation
v. preload
v. premature (VP, Vp)
v. premature beat (VPB)
v. premature complex (VPC)
v. premature contraction (VPC)
v. premature contraction threshold (VPCT)
v. premature depolarization (VPD)
v. pressure (PV)
v. pressure-volume loop
v. pulse amplitude
v. pulse width
v. puncture
v. radial dysplasia (VRD)
v. rale (VR)
v. reduction surgery
v. reentry
v. relaxation
v. remodeling
v. reserve
v. residual volume (VRV)
v. response
v. restoration surgery
v. resynchronization system
v. resynchronization therapy
v. resynchronizer
v. rhythm (VR)
right v. (RV)
v. safety pacing
v. sensing configuration
v. sensitivity
v. septal defect (VSD)
v. septal defect murmur
v. septal defect vegetation
v. septal heart defect (VSHD)
v. septal rupture
v. septum (VS)
v. situs solitus
v. standstill
v. stroke work (VSW)
v. stroke work index
v. synchronous pulse generator
v. systole
v. systolic impairment
v. systolic stiffness
v. tachyarrhythmia (VTA)
v. tachycardia (VT)
v. tachycardia cycle length (VTCL)
v. tachycardia event (VTE)
v. tachycardia/ventricular fibrillation (VT/VF)

v. thrombus
v. triggered (VVT)
v. triggered pulse generator
v. vein
v. volume
v. volume constant (vvk)
v. wall contractility
v. wall motion (VWM)
v. wall shortening
v. wall thinning
v. wave
ventricular-based pacing
ventricularis
crista v.
ventricularization
ventricular-programmed stimulation
ventriculectomy
ventriculoarterial
v. concordance
v. coupling
v. discordance
ventriculoatrial (VA)
v. conduction (VAC)
v. effective refractory period
sequential v. (SVA)
v. shunt (VAS)
v. shunt catheter
ventriculocyte
ventriculogram
left v. (LV-gram)
ventriculogram-derived ejection fraction
ventriculographic ejection fraction
ventriculography
biplane v.
v. catheter
contrast v. (CV)
contrast left v.
equilibrium multigated
radionuclide v.
left v.
quantitative left v.
radionuclide v. (RNV, RNVG)
rest-exercise equilibrium
radionuclide v.
tomographic radionuclide v.
ventriculojugular (VJ)
ventriculomegaly (VM, VML)
ventriculometry (VM)
ventriculophasic
ventriculoplasty
ventriculopuncture
ventriculoradial dysplasia
ventriculoscopy
ventriculotomy
encircling endocardial v.
endocardial v. (ECV)
partial encircling endocardial v.
ventriculus laryngis

Ventritex
V. Angstrom MD implantable
cardioverter-defibrillator
V. Cadence ICD
V. Cadence implantable
cardioverter-defibrillator
V. Contour
V. TVL system
ventroanterior (VA)
ventrolateral medulla (VLM)
Ventstream nebulizer
Venture demand oxygen delivery device
Venturi
V. effect
V. exhalation assist
V. force
V. jet adapter
V. mask
V. phenomenon
V. tube
V. ventilator
V. wave
venule
venulitis
cutaneous necrotizing v.
VePesid
V. injection
V. Oral
vera
polycythemia v.
verapamil
v. HCl
v. hydrochloride
PPR v.
trandolapril and v.
verapamil-sensitive
veratridine
verbal amnesia
Verhoeff
V. elastica stain
V. tissue elastin stain
Veriflex
V. cardiac device
V. stent
VerifyNow
V. aspirin assay
V. test
Veripath peripheral guiding catheter
Veris MR vital signs physiological monitor
vermicular pulse
vermiculite
verminous
v. aneurysm
v. bronchitis
Vermox
vernal
v. edema
v. edema of lung

V

815

Vernet syndrome
Verneuil canal
veronii
    Aeromonas v.
VERP
    ventricular effective refractory period
verruca, pl. **verrucae**
verrucosa
    arteritis v.
    Phialophora v.
verrucous
    v. carcinoma
    v. carditis
    v. endocarditis
    v. vegetation
verruga peruana
Versacaps
VersaLab APM2 for Twins
VersaStep laparoscopy system
Versatrax II 7000A pacemaker
versicolor
    Aspergillus v.
version
    Ferrans and Powers Quality of
      Life Index, Cardiac V.
Verstraeten bruit
vertebra, pl. **vertebrae**
    cervical v. (CV)
vertebral
    v. artery (VA)
    v. artery bypass graft
    v. defects, imperforate anus,
      transesophageal fistula, radial and
      renal dysplasia (VATER)
    v. endarterectomy
    v. part
    v. part of costal surface of lung
    v. part of diaphragm
    v., vascular, anal, cardiac,
      tracheoesophageal, renal, limb
      anomalies (VACTERL)
vertebrobasilar
    v. occlusive disease
    v. territory ischemia (VBI)
    v. TIA
vertebrocostal trigone
vertical
    v. deceleration
    v. deceleration mechanism
    v. heart
    v. integration
    v. long axis
    v. long-axis tomogram
    v. long-axis view
    v. VAS
vertigo
    laryngeal v.
    rotary v.

very
    v. high density lipoprotein (VHDL)
    v. long chain fatty acid (VLCFA)
    v. low calorie diet (VLCD)
    v. low density lipoprotein (VLDL)
    v. low density lipoprotein receptor
      (VLDLR)
    v. low density lipoprotein-
      triglyceride complex (VLDL-TG)
vesicant
vesicle
    air v.
    brush border membrane v.
      (BBMV)
    intermediary v.
    malpighian v.
vesicular
    v. breath sounds
    v. bronchiolitis
    v. bronchitis
    v. emphysema
    v. fluid
    v. monoamine transformer (VMAT)
    v. murmur
    v. rale
vesicular-vacuolar organelle (VVO)
vesiculobronchial
vesiculobullous
vesiculocavernous respiration
vesnarinone
vessel
    absorbent v.
    afferent v.
    anastomotic v.
    1-v. angioplasty
    aortic arch v.
    blood v. (BV)
    bouquet of v.'s
    branch v.
    capacitance v.
    v. clamp
    codominant v.
    collateral v.
    collateralizing v.
    conductance v.
    congenitally corrected transposition
      of great v.'s (CC-TGA)
    corner v.
    coronary conduit v.
    3-v. coronary disease
    coronary resistance v.
    corrected transposition of great v.'s
    v. dilator
    feeder v.
    femoral v.
    ghost v.
    grafted v.
    great v.
    infarct-related v.

intercostal mammary v.
internal mammary v.
intraacinar v.
large v.
v. lumen
mammary v.
native v.
nondominant v.
v. occlusion system
P/D v.
polytef artificial v.
preacinar v.
prearteriolar v.
proximal and distal portion of v.
recruitable collateral v.
renal blood v.
resistance v.
restenotic small coronary v.
retinal v.
small v. (SV)
small coronary v.
v. spasm
splanchnic v.
subclavian v.
target v.
thoracic v.
tortuous v.
transposition of great v.'s (TGV)
v. trauma
v. wall movement
Vesseloops rubber band
vessel-sizing catheter
vest
Bremer AirFlo V.
cardiac v.
cooling v.
Mark VII cooling v.
ThAIRapy v.
VEST ambulatory ventricular function monitor
vestibula (*pl. of* vestibulum)
vestibular
v. fold
v. laryngitis
v. ligament
vestibule
esophagogastric v.
gastroesophageal v.
v. of larynx
Sibson v.
vestibulum, pl. **vestibula**
v. laryngis
rima v.
vestigial
v. fold
v. structure
VET
ventricular ejection time

veteran
V.'s Administration (VA)
V.'s Affairs Medical Center
V.'s Affairs Medical Center
scoring system
V.'s Affairs Non-Q-Wave Infarction
Strategies in Hospital
V.'s Specific Activity Questionnaire
(VSAQ)
VE/VCO$_2$
ventilation/carbon dioxide production
VEX treadmill test
VF
left leg electrode for electrocardiogram
ventricular fibrillation
ventricular fluid
ventricular flutter
ventricular function
VF electrode
R-on-T-initiated VF
VFA
viral-free antigen
volatile fatty acid
VFC
venous flow controller
ventricular function curve
Actis VFC
VFI
venous filling index
V-Flex
V-F. FMJ stent
V-F. Plus stent
VF/VT
ventricular fibrillation/ventricular
tachycardia
VG
ventricular gallop
VGM
venous graft myringoplasty
VH
ventricular hypertrophy
VHC
valved holding chamber
AeroChamber VHC
VHD
valvular heart disease
vascular hemostatic device
VasoSeal VHD
VHDL
very high density lipoprotein
Vhigh
high regional wall motion velocity
V-H interval
VHR
ventricular heart rate
Viabahn
V. covered stent
V. endoprosthesis stent-graft

V

viability
    v. identification with dipyridamole-dobutamine administration (VIDA)
    v. index
    myocardial v.
viable
    v. endocardium
    v. myocardium
Viagra
Viagraph ECG system
vial
Viamonte-Hobbs dye injector
Vibracare percussor
Vibramycin
    V. injection
    V. Oral
vibrans
    pulsus v.
Vibra-Tabs
vibration
    chest percussion and v.
    v. disease
    postural drainage, percussion, v. (PDPV)
vibrational angioplasty
Vibrio
    V. cholerae
    V. parahaemolyticus
vibrissa, pl. **vibrissae**
vibrocardiogram
vicarious respiration
VICD, V-ICD
    ventricular implantable cardioverter-defibrillator
Vicia
    V. sativa
    V. sativa asthma
Vicks
    V. 44D Cough & Head Congestion
    V. Formula 44
    V. Formula 44 Pediatric Formula
    V. Pediatric Formula 44E
Vicodin
Victoria influenza
VIDA
    viability identification with dipyridamole-dobutamine administration
    myocardial VIDA
    VIDA stress echocardiography
Vidas D-dimer exclusion assay
video
    v. camera
    v. densitometry
    v. imaging
    v. loop
    v. monitor
    v. system
    v. thoracotomy

videoangiography
    digital v.
video-assisted
    v.-a. diagnostic thoracoscopic technique
    v.-a. endoscopic guidance
    v.-a. thoracic surgery (VATS)
    v.-a. thoracic surgical lung biopsy
    v.-a. thoracic surgical non-rib-spreading lobectomy (VNSSL)
    v.-a. thoracoscopic surgery (VATS)
    v.-a. thoracoscopic thymectomy
    v.-a. thoracoscopy (VAT, VATS)
videobronchoscope
videodensitometric
    v. analysis system
    v. myocardial textural analysis
videodensitometry
videohydrothoracoscope
videointensity
videomorphometry
videostroboscopic endoscopy
videotape recorder
videothoracoscopic
    v. operator staging (VOS)
    v. pericardial window
videothoracoscopy
Videx Oral
Vienna
    V. TAH
    V. total artificial heart
Vieussens
    arc of V.
    circle of V.
    valve of V.
    V. valve
view
    A2C, A4C v.
    apical 2-chamber v.
    apical 4-chamber v.
    Baltaxe v.
    caudocranial hemiaxial v.
    2-chamber v.
    4-chamber v.
    5-chamber v.
    cine v.
    coned-down v.
    craniocaudal v.
    Doppler 2-chamber v. (D2CV)
    Doppler 4-chamber v. (D4CV)
    en bloc face v.
    expiratory v.
    field of v. (FOV)
    first-pass v.
    gated v.
    hemiaxial v.
    horizontal long-axis v.
    ice-pick v.
    inspiratory v.

laid-back v.
lateral v.
left portal v. (LPV)
long axial oblique v.
long-axis v.
orthogonal v.
parasternal long-axis v.
parasternal short-axis v.
RAO v.
resting parasternal long-axis v.
resting parasternal short-axis v.
sagittal v.
scout v.
short-axis parasternal v.
sitting-up v.
spider x-ray v.
subcostal right ventricle v.
suprasternal v.
swimmer's v.
vertical long-axis v.
weeping willow v.
view-aliasing artifact
Viggo Spectramed catheter
vigilance
care v. (CV)
V. CCO/SvO₂/CEDV monitor
V. monitoring system
v. response
Vigilon dressing
Vigor DR pacemaker
Viking
V. Bard catheter
V. coronary guiding catheter
VILI
ventilator-induced lung injury
Villaret syndrome
villosa
pericarditis v.
villus, pl. **villi**
pleural villi
villi pleurales
Vim-Silverman needle
vinblastine sulfate
vinca alkaloid
Vincasar
V. PFS
V. PFS injection
Vincent angina
vincristine
cyclophosphamide, doxorubicin, v. (CAV)
v. sulfate
vinculum linguae
vindesine, cisplatin, lomustine, cyclophosphamide (VCPC)
Vineberg cardiac revascularization procedure
vineyard sprayer's lung

Vingmed
V. CFM 800 echocardiographic system
V. CFM 750 transducer
V. System Five device
vinorelbine tartrate
vinyl chloride
viomycin
Vioxx
VIP
vasoactive intestinal peptide
vasoinhibitory peptide
venous impedance plethysmography
ventricular inotropic parameter
V.I.P. Bird volume monitor
Viprinex
Viracept
viral
v. antigen assay
v. bronchiolitis
v. capsid antigen (VCA)
v. cardiomyopathy
v. hepatitis
v. myocarditis (VM)
v. pericarditis
v. pneumonia
v. respiratory infection
v. rhinosinusitis
v. vector
v. wheezing
viral-free antigen (VFA)
Viramune
Virazole Aerosol
Virchow-Robin space
Virchow triad
Virgo anticardiolipin screening ELISA test kit
viridans
Aerococcus v.
Streptococcus v.
viridans endocarditis
viridis
Thermoactinomyces v.
Virilon
Viringe vascular access flush device
Virtis blender
virtual bronchoscopy (VB)
Virtuoso LX Smart CPAP system
virulence
virus
adeno-associated v. (AAV)
aerosolized v.
Amapari v.
Andes v.
Arenaviridae v.
Astroviridae v.
avian influenza v. (AIV)
avian influenza A (H5N1) v.
Bayou v.

virus *(continued)*
  Black Creek Canal v.
  v. bronchopneumonia
  CA v.
  Calciviridae v.
  Coe v.
  Columbia SK v.
  Coronaviridae v.
  coxsackie A, B, B3, B4 v.
  croup-associated v.
  Ebola v.
  ECHO v.
  EMC v.
  encephalomyocarditis v.
  enteric cytopathogenic human
    orphan v.
  Epstein-Barr v. (EBV)
  Filoviridae v.
  Hantaan v.
  herpes simplex v. (HSV)
  human immunodeficiency v. (HIV)
  human T-cell lymphotropic v.
    (HTLV)
  influenza A, B, C v.
  Juquitiba v.
  Kotonkan v.
  Laguna Negra v.
  Lassa v.
  Lipovnik v.
  Marburg v.
  Mayaro v.
  Moloney murine leukemia v.
    (MoMLV)
  Muerto Canyon v.
  Nipah v. (NiV)
  Orthomyxoviridae v.
  parainfluenza v. (PIV)
  parainfluenza v. type 1 (PIV-1)
  parainfluenza v. type 2 (PIV-2)
  parainfluenza v. type 3 (PIV-3)
  parainfluenza v. type 4 (PIV-4)
  Paramyxoviridae v.
  Picornaviridae v.
  REO v.
  respiratory syncytial v. (RSV)
  Rift Valley fever v.
  Ross River v.
  Rous sarcoma v. (RSV)
  Semliki Forest v.
  Sendai v.
  simian v. 40 (SV40)
  Sindbis v.
  Sin Nombre v. (SNV)
  syncytial v.
  Togaviridae v.
  U v.
  varicella-zoster v. (VZV, VZ)
  West Nile v.

VIS
  venous insufficiency syndrome
visa
    V. II ST PTCA balloon catheter
    V. Iris system
viscera (*pl. of* viscus)
visceral
  v. heterotaxy
  v. larva migrans
  v. peel
  v. pericardiectomy
  v. pericardium
  v. pleura
  v. pleurisy
  v. syncope
visceralis
  pleura v.
visceroatrial
  v. situs ambiguus
  v. situs inversus
  v. situs solitus
viscerobronchial cardiovascular anomaly
viscerocardiac reflex
visceropleural
viscid
  v. mucus
  v. sputum
viscidosis
viscoelastic fluid
viscoelasticity
  sputum v.
viscometer
  Brookfield v.
  Ostwald v.
viscosity
  blood v. (BlV)
  mucus v.
  plasma v. (PV)
viscous drag
viscus, pl. **viscera**
  hollow v.
vise
  hemodynamic v.
  torque v.
vision
    V. bare-metal stent
    V. blood cardioplegia system
    V. PTCA catheter
Visipaque
Visov test
vista
    V. Brite Tip IG introducer guide
    V. Brite Tip large lumen guiding
      catheter
    V. 4, T, TRS pacemaker
Vistaril
    V. Injection
    V. Oral
VISTA software

Vistide
visual
v. amnesia
v. analog scale (VAS)
visualization
far-field v.
fluoroscopic v.
near-field v.
noninvasive v.
suboptimal v.
visualized
suboptimally v.
visually evoked flow response (VEFR)
visuospatial neglect
VitaCuff device
Vitagraft vascular graft
vital
v. capacity (VC)
v. exhaustion
v. signs
Vitallium
Vitalograph
V. Bacterial/Viral Filter
V. BreathCO Monitor
V. 2120 handheld recording
spirometer
V. pulmonary monitor
Vitalometer test
Vitalor
V. incentive spirometer
V. screening pulmonary function
test
Vital-Port Infusion Pal
Vital-Ryder microvascular needle holder
VitalSAT pulse oximeter
vitamin
v. B, B₁, B₆, B₁₂, C, D, E, K
v. K antagonist
Vitatron
V. catheter electrode
V. Diamond ICD
V. Diamond II pacemaker
V. lead
V. pacing system
V. Selection AFm
Vitek catheter
vitellogenin
Vitesse
V. E catheter
V. 0.9-mm catheter
vitiated air
Vitrasert
vitrector
vitreous
v. fiber
v. opacity
vitro
in v.
vitronectin

Vitros analyzer
viva
Air V.
Vivactil
Viva Primo balloon catheter
vivax
Plasmodium v.
Vivid 7 cardiac ultrasound machine
vivo
ex v.
in v.
Vivonex
V. Moss tube
V. Plus nutritional supplement
VixOne small-volume nebulizer
VJ
ventriculojugular
VL
left arm electrode for electrocardiogram
VL electrode
VLCD
very low calorie diet
VLCFA
very long chain fatty acid
VLDL
very low density lipoprotein
VLDLR
very low density lipoprotein receptor
VLDL-TG
very low density lipoprotein-triglyceride
complex
V₁-like ambulatory lead syndrome
V₅-like ambulatory lead syndrome
VLM
ventrolateral medulla
VLP
ventricular late potential
VLS
vascular leak syndrome
VM
Valsalva maneuver
vasomotor
ventriculomegaly
ventriculometry
viral myocarditis
VMAT
vesicular monoamine transformer
Vmax (*var. of* V_MAX)
Doppler peak flow velocity
VMC
vasomotor center
VMCG
vector magnetocardiogram
VMF
vasomotor flushing
VML
ventriculomegaly
VMR
vasomotor response

821

VMT
vasomotor tonus
VNSSL
video-assisted thoracic surgical non-rib-
spreading lobectomy
VNUS
VNUS Closure
catheter/radiofrequency generator
VNUS Closure system
VO₂
oxygen uptake peak VO₂
oxygen uptake
VOC
volatile organic compound
vocal
v. cord
v. cord adduction
v. cord dysfunction (VCD)
v. fremitus
v. process
vocalis
chorda v.
rima v.
vocational rehabilitation
VOD
venoocclusive disease
Voda guiding catheter
Vogt-Koyanagi-Harada syndrome
voice
amphoric v.
bronchial v.
v. button
cavernous v.
double v.
eunuchoid v.
hot potato v.
voix de Polichinelle
volatile
v. fatty acid (VFA)
v. organic compound (VOC)
Voldyne 5000 volumetric exerciser
Volkmann ischemic paralysis
Vollmer test
Volmax
volt (V)
electron v. (eV)
kiloelectron v. (keV)
megaelectron v. (MeV)
voltage
battery v.
Cornell v.
v. criteria
v. equilibrium
Gubner-Ungerleider v.
pacemaker output v.
root-mean-square v.
Sokolow-Lyon v.
transmembrane v.

voltage-dependent
v.-d. block
v.-d. calcium channel
voltage-gated channel
voltage-sensitive calcium channel (VSCC)
volume (V)
alveolar v. (VA)
aortic valve stroke v. (AVSV)
blood v. (BLV, BlV)
calculated minute v.
cardiac v. (CV)
cardiopulmonary blood v. (CPBV)
central blood v. (CBV)
central circulating blood v. (CCBV)
cerebral red blood cell v. (CRCV)
circulating blood v. (CBV)
circulation v.
closing v. (CV)
compressible v.
conductance stroke v.
consolidated lung v.
v. contraction
v. control (VC)
v. controller
corrected blood v. (CBV)
v. depletion
v. of distribution
v. of distribution effect
dP/dt$_{MAX}$ end-diastolic v.
effective arterial blood v. (EABV)
effective blood v. (EBV)
effective circulating blood v. (ECBV)
effort-independent lung v.
ejected v. (EV)
elastic equilibrium v. (EEV)
embolic v.
end-diastolic v. (EDV)
end-expiratory lung v. (EELV)
end-inspiratory lung v. (EILV)
end-systolic v. (ESV)
estimated blood v. (EBV)
v. expansion
expectorated sputum v.
expiratory reserve v. (ERV)
extracorporeal v. (ECV)
forced expiratory v. (FEV)
forward stroke v. (FSV)
frequency to tidal v. (f/VT)
heart v. (HV)
v. heating
high-frequency breath v.
high lung v.
v. infusion
inspiratory reserve v. (IRV)
intravascular v.
left atrial active emptying v.

left atrial end-diastolic v. (LAEDV)
left atrial end-systolic v. (LAESV)
left atrial maximal v.
left atrial minimal v.
left heart blood v. (LHBV)
left ventricular v. (LVV)
left ventricular diastolic v. (LVDP, LVDV)
left ventricular end-diastolic v. (LVEDV)
left ventricular end-systolic v. (LVESV)
left ventricular infarct v. (LVIV)
left ventricular stroke v. (LVSV)
v. load hypertrophy
v. loading
v. loop
v. loss
lung v.
lung blood v. (LBV)
mandatory minute v. (MMV)
maximal expiratory flow v. (MEFV)
mean corpuscular v. (MCV)
minute v.
v. overload
v. oxygen consumption (VO₂max)
v. to peak expiratory flow and total expiratory volume (VPTEF/VT)
planimetry v.
plaque v.
plasma v.
pressure v. (PV)
presystolic pressure and v.
pulmonary blood v. (PBV)
pulmonary blood mixing v. (PBMV)
pulmonary capillary blood v. (Vc)
ratio of tidal expiratory and inspiratory flow at 50% of tidal v. (TEF₅₀/TIF₅₀)
regurgitant v. (RV, RVol)
relative cardiac v.
residual v. (RV)
respiratory minute v.
resting stroke v.
resting tidal v.
v. resuscitation
right heart mixing v. (RHMV)
right ventricular v. (RVV)
right ventricular diastolic v. (RVDV)
right ventricular end-diastolic v. (RVEDV)
right ventricular end-systolic v. (RVESV)
right ventricular stroke v. (RVSV)
Simpson rule for ventricular v.

sputum v.
static lung v.
v. stiffness
stroke v. (SV)
subphysiological v.
v. thickness index (VTI)
thoracic v.
thoracic gas v. (TGV, V_TG)
tidal v. (TV, V_T, Vt)
tidal breathing flow v. (TBFV)
tidal expiratory v. (TV_E)
tidal expiratory flow at 25% of tidal v. (TEF₂₅)
tidal expiratory flow at 50% of tidal v. (TEF₅₀)
tidal expiratory flow at 75% of tidal v. (TEF₇₅)
tidal inspiratory v. (TV_I)
tidal inspiratory flow at 50% of tidal v. (TIF₅₀)
timed forced expiratory v.
total blood v. (TBV)
total right ventricular v. (TRVV)
trapped gas v.
urine v.
venous v. (VV)
v. ventilator
ventricular v.
ventricular end-diastolic v. (VDV)
ventricular residual v. (VRV)
volume to peak expiratory flow and total expiratory v. (VPTEF/VT)

volume-assured pressure support (VAPS)
volume-challenge test
volume-controlled
    v.-c. respirator
    v.-c. ventilation (VCV)
volume-cycled
    v.-c. decelerating-flow ventilation (VCDF)
    v.-c. ventilator
volume-displacement
    v.-d. plethysmograph
    v.-d. spirometer
volume-overloaded left ventricle
volumeter
volume-time curve
volumetric
    v. capnogram
    v. diffusive respirator (VDR)
    v. infusion pump
    v. lung depth (Vp)
volutrauma
volvulus
    Onchocerca v.
VO₂max
    aerobic capacity

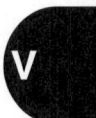

VO₂max *(continued)*
  oxygen consumption
  oxygen consumption per minute
  peak exercise oxygen consumption
  volume oxygen consumption
von
    v. Claus chronometric method
    v. Recklinghausen disease
    v. Recklinghausen syndrome
    v. Recklinghausen test
    v. Reyn criteria
    v. Willebrand disease
    v. Willebrand factor (vWF)
    v. Willebrand protein (vWP)
VOO
  ventricular asynchronous
    VOO pacemaker
    VOO pacing
voodoo death
Voorhees bag
VOP
  vasoocclusive pain
  venous occlusion plethysmography
voriconazole
vortex
    v. cordis
    v. effect catheter
    v. flow
VOS
  videothoracoscopic operator staging
VoSpire ER
voxel gray scale
VP
  vascular profiling
  vasopressin
  venous pressure
  ventricular pacing
  ventricular pericardium
  ventricular premature
    VP beat
Vp
  ventricular premature
  volumetric lung depth
V-Pace transluminal pacing lead
VPAP
  variable positive airway pressure
    VPAP II ST-A bilevel flow
      generator
    VPAP II ST ventilatory support
      system
VPB
  ventricular premature beat
VPC
  ventricular premature complex
  ventricular premature contraction
VPCT
  ventricular premature contraction
    threshold

VPD
  ventricular premature depolarization
VPF
  vascular permeability factor
VPGSS
  venous pressure gradient support
    stockings
VPI
  vasopeptidase inhibitor
VPR
  ventricular paced rhythm
VPTEF/VT
  volume to peak expiratory flow and total
    expiratory volume
VPW pattern
$\dot{V}/\dot{Q}$
  ventilation/perfusion
    $\dot{V}/\dot{Q}$ defect
    $\dot{V}/\dot{Q}$ lung scan
    $\dot{V}/\dot{Q}$ mismatch
    $\dot{V}/\dot{Q}$ quotient
VQI
  ventricular perfusion index
VR
  right arm electrode for electrocardiogram
  valve replacement
  vascular resistance
  velocity ratio
  venous reflux
  venous return
  ventricular rale
  ventricular rhythm
    VR electrode
VRD
  ventricular radial dysplasia
Vroman effect
VRV
  ventricular residual volume
VS
  venesection
  ventricular septum
Vs
  venesection
VSA
  vasospastic angina
VSAQ
  Veterans Specific Activity Questionnaire
VSCC
  voltage-sensitive calcium channel
VScore with AutoGate cardiac imaging
VSD
  ventricular septal defect
    doubly committed VSD
    Eisenmenger VSD
    injury VSD
    inlet VSD
    outlet VSD
    pinhole VSD
    restrictive VSD

subpulmonary VSD
trabecular VSD

VSFP
venous stop flow pressure

VSHD
ventricular septal heart defect

V-slope method

VSMC
vascular smooth muscle cell

V-Star
PhotoGenica V-S.

VSW
ventricular stroke work

Vsys
systolic wall motion velocity

Vt
tidal volume

VT
ventricular tachycardia
VT Mercury Vac organic mercury
vacuum cleaner
VT 1000 neonatal workstation
R-on-T-initiated nonsustained VT

VTA
ventricular tachyarrhythmia

V-Tam T shirt monitor

VTCL
ventricular tachycardia cycle length

VTE
venous thromboembolism
ventricular tachycardia event

VTI
volume thickness index
VTI oxygen monitor with
disposable polarographic oxygen
sensor

VTK catheter

VTS
variable thickness strut
VTS technology

VT/VF
ventricular tachycardia/ventricular
fibrillation

Vueport
V. balloon occlusion guiding
catheter
V. balloon technology

vulgaris
Proteus v.
Thermoactinomyces v.

vulnerability
plaque v.

vulnerable
v. myocardium

v. period
v. phase
v. plaque

Vumon injection

VV
venous volume
venovenous

V1-V6
ventral lead 1–6
V1-V6 EKG leads

V-Vac suction apparatus

VVD
ventricular demand-triggered
VVD mode
VVD pacemaker
VVD pacing

VVDL
venovenous double-lumen
VVDL catheter

VVI
ventricular inhibited
VVI pacemaker
VVI pacing

VVIR
VVIR mode
VVIR pacemaker
VVIR pacing

VVI-RR pacing

VVI/VVIR pacing

vvk
ventricular volume constant

VVO
vesicular-vacuolar organelle

VVS
vasovagal syncope

VVT
ventricular triggered
VVT mode
VVT pacemaker
VVT pacing

VW
vascular wall

vWF
von Willebrand factor

VWM
ventricular wall motion

vWP
von Willebrand protein

VX nerve gas

Vytorin

VZIG
varicella-zoster immunoglobulin

VZV, VZ
varicella-zoster virus

V

W

W pattern
W pattern on right atrial waveform
W wave on echocardiogram

Waardenburg syndrome
Wada test
wadsworthensis
    Sutterella w.
wadsworthii
    Legionella w.
waist
    cardiac w.
    w. of catheter
    w. of heart
    hypertriglyceridemic w.
waisting of balloon
waist-to-hip ratio (WHR)
wake after sleep onset time (WASO)
Waldenström macroglobulinemia
Waldeyer
    W. throat ring
    W. tonsillar ring
Waldhausen subclavian flap technique
walk
    w. distance
    w. distance test
    shuttle test w.
Walkabout oxygen conserver
WalkCare slippers
Walker-Murdoch wrist sign
walking
    nocturnal w.
    w. pneumonia
    w. ventilation test
walk-through angina
wall
    w. amplitude
    anterior w. (AW)
    anterior aortic w. (AAW)
    anterobasal w.
    aortic posterior w. (AOPW, AoPW)
    chest w.
    distal lateral w.
    free w.
    friable w.
    heart w.
    inferobasal w.
    inner w. (IW)
    lateral w. (LW)
    left atrial w. (LAW)
    left atrial posterior w. (LAPW)
    left ventricular w. (LVW)
    left ventricular posterior w. (LVPW)

membranous w.
w. motion (WM)
w. motion abnormality (WMA)
w. motion analysis (WMA)
w. motion index (WMI)
w. motion score
w. motion score index (WMSI)
w. motion velocity
posterior w. (PW)
posteroseptal w.
right atrial w. (RAW)
right atrial free w. (RAFW)
right ventricle anterior w. (RVAW)
right ventricular w. (RVW)
w. stress
w. structure
subacute ventricular free w.
w. tension
w. thickening
w. thickness (WT)
w. tracking
w. tracking system
vascular w. (VW)

Wallace Flexihub central venous pressure cannula
Wallenberg syndrome
Wallerian degeneration (WD)
Wallgraft
    W. stent
    W. tracheobronchial endoprosthesis
Wallstent
    W. endoprosthesis with Unistep Plus delivery system
    W. flexible, self-expanding wire-mesh stent
    Magic W.
    W. Magic stent
    W. Monorail carotid stent
    Schneider W.
    W. spring-loaded stent
    W. venous endoprosthesis
    W. venous endoprosthesis with Unistep
    W. with Unistep
Walter Reed classification
waltersii
    Legionella w.
wand
    light w.
wandering
    w. atrial pacemaker (WAP)
    w. baseline
    w. goiter
    w. heart

W

wandering (continued)
    w. pacemaker
    w. pneumonia
Wangiella dermatitidis
Wang transbronchial needle
waning
    waxing and w.
WAP
    wandering atrial pacemaker
ward
    general w.
Ward-Romano syndrome
Wardrop method
warfarin
    w. dose index (WDI)
    w. sodium
    w. therapy
warfarin-aspirin symptomatic intracranial disease (WASID)
Warfilone
warm
    w. heparinized saline flush
    w. nodule
warmer
    blood w.
warm-up phenomenon
warmup angina
warning arrhythmia
Warthin-Starry-staining bacillus
wash
    w. bath
    ENT w.
    nasopharyngeal w.
washing
    bronchial w.
    bronchoalveolar w.
    bronchopulmonary w.
    w.'s and brushings
    lung w.
washout
    w. cannula
    helium w.
    w. period
    w. phase
    w. phenomenon
    thallium w.
WASID
    warfarin-aspirin symptomatic intracranial disease
WASO
    wake after sleep onset time
Wasserman
    W. needle
    W. number
Wasserman-positive pulmonary infiltrate
wasted ventilation
wasting
    potassium w.

salt w.
    w. syndrome
WAT
    word association test
watch
    Pulse Pro heart rate monitor w.
water
    w. brash
    carmustine-impregnated w.
    w. channel
    w. column resistor
    dextrose 5% in w. (D5W, D-5-W, D_5W)
    extravascular lung w. (EVLW)
    feet of sea w. (fsw)
    w. hammer pulse
    w. lily sign
    lung w.
    w. retention
    w. vapor pressure
water-bottle heart
waterfall effect
water-gurgle test
water-hammer pulse
Waterman bronchoscope
watermelon seeding effect
waterproof tape
water-seal
    w.-s. chest tube
    w.-s. suction drainage
water-sealed spirometer
watershed
    w. infarct
    w. infarction
    w. pattern
    w. region
Waters projection
Waterston
    W. anastomosis
    W. anastomosis for congenital pulmonary stenosis
    W. groove
    W. operation
    W. shunt
Waterston-Cooley
    W.-C. procedure
    W.-C. pulmonary artery shunt
watertight seal
waterwheel
    w. murmur
    w. sound
water-whistle sound
Watson
    W. heart valve holder
    W. syndrome
watt-second (WS)
wave
    A w.
    a w.

A larger than V w.
w. amplitude
w. analyzer
arterial w.
atrial repolarization w.
augmented V w.
bifid P w.
blast w.
brain w.
C w.
cannon w.
catacrotic w.
catadicrotic w.
constant tilt w.
w. coronary event
Corrigan w.
CV w.
D w.
deep pathologic Q w.
delta w.
depolarization w.
diastolic w.
dicrotic w.
diphasic P, T w.
duration of ECG w.
duration of P w.
E w.
early systolic w.
ECG w.
electrocardiographic fibrillatory w.
epsilon w.
E wave to A w. (E:A)
excitation w.
F w.
f w.
ff w.'s
fibrillary w.
fibrillatory w.
flattened T w.
flipped T w.
flutter w.
flutter-fibrillation w.
giant a w.
giant TU fusion w.
giant T, V w.
H w.
high R w.
hyperacute T w.
inverted T w.
isolated T w.
J w.
Mayer w.
Minnesota criteria for high R w.
negative deflection that follows
  R w. (S)
negative T, U w.
normalization of inverted T w.
notched P, S w.
NSSTT w.

w. number
Osborne (J) w.
overflow w.
P w.
palpable A w.
pathologic Q w.
peaked P w.
percussion w.
peristaltic w. (PW)
polymorphic slow w.
P-on-T w.
portion of segment between end of
  S wave and beginning of T w.
  (ST)
posterior Q w.
postextrasystolic T w.
precordial A w.
pressure w. (PW)
prominent U w.
propagation of R w.
PRS w.
pseudonormalization of T w.
pseudo R' w.
pseudo S w.
pulse w. (PW)
Q w.
QS w.
R w.
R' w.
rapid filling w.
recoil w.
regurgitant w.
retraction w.
retrograde P w.
RF w.
S w.
S' w.
sawtooth P w.
scroll reentrant w.
seismic w.
shallow pathologic Q w.
sine w.
slow filling w.
slurred R w.
small P w.
spike w. (SW, S/W)
w. spike
spiral reentrant w.
ST w.
standardization w.
stationary arterial w.
ST-T w.
systolic reflection w.
systolic S w.
T w.
Ta w.
tall T w.
tidal w.
transient abnormal Q w. (TAQW)

W

wave *(continued)*
    U w.
    undulating deflection that follows T w.
    upright T w.
    V w.
    venous Corrigan w.
    ventricular w.
    Venturi w.
    W. VM200 ventilator
    x w.
    X descent of A w.
    y w.
    Y descent w.

waveform
    artery w.
    A-wave spectral velocity w.
    biphasic defibrillation w. (BDW)
    blunted w.
    CO_2 w.
    dampened w.
    defibrillation w.
    displacement w.
    distention w.
    Edmark monophasic w.
    E-wave spectral velocity w.
    flow-delivery w.
    forward pressure w.
    Gurvich biphasic w.
    incident pressure w.
    Lown-Edmark w.
    monophasic defibrillation w. (MDW)
    M pattern on right atrial w.
    nonsinusoidal w.
    pressure w.
    quasisinusoidal w.
    rectilinear biphasic w.
    reentry w.
    reflected pressure w.
    shock w.
    spectral w.
    W pattern on right atrial w.

wavelength (WL)
    w. of reentry

WaveMap intracoronary blood pressure measurement system

wavenumber

waveshape

wave-speed mechanism

WaveWire intracoronary blood pressure measurement system

wavy
    w. fiber
    w. respiration

waxing
    w. and waning
    w. and waning chest pain
    w. and waning in intensity

wax-matrix technique

way
    4-W. Long Acting Nasal Solution
    3-w. stopcock

WCD
    wearable cardioverter-defibrillator
    WCD 2000 System
    WCD 2000 system wearable cardioverter-defibrillator

WD
    Wallerian degeneration

WDI
    warfarin dose index

weakness

wean

weaning
    w. index (WI)
    w. protocol
    terminal w.
    T-piece w.
    ventilator w.

wearable
    w. cardioverter-defibrillator (WCD)
    w. cardioverter-defibrillator device
    w. defibrillator

wear-and-tear lesion

Weavenit
    W. patch graft
    W. prosthesis

web
    congenital coronary ostia w.
    esophageal w.
    laryngeal w.
    pulmonary arterial w.
    venous w.

Weber-Christian disease

Weber experiment

Weber-Janicki cardiopulmonary exercise protocol

Weber-Osler-Rendu syndrome

web-spacer

Webster
    W. halo catheter
    W. orthogonal electrode catheter

Wedensky
    W. effect
    W. modulated signal-averaged electrocardiogram

wedge
    w. angiogram
    arterial w.
    w. biopsy
    w. excision
    w. infiltrate
    mediastinal w.
    w. pressure (WP)
    w. pressure balloon catheter
    pulmonary w. (PW)
    w. pulmonary angiography

pulmonary artery w. (PAW)
pulmonary capillary w. (PCW)
w. resection
w. spirometer
Weeks bacillus
weeping
w. dermatitis
w. fig asthma
w. willow view
Wegener
W. granulomatosis (WG)
W. nodule
Weibel-Palade bodies
Weigert-van Gieson stain
weight
heart w. (HW)
weighted ball resistor
Weil disease
Weil-Felix reaction
Weill sign
Weinberg test
Weir method
Weisfeldt and Becker 3-phase model
Weiss logarithmic method
Weitzman criteria
Welch
W. Allyn PneumoCheck spirometer
W. Allyn/Schiller AT-1 3-channel
ECG
W. Allyn/Schiller AT-10 Exercise
Testing system
W. Allyn/Schiller AT-2 full-size
ECG
W. Allyn/Schiller AT-10 hospital
grade ECG
W. Allyn/Schiller AT-2*plus* full-size
ECG
W. Allyn/Schiller MS-3 pocket-size
ECG
W. Allyn/Schiller SP-1 budget
spirometry
W. Allyn/Schiller SP-10 diagnostic
spirometry
WelChol
Welcker method
welder's
w. lung
w. siderosis
welding
spot w.
well
pericardial w.
well-being
clinical w.-b.
Shwachman score of clinical w.-b.
well-differentiated carcinoma
Wenckebach
W. atrioventricular block
W. A-V block

W. cycle
W. cycle length
W. disease
W. exit block
W. period
W. periodicity
W. periodicity block
W. phenomenon
W. sign
Werlhof disease
Werner syndrome
Wernicke aphasia
Wessex prosthetic valve
west
W. Nile virus
W. syndrome
W. zone 1-3
Westaby tracheobronchial silicone stent
Westberg space
Westergren
W. erythrocyte sedimentation rate
W. method
westermani
Paragonimus w.
Westermark sign
western
W. blot
W. red cedar
Westminster drug-free protocol
Westrim LA
wet
w. beriberi
w. cough
w. lung
w. nebulization
w. pleurisy
w. rale
w. swallow
wet-to-dry dressing
Wexler arterial bypass catheter
WG
Wegener granulomatosis
whale's
w. tail angiographic landmark
w. tail angiographic landmark of
left anterior descending coronary
artery bifurcation
wheal and flare
Wheatstone bridge
wheat weevil disease
wheeze
asthmatoid w.
asthmoid w.
monophonic w.
wheezing
bronchial w.
early w.
emotional laryngeal w.
exercise-associated w.

W

wheezing *(continued)*
  expiratory w.
  laryngeal w.
  nonatopic w.
  transient early w.
  viral w.
  workplace-related w.
wheezy bronchitis
WHI
  Women's Health Initiative
whiff test
whip
  catheter w.
whipping
  systolic w.
Whipple disease
whippleii
  Tropheryma w.
whisker plot
whisper
  W. guidewire
  W. Mist humidifier
whispered
  w. bronchophony
  w. pectoriloquy
whispering
  w. pectoriloquy
  w. resonance
whistle
  box of w.'s
  coaching w.
whistling rale
white
  w. asphyxia
  w. blood cell count
  w. clot syndrome
  w. coat hypertension
  w. coronary thrombus
  w. light bronchoscopy (WLB)
  w. line
  w. lung
  w. matter (WM)
  w. matter hyperintensity (WMHI)
  w. plaque
  w. pneumonia
  w. spot
  w. sputum
  W. system
  w. thrombus
  W. vessel sizing catheter
white-coat
  w.-c. angina
  w.-c. effect
Whitfield ointment
WHO
  World Health Organization
WHO/Fredrickson
  WHO/F. classification

WHO/F. classification of primary
  hyperlipidemia
whole
  w. blood aggregometer
  w. blood buffer base
  w. blood cardioplegia
whole-body
  w.-b. amyloid load
  w.-b. hyperthermia
whole-grain food
Wholey
  W. Hi-Torque Floppy guidewire
  W. Hi-Torque modified J
    guidewire
  W. Hi-Torque standard guidewire
  W. wire
whoop
  precordial w.
  systolic w.
whooping
  w. cough
  w. murmur
whorled
whorling of myocardial cell
whorl motion
WHR
  waist-to-hip ratio
    WHR for upper body obesity
WI
  weaning index
WI-38 cell
Wichmann asthma
Wickwitz esophageal stricture
Widal-Abrami-Lermoyez triad
Widal test
wide
  w. complex rhythm
  w. QRS tachycardia
widely split second sound
wide-necked aneurysm
widened
  mediastinal w.
widening
  luminal w.
  mediastinal w.
  w. of pulse pressure
wide-open breath
Wideroe test
width
  atrial pulse w.
  Doppler PR jet w.
  pulse w.
  ventricular pulse w.
Wiener filter
Wiggle coronary guidewire
Wigle scale
Wigraine

Wiktor
    W. balloon expandable coronary stent
    W. GX coronary stent
    W. GX Hepamed coated coronary stent system
    W. Prime coronary stent system
Wiktor-I implantable stent
wild-type protein
Wilhelmy balance
Wilkie disease
Wilkins echocardiographic score
Wilks lambda criterion
Wilks-Schapiro test
Willebrand-Jürgens syndrome
Willett-Stampfer method
William
    W. Harvey arterial blood filter
    W. Harvey cardiotomy reservoir
    W. test
Williams
    W. phenomenon
    W. sign
    W. syndrome
    W. tracheal tone
Williams-Campbell syndrome
Williamson sign
Willis
    circle of W. (CW)
Wilms thoracoplasty
Wilson
    W. block
    W. central terminal
    W. disease
    W. lead
Wilson-Cook papillotome
Wilson-Kimmelsteil disease
Wilson-Mikity syndrome
Wilson-White method
Wilton
    W. Webster coronary sinus thermodilution catheter
    W. Webster thermodilution flow and pacing catheter
windkessel
    w. effect
    w. model
window
    acoustic w.
    aortic w.
    aortopulmonary w. (APW)
    Blackman w.
    cycle length w.
    Hanning w.
    imaging w.
    parasternal w.
    pericardial w.
    pleuropericardial w.
    pulmonary parenchymal w.

    subxiphoid w.
    tachycardia w.
    transthoracic acoustic w.
    videothoracoscopic pericardial w.
windowed balloon
windpipe
windsock
    w. aneurysm
    w. morphology
    w. sign
winged baseplate
Wingspan stent system
Winiwarter-Buerger disease
Winpred
Winslow test
Winstrol
winter
    w. bronchitis
    w. cough
    w. vomiting disease
Wintrich sign
Wintrobe sedimentation rate
wire (*See also* guidewire)
    all track w. (ATW)
    Amplatz tapered movable core w.
    Amplatz torque w.
    Asahi Light w.
    atrial pacing w.
    ATW marker w.
    biventricular pacing w.
    Choice PT plus w.
    control w.
    coronary w.
    crenulated tantalum w.
    delivery w.
    dock w.
    docking w.
    Doppler velocity w.
    Eder-Puestow w.
    endocardial w.
    extra-flexible w.
    flow w.
    w. guide
    Hancock temporary cardiac pacing w.
    Hi-Torque balance middleweight universal guide w.
    w. holder
    w. insertion
    intracoronary Doppler flow w.
    J exchange w.
    J retention w.
    Katzen infusion w.
    Linx extension w.
    Lunderquist exchange w.
    magnet w.
    Medi-Tech w.
    w. mesh self-expandable stent
    noodle w.

W

wire *(continued)*
    olive-tipped Magnum w.
    pacemaker w. (PMW)
    platinum w.
    pressure guide pressure w.
    pusher w.
    Radifocus w.
    Shinobi w.
    Stabilizer marker w.
    w. stylet
    tantalum w.
    tip-deflecting w.
    Wholey w.
wire-loop lesion
wire-wound endotracheal tube
wiring
    copper w.
    sternal w.
    w. of sternum
wiry pulse
Wiseguide catheter
Wiskott-Aldrich syndrome
wispish intraluminal frond
Wizard disposable inflation device
Wizdom
    W. PTCA steerable guidewire
    W. ST steerable guidewire
WL
    wavelength
WLB
    white light bronchoscopy
WM
    wall motion
    white matter
WMA
    wall motion abnormality
    wall motion analysis
Wmax
    peak work rate
WMFT
    Wolf Motor Function Test
WMHI
    white matter hyperintensity
WMI
    wall motion index
WMSI
    wall motion score index
WOB
    work of breathing
Wobenzym tablet
Woillez disease
Wolff-Parkinson-White (WPW)
    W.-P.-W. bypass tract
    W.-P.-W. reentrant tachycardia
    W.-P.-W. syndrome
Wolfina
Wolf Motor Function Test (WMFT)
wollastonite

Wolman
    W. disease
    W. xanthomatosis
Womack procedure
Women's Health Initiative (WHI)
wood
    W. classification
    W. lamp
    w. pulp worker's lung
    w. pulp worker's lung disease
    w. smoke
    W. unit
    W. units index
wooden resonance
wooden-shoe heart
Woodworth phenomenon
woody
    w. edema
    w. thyroiditis
Wooler-type annuloplasty
woolsorter's
    w. disease
    w. pneumonia
word association test (WAT)
work
    w. of breathing (WOB)
    w. capacity
    cardiac w. (CW)
    w. effect
    left ventricular w. (LVW)
    left ventricular stroke w. (LVSW)
    w. rate
    w. rate increment
    w. rehabilitation
    right ventricular stroke w. (RVSW)
    w. status
    stroke w. (SW, S/W)
    w. threshold
    ventricular stroke w. (VSW)
work-aggravated asthma
workhorse balloon
WorkHorse II PTA balloon catheter
workload
    peak w.
workplace exposure
workplace-related
    w.-r. cough
    w.-r. dyspnea
    w.-r. wheezing
work-related
    w.-r. asthma
    w.-r. bronchial hyperreactivity
worksite challenge test
workstation
    EnSite 3000 electrophysiology w.
    VT 1000 neonatal w.
World Health Organization (WHO)
worsening
    paradoxical w.

wound
    blowing w.
    bullet w.
    w. closure
    entrance w.
    exit w.
    gunshot w.
    knife w.
    stab w.
    sucking chest w.
    W. VAC

woven
    w. coronary artery disease
    w. Dacron catheter
    w. Dacron fabric graft
    w. Dacron tube graft
    w. Teflon
    w. Teflon prosthesis

woven-tube vascular graft prosthesis

WP
    wedge pressure

WPW
    Wolff-Parkinson-White
    WPW syndrome

wrap
    cardiac muscle w.
    no-phase w.
    omental w.

wrap-around ghosting artifact

wrapping
    w. of abdominal aortic aneurysm
    aneurysm w.

wrecking ball effect

Wright
    W. peak flow
    W. respirometer
    W. spirometer
    W. stain
    W. syndrome

Wright-Giemsa stain

wringer wrap configuration

Wrisberg ganglion

wrist positioning splint

WS
    watt-second

W-strain tuberculosis

WT
    wall thickness

Wuchereria bancrofti

Wu-Hoak hypothesis

Wyamine Sulfate

Wycillin injection

Wylie
    W. carotid artery clamp
    W. endarterectomy set
    W. vascular clamp

W

X

X depression of jugular venous pulse
X descent of A wave
X descent of jugular venous pulse
phospholipid-bound activated factor X (Fxa)
X recordings
X wave of Ohnell
X, Y depression
X, Y descent
X, Y, Z axis

Xact

X. carotid stent
X. carotid stent system

xamoterol
xanthelasma
xanthine

x. oxidase
x. oxidase reaction

xanthinol niacinate
xanthogranuloma
xanthoma

cutaneous x.
eruptive x.
palmar x.
planar x.
x. regression
x. striatum palmare
x. tendinosum
tendinous x.
tuberoeruptive x.
tuberous x.

xanthomatosis

Wolman x.

xanthomatous
Xanthomonas maltophilia
Xceed self-expanding stent
Xcelerant delivery system
X-Cell cardiac bioprosthesis
Xcelon nylon
Xcelovair
X-descent trough
Xe

xenon

^{127}Xe

xenon-127

^{133}Xe

xenon-133

XeCl excimer laser
XECT

xenon-enhanced computed tomography

Xeloda
xemilofiban
Xenical

xenoantibody
xenobiotic
xenodiagnosis
xenogeneic
xenograft

Ionescu-Shiley pericardial x.
porcine x.
stentless porcine x.

xenon (Xe)

x. chloride
x. chloride excimer laser
x. lung ventilation imaging
x. washout technique

xenon-127 (^{127}Xe)
xenon-133 (^{133}Xe)
xenon-enhanced computed tomography (XECT)
xenopi

Mycobacterium x.
Mycoplasma x.

Xenopus

X. *laevis*
X. oocyte
X. *tropicalis*

Xenotech prosthetic valve
xenotransplant
Xeroform gauze
xerosis
X-gal-positive cell
Xience V everolimus eluting coronary stent
Xillix LIFE-Lung system
ximelagatran
xinafoate

salmeterol x.

xipamide
xiphisternal

x. crunching sound
x. process

xiphisternum
xiphocostal
xiphodynia
xiphoid

x. angle
x. cartilage
x. process

xiphoiditis
xiphosternal junction
x-irradiate
x-irradiation
XL

extended release
InnoPran XL
Procardia XL
Toprol XL

X

XLAS
  X-linked aqueductal stenosis
XLCM
  X-linked dilated cardiomyopathy
X-linked
  X-l. aqueductal stenosis (XLAS)
  X-l. dilated cardiomyopathy
  (XLCM)
XMI thrombectomy catheter
Xolair
Xopenex inhalation solution
XO syndrome
Xpeedior t120 catheter
X-Press
  X.-P. suture-mediated device
  X.-P. vascular closure system
XR
  extended release
  Dilacor XR
x-ray (*See also* radiograph)
  babygram x-r.
  x-r. beam filtration
  x-r. beam hardening
  chest x-r. (CX, CXR, CxR)
  x-r. cine computed tomography
  x-r. energy microprobe analysis
  x-r. generator
  Infinix NB-i vascular x-r.
  scanning-beam digital x-r.
  x-r. scatter collimation
  sinus x-r.
  x-r. tube

x-ray-guided recanalization
XRT
  radiotherapy
X-Scribe
  X-S. stress test
  X-S. stress testing system
X-Sept
  X-S. transition catheter
  X-S. transseptal sheath
X-Sizer single-use catheter system
XT
  extended release
  Cartia XT
  Diltia XT
  XT radiopaque coronary stent
X-Trode stent
x wave
XXXX syndrome
XXXY syndrome
xylene
Xylocaine
  X. Oral
  X. Topical Ointment
  X. Topical Solution
Xylocard
xylol pulse indicator
xylosoxidans
  Achromobacter x.
  Alcaligenes x.
Xyrem
XYZ lead system

Y

Y connector
Y coupler
Y depression of jugular venous pulse
Y descent of jugular venous pulse
Y descent wave
Y graft
Y stent
Y stenting
Y technique
Y wave pressure on right atrial catheterization

Yacoub and Radley-Smith classification
YAG

yttrium-aluminum-garnet
YAG laser

Yamaguchi disease
Yankauer

Y. bronchoscope
Y. pharyngeal speculum

Yasargil carotid clamp
Yates correction
yaws
Y-composite arterial graft
Y-descent trough
Yeager formula
year

disability-adjusted life y. (DALY)

yellow

y. cross

y. fever
y. hepatization
Y. IRIS system
y. nail syndrome (YNS)
y. plaque
y. sputum

yellowish-green sputum
Yentl syndrome
Yersinia

Y. enterocolitica
Y. pestis
Y. pseudotuberculosis

Yesavage score
YNS

yellow nail syndrome

Yodoxin
yohimbine hydrochloride
Youden index
Youlten nasal inspiratory peak flowmeter
Youman-Parlett test
young

Y. modulus
Y. syndrome

Y-shaped

Y-s. bifurcation
Y-s. graft

YSI 4000 telethermometer
yttrium-aluminum-garnet (YAG)
y wave

Y

Z

Z band
Z cardiac catheter
Z line
Z mutation
Z point
Z point pressure on left atrial
   catheterization
Z point pressure on right atrial
   catheterization
Z score
Z score weight-Z score height
Z stent
zabicipril
Zaditen
zafirlukast
Zagam Respipac
Zahn
Z. lines
pocket of Z.
Zaire subtype
zalcitabine
Zalkind lung retractor
Zamboni disease
Zanaflex
zanamivir
Zang space
Zanosar
zardaverine asthma
Zaroxolyn
zatebradine
Zavala
Z. lung biopsy needle
Z. technique
ZCV
Zynergy CardioVascular Inc.
Zebeta
zebra artifact
ZEEP
zero end-expiratory pressure
ZEEP PV curve
Zemaira
Zemuron
Zenapax
Zener diode
Zenith AAA endovascular graft system
Zenker diverticulum
Zenotech graft material
Zephrex
Zerit
zero
z. amplitude
z. diastolic blood pressure
z. end-expiratory pressure (ZEEP)

z. end-inspiratory pressure
z. velocity line
zero-flow pressure (Pzf, ZFP)
zero-order kinetics
Zestoretic
Zestril
Zeta stent
Zetia
Zeus system
ZFP
zero-flow pressure
Z-Gly-Gly-Arg-AMC
fluorogenic thrombin substrate Z-
   G.-G.-A.-AMC
Ziac
Ziagen
zidovudine and lamivudine
Ziehl-Neelsen stain
zigzag stent
Zilactin-L
zileuton
Zilver
Z. self-expanding stent
Z. vascular stent
Zimmer antiembolism support stockings
Zimmermann arch
Zinacef injection
zinc
z. chloride
z. finger gene
z. fume fever
z. gelatin
z. protoporphyrin
Zinecard
ZIP
zoster immune plasma
zipper
Z. antidisconnect device
z. scar
zirconium tetrachloride
Zithromax Z-Pak
ZK-EPO
ZK-Epothilone
ZK-Epothilone (ZK-EPO)
Z-Med catheter
Zocor
zofenopril
zofenoprilic acid
Zofran
Zoladex implant
Zoll
Z. NTP 1000 noninvasive
   pacemaker
Z. PD 1200 external defibrillator

Z

Zollinger-Gilmore intraluminal vein stripper
zolmitriptan
zolpidem tartrate
ZoMaxx drug-eluting stent
zonal predominance
zone
  border z.
  echo z.
  Fraunhofer z.
  Fresnel z.
  H z.
  Head z.
  ischemic z.
  midlung z.
  myocardial border z.
  periinfarction z.
  z. 1 phenomenon
  posterior upper lung z.
  protective z.
  safe z.
  slow z.
  sonolucent z.
  subcostal z.
  subendocardial z.
  tendinous z.
  z. therapy
  transitional cell z.
  upper lung z.
  vascular z.
  West z. 1-3

zoom
  acquisition z. (AZ)
zopolrestat
ZORprin
zoster
  herpes z.
  z. immune plasma (ZIP)
Zosyn
Z-Pak
  Zithromax Z-P.
ZT
  Zwolle trial
Zuckerkandl bodies
Zuma coronary guiding catheter
Zwenger test
Zwolle trial (ZT)
Zyban
Zydone
Zygomycetes
zygomycosis
zymogen
zymography
  gelatin z.
  in situ z.
  substrate gel z.
Zynergy CardioVascular Inc. (ZCV)
Zyrtec
Zyvox

Contents: The Appendices

Appendix 1
Illustrations

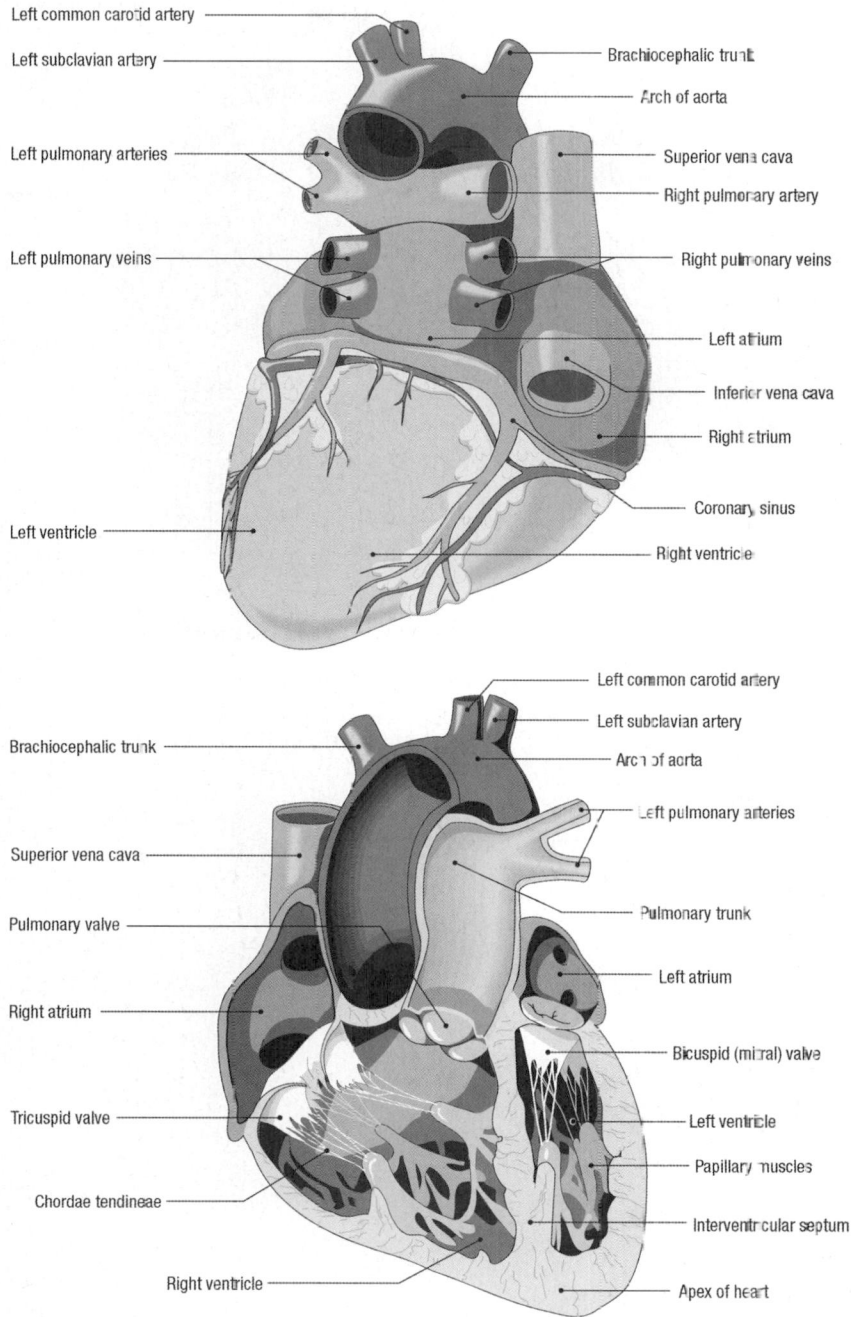

Figure 1. The relationship of the great vessels of heart. (Top) posterior view, (bottom) coronal view.

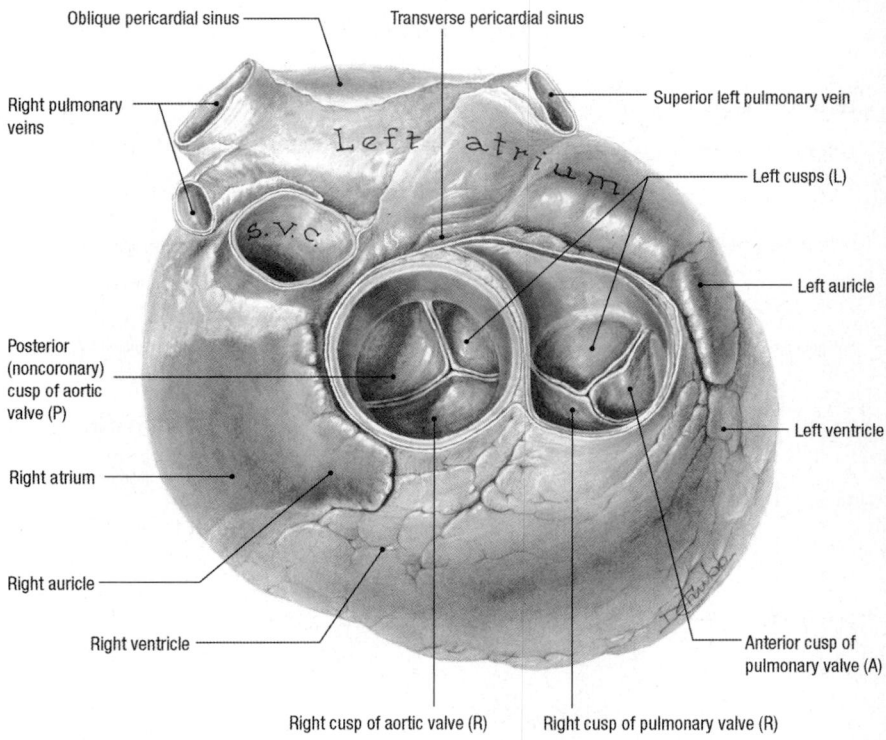

Oblique pericardial sinus
Transverse pericardial sinus
Right pulmonary veins
Superior left pulmonary vein
Left atrium
Left cusps (L)
S.V.C.
Left auricle
Posterior (noncoronary) cusp of aortic valve (P)
Left ventricle
Right atrium
Right auricle
Right ventricle
Anterior cusp of pulmonary valve (A)
Right cusp of aortic valve (R)
Right cusp of pulmonary valve (R)

Figure 2. Excised heart, superior view.

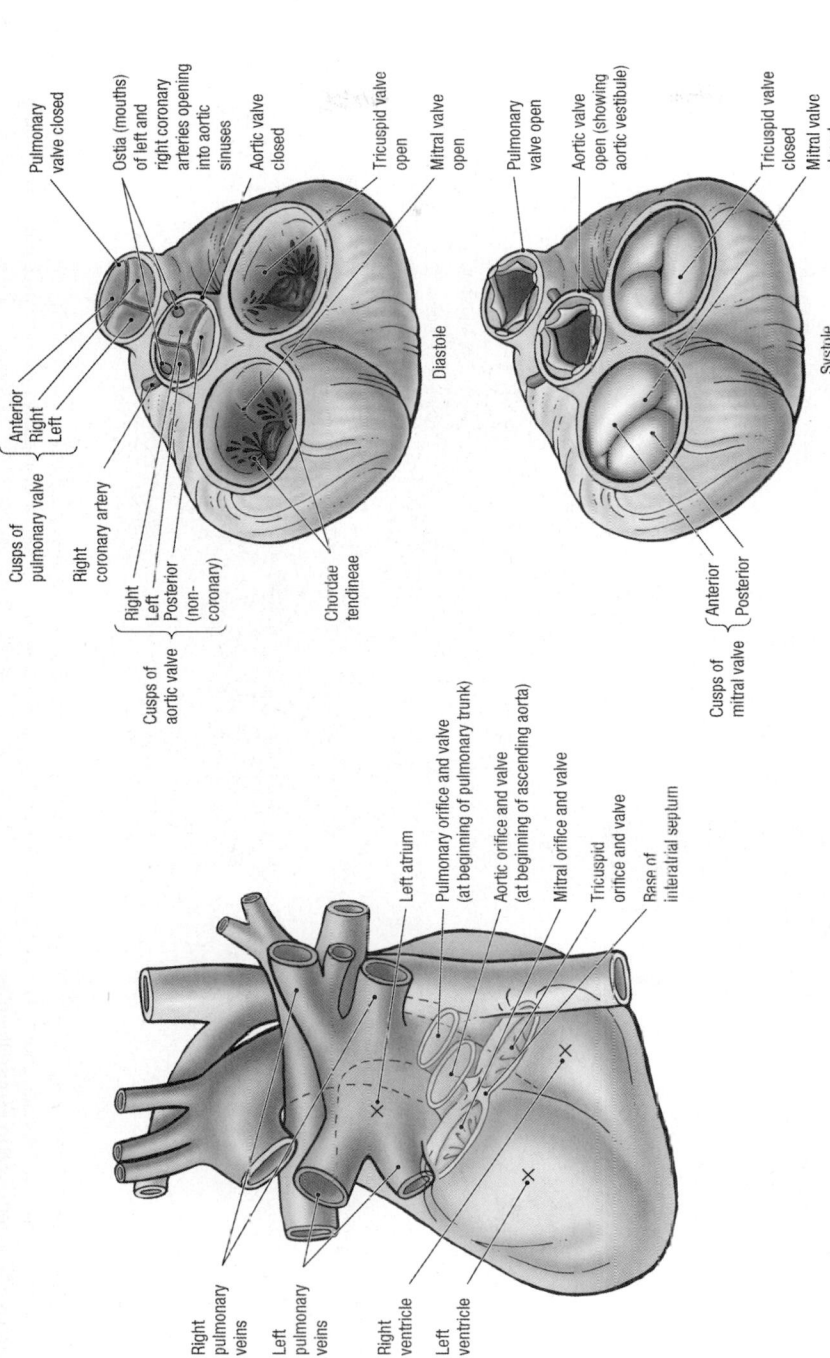

Figure 3. Valves of the heart and great vessels. At the beginning of diastole (ventricular filling), the aortic and pulmonary valves are closed; shortly thereafter, the tricuspid and mitral valves open. Shortly after systole (ventricular emptying) begins, the tricuspid and mitral valves close and the aortic and pulmonary valves open.

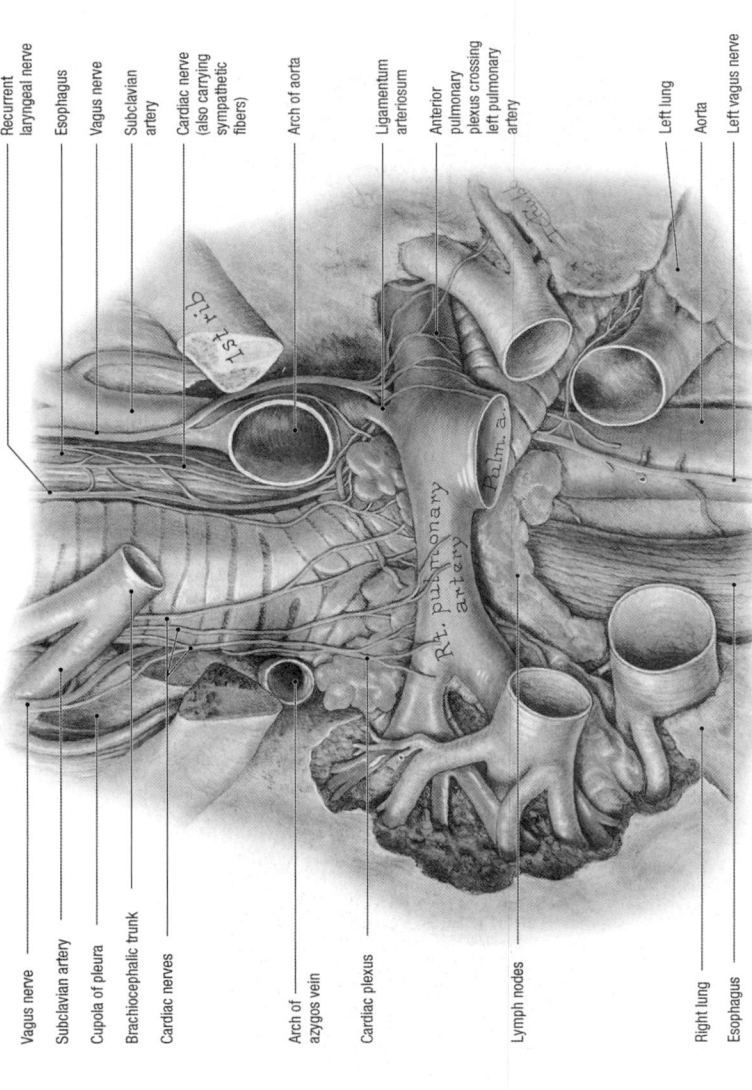

Recurrent laryngeal nerve

Esophagus

Vagus nerve

Subclavian artery

Cardiac nerve (also carrying sympathetic fibers)

Arch of aorta

Ligamentum arteriosum

Anterior pulmonary plexus crossing left pulmonary artery

Left lung

Aorta

Left vagus nerve

Vagus nerve

Subclavian artery

Cupola of pleura

Brachiocephalic trunk

Cardiac nerves

Arch of azygos vein

Cardiac plexus

Lymph nodes

Right lung

Esophagus

1st rib

Rt. pulmonary artery

Pul. a.

Figure 4. Dissection of the superior mediastinum. Observe the cardiac branches of the vagus and sympathetic nerves running down the sides of the trachea and forming the cardiac plexus. Although shown lying on the trachea, the primary relationship of the cardiac plexus is to the ascending aorta and pulmonary trunks, which have been removed to expose the plexus.

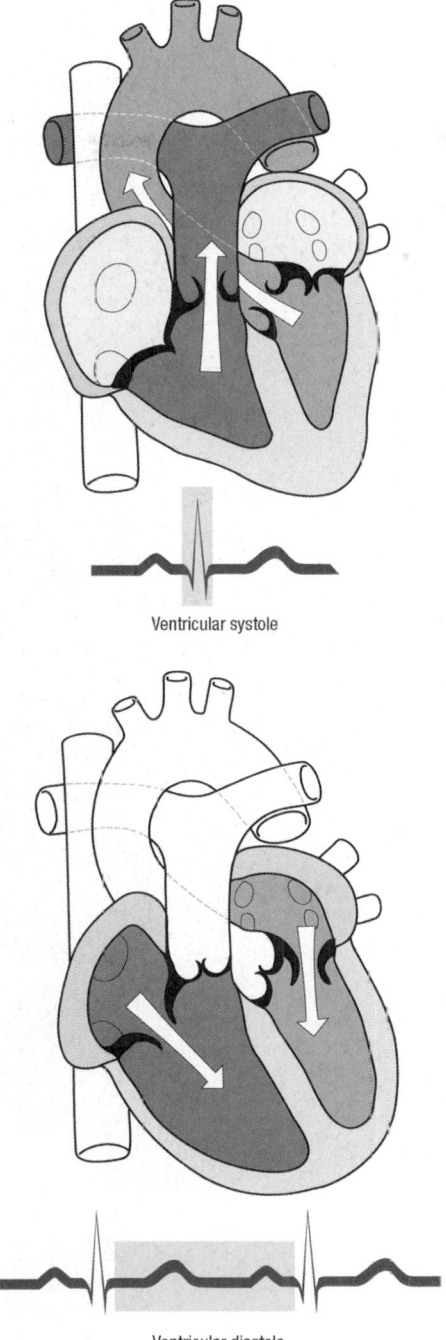

Ventricular systole

Ventricular diastole

Figure 5. The cardiac cycle.

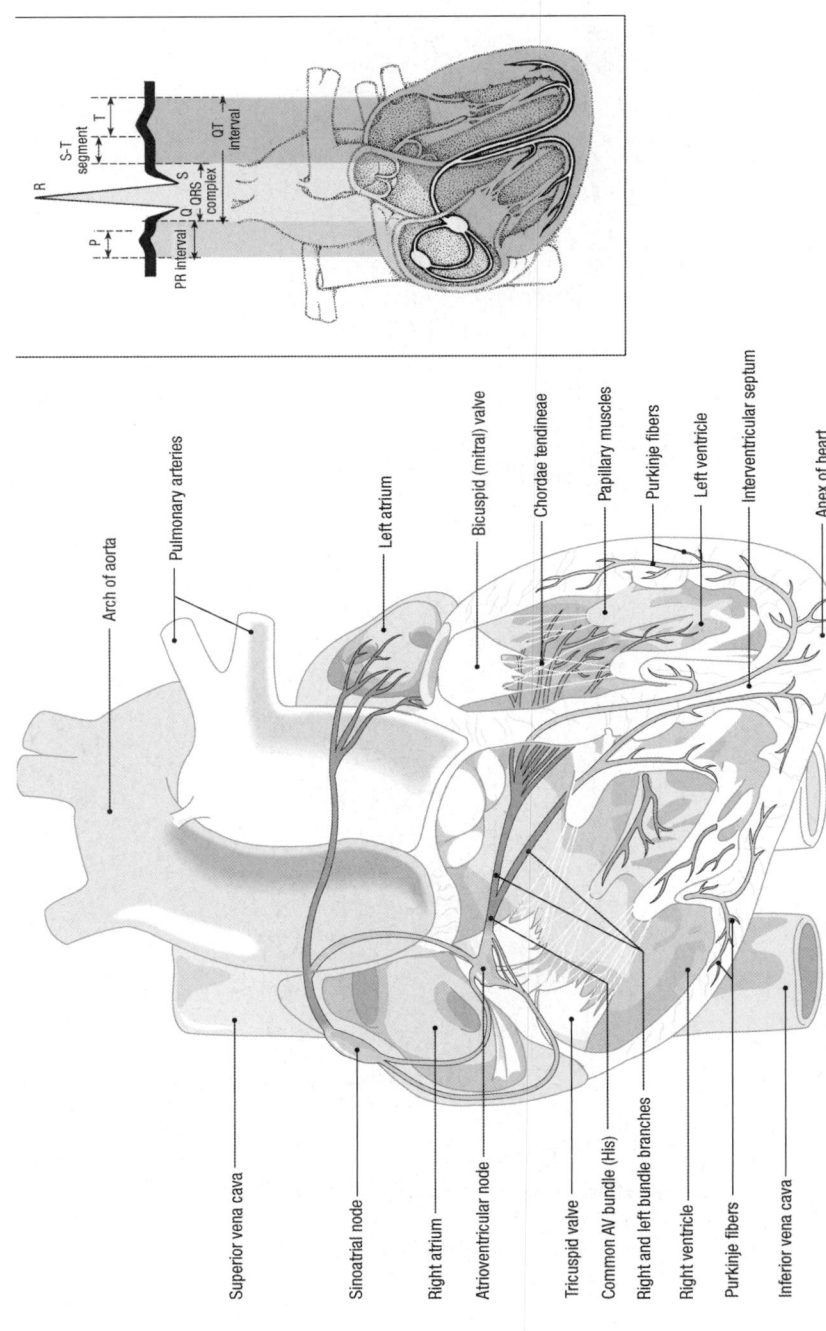

Figure 6. Conducting system of the heart. (Inset) an electrical picture of the heart is represented by positive and negative deflections on a graph labeled with the letters P, Q, R, S, and T, corresponding to the events of the cardiac cycle.

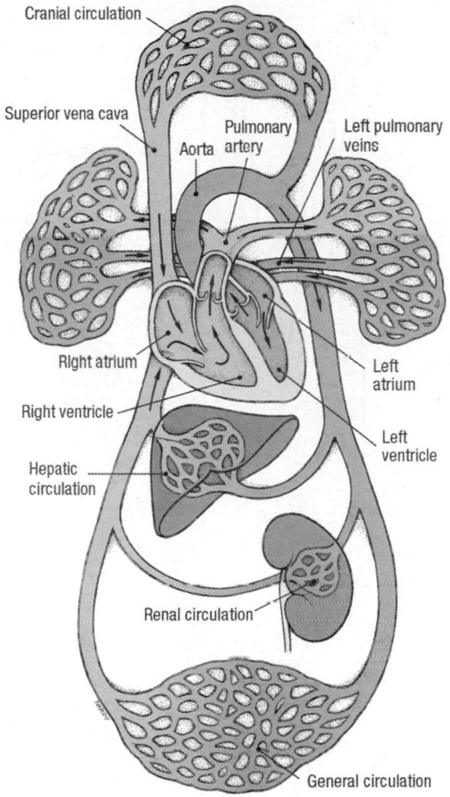

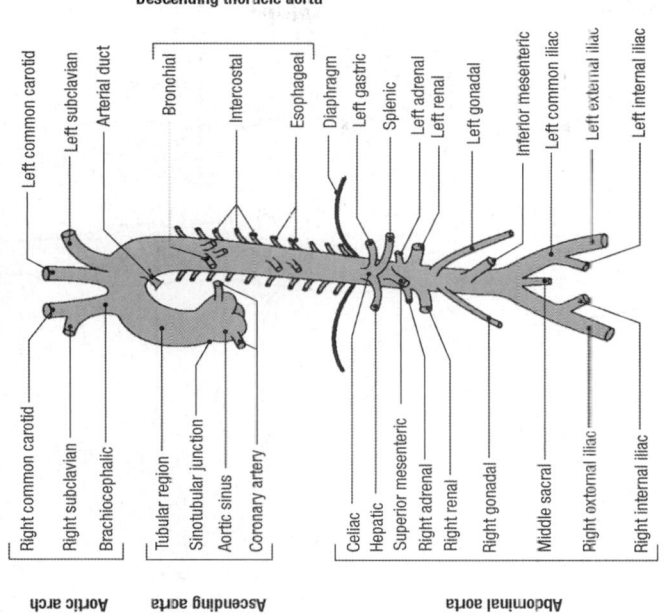

Descending thoracic aorta

Left common carotid
Left subclavian
Arterial duct
Bronchial
Intercostal
Esophageal
Diaphragm
Left gastric
Splenic
Left adrenal
Left renal
Left gonadal
Inferior mesenteric
Left common iliac
Left external iliac
Left internal iliac

Right common carotid
Right subclavian
Brachiocephalic
Tubular region
Sinotubular junction
Aortic sinus
Coronary artery
Celiac
Hepatic
Superior mesenteric
Right adrenal
Right renal
Right gonadal
Middle sacral
Right external iliac
Right internal iliac

Aortic arch
Ascending aorta
Abdominal aorta

Figure 8. Systemic circulation: through the body, from the left ventricle to the right atrium.

Left pulmonary veins
Left atrium
Left ventricle
Pulmonary artery
Aorta
General circulation
Renal circulation
Cranial circulation
Superior vena cava
Right atrium
Right ventricle
Hepatic circulation

Figure 7. Pulmonary circulation: through the lungs, from the right ventricle to the left atrium.

A7

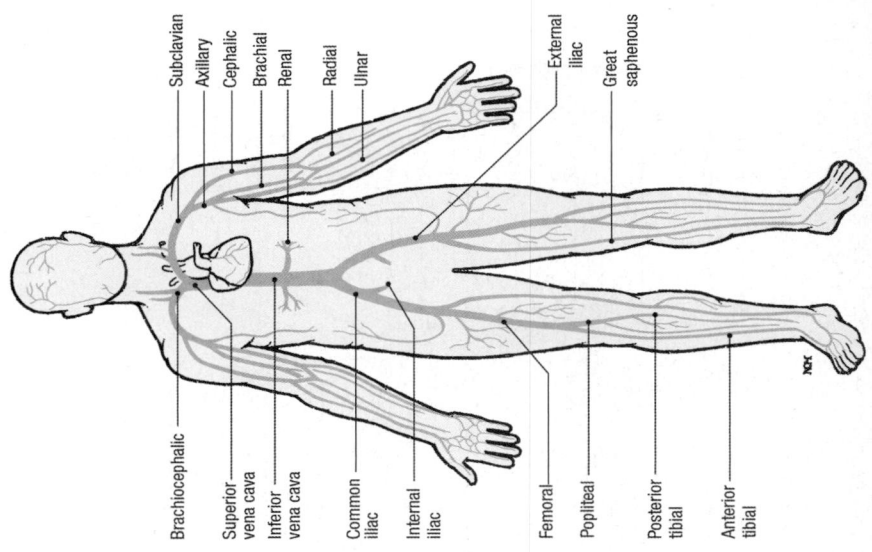

Figure 10. Major veins of the body.

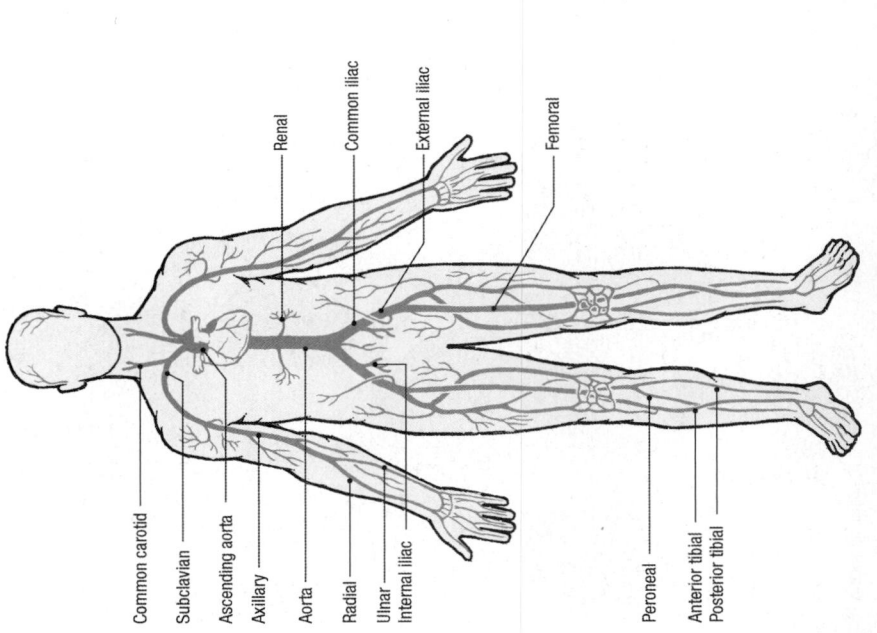

Figure 9. Major arteries of the body.

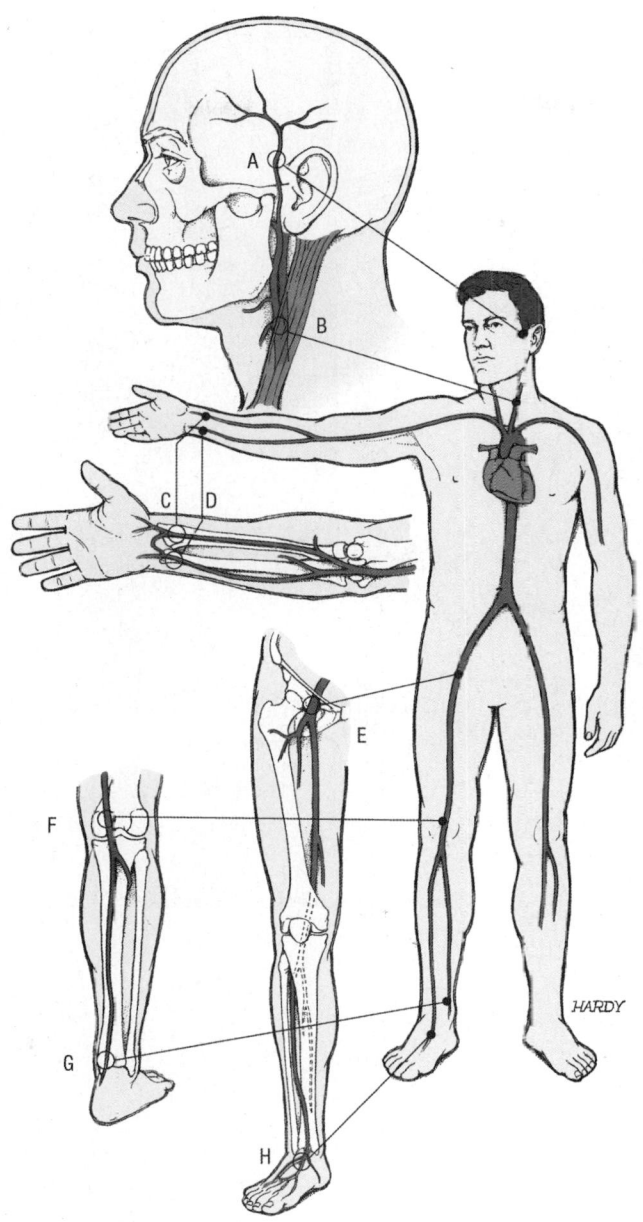

Figure 11. Peripheral pulses: (A) temporal, (B) carotid, (C) radial, (D) ulnar, (E) femoral, (F) popliteal, (G) posterior tibial, (H) dorsalis pedis.

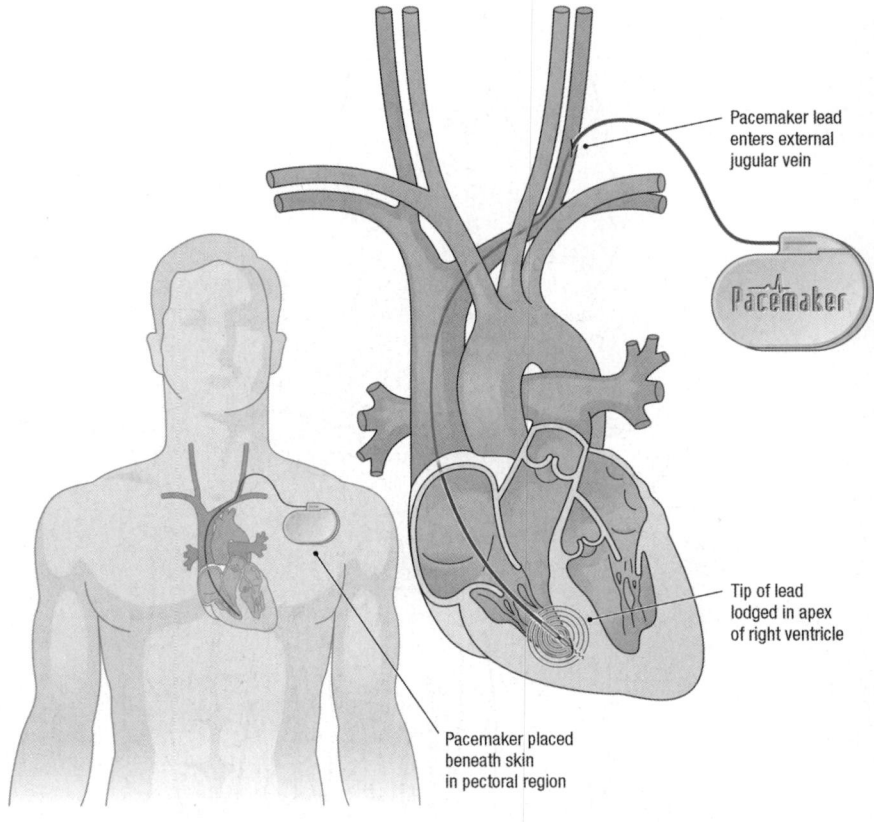

Figure 12. Placement of a pacemaker.

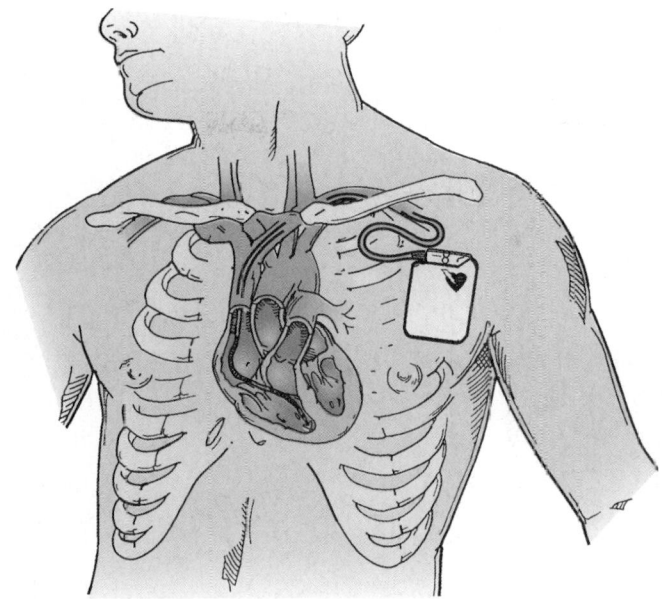

Figure 13. The implantable cardioverter defibrillator (ICD) mechanical system consists of a generator and a sensing/pacing/defibrillating electrode. Two epicardial patches may also be used.

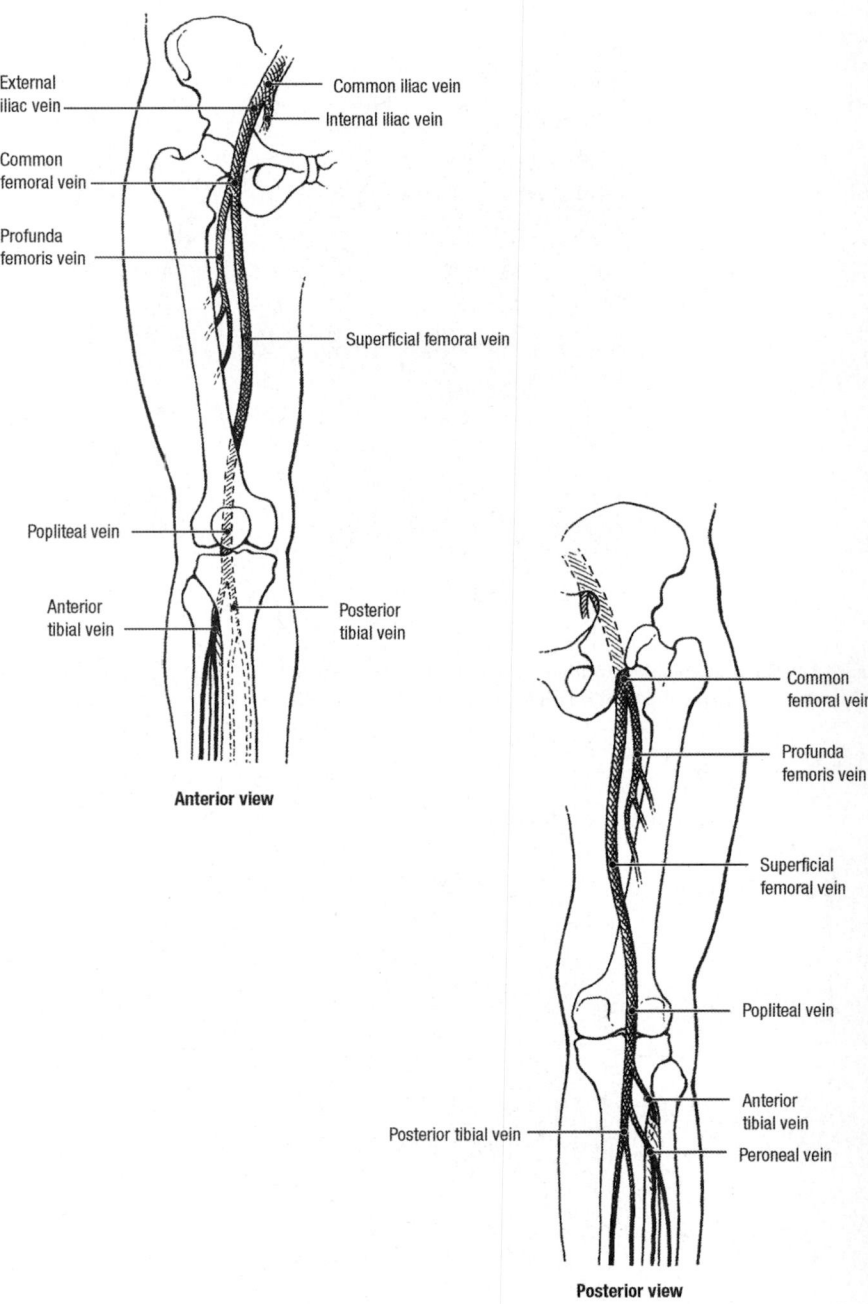

Figure 14. Anatomy of the deep venous system of the right lower limb. (Top) anterior view, (bottom) posterior view.

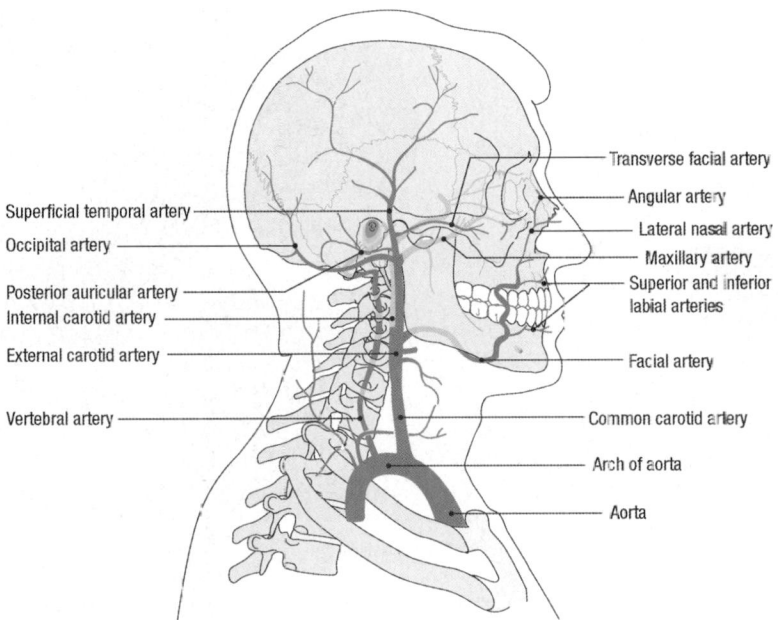

Transverse facial artery

Angular artery

Lateral nasal artery

Maxillary artery

Superior and inferior labial arteries

Superficial temporal artery

Occipital artery

Posterior auricular artery

Internal carotid artery

External carotid artery

Facial artery

Vertebral artery

Common carotid artery

Arch of aorta

Aorta

Figure 15. Arteries of the head and neck.

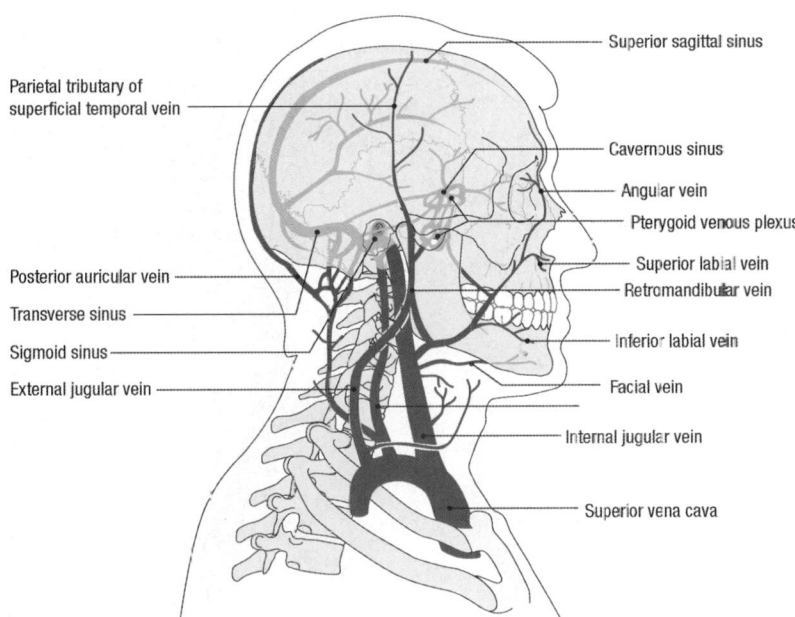

Superior sagittal sinus

Parietal tributary of superficial temporal vein

Cavernous sinus

Angular vein

Pterygoid venous plexus

Superior labial vein

Retromandibular vein

Posterior auricular vein

Transverse sinus

Sigmoid sinus

External jugular vein

Inferior labial vein

Facial vein

Internal jugular vein

Superior vena cava

Figure 16. Veins of the head and neck.

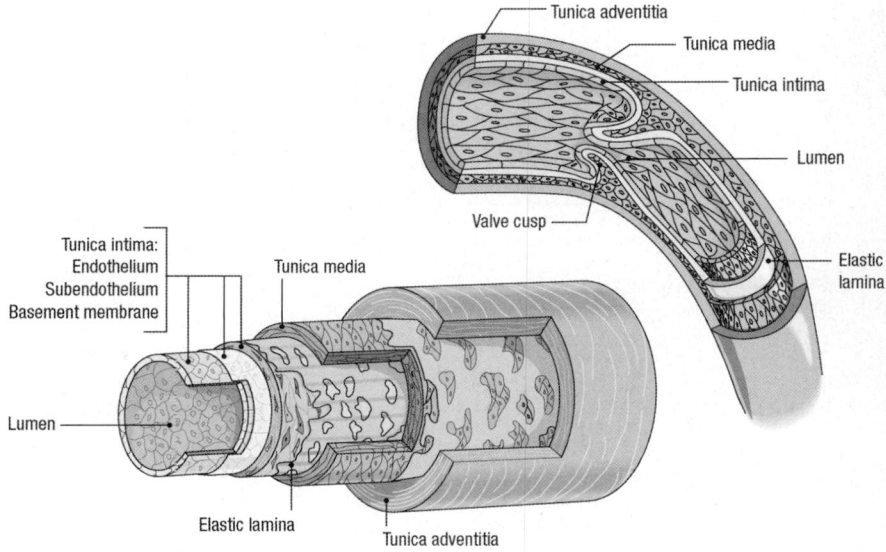

Figure 17. Structure of blood vessels. The walls of blood vessels are constructed of three concentric coats (Latin tunicae). With less muscle, veins (right) are thinner walled than their companion arteries (left) and have wide lumens (Latin lumina) that usually appear flattened in tissue sections.

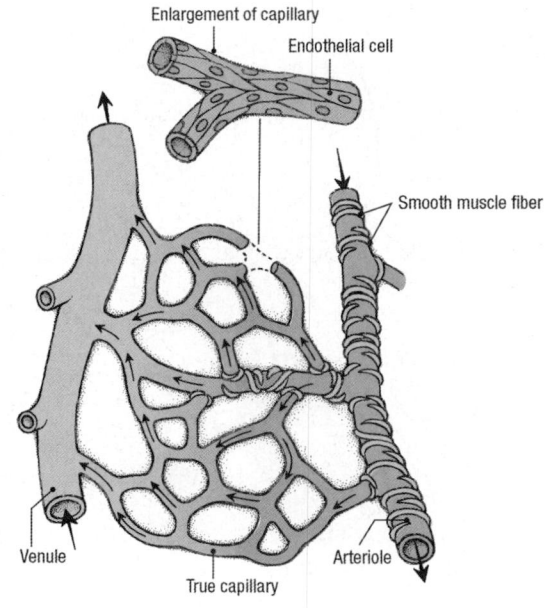

Figure 18. Capillary bed.

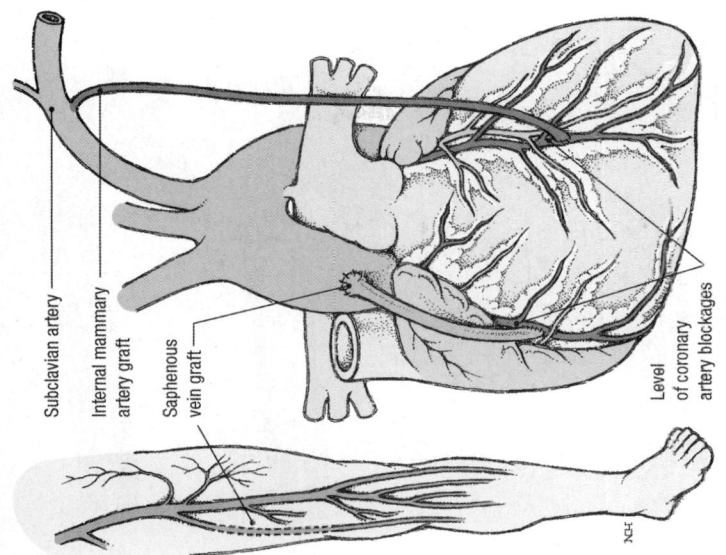

Figure 20. Aneurysm.

Subclavian artery

Internal mammary artery graft

Saphenous vein graft

Level of coronary artery blockages

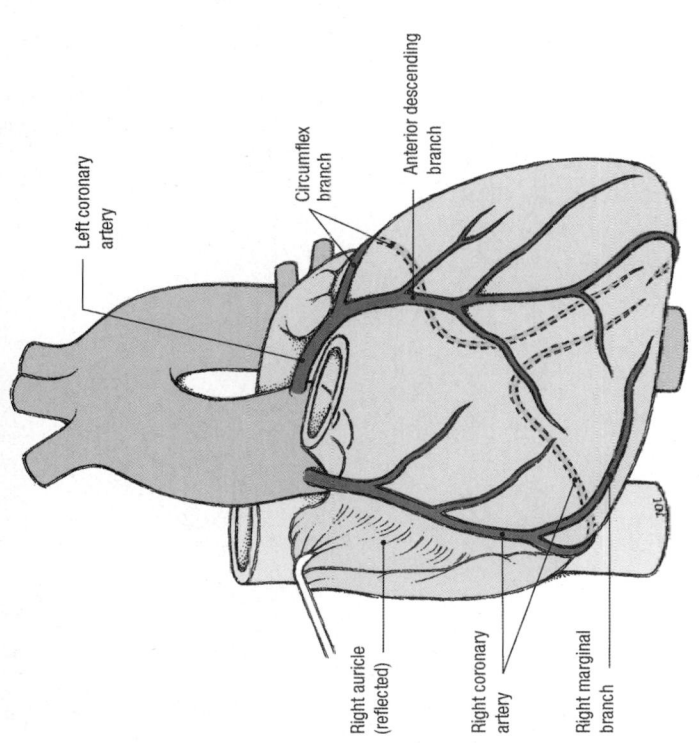

Figure 19. Coronary arteries.

Left coronary artery

Circumflex branch

Anterior descending branch

Right auricle (reflected)

Right coronary artery

Right marginal branch

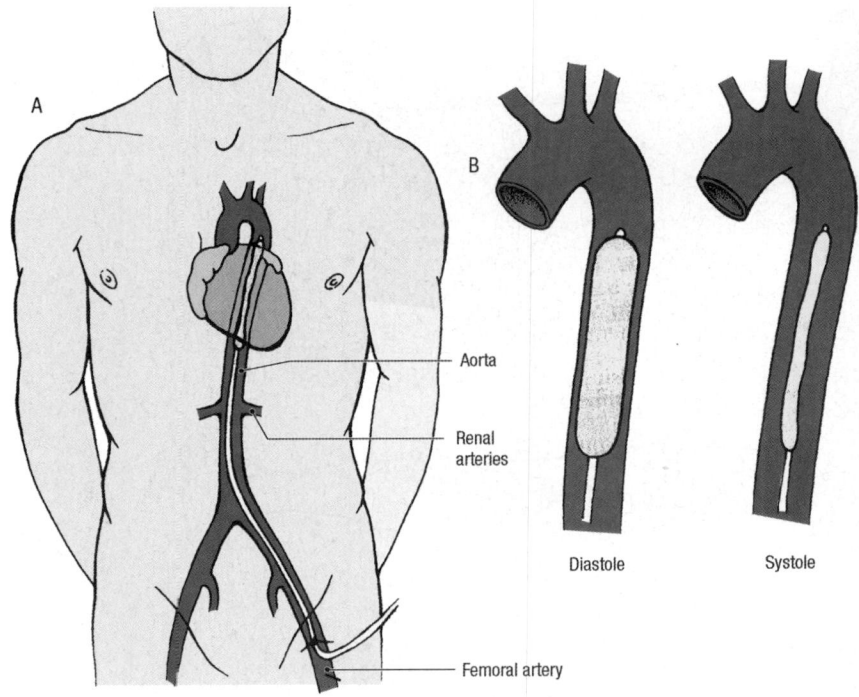

Figure 21. Counterpulsation. (A) Introduction of the intraaortic balloon catheter via the femoral artery. (B) The intraaortic balloon pump augments diastole, resulting in increased perfusion of the coronary arteries and myocardium and a decrease in the left ventricular work load.

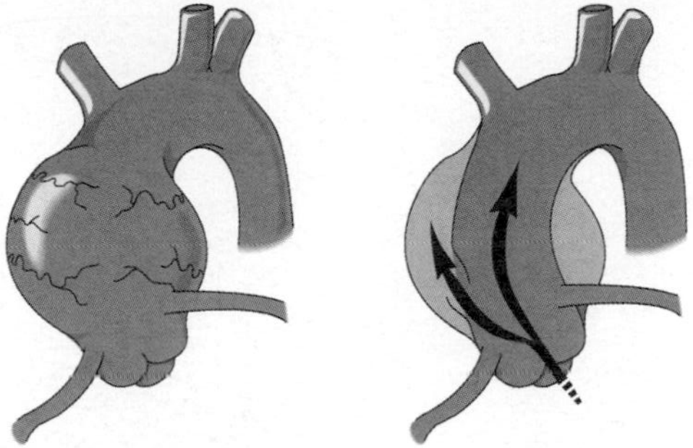

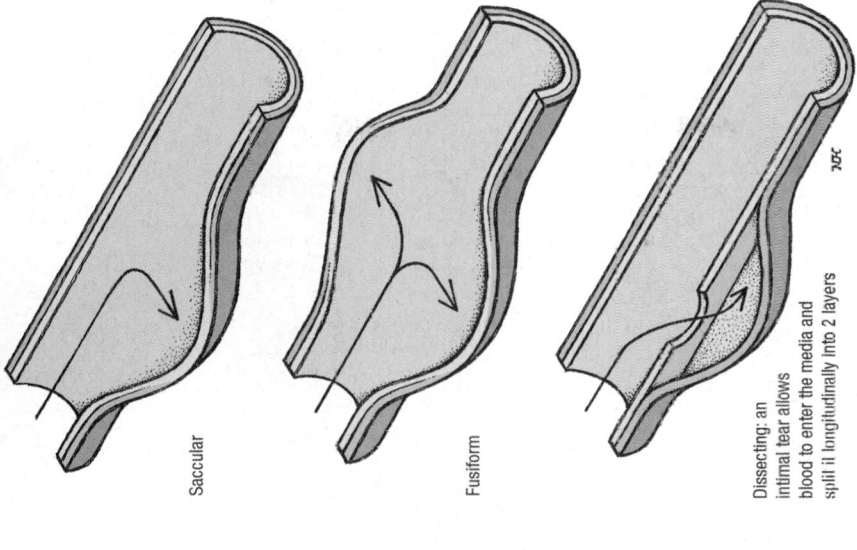

Saccular

Fusiform

Dissecting: an intimal tear allows blood to enter the media and split it longitudinally into 2 layers

Figure 24. Aneurysm.

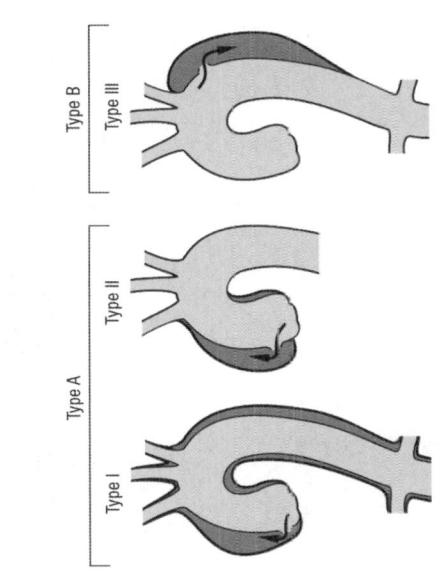

Figure 22. Different types of aortic aneurysms. (Left) ascending aortic aneurysm, (right) aortic dissection.

Type A

Type I

Type II

Type B

Type III

Figure 23. Aneurysms affecting the descending aorta: Stanford classification, Type A and Type B; deBakey classification, Types I, II, III.

A17

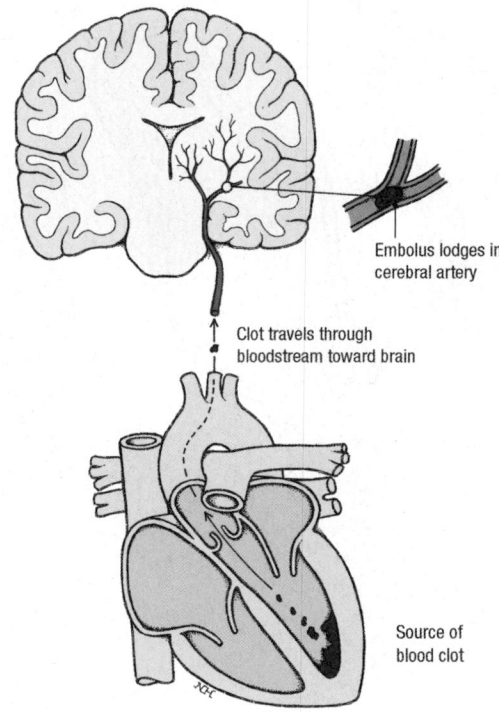

Figure 25. Embolism (embolus arising from a mural thrombus of the left ventricle).

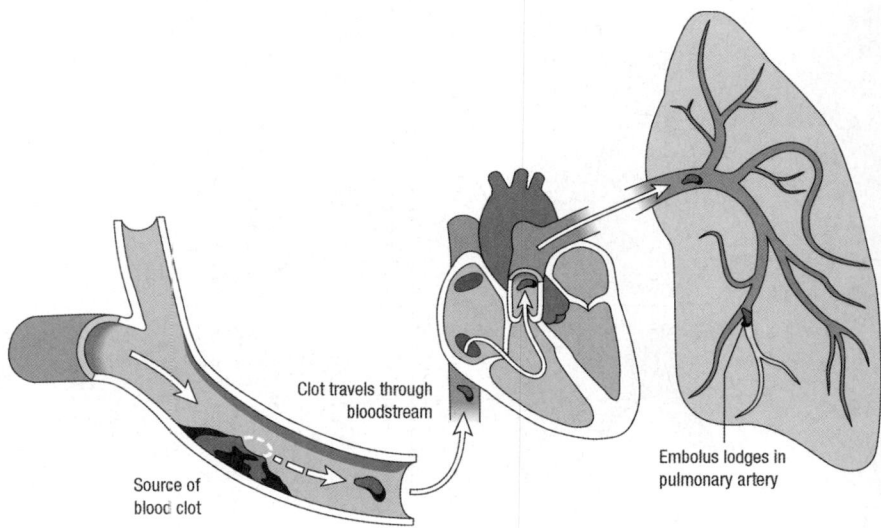

Figure 26. Embolism (embolus arising from thrombus in distal vein).

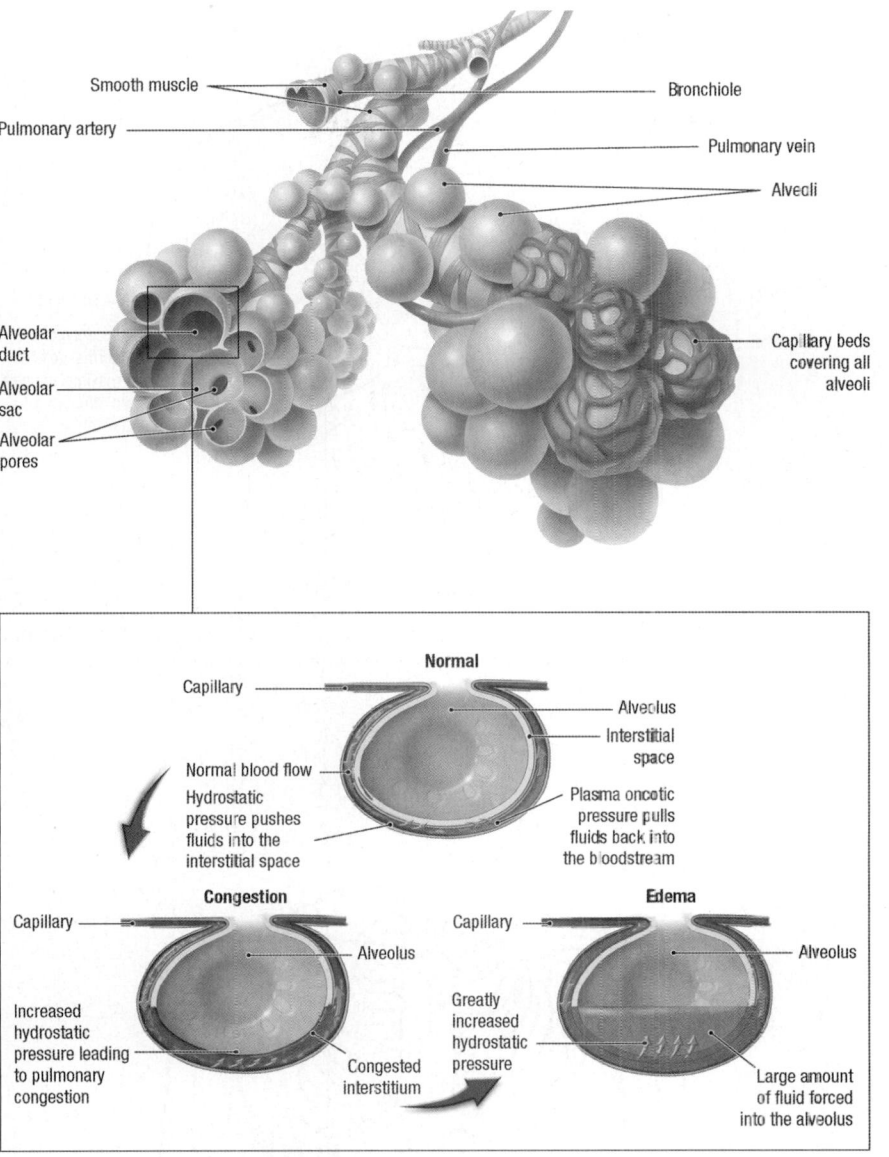

Figure 27. Normal alveoli and how pulmonary edema develops.

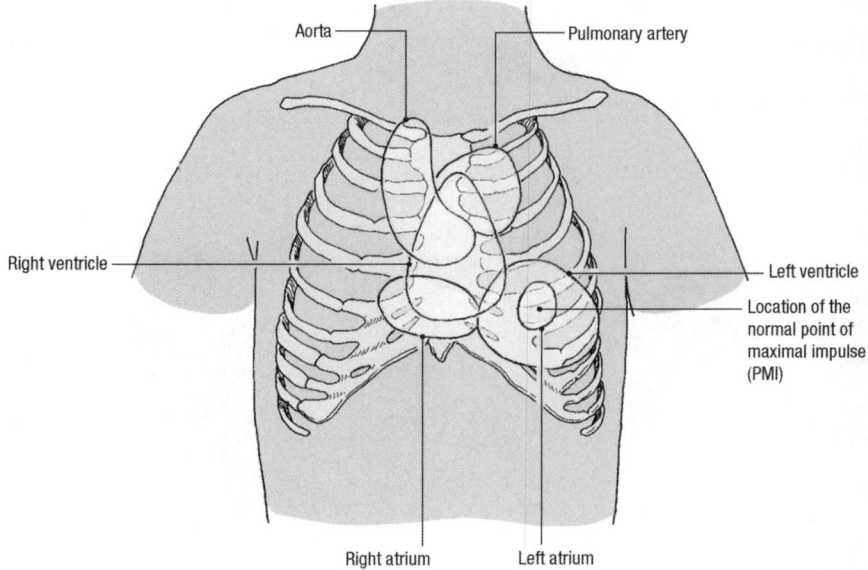

Figure 28. Auscultation points for cardiovascular structures. The sound generated by cardiovascular structures will be transmitted to areas of the chest wall that they most closely approximate.

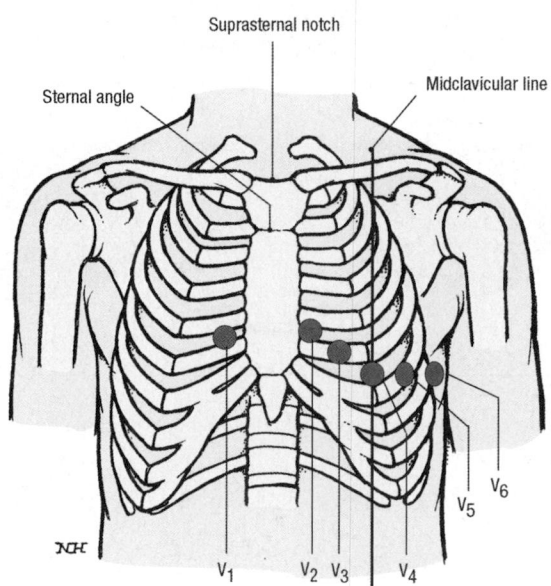

Figure 29. Electrocardiogram (ECG) lead placement: landmarks for chest lead placement.

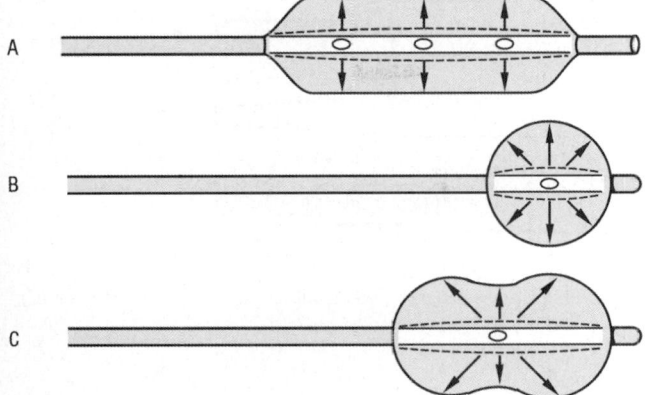

A

B

C

Figure 30. Three types of balloon catheters: (A) Gruentzig double-lumen dilation catheter, (B) Fogarty protrusion catheter, (C) double-bellied balloon catheter used to expand valves.

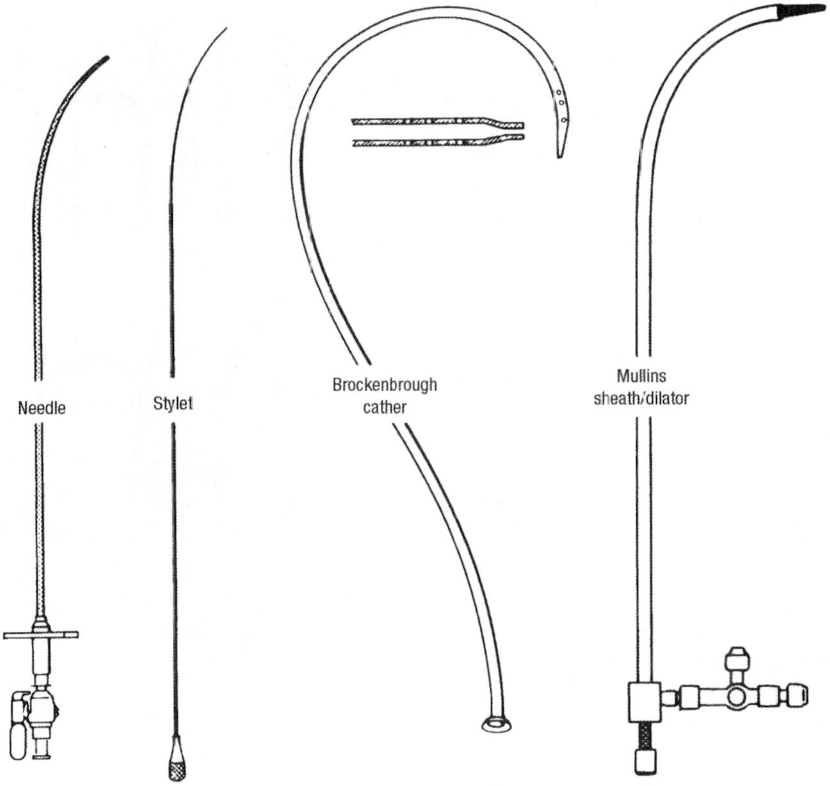

Needle   Stylet   Brockenbrough cather   Mullins sheath/dilator

A   B   C   D

Figure 31. Equipment for transseptal puncture: (A) the Brockenbrough needle; (B) Bing stylet used in conjunction with the following: (C) Brockenbrough catheter, (D) Mullins sheath/dilator system.

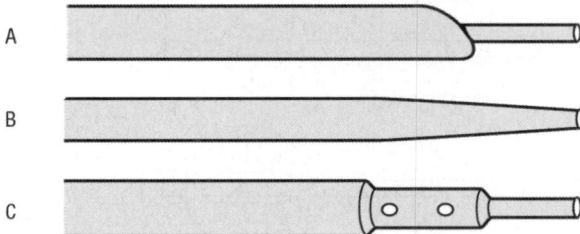

Figure 32. Catheters used to widen vessel stenosis in a stepwise manner: (A) Dotter, (B) Zeitler, (C) Andel.

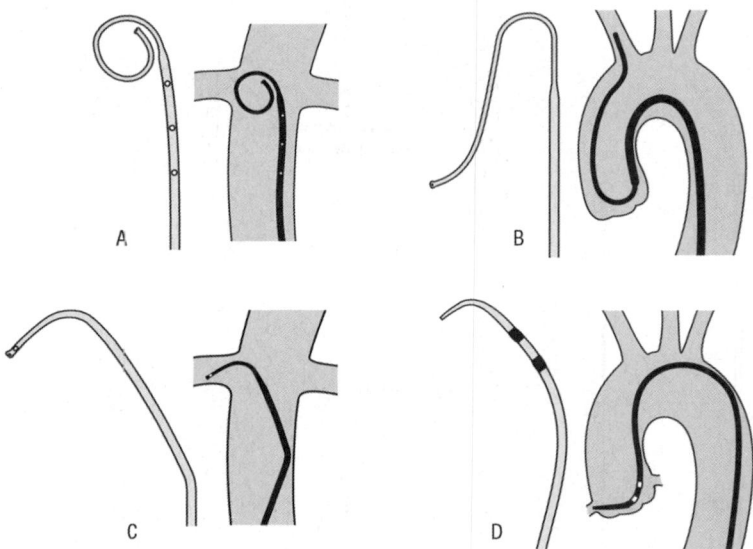

Figure 33. Various angiography catheters: (A) aorta catheter with side holes, (B) side-bending cerebral catheter (sidewinder), (C) side-bending catheter for selective viewing of visceral vessels, (D) Judkins coronary catheter.

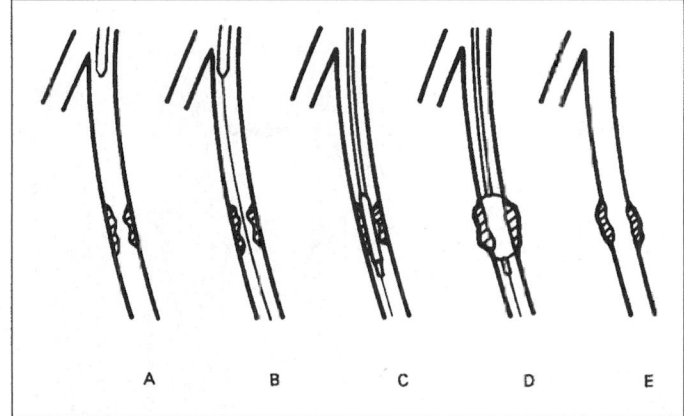

Figure 34. Balloon angioplasty. (A) Focal stenosis in superficial femoral artery, (B) Lesion is crossed with a catheter-guidewire combination, (C) Using IA DSA road-mapping or external markers, lesion is localized and balloon is positioned across it under fluoroscopic guidance, (D) When "waist" on balloon is resolved, it is deflated and safety-access 0.025-in. guidewire is introduced through hemostatic Y-connector (attached to hub). Balloon-catheter is retracted with wire across PTA site. With this setup, one can perform angiogram or "pull-back" pressure gradient without having to recross lesion, (E) When result is satisfactory, final angiogram is performed after safety wire is removed. Angioplasty tears circumferential fibers in vessel wall, increasing lumen area—plaques themselves are generally incompressible.

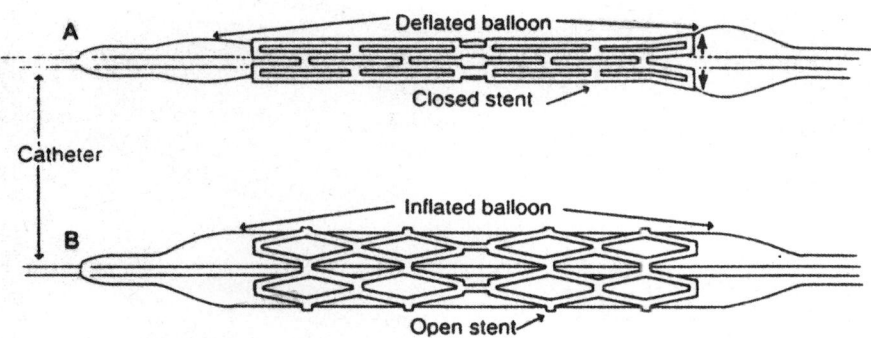

Figure 35. Intracoronary artery stent. (A) Stent closed, before balloon inflation. (B) Stent open, balloon inflated; stent will remain expanded after balloon is deflated and removed.

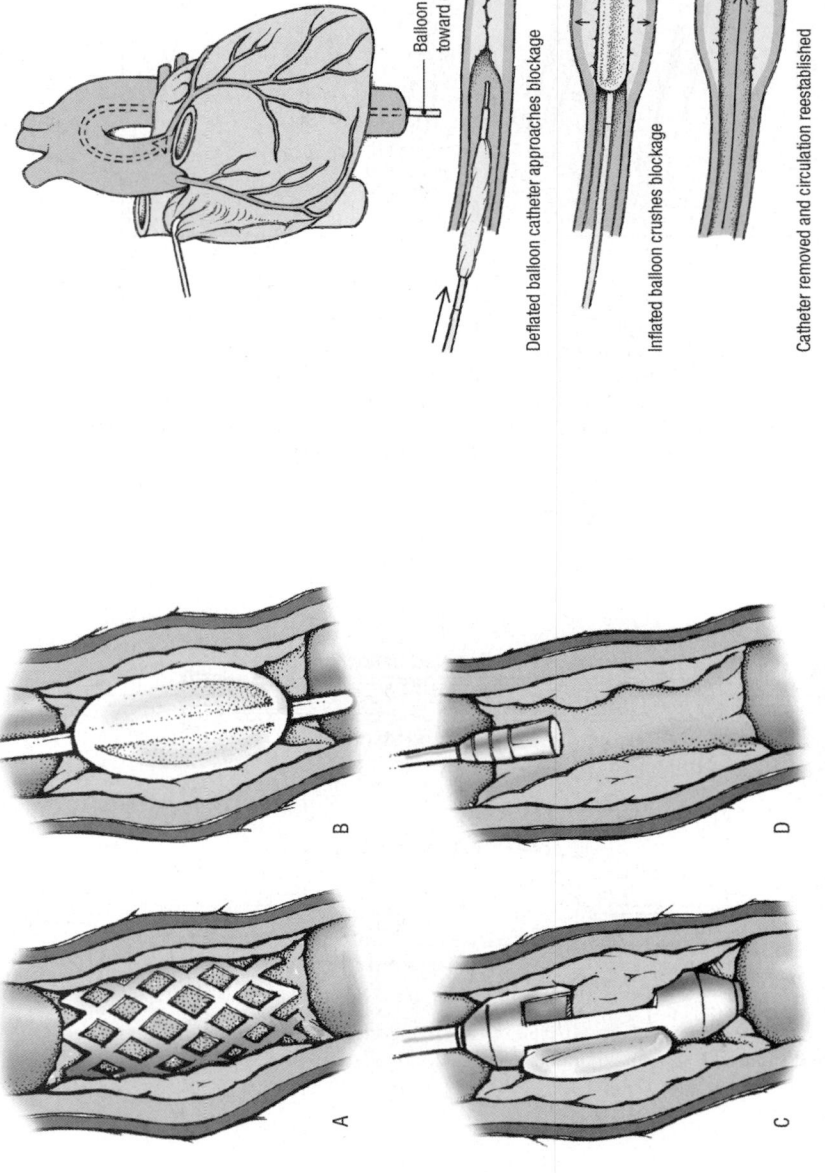

Figure 37. Percutaneous transluminal angioplasty.

Balloon catheter headed toward coronary artery

Deflated balloon catheter approaches blockage

Inflated balloon crushes blockage

Catheter removed and circulation reestablished

Figure 36. Close-up views of coronary arteries showing a variety of procedures to improve blood supply to the heart: (A) stent, (B) balloon angioplasty, (C) atherectomy, (D) laser ablation.

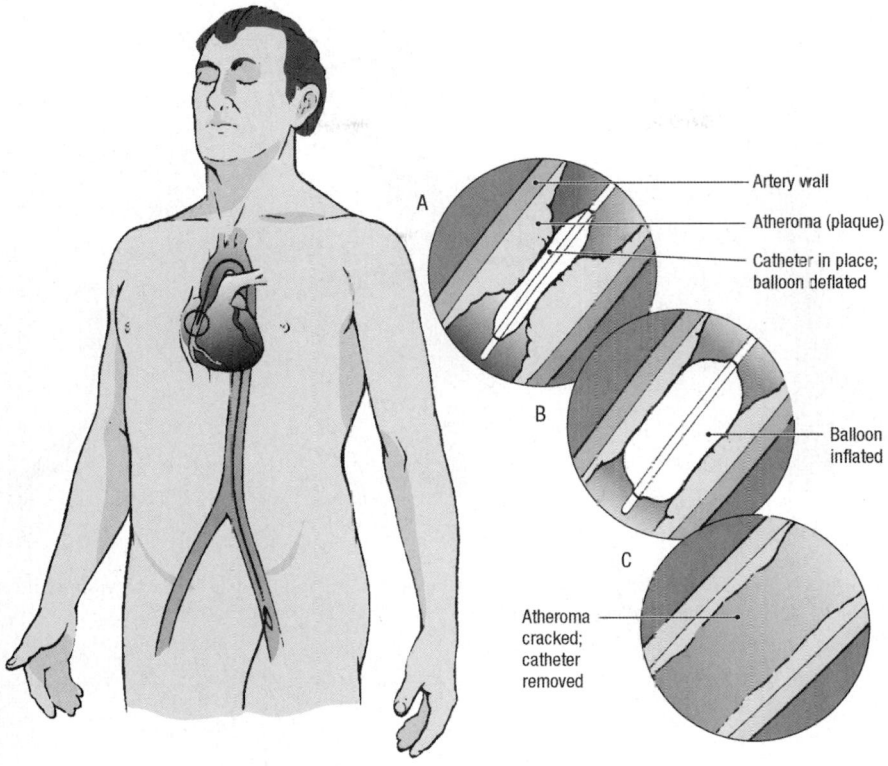

Figure 38. Percutaneous transluminal coronary angioplasty. (A) A balloon-tipped catheter is passed into the affected coronary artery and placed within the area of the atheroma (plaque). (B) The balloon is then rapidly inflated and deflated with controlled pressure. (C) After the atheroma is cracked, the catheter is removed, and blood flow improves.

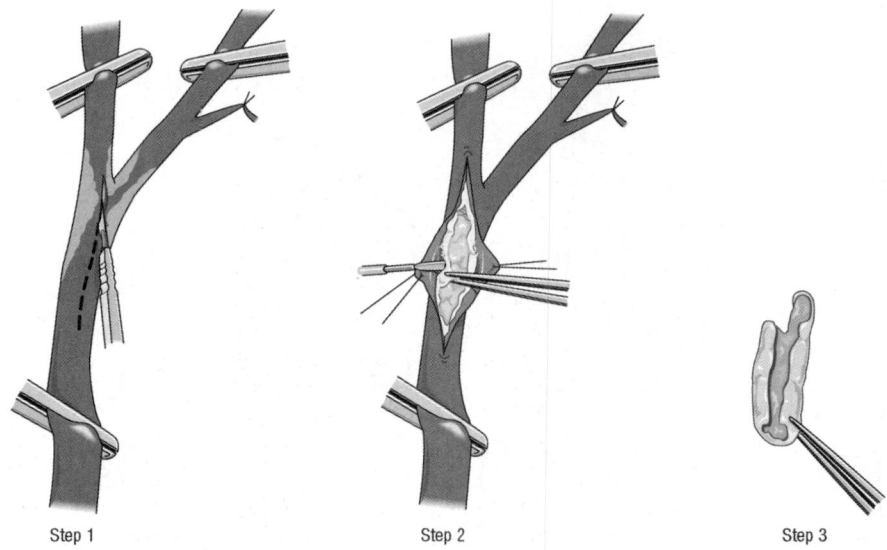

Step 1   Step 2   Step 3

Figure 39. An endarterectomy where diseased endothelium and media of an artery are removed so as to leave a smooth lining.

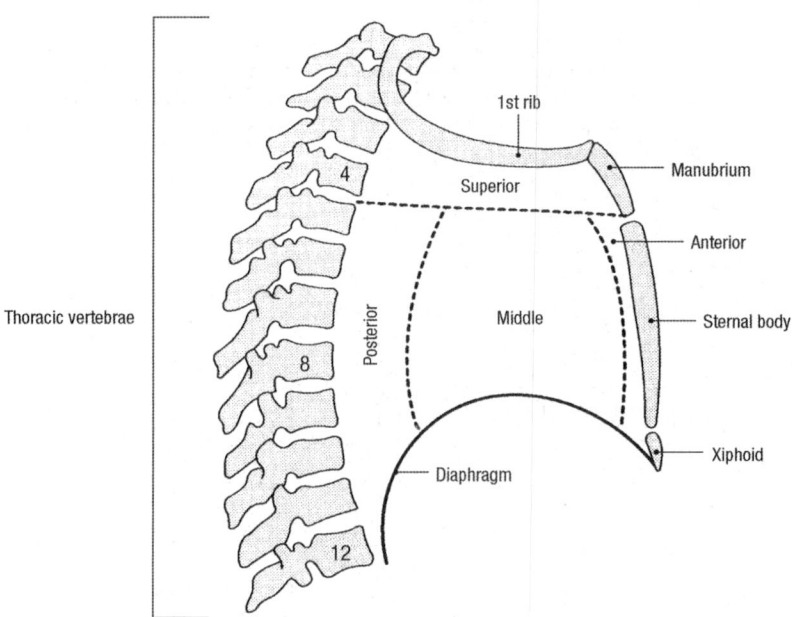

Figure 40. Mediastinum shown schematically. Viewed from a right lateral perspective, the mediastinum has four divisions: superior, posterior, middle, and anterior.

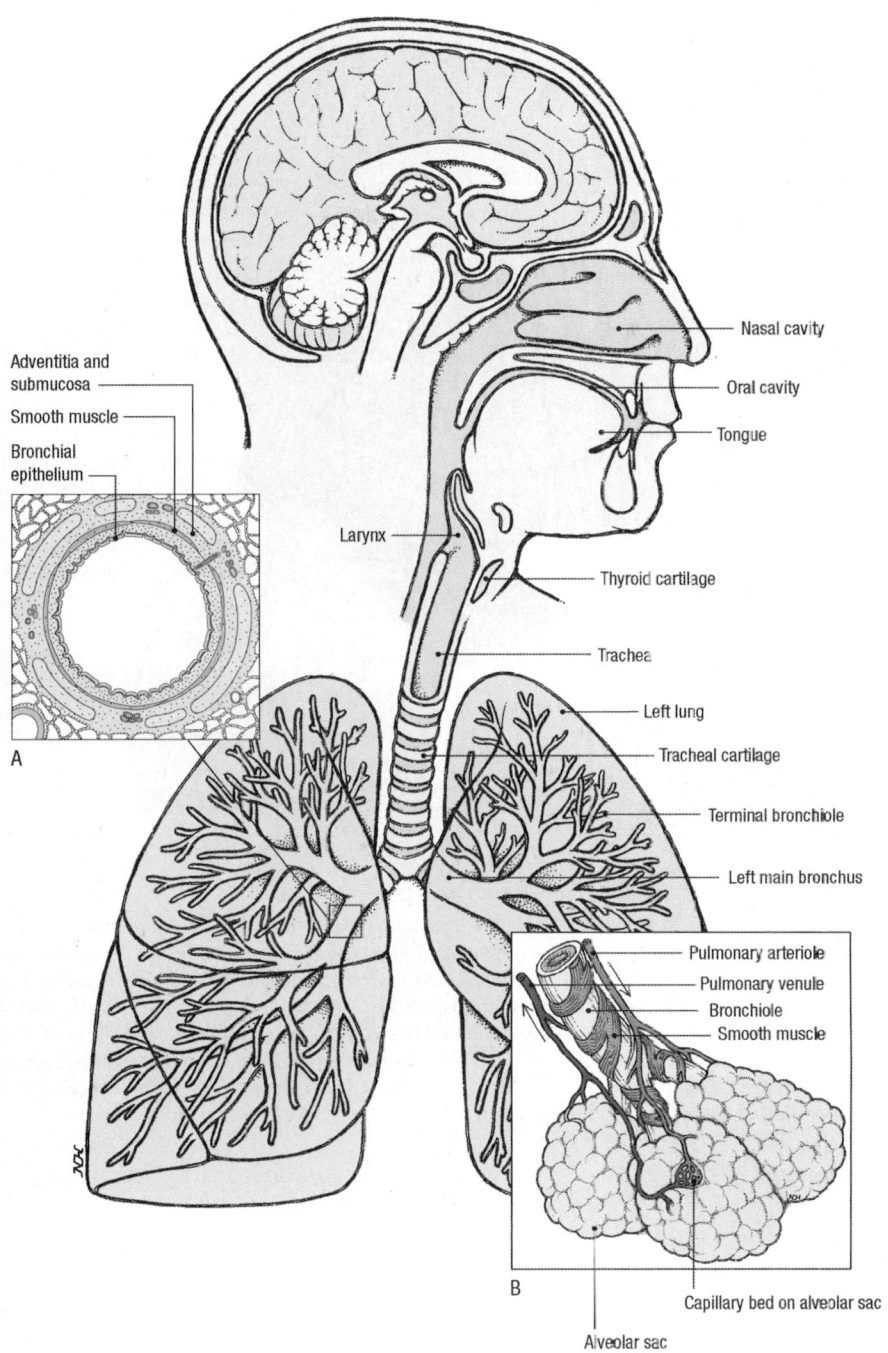

Figure 41. Lungs and respiratory anatomy. (A) intrapulmonary bronchus, (B) pulmonary alveolus.

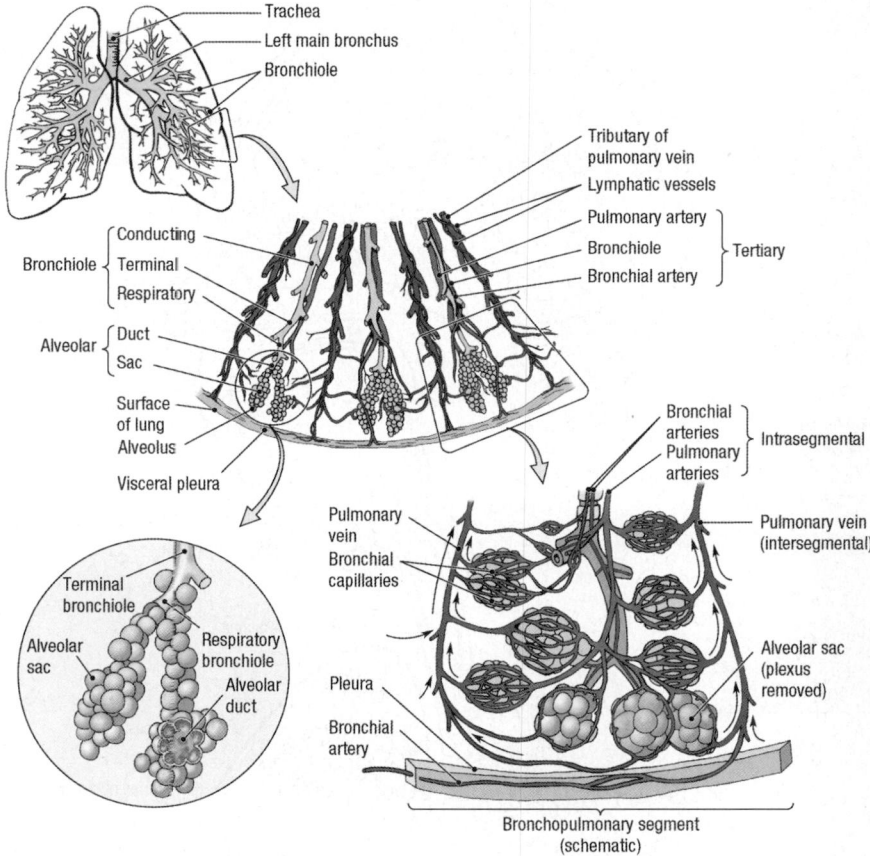

Figure 42. Structure of the lungs. The bronchopulmonary segment is the structural unit of the lung. Some 15 or more generations after the segmental bronchus, each terminal bronchiole gives rise to several generations of respiratory bronchioles, and each respiratory bronchiole gives rise to 5 or 6 alveolar sacs lined by alveoli, which are the basic structures for gas exchange. Each intrasegmental pulmonary artery, carrying poorly oxygenated blood, ends in a capillary plexus in the walls of the alveolar sacs and alveoli, where O_2 and CO_2 are exchanged. The pulmonary veins arise from the pulmonary capillaries draining toward and coursing in the septa between adjacent segments to carry well-oxygenated blood to the heart.

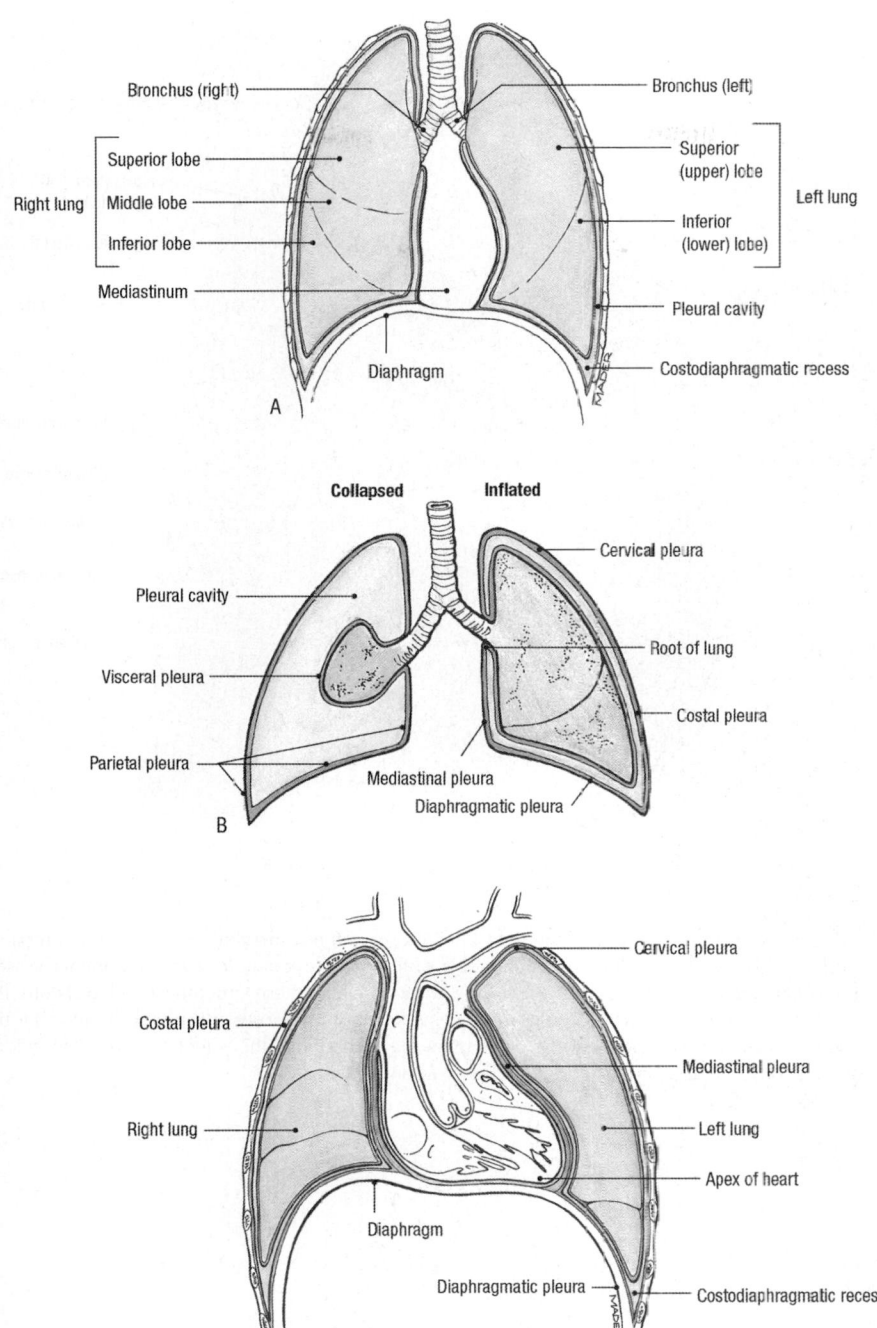

Figure 43. Respiratory system: (A) overview, (B) pleural cavity and pleura, (C) coronal section through heart and lungs.

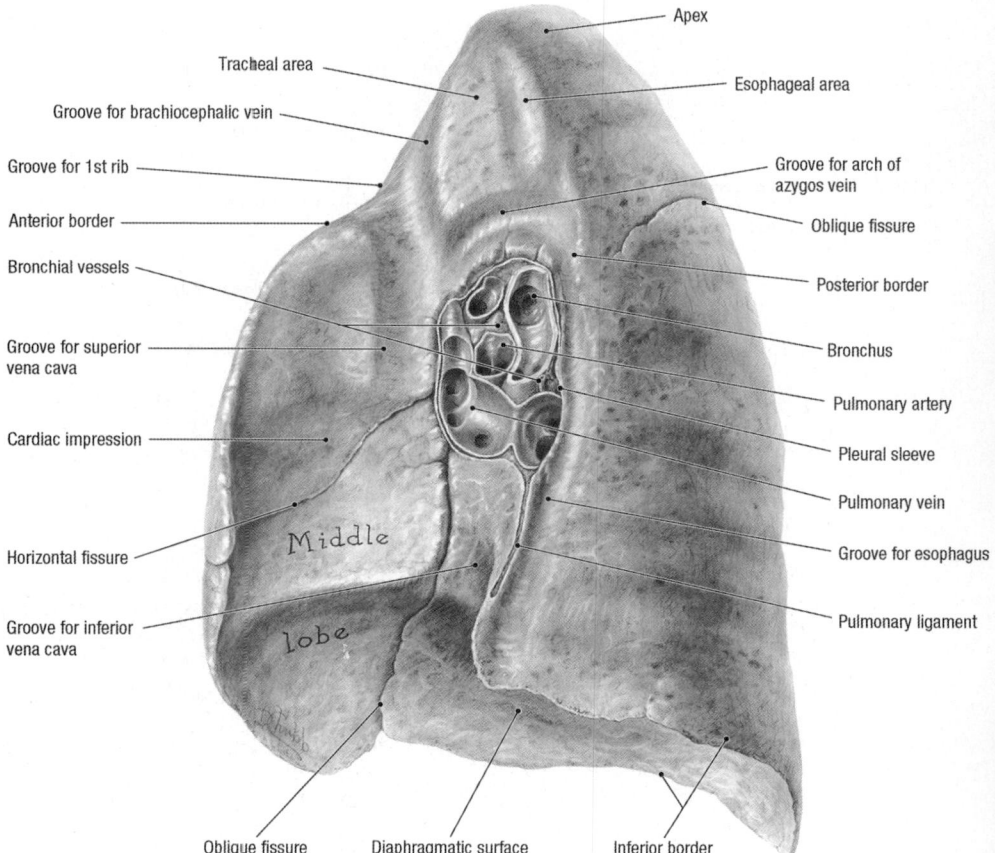

Apex

Tracheal area

Esophageal area

Groove for brachiocephalic vein

Groove for 1st rib

Groove for arch of
azygos vein

Anterior border

Oblique fissure

Bronchial vessels

Posterior border

Groove for superior
vena cava

Bronchus

Cardiac impression

Pulmonary artery

Pleural sleeve

Pulmonary vein

Horizontal fissure

Groove for esophagus

Groove for inferior
vena cava

Pulmonary ligament

Middle

lobe

Oblique fissure

Diaphragmatic surface

Inferior border

Figure 44. Mediastinal surface of the right lung. Observe the somewhat pear-shaped depression, the hilum (doorway) of the lung near the center of this surface, containing the pulmonary vessels and bronchi that constitute the root of the lung, through which these structures (cut here) enter the lung. At the hilum, note that the pulmonary veins lie most anteriorly and inferiorly and that the bronchus is central and posteriorly placed. In the right lung, the superior lobar (eparterial) bronchus may occur superior to the pulmonary artery.

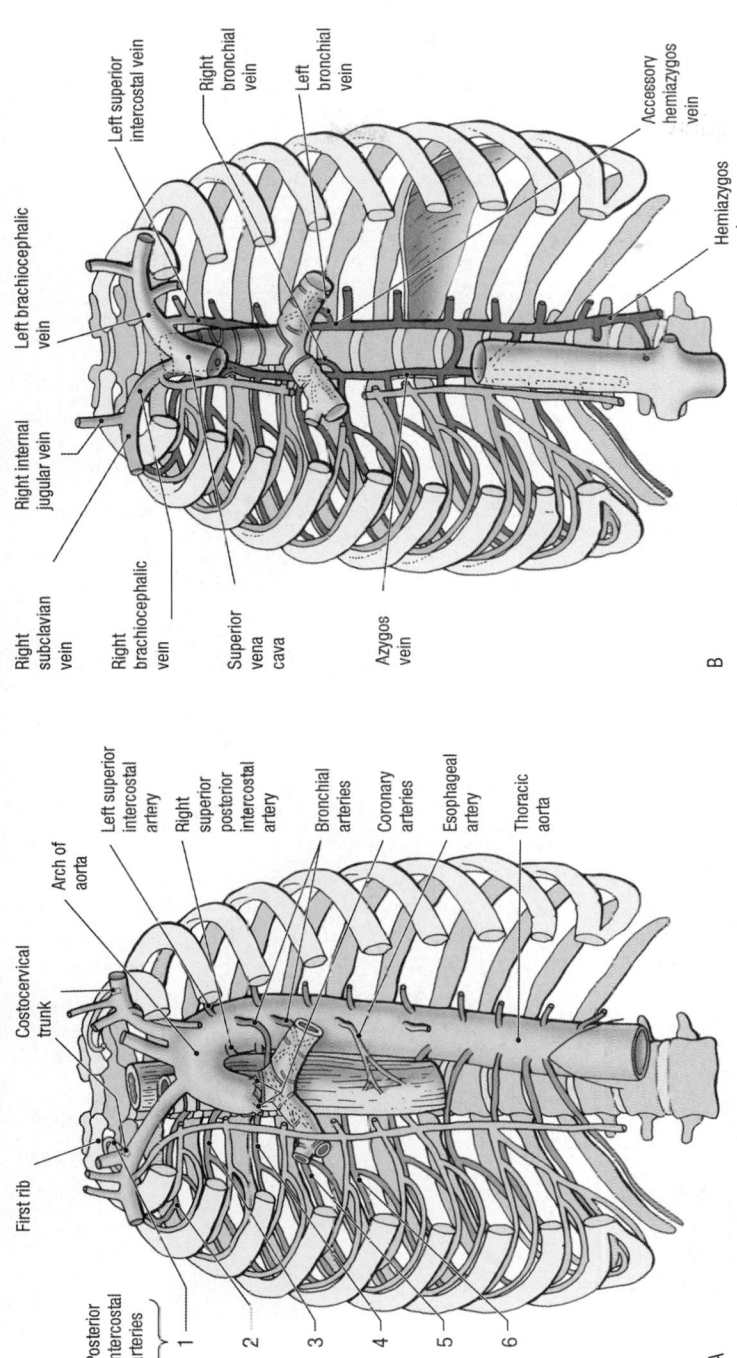

Figure 45. Bronchial arteries and veins. (A) The bronchial arteries supply blood for the nutrition of the supporting tissues of the lungs and visceral pleura. These arteries arise from the thoracic aorta but the origin of the right bronchial artery is variable. It may arise from (a) a superior posterior intercostal artery; (b) a common trunk from the thoracic aorta with the right third posterior intercostal artery; or (c) the left superior bronchial artery. (B) The bronchial veins drain some of the blood supplied to the lungs by the bronchial arteries; the rest is drained by the pulmonary veins. The right bronchial vein drains into the azygos vein and the left bronchial vein drains into the accessory hemiazygos vein or the left superior intercostal vein.

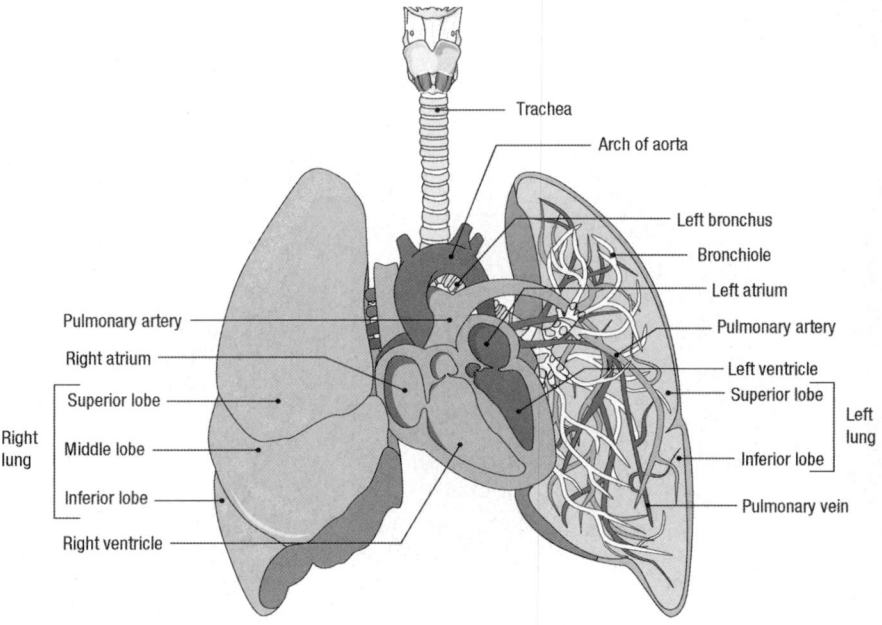

Figure 46. Cardiopulmonary system shown with cutaway of heart and left lung revealing internal anatomy.

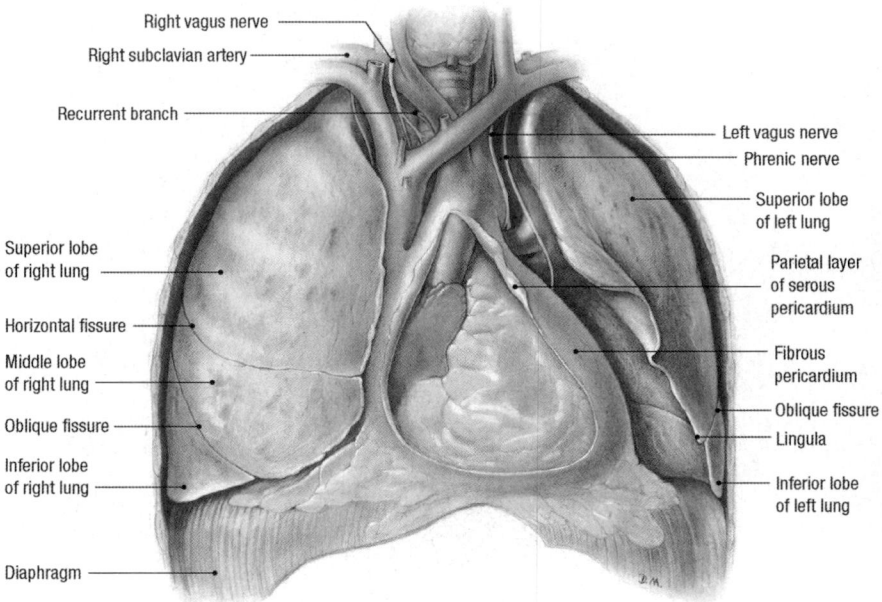

Figure 47. Thoracic contents in situ, anterior view.

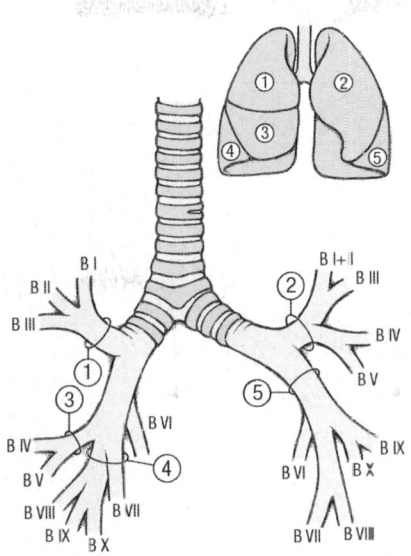

Figure 48. Segmental bronchi: right lung: (B I) apical, (B II) posterior, (B III) anterior, (B IV) lateral, (B V) medial, (B VI) apical, (B VII) medial basal, (B VIII) anterior basal, (B IX) lateral basal, (B X) posterior basal; left lung: (B I+II) apicoposterior, (B III) anterior, (B IV) superior lingular, (B V) inferior lingular, (B VI) apical, (B VII) medial basal, (B VIII) anterior basal, (B IX) lateral basal, (B X) posterior basal; lobes of lungs supplied: (1) right superior, (2) left superior, (3) right middle, (4) right inferior, (5) left inferior.

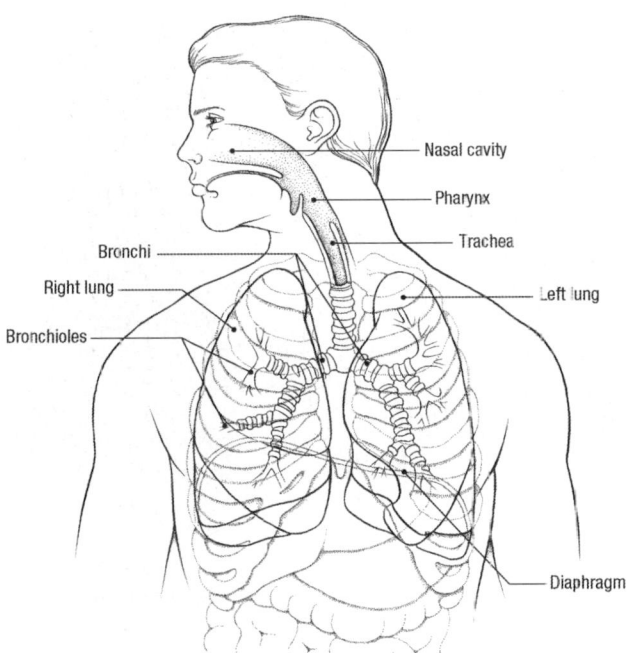

Figure 49. Anterior view of the male figure showing the main features of the respiratory system.

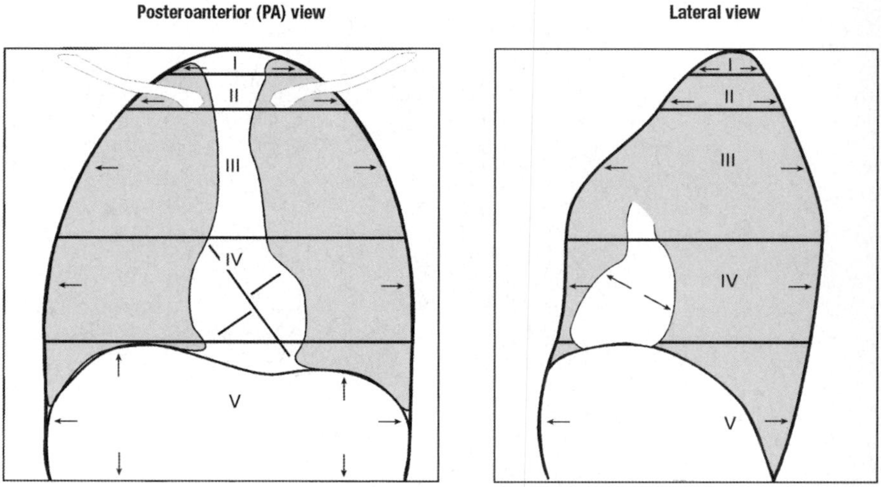

Posteroanterior (PA) view

Lateral view

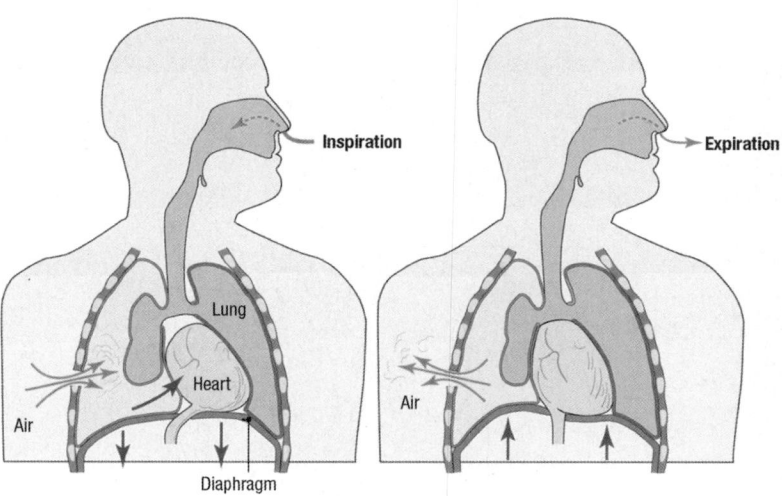

Figure 50. Posteroanterior (PA) and lateral chest films at full inspirations are divided into five (I-V) elliptical segments for measurement of total lung capacity.

Inspiration

Expiration

Lung

Heart

Air

Air

Diaphragm

Figure 51. Left illustration shows how the heart and lungs are affected during inspiration in a person with pneumothorax. Right illustration shows how the heart and lungs are affected during expiration in a person with pneumothorax.

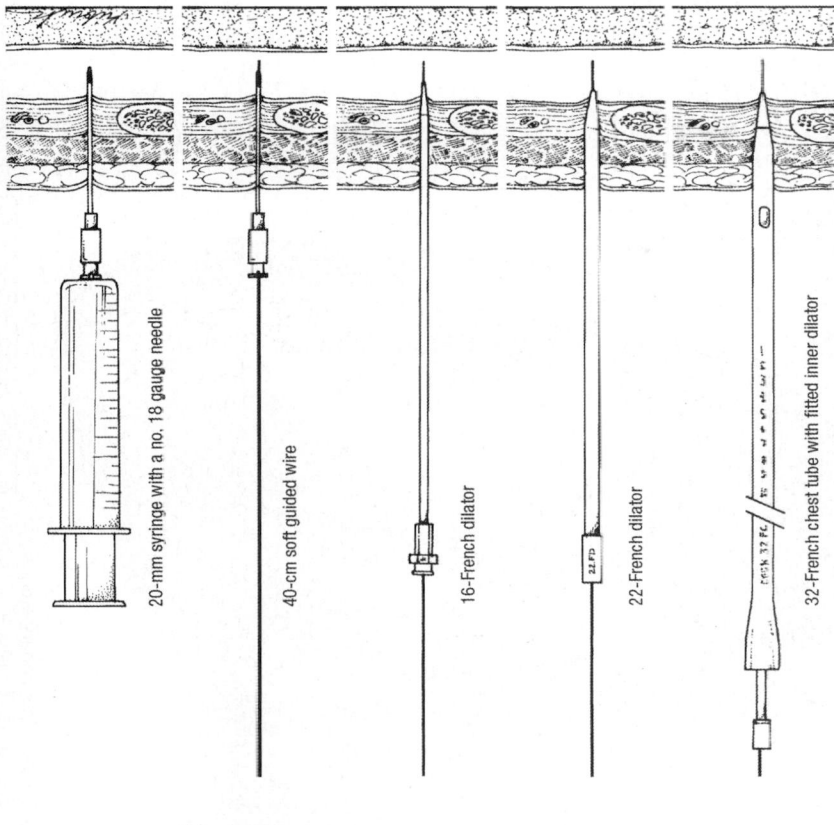

20-mm syringe with a no. 18 gauge needle

40-cm soft guided wire

16-French dilator

22-French dilator

32-French chest tube with fitted inner dilator

Figure 53. Chest tube insertion for thoracoscopy. Prior to initiating the syringe insertion, a local anesthetic is administered. Patient discomfort is minimal with use of the graduated size in dilator diameters.

swelling of mucosa

constriction of muscularis

excessive, abnormally thick mucus

normal bronchiole

bronchiole with asthma

Figure 52. Asthma: changes in bronchiole during asthma attack.

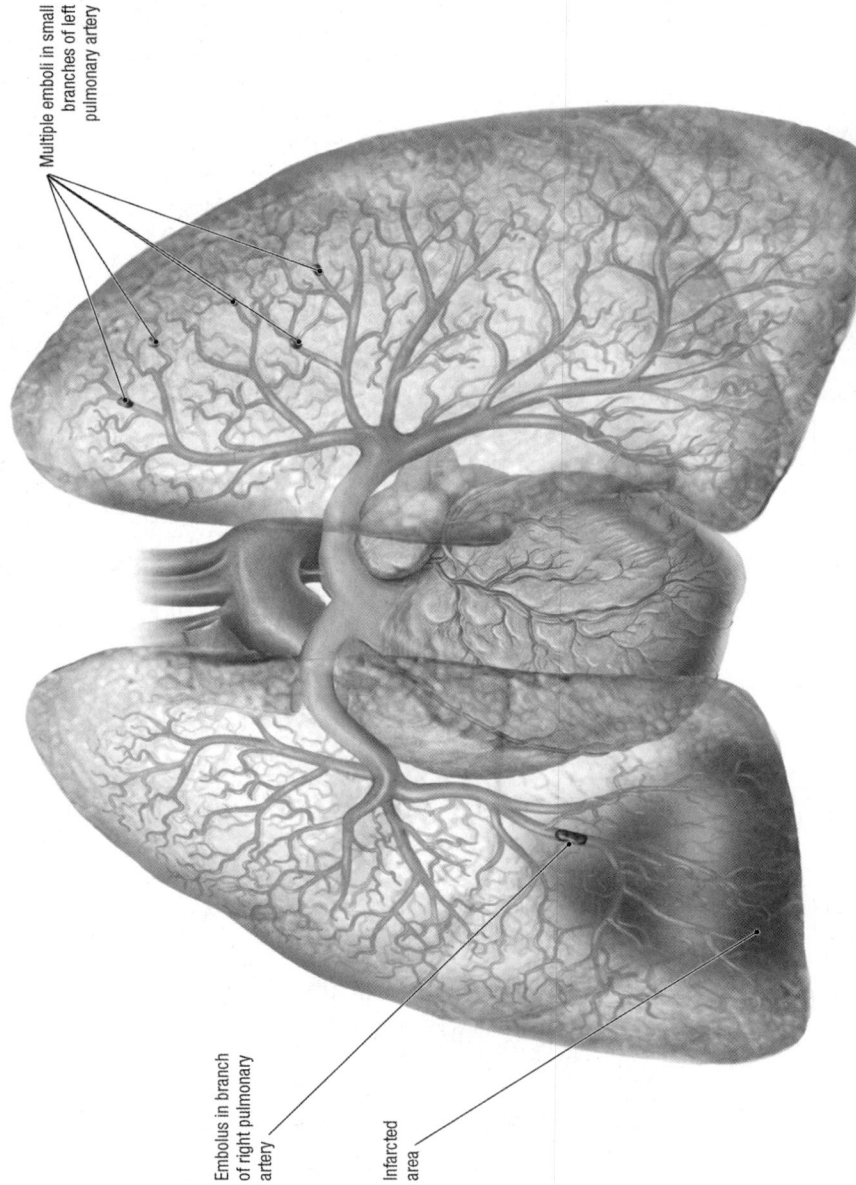

Multiple emboli in small branches of left pulmonary artery

Embolus in branch of right pulmonary artery

Infarcted area

Figure 54. Sites of pulmonary emboli.

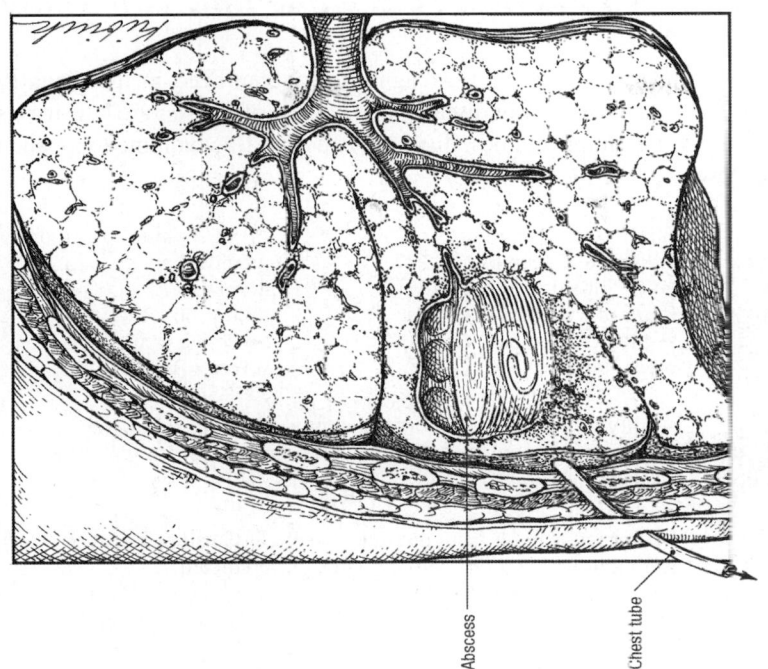

Figure 56. Chest tube placed through thoracic wall into lung in order to drain abscess.

Abscess

Chest tube

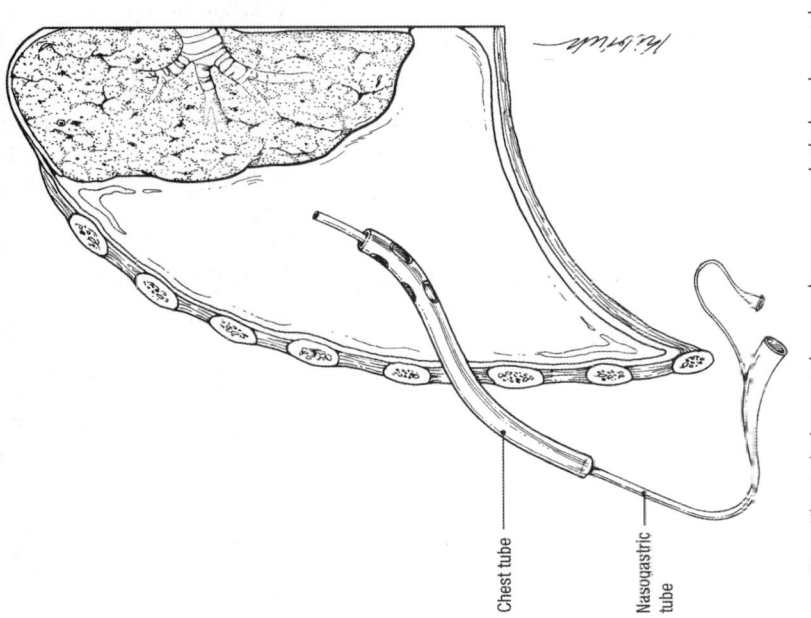

Figure 55. Chest drainage tube can become occluded and must be replaced. Using the nasogastric tube as a guide, the new chest tube is inserted over it and into the thoracic cavity.

Chest tube

Nasogastric tube

Pulmonary Function Test Table and Lab Values

Pulmonary function tests (PFTs) are diagnostic tools utilized in the diagnosis of obstructive and restrictive airway diseases and consist of 6 tests: airflow, maximum voluntary ventilation, lung volumes, diffusion capacity, flow volume loop, and arterial blood gases.

1. airflow	a. FEV1 (forced expiratory volume in 1 second) b. FVC (forced vital capacity) c. Ratio of FEV1/FVC equals % predicted; actual equals % predicted.	FEV1% values based on % of predicted: normal = 75–100% mild = 60–75% moderate = 50–60% severe = <50%
2. maximum voluntary ventilation	Ability to breathe in and out as hard and fast as possible for 10 seconds (liters/min).	Number should be approximately 40 times the FEV1.
3. lung volumes	Performed using helium dilution technique or body plethysmography. Key lung volume is total lung capacity (TLC).	TLC values based on % of predicted; restriction = <80% hyperinflation = >120%
4. diffusion capacity	Diffusion capacity of the lungs for carbon monoxide (DLCO).	Results based on the % of predicted; nonsmoker normal = <1.5 (arterial and venous) smoker normal = 1.5–5 (arterial and venous)
5. flow volume loop	Graphic display of simultaneously obtained lung volume versus airflow. Forced vital capacity (FVC) followed by forced inspiratory capacity (FIVC) maneuvers.	Flow rates are measured at 25%, 50% and 75% points.
6. arterial blood gases	Arterial blood gas (ABG) measures levels of oxygen and carbon dioxide in the blood.	

Arterial and Venous Blood Gas Normal Lab Values

Abbreviation	Description	Normal Lab Value
AVO_2	arteriovenous oxygen	3.5–5.0 vol %
BE or BD	base excess or base deficit	±3 mEq/L
CO	carbon monoxide	nonsmoker: <1.5 (arterial) nonsmoker: <1.5 (venous) smoker: 1.5–5 (arterial) smoker: 1.5–5 (venous)
COHb	carboxyhemoglobin	<1.5%
ctHb	concentration of total hemoglobin in blood	males: 14.0–18.0 g/dL females: 12.0–16.0 g/dL
ctO_2Hb	concentration of O2 in hemoglobin	15–23 vol%
HCO_3	plasma bicarbonate; an indicator of the metabolic acid-base status	male: 23–29 mmol/L (arterial) male: 25–30 mmol/L (venous) female: 20–29 mmol/L (arterial) female: 23–28 mmol/L (venous)
HHb	deoxyhemoglobin	<2.0%
MetHb	methemoglobin	<1.5%
O_2	oxygen	15–23 vol% (arterial) 15–23% vol% (venous)
O_2Hb	oxyhemoglobin	95–97 (arterial) 40–70 (venous)
P_{50}	partial pressure of O_2 at 50% of saturation	25.0–29.0 mmHg
PCO_2	partial pressure (P) of carbon dioxide (CO_2)	36–46 mmHg (arterial) 40–52 mmHg (venous)
pH	alkalinity or acidity of blood	7.35–7.46 (arterial) 7.33–7.40 (venous)
PO_2	partial pressure (P) of oxygen (O_2)	74–109 mmHg (arterial) 25–44 mmHg (venous)
SaO_2	percentage of available hemoglobin that is saturated (Sa) with oxygen (O_2)	94–100%

Pulmonary Function Terms

air trapping

airway resistance (RAW, R (AW), R_{aw})

airways hyperreactivity (AHR)

airways hyperresponsiveness (AHR)

airways obstruction (AO)

body plethysmograph

breath excretion test

breath holding test

bronchial challenge test

bronchoprovocation test

carbon monoxide diffusing capacity (DLCO, DL_{CO}, D_{CO})

exercise-induced bronchospasm (EIB)

expiratory reserve volume (ERV)

flow-sensing spirometer

flow-volume loop

forced expiration

forced expiratory capacity (FEC)

forced expiratory flow (FEF)

forced expiratory flow after 50% of vital capacity has been expelled (FEF50)

forced expiratory maneuver

forced expiratory spirogram (FES)

forced expiratory technique

forced expiratory time (FET)

forced expiratory volume (FEV)

forced expiratory volume in 1 second (FEV_1, FEV-1)

forced expiratory volume in 1 second to forced vital capacity ratio (FEV_1/FVC)

forced inspiration

forced inspiratory vital capacity (FIVC)

forced midexpiratory flow (FMF)

forced respiration

forced vital capacity (FVC)

fraction of inspired oxygen (FIO_2, FiO2, FiO_2)

functional residual capacity (FRC)

helium dilution study

hyperinflation

inhalation challenge test

inspiratory airflow

inspiratory capacity (IC)

inspiratory flow rate

inspiratory reserve volume (IRV)

inspiratory to expiratory ratio (I:E)

inspiratory vital capacity (IVC)

maximal breathing capacity (MBC)

maximal expiratory flow rate (MEFR)

maximal expiratory flow volume (MEFV)

maximal expiratory pressure (MEP)

maximal forced expiratory flow (FEFmax)

maximal inspiratory flow rate (MIFR)

maximal inspiratory pressure (MIP)

maximal midexpiratory flow rate (MMFR, MMEFR)

maximal ventilation (MV)

maximal ventilation rate (MVR)

maximal voluntary ventilation (MVV)

maximum breathing capacity (MBC)

maximum expiratory airflow-static lung elastic recoil pressure (MFSR)

maximum expiratory flow at 50% vital capacity (MEF50)

mean airway pressure (MAP)

mean forced expiratory flow rate ($FEF_{25-75\%}$)

mean forced midexpiratory flow

mean inspiratory flow (MIF)

nitrogen washout

oxygen challenge test

oxygen consumption (VO2)

oxygen saturation measured by pulse oximetry (SpO_2)

peak airway pressure (Ppeak)

peak expiratory flow (PEF)

peak expiratory flow rate (PEFR)

peak flowmeter (PFM)

peak inspiratory flow (PIF)
peak inspiratory flow rate (PIFR)
peak inspiratory pressure (PIP)
peak tidal expiratory flow (PTEF)
peak tidal inspiratory flow (PTIF)
plethysmography
positive airway pressure (PAP)
pulmonary function test (PFT)
ratio of expiratory flow to inspiratory flow at 50% of forced vital capacity (FEF_{50}/FIF_{50})
residual volume (RV)
residual volume determination
residual volume to total lung capacity ratio (RV/TLC)
respiratory distress syndrome (RDS)

respiratory disturbance index (RDI)
respiratory exchange ratio (RER)
respiratory inductive plethysmography (RIP)
respiratory quotient (RQ)
single-breath nitrogen washout (SBN2)
slow vital capacity (SVC)
spirogram
spirometry
split-function lung test
static lung compliance
thoracic gas volume (VTG)
tidal volume (VT)
total lung capacity (TLC)
vital capacity (VC)
volume displacement spirometer

Ventilation Terms

adaptive support ventilation (ASV)
airway pressure release ventilation
  (APRV)
artificial ventilation
assist control (AC)
assist-control ventilation (ACV)
assist-control mode ventilation
assisted ventilation
assisted mechanical ventilation (AMV)
backup ventilation (BUV)
bag ventilation
bilevel positive airway pressure
  (BiPAP)
continuous-flow ventilation
continuous mandatory ventilation
continuous positive airway pressure
  (CPAP)
continuous positive pressure ventilation
  (CPPV)
continuous spontaneous ventilation
  (CSV)
controlled ventilation
controlled mechanical ventilation
  (CMV)
control mode ventilation
conventional ventilation (CV)
forced mandatory intermittent
  ventilation (FMIV)
fractional inspired oxygen (FIO2)
high-frequency ventilation (HFV)
high-frequency jet ventilation (HFJV)
high-frequency oscillatory ventilation
high-frequency percussive ventilation
high-frequency positive pressure
  ventilation (HFPPV)
intermittent demand ventilation (IDV)
intermittent mandatory ventilation
  (IMV)

intermittent mechanical ventilation
  (IMV)
intermittent percussive ventilation
  (IPV)
intermittent positive pressure ventilation
  (IPPV)
intrapulmonary percussive ventilation
  (IPV)
inverse-ratio ventilation
jet ventilation
maximal voluntary ventilation (MVV)
mechanical ventilation (MV)
negative end-expiratory pressure
  (NEEP)
negative pressure ventilation (NPV)
noninvasive ventilation (NIV)
noninvasive mechanical ventilation
noninvasive positive pressure
  ventilation (NIPPV, NPPV)
peak inspiratory pressure (PIP)
positive airway pressure ventilation
  (PAPV)
positive end-expiratory pressure (PEEP)
positive pressure ventilator
pressure support ventilation (PSV)
pressure cycled ventilator
synchronized intermittent mandatory
  ventilation (SIMV)
tidal volume (VT)
time-cycled ventilator
ultrahigh frequency ventilation
ventilation meter
ventilator dependency
volume-controlled ventilation (VCV)
volume-cycled decelerating-flow
  ventilation (VCDF)
volume-cycled ventilator

Sample Reports and Dictation

ANGIOGRAPHY AND STENTING OF LEFT ANTERIOR DESCENDING ARTERY

DIAGNOSES
1. Coronary artery disease with recent hospitalization for anterior ST-elevation myocardial infarction, treated by thrombolysis using TNKase.
2. Successful angioplasty and stenting of the mid left anterior descending artery with placement of a bare-metal stent.
3. Previous history of obesity, hypertension, hypercholesterolemia, smoking, and family history of premature coronary artery disease.

CLINICAL SUMMARY: I saw the patient before her angiogram today. As you know, she is a 51-year-old female with past medical history of hypertension, hypercholesterolemia, and smoking and family history of premature coronary artery disease, who presented to hospital after symptoms of crescendo angina for 2 weeks and prolonged episode of chest pain for several hours prior to admission. In the emergency room, she was found to have anterior myocardial infarction, and in view of ongoing chest pain, she was treated by thrombolysis using TNKase. Her post-MI course was complicated with some nonsustained ventricular tachycardia and mild congestive heart failure, treated by diuresis. Her electrocardiogram developed anterior Q waves and anterolateral T-wave inversions. In view of these findings, she was referred for angiogram and possible angioplasty.

After informed consent, we obtained arterial access in the right femoral artery and used Judkins catheters for coronary angiography. This was completed without undue event. The results are as follows:
1. Left main coronary artery was angiographically normal.
2. Left anterior descending artery had mild luminal irregularities in its proximal segment and a significant culprit 80% stenosis in its midsegment. The distal LAD had mild disease.
3. The left circumflex artery had mild disease and its first obtuse marginal branch had a 50% lesion in its proximal segment.
4. The right coronary artery had mild disease, but no hemodynamically significant lesions were present.
5. Left ventricular angiography showed left ventricular end-diastolic pressure of 30 and anterolateral akinesia. The left ventricular systolic function was markedly decreased, and estimated ejection fraction was about 30%.

In view of these findings, we decided to proceed with angioplasty of the LAD. We used an EBU 4.0 guide, crossed the lesion with a Wizdom guidewire and dilated it with 3.0 x 11 balloon at 10 atmospheres. Then we placed a 3.0 x 15 Driver stent that was deployed at 18 atmospheres. The followup angiography showed excellent result with no residual stenosis and TIMI 3 flow in the distal vessel. The patient was also treated with intravenous Integrilin infusion that will be continued for the next 18 hours. The right femoral access site was closed using an Angio-Seal device without any event.

If the patient remains stable, she will be transferred back to her referring hospital in 48 hours for further management.

COMMENTS AND SUGGESTIONS
1. Coronary artery disease with recent hospitalization for anterior infarction.
2. Successful angioplasty and stenting of the mid-LAD with placement of a bare-metal stent.
3. She is advised to take aspirin 325 mg p.o. once a day and Plavix 75 mg p.o. once a day for the next 30 days to prevent stent thrombosis.
4. She will be transferred back under your care for further management.

ANGIOPLASTY AND STENTING USING CRUSH TECHNIQUE

DIAGNOSES
1. Coronary artery disease. Recent hospitalization for a non-ST elevation myocardial infarction, complicated by acute pulmonary edema.
2. Successful angioplasty and stenting of the mid right coronary artery with placement of a Taxus paclitaxel-eluting stent.
3. Successful angioplasty and stenting of the distal right coronary artery involving the origin of the posterior descending artery branch with placement of Taxus paclitaxel-eluting stents with crush technique.

CLINICAL SUMMARY: I saw the patient before his angioplastic procedure today. As you know, he is a 75-year-old gentleman with past medical history of type 2 diabetes, hypercholesterolemia, and remote smoking who was in his usual state of health until he was admitted with acute pulmonary edema and was treated by BiPAP. He also was found to have a non-ST elevation myocardial infarction by elevated troponin levels. His post-MI course was uncomplicated, and he was subjected to cardiac catheterization. The coronary angiogram demonstrated angiographically normal left main coronary artery, mild disease of the left anterior descending artery, moderate disease of the first diagonal branch of the LAD, moderate disease of the left circumflex artery, a significant 70% lesion in the mid right coronary artery, and an 80% lesion at the ostium of the PDA branch. There were moderate calcifications noted in the coronary system. He had grade 3 left ventricular systolic function with anterolateral and inferior hypokinesia. In view of these findings, he was referred for angioplasty of the right coronary artery.

After informed consent, we obtained arterial access in the right femoral artery and used a 7-French AR-2 guiding catheter. We placed a Wizdom guidewire in the posterolateral branch of the RCA and a Whisper guidewire in the PDA branch of the RCA. First we dilated the mid-RCA lesion with a 2.5 x 15 balloon at 15 atmospheres. Then we dilated the ostial PDA lesion with a 2.5 x 12 balloon at 12 atmospheres. Then we advanced a 2.75 x 16 stent in the PDA branch of the RCA and a 3.5 x 16 stent in the posterolateral branch. These stents were deployed using crush technique. Then we had significant difficulty recrossing the PDA stent for post dilatation. Finally, we were able to cross back into the PDA branch with the Whisper guidewire and first dilated it with a 1.5 x 11 Mercury balloon. Then we used a 2.0 x 11 Mercury balloon in the PDA stent that was inflated up to 20 atmospheres. Then we placed a 2.75 x 13 PowerSail in the PDA branch and a 3.5 x 13 PowerSail in the posterolateral stent. Both of these balloons were simultaneously inflated for up to 14 atmospheres using kissing stent technique. The final angiogram showed excellent result with no residual stenosis and TIMI 3 flow in the distal vessel.

Then we wanted to place a 3.5 x 28 Taxus paclitaxel-eluting stent in the mid-RCA but we could not advance the stent to the desired location. We postdilated the mid lesion first with a 3.25 x 20 Quantum balloon at 20 atmospheres and then further postdilated this lesion with a 3.5 x 15 PowerSail balloon at 20 atmospheres. Then we had to change the guidewire to a balanced heavy-weight guidewire, and finally we were successfully able to place a 3.5 x 28 Taxus paclitaxel-eluting stent in the mid-RCA that was inflated up to 16 atmospheres. The final angiography showed excellent results with no residual stenosis and TIMI 3 flow in the distal vessel. There were no complications during this procedure. The patient was also treated with intravenous ReoPro infusion that will be continued for next 12 hours. An 8-French Angio-Seal was placed in the right femoral artery without an event.

Anticipating the patient experiences a stable hospital course, he will be transferred back to his referring hospital in 48 hours.

COMMENTS AND SUGGESTIONS
1. Coronary artery disease with recent hospitalization for non-ST elevation myocardial infarction complicated by pulmonary edema.
2. Successful angioplasty and stenting of the mid-RCA with placement of a Taxus stent.
3. Successful angioplasty and stenting of the distal RCA, origin of the PDA branch, and posterolateral branch with placement of Taxus stents with crush technique.
4. The patient is advised to take aspirin 325 mg p.o. once a day and Plavix 75 mg p.o. once a day for the next 12 months to prevent stent thrombosis.

CARDIOVERSION

PROCEDURE PERFORMED: Cardioversion.

INDICATIONS FOR PROCEDURE: Atrial fibrillation.

DESCRIPTION OF PROCEDURE: The patient was consented. She was sedated by the anesthesiologist. She was shocked at 100 J on a biphasic machine with only 1 attempt. She promptly cardioverted to sinus rhythm. The patient tolerated the procedure well without complications and was discharged to home.

CHEST PAIN CARDIOLOGY CONSULTATION

REASON FOR ADMISSION: The patient is a 65-year-old gentleman who presents to the hospital with chest pain.

REASON FOR CONSULTATION: I was asked to evaluate the patient's chest pain and cardiac function.

HISTORY OF PRESENT ILLNESS: The patient states he has had no prior chest pain or cardiac problems. He was in his usual state of health yesterday, when he suddenly developed onset of retrosternal chest pressure. This pressure did not radiate, but the patient did experience diaphoresis at the time of the chest discomfort. He had no nausea or vomiting. The pain was described as relatively severe and was rated a 6/10 by the patient.

An electrocardiogram in the emergency room showed sinus rhythm with nonspecific T-wave changes in leads V2, V3, and aVL. There was no ischemia noted. The patient's first set of cardiac enzymes was normal.

The patient was given sublingual nitroglycerin in the emergency room, and at the time of my evaluation states he is pain free. The telemetry monitor reveals a sinus rhythm.

PAST MEDICAL HISTORY: The patient has a history of emphysema and chronic obstructive pulmonary disease. He also has type 2 diabetes mellitus.

PAST SURGICAL HISTORY: History of tonsillectomy as a child and appendectomy 10 years ago.

CARDIAC RISK FACTORS: The patient quit smoking more than 15 years ago. He used to smoke 1 pack per day. The patient's cholesterol level has been slightly elevated for the last several years. The patient does have an aunt with a heart condition, but he cannot state the exact nature of that condition. The patient has never been told he has hypertension.

MEDICATIONS: None. The patient's diabetes mellitus is diet controlled.

PHYSICAL EXAMINATION

GENERAL: This is a pleasant gentleman in no apparent distress at the present time.

VITAL SIGNS: Blood pressure 125/68, pulse 72, respiratory rate 16, and temperature 98.6.

HEENT: Atraumatic, normocephalic. Pupils equal, round, and reactive to light and accommodation. Extraocular movements are intact.

NECK: Supple. No jugular venous distention.

LUNG: Clear to auscultation.

HEART: Regular rate and rhythm. No gallop or murmur heard.

ABDOMEN: Soft and nontender. Liver and spleen not palpable.

EXTREMITIES: Warm and dry. No cyanosis, clubbing, or edema.

NEUROLOGIC: Cranial nerves II through XII are intact.

IMPRESSION: The patient is a gentleman who presents with chest discomfort, found to have nonspecific changes on electrocardiogram in the emergency room. His enzymes have been normal thus far. The patient's cardiac risk factors are diabetes mellitus and tobacco use in the past.

PLAN: I will place the patient on a rule-out myocardial infarction protocol. If he rules out for a myocardial infarction, I would recommend the patient undergo a stress test tomorrow. Further recommendations will be based on the results of these studies.

CORONARY ANGIOPLASTY: 3-VESSEL

SUMMARY: I performed coronary angioplasty on the patient, who is a 77-year-old woman admitted with prolonged episodes of chest pain. The troponin was above 40.

She had a non-ST segment elevation myocardial infarction. Her ECG showed tall R waves in leads V1 and V2 with some T-wave inversion in V5-V6, consistent with possibly posterior wall myocardial infarction. She subsequently underwent coronary angiography. This showed triple-vessel disease. There were significant lesions in the distal RCA and the midcircumflex (which was likely the culprit vessel), and a moderate lesion in the proximal mid-LAD (which was quite a long lesion).

She had a 2D echo, which showed grade 2 left ventricular function. The midlateral wall was hypokinetic, and the entire posterior wall was akinetic.

She appears to be a recently diagnosed diabetic. Her hemoglobin A1c was 6.8%. Her random blood sugars have been high. She has hypercholesterolemia and is on medication. Her most recent cholesterol value showed a total cholesterol of 4.80, triglyceride 1.34, HDL 1.25, and LDL 2.93 with a cholesterol-to-HDL ratio of 3.84. She is a nonsmoker. She does have history, as well, of hypertension.

Past surgical history includes hysterectomy and cataract surgery.

Her current medications include Plavix (which was started a few days ago), enteric-coated aspirin, Lipitor 40 mg daily, metoprolol 50 mg b.i.d., Altace 2.5 mg b.i.d., and Pantoloc 40 mg daily. She also has been on enoxaparin.

On examination, blood pressure was 120/60, heart rate 70 beats per minute and regular, and chest was clear. Cardiovascular examination was normal. No extra heart sounds or murmurs were heard. Peripheral pulses were palpable.

A 12-lead ECG showed sinus rhythm at 73 beats per minute. There were tall R waves in V1 and V2.

A coronary angioplasty was performed. The right femoral artery approach was used. Initially we did the lesion in the distal right coronary artery. After crossing the stenosis with a guidewire, dilated with a 2.5-mm balloon, then placed in a 2.5-mm diameter, 15-mm length Minivision stent. This gave an excellent angiographic result with no residual stenosis. There was TIMI 3 flow.

We then proceeded to do lesions in the circumflex and LAD. The circumflex was crossed with a guidewire and then predilated with a 2.5-mm balloon. We then placed a 3.0-mm diameter, 17-mm length Exulter stent, post-dilated inside the stent with a 3.0-mm balloon at high pressure. This gave an excellent angiographic result in the midcircumflex with a reduction in stenosis from 90% to 0%. There was TIMI 3 flow.

The last lesion was done in the proximal LAD. In fact this was a long segment of disease; most of the time was about 50% and went to about 70% at its more severe part. It was predilated with a 2.5-mm balloon. We then placed a 3.0-mm diameter,

32-mm length Taxus stent, which was a paclitaxel drug-eluting stent, postdilated inside the stent with a 3.0-mm balloon at high pressure. This gave an excellent angiographic result with no residual stenosis. There was TIMI 3 flow in the distal vessel.

The procedure was done under Integrilin. An Angio-Seal device was placed on the right femoral area at the end of the case. The procedure was well tolerated.

SUMMARY

She has undergone triple-vessel stenting with a drug-eluting stent in the LAD and bare-metal stent in the midcircumflex and distal RCA. The procedure was well tolerated. She will need to stay on Plavix for at least 1 year and long-term aspirin therapy. In addition, she will need further followup of her blood sugars, which were a little elevated on her recent hospitalization.

CORONARY ANGIOPLASTY: 2-VESSEL

PREOPERATIVE DIAGNOSIS: Two-vessel coronary artery disease.

POSTOPERATIVE DIAGNOSIS: Two-vessel coronary artery disease.

PROCEDURE PERFORMED: Coronary angioplasty.

HISTORY AND INDICATIONS FOR PROCEDURE: This 67-year-old male was referred for cardiac catheterization, which revealed 2-vessel coronary disease suitable for angioplasty which we performed today.

The patient has had angina for a couple months. Stress testing was positive. There is a family history of heart disease, but he has not been a smoker. His blood pressure has been up recently. He has enjoyed pretty good health otherwise.

Procedure: We performed the procedure today through the right femoral artery. We used a 7-French guide because we knew we were going to have some issues with tortuosity in the right coronary artery.

We first approached the LAD lesion, which was not easy in itself. This was a calcified lesion which did not dilate readily. With high pressure inflations, we did predilate the lesion nicely and then implanted a 3-mm stent that was 24-mm long. We postdilated the stent with a 3.25-mm high-pressure balloon, and the final result was excellent. I was a little concerned about the distal end of the stent. I wondered if there was a small dissection there, so we performed intracoronary vascular ultrasound, and this, indeed, showed that there was no dissection, and the stent was well deployed.

The right coronary artery was very tortuous. We used an AL-1 guide catheter, which was again a 7-French catheter, for extra support. We put a guidewire through the lesion. Because the vessel was so tortuous, we ended up with some invagination of the endothelium in the proximal segment. This has been called the "accordion effect." We then deployed a stent which was 16-mm long and 3.25 mm in diameter in the end lesion. The final result was excellent. We then pulled the guidewire back and repeated the angiogram, and the accordion effect had disappeared. I was pleased with the result. There was other plaque in this right coronary artery which amounts to several 40% lesions, but there was no other major obstruction. I should state that both of these stents were bare-metal stents.

The groin was closed with a closure device. He will be going home tomorrow on aspirin and Plavix. It has been our practice, even with 2 metal stents, to leave these patients on Plavix for 1 year.

CPAP TITRATION SLEEP STUDY

CLINICAL HISTORY: The patient is a 54-year-old gentleman with a previously documented obstructive sleep apnea syndrome. The purpose of this study was to document in the sleep lab the patient's response to a therapeutic trial of nasal CPAP.

TECHNICAL RECORDING SUMMARY: Sleep stages were monitored using 2 EEG leads, 2 EOG leads, and 1 submental EMG lead. Respirations were monitored using oral and nasal thermistors, respiratory belts, pulse oximetry, and snoring microphone. ECG was monitored throughout the study. Leg movements were monitored using surface EMG electrodes.

POLYSOMNOGRAPHIC SUMMARY — CPAP TITRATION

SLEEP CONTINUITY AND SLEEP ARCHITECTURE: As outlined on accompanying sleep report summary.

CPAP TITRATION: The study was started at 4 cm of water pressure. It was gradually increased in an attempt to ablate snoring, to assure adequate air flow, to prevent desaturations, and to achieve consolidated sleep. It was found that at a CPAP level of 10 cm of water pressure all of these objectives were met.

ECG / HEART RATE: ECG showed normal sinus rhythm with isolated premature ventricular contractions.

PERIODIC LIMB MOVEMENTS: There were no periodic leg movements seen.

DIAGNOSTIC IMPRESSION: This overnight sleep study showed an excellent therapeutic response to nasal CPAP.

RECOMMENDATIONS: It would be recommended that the patient be started on nasal CPAP at 10 cm of water pressure with inline heated humidification to minimize nasal complications via small nasal pillows.

Weight reduction, avoidance of alcohol at bedtime, and treatment of nasal congestion and underlying hypothyroidism may also be helpful, if clinically indicated.

DOUBLE CORONARY BYPASS AND HEMODIALYSIS

PREOPERATIVE DIAGNOSIS: Coronary artery disease.

POSTOPERATIVE DIAGNOSIS: Coronary artery disease.

PROCEDURE PERFORMED: Double coronary bypass and hemodialysis, reoperation.

CLINICAL SUMMARY: This gentleman is now 64 years old. In 1982, he presented with a myocardial infarction followed by exertional angina. Eventually, in 1984, he was admitted and underwent triple coronary bypass. He did very well afterward and was followed on a regular basis. Recurrence of angina a few years ago put him back on antianginal therapy, but the symptoms were minimal and the patient continued to function well.

Because of worsening of his condition 18 months ago, the patient was admitted and had coronary artery angiogram which identified total occlusion of all the grafts except for the LAD, which presented not only an excellent flow but collateral supply to the circumflex and occluded right. The left ventricular function was fair. Attempt at reopening the circumflex had a very short success, and eventually the patient was left on antianginal therapy. The patient was hesitant about having a second surgery; however, he reconsidered when he required admission with unstable angina while traveling abroad. After stabilization of his unstable condition, a repeat angiogram confirmed again the fact that the LAD graft was the only structure still patent and arrangements were made for revascularization.

PROCEDURE: The patient was taken to the operating room and placed in the supine position. General anesthesia was induced. The patient was intubated and Swan-Ganz, arterial line, and Foley catheter inserted. Then the chest and both legs were prepped and draped in usual fashion. The TEE probe confirmed the inferior hypokinesis. Using the oscillating saw, the previous sternotomy was reopened while the distal half of the right saphenous vein was harvested. This presented with a regular caliber and suitable for grafting. The incision in the leg was closed in usual fashion. Progressively, the pericardium was freed from the right ventricle, right atrium, and the aorta. Heparin was given and the heart cannulated. Antegrade and retrograde cardioplegia were used. The patient was put on cardiopulmonary bypass and the aorta cross-clamped. Half a liter of antegrade cardioplegia was given followed by half a liter of retrograde cardioplegia. The distal right was opened. Unfortunately, once it was opened, the PDA offered a caliber of only 1.25 mm, and we realized that there was also some distal disease at that level. Since the vessel was open, it was decided to bypass using a segment of saphenous vein.

The proximal portion of this anastomosis was performed on the aorta under complete cross-clamp with retrograde cardioplegia flowing. The same procedure was carried out at the level of the largest obtuse marginal branch, which this time offered a caliber of 2 mm. The proximal anastomosis was also performed under complete cross-clamp with cardioplegia running and the patient being rewarmed.

The aorta was unclamped and resumed spontaneously normal sinus rhythm. The patient was then noticed to have hyperkalemia, for which hemodialysis was initiated during pump time. Once the potassium reached acceptable value (below 6), the patient was taken off bypass easily. The heart was decannulated and pursestring attached. Heparin was reversed using protamine. Two pacer wires and one drain were left in place. Prior to closure, a flow study of the graft was performed. Not surprisingly, the right graft offered a dismal flow at less than 10 mL, while the obtuse marginal graft offered a flow between 30-35 mL a minute.

Hemostasis was performed on the sternum in usual fashion. The skin was closed in the usual fashion.

Total pump run time was 90 minutes with a cross-clamp time of 52 minutes and the cardiac index above 3.

INTRACORONARY VASCULAR ULTRASOUND CONSULTATION

REASON FOR CONSULTATION: Intracoronary vascular ultrasound interrogation of proximal left anterior descending artery, followed by stent implantation.

CLINICAL NOTE: The patient is a 47-year-old gentleman who was transferred to our hospital after suffering a non-ST-elevation myocardial infarction. The patient has a very short cardiac history, which began when he experienced chest pain while cleaning his truck. The chest pain at that time lasted for 1 hour. Since that first episode, he suffered recurrent episodes, which were brought on by minimal activity. He did not experience any rest pains. He experienced a second prolonged episode of chest pain, and he presented to an outside emergency department. The initial blood work on presentation showed a slight elevation of serum troponin to 0.24. The electrocardiogram on presentation showed marked ST- and T-wave abnormalities in the anterolateral leads. Diagnostic coronary angiography was performed. Diagnostic images showed a normal left main coronary artery. The circumflex was free of disease. The LAD showed an unusual linear filling defect just after its origin with the rest of the LAD being free of disease. The right coronary artery was normal. The patient was then transferred for further management. Since his initial presentation to the outside institution, the patient has experienced recurrences of his chest discomfort.

The patient's only cardiac risk factor is cigarette smoking. He does not suffer from hypertension, hyperlipidemia, or diabetes. There is no family history of premature coronary artery disease.

The patient was taken to the catheterization laboratory for IVUS interrogation. Arterial access was obtained through the right femoral artery. Diagnostic images of the proximal segment of the LAD once again showed the unusual linear filling abnormality. IVUS images showed an eccentric soft plaque at the site of the filling defect. The area of stenosis at this site was 50%. The area of the LAD at the stenosis was 5.3 mm2.

We elected to proceed with coronary stenting due to the patient's clinical indications. The lesion in the proximal LAD was direct stented with a 3.5 x 8-mm Taxus paclitaxel-eluting stent. The final angiographic result was excellent. Integrilin was started in the catheterization laboratory and should be continued for 18 hours after this procedure.

The patient was transferred back to the CCU, feeling well and in good spirits. On discharge from the hospital, in addition to his other cardioactive medications, he should be given a prescription for clopidogrel 75 mg every day which he should be instructed to continue for 1 year after this procedure.

MEDIPORT INSERTION

PREOPERATIVE DIAGNOSIS: Nasopharyngeal carcinoma.

POSTOPERATIVE DIAGNOSIS: Nasopharyngeal carcinoma.

OPERATION: MediPort insertion.

ANESTHEIA: General and 0.5% Marcaine local.

DESCRIPTION OF OPERATION: The patient was brought to the operating room and placed on the table in the supine position. General LMA anesthesia was induced. The right side of the neck and chest were washed and prepped with Betadine and draped in sterile fashion. A subcutaneous injection of Marcaine was given. A transverse right neck incision was made about 1 cm in length overlying the easily visible external jugular vein. The external jugular was dissected out and ligated with 4-0 silk. The catheter, a 6.6-French silastic catheter, was flushed with saline and through venotomy in the external jugular vein passed centrally with the tip in the superior vena cava near its junction with the right atrium. There was good blood return and easy flushing with saline. A separate transverse skin incision was made in the right infraclavicular area and a flap created inferiorly to create a pocket raising subcutaneous tissue off the pectoralis major fascia. Cautery was used for hemostasis. A MediPort was placed in the pocket and noted to fit comfortably. It was flushed with saline and then sutured to the pectoralis major fascia with 4-point fixation using 2-0 Ethibond. A tunneler was used to connect the 2 incisions and, being certain there were no kinks in the catheter, was pulled into the lower incision and, using the small white connecting device, was connected to the MediPort. Again the system was tested with saline and noted to have good blood return and flushing easily. Fluoroscopy was used throughout to be certain there were no kinks and to be certain of the position of the catheter. With everything in good position and fully functional, the system was heparinized with heparin lock solution of 100 units per mL of heparin. Layered closure was carried out closing the platysma on the neck and Scarpa fascia on the chest with interrupted 4-0 Vicryl, and the skin incisions were closed with subcuticular sutures of 5-0 Vicryl. Mastisol and Steri-Strips were applied.

The patient was awoken from anesthesia and brought to the recovery room, having tolerated the procedure well. All counts were correct. No complications were encountered.

MEDIPORT REMOVAL

PREOPERATIVE DIAGNOSIS: Nasopharyngeal carcinoma.

POSTOPERATIVE DIAGNOSIS: Nasopharyngeal carcinoma.

OPERATION: MediPort removal.

ANESTHESIA: General LMA and 0.5% Marcaine local.

DESCRIPTION OF PROCEDURE: The patient was brought to the operating room and placed on the table in the supine position. General LMA anesthesia was induced. The right side of the neck and anterior chest were washed and then prepped with Betadine and draped in sterile fashion. A subcutaneous injection of Marcaine was given. An ellipse was done surrounding the old scar and excised for cosmetic purposes. The pseudosheath around the tubing was opened and the MediPort tubing was removed in its entirety without any difficulty. The pseudosheath was suture ligated with 4-0 Vicryl. The MediPort and associated sutures were dissected out using cautery for hemostasis. It was removed in its entirety, leaving no foreign material behind. With good hemostasis in the pocket, the subcutaneous tissues were closed with interrupted 4-0 Vicryl. The skin was closed with a running subcuticular suture of 5-0 Vicryl. Mastisol and Steri-Strips were applied.

The patient was awoken from anesthesia and brought to recovery room having tolerated the procedure well. All counts were correct.

METHACHOLINE CHALLENGE PFT REPORT

Interpretation: SVC and FVC are normal. FEV1 is normal as a percentage of predicted and normal as a percentage of FVC. Midexpiratory flow and MVV are normal. The expiratory portion of the flow volume loop is normal. Peak expiratory flow and expiratory flows, at 50% and 75% of FVC, are normal. Inspiratory flows exceed expiratory flows at the corresponding lung volumes. TLC, FRC, RV, and RV/TLC ratio are normal.

There is no definitive evidence on baseline testing of either an obstructive or restrictive ventilatory defect.

After 200 cumulative units of methacholine aerosol, there was a 23% reduction in FEV1, indicating a bronchospastic response to a cholinergic challenge.

IMPRESSION: Findings are consistent with heightened airways responsiveness; the diagnosis of asthma is usually made with a greater degree of airway responsiveness.

MULTIPLE SLEEP LATENCY TEST

CLINICAL HISTORY: The patient is a 53-year-old woman studied because of a history of profound daytime fatigue and hypersomnolence.

TECHNICAL RECORDING SUMMARY: Sleep stages were monitored using 2 EEG leads, 2 EOG leads, and 1 submental EMG lead. Respirations were monitored using oral and nasal thermistors, nasal pressure transducer, respiratory belts, pulse oximetry, and snoring microphone. ECG was monitored throughout the study. Leg movements were monitored using surface EMG electrodes. The multiple sleep latency test consisted of five 20-minute naps separated by 2-hour intervals with measurements of latency to first onset of sleep, as well as assessment of sleep onset REM activity.

POLYSOMNOGRAPHIC SUMMARY

SLEEP CONTINUITY AND SLEEP ARCHITECTURE: Sleep architecture was notable for showing normal distribution of sleep stages, although sleep efficiency was reduced at 85%; and there was an excess of wake time. There were frequent spontaneous arousals not associated with respiratory events, although there were frequent periodic limb movements seen.

RESPIRATORY MEASURES: Throughout the night, there were no significant obstructive apneas-hypopneas seen. The lowest oxygen saturation obtained was 89% with a baseline oxygen saturation of 99%. There did not appear to be any positional component to the respiratory events. There was mild snoring audible throughout the study.

ECG/HEART RATE: ECG showed normal sinus rhythm throughout, with no ventricular ectopy noted.

PERIODIC LIMB MOVEMENTS: There were 132 periodic leg movements seen, 39 of which were associated with a transient arousal, for a periodic limb movement arousal index of 6 events per hour of sleep.

Subsequent multiple sleep latency test consisted of 5 naps. Sleep latency tests were as follows:

Multiple Sleep Latency Test
Nap #1   Sleep Latency: 4.5 minutes.
Nap #2   Sleep Latency: 4.5 minutes.
Nap #3   Sleep Latency: 1.5 minutes.
Nap #4   Sleep Latency: 1.5 minutes.
Nap #5   Sleep Latency: 2.5 minutes.

No REM sleep was seen on any of the naps, and the mean sleep latency was 3.4 minutes.

DIAGNOSTIC IMPRESSION: The overnight sleep study showed evidence of mild snoring and periodic limb movement disorder. The subsequent multiple sleep latency test showed evidence of severe hypersomnolence, although there was no evidence of REM sleep seen, thus a diagnosis of narcolepsy cannot be definitively established.

Hypersomnolence can be seen with periodic limb movement disorder, although it would be unusual with this degree of nocturnal myoclonus.

RECOMMENDATIONS: Based on the results of this study, periodic limb movements may be treated with Mirapex, Sinemet, clonazepam, and codeine at bedtime. Avoidance of stimulants, such as caffeine, may be beneficial. If daytime fatigue and hypersomnolence continue to be significant problems despite treatment of leg movements, then consideration should be given to treating profound hypersomnolence with either Provigil or Ritalin for presumed idiopathic central hypersomnolence.

Weight reduction, avoidance of alcohol at bedtime, treatment of nasal congestion, and underlying hypothyroidism may also be helpful, if clinically indicated.

PACEMAKER ANALYSIS

PACEMAKER ANALYSIS: Type: Medtronic Kappa 901. Battery Voltage: 2.77 volts. Battery Impedance: 372 ohms. Atrial Lead Impedance: 461 ohms. Ventricular Lead Impedance: 764 ohms. Measured Ventricular Capture Threshold: 0.37 volts at 0.4 milliseconds. Minimum P-wave amplitude was 1.0 millivolts. There were 13 mode-switching episodes, the longest lasting over 5 hours. Forty nine percent (49%) of the events were atrially sensed and ventricularly paced; 37% of the events were atrially and ventricularly paced. Heart rate histogram shows that most of the events occurred at the lower pacing rate. Pacing mode is DDDR. Lower Pacing Rate: 50 ppm. Maximum Tracking Rate: 115 ppm. The atrial and ventricular pulse amplitudes were 2.5 volts. No changes were made in pacing parameters today.

PACEMAKER ANALYSIS: Type: St. Jude Identity ADX. Pacing Mode: DDD. Lower Pacing Rate: 60 ppm. Maximum Tracking Rate: 110 ppm. Battery Voltage: 2.75 volts. Battery Current: 10 microamps. Battery Impedance: 2.4 ohms. Atrial Lead Impedance: 491 ohms. Ventricular Lead Impedance: 500 ohms. Sixty percent (60%) of the events were atrially and ventricularly sensed. Sixteen percent (16%) of the events were atrially and ventricularly paced. Thirty percent (30%) of the accounts were paced in the atrium and 14% were paced in the ventricle. Heart rate histogram showed good heart rate distribution. Ventricular auto capture threshold was turned on. Automatic pulse amplitude of 4.5 volts. E/R Sensitivity: 2.3 millivolts. Ventricular pulse configuration was switched to unipolar. There were 2 episodes of rapid atrial rate, which lasted less than 1 minute. Atrial Capture Threshold: 0.5 volts at 0.5 milliseconds. Ventricular Capture Threshold: 0.5 volts at 0.5 milliseconds. Measured evoked response was 5.87 millivolts. The measured lead polarization was 0.39 volts. No other changes were made in pacing parameters. The patient will have repeat pacemaker analysis in 6 months.

PACEMAKER INSERTION: INSERTION OF NEW PACEMAKER ON THE RIGHT, REMOVAL OF INFECTED AND ERODED LEFT PACEMAKER GENERATOR

PREOPERATIVE DIAGNOSIS: Eroded left pacemaker generator.

POSTOPERATIVE DIAGNOSIS: Eroded left pacemaker generator.

PROCEDURE PERFORMED: Insertion of new pacemaker on the right and removal of infected and eroded left pacemaker generator.

INDICATIONS: This pleasant older lady, who had her pacemaker generator changed a few years ago, came in with the pacemaker generator eroding through the skin on the left anterolateral chest wall.

FINDINGS: The patient appeared to be more or less dependent on her pacemaker, so we left the old one in and left the lead in place because we knew there would be little or no chance for removing this successfully. Instead, we went directly to placing a new right-sided pacemaker first. The right heart configuration was normal, and it was easy to find good position for a single-chamber lead in the right ventricle. We removed the old generator by excising the thinned-out skin on top of the generator and dissecting out some of the cavity that it was sitting in and removing the generator with skin intact. The leads were removed and cleaned up, and Silastic caps were placed on the exposed ends of the lead. These were tied in place with 3-0 Prolene. The cavity on the left side was then débrided up and closed.

DESCRIPTION OF PROCEDURE: With the patient under general endotracheal anesthesia, prepped and draped in the usual manner, a small incision was made in the upper outer right chest and was carried down to the fascia. The deltopectoral groove was explored, but no cephalic vein was found, so a single subclavian stab was made and the introducer wire, dilator, and peel-away sheath were passed into the central venous system. The dilator and the wire were removed, and the lead (an Intermedics 4457 model lead) was placed into the central venous system and it was passed into the right heart without trouble. Once we noted good position and good pacing parameters, we sewed it in place at the pectoralis fascia with the supplied silastic cuff and 3-0 Prolene.

REGULAR PFT REPORT

INTERPRETATION: SVC and FVC are normal. FEV1 is normal as a percentage of predicted and normal as a percentage of FVC. Midexpiratory flow and MVV are normal. The expiratory portion of the flow volume loop is irregular, indicating variable effort; peak expiratory flow and expiratory flows at 50% and 75% of FVC are normal. Inspiratory flows exceed expiratory flows at the corresponding lung volumes. TLC, FRC, RV, and RV/TLC ratio are all increased. Single breath diffusing capacity for carbon monoxide is normal.

There is no definitive evidence on baseline testing of either an obstructive or restrictive ventilatory defect. The normal diffusion argues any significant loss in alveolar capillary surface area and implies normal gas exchange.

After 6 inhalations (540 mcg) of an albuterol MDI, there were statistically insignificant changes in FVC, FEV1, and midexpiratory flow, indicating a lack of response to a bronchodilator challenge. With the patient in a sitting position, breathing room air, O2 saturation as measured by oximetry was 96%. The patient's resting heart rate was 78 BPM. The patient ambulated for 150 feet. At the highest work load, the O2 saturation was 96%. The patient's heart rate went up to 93.

IMPRESSION: Findings are consistent with normal pulmonary function testing for a patient of this age. There is no evidence of rest or submaximal exercise desaturation.

REGULAR SLEEP STUDY

CLINICAL HISTORY: The patient is a 37-year-old gentleman studied because of a history of snoring, daytime fatigue, and hypersomnolence.

TECHNICAL RECORDING SUMMARY: Sleep stages were monitored using 2 EEG leads, 2 EOG leads, and 1 submental EMG lead. Respirations were monitored using oral and nasal thermistors, respiratory belts, pulse oximetry, and snoring microphone. ECG was monitored throughout the study. Leg movements were monitored using surface EMG electrodes.

POLYSOMNOGRAPHIC SUMMARY

SLEEP CONTINUITY AND SLEEP ARCHITECTURE: As outlined on accompanying sleep report summary.

RESPIRATORY MEASURES: Throughout the night, there were 119 obstructive apneas-hypopneas seen, all of which were associated with a transient arousal for an apnea-hypopnea index of 23 events per hour of sleep. The lowest oxygen saturation obtained was 86% with a baseline oxygen saturation of 99%. There was no positional component to the respiratory events. There was moderately loud snoring audible throughout the study.

ECG/HEART RATE: ECG showed normal sinus rhythm throughout with no ventricular ectopy noted.

PERIODIC LIMB MOVEMENTS: There were no significant periodic leg movements seen.

DIAGNOSTIC IMPRESSION: This overnight sleep study showed a moderate degree of obstructive sleep apnea syndrome.

RECOMMENDATIONS: Based on the results of this sleep study, reasonable therapeutic options would include a trial of nasal CPAP, use of a mandibular retainer, and consideration of upper airway surgery.

Weight reduction, avoidance of alcohol at bedtime, and treatment of nasal congestion and underlying hypothyroidism may also be helpful, if clinically indicated.

RIGHT CAROTID ENDARTERECTOMY WITH DACRON PATCH

PREOPERATIVE DIAGNOSIS: Asymptomatic high-grade right internal carotid artery stenosis.

POSTOPERATIVE DIAGNOSIS: Asymptomatic high-grade right internal carotid artery stenosis.

OPERATION: Right carotid endarterectomy with Dacron patch.

ANESTHESIA: General.

INDICATIONS FOR PROCEDURE: The patient is a 65-year-old gentleman who was noted to have high-grade carotid artery stenosis on duplex, and this was confirmed by MRA. He was medically cleared and brought to the operating room for the above procedure after informed consent was obtained.

INTRAOPERATIVE FINDINGS: A high-grade stenosis was noted with severe plaque at the origin of the right internal carotid artery, and the artery proximally and distally was widely patent.

PROCEDURE: The patient was brought to the operating room and placed supine on the operating table. General anesthesia was induced, he was intubated, and an arterial line was inserted. His head was turned to the left and his lower face, neck and upper chest were prepped with Betadine and draped in the usual sterile fashion. An incision was made along the anterior border of the sternocleidomastoid muscle. The platysma was divided and the sternocleidomastoid was reflected laterally. The common carotid artery was identified, skeletonized, and looped. The facial vein was ligated and divided. The carotid bulb was identified and the internal carotid artery was identified, skeletonized, and looped distally. The external carotid and superior thyroid arteries were then looped. The patient was administered heparin, and during this time, the carotid bulb was dissected.

After completion of this dissection and adequate time for anticoagulation, a clamp was placed on the internal carotid artery distally and on the common carotid artery proximally, and the loops pulled up on the other 2 vessels. The arteriotomy was created on the common carotid artery and extended through the plaque into the internal carotid artery distally. A Javid shunt was inserted into the internal carotid artery distally, back bleeding was fair, and the shunt was then placed in the common carotid artery. An endarterectomy was performed in a standard fashion; plaque was elevated on both sides. It was cut from the common carotid artery proximally, feathered from the internal artery distally, and everted from the external carotid artery. Good endpoint on the internal carotid artery was achieved. One tacking suture was required. Fragments of loose debris were removed until a smooth luminal surface was achieved. Once we were happy with this, the closure was begun.

Closure was done with a patch. This was a Dacron patch, sutured at the distal end of the arteriotomy, tied down, and, in a running fashion, sutured around both sides. Before completion, the shunt was removed. Back bleeding and inflow were noted to be good. The loop was released from the external carotid artery. This ce-aired the artery. The closure was completed, and the clamp was first released from the common carotid artery. This flushed any debris into the external carotid system. The clamp was then released from the internal carotid artery. Two bleeding points required separate sutures, and then hemostasis was adequate. Once we were happy that hemostasis was adequate, we proceeded with closure. A Jackson-Pratt drain was placed through a separate stab wound and sutured in place. The platysma was approximated with Vicryl. The skin was approximated with Monocryl. Steri-Strips and a sterile dressing were applied.

The patient tolerated the procedure well. There were no intraoperative complications. All counts were correct at the end of the procedure. He was awakened in the operating room and noted to be neurologically intact. He was transferred to the recovery room in a stable condition and extubated.

ESTIMATED BLOOD LOSS: 200 mL.

SPECIMEN: Carotid plaque.

Sample Reports and Dictation

Split Study with CPAP Titration

Clinical History: The patient is a 42-year-old gentleman studied because of a history of snoring, daytime fatigue, and hypersomnolence.

Technical Recording Summary: Sleep stages were monitored using 2 EEG leads, 2 EOG leads, and 1 submental EMG lead. Respirations were monitored using oral and nasal thermistors, respiratory belts, pulse oximetry, and snoring microphone. ECG was monitored throughout the study. Leg movements were monitored using surface EMG electrodes.

Polysomnographic Summary — Split Study with CPAP Titration

Sleep Continuity and Sleep Architecture: As outlined on accompanying sleep report summary.

Respiratory Measures: During the initial portion of the study, there were 94 apneas-hypopneas seen for an apnea-hypopnea index of 50 events per hour of sleep. The lowest oxygen saturation obtained was 79% with a baseline of 99%. There was loud snoring audible during the initial portion of the study.

CPAP Titration: Because of the presence of significant obstructive sleep apnea syndrome, the patient was started on a therapeutic trial of nasal CPAP at 1:42 A.M. which was titrated to 13 cm of water pressure.

ECG/Heart Rate: ECG showed normal sinus rhythm throughout with no ventricular ectopy noted.

Periodic Limb Movements: There were no periodic leg movements seen.

Diagnostic Impression: This overnight sleep study showed a severe degree of obstructive sleep apnea syndrome during the initial portion of the study. Subsequently, there was an excellent therapeutic response to nasal CPAP.

Recommendations: It would be recommended that the patient be started on nasal CPAP at 13 cm of water pressure with inline heated humidification to minimize nasal complications via a medium Respironics Contour Deluxe mask.

Weight reduction, avoidance of alcohol at bedtime, and treatment of nasal congestion and underlying hypothyroidism may also be helpful, if clinically indicated.

THORASCOPIC MICROWAVE MAZE PROCEDURE

PREOPERATIVE DIAGNOSIS: Paroxysmal atrial fibrillation.

POSTOPERATIVE DIAGNOSIS: Paroxysmal atrial fibrillation.

OPERATION: Thoracoscopic microwave Maze procedure.

ANESTHESIA: General endotracheal.

INDICATIONS: The patient is a 58-year-old man with a 2-year history of paroxysmal atrial fibrillation. He has tried amiodarone and other antiarrhythmic drugs, but none has been successful, until Tikosyn. Although this drug works, he cannot fly as a commercial pilot on it because of FAA regulations. He referred himself for consultation and now wishes to have an ablation performed. The risks and benefits were explained to the patient, who agreed to proceed.

NARRATIVE: The patient was brought to the operating room and placed on the operating table in the supine position, where general endotracheal anesthesia was induced without incident. A double-lumen endotracheal tube was positioned and monitoring lines placed. The chest, abdomen, and groin were prepped and draped in the usual sterile fashion and the right lung deflated.

Two 5-mm and one 10-mm ports were made in the chest, in the midaxillary 4th and 5th intercostal spaces and in the 6th midclavicular space, respectively. The pericardium was opened sharply just anterior to the phrenic nerve, from the superior vena cavaSVC to the inferior vena cavaIVC. The IVC and SVC were dissected out and the retrocaval spaces probed to confirm continuity with the oblique and transverse sinuses, respectively. A 14-French Rob-Nel catheter was placed in each space, going from right to left, behind each cava. The thoracoscopic instruments were removed and the right lung reinflated.

The left lung was deflated and the same ports were created, with the addition of a fourth 5-mm port in the posterior axillary line at the 4th interspace. The left pericardium was opened and the left atrial appendage identified. The superior Rob-Nel catheter was retrieved and its tip delivered out of the chest, where a suture "tag" was placed on it. We then retrieved the inferior catheter. The Guidant Flex 10 ablation probe was then fed into the right chest through the 10-mm port and around the pulmonary veins under direct vision from the left side. It was positioned correctly posterior to the left atrial appendage. A total of 9 lesions were then made to completely encircle the pulmonary veins at 65 watts/lesion and 90 seconds/lesion. A completely encircling lesion was visually confirmed. We then ablated the base of the left atrial appendage to its tip by repositioning the probe.

We then turned our attention to the left appendage, which was amputated at its base with a Power Medical SurgAssist SLC55G stapler. We confirmed that there was no bleeding. TEE showed a small residual sac. Another attempt was made to staple closer to the base, but this resulted in lateral ischemia and hypotension, likely because of pressure on the left circumflex, so we stopped this attempt. Two 28-French chest tubes were then placed, one in each pleural space, and the lungs reinflated.

All instruments were removed and the port sites closed with sutures. Lidocaine 1% 40 mL and 0.5% Marcaine mix was infiltrated into the chest tube and trocar sites. The patient was awoken and extubated in the operating room uneventfully. He was then transferred to the cardiothoracic intensive care unit in stable condition. All sponge and instrument counts were correct at the end of the case, and there were no known complications. As the attending physician, I was present for the entire procedure.

TRANSESOPHAGEAL ECHOCARDIOGRAM

INTERPRETATION: The risks and benefits of the procedure were explained to the patient, and consent was signed. The patient was sedated with IV Versed and fentanyl. Posterior pharynx was anesthetized with Hurricane spray. TEE probe was passed to 40 cm without difficulty. The 4 cardiac valves, common cardiac chambers, left atrial appendage, thoracic aorta, and left atrial appendage were interrogated. The thoracic aorta was not visualized, as the patient began regurgitating during the last portion of the test.

There was global hypokinesis of the left ventricle with more severe anteroseptal hypokinesis. The estimated ejection fraction was 35% to 40%. Left atrium appeared enlarged. The cardiac valves appeared structurally normal. There was moderate to severe mitral regurgitation. Reversal of flow within the pulmonary veins was not identified. There was mild aortic insufficiency. There was mild pulmonic insufficiency. There was mild tricuspid regurgitation. No significant stenosis of the cardiac valves was appreciated. A thrombus was not appreciated within the left atrial appendage. There was no evidence of an atrial septal defect by color Doppler study. No immediate complications were identified.

CONCLUSIONS
1. Global hypokinesis of the left ventricle with more severe anteroseptal hypokinesis.
2. Moderate reduction of the left ventricular systolic function.
3. Moderate to severe mitral regurgitation.
4. Mild aortic insufficiency.
5. Mild tricuspid regurgitation.

Common Terms by Procedure

ANGIOGRAPHY AND STENTING OF LEFT ANTERIOR DESCENDING ARTERY

akinesia
angiogram
angioplasty
Angio-Seal device
atmospheres
balloon
bare-metal stent
circumflex artery
congestive heart failure
coronary artery
coronary artery disease
crescendo angina
descending artery
diuresis
Driver stent
EBU 4.0 guide
ejection fraction
electrocardiogram
femoral artery
hypercholesterolemia
hypertension
Integrilin
Judkins catheter
left anterior descending artery (LAD)
left ventricular end-diastolic pressure (LVEDP)
lesion
myocardial infarction
obtuse marginal (OM)
OM branch
Plavix
Q wave
stenosis
stenting
systolic function
tenecteplase (TNKase)
thrombolysis
thrombosis
TIMI 3 flow
transmural inferior myocardial infarction (TIMI)
T-wave inversion
ventricular tachycardia
Wizdom guidewire

ANGIOPLASTY AND STENTING USING CRUSH TECHNIQUE

acute pulmonary edema
angioplasty
atmospheres
balloon
bilevel positive airway pressure (BiPAP)
calcifications
cardiac catheterization
circumflex artery
coronary angiogram
coronary artery
coronary artery disease
crush technique
diagonal branch
dilatation
femoral artery
8-French Angio-Seal
7-French AR2 guiding catheter
guidewire
hypercholesterolemia
hypokinesia
intravenous ReoPro infusion
kissing stent technique
lesion
Mercury balloon
non-ST-elevation myocardial infarction
ostial
ostium

PDA branch
Plavix
posterior descending artery (PDA)
PowerSail balloon
pulmonary edema
Quantum balloon
right coronary artery (RCA)
stenosis
stent
stenting
Taxus paclitaxel-eluting stent
Taxus stent
Thrombosis
TIMI 3
transmural inferior myocardial
    infarction (TIMI)
troponin
ventricular systolic function
vessel
Whisper guidewire

CARDIOVERSION
anesthesiologist
atrial fibrillation
biphasic machine
cardioversion
100-J shock
shocked
sinus rhythm

CHEST PAIN CARDIOLOGY CONSULTATION
cardiac enzyme
cardiac function
cardiac risk factor
chest pain
chest pressure
cholesterol
chronic obstructive pulmonary disease
diaphoresis
electrocardiogram
emphysema
hypertension
ischemia

leads V2, V3, and aVL
myocardial infarction
nonspecific T-wave changes
rule-out myocardial infarction protocol
sinus rhythm
stress test
sublingual nitroglycerin
telemetry monitor

CORONARY ANGIOPLASTY: 3-VESSEL
akinetic
Angio-Seal device
aspirin therapy
balloon
bare-metal stent
chest pain
cholesterol
circumflex
coronary angioplasty
coronary artery
distal RCA
2D echo
electrocardiogram (ECG)
12-lead ECG
Exulter stent
femoral artery
grade 2 left ventricular function
guidewire
high-density lipoprotein (HDL)
hypercholesterolemia
hypertension
hypokinetic
Integrilin
leads V1, V2
left anterior descending artery (LAD)
lesion
low-density lipoprotein (LDL)
mid lateral wall
midcircumflex
Minivision stent
myocardial infarction
non-ST segment
paclitaxel drug-eluting stent

Plavix
proximal mid LAD
R wave
right coronary artery (RCA)
sinus rhythm
stenosis
Taxus stent
TIMI 3 flow
transmural inferior myocardial
 infarction (TIMI)
triglyceride
triple-vessel disease
troponin
T-wave inversion
vessel

CORONARY
ANGIOPLASTY: 2-VESSEL

accordion effect
AL1 guide catheter
angina
angiogram
angioplasty
aspirin
bare-metal stent
calcified lesion
cardiac catheterization
7-French catheter
closure device
coronary angioplasty
coronary artery
coronary artery disease
deploy
dilate
dissection
endothelium
femoral artery
groin
7-French guide
guidewire
heart disease
high-pressure balloon
intracoronary vascular ultrasound
 (IVUS)

invagination
LAD lesion
left anterior descending artery (LAD)
lesion
obstruction
plaque
Plavix
stent
stress testing
tortuosity
tortuous
vessel

CPAP TITRATION
SLEEP STUDY

ablate
air flow
continuous positive airway pressure
 (CPAP)
CPAP titration
desaturation
electrocardiogram (ECG)
electroencephalogram (EEG)
EEG lead
ECG
electrode
electrooculogram (EOG)
electromyogram (EMG)
EMG lead
EOG lead
heated humidification
nasal CPAP
nasal pillow
nasal thermistor
normal sinus rhythm
obstructive sleep apnea syndrome
oral thermistor
polysomnographic
premature ventricular contractions
pulse oximetry
respirations
respiratory belt
sleep lab
sleep stage

Common Terms
by Procedure

snoring microphone
therapeutic trial
water pressure

DOUBLE CORONARY BYPASS AND HEMODIALYSIS

anastomosis
antegrade cardioplegia
antianginal therapy
aorta
arterial line
atrium
bypass
caliber
cannulate
cardiac index
cardiopulmonary bypass
collateral supply
coronary artery angiogram
coronary artery disease
coronary bypass
cross-clamp
decannulated
drain
exertional angina
flow
flow study
Foley catheter
general anesthesia
graft
hemodialysis
heparin
hyperkalemia
hypokinesis
intubate
LAD graft
left anterior descending artery (LAD)
left ventricular function
myocardial infarction (MI)
normal sinus rhythm
obtuse marginal branch
oscillating saw
pacer wires

pericardium
posterior descending artery (PDA)
potassium
protamine
pump time
pursestring
retrograde cardioplegia
revascularization
rewarmed
saphenous vein
stabilization
sternotomy
sternum
supine position
Swan-Ganz
TEE probe
total occlusion
transesophageal echocardiography
   (TEE)
unstable angina
ventricle

INTRACORONARY VASCULAR ULTRASOUND CONSULTATION

anterolateral lead
arterial access
cardiac care unit (CCU)
cardiac risk factor
cardioactive medications
catheterization laboratory
chest discomfort
chest pain
circumflex
clinical indication
clopidogrel
coronary artery
coronary stenting
diagnostic coronary angiography
diagnostic images
electrocardiogram
femoral artery
hyperlipidemia
hypertension

Integrilin
intracoronary vascular ultrasound
    (IVUS)
IVUS interrogation
left anterior descending artery (LAD)
lesion
linear filling defect
non-ST-elevation myocardial infarction
premature coronary artery disease
proximal LAD
proximal segment
serum troponin
soft plaque
ST- and T-wave abnormalities
stenosis
stent implantation
Taxus paclitaxel-eluting stent

platysma
pocket
right atrium
saline
Scarpa fascia
4-0 silk
sterile fashion
Steri-Strips
subcutaneous injection
subcutaneous tissue
subcuticular sutures
superior vena cava
supine position
transverse skin incision
tunneler
venotomy
5-0 Vicryl

MEDIPORT INSERTION
anesthesia
Betadine
blood return
catheter
cautery
easy flushing
2-0 Ethibond
external jugular vein
flap
fluoroscopy
4-point fixation
6.6-French silastic catheter
hemostasis
heparin lock solution
heparinized
infraclavicular area
interrupted 4-0 Vicryl
laryngeal mask airway (LMA)
layered closure
LMA anesthesia
Marcaine
Mastisol
MediPort
nasopharyngeal carcinoma
pectoralis major fascia

MEDIPORT REMOVAL
Betadine
cautery
dissected out
ellipse
hemostasis
interrupted 4-0 Vicryl
laryngeal mask airway (LMA)
LMA anesthesia
Marcaine
Mastisol
MediPort
MediPort tubing
nasopharyngeal carcinoma
pocket
pseudosheath
running subcuticular suture
sterile fashion
Steri-Strips
subcutaneous injection
subcutaneous tissues
supine position
suture ligated
sutures
4-0 Vicryl
5-0 Vicryl

METHACHOLINE CHALLENGE PFT REPORT

asthma
bronchospastic response
cholinergic challenge
flow volume loop
forced expiratory volume in 1 second (FEV1)
forced vital capacity (FVC)
functional residual capacity (FRC)
heightened airways responsiveness
inspiratory flow
maximum volume ventilation (MVV)
methacholine aerosol
midexpiratory flow
obstructive ventilatory defect
peak expiratory flow
percentage of predicted
residual volume (RV)
restrictive ventilatory defect
RV/TLC ratio
slow vital capacity (SVC)
total lung capacity (TLC)

MULTIPLE SLEEP LATENCY TEST

caffeine
clonazepam
codeine
daytime fatigue
EEG lead
electrocardiogram (ECG)
electroencephalogram (EEG)
electromyogram (EMG)
electrooculogram (EOG)
EOG lead
excess of wake time
fatigue
hypersomnolence
hypopnea
idiopathic central hypersomnolence
interval
leg movements
limb movement arousal index

mean sleep latency
Mirapex
multiple sleep latency test
nap
narcolepsy
nasal pressure transducer
nasal thermistor
nocturnal myoclonus
normal sinus rhythm
obstructive apnea
oral thermistor
overnight sleep study
oxygen saturation
periodic limb movement
positional component
profound hypersomnolence
Provigil
pulse oximetry
rapid eye movement (REM)
REM activity
REM sleep
respirations
respiratory belt
respiratory event
respiratory measures
Ritalin
Sinemet
sleep architecture
sleep continuity
sleep efficiency
sleep stage
snoring
snoring microphone
spontaneous arousal
stimulants
submental EMG
surface EMG electrode
transient arousal
ventricular ectopy

PACEMAKER ANALYSIS

atrial capture threshold
atrial lead impedance
atrial pulse amplitude

atrially sensed
atrium
automatic pulse amplitude
battery impedance
battery voltage
DDDR pacing
E/R sensitivity
event
evoked response
heart rate distribution
heart rate histogram
maximum tracking rate
measured lead polarization
Medtronic Kappa 901
millivolts
minimum Pwave amplitude
mode-switching episodes
ohms
pacing mode
pacing parameters
pacing rate
rapid atrial rate
St. Jude Identity ADX
unipolar
ventricle
ventricular auto capture threshold
ventricular capture threshold
ventricular lead impedance
ventricular pulse amplitude
ventricular pulse configuration
ventricularly paced
volts

PACEMAKER INSERTION: INSERTION OF NEW PACEMAKER ON THE RIGHT, REMOVAL OF INFECTED AND ERODED LEFT PACEMAKER GENERATOR

cavity
central venous system
cephalic vein

chest wall
débrided up
deltopectoral groove
dilator
erode
fascia
general endotracheal anesthesia
Intermedics 4457 model lead
introducer wire
lead
left pacemaker generator
pacing parameters
pectoralis fascia
peel-away sheath
prepped and draped
3-0 Prolene
right heart configuration
right ventricle
right-sided pacemaker
Silastic cap
silastic cuff
single subclavian stab
single-chamber lead

REGULAR PFT REPORT

albuterol MDI
alveolar capillary surface area
bronchodilator challenge
expiratory portion
flow volume loop
forced expiratory volume in 1 second (FEV1)
forced vital capacity (FVC)
functional residual capacity (FRC)
maximum volume ventilation (MVV)
midexpiratory flow
normal diffusion
normal gas exchange
O_2 saturation
obstructive ventilatory defect
oximetry
peak expiratory flow
percentage of FVC
percentage of predicted

residual volume (RV)
resting heart rate
restrictive ventilatory defect
room air
RV/TLC ratio
single breath diffusing capacity for
    carbon monoxide
slow vital capacity (SVC)
submaximal exercise desaturation
total lung capacity (TLC)
variable effort

REGULAR SLEEP STUDY
apnea-hypopnea index
baseline oxygen saturation
continuous positive airway pressure
    (CPAP)
EEG lead
electrocardiogram (ECG)
electroencephalogram (EEG)
electromyogram (EMG)
electrooculogram (EOG)
EMG electrode
EOG lead
events per hour
fatigue
heart rate
hypersomnolence
leg movement
mandibular retainer
moderately loud snoring
nasal CPAP
nasal thermistor
normal sinus rhythm
obstructive apnea
obstructive hypopnea
obstructive sleep apnea syndrome
oral thermistor
overnight sleep study
oxygen saturation
periodic limb movement
positional component
pulse oximetry
respirations

respiratory belt
respiratory event
respiratory measures
sleep architecture
sleep continuity
sleep report summary
sleep stages
snoring microphone
submental EMG lead
transient arousal
upper airway surgery
ventricular ectopy

RIGHT CAROTID ENDARTERECTOMY WITH DACRON PATCH
anticoagulation
arterial line
arteriotomy
back bleeding
Betadine
carotid bulb
carotid endarterectomy
carotid plaque
common carotid artery
Dacron patch
de-aired
dissection
duplex
endarterectomy
endpoint
external carotid artery
facial vein
general anesthesia
hemostasis
heparin
high-grade carotid artery stenosis
inflow
internal carotid artery
intubate
Jackson-Pratt drain
Javid shunt
ligated and divided
looped

loose debris
magnetic resonance angiography
  (MRA)
Monocryl
neurologically intact
plaque
platysma
shunt
skeletonized
smooth luminal surface
stab wound
sterile dressing
sterile fashion
Steri-Strips
sternocleidomastoid muscle
superior thyroid artery
tacking suture
vessel
Vicryl

SPLIT STUDY WITH CPAP TITRATION

apnea
apnea-hypopnea index
continuous positive airway pressure
  (CPAP)
CPAP titration
daytime fatigue
EEG lead
electrocardiogram (ECG)
electroencephalogram (EEG)
electromyogram (EMG)
electrooculogram (EOG)
EMG electrodes
EOG lead
events per hour of sleep
heart rate
hypersomnolence
hypopnea
inline heated humidification
leg movements
nasal CPAP
nasal thermistor
normal sinus rhythm

obstructive sleep apnea syndrome
oral thermistor
overnight sleep study
oxygen saturation
periodic limb movements
pulse oximetry
respirations
respiratory belt
respiratory measures
Respironics Contour Deluxe mask
sleep architecture
sleep continuity
sleep report summary
sleep stages
snoring
snoring microphone
submental EMG lead
therapeutic response
titration
ventricular ectopy
water pressure

THORASCOPIC MICROWAVE MAZE PROCEDURE

ablation
amiodarone
atrial appendage
cardiothoracic intensive care unit
  (CTICU)
chest tube
completely encircling lesion
double-lumen ET tube
extubated
14-French Rob-Nel catheter
28-French chest tube
general endotracheal anesthesia
Guidant Flex 10 ablation probe
hypotension
inferior vena cava (IVC)
intercostal space
ischemia
left circumflex coronary artery (LCX)
lesion

Lidocaine and Marcaine mix
midclavicular space
monitoring lines
oblique sinus
paroxysmal atrial fibrillation
pericardium
phrenic nerve
pleural space
port sites
Power Medical SurgAssist SLC55G
    stapler
pulmonary vein
residual sac
retrocaval space probed
seconds/lesion
sterile fashion
superior vena cava (SVC)
supine position
suture
thoracoscopic instrument
thoracoscopic microwave Maze
    procedure
Tikosyn
transesophageal echocardiography
    (TEE)
transverse sinus
trocar site
watts/lesion

TRANSESOPHAGEAL ECHOCARDIOGRAM

anteroseptal hypokinesis
aortic insufficiency
atrial appendage
atrial septal defect
atrium
cardiac valve
color Doppler study
common cardiac chamber
ejection fraction
fentanyl
global hypokinesis
Hurricaine spray
mitral regurgitation
pharynx
pulmonary vein
pulmonic insufficiency
reversal of flow
stenosis
TEE probe
thoracic aorta
thrombus
transesophageal echocardiography
    (TEE)
tricuspid regurgitation
ventricle
Versed

Cardiology Trials and Studies

AASK
African American Study of Kidney Disease and Hypertension Pilot study

ABACAS
Adjunctive Balloon Angioplasty Following Coronary Atherectomy Study

ABC
Alpha Beta Canadian trial

ACAD
Azithromycin Coronary Artery Disease study

ACADEMIC
Azithromycin in Coronary Artery Disease Elimination of Myocardial Infection with Chlamydia

ACAS
Asymptomatic Carotid Atherosclerosis Study

ACCEPT
Accupril Canadian Clinical Evaluation and Patient Teaching
American College of Cardiology Evaluation of Preventive Therapies

ACCESS
A Comparison of Percutaneous Entry Sites for Coronary Angioplasty
Atorvastatin Comparative Cholesterol Efficacy and Safety Study

ACCT
Amlodipine Cardiovascular Community Trial

ACES
Alternans Cardiac Electrical Safety Study
Azithromycin and Coronary Events Study

ACHIEVE
Accupril congestive heart failure investigation and economic variable evaluation

ACIP
Asymptomatic Cardiac Ischemic Pilot trial

ACME
Angioplasty Compared to Medicine study

ACP
Asymptomatic Cardiac Ischemia Pilot

ACRE
Appropriateness of Coronary Revascularization study

ACT
Angioplasty Compliance Trial
Attacking Claudication with Ticlopidine study

ACTION
A Coronary Disease Trial Investigating Outcome with Nifedipine GITS

ACTIVATE
ACAT IntraVascular Atherosclerosis Treatment Evaluation

ACTIVE
Atrial Fibrillation Clopidogrel Trial with Irbesartan for the prevention of
   Vascular Events

ACTS
American-Canadian Thrombosis Study

ACUITY Timing Trial
Acute Catheterization and Urgent Intervention Triage Strategy trial

ACUTE
Analysis of Coronary Ultrasound Thrombolysis Endpoints
Assessment of Cardioversion Utilizing Transesophageal Echocardiography
   pilot study

ADAPTS
Acute Directional Atherectomy Prior to Stenting

ADEG
Antiarrhythmic Drug Evaluation Group trial

ADEP
Atherosclerotic Disease Evolution by Picotamide study

AMETHYST
Assessment of Medtronic AVE Interceptor Saphenous Vein Graft Filter
   System Trial

ADMIRAL
Abciximab before Direct Angioplasty and Stenting in Myocardial Infarction
   Regarding Acute and Long-term Followup Trial

ADMIRE
AMP 579 Delivery for Myocardial Infarction Reduction trial

ADMIT
Arterial Disease Multiple Intervention Trial

ADOPT
Accupril Decision on Pharmacotherapy Trial

AFASAK
Atrial Fibrillation Aspirin Anticoagulation trial

AFCAPS
Air Force Coronary Atherosclerosis Prevention Study

AFCAPS/TexCAPS
C-reactive Protein Substudy: Air Force/Texas Coronary Atherosclerosis
    Prevention Study

AFFIRM
Atrial Fibrillation Follow-Up Investigation of Rhythm Management study

AFI
Atrial Fibrillation Investigators study

AFIB
Atrial Fibrillation Investigation with Bidisomide trial

AFIRME
Antagonist of the Fibrinogen Receptor After Myocardial Events study

AFIST II
Atrial Fibrillation Suppression Trial II

AFTER
Anistreplase Following Thrombolysis Effect on Reocclusion study
Aspirin/Anticoagulants Following Thrombolysis with Eminase Results study

AIMI
AngioJet in Acute Myocardial Infarction trial

AIMS
Acylated Plasminogen-Streptokinase Activator Complex Intervention
    Mortality Study

AIREX
Acute Infarction Ramipril Efficacy Extension study

AITIA
Aspirin in Transient Ischemic Attacks study

AITIAIS
Aspirin in Transient Ischemic Attacks Italian Study

ALDUSA
Aspirin Low Dosage in Unstable Angina study

ALERT
Amiodarone Versus Lidocaine Inpatient Emergency Resuscitation Trial

ALIVE
Adenosine Lidocaine Infarct Zone Viability Enhancement trial
Amiodarone Versus Lidocaine In Prehospital Refractory Ventricular Fibrillation
    study
Azimilide Postinfarction Survival Evaluation trial

ALL
Antihypertensive and Lipid Lowering study

ALLHAT
Antihypertensive and Lipid-lowering Treatment to Prevent Heart Attack Trial

AMI
Argatroban in Myocardial Infarction study

AMI-SK trial
Acute Myocardial Infarction-Streptokinase trial

AMICUS
Austrian Multicenter Isradipine Cum Spirapril Study

AMIGO trial
Atherectomy before Multilink Improves Lumen Gain and Clinical Outcomes trial

AMISTAD
Acute Myocardial Infarction Study of Adenosine trial

AMPI
ASPAC in acute myocardial infarction placebo controlled investigation

AMRO
Amsterdam-Rotterdam trial comparing excimer laser and percutaneous transluminal coronary angioplasty

AMT
Adenosine Scan Multicenter Trial

ANBP
Australian National Blood Pressure trial

ANS
American Nimodipine Study

ANTENOX
Switch to Oral Anticoagulant from Enoxaparin in Treatment of Acute Deep Venous Thrombosis Study

ANZ
Australia and New Zealand heart failure collaborative study

APAMIT
Asia-Pacific Acute Myocardial Infarction Trial

APIS
Antihypertensive Patch, Italian Study

APLAUD
Antiplatelet Useful Dose trial

APPI
Active Persantine in Postischemic Injury study

APPROACH
Alberta Provincial Project For Outcomes Assessment in Coronary Heart Disease

APRAIS
Acute Phase Reactions and Ischemic Coronary Syndromes Study

APRAISE
Antisense To Prevent Restenosis After Intervention Stent Evaluation

APRICOT
Antithrombotics in the Prevention of Reocclusion in Coronary Thrombolysis Trial
Aspirin Versus Coumadin in the Prevention of Reocclusion and Recurrent Ischemia
  After Successful Thrombolysis Trial

APSIS
Angina Prognosis Study in Stockholm
Angina Prognosis Study with Isoptin and Seloken

APTH
Ambulatory Blood Pressure Monitoring and Treatment of Hypertension

ARCH
Amiodarone Reduces Coronary Artery Bypass Grafting Hospitalization trial

ARCHeR trial
ACCULINK for Revascularization of Carotids in High-Risk Patients

ARCOS
Auckland Region Coronary or Stroke Study

ARCS
Atherosclerosis Risk in Communities Study

ARGAMI
Argatroban Compared with Heparin in Myocardial Infarction Treated with
  Recombinant Tissue Plasminogen Activator

ARIS
Anturan Reinfarction Italian Study

ARREST
Amiodarone in Out-of-Hospital Resuscitation of Refractory Sustained Ventricular
  Tachyarrhythmia Study

ARS
Amsterdam Resuscitation Study
Atherogenic Risk Study

ART
AngioJet Rapid Thrombectomy Catheter study

ARTIST
Angioplasty Versus Rotational Atherectomy for Treatment of Diffuse In-stent
  Restenosis Trial

ARTISTIC
AngioRad Radiation Technology for In-stent Restenosis Trial in Coronaries

ARTS
Arterial Revascularization Therapies Study

ASAAC
Acetylsalicylic Acid versus Anticoagulants study

ASAP
Acetylsalicylic Acid Persantine study
Azimilide Supraventricular Arrhythmia Program trial

ASCOT
Anglo Scandinavian Cardiac Outcomes Trial

ASDOS
Atrial Septal Defect Occlusion System Study

ASENOX
Accelerated Streptokinase and Enoxaparin trial

ASIS
American Study of Infarct Survival
Angina And Silent Ischemia Study

ASPS
Australian Swedish Pindolol Study

ASSENT-3 Trial
Assessment of the Safety of a New Thrombolytic 3 trial

ASSET
Anglo Scandinavian Study of Early Thrombosis
Atorvastatin Simvastatin Safety and Efficacy Trial

ASSURE
A Stent Versus Stent Ultrasound Remodeling Evaluation

ATACS
Antithrombotic Therapy in Acute Coronary Syndromes trial

ATEST
Atenolol and Streptokinase Trial

ATIAIS
Anturan Transient Ischemic Attack Italian Study

ATIME
Accupril Titration Intervention Management Interval Management Evaluation

ATLANTIC
angina treatment, lasers and normal therapy in comparison

ATLAS
Acolysis During Treatment of Lesions Affecting Saphenous Vein Bypass Grafts

ATLAST
Antiplatelet Therapy Versus Lovenox Plus Antiplatelet Therapy for Patients with Increased Risk of Stent Thrombosis
Aspirin/Ticlopidine Versus Low-Molecular Weight Heparin/Aspirin/Ticlopidine Stent Trial

ATMA
Amiodarone Trials Meta Analysis

ATRAMI
Autonomic Tone And Reflexes After Myocardial Infarction trial

ATTMH
Australian Therapeutic Trial of Mild Hypertension

AVERT
Atorvastatin Versus Revascularization Treatment Trial

AVID Trial
Angiography Versus Intravascular Ultrasound Directed Trial
prophylactic amiodarone versus implantable defibrillator therapy trial

AWESOME
Angina with Extremely Serious Operative Mortality Evaluation

BAATAF
Boston Area Anticoagulation Trial for Atrial Fibrillation

BACUS
Balloon Angioplasty Compliance Ultrasound Study

BADE
Bioimpedance as an Adjunct to Dobutamine Echocardiography study

BAHAMA
Baragwanath Hypertension Ambulatory Blood Pressure Monitoring Multiarm study

BARASTER
Balloon Angioplasty Versus Rotational Atherectomy for Stent Restenosis

BARI
Bypass Angioplasty Revascularization Investigation

BASC
Blood Pressure in Acute Stroke Collaboration

BBPP
Beta-blocker Pooling Project

BCAPS
Beta-blocker Cholesterol-Lowering Asymptomatic Plaque Study

BCSP
Bavarian Cholesterol Screening Project

BEACH
Boston Scientific/EPI: A Carotid Stenting Trial for High-Risk Surgical Patients

BENESTENT
Belgian-Netherlands Stent study

BEPS
Belgian Eminase Prehospital Study

BERT
Beta Energy Restenosis Trial

BESMART
BeStent in Small Arteries study

BESS
Berlin Pacemaker Study On Syncope

BESSAMI
Berlin Stent Study in Acute Myocardial Infarction

BEST
Beta-Cath System Trial
Medtronic BeStent coronary stent versus Palmaz-Schatz coronary stent

BET
Benefit Evaluation of Direct Coronary Stenting

BHACAS
Beating Heart Against Cardioplegic Arrest Studies

BHS
Bogalusa Heart Study
Brisighella Heart Study

BIGMAC
Beaumont interventional group, Mevacor, ACE inhibitor, colchicine restenosis trial
Bidirectional Gantry Multiarray Coil study

BIOMACS
Biochemical Markers of Acute Coronary Syndromes Study

BIP
Bezafibrate Infarction Prevention study

BIRD
Bolus versus Infusion Rescupase Development study

BISTRO
Boehringer Ingelheim Study in Thrombosis

BLASP
Barbados Low-dose Aspirin Study in Pregnancy

BMS
Belfast Metoprolol Study

BNS
Belfast Nifedipine Study

BOAT
Balloon Angioplasty Versus Optimal Atherectomy Trial

BOILER
Balloon Occlusive Intravascular Lysis Enhanced Recanalization Strategy study

BOSS
Balloon Optimization versus Stent Study

BPEG
British Packing and Electrophysiology Group study

BPSMC
blood pressure study in Mexican children

BRESUS
British Hospital Resuscitation Study

BRH
British Regional Heart study

BRHS
British Regional Heart Study

BRIE
Beta Radiation in Europe

BRITE II
Beta Radiation to Reduce In-stent Restenosis II

CAASET
Canadian Amlodipine and Atenolol Stress Echo Trial

CABADAS
Prevention of Coronary Artery Bypass Graft Occlusion by Aspirin, Dipyridamole and Acenocoumarol Study

CABRI
Coronary Angioplasty versus Bypass Revascularization Investigation

CACTIS
Comparison of Aspirin with Clopidogrel or Ticlopidine in Stents Trial

CADHYP
Coronary Artery Disease in Hypertension study

CADILLAC
Controlled Abciximab and Device Investigation to Lower Late Angioplasty Complications

CADRES
Coronary Artery Descriptors and Restenosis Study

CAFA
Canadian Atrial Fibrillation Anticoagulation study

CAFE
Coronary Artery Flow Evaluation

CAMCAT
Canadian Multicenter Clentiazem Angina Trial

CAPARES
Coronary Angioplasty Amlodipine In Restenosis Trial

CAPAS
Cutting Balloon Angioplasty versus Plain Old Balloon Angioplasty Randomized Study

CAPE
Circadian Antiischemia Program in Europe

CAPERNET
Carotid Artery Revascularization Using the Boston Scientific EPI FilterWire EX and EndoTex NexStent

CAPITOL
Captopril Postinfarction Tolerance Trial

CAPP
Captopril Prevention Project study
Concerted Action Polyp Prevention study

CAPPHY
Captopril Primary Prevention in Hypertension study

CAPPP
Captopril Prevention Project

CAPRICORN
Carvedilol Postinfarct Survival Controlled Evaluation

CAPRIE
Clopidogrel Versus Aspirin in Patients at Risk for Ischemic Events

CAPTIN
Captopril Before Reperfusion in Acute Myocardial Infarction
Captopril Plus Tissue Plasminogen Activator Following Acute Myocardial
  Infarction

CAPTIVE
CardioShield Application Protects during Transluminal Intervention of Vein Grafts
  by Reducing Emboli trial

CAPTURE
C7E3 Antiplatelet Therapy in Unstable Refractory Angina trial
Chimeric Antiplatelet Therapy in Unstable Angina Refractory to Standard
  Treatment trial

CARAT
Coronary Angioplasty and Rotational Atherectomy Trial

CARDIAC
Cardiovascular Disease and Alimentary Comparison study

CARD PORT
Cardiac Arrhythmia and Risk of Death Patient Outcome Research Team

CARE
Carvedilol Arthrectomy Restenosis trial
Cholesterol and Recurrent Events study

CARMEN
Carvedilol Angiotensin Converting Enzyme Inhibitors Remodeling Mild Heart
  Failure Evaluation

CARPORT
Coronary Artery Restenosis Prevention on Repeated Thromboxane A2-Receptor
  Antagonism study

CARS
Coronary Artery Regression Study
Coumadin Aspirin Reinfarction Study

CART
Colchicine Angioplasty Restenosis Trial

CASCO
Calcium Sensitization in Congestive Heart Failure

CASH
Cardiac Arrest Study, Hamburg
Consensus Action on Salt and Hypertension

CASIS
Canadian Amlodipine/Atenolol in Silent Ischemia Study
Coronary Artery Stent Implantation Study
Coronary Artery Surgery Study

CASSIS
Czech and Slovak Spirapril Intervention Study

CASTEL
Cardiovascular Study in the Elderly

CASTOR
Coronary Angioscopic Study of Restenosis

CAT
Cardiomyopathy Trial
Coronary Angioplasty Trial

CATCH
Child and Adolescent Trial for Cardiovascular Heath
Community Action to Control High Blood Pressure

CAVA
Coronary Atherectomy Versus Angioplasty study

CAVATAS
Carotid and Vertebral Artery Transluminal Angioplasty Study

CAVEAT
Coronary Angioplasty Versus Excisional Atherectomy Trial

CBASS
Cutting Balloon Angioplasty for Small Size Vessels trial

CCAT
Canadian Coronary Atherectomy Trial

CCCCP
Comprehensive Cardiovascular Community Control Program

CCHAT
Canadian Cozaar, Hyzaar and Amlodipine Trial

CCHD
Caerphilly Collaborative Heart Disease study

CCHP
Corpus Christi Heart Project

CCHS
Copenhagen City Heart Study

CCP
Cooperative Cardiovascular Project

CCRT
Cardiac Catheter Reuse Trial

CCS
Chinese Cardiac Study

CCT
Chinese Captopril Trial

CDP
Coronary Drug Project

CDPAS
Coronary Disease Prevention with Aspirin Study
Coronary Drug Project Aspirin Study

CEDARS
Comprehensive Evaluation of Defibrillators and Resuscitative Shock study

CEI-AMI
Converting Enzyme Inhibitor treatment of patients in China with Acute Myocardial
   Infarction

CELL
Cost Effectiveness of Lipid Lowering study

CERT
Cardiovascular Event Reduction Trial

CESAR
Centralised European Studies in Angina Research

CESARZ
Clinical European Studies in Angina and Revascularization

CESNA
Comparative Efficacy and Safety of Nisoldipine and Amlodipine in hypertension

CESNA-II
Comparative Efficacy and Safety of Nisoldipine and Amlodipine in hypertension
   with ischemic heart disease

CESNA-III
Comparative Efficacy and Safety of Nisoldipine extended release and Amlodipine
   in African-American patients with hypertension

CHAD
Cholesterol, Hypertension and Diabetes study

CHAMP
Cardiac Hospitalization Atherosclerosis Management Program

CHANGE
Chronic Heart Failure and Graded Exercise study

CHARM
Candesartan in Heart failure Assessment in Reduction of Mortality

CHEAPER
Confirmation that Heparin is an Alternative to Promote Early Reperfusion in Acute Myocardial Infarction study

CHEER
Chest Pain Evaluation in Emergency Room trial

CHEPER
Chest Pain Evaluation Registry study

CHF-IES
Congestive Heart Failure, Italian Epidemiological Study

CHIP
Coronary Health Improvement Project

CHIVAS
Coronary Heart Disease Stenting In Small Vessels versus Balloon Angioplasty Study

CHOICE
Caring for Hypertension on Initiation Cost and Effectiveness study
Congestive Heart Failure Mortality Investigation on Carvedilol's Efficacy

CHOICES
Coronary Heart Disease, Osteoporosis Interventions, and Community Evaluation Studies

CHRISTMAS
Carvedilol Hibernation Reversible Ischemia Trial: Marker of Success

CHS
Cardiovascular Health Study
Charleston Heart Study
Congenital Heart Surgeons Society Study
Copenhagen City Heart Study
Coronary Heart Study

CIAIT
Chinese Infarction Angiotensin Converting Enzyme Inhibitor Trial

CIDS
Canadian Internal Defibrillator Study

CIS
Coronary Intervention Study

CITTS
Central Illinois Thrombolytic Therapy Study

CLASP
Collaborative Low-dose Aspirin Study in Pregnancy

CLASSICS
Clopidogrel Aspirin Stent Interventional Cooperative Study

CLEOPAD
Clopidogrel in Peripheral Artery Disease study

CLIP
Cholesterol-lowering intervention program

CLOT
Clinical Perspectives on Lysis of Thrombi study

CLOUT
Core Laboratory Ultrasound Analysis

COAST Trial
Heparin-Coated Stents in Small Coronary Arteries Trial

COAT
Cooperative Osaka Adenosine Trial

COBRA
Comparison Of Balloon versus Rotational Angioplasty

COLTS
Coronary Observational Long-Term Study

COMBAT
Conventional versus Multisite Pacing for Bradyarrhythmia Therapy

COMET
Carvedilol or Metoprolol European Trial
Carvedilol or Metoprolol Evaluation Trial

COMMIT
Comprehensive Multidisciplinary Interventional Trial for Regression of Coronary Heart Disease

COMPARE
Randomized Comparison of Platelet Inhibition with Abciximab, Tirofiban, and Eptifibatide during Percutaneous Coronary Intervention in Acute Coronary Syndromes

COMPASS
Cilostazol or Multilink for Percutaneous Transluminal Coronary Angioplasty Small Vessel Study

CONSENSUS
Cooperative North Scandinavian Enalapril Survival Study

CONVINCE
Controlled Onset Verapamil Investigation for Cardiovascular Endpoints study

COPERNICUS
Carvedilol Prospective Randomized Cumulative Survival trial

CORALI
Coronarography Plus Alimentation trial

CORDIS-MICA
Cordis MiniCrown Stent in Small Coronary Arteries

CORGENE
Coronary Disease and Angiotensin Converting Enzyme I/D Genotype study

CORIS
Coronary Risk Factor Study

CORRECT
Complete versus Restrictive Revascularization by Coronary Angioplasty Trial

CORSICA
Chronic Occlusion Revascularization with Stent Implantation versus Coronary Angioplasty study

CORTES
Clivarin Assessment of Regression of Thrombosis Efficacy and Safety Study

COST
Cardiac Output Study Technology

COTAIM
Continuation of Trial Antihypertensive Interventions and Management

COURAGE
Clinical Outcomes Utilizing Revascularization and Aggressive Drug Evaluation

COURT
Contrast Media Utilization in High Risk Percutaneous Transluminal Coronary Angioplasty Trial

CPAS
Canadian Prinivil Atenolol Study

CPEP
Chicago Coronary Prevention Evaluation Program

CPHRP
Coronary Prevention and Hypertension Research Project

C-PORT
Cardiovascular Patient Outcomes Research Team Trial

CPPT
Coronary Primary Prevention Trial

CPRG
Coronary Prevention Research Group

CRAC
Compliance-related Angioplasty Complications study

CRAF
Canadian Registry of Atrial Fibrillation

CRAFT
Catheterization Rescue Angioplasty Following Thrombolysis Trial
Controlled Randomized Atrial Fibrillation Trial

CREATE
Carotid Revascularization Endarterectomy versus Stent trial
Cholesterol Research Education and Treatment Evaluation

CREDO
Clopidogrel Reduction of Events During Extended Observation study

CREW
Coronary Regression with Estrogen in Women study

CRIS
Calcium Antagonist Reinfarction Italian Study

CRISP
Cholesterol Reduction in Seniors Program Pilot study

CRIYFS
Cardiovascular Risk in Young Finns Study

CRUISE
Can Routine Ultrasound Influence Stent Expansion study
Coronary Revascularization Using Integrilin and Single bolus Enoxaparin

CRUSADE
Coronary Reserve Utilization for Stent Angiography Doppler Endpoint study
Coronary Revascularization Ultrasound Angioplasty Device trial

CSCHDS
Caerphilly and Speedwell Collaborative Heart Disease Studies

CSGTEI
Collaborative Study Group Trial on the Effect of Irbesartan

C-SIRIUS
Canadian Sirolimus-Eluting Stent in Coronary Lesions Study

C-SMART
Cardiomyoplasty Skeletal Muscle Assist Randomized Trial

CTA
Committee on Thrombolytic Agents

CTAF
Canadian trial of atrial fibrillation

CTOPP
Canadian trial of physiological pacing

CTRD
Cardiac Transplant Research Database

CTS
Collaborative Transplant Study

CTSP
cooperative triglyceride standardization program

CUBA
Cutting Balloon versus Conventional Balloon Angioplasty study

CUBS
Clinical Utility Baseline trial

CURE
Clopidogrel in Unstable Anginal to Prevent Recurrent Ischemic Events trial
Columbia University Restenosis Elimination trial

CVIR
Cardiovascular Information Registry

CYCAZAREM
Cyclophosphamide versus Azathioprine during Remission of Systemic Vasculitis trial

DAAF
Digoxin in Acute Atrial Fibrillation study

DAIS
Diabetes Atherosclerosis Intervention Study

DAMAD
diabetic microangiopathy modification with aspirin versus dipyridamole

DANAMI
Danish Multicenter Study of Acute Myocardial Infarction

DANSTENT
Danish Multicenter Stent Study

DAPPAF
Dual-site Atrial Pacing for Prevention of Atrial Fibrillation trial

DART
Diet and Reinfarction Trial
Dilation versus Ablation Revascularization Trial

DATA
Diltiazem as Adjunctive Therapy to Activase study

DATOS
Diet and Antismoking Trial of Oslo Study

DAVIT
Danish Verapamil Infarction Trial

DBLE
Double Bolus Lytic Efficacy trial

DDDD-CAT
Drug Delivery Device Dispatch in Coronary Angioplasty Trial

DEBATE
Doppler Endpoints Balloon Angioplasty Trial, Europe

DEER
Diet and Exercise in Elevated Risk trial

DEFIBRILAT
Defibrillator as Bridge to Later Transplantation study

DELIVER
The RX Achieve Drug-eluting Coronary Stent System in the Treatment of Patients
    with de novo Native Coronary Lesions

DES
Danish Enoxaparin Study

DESIRE
Debulking and Stenting in Restenosis Elimination trial

DESTINI
Doppler Endpoint Stent International Investigation
Duke University Clinical Cardiology Study Elective Stent Trial: a Cost
    Containment Initiative

DHAOS
Dutch Hypertension and Offspring Study

DHCCP
Department of Health and Social Security Hypertension Care Computing Project

DHFS
Diet-Heart Feasibility Study

DIAMOND
Danish Investigation of Arrhythmia and Mortality on Dofetilide

DIAMOND-CHF
Danish Investigation of Arrhythmia and Mortality on Dofetilide in Congestive
    Heart Failure

DIAMOND-MI
Danish Investigation of Arrhythmia and Mortality on Dofetilide in Myocardial Infarction

DiDi
Diltiazem in Dilated Cardiomyopathy trial

DIGAF
Digoxin in Atrial Fibrillation study

DIGAMI
Diabetes Mellitus-Insulin Glucose Infusion in Acute Myocardial Infarction

DIG-CAPTOPRIL
Canadian Digoxin Captopril Study

DILCACOMP
Diltiazem Captopril Comparative study

DILDURANG
Diltiazem Duration in Angina study

DILPLACOMP
Diltiazem Placebo Comparative trial

DIMT
Dutch Ibopamine Multicenter Trial

DIRECT
Direct Myocardial Revascularization in Regeneration of Endomyocardial Channels Trial

DIRS
Dutch Invasive Reperfusion Study

DISCO
Direct Stenting of Coronary Artery trial

DISH
Dietary Intervention Study of Hypertension

DISTINCT
Biocompatibles BiodivYsio Stent In Randomized Control Trial

DISTRESS
Dispatch Stent Restenosis Study

DOMIOS
Determinants of Myocardial Infarction Onset Study

DOUBLE
Double Bolus Lytic Efficacy trial

DOUBTLESS
Doppler and Ultrasound-Guided Balloon Therapeutics for Coronary Lesions Study

DPR
Dietary Prevention of Recurrent Myocardial Infarction

DRASTIC
Dutch Renal Artery Stenosis Intervention Cooperative

DRS
Diltiazem Reinfarction Study

DSMA
Diet and Stress Management in Angina

DUCCS
Duke University Clinical Cardiology Study

DUTCH-TIA
Dutch transient ischemic attack study

DVT
Danish Verapamil Trial

EAFT
European Atrial Fibrillation Trial

EAGAR
Estrogen and Graft Atherosclerosis Research Trial

EARS
European Atherosclerosis Research Study

EAS
Edinburgh Artery Study

EASI
European Antiplatelet Stent Investigation
Emory Angioplasty versus Surgery Trial

ECAA
European Concerted Action on Anticoagulation Study

ECAP
European Concerted Action Project

ECAT
European Concerted Action on Thrombosis and Disabilities study

ECAT AP
European Concerted Action on Thrombosis: Angina Pectoris study

ECCE
Effects of Captopril on Cardiopulmonary Exercise study

ECRIS
EndoCoronary-Rhenium-Irradiation Study

ECSG
European Cooperative Study Group

ECSS
European Coronary Surgery Study

EDIC
Echocardiography Dobutamine International Cooperative study

EDIT
Early Defibrillator Implantation Trial

EDRES
Effects of Debulking on Restenosis trial

EFERF
Enalapril Felodipine Extended Release Factorial study

EFICAT
Ejection Fraction in Carvedilol-Treated Transplant Candidates study

EFS
European Fraxiparine Study

EHVT
Edinburgh Heart Valve Trial

EIHDW
Evaluation of Ischemic Heart Disease in Women Study

EIS
European Infarction Study

ELAT
Embolism in Left Atrial Thrombi study

ELCA
Excimer Laser Coronary Angioplasty Registry

ELHE
Evaluation of losartan in hemodialysis study

ELITE
Evaluation of Losartan in the Elderly Study

ELSA
European Lacidipine Study on Atherosclerosis
European Longitudinal Study on Aging

ELVD
Exercise in Left Ventricular Dysfunction trial

ELVD-CHF
Exercise in Left Ventricular Dysfunction and Chronic Heart Failure trial

EMERALD
European and Australian Multicenter Evaluation Research on Atrial Fibrillation
   Dofetilide
Enhanced Myocardial Efficacy and Recovery by Aspiration of Liberalized
   Debris trial

EMIAT
European Myocardial Infarction Amiodarone Trial
European Myocardial Infarction Arrhythmia Trial

EMIP
European Myocardial Infarction Project

EMIP-FR
European Myocardial Infarction Project, Free Radicals

EMPAR
Enoxaparin MaxEPA Prevention of Angioplasty Restenosis study

EMPIRE
Economics of Myocardial Perfusion Imaging in Europe study

ENASA
Enoxaparin and/or Aspirin in Unstable Angina trial

ENCORE
Evaluation of Nifedipine and Cerivastatin on Recovery of Endothelial Function
   trial

ENDPT
Evaluation of Doppler Parameters During Percutaneous Transluminal Coronary
   Angioplasty

ENOXART
Enoxaparin in Arterial Surgery study

ENRICAD
Enhancing Recovery in Coronary Artery Disease trial

ENRICHD
Enhancing Recovery in Coronary Heart Disease Patients trial

ENTICES
Enoxaparin and Ticlopidine After Elective Stenting study

EPIC
Echocardiography Persantine International Cooperative study
Echo Persantine Italian Cooperative study
Evaluation of 7E3 for the Prevention of Ischemic Complications

EPIDS
Early Postmyocardial Infarction Intravenous Dipyridamole study

EPILOG
Evaluation of Percutaneous Transluminal Coronary Angioplasty to Improve Long-term Outcome with Abciximab Glycoprotein IIb/IIIa Blockade Trial

EPISTENT
Epilog Stent trial

EPISTENT
Evaluation of Platelet IIb/IIIa Inhibition in Stenting

EPRCSS
European Prospective Randomized Coronary Surgery Study

EQUIPP
Evaluation of Quinapril in Primary Practice trial

ERA
Estrogen Replacement in Atherosclerosis study

ERAC
Argentine Randomized Trial of Percutaneous Transluminal Coronary Angioplasty versus Coronary Artery Bypass Surgery in Multivessel Disease

ERACI II
Argentine Randomized Trial of Percutaneous Transluminal Coronary Angioplasty versus Coronary Artery Bypass Surgery in Multivessel Disease II

ERASER
Evaluation of ReoPro and Stenting to Eliminate Restenosis trial

ERBAC
Excimer Rotational Balloon Angioplasty Comparison
Excimer, Rotablator, Balloon Angioplasty For Complex Lesions study

ERNST
European Resuscitation Nimodipine Study

ESBY
electrical stimulation versus coronary artery bypass study

ESCALAT
Efegatran And Streptokinase to Canalize Arteries Like Accelerated Tissue Plasminogen Activator study

ESCAMI
Evaluation of the Safety and Cardioprotective Effects of Eniporide in Acute Myocardial Infarction

ESCOBAR
Emergency Stenting Compared to Conventional Balloon Angioplasty
Randomized trial

ESETCID
European Study Of Epidemiology And Treatment Of Cardiac Inflammatory
Diseases

E-SIRIUS
European Sirolimus-Eluting Stent in Coronary Lesions

ESMIR
Echocardiographic Selection of Patients for Mitral Regurgitation study

ESPRIM
European Study Prevention Research of Infarct with Molsidomine

ESPRIT
European Study of the Prevention of Reocclusion after Initial Thrombolysis

ESSENCE
Efficacy Safety Subcutaneous Enoxaparin in Non-Q Wave Coronary Events study

ESSEX
European Scimed Stent Experience

ESVEM
Electrophysiologic Study versus Electrocardiographic Monitoring

EURAMIC
European Community Multicenter Study on Antioxidants, Myocardial Infarction
and Breast Cancer

EURID
European Registry for Implantable Cardioverter Defibrillators

EURO-ART
European AngioJet Rapid Thrombectomy study

EUROCARE
European Carvedilol Restenosis trial

EUROCARDI
European Concerted Action for the Rapid Diagnosis of Myocardial Infarction

EURO-DIRECT
European Direct Myocardial Revascularization in Regeneration of Endomyocardial
Channels trial

EUROPA
European trial of reduction of cardiac events with perindopril in stable coronary
artery disease

EUROSCOP
European Registry Society Study of Chronic Obstructive Pulmonary Diseases

EUROWINTER
European study on cold exposure and winter mortality from ischemic heart disease

EVADE
experience with left ventricular assist device with exercise trial

EVAR trial 1 and 2
Endovascular Aneurysm Repair Trial 1 and 2

EVET
Enoxaparin versus Tinzaparin

EWA
Estrogen in Women with Atherosclerosis study

EWGCP
European Working Group on Cardiac Pacing

EWPHE
European Working Party on Hypertension in the Elderly

EWR
European Wallstent Registry

EXACTO
Excimer Laser Angioplasty in Coronary Total Occlusion study

EXCEL
Expanded Clinical Evaluation of Lovastatin trial

EXCITE
Evaluation of Oral Xemilofiban in Controlling Thrombotic Events

EXPAPS
Exeter Primary Angioplasty Pilot Study

EXTRA
Evaluation of XT Stent for Restenosis of Native Arteries

EXTRACT
Enoxaparin and Thrombolysis Reperfusion for Acute Myocardial Infarction
   Treatment

FACET
Flosequinan Angiotensin Converting Enzyme Inhibitor Trial
Fosinopril versus Amlodipine Cardiovascular Events Trial

FACIT
Folate After Coronary Intervention Trial

FACTS
Functional Angiometric Correlation with Thallium Scintigraphy trial

FANTASTIC
Full Anticoagulation versus Ticlopidine Plus Aspirin After Stent Implantation
Study

FAP
Fibrinolytics versus Primary Angioplasty Trial

FAPIS
Flecainide and Propafenone Italian Study

FAPS
Felodipine Atherosclerosis Prevention Study
French Aortic Plaque Study

FASTEST
Femoral Artery Stent Study

FAST-MI
Field Ambulance Study of Thrombolysis in Myocardial Infarction

FATIMA
Fraxiparin Anticoagulant Therapy in Myocardial Infarction Study in Amsterdam

FATS
Familial Atherosclerosis Treatment Study

FEMINA
Felodipine ER and Metoprolol CR in the Treatment of Patients with Stable
Angina Pectoris

FEST
Fosinopril Efficacy/Safety Trial
Fosinopril on Exercise Tolerance Study

FHRS
Familial Hypercholesterolemia Regression Study

FHS
Family Heart Study
Framingham Heart Study

FIELD
Fenofibrate Intervention and Event Lowering in Diabetes trial

FIG
Flosequinan Investigator Group

FIM study
First-in-Man study

FINESS
First International New Intravascular Rigid-Flex Endovascular Stent Study

FINMONICA
Finnish monitoring trends and determinants in cardiovascular diseases

FINRISK
Finland Cardiovascular Risk study

FIRE
FilterWire EX Randomized Evaluation trial

FIRST
Flolan International Randomized Survival Trial

FISH
Finnish Isradipine Study in Hypertension

FLARE
Fluvastatin Angioplasty Restenosis trial

FLEQUIN
Flecainide Compared to Oral Quinidine study

FLUENT
Fluvastatin Long-term Extension Trial

FMS
Fragmin Multicenter Study

FMT
Fragmin Multicenter Trial

FORECAST
fractional flow reserve or relative fractional velocity reserve evaluation of coronary
   artery stenosis versus thallium

FORT
Fish Oil Restenosis Trial

FOS
Framingham Offspring Study

FOSS
Framingham Offspring, Spouse Study

FRAMI
Fragmin in Acute Myocardial Infarction study

FRAXIDIS
Fraxiparine in Post-Hospital Discharge study

FRAXIS
Fraxiparine in Ischemic Syndromes study

FRAXODI
Fraxiparine Once Daily Injection study

FREEDOM
Future Revascularization Evaluation in Patients with Diabetes Mellitus

FRESCO
Florence Randomized Elective Stenting in Acute Coronary Occlusion study

FRIC
Fragmin in unstable coronary artery disease trial

FRISC
Fast Revascularization during InStability in Coronary artery disease
Fragmin during InStability in Coronary artery disease trial

FRISC II
Fragmin and/or Fast Revascularization during InStability in Coronary artery
  disease trial

FROG
French Rotablator group study

FROST
French Optimal Stenting Trial

FTC
Fibrinolysis Trialists Collaboration

FTT
Fibrinolytic Therapy Trialist Collaboration

GABI
German Angioplasty Bypass Intervention trial
German Angioplasty Bypass Surgery Investigation

GAMIS
German-Austrian Myocardial Infarction Study

GARS
German-Austrian Reinfarction Study

GCP
German Cardiovascular Prevention study

GDCMS
German Dilated Cardiomyopathy Study

GEART
Gemfibrozil Atherosclerosis Regression Trial

GELIA
German Experience with Low-Intensity Anticoagulation

GIPSI
Gradual Inflation at Optimum Pressure versus Stent Implantation study

GISSI
Grupo Italiano per lo Studio della Streptochinasi Nell'infarto Miocardico (Effectiveness of Intravenous Thrombolytic Treatment in Acute Myocardial Infarction)

GMT
Göteborg Metoprolol Trial

GR II
Gianturco Roubin Second-generation Coronary Stent Trial

GRACE
Gianturco Roubin Stent in Acute Closure Evaluation
Global Registry of Acute Coronary Events

GRAMI
Gianturco Roubin Second-Generation Coronary Stent in Acute Coronary Infarction

GRASP
Glaxo Restenosis and Symptoms Project

GREAT
Grampian Region Early Anistreplase Trial

GRECO
German Recanalization of Coronary Occlusion Trial
German Recombinant Plasminogen Activator Study

GUARANTEE
Global Unstable Angina Registry and Treatment Evaluation
Gruppo Italiano per lo Studio della Streptochinasi nell'Infarcto Miocardico 3

GUARD
Saphenous Vein Graft Intervention Using AngioGuard for Reduction of Distal Embolization

GUARDIAN
Guard During Ischemia Against Necrosis

GUIDE
Guidance by Ultrasound Imaging for Decision Endpoints trial

GUIDE II
Guidance by Ultrasound Imaging for Decision Endpoints II trial

GUSTO-I
Global Utilization of Streptokinase and Tissue Plasminogen Activator for Occluded coronary arteries trial

GUSTO-IIa
Global Use of Strategies to Open Occluded Coronary Arteries

GUSTO-IIb
Global Use of Strategies to Open Occluded Arteries in Acute Coronary
Syndromes trial

GUSTO-III
Global Use of Strategies to Open Occluded Coronary Arteries trial

GUSTO-IV
Global use of Streptokinase and Tissue Plasminogen Activator for Occluded
Arteries trial

HAL
Heart Attacks in London study

HALF
Homocysteine, Atherosclerosis, Lipid and Familial hypercholesterolemia study

HALT
Hypertension And Lipid Trial

HALT MI
Hu23F2G anti-adhesion to limit cytotoxic injury following acute myocardial
infarction study

HAMIT
Heparin in Acute Myocardial Infarction trial

HANE
Hydrochlorothiazide, Atenolol, Nitrendipine, and Enalapril study

HAPI
Heparin as an Alternative to Promote Patency in Acute Mocardial Infarction Study

HAPORT
Heart Attack Patient Outcome Research Team study

HAPPHY
Heart Attack Primary Prevention in Hypertension

HAROLD
Hypertension and Ambulatory Recording in the Old

HARP
Harvard Atherosclerosis Reversibility Project

HART
Heparin-Aspirin Reperfusion Trial
Hypertension Audit of Risk Factor Therapy Study

HART II
Heparin and Reperfusion Therapies Study

HARVEST
Hypertension and Ambulatory Recording Venetia Study

HAS
Hirulog angioplasty study, hypertensive arteriosclerotic

HASI
Hirulog Angioplasty Study Investigators

HATS
HDL-atherosclerosis treatment study

HDDRISC
Heart Disease and Diabetes Risk Indicators in a Screened Cohort Study

HDES
Heidelberg Diet and Exercise Study

HDFP
Hypertension Detection and Followup Program

HDS
Hypertension in Diabetes Study

HEART
Hyperlipidemia, Epidemiology, Atherosclerosis Risk Factor Trial

HELP
Heart European Leaders Panel study

HELPS
HydroCoil Endovascular Aneurysm Occlusion and Pacing Study

HELPS
Hypertension, Exercise and Lifestyle Programs for Seniors study

HELVETICA
Hirudin in European Restenosis Prevention Trial versus Heparin Treatment in Percutaneous Transluminal Coronary Angioplasty

HEMOSTAT
Hemostasis with Prostar XL versus Angio-Seal after Coronary Intervention Trial

HEP
Hypertension in Elderly Persons trial

HERO
Hirulog Early Reperfusion/Occlusion study

HEROICS
How Effective are Revascularization Options in Cardiogenic Shock trial

HERS
Heart and Estrogen-Progestin Replacement Study

HHP
Honolulu Heart Program

HHS
Helsinki Heart Study
Honolulu Heart Study

HIC
Heart Information Center

HINT
Holland Interuniversity Nifedipine/Metoprolol Trial

HIPOS
Hypertension In Pregnancy: Offspring Study

HIPS
Heparin Delivery with InfusaSleeve Catheter Prior to Stent Implantation Study
Heparin Infusion Prior to Stenting Study

HIRMIT
High-Risk Myocardial Ischemia Trial

HIS
Hungarian Isradipine Study

HIT
High-density Lipoprotein Cholesterol Intervention Trial
Hirudin for the Improvement of Thrombolysis Study

HIT-SK
Hirudin for the Improvement of Thrombolysis with Streptokinase

HOCAP
Hypertrophic Obstructive Cardiomyopathy Ablation Pacing study

HOPE
Hypertensive Old People in Edinburgh study
Heart Outcomes and Prevention Evaluation

HOT
Hypertension Optimal Treatment study

HOT MI
Hyperbaric Oxygen and Thrombolysis in Myocardial Infarction study

HPT
Hypertension Prevention Trial

Hy-C
Hydralazine versus Captopril Trial

HYNON
Hypertension Non-drug Treatment Cooperative study

HyperGEN
Hypertension Genetic Epidemiology Network Study

HYPPOS
Hypertensive Population Survey

HYPREN
Hypertension Under Prazosin and Enalapril study

HYSTENOX
Enoxaparin Following Hysterectomy study

HYVET
Hypertension in the Very Elderly Trial

IAMA
Infection in Atherosclerosis and use of Macrolide Antibiotics Study

IAP
International Atherosclerosis Project

IARG
International Anticoagulant Review Group study

ICARIS
Intervention Cardiology Risk Stratification study

ICIN
Intracoronary Streptokinase Trial of the Interuniversity Cardiology Institute of the
  Netherlands

IDCS
Idiopathic Dilated Cardiomyopathy Study

IDHS
Indian Diet Heart Study

IDHPORT
Ischemic Heart Disease Patient Outcomes Research Team

IHD SDP
Ischemic Heart Disease Shared Decision Making Program

IIHD
Israeli Ischemic Heart Disease study

IIUK
Intraoperative Intraarterial Urokinase study

ILRCFS
Iowa Lipid Research Clinics Family Study

IMAGE
International Metoprolol/Nifedipine Anginal Exercise trial
International Multicenter Angina Exercise study
International Multicenter Aprotinin Graft Patency Experience trial

IMEP
Investigation in Menopausal Women of the Effect of Estradiol and Progesterone on Cardiovascular Risk Factors

IMPACT
Integrilin to Minimize Platelet Aggregation and Coronary Thrombosis trial
International Mexiletine and Placebo Antiarrhythmia Coronary Trial

IMPACT-II
Integrilin to Minimize Platelet Aggregation and Coronary Thrombosis trial

IMPACT-AMI
Integrilin to Minimize Platelet Aggregation and Coronary Thrombosis, Acute Myocardial Infarction trial

IMPACT-stent
Integrilin to Minimize Platelet Aggregation and Coronary Thrombosis in Stenting trial

IMPRESS
Intramural Low Molecular Weight Heparin for Prevention of Restenosis Study

IMPROVED
Introduction of Mycophenolate Mofetil and Reduction of Cyclosporine Valuable in Renal Dysfunction after Heart Transplantation Study

IN-CHF
Italian Network Congestive Heart Failure

INDANA
Individual Data Analysis of Antihypertensive Intervention Trials

INHIBIT
Intimal Hyperplasia Inhibition with Beta In-stent Trial

INJECT
International Joint Efficacy Comparison of Thrombolytics trial

INLINIS
Ireland-Netherlands Lisinopril, Nifedipine Study

INROAD
In-stent Restenosis Optimal Angioplasty Device trial

INTERHEART study
Cardiovascular Disease Study

ISAR-COOL
Intracoronary Stenting with Antithrombotic Cooling-Off study

ISAR-REACT
Intracoronary Stenting and Antithrombotic Regimen-Rapid Early Action for Coronary Treatment

ISAR-SMART
Intracoronary Stenting or Angioplasty for Restenosis Reduction in Small Arteries

INSIGHT
International Nifedipine Study Intervention as a Hoal in Hypertension Treatment

INSPIRE
Increasing Participation in Cardiac Rehabilitation
Intravascular Ultrasound Study Predictor of Restenosis trial

INTACT
International Nifedipine Trial on antiatherosclerotic therapy

INTEGRITI
Integrelin and Tenecteplase in Acute Myocardial Infarction

INTERACT
Integrilin and Enoxaparin Randomized Assessment of Acute Coronary Syndrome
    Treatment

INTERCEPT
Incomplete Infarction Trial of European Research Collaborators Evaluating
    Prognosis Post-thrombolysis

INTERMAP
International Study of Macronutrients and Blood Pressure

INTERSALT
International Study of Salt and Blood Pressure

INTIMA
Infusion of Tissue Plasminogen Activator in Myocardial Infarction at the Acute
    Phase Study

In-TIME
Intravenous Lanoteplase for Treating Infarcting Myocardium Early trial

INTRO-AMI
Integrilin and reduced dose of thrombolysis in acute myocardial infarction

INVEST
International Verapamil SR/Trandolapril study

IPPHS
International Primary Pulmonary Hypertension Study

IPPPSH
International Prospective Primary Prevention Study in Hypertension

IRAD
International Registry of Aortic Dissection

IRAS
Insulin Resistance Atherosclerosis Study

IRBOT
Oral Glycoprotein IIb/IIIa Receptor Blockade to Inhibit Thrombosis Trial

IRIS
Isostent for Reperfusion Intervention study

IRS
Invasive Reperfusion Study

ISAM
Intravenous Streptokinase in Acute Myocardial Infarction Trial

ISAR
Intracoronary Stenting and Antithrombotic Regimen trial

ISCAB
Israeli Coronary Artery Bypass study

ISCOAT
Italian Study on Complications of Oral Anticoagulant Therapy

ISHT
International Society for Heart Transplantation Registry

ISIS
International Study of Infarct Survival

ITPASMT
International Tissue Plasminogen Activator/Streptokinase Mortality Trial

ITS
Israeli thrombolytic survey

IVUS/QCA
Intravascular Ultrasound Quantitative Coronary Angiography study

JELIS
Japan Eicosapentaenoic Acid (EPA) Lipid Intervention Study

JIMI
Japanese Intervention Trial in Myocardial Infarction

JLRCPS
Jerusalem Lipid Research Clinic Prevalence Study

JNC-V
Fifth Report of the Joint National Committee on Detection, Evaluation and
   Treatment of High Blood Pressure

JNC-VI
Sixth Report of the Joint National Committee on Detection, Evaluation and
   Treatment of High Blood Pressure

JUMBO
Joint Utilization of Medications to Block platelets Optimally

KAMI
Koch Acute Myocardial Infarction study

KAMIT
Kentucky Acute Myocardial Infarction Trial

KAPS
Kuopio Atherosclerosis Prevention Study

KAT
Kuopio Angioplasty Gene Transfer Trial

KIHD
Kuopio Ischemic Heart Disease Risk Factor study

KISS
Kobe Idiopathic Cardiomyopathy Survival Study

KUMIS
Kumamoto University Myocardial Infarction Study

KYSMI
Kyoto Shiga Myocardial Infarction study

LAPIS
Late Potentials In Myocardial Infarction Study

LARA
Low-dose Aspirin Trial on Restenosis after Angioplasty

LARS
Laser Angioplasty in Restenosed Stents trial

LASAR
Local Alcohol and Stent Against Restenosis trial

LASMAL-I
Latin American Small Vessel Randomized study

LASTLHY
Latin American study of lacidipine in hypertension

LATE
Late Assessment of Thrombolytic Efficacy trial

LAVA
Laser Angioplasty versus Angioplasty
Leiden Artificial Valves and Anticoagulation study

LBS
Lübeck Blood Pressure Study

L-CAPS
Low-density Lipoprotein Coronary Atherosclerosis Prospective Study

LCAS
Lipoprotein And Coronary Atherosclerosis Study

LEET
Low-Energy Endotak Trial

LET
Losartan Effectiveness and Tolerability study

LHIPS
Local Heparin Infusion Pre-stenting trial

LHS
Losartan Hemodynamic Study

LHT
Lifestyle Heart Trial

LIFE
Losartan Intervention for Endpoint Reduction in Hypertension trial

LIHPS
Local Delivery of Heparin in Stenting for Suboptimal Result or Threatened
   Closure Post-percutaneous Transluminal Coronary Angioplasty Using the Local
   Med InfusaSleeve

LIMIT
Leicester Intravenous Magnesium Intervention Trial

LIMIT-AMI
Double Blind, Placebo Controlled, Multicenter Angiographic Trial of rhuMAb
   CD18 in Acute Myocardial Infarction

LIMITS
Liquaemin in myocardial infarction during thrombolysis with saruplase trial

LIPID
Long-term Intervention with Pravastatin in Ischemic Disease Trial

LIPS
Lescol Intervention Prevention Study

LISA
Lescol in Severe Atherosclerosis trial

LIT
Leiden intervention trial with vegetarian diet for coronary atherosclerosis
Lopressor Intervention Trial

LIVE
Left Ventricular Hypertrophy Indapamide versus Enalapril trial

LOMIR-MCT-IL
Lomir (isradipine) Multicenter Study in Israel

LOT
Long-term Outcome After Thrombolysis study

LPS
Lovastatin Pravastatin Study

LRC-CDPT
Lipid Research Clinics Coronary Drugs Project Trial

LRC-CPPT
Lipid Research Clinics Coronary Primary Prevention Trial

LRC-MFS
Lipid Research Clinics Mortality Followup Study

LRT
Lovastatin Restenosis Trial

L-TAP
Lipid Treatment Assessment Project

MAAS
Multicenter Antiatherosclerosis Study
Multicenter Anti-Atheroma Study

MABIS
Munich and Berlin Infarction Study

MACAS
Marburg Cardiomyopathy Study

MADAM
Moexipril as Antihypertensive Drug After Menopause study

MADIT/CES
Multicenter Automatic Defibrillator Implantation Trial Cost Effectiveness Study

MAGIC
Magnesium in Cardiac Arrest trial
Magnesium in Coronaries trial

MAGICA
Magnesium in Cardiac Arrhythmia trial

MAJIC
Mayo Japan Investigation on Chronic Total Occlusion

MAPHY
Metoprolol Atherosclerosis Prevention in Hypertension Study

MAPPET
Management Strategies and Prognosis in Pulmonary Embolism Trial

MAPS
Multivessel Angioplasty Prognosis Study

MARCATOR
Multicenter American Research Trial with Cilazapril after Angioplasty to Prevent Transluminal Coronary Obstruction and Restenosis

MARISA
Monotherapy Assessment of Ranolazine in Stable Angina trial

MARS
Monitored Atherosclerosis Regression Study

MASS
Medicine, Angioplasty, or Surgery Study

MAST
Managing Anticoagulation Services Trial

MATE
Medicine versus Angiography for Thrombolytic Exclusions trial

MATH
Modern Approach to Treatment of Hypertension study

MATTIS
Multicenter Aspirin and Ticlopidine Trials After Intracoronary Stenting study

MAVERIC
Midlands Trial of Empirical Amiodarone versus Electrophysiological Guided Intervention and Cardioverter Implant in Ventricular Arrhythmias

MBVT
Munich and Berlin Trial for Sustained Ventricular Tachyarrhythmias

MCBIT
Munich Coronary Bypass Intervention Trial

MCS
Minnesota Coronary Survey

MCSDT
Minnesota Coronary Survey Dietary Trial

McSPI
Multicenter Study of Perioperative Ischemia

MDC
Metoprolol in Dilated Cardiomyopathy trial
Multicenter Dilated Cardiomyopathy trial

MDIPT
Multicenter Diltiazem Postinfarction Trial

MEADOW
Method Alternative, Distal Occlusion and Washout in Saphenous Vein Graft study

MEGA
Management of Elevated Cholesterol in the Primary Prevention Group of Adult Japanese Study

MEHP
Metoprolol in Elderly Hypertensive Patients study

MELODHY
Metoprolol Low Dose in Hypertension study

MENTOR
Medtronic Wiktor Hepamed stent trial

MERCATOR
Multicenter European Research Trial with Cilazapril after Angioplasty to Prevent Transluminal Coronary Obstruction and Restenosis

MERIT-HF
Metoprolol Controlled-Release Randomized Intervention Trial in Heart Failure

MESA
Marshfield Epidemiologic Study Area

MEXIS
Metoprolol and Xamoterol Infarction Study

M-HART
Montreal Heart Attack Readjustment Trial

M-HEART
Multihospital Eastern Atlantic Restenosis Trial

MHFT
Munich Mild Heart Failure Trial

MHHP
Minnesota Heart Health Program

MHHS
Minnesota Heart Health Survey

MHS
Minnesota Heart Survey

MIAMI
Metoprolol in Acute Myocardial Infarction study

MICOL
Multicenter Italian Study of Cholesterol

MICRO-HOPE
Microalbuminuria, Cardiovascular and Renal Outcomes, Heart Outcomes
  Prevention Evaluation

MICS
Myocardial Infarction Cost Study

MIDAS
Multicenter Isradipine Diuretic Atherosclerosis Study
Myocardial Infarction Data Acquisition System Study

MILIS
Multicenter Investigation of the Limitations of Infarct Size

MIMS
Migraine and Myocardial Ischemia Study

MINT
Myocardial Infarction with Novastan and Tissue Plasminogen Activator study

MIOS
Myocardial Infarction Onset Study

MIRACL
Myocardial Ischemia Reduction with Acute Cholesterol Lowering trial

MIRRACLE
Myocardial Infarction Risk Recognition and Conversion of Life-Threatening
  Events into Survival trial

MIRSA
Multicenter International Randomized Study of Angina Pectoris

MiSAD
Milan Study on Atherosclerosis and Diabetes

MISNES
Multicenter Italian Study on Neonatal Electrocardiography and Sudden Infant
  Death Syndrome

MIST
Mibefradil Ischemia Suppression Trial
Multicenter Isradipine Salt Trial

MITI
Myocardial Infarction Triage and Intervention project

MITRA
Maximal Individual Therapy in Acute Myocardial Infarction

MLCCHF
Multicenter Lisinopril Captopril Congestive Heart Failure study

MMIRG
Multicenter Myocardial Ischemia Research Group

MMTT
Multicenter Myocarditis Treatment Trial

MOCHA
Multicenter Oral Carvedilol in Heart Failure Assessment

MONICA
Monitoring Trends and Determinants in Cardiovascular Diseases

MOST
Mode Selection Trial in Sinus Node Dysfunction

M-PATHY
Multicenter Study of Pacing Therapy for Hypertrophic Cardiomyopathy

MPIP
Multicenter Postinfarction Program

MPPCD
Multifactorial Primary Prevention of Cardiovascular Diseases study

MPRG
Multicenter Postinfarction Research Group

MRC/BHF
Medical Research Council, British Heart Foundation Protection Study

MRFIT
Multiple Risk Factor Intervention Trial

MR-PET
Magnetic Resonance versus Positron Emission Tomography for Detection of Myocardial Viability Study

MSHT
Mount Sinai Hypertension Trial

MSMI
Multicenter Study of Myocardial Ischemia

MSSMI
Multicenter Study of Silent Myocardial Ischemia

MTT
Myocarditis Treatment Trial

MUSIC
Multicenter Ultrasound during Stent Implantation in Coronary Arteries study
Multicenter Ultrasound Stent in Coronary Artery Disease study
Multicenter Ultrasound Study in Coronaries

MUST
Multicenter Stent study
Multicenter Stents Ticlopidine study
Multicenter Ultrasound Study with Ticlid

MUST-EECP
Multicenter Study of Enhanced External Counterpulsation

MUSTIC
Multisite Stimulation in Cardiac Insufficiency
Multisite Stimulation in Cardiomyopathy

MUSTT
Multicenter Unstable Tachycardia Trial
Multicenter Unsustained Tachycardia Trial

NACI
New Applications for Coronary Interventions Registry
New Approaches to Coronary Interventions Registry

NACI DCA
New Approaches to Coronary Interventions Registry Directional Coronary
    Atherectomy Study

NACPTAR
North American Cerebral Transluminal Angioplasty Registration

NAMIS
Nifedipine Angina Myocardial Infarction Study

NASCET
North American Symptomatic Carotid Endarterectomy Trial

N-CAP
Nifedipine Gastrointestinal Therapeutic System Circadian Antiischemic Program

NDHS
National Diet-Heart Study

NEAT
Neurohumoral Effects in Acute Myocardial Infarction of Trandolapril Study

NEET
Nordic Enalapril Exercise Trial

NEWDILTIL
New Diltiazem versus Tildiem study

NEXT
New European XT Stent Registry

NHAAP
National Heart Attack Alert Program

NHBPCC
National High Blood Pressure Coordinating Committee

NHBPEP
National High Blood Pressure Education Program

NHLBI II
National Heart, Lung, and Blood Institute Type II Coronary Intervention Study

NHLBI-ICD
National Heart, Lung, and Blood Institute Implantable Cardioverter Defibrillator trial

NHLBI-PTCA
National Heart, Lung, and Blood Institute Percutaneous Transluminal Coronary Angioplasty Registry

NHLBITS
National Heart, Lung, and Blood Institute Twin Study

NHP
National Hypertension Project (Egypt)

NHS-1
First Natural History Study of Congenital Heart Defects

NHS-2
Second Natural History Study of Congenital Heart Defects

NICE 3
National Investigators Collaboration on Enoxaparin 3

NICOLE
Nisoldipine In Coronary Artery Disease in Leuven

Ni-Hon-San
Nipponese in Honolulu and San Francisco trial

NIHS
National Institute of Hypertension Studies

NIR
New Intravascular Rigid Stent Trial

NIRVANA
NIR Vascular Advanced North American trial

NNLIT
North Norwegian Lidocaine Intervention Trial

NNMT
Norwegian Nifedipine Multicenter Trial

NORDIL
Nordic Diltiazem study

NOWIS
North-Wurttemberg Infarction Study

NPHS
Northwick Park Heart Study

NRICR
National Registry for In-Hospital Cardiopulmonary Resuscitation

NUAPS
National Unstable Angina Pectoris Study

OARS
Optimal Atherectomy Restenosis Study

OASIS
Organization to Assess Strategies for Ischemic Syndromes

OAT
Ochanomizu Aspirin Trial
Occluded Artery Trial
Open Artery Trial

OCBAS
Optimal Coronary Balloon Angioplasty versus Stent trial
Optimal Coronary Balloon Angioplasty with Provisional Stenting versus Primary
    Stent trial

OCS
Oxford Cholesterol Study

OD1
Organ Disease 1 Coronary Atherosclerosis Multicenter Study

ODES
Oslo Diet and Exercise Study

OHS
Oslo Hypertension Study

OHT
Oslo Heart Trial

OIS
Oslo Ischemia Study

OmniHeart
Optimal Macronutrient Intake Trial to Prevent Heart Disease

OPTICUS
Optimization with Intracoronary Ultrasound to Reduce Stent Restenosis Trial

OPTIMAAL
Optimal Therapy in Myocardial Infarction with the Angiotensin II Antagonist Losartan study

OPTIME
Outcomes of a Prospective Trial of Intravenous Milrinone for Exacerbations

OPTIME CHF
Outcomes of a Prospective Trial of Intravenous Milrinone for Exacerbations of Chronic Heart Failure

OPUS
Orbofiban in Patients with Unstable Coronary Syndromes study

OSCAR
Olive oil, Safflower oil, Canola oil And Rapeseed oil dietary study

OSDAT
Oslo Study Diet and Antismoking Trial

OSIRIS
Optimization Study of Infarct Reperfusion Investigated by ST Monitoring

OSTI
Optimal Stent Implantation Trial

OUTCLAS
Outpatient Coronary Low Profile Angioplasty Study

OXMIS
Oxford Myocardial Infarction Incidence Study

PA3
Atrial Pacing Periablation for Paroxysmal Atrial Fibrillation Trial

PAC-A-TACH
pacemaker atrial tachycardia trial

PACCO
Pulmonary Artery Catheterization and Clinical Outcomes study

PACCS
Prospective Army Coronary Calcium Study

PACE
Pacing and Clinical Electrophysiology study
Prevention with Low-dose Aspirin of Cardiovascular Diseases in the Elderly Study

PACK
Prevention of Atherosclerotic Complications with Ketanserin study

PACT
Plasminogen Activator Angioplasty Compatibility Trial
Plasminogen Activator Coronary Angioplasty Trial
Prehospital Application of Coronary Thrombolysis Study
Prospective Acute Coronary Syndrome Trial
Prourokinase in Acute Coronary Thrombosis Study

PAD
Public Access Defibrillation trial

PAD-I
Public Access Defibrillation I trial

PAFAC
Prevention of Atrial Fibrillation After Cardioversion study

PAFIT
Paroxysmal Atrial Fibrillation Italian Trial

PAFT
Propafenone Atrial Fibrillation Trial

PAIMS
Plasminogen Activator Italian Multicenter Study

PAIS
Pravastatin in Acute Ischemic Syndromes study

PAIVS
Pulmonary Atresia with Intact Ventricular Septum collaborative study

PAMI
Primary Angioplasty in Myocardial Infarction trial

PARADIGM
Platelet Aggregation Receptor Antagonist Dose Investigation for Perfusion Gain in
   Myocardial Infarction study

PARADISE
Platelet IIb/IIIa Antagonism for the Reduction of Acute Coronary Events Dose
   Investigation and Safety Evaluation study

PARAGON
Platelet IIb/IIIa Antagonist for the Reduction of Acute Coronary Syndrome Events
   in a Global Organization Network

PARAT
Prevention of Arterial Restenosis Angiographic Trial

PARIS
Persantine and Aspirin Reinfarction Study

PARK
Postangioplasty Restenosis Ketanserin study
Prevention of Angioplasty Reocclusion with Ketanserin trial

PART
Prevention of Atherosclerosis with Ramipril Therapy trial
Probucol Angioplasty Restenosis Trial

PART-1
Predictors of Atherosclerosis Risk and Thrombosis trial

PART-2
Predictors of Atherosclerosis Risk and Thrombosis trial

PAS
Paragon (stent) elective or acute stent trial
Polish Amiodarone Study

PASE
Pacemaker Selection in the Elderly trial

PASS
Practical Applicability of Saruplase Study
Prehospital Applicability of Saruplase Study

PASTA
percutaneous ambulatory stent trial
primary angioplasty versus stent implantation in acute myocardial infarction trial

PAD
Polish amiodarone trial

PARIS
Peripheral Artery Radiation Investigation Study

PATAF
prevention of arterial thromboembolism in nonvalvular atrial fibrillation study
primary prevention of arterial thromboembolic processes in atrial fibrillation trial

PATE
Pravastatin Antiatherosclerosis Trial in the Elderly

PATENT
Prourokinase and Tissue Plasminogen Activator Enhancement of Thrombolysis
  Trial

PATHS
Prevention and Treatment of Hypertension Study

PATS
Poststroke Antihypertensive Treatment Study
Prehospital Administration of Tissue Plasminogen Activator Study

P2C2 HIV
Pediatric Pulmonary and Cardiac Complications of Vertically Transmitted HIV
  Infection Study

PCMR
Pediatric Cardiomyopathy Registry

PCS
Prevention of Coronary Atherosclerosis Study

PDAY
Pathological Determinants of Atherosclerosis in Youth study

PDAY/RFEHA
Pathobiological Determinants of Atherosclerosis in Youth/Risk Factors in Early
  Human Atherogenesis study

PEACH
Physiologic Evaluation After Coronary Hyperemia trial

PECTE
Pulmonary Embolism Colfarit Trial in the Elderly

PEGASUS
Percutaneous Endarterectomy, the Goal of Atherectomy Successfully Guided by
  UltraSound trial

PEPCI
Pharmacokinetics of Enoxaparin in Patients undergoing Percutaneous Coronary
  Intervention

PEPP
Pregnancy Exposures and Preeclampsia Prevention project

PERFEXT
Perfusion, Performance, Exercise Trial

PERM
Prospective Evaluation of Perfusion Markers study

PHARM
Pharmacist in Heart Failure: Assessment, Recommendation and Monitoring Study

PHASE
Prehospital Arrest Survival Evaluation

PHHP
Pawtucket Heart Health Program

PHYLLIS
Plaque Hypertension Lipid-Lowering Italian Study

PICO
Pimobendan in Congestive Heart Failure study

PICS
Pacing in Cardiomyopathy Study

PICTURE
Post-Intracoronary Treatment Ultrasound Results Evaluation study

PIG
Polaris Investigator Group

PILOT
Polish Intramural Low Molecular Weight Heparin Outpatient Stent Trial

PIOPED
Prospective Investigation of Pulmonary Embolism Diagnosis Data Base

PISA-PED
Prospective Investigative Study of Acute Pulmonary Embolism Diagnosis

PLAC
Pravastatin Limitation in Atherosclerosis in the Coronary Arteries Study

PLAC-2
Pravastatin, Lipids and Atherosclerosis in the Carotid Arteries Study

PLEXES
Pacing Lead Explant with Excimer Sheath Study

PLM
Prevention of Mortality with Low-molecular Weight Heparin in Medical Patients Study

PLOSA
Physiologic Low-stress Angioplasty Trial

PLS
Postsurgery Logiparin Study

PMNSG
Pravastatin Multinational Study Group

PMS
Pravastatin Multinational Study

POLARIS
Polymorphisms and Risk of Ischemic Stroke

POLISH
Polish Investigators to Evaluate the Effect of Amiodarone on Mortality after Myocardial Infarction

Pol-MONICA
Polish Monitoring Trends and Determinants in Cardiovascular Diseases Study

POLONIA
Polish-American Local Lovenox-NIR Stent Assessment Study

POSCH
Program on Surgical Control of Hyperlipidemia

POSSUM
physiological and operative severity score for the enumeration of morbidity and
    mortality study

POST
Predictors and Outcomes of Stent Thrombosis Study
Prevention of Syncope Trial

POST-CABG
Postcoronary Artery Bypass Graft study

PPP
Prospective Pravastatin Pooling project

PPS
Paris Prospective Study

PQRST
Probucol Quantitative Regression Swedish Trial

PRACTICAL
Placebo-controlled Randomized ACE Inhibition Comparative Trial in Cardiac
    Infarction and Left Ventricular Function

PRAGUE
Primary Angioplasty after Transfer of Patients from General Community Hospitals
    to Catheterization Units with or without Emergency Thrombolytic infusion Study

PRAISE
Prospective Randomized Amlodipine Survival Evaluation

PREDICT
Prospective Randomized Evaluation of Diltiazem CD Trial

PREFACE
Pravastatin-related Effects Following Angioplasty on Coronary Endothelium study

PREFER
Patient Randomized to Either Femoral or Radial Catheterization

PREMIS
Prehospital Myocardial Infarction Study

PRESERVE
Prospective Randomized Enalapril Study Evaluating Regression of Ventricular
    Enlargement

PREVEND IT
Prevention of Renal and Vascular Endstage Disease Intervention Trial

PREVENT
Prevention of Recurrent Venous Thromboembolism
Proliferation Reduction Using Vascular Energy Trial
Prospective Randomized Evaluation of the Vascular Effects of Norvasc Trial

PRIDE
platelet aggregation and receptor occupancy with Integrilin-A dynamic evaluation
    study
Primary Implantable Defibrillator Study

PRIME
Promotion of Reperfusion by Inhibition of Thrombin during Myocardial Infarction
    Evaluation study
Promotion of reperfusion in myocardial infarction evolution study
Prospective Randomized Ibopamine Mortality Evaluation study
Prospective Randomized Study of Ibopamine on Mortality and Efficacy in Heart
    Failure

PRIMI
Prourokinase in Myocardial Infarction Trial

PRIMO-CABG
Pexelizumab for the Reduction of Infarction and Mortality in Coronary Artery
    Bypass Graft Surgery Study

PRINCE
Pravastatin Inflammation/CRP Evaluation

PRISM
Platelet Receptor Inhibition in Ischemic Syndrome Management study

PRISM-PLUS
Platelet Receptor Inhibition in Ischemic Syndrome Management in Patients
    Limited by Unstable Signs and Symptoms Study

PROBE
Prospective, Randomized, Open Blinded Endpoint Trial
Prospective Randomized, Open Trial with Blinded Endpoint Evaluation

PROCAM
Prospective Cardiovascular Münster Study

PROMISE
Prospective Randomized Milrinone Survival Evaluation study

PROSPECT
Proscar Safety Plus Efficacy Canadian Two-year Study

PROSPER
Prospective Study of Pravastatin in the Elderly at Risk

PROTECT
Prospective Reinfarction in the Thrombolytic Era Cardizem-CD Trial

PROVED
Prospective Randomized Study of Ventricular Failure and the Efficacy of Digoxin

PROVE IT
Pravastatin or Atorvastatin Evaluation and Infection Therapy

PROVE IT-TIMI 22
Pravastatin or Atorvastatin Evaluation and Infection Therapy-Thrombolysis in
    Myocardial Infarction 22 trial

PSAAMI
Primary Stenting versus Angioplasty in Acute Myocardial Infarction trial

PSTAF
Pilsicainide Suppression Trial of Atrial Fibrillation

PURSUIT
Platelet Glycoprotein IIb/IIIa Underpinning the Receptor for Suppression of
    Unstable Ischemia Trial
Platelet Glycoprotein IIb/IIIa in Unstable Angina, Receptor Suppression Using
    Integrilin Therapy

QCS
Quebec Cardiovascular Study

QHFT
Quinapril Heart Failure Trial

QOLHS
Quality Of Life Hypertension Study

QUADS
Quinapril Australian Dosing Study

QUASAR
Quinapril Antiischemia and Symptoms of Angina Reduction trial

QUEXTRA
Quantitative Exercise Testing and Angiography Study

QUEST
Quebec's gender specific modulation of cytochrome P450s mediated
    cardiovascular drugs metabolism study

QUIET
Quinapril Ischemic Event Trial

RAALLT
Reversal of Atherosclerosis with Aggressive Lipid Lowering Trial

RAAMI
Randomized Angiographic Trial of Alteplase in Myocardial Infarction
Rapid Administration of Alteplase in Myocardial Infarction trial

RAAS
Randomized Angiotensin II Receptor Antagonist, Angiotensin-converting Enzyme
 Inhibitor Study

RACE
Ramipril Cardioprotective Evaluation trial
Rate Control versus Electrical Cardioversion for Persistent Atrial Fibrillation study

RADIANCE
Randomized Assessment of Digoxin on Inhibitors of Angiotensin-Converting
 Enzyme study

RAFT
Recurrent Atrial Fibrillation Trial
Rythmol-SR Atrial Fibrillation Trial

RALES
Randomized Aldactone Evaluation Study

RaMI
Ravenna myocardial infarction trial

RAMIT
Ravenna myocardial infarction trial

RAPID
Recombinant Plasminogen Activator Angiographic Phase II International Dose
 Finding Study
Regional Arizona Prehospital Infarction Diagnosis Study
Reteplase Angiographic Patency International Dose-ranging Study

RAPT
Ridogrel versus Aspirin Potency Trial

RAVES
Reduced Anticoagulation in Saphenous Vein Graft Stent Trial
Reduced Anticoagulation Vein Graft Study

REACH
Research on Endothelin Antagonism in Chronic Heart Failure
Resource Utilization in Congestive Heart Failure Study

RECREATE
Rescue of Closed Arteries Treated by Stent for Threatened or Abrupt Closure Study

REDUCE
Randomized Double-blind Unfractionated Heparin and Placebo-controlled
 Multicenter Trial

Restenosis Reduction by Cutting Balloon Evaluation Study

REFLECT-1
Randomized Evaluation of Flosequinan on Exercise Tolerance, Initial Efficacy Trial

REFLECT-2
Randomized Evaluation of Flosequinan on Exercise Tolerance, Dose Response Study

REFLEX
Restenosis Rates with Flexible GFX Stents Study

REFSA
Randomized European Femoral Stent versus Angioplasty Trial

REMATCH trial
Randomized Evaluation of Mechanical Assistance in the Treatment of Congestive
  Heart Failure trial

RENEWAL
Randomized Trial of Endoluminal Reconstruction Using the NIR Stent or
  Wallstent in Angioplasty of Long Segment Disease

RENO
Radiation in Europe Novoste

REPAIR
Reperfusion in Acute Infarction, Rotterdam Study

REPLACE-2
Randomized Evaluation in PCI Linking Angiomax to Reduced Clinical Events trial

RES
Reproducibility Echocardiography Study

RESCUE
Randomized Evaluation of Salvage Angioplasty with Combined Utilization of
  Endpoints Trial

RESCUT
Restenosis Cutting Balloon Evaluation

RESEARCH
Rapamycin-Eluting Stent Evaluated at Rotterdam Cardiology Hospital trial

RESIST
Restenosis after Intravascular Ultrasound-guided Stenting Study

REST
Restenosis Stent Trial

RESTORE
Randomized Efficacy Study of Tirofiban for Outcomes and Restenosis trial

RETA
Registry for the Endovascular Treatment of Aneurysms

REVERSAL
Reversal of Atherosclerosis with Aggressive Lipid Lowering

RIGHT
Cerivastatin Gemfibrozil Hyperlipidemia Treatment Study

RISC
Research Group on Instability in Coronary Artery Disease Study

RITA
Randomized Intervention Treatment of Angina (UK)

RITED
Italian Registry of Echo-dobutamine Tests

ROBUST
Recanalization of Occluded Bypass Graft with Prolonged Urokinase Infusion Site Trial

ROCKET
Regionally Organized Cardiac Key European Trial

ROMIO
Rule Out Myocardial Infarct Observation study

ROSETTA
Routine versus Selective Exercise Treadmill Test After Angioplasty trial

ROSTER
Rotational Atherectomy versus Balloon Angioplasty for In-stent Restenosis Trial

ROTASTENT
Rotational Atherectomy with Adjunctive Stenting Trial

RS
Reykjavik Study

RUTH
Raloxifene Use for the Heart Study

4S
Scandinavian Simvastatin Survival Study Group

SABER
Stent-Assisted Balloon Angioplasty and its Effects on Restenosis study

SAFE-PACE
Syncope and Falls in the Elderly, Role of Pacemaker Study

SAFER
Saphenous Vein Graft Angioplasty Free of Emboli Randomized Trial

SAFIRE-D
Symptomatic Atrial Fibrillation Investigation and Randomized Evaluation of Dofetilide Study

SAGES
Signal-Averaged Electrocardiographic Study

SAHCS
Streptokinase, Aspirin, Heparin Collaborative Study

SAHS
San Antonio Heart Study

SALAD
Surgery versus Angioplasty for Proximal Left Anterior Descending Coronary Artery Stenosis trial

SALT
Swedish Aspirin in Low dose Trial

SALT 1 and 2
Study of Ascending Levels of Tolvaptan in Hyponatremia 1 and 2

SALTS
Strategic Alternatives with Ticlopidine in Stenting Study

SAMI
Streptokinase and Angioplasty in Myocardial Infarction trial
Streptokinase in Acute Myocardial Infarction Study

SAMII
Survey of Acute Myocardial Ischemia and Infarction study

SAMIT
Streptokinase and Angioplasty Myocardial Infarction Trial

SAMPLE
Study on Ambulatory Monitoring of Pressure and Lisinopril Evaluation

SAPAT
Swedish Angina Pectoris Aspirin Trial

SAPPHIRE
Stanford Asian Pacific program in hypertension and insulin resistance
Stenting and Angioplasty with Protection in Patients at High Risk of Endarterectomy

SAPS
San Antonio Rotablator Study

SAS
Scandinavian Angiopeptin Study

SAT
Saruplase Alteplase Study

SATE
Safety Antiarrhythmic Trial Evaluation

SAVE
Survival and Ventricular Enlargement trial

SCAMP
Stanford Coronary Artery Monitoring Project

SCAT
Simvastatin and enalapril Coronary Atherosclerosis Trial

SCD-HeFT
Sudden Cardiac Death in Heart Failure
Trial of Prophylactic Amiodarone versus Implantable Defibrillator Therapy

SCIV
Subcutaneous versus Intravenous Heparin in Deep Venous Thrombosis Study

SCORES
Stent Comparative Restenosis trial

SCRIP
Stanford Coronary Risk Intervention Project

SCRIPPS
Scripps Coronary Radiation to Inhibit Proliferation Poststenting Study

SEARCH
Study of the Effectiveness of Additional Reductions of Cholesterol and
  Homocysteine

SECURE
Study to Evaluate Carotid Ultrasound Changes in patients treated with Ramipril
  and vitamin E

SECURITY
Study to Evaluate the Neuroshield Bare Wire Cerebral Protection System and
  X.act Stent in Patients at High Risk for Carotid Endarterectomy

SELCA
Smooth Excimer Laser Coronary Angioplasty study

SENDCAP
St. Mary's Ealing, Northwick Park diabetes cardiovascular prevention study

SESAM
Study in Europe of Saruplase and Alteplase in Myocardial infarction

SHARE
Study of Heart Assessment and Risk in Ethnic Groups

SHARP
Scottish Heart and Arterial Disease Risk Prevention program
Subcutaneous Heparin in Angioplasty Restenosis Prevention trial

SHEP
Systolic Hypertension in the Elderly Program

SHHS
Scottish Heart Health Study
Sleep Heart Health Study

SHIPS
Shiga Pravastatin Study

SHOCK
Should we Emergently Revascularize Occluded Coronaries for Cardiogenic Shock, International Randomized Trial

SHOT
Shunt Occlusion Trial

SHP
Skaraborg Hypertension Project

SHS
Strong Heart Study

SHVRC
Shiley Heart Valve Research Center project

SIAM
Streptokinase in Acute Myocardial Infarction study

SICCO
Stenting in Chronic Coronary Occlusion study

SIHDSPS
Stockholm Ischemic Heart Disease Secondary Prevention Study

SIMA
Stenting versus Internal Mammary Artery for Single Left Anterior Descending Arterial Lesion Trial

SIPS
Strategy for Intracoronary Ultrasound-guided Percutaneous Transluminal Coronary Angioplasty and Stenting Trial

SIRIUS
Sirolimus-Eluting Stent in Coronary Lesions trial
Sirolimus-Coated Stent in Treatment of Patients with De Novo Coronary Artery Lesions trial

SIROCCO
Sirolimus Coated Cordis SMART Nitinol Self-expandable Stent for Treatment of Obstructive Superficial Femoral Artery Disease trial

SISA
Stenting in Small Arteries trial

SISAMI
Silent Ischemia in Survivors of Acute Myocardial Infarction study

SISCA
Stenting in Small Coronary Arteries trial

SISH
Stage I Systolic Hypertension in the Elderly Study

SISTEMI
Southern Italian Study on Thrombolysis Early in Myocardial Infarction

SKDAMI
Streptokinase Plus Desmopressin in Acute Myocardial Infarction Study

SKHYDIP
Skara Hypertension and Diabetes Project

SMART
Self-measurement for Assessment of the Response to Trandolapril Study
Study of Medicine versus Angioplasty Reperfusion Trial
Study of Microstent's Ability to Limit Restenosis Trial

SMARTT
Serum Markers, Acute Myocardial Infarction and Rapid Treatment Trial

SMASH
Swiss multicenter evaluation of early angioplasty for shock

SMILE
Survival of Myocardial Infarction, Long-term Evaluation study

SMISS
Silent Myocardial Ischemia Stress Study

SMS
Simvastatin Multicenter Study

SMT
Stockholm Metoprolol Trial

SNAP
Study of Nitroglycerin and Chest Pain

SNaP
Study of Sodium and Blood Pressure

SNAPE
Study of Nicorandil in Angina Pectoris in the Elderly

SOAR
Safety of Orbofiban in Acute coronary Research study

SOCIAIDS
Study of Cardiac Involvement in Acquired Immunodeficiency Syndrome

SOCRATES
Study of Coronary Revascularization and Therapeutic Evaluations

SOLD
Stenting after Optimal Lesion Debulking Trial

SOLVD
Studies of Left Ventricular Dysfunction

SoS
Stent or Surgery study

SPACTO
Stent versus Percutaneous Angioplasty in Chronic Total Occlusion Trial

SPAF TEE
Stroke Prevention in Atrial Fibrillation, Transesophageal Echo study

SPICE
Study of Patients Intolerant to Converting Enzyme Inhibitors

SPICED TEAS
Study of Pacemakers and Implantable Cardioverter Defibrillator Triggering by Electronic Article Surveillance Devices

SPINAF
Stroke Prevention in Nonrheumatic Atrial Fibrillation study

SPIR
Study of Perioperative Ischemia Research

SPIRIT
Salvage from Perindopril in Reperfused Infarction Trial
Stroke Prevention in Reversible Ischemia Trial

SPORT
Stenting Post Rotational Atherectomy Trial

SPRINT
Secondary Prevention of Reinfarction Israeli Nifedipine Trial

SPRS
Sixty Plus Reinfarction Study

SPRT
Sixty Plus Reinfarction Trial

STAMI
Stenting for Acute Myocardial Infarction study

STAMP
Systemic Thrombolysis in Acute Myocardial Infarction with Prourokinase and Urokinase trial

STARS
Stent Anticoagulation Regimen Study
Stent Antithrombolytic Regimen Study
Stent Anticoagulation Restenosis Study
St. Thomas Atherosclerosis Regression Study

START
Saruplase and Taprostene Acute Reocclusion Trial
St. Thomas Atherosclerosis Regression Trial
Stent versus Angioplasty Restenosis Trial
stent versus directional coronary atherectomy randomized trial

STAT
Stent Thrombosis After Ticlopidine study

STATRS
Stent Antithrombotic Regimen Study

STENT-BY
Stent versus Bypass Surgery for Vessels Undergoing Abrupt Closure Trial

STENTIM
Stenting in Acute Myocardial Infarction Study

STENT PAMI
Stent Primary Angioplasty for Myocardial Infarction

STEP
Study of Taprostene in Elective Percutaneous Transluminal Coronary Angioplasty

STEPHY
Starnberg Trial on Epidemiology of Parkinsonism and Hypertension in the Elderly

STEPS
Significance of Transesophageal Electrocardiographic findings in Prevention of Stroke study

STEREO
Stents and ReoPro Trial
Strut Thickness Effect on Restenosis Outcome

STIMIS
Study of Time Intervals in Myocardial Ischemic Syndromes

STIMS
Swedish Ticlodipine Multicenter Study

STONE
Shanghai Trial of Nifedipine in the Elderly

STOP
Shunt Thrombotic Occlusion Prevention by Picotamide Study
Stenting for Total Occlusion and Restenosis Prevention Study
Study of Hypertension in the Elderly (Sweden)
Swedish Trial in Old Patients with Hypertension

STOPAMI-4 study
Randomized Trial of Coronary Stenting versus Balloon Angioplasty as a Rescue
    Intervention after Failed Thrombolysis

STOP 2
Swedish Trial in Old Patients with Hypertension 2

STOP-AF
Systematic Trial of Pacing to Prevent Atrial Fibrillation

STOP-hypertension
Swedish Trial in Older Patients with Hypertension

STRATAS
Study to Determine Rotablator and Transluminal Angioplasty Strategy

STRESS
Stent Restenosis Study

STRETCH
Symptom Tolerability Response to Exercise Trial of Candesartan Cilexetil in
    Patients with Heart Failure

STRIP
Special Turku Coronary Risk Factor Intervention Project

SURE
Serial Ultrasound Analysis of Restenosis Study

SUSHI
Stent Use is Superior for Hospitalized Infarction Patients study

SUTAMI
Saruplase and Urokinase in the Treatment of Acute Myocardial Infarction trial

SVTS
Sotalol Ventricular Tachycardia Study

SWEET
Square Wave Endurance Exercise Trial

SWISH
Swedish Isradipine Study in Hypertension

SWISSI
Swiss Interventional Study in Silent Ischemia

SYMPHONY
Sibrafiban versus Aspirin to Yield Maximum Protection from Ischemic Heart Events Postacute Coronary Syndromes Trial

SYNBIAPACE
Synchronous Biatrial Pacing Therapy Study

SYNERGY
Superior Yield of the New Strategy of Enoxaparin, Revascularization and Glycoprotein IIb/IIIa Inhibitors

SYST-CHINA
Systolic Hypertension in Elderly Chinese Trial

SYST-EUR
Systolic Hypertension in Europeans Study

TACS
Thrombolysis and Angioplasty in Cardiogenic Shock study

TACT
Ticlopidine Angioplasty Coronary Trial
Ticlopidine versus Placebo for Prevention of Acute Closure after Angioplasty Trial

TACTICS
Thrombolysis and Counterpulsation to Improve Cardiogenic Shock Survival Trial

TACTICS-TIMI 18
Treat Angina with Aggrastat and Determine Cost of Therapy with an Invasive or Conservative Strategy-Thrombolysis In Myocardial Infarction 18 trial

TAIM
Trial of Antihypertensive Intervention and Management

TAM
Total Atherosclerosis Management study

TAMI
Thrombolysis and Angioplasty in Myocardial Infarction study

TARGET
Do Tirofiban and ReoPro Give Similar Efficacy? trial

TASC
Trial of Angioplasty and Stents in Canada

TASH
Transcoronary Ablation of Septum Hypertrophy study

TASMAN
Thrombolysis Anticoagulant Study, Mediterranean, Australia, New Zealand

TASS
Ticlopidine Aspirin Stroke Study

TASTE
Ticlopidine Aspirin Stent Evaluation

TAUSA
Thrombolysis and Angioplasty in Unstable Angina trial

TAXUS II
Paclitaxel-eluting Stent Study

TCI
To Come In (open heart surgery program at Cleveland Clinic)

TEAHAT
Thrombolysis Early in Acute Heart Attack Trial

TEAM
Thrombolytic Trial of Eminase in Acute Myocardial Infarction

TECBEST
Transluminal Extraction Catheter Before Stent study

TECSS
The European Coronary Surgery Study

TENACITY
Tirofiban Evaluation of Novel Dosing versus Abciximab with Clopidogrel and
Inhibition of Thrombin Study

TEST
Timolol, Encainide, Sotalol Trial

THAMES
Tenormin in Hypertension and Myocardial Ischemia Epidemiological Study

THAT
Thrombolysis in Acute Myocardial Infarction Trial

THIS
Tissue Plasminogen Activator Heparin Interaction Study

THRIVE
Thrombin Inhibitor in Venous Thromboembolism

THS
Tromso Heart Study
Turkish Heart Study

TIBBS
Total Ischemic Burden Bisoprolol Study

TIBET
Total Ischemic Burden European Trial

TICO
Thrombolysis in Coronary Occlusion Study

TIG
Thrombosis Interest Group study

TIM
Triflusal in Myocardial Infarction Study

TIME
Treatment of Infarcting Myocardium Early Trial

TIMED
Trials to Investigate Morning versus Evening Dosing (Nisoldipine in Hypertension)

TIMI IIIA
Thrombolysis In Myocardial Ischemia Trial

TIMI IIIB
Thrombolysis In Myocardial Infarction Trial

TIMI-7
Thrombin Inhibition In Myocardial ischemia trial

TIMI-9
Thrombolysis and Thrombin Inhibition in Myocardial Infarction Trial

TIMIKO
Thrombolysis in Myocardial Infarction in Korea Study

TIMS
Tertatolol International Multicentre study

TIPE
Thrombolysis in Pulmonary Embolism study

TIPS
Transjugular Intrahepatic Portacaval Shunt study

TOAT
The Open Artery Trial

TOCC
Total Occlusion of Coronary Arteries, Chronic Study

TOHP
Trial of Hypertension Prevention study

TOLC
Treatment of Low-density Lipoprotein-bound Cholesterol Study

TOMHS
Treatment of Mild Hypertension Study

TOMIIS
Total Occlusion Postmyocardial Infarction Intervention Study

TOP
Thrombolysis in Old Patients study

TOPAS
Thrombolysis or Peripheral Artery Surgery study

TOPLIT
Transluminal Extraction Catheter or Percutaneous Transluminal Coronary
Angioplasty in Thrombus Study

TOPS
Thrombolysis in Old Patients Study
Treatment of Postthrombolytic Stenosis study

TOSCA
Total Occlusion Study in Canada

TOTAL
Total Occlusion Trial with Angioplasty by using Laser guidewire

TPASK
Tissue Plasminogen Activator versus Streptokinase trial

TPAT
Tissue Plasminogen Activator, Toronto Trial

TPI
Thrombolytic Predictive Instrument project

TRACE
Trandolapril Cardiac Evaluation Trial

TRANDA
Trandolapril Andalusian Study

TRANSFAIR
Transfatty Acids in Food in Europe Study

TRAP
Twin Reversed Arterial Perfusion study

TRAPIST
Trapidil versus Placebo to Prevent In-stent Intimal Hyperplasia Study

TREAT
Tranilast Restenosis Following Angioplasty Trial

TRENT
Trial of Early Nifedipine Treatment of Acute Myocardial Infarction

TRIC
Thrombolysis with Recombinant Tissue Plasminogen Activator During Instability in Coronary Artery Disease Trial

TRIM
Thrombin Inhibition in Myocardial Ischemia Study

TRIMM
Triggers and Mechanisms of Myocardial Infarction study

TROPHY
Treatment Effects of Lisinopril versus Hydrochlorothiazide in Obese Patients with Hypertension Trial
Treatment of Obese Patients with Hypertension Trial
Trial of Preventing Hypertension

TTOPP
Thrombolytic Therapy in Older Patient Population study

TUCC
Tissue Plasminogen Activator/Urokinase Comparison in China Study

TULIP
Thrombocyte Activity Evaluation in the Study to Determine the Effect of the Ultrasound Guidance of Long Intracoronary Stent Placement

TWISTER
Trial of Within-Stent Treatment of Endoluminal Restenosis

UCARE, U-CARE
Unexplained Cardiac Arrest Registry of Europe

UD-AHF
UD-CG 115 BS in Acute Heart Failure study

UKCSG
United Kingdom Collaborative Study Group (timolol trial)

UKHAS
United Kingdom Heart Attack Study

UKHEART
United Kingdom heart failure evaluation and assessment of risk trial

UK in USA
Urokinase in Unstable Angina Study

UKNCSPAIVS
United Kingdom national collaborative study of pulmonary atresia with intact ventricular septum

UKPACE
United Kingdom Pacing and Cardiovascular Events study
United Kingdom Pacing and Clinical Events study

UKSAT
United Kingdom Small Aneurysm Trial

UK-TIA
United Kingdom Transient Ischemic Attack trial (aspirin trial)

ULTRA
Utilizing GFX 2.5 Stent in Small Diameter Arteries

UNASEM
Unstable Angina Study using Eminase

UNRPCA
Use of Nicardipine to Retard the Progression of Coronary Atherosclerosis trial

UNSA
Unstable Angina Study

UPET
Urokinase Pulmonary Embolism Trial

UPSIZE
Ultrasound-controlled Percutaneous Transluminal Coronary Angioplasty with Optimal Balloon Size Study

URALMI
Urokinase and Alteplase in Myocardial Infarction study

USPET
Urokinase Streptokinase Pulmonary Embolism Trial

UTOPIA
Utilization of Platelet Inhibition in Angina Trial

VACA
Valvuloplasty and Angioplasty in Congenital Anomalies Registry

VA-HIT
Veterans Affairs high-density lipoprotein intervention trial

Val-HeFT
Valsartan Heart Failure Trial

Val-HeFT Echocardiographic Study
Valsartan Benefits Left Ventricular Structure and Function in Heart Failure

VALIANT
Valsartan in Acute Myocardial Infarction Study

VALUE
Valsartan Antihypertensive Long-term Use Evaluation

VANQWISH
Veterans Affairs Non-Q-Wave Infarction Strategies In-hospital study

VAS
Verapamil Angioplasty Study

VASIS
Vasovagal Syncope International Study

VASPNAF
Veterans Administration stroke prevention in nonrheumatic atrial fibrillation study

VEGAS
Vein Graft AngioJet Study

VERDI
Verapamil versus Diuretics Trial

VERDICT
Verapamil Digoxin Cardioversion Trial

VHAS
Verapamil in Hypertension Atherosclerosis Study

V-HeFT
Vasodilator Heart Failure Trial
Veterans Administration Heart Failure Trial

VIGOUR
Virtual Coordinating Center for Global Collaborative Cardiovascular Research

VITA
Vicenza Thrombophilia and Atherosclerosis project

VOTE
Value of Transesophageal Echocardiography study

VPS
Vasovagal Pacemaker Study

VPS II
Second Vasovagal Pacemaker Study

VT-MASS
Metoprolol and Sotalol for Sustained Ventricular Tachycardia Study

WACS
Women's Atherosclerosis Cardiovascular Study

WAFUS
Warfarin Anticoagulation Followup Study

WALLSTENT-CABG
Wallstent European Study on Stenting for Coronary Artery Bypass Grafts

WARIS
Warfarin Reinfarction Study

WARIS II
Warfarin-Aspirin Reinfarction Study, Norwegian

WASH
Warfarin-Aspirin Study of Heart Failure

WATCH
Warfarin Antiplatelet Trial in Chronic Heart Failure
Worcester-Area Trial for Counseling in Hyperlipidemia

WCUS
Wiktor Stent and Cutting Balloon Angioplasty Study

WELL-HART
Women's Estrogen/Progestin and Lipid-Lowering Hormone Atherosclerosis
Regression Trial

WEST
Western European Stent Trial

WHAS
Women's Heart Attack Study

WHAT
Worcester Heart Attack Trial

WHO-ISH
World Health Organization/International Society of Hypertension Survey

WHS
Women's Health Study

WHT
Women's Heart Trial

WIN
Wallstent in Native Vessel Study

WINS
Wallstent in Saphenous Vein Grafts Study

WISE
Women's Ischemic Syndrome Evaluation

WOLF
Work, Lipids, Fibrinogen Study

WOOFS
Warfarin Optimized Outpatient Followup Study

WOSCOPS
West of Scotland Coronary Prevention Study: prevention of coronary heart disease with pravastatin in men with hypercholesterolemia

WRIST
Washington Radiation for In-Stent Restenosis Trial

WWICT
Western Washington Intracoronary Streptokinase Trial

WWISK
Western Washington Intracoronary Streptokinase trial

WWIST
Western Washington Intravenous Streptokinase Trial

WWIV
Western Washington Intravascular Streptokinase trial

WWIVSK
Western Washington Intravenous Streptokinase trial

WWSIMIT
Western Washington Streptokinase in Myocardial Infarction Trials

XAD
External Atrial Defibrillation trial

X-TRACT
X-Sizer for Treatment of Thrombus and Atherosclerosis in Coronary Interventions trial

YCVDS
Yugoslavia Cardiovascular Disease Study

ZWOLLE
Primary Coronary Angioplasty Compared with Intravenous Streptokinase Study

Drugs by Indication

ACUTE CORONARY SYNDROME
Antiplatelet Agent
  Aggrastat® [US/Can]
  eptifibatide
  Integrilin® [US/Can]
  tirofiban

ADAMS-STOKES SYNDROME
Adrenergic Agonist Agent
  Adrenalin® [US/Can]
  epinephrine
  EpiPen® [US/Can]
  EpiPen® Jr [US/Can]
  isoproterenol
  Isuprel® [US]
  Primatene® Mist [US-OTC]
  Raphon [US-OTC]
  S2® [US-OTC]
  Twinject™ [US]

ALVEOLAR PROTEINOSIS
Antithyroid Agent
  Iosat™ [US-OTC]
  Pima® [US]
  potassium iodide
  SSKI® [US]
  ThyroSafe™ [US-OTC]
  ThyroShield™ [US-OTC]

ANESTHESIA (GENERAL)
Barbiturate
  Brevital® [Can]
  Brevital® Sodium [US]
  methohexital
General Anesthetic
  Amidate® [US/Can]
  Compound 347™ [US]
  desflurane
  Diprivan® [US/Can]
  enflurane
  Ethrane® [US]
  etomidate
  Forane® [US]
  halothane
  isoflurane
  Ketalar® [US/Can]
  ketamine
  Ketamine Hydrochloride Injection, USP [Can]
  propofol
  sevoflurane
  Sevorane™ [Can]
  Suprane® [US/Can]
  Terrell™ [US]
  Ultane® [US]

ANESTHESIA (LOCAL)
  Alcaine® [US/Can]
  Americaine® [US-OTC]
  Ametop™ [Can]
  Anestacon® [US]
  Anusol® Ointment [US-OTC]
  articaine and epinephrine
  Astracaine® [Can]
  Astracaine® Forte [Can]
  Band-Aid® Hurt-Free™ Antiseptic Wash [US-OTC]
  benzocaine
  benzocaine, butyl aminobenzoate, tetracaine, and benzalkonium chloride
  Benzodent® [US-OTC]
  Betacaine® [Can]
  bupivacaine
  bupivacaine and epinephrine
  Burnamycin [US-OTC]
  Caladryl® Clear [US-OTC]
  CalaMycin® Cool and Clear [US-OTC]

Callergy Clear [US-OTC]
Carbocaine® [US/Can]
Carbocaine® 2% with Neo-
  Cobefrin® [US]
Cepacol® Sore Throat [US-OTC]
Cetacaine® [US]
cetylpyridinium
chloroprocaine
Citanest® Plain [US/Can]
cocaine
Curasore [US-OTC]
Cylex® [US-OTC]
C_pacol® Dual Action Maximum
  Strength [US-OTC]
Dentapaine [US-OTC]
Dermoplast® Antibacterial
  [US-OTC]
Dermoplast® Pain Relieving
  [US-OTC]
Detane® [US-OTC]
dibucaine
Diocaine® [Can]
Duocaine™ [US]
dyclonine
ethyl chloride
ethyl chloride and
  dichlorotetrafluoroethane
Flucaine® [US]
Fluoracaine® [US]
Fluro-Ethyl® [US]
Foille® [US-OTC]
Gebauer's Ethyl Chloride® [US]
  hexylresorcinol
Hurricaine® [US-OTC]
L-M-X™ 4 [US-OTC]
L-M-X™ 5 [US-OTC]
Lanacane® [US-OTC]
Lanacane® Maximum Strength
  [US-OTC]
LidaMantle® [US]
lidocaine
lidocaine and bupivacaine
lidocaine and epinephrine
Lidodan™ [Can]

Lidoderm® [US/Can]
LidoSite™ [US]
LTA® 360 [US]
Marcaine® [US/Can]
Marcaine® Spinal [US]
Marcaine® with Epinephrine [US]
mepivacaine
mepivacaine and levonordefrin
Mycinettes® [US-OTC]
Naropin® [US/Can]
Nesacaine® [US]
Nesacaine®-CE [Can]
Nesacaine®-MPF [US]
Novocain® [US]
Nupercainal® [US-OTC]
Ophthetic® [US]
Oticaine [US]
Otocaine™ [US]
Polocaine® [US/Can]
Polocaine® 2% and Levonordefrin
  1:20,000 [Can]
Polocaine® Dental [US]
Polocaine® MPF [US]
Pontocaine® [US/Can]
Pontocaine® Niphanoid® [US]
Pontocaine® With Dextrose [US]
pramoxine
Prax® [US-OTC]
Premjact® [US-OTC]
prilocaine
procaine
proparacaine
proparacaine and fluorescein
ropivacaine
Sarna® Sensitive [US]
Sensorcaine® [US/Can]
Sensorcaine®-MPF [US]
Sensorcaine®-MPF with Epinephrine
  [US]
Sensorcaine® with Epinephrine
  [US/Can]
Septanest® N [Can]
Septanest® SP [Can]
Septocaine® [US]

S.T. 37® [US-OTC]
Sting-Kill [US-OTC]
Tanac® [US-OTC]
tetracaine
tetracaine and dextrose
Thorets [US-OTC]
Topicaine® [US-OTC]
Trocaine® [US-OTC]
Tronolane® [US-OTC]
Ultracaine® D-S [Can]
Ultracaine® D-S Forte [Can]
Xylocaine® [US/Can]
Xylocaine® MPF [US]
Xylocaine® MPF With Epinephrine
  [US]
Xylocaine® Viscous [US]
Xylocaine® With Epinephrine
  [US/Can]
Xylocard® [Can]
Zilactin® [Can]
Zilactin-L® [US-OTC]
Zilactin®-B [US-OTC/Can]
Zilactin Baby® [Can]
Zilactin Toothache and Gum Pain®
  [US-OTC]
Zorcaine™ [US]

ANGINA PECTORIS

Antiarrhythmic Agent, Class II
  acebutolol
  Apo-Acebutolol® [Can]
  Apo-Propranolol® [Can]
  Gen-Acebutolol [Can]
  Inderal® [US/Can]
  Inderal® LA [US/Can]
  InnoPran XL™ [US]
  Monitan® [Can]
  Novo-Acebutolol [Can]
  Novo-Pranol [Can]
  Nu-Acebutolol [Can]
  Nu-Propranolol [Can]
  propranolol
  Propranolol Hydrochloride Injection,
    USP [Can]

Rhotral [Can]
Rhoxal-acebutolol [Can]
Sandoz-Acebutolol [Can]
Sectral® [US/Can]
Antiarrhythmic Agent, Class IV
  Alti-Verapamil [Can]
  Apo-Verap® [Can]
  Apo-Verap® SR [Can]
  Calan® [US/Can]
  Calan® SR [US]
  Chronovera® [Can]
  Covera® [Can]
  Covera-HS® [US/Can]
  Gen-Verapamil [Can]
  Gen-Verapamil SR [Can]
  Isoptin® SR [US/Can]
  Novo-Veramil SR [Can]
  Nu-Verap [Can]
  Riva-Verapamil SR [Can]
  verapamil
  Verapamil Hydrochloride Injection,
    USP [Can]
  Verelan® [US]
  Verelan® PM [US]
Antilipemic Agent, HMG-CoA
  Reductase Inhibitor
  amlodipine and atorvastatin
  Caduet® [US/Can]
Calcium Channel Blocker
  Adalat® XL® [Can]
  Adalat® CC [US]
  Afeditab™ CR [US]
  Alti-Diltiazem CD [Can]
  Alti-Verapamil [Can]
  amlodipine
  amlodipine and atorvastatin
  Apo-Diltiaz® [Can]
  Apo-Diltiaz CD® [Can]
  Apo-Diltiaz® Injectable [Can]
  Apo-Diltiaz SR® [Can]
  Apo-Nifed® [Can]
  Apo-Nifed PA® [Can]
  Apo-Verap® [Can]
  Apo-Verap® SR [Can]

Caduet® [US/Can]
Calan® [US/Can]
Calan® SR [US]
Cardene® [US]
Cardene® I.V. [US]
Cardene® SR [US]
Cardizem® [US/Can]
Cardizem® CD [US/Can]
Cardizem® LA [US]
Cardizem® SR [Can]
Cartia XT™ [US]
Chronovera® [Can]
Covera® [Can]
Covera-HS® [US/Can]
Dilacor® XR [US]
Diltia XT® [US]
diltiazem
Diltiazem HCl ER® [Can]
Diltiazem Hydrochloride Injection
    [Can]
felodipine
Gen-Diltiazem [Can]
Gen-Diltiazem CD [Can]
Gen-Verapamil [Can]
Gen-Verapamil SR [Can]
Isoptin® SR [US/Can]
Med-Diltiazem [Can]
nicardipine
Nifediac™ CC [US]
Nifedical™ XL [US]
nifedipine
Norvasc® [US/Can]
Novo-Diltazem [Can]
Novo-Diltazem-CD [Can]
Novo-Diltiazem HCl ER [Can]
Novo-Nifedin [Can]
Novo-Veramil SR [Can]
Nu-Diltiaz [Can]
Nu-Diltiaz-CD [Can]
Nu-Nifed [Can]
Nu-Verap [Can]
Plendil® [US/Can]
Procardia® [US/Can]
Procardia XL® [US]

ratio-Diltiazem CD [Can]
Renedil® [Can]
Rhoxal-diltiazem CD [Can]
Rhoxal-diltiazem SR [Can]
Rhoxal-diltiazem T [Can]
Riva-Verapamil SR [Can]
Sandoz-Diltiazem CD [Can]
Sandoz-Diltiazem T [Can]
Syn-Diltiazem® [Can]
Taztia XT™ [US]
Tiazac® [US/Can]
Tiazac® XC [Can]
verapamil
Verapamil Hydrochloride Injection,
    USP [Can]
Verelan® [US]
Verelan® PM [US]
Cardiovascular Agent, Miscellaneous
    Ranexa™ [US]
    ranolazine
Vasodilator
    amyl nitrite
    Apo-Dipyridamole FC® [Can]
    Apo-ISDN® [Can]
    Apo-ISMN [Can]
    Cedocard®-SR [Can]
    Coronex® [Can]
    Dilatrate®-SR [US]
    dipyridamole
    Gen-Nitro [Can]
    Imdur® [US/Can]
    Ismo® [US]
    Isochron™ [US]
    Isordil® [US]
    isosorbide dinitrate
    isosorbide mononitrate
    Minitran™ [US/Can]
    Monoket® [US]
    Nitrek® [US]
    Nitro-Bid® [US]
    Nitro-Dur® [US/Can]
    nitroglycerin
    Nitrol® [Can]
    Nitrolingual® [US]

NitroQuick® [US]
Nitrostat® [US/Can]
NitroTime® [US]
Novo-Sorbide [Can]
Persantine® [US/Can]
PMS-Isosorbide [Can]
Rho-Nitro [Can]
Transderm-Nitro® [Can]
Trinipatch® 0.2 [Can]
Trinipatch® 0.4 [Can]
Trinipatch® 0.6 [Can]

ANGIOEDEMA (HEREDITARY)
Anabolic Steroid
  stanozolol
  Winstrol® [US]
Androgen
  Cyclomen® [Can]
  danazol
  Danocrine® [Can]

ARRHYTHMIAS
Antiarrhythmic Agent, Class I
  Ethmozine® [US/Can]
  moricizine
Antiarrhythmic Agent, Class I-A
  Apo-Procainamide® [Can]
  Apo-Quinidine® [Can]
  BioQuin® Durules™ [Can]
  disopyramide
  Norpace® [US/Can]
  Norpace® CR [US]
  Novo-Quinidin [Can]
  procainamide
  Procainamide Hydrochloride Injection, USP [Can]
  Procanbid® [US]
  Procan® SR [Can]
  Quinate® [Can]
  quinidine
  Rythmodan® [Can]
  Rythmodan®-LA [Can]

Antiarrhythmic Agent, Class I-B
  Anestacon® [US]
  Band-Aid® Hurt-Free™ Antiseptic Wash [US-OTC]
  Betacaine® [Can]
  Burnamycin [US-OTC]
  Burn Jel [US-OTC]
  Burn-O-Jel [US-OTC]
  Dilantin® [US/Can]
  L-M-X™ 4 [US-OTC]
  L-M-X™ 5 [US-OTC]
  LidaMantle® [US]
  lidocaine
  Lidodan™ [Can]
  Lidoderm® [US/Can]
  LTA® 360 [US]
  mexiletine
  Novo-Mexiletine [Can]
  Phenytek™ [US]
  phenytoin
  Premjact® [US-OTC]
  Topicaine® [US-OTC]
  Xylocaine® [US/Can]
  Xylocaine® MPF [US]
  Xylocaine® Viscous [US]
  Xylocard® [Can]
  Zilactin® [Can]
  Zilactin-L® [US-OTC]
Antiarrhythmic Agent, Class I-C
  Apo-Flecainide® [Can]
  Apo-Propafenone® [Can]
  flecainide
  propafenone
  Rythmol® [US]
  Rythmol® Gen-Propafenone [Can]
  Rythmol® SR [US]
  Tambocor™ [US/Can]
Antiarrhythmic Agent, Class II
  acebutolol
  Alti-Sotalol [Can]
  Apo-Acebutolol® [Can]
  Apo-Propranolol® [Can]
  Apo-Sotalol® [Can]
  Betapace® [US]

Betapace AF® [US/Can]
Brevibloc® [US/Can]
CO Sotalol [Can]
esmolol
Gen-Acebutolol [Can]
Gen-Sotalol [Can]
Inderal® [US/Can]
Inderal® LA [US/Can]
InnoPran XL™ [US]
Lin-Sotalol [Can]
Monitan® [Can]
Novo-Acebutolol [Can]
Novo-Pranol [Can]
Novo-Sotalol [Can]
Nu-Acebutolol [Can]
Nu-Propranolol [Can]
Nu-Sotalol [Can]
PMS-Sotalol [Can]
propranolol
Propranolol Hydrochloride Injection, USP [Can]
Rho®-Sotalol [Can]
Rhotral [Can]
Rhoxal-acebutolol [Can]
Riva-Sotalol [Can]
Rylosol [Can]
Sandoz-Acebutolol [Can]
Sectral® [US/Can]
Sorine® [US]
Sotacor® [Can]
sotalol

Antiarrhythmic Agent, Class III
Alti-Amiodarone [Can]
Alti-Sotalol [Can]
amiodarone
Amiodarone Hydrochloride for Injection® [Can]
Apo-Amiodarone® [Can]
Apo-Sotalol® [Can]
Betapace® [US]
Betapace AF® [US/Can]
Cordarone® [US/Can]
Corvert® [US]
CO Sotalol [Can]

dofetilide
Gen-Amiodarone [Can]
Gen-Sotalol [Can]
ibutilide
Lin-Sotalol [Can]
Novo-Amiodarone [Can]
Novo-Sotalol [Can]
Nu-Sotalol [Can]
Pacerone® [US]
PMS-Sotalol [Can]
Rho®-Sotalol [Can]
Rhoxal-amiodarone [Can]
Riva-Sotalol [Can]
Rylosol [Can]
Sandoz-Amiodarone [Can]
Sorine® [US]
Sotacor® [Can]
sotalol
Tikosyn™ [US/Can]

Antiarrhythmic Agent, Class IV
Alti-Verapamil [Can]
Apo-Verap® [Can]
Apo-Verap® SR [Can]
Calan® [US/Can]
Calan® SR [US]
Chronovera® [Can]
Covera® [Can]
Covera-HS® [US/Can]
Gen-Verapamil [Can]
Gen-Verapamil SR [Can]
Isoptin® SR [US/Can]
Novo-Veramil SR [Can]
Nu-Verap [Can]
Riva-Verapamil SR [Can]
verapamil
Verapamil Hydrochloride Injection, USP [Can]
Verelan® [US]
Verelan® PM [US]

Antiarrhythmic Agent, Miscellaneous
Digitek® [US]
digoxin
Digoxin CSD [Can]
Lanoxicaps® [US/Can]

Lanoxin® [US/Can]
Novo-Digoxin [Can]
Pediatric Digoxin CSD [Can]

ASCITES
Diuretic, Loop
Apo-Furosemide® [Can]
bumetanide
Bumex® [US/Can]
Burinex® [Can]
Demadex® [US]
Edecrin® [US/Can]
ethacrynic acid
furosemide
Furosemide Injection, USP [Can]
Furosemide Special [Can]
Lasix® [US/Can]
Lasix® Special [Can]
Novo-Semide [Can]
torsemide
Diuretic, Miscellaneous
Apo-Chlorthalidone® [Can]
Apo-Indapamide® [Can]
chlorthalidone
Gen-Indapamide [Can]
indapamide
Lozide® [Can]
Lozol® [US/Can]
metolazone
Mykrox® [Can]
Novo-Indapamide [Can]
Nu-Indapamide [Can]
PMS-Indapamide [Can]
Thalitone® [US]
Zaroxolyn® [US/Can]
Diuretic, Potassium Sparing
Aldactone® [US/Can]
Novo-Spiroton [Can]
spironolactone
Diuretic, Thiazide
Apo-Hydro® [Can]
Aquatensen® [Can]
chlorothiazide
Diuril® [US/Can]
Enduron® [Can]
hydrochlorothiazide
methyclothiazide
Microzide™ [US]
Novo-Hydrazide [Can]
PMS-Hydrochlorothiazide [Can]

ASPERGILLOSIS
Antifungal Agent
Abelcet® [US/Can]
Amphocin® [US]
Amphotec® [US/Can]
amphotericin B cholesteryl sulfate
complex
amphotericin B (conventional)
amphotericin B lipid complex
Ancobon® [US/Can]
flucytosine
Fungizone® [Can]
VFEND® [US/Can]
voriconazole
Antifungal Agent, Systemic
AmBisome® [US/Can]
amphotericin B liposomal
Cancidas® [US/Can]
caspofungin

ASTHMA
Adrenal Corticosteroid
Apo-Beclomethasone® [Can]
Apo-Dexamethasone® [Can]
Azmacort® [US]
beclomethasone
Beconase® AQ [US]
Decadron® [US]
Dexamethasone Intensol® [US]
dexamethasone (systemic)
Dexasone® [Can]
DexPak® TaperPak® [US]
Diodex® [Can]
Flovent® Diskus® [Can]
Flovent® HFA [US/Can]
fluticasone (oral inhalation)
Gen-Beclo [Can]

Nu-Beclomethasone [Can]
PMS-Dexamethasone [Can]
Propaderm® [Can]
QVAR® [US/Can]
Rivanase AQ [Can]
triamcinolone (inhalation, oral)
Vanceril® AEM [Can]
Adrenergic Agonist Agent
    AccuNeb® [US]
    Adrenalin® [US/Can]
    Airomir [Can]
    albuterol
    Alti-Salbutamol [Can]
    Alupent® [US]
    Apo-Orciprenaline® [Can]
    Apo-Salvent® [Can]
    Apo-Salvent® CFC Free [Can]
    Apo-Salvent® Respirator Solution
        [Can]
    Apo-Salvent® Sterules [Can]
    Brethine® [US]
    Bricanyl® [Can]
    ephedrine
    epinephrine
    EpiPen® [US/Can]
    EpiPen® Jr [US/Can]
    Gen-Salbutamol [Can]
    isoproterenol
    Isuprel® [US]
    Levophed® [US/Can]
    Maxair™ Autohaler™ [US]
    metaproterenol
    norepinephrine
    pirbuterol
    PMS-Salbutamol [Can]
    Pretz-D® [US-OTC]
    Primatene® Mist [US-OTC]
    ProAir™ HFA [US]
    Proventil® [US]
    Proventil® HFA [US]
    Raphon [US-OTC]
    ratio-Inspra-Sal [Can]
    Ratio-Orciprenaline® [Can]
    ratio-Salbutamol [Can]

Rhoxal-salbutamol [Can]
S2® [US-OTC]
Salbu-2 [Can]
Salbu-4 [Can]
salmeterol
Serevent® [Can]
Serevent® Diskus® [US]
Tanta-Orciprenaline® [Can]
terbutaline
Twinject™ [US]
Ventolin® [Can]
Ventolin® Diskus [Can]
Ventolin® HFA [US/Can]
Ventrodisk [Can]
VoSpire ER® [US]
Anticholinergic Agent
    Alti-Ipratropium [Can]
    Apo-Ipravent® [Can]
    Atrovent® [US/Can]
    Atrovent® HFA [US/Can]
    Gen-Ipratropium [Can]
    ipratropium
    Novo-Ipramide [Can]
    Nu-Ipratropium [Can]
    PMS-Ipratropium [Can]
Beta2-Adrenergic Agonist Agent
    Advair Diskus® [US/Can]
    Berotec® [Can]
    budesonide and formoterol
        (Canada only)
    fenoterol (Canada only)
    fluticasone and salmeterol
    Foradil® [Can]
    Foradil® Aerolizer™ [US]
    formoterol
    Oxeze® Turbuhaler® [Can]
    Symbicort® [Can]
Corticosteroid, Inhalant
    Advair Diskus® [US/Can]
    fluticasone and salmeterol
Corticosteroid, Inhalant (Oral)
    budesonide and formoterol (Canada
        only)
    Symbicort® [Can]

Leukotriene Receptor Antagonist
  Accolate® [US/Can]
  montelukast
  Singulair® [US/Can]
  zafirlukast
Mast Cell Stabilizer
  Apo-Cromolyn® [Can]
  Crolom® [US]
  cromolyn sodium
  Gastrocrom® [US]
  Intal® [US/Can]
  Nalcrom® [Can]
  NasalCrom® [US-OTC]
  nedocromil (inhalation)
  Nu-Cromolyn [Can]
  Opticrom® [US/Can]
  Tilade® [US/Can]
Monoclonal Antibody
  omalizumab
  Xolair® [US/Can]
Theophylline Derivative
  aminophylline
  Apo-Theo LA® [Can]
  Dilor® [Can]
  Dylix [US]
  dyphylline
  Elixophyllin® [US]
  Elixophyllin-GG® [US]
  Lufyllin® [US/Can]
  Novo-Theophyl SR [Can]
  Phyllocontin® [Can]
  Phyllocontin®-350 [Can]
  PMS-Theophylline [Can]
  Pulmophylline [Can]
  ratio-Theo-Bronc [Can]
  Theo-24® [US]
  TheoCap™ [US]
  Theochron® [US]
  Theochron® SR [Can]
  Theolair™ [Can]
  theophylline
  theophylline and guaifenesin
  Uniphyl® [US]
  Uniphyl® SRT [Can]

ASTHMA (DIAGNOSTIC)
Diagnostic Agent
  methacholine
  Methacholine Omega [Can]
  Provocholine® [US/Can]

ATELECTASIS
Antithyroid Agent
  Iosat™ [US-OTC]
  Pima® [US]
  potassium iodide
  SSKI® [US]
  ThyroSafe™ [US-OTC]
  ThyroShield™ [US-OTC
Expectorant
  Iosat™ [US-OTC]
  Pima® [US]
  potassium iodide
  SSKI® [US]
  ThyroSafe™ [US-OTC]
  ThyroShield™ [US-OTC]
Mucolytic Agent
  Acetadote® [US]
  acetylcysteine
  Acetylcysteine Solution [Can]
  Mucomyst® [Can]
  Parvolex® [Can]

BACTERIAL ENDOCARDITIS (PROPHYLAXIS)
Aminoglycoside (Antibiotic)
  Alcomicin® [Can]
  Diogent® [Can]
  Garamycin® [Can]
  Gentak® [US]
  gentamicin
  Gentamicin Injection, USP [Can]
  SAB-Gentamicin [Can]
Antibiotic, Miscellaneous
  Alti-Clindamycin [Can]
  Apo-Clindamycin® [Can]
  Cleocin® [US]

Cleocin HCl® [US]
Cleocin Pediatric® [US]
Cleocin Phosphate® [US]
Cleocin T® [US]
Clindagel® [US]
ClindaMax™ [US]
clindamycin
Clindamycin Injection, USP [Can]
Clindesse™ [US]
Clindets® [US]
Clindoxyl® [Can]
Dalacin® C [Can]
Dalacin® T [Can]
Dalacin® Vaginal [Can]
Evoclin™ [US]
Novo-Clindamycin [Can]
Taro-Clindamycin [Can]
Vancocin® [US/Can]
vancomycin
Cephalosporin (First Generation)
Apo-Cefadroxil® [Can]
Apo-Cephalex® [Can]
Biocef® [US]
cefadroxil
cephalexin
Duricef® [US/Can]
Keflex® [US]
Keftab® [Can]
Novo-Cefadroxil [Can]
Novo-Lexin [Can]
Nu-Cephalex [Can]
Macrolide (Antibiotic)
Apo-Azithromycin® [Can]
azithromycin
Biaxin® [US/Can]
Biaxin® XL [US/Can]
clarithromycin
CO Azithromycin [Can]
GMD-Azithromycin [Can]
Novo-Azithromycin [Can]
PMS-Azithromycin [Can]
ratio-Azithromycin [Can]
ratio-Clarithromycin [Can]
Sandoz-Azithromycin [Can]

Zithromax® [US/Can]
Zmax™ [US]
Penicillin
amoxicillin
Amoxil® [US]
ampicillin
Apo-Amoxi® [Can]
Apo-Ampi® [Can]
Apo-Pen VK® [Can]
Gen-Amoxicillin [Can]
Lin-Amox [Can]
Novamoxin® [Can]
Novo-Ampicillin [Can]
Novo-Pen-VK [Can]
Nu-Amoxi [Can]
Nu-Ampi [Can]
Nu-Pen-VK [Can]
penicillin V potassium
PHL-Amoxicillin [Can]
PMS-Amoxicillin [Can]
Veetids® [US]

BLASTOMYCOSIS

Antifungal Agent
Apo-Ketoconazole® [Can]
itraconazole
ketoconazole
Ketoderm® [Can]
Nizoral® [US]
Nizoral® A-D [US-OTC]
Novo-Ketoconazole [Can]
Sporanox® [US/Can]

BRONCHIECTASIS

Adrenergic Agonist Agent
AccuNeb® [US]
Adrenalin® [US/Can]
Airomir [Can]
albuterol
Alti-Salbutamol [Can]
Alupent® [US]
Apo-Orciprenaline® [Can]
Apo-Salvent® [Can]
Apo-Salvent® CFC Free [Can]

Apo-Salvent® Respirator Solution [Can]
Apo-Salvent® Sterules [Can]
Brethine® [US]
Bricanyl® [Can]
ephedrine
epinephrine
EpiPen® [US/Can]
EpiPen® Jr [US/Can]
Gen-Salbutamol [Can]
isoproterenol
Isuprel® [US]
metaproterenol
PMS-Salbutamol [Can]
Pretz-D® [US-OTC]
Primatene® Mist [US-OTC]
ProAir™ HFA [US]
Proventil® [US]
Proventil® HFA [US]
Raphon [US-OTC]
ratio-Inspra-Sal [Can]
Ratio-Orciprenaline® [Can]
ratio-Salbutamol [Can]
Rhoxal-salbutamol [Can]
S2® [US-OTC]
Salbu-2 [Can]
Salbu-4 [Can]
Tanta-Orciprenaline® [Can]
terbutaline
Twinject™ [US]
Ventolin® [Can]
Ventolin® Diskus [Can]
Ventolin® HFA [US/Can]
Ventrodisk [Can]
VoSpire ER® [US]
Mucolytic Agent
Acetadote® [US]
acetylcysteine
Acetylcysteine Solution [Can]
Mucomyst® [Can]
Parvolex® [Can]

BRONCHIOLITIS
Antiviral Agent

Copegus® [US]
Rebetol® [US]
Ribasphere™ [US]
ribavirin
Virazole® [US/Can]

BRONCHITIS
Adrenergic Agonist Agent
AccuNeb® [US]
Adrenalin® [US/Can]
Airomir [Can]
albuterol
Alti-Salbutamol [Can]
Apo-Salvent® [Can]
Apo-Salvent® CFC Free [Can]
Apo-Salvent® Respirator Solution [Can]
Apo-Salvent® Sterules [Can]
ephedrine
epinephrine
EpiPen® [US/Can]
EpiPen® Jr [US/Can]
Gen-Salbutamol [Can]
isoproterenol
Isuprel® [US]
PMS-Salbutamol [Can]
Pretz-D® [US-OTC]
Primatene® Mist [US-OTC]
ProAir™ HFA [US]
Proventil® [US]
Proventil® HFA [US]
Raphon [US-OTC]
ratio-Inspra-Sal [Can]
ratio-Salbutamol [Can]
Rhoxal-salbutamol [Can]
S2® [US-OTC]
Salbu-2 [Can]
Salbu-4 [Can]
Twinject™ [US]
Ventolin® [Can]
Ventolin® Diskus [Can]
Ventolin® HFA [US/Can]
Ventrodisk [Can]
VoSpire ER® [US]

Antibiotic, Cephalosporin
  cefditoren
  Spectracef™ [US]
Antibiotic, Quinolone
  Avelox® [US/Can]
  Avelox® I.V. [US/Can]
  Factive® [US]
  gemifloxacin
  moxifloxacin
  Vigamox™ [US/Can]
Anticholinergic Agent
  Spiriva® [US/Can]
  tiotropium
Antihistamine/Antitussive
  carbetapentane and chlorpheniramine
  Tannate 12 S [US]
  Tannic-12 [US]
  Tannic-12 S [US]
  Tannihist-12 RF [US]
  Tussi-12® [US]
  Tussi-12 S™ [US]
  Tussizone-12 RF™ [US]
Cephalosporin (Third Generation)
  cefdinir
  Omnicef® [US/Can]
Mucolytic Agent
  Acetadote® [US]
  acetylcysteine
  Acetylcysteine Solution [Can]
  Mucomyst® [Can]
  Parvolex® [Can]
Theophylline Derivative
  aminophylline
  Apo-Theo LA® [Can]
  Dilor® [Can]
  Dylix [US]
  dyphylline
  Elixophyllin® [US]
  Elixophyllin-GG® [US]
  Lufyllin® [US/Can]
  Novo-Theophyl SR [Can]
  Phyllocontin® [Can]
  Phyllocontin®-350 [Can]

PMS-Theophylline [Can]
Pulmophylline [Can]
ratio-Theo-Bronc [Can]
Theo-24® [US]
TheoCap™ [US]
Theochron® [US]
Theochron® SR [Can]
Theolair™ [Can]
theophylline
theophylline and guaifenesin
Uniphyl® [US]
Uniphyl® SRT [Can]

BRONCHOSPASM

Adrenergic Agonist Agent
  AccuNeb® [US]
  Adrenalin® [US/Can]
  Airomir [Can]
  albuterol
  Alti-Salbutamol [Can]
  Alupent® [US]
  Apo-Orciprenaline® [Can]
  Apo-Salvent® [Can]
  Apo-Salvent® CFC Free [Can]
  Apo-Salvent® Respirator Solution
    [Can]
  Apo-Salvent® Sterules [Can]
  Brethine® [US]
  Bricanyl® [Can]
  ephedrine
  epinephrine
  EpiPen® [US/Can]
  EpiPen® Jr [US/Can]
  Gen-Salbutamol [Can]
  isoproterenol
  Isuprel® [US]
  levalbuterol
  Maxair™ Autohaler™ [US]
  metaproterenol
  pirbuterol
  PMS-Salbutamol [Can]
  Pretz-D® [US-OTC]
  Primatene® Mist [US-OTC]

ProAir™ HFA [US]
Proventil® [US]
Proventil® HFA [US]
Raphon [US-OTC]
ratio-Inspra-Sal [Can]
Ratio-Orciprenaline® [Can]
ratio-Salbutamol [Can]
Rhoxal-salbutamol [Can]
S2® [US-OTC]
Salbu-2 [Can]
Salbu-4 [Can]
salmeterol
Serevent® [Can]
Serevent® Diskus® [US]
Tanta-Orciprenaline® [Can]
terbutaline
Twinject™ [US]
Ventolin® [Can]
Ventolin® Diskus [Can]
Ventolin® HFA [US/Can]
Ventrodisk [Can]
VoSpire ER® [US]
Xopenex® [US/Can]
Xopenex HFA™ [US]
Anticholinergic Agent
AtroPen® [US]
atropine
Atropine-Care® [US]
Dioptic's Atropine Solution [Can]
Isopto® Atropine [US/Can]
Sal-Tropine™ [US]
Beta2-Adrenergic Agonist Agent
Foradil® [Can]
Foradil® Aerolizer™ [US]
formoterol
levalbuterol
Oxeze® Turbuhaler® [Can]
Xopenex® [US/Can]
Xopenex HFA™ [US]
Bronchodilator
levalbuterol
Xopenex® [US/Can]
Xopenex HFA™ [US]

Mast Cell Stabilizer
Apo-Cromolyn® [Can]
Crolom® [US]
cromolyn sodium
Intal® [US/Can]
Nalcrom® [Can]
NasalCrom® [US-OTC]
Nu-Cromolyn [Can]
Opticrom® [US/Can]

CACHEXIA
Antineoplastic Agent
Apo-Megestrol® [Can]
Megace® [US/Can]
Megace® ES [US]
Megace® OS [Can]
megestrol
Nu-Megestrol [Can]

CALCIUM CHANNEL BLOCKER TOXICITY
Electrolyte Supplement, Oral
calcium gluconate

CARDIAC DECOMPENSATION
Adrenergic Agonist Agent
dobutamine
Dobutamine Injection, USP [Can]
Dobutrex® [Can]

CARDIOGENIC SHOCK
Adrenergic Agonist Agent
dobutamine
Dobutamine Injection, USP [Can]
Dobutrex® [Can]
dopamine
Antiarrhythmic Agent, Miscellaneous
Digitek® [US]
digoxin
Digoxin CSD [Can]
Lanoxicaps® [US/Can]

Lanoxin® [US/Can]
Novo-Digoxin [Can]
Pediatric Digoxin CSD [Can]
Cardiac Glycoside
Digitek® [US]
digoxin
Digoxin CSD [Can]
Lanoxicaps® [US/Can]
Lanoxin® [US/Can]
Novo-Digoxin [Can]
Pediatric Digoxin CSD [Can]

CARDIOMYOPATHY

Cardiovascular Agent, Other
dexrazoxane
Zinecard® [US/Can]

CEREBROVASCULAR ACCIDENT (CVA)

Antiplatelet Agent
Alti-Ticlopidine [Can]
Apo-Ticlopidine® [Can]
Asaphen [Can]
Asaphen E.C. [Can]
Ascriptin® [US-OTC]
Ascriptin® Extra Strength [US-OTC]
Aspercin [US-OTC]
Aspercin Extra [US-OTC]
aspirin
Bayer® Aspirin [US-OTC]
Bayer® Aspirin Extra Strength
    [US-OTC]
Bayer® Aspirin Regimen Adult Low
    Strength [US-OTC]
Bayer® Aspirin Regimen Children's
    [US-OTC]
Bayer® Aspirin Regimen Regular
    Strength [US-OTC]
Bayer® Extra Strength Arthritis Pain
    Regimen [US-OTC]
Bayer® Plus Extra Strength
    [US-OTC]
Bayer® Women's Aspirin Plus
    Calcium [US-OTC]

Bufferin® [US-OTC]
Bufferin® Extra Strength [US-OTC]
Buffinol [US-OTC]
Buffinol Extra [US-OTC]
Easprin® [US]
Ecotrin® [US-OTC]
Ecotrin® Low Strength [US-OTC]
Ecotrin® Maximum Strength
    [US-OTC]
Entrophen® [Can]
Gen-Ticlopidine [Can]
Halfprin® [US-OTC]
Novasen [Can]
Novo-Ticlopidine [Can]
Nu-Ticlopidine [Can]
Rhoxal-ticlopidine [Can]
Sandoz-Ticlopidine [Can]
St. Joseph® Adult Aspirin [US-OTC]
Sureprin 81™ [US-OTC]
Ticlid® [US/Can]
ticlopidine
ZORprin® [US]
Fibrinolytic Agent
Activase® [US]
Activase® rt-PA [Can]
alteplase
Cathflo™ Activase® [US/Can]

CHRONIC OBSTRUCTIVE PULMONARY DISEASE (COPD)

Adrenergic Agonist Agent
AccuNeb® [US]
Airomir [Can]
albuterol
Alti-Salbutamol [Can]
Alupent® [US]
Apo-Orciprenaline® [Can]
Apo-Salvent® [Can] Apo-Salvent®
    CFC Free [Can]
Apo-Salvent® Respirator Solution
    [Can]
Apo-Salvent® Sterules [Can]
Gen-Salbutamol [Can]

isoproterenol
Isuprel® [US]
metaproterenol
PMS-Salbutamol [Can]
ProAir™ HFA [US]
Proventil® [US]
Proventil® HFA [US]
ratio-Inspra-Sal [Can]
Ratio-Orciprenaline® [Can]
ratio-Salbutamol [Can]
Rhoxal-salbutamol [Can]
Salbu-2 [Can]
Salbu-4 [Can]
Tanta-Orciprenaline® [Can]
Ventolin® [Can]
Ventolin® Diskus [Can]
Ventolin® HFA [US/Can]
Ventrodisk [Can]
VoSpire ER® [US]
Anticholinergic Agent
Alti-Ipratropium [Can]
Apo-Ipravent® [Can]
Atrovent® [US/Can]
Atrovent® HFA [US/Can]
Gen-Ipratropium [Can]
ipratropium
Novo-Ipramide [Can]
Nu-Ipratropium [Can]
PMS-Ipratropium [Can]
Antithyroid Agent
Iosat™ [US-OTC]
Pima® [US]
potassium iodide
SSKI® [US]
ThyroSafe™ [US-OTC]
ThyroShield™ [US-OTC]
Bronchodilator
CO Ipra-Sal [Can]
Combivent® [US/Can]
DuoNeb™ [US]
Gen-Combo Sterinebs [Can]
ipratropium and albuterol
Expectorant
Iosat™ [US-OTC]

Pima® [US]
potassium iodide
SSKI® [US]
ThyroSafe™ [US-OTC]
ThyroShield™ [US-OTC]
Theophylline Derivative
aminophylline
Apo-Theo LA® [Can]
Dilor® [Can]
Dylix [US]
dyphylline
Elixophyllin® [US]
Elixophyllin-GG® [US]
Lufyllin® [US/Can]
Novo-Theophyl SR [Can]
Phyllocontin® [Can]
Phyllocontin®-350 [Can]
PMS-Theophylline [Can]
Pulmophylline [Can]
ratio-Theo-Bronc [Can]
Theo-24® [US]
TheoCap™ [US]
Theochron® [US]
Theochron® SR [Can]
Theolair™ [Can]
theophylline
theophylline and guaifenesin
Uniphyl® [US]
Uniphyl® SRT [Can]

COCCIDIOIDOMYCOSIS
Antifungal Agent
Apo-Ketoconazole® [Can]
ketoconazole
Ketoderm® [Can]
Nizoral® [US]
Nizoral® A-D [US-OTC]
Novo-Ketoconazole [Can]

CONGESTIVE HEART FAILURE
Adrenergic Agonist Agent
dopamine

inamrinone
Alpha-Adrenergic Blocking Agent
  Apo-Prazo® [Can]
  Minipress® [US/Can]
  Novo-Prazin [Can]
  Nu-Prazo [Can]
  prazosin
Angiotensin-Converting Enzyme (ACE)
  Inhibitor
  Accupril® [US/Can]
  Altace® [US/Can]
  Alti-Captopril [Can]
  Apo-Capto® [Can]
  Apo-Fosinopril® [Can]
  Apo-Lisinopril® [Can]
  Capoten® [US/Can]
  captopril
  cilazapril (Canada only)
  enalapril
  fosinopril
  Gen-Captopril [Can]
  Inhibace® [Can]
  lisinopril
  Mavik® [US/Can]
  Monopril® [US/Can]
  Novo-Captopril [Can]
  Novo-Cilazapril [Can]
  Novo-Fosinopril [Can]
  Nu-Capto [Can]
  PMS-Captopril [Can]
  Prinivil® [US/Can]
  quinapril
  ramipril
  ratio-Fosinopril [Can]
  Riva-Rosinopril [Can]
  trandolapril
  Vasotec® [US/Can]
  Zestril® [US/Can]
Beta-Adrenergic Blocker
  Apo-Carvedilol® [Can]
  carvedilol
  Coreg® [US/Can]
  Novo-Carvedilol [Can]

  PMS-Carvedilol [Can]
  RAN™-Carvedilol [Can]
  ratio-Carvedilol [Can]
Cardiac Glycoside
  Digitek® [US]
  digoxin
  Digoxin CSD [Can]
  Lanoxicaps® [US/Can]
  Lanoxin® [US/Can]
  Novo-Digoxin [Can]
  Pediatric Digoxin CSD [Can]
Cardiovascular Agent, Other
  milrinone
  Milrinone Lactate Injection [Can]
  Primacor® [US]
Diuretic, Loop
  Apo-Furosemide® [Can]
  bumetanide
  Bumex® [US/Can]
  Burinex® [Can]
  Demadex® [US]
  furosemide
  Furosemide Injection, USP [Can]
  Furosemide Special [Can]
  Lasix® [US/Can]
  Lasix® Special [Can]
  Novo-Semide [Can]
  torsemide
Diuretic, Potassium Sparing
  amiloride
  Apo-Amiloride® [Can]
  Dyrenium® [US]
  triamterene
Natriuretic Peptide, B-type, Human
  Natrecor® [US]
  nesiritide
Vasodilator
  Apo-Hydralazine® [Can]
  Apresoline® [Can]
  BiDil® [US]
  Gen-Nitro [Can]
  hydralazine
  isosorbide dinitrate and hydralazine

Minitran™ [US/Can]
Natrecor® [US]
nesiritide
Nitrek® [US]
Nitro-Bid® [US]
Nitro-Dur® [US/Can]
nitroglycerin
Nitrol® [Can]
Nitrolingual® [US]
Nitropress® [US]
nitroprusside
NitroQuick® [US]
Nitrostat® [US/Can]
NitroTime® [US]
Novo-Hylazin [Can]
Nu-Hydral [Can]
Rho-Nitro [Can]
Transderm-Nitro® [Can]
Trinipatch® 0.2 [Can]
Trinipatch® 0.4 [Can]
\Trinipatch® 0.6 [Can]

COUGH

Antihistamine/Antitussive
  hydrocodone and chlorpheniramine
  HyTan™ [US]
  promethazine and codeine
  promethazine and dextromethorphan
  Tussionex® [US]
Antihistamine/Decongestant/Antitussive
  Alka-Seltzer® Plus® Cold and
  Cough [US-OTC]
  AllanVan-DM [US]
  Atuss® HD [US]
  Carbaphen 12® [US]
  Carbaphen 12 Ped® [US]
  carbetapentane, phenylephrine, and
    chlorpheniramine
  carbinoxamine, pseudoephedrine,
    and dextromethorphan
  chlorpheniramine, ephedrine,
    phenylephrine, and carbetapentane

chlorpheniramine, phenylephrine,
  and dextromethorphan
chlorpheniramine, phenylephrine,
  codeine, and potassium iodide
chlorpheniramine, pseudoephedrine,
  and codeine
chlorpheniramine, pseudoephedrine,
  and dextromethorphan
CoActifed® [Can]
Codal-DM [US-OTC]
Codimal® DM [US-OTC]
Codituss DM [US-OTC]
Coldcough HC [US]
Coldtuss DR [US]
Cordron-HC [US]
Corfen DM [US]
Coughtuss [US]
Covan® [Can]
Cytuss HC [US]
Dec-Chlorphen DM [US]
De-Chlor DM [US]
De-Chlor DR [US]
De-Chlor HC [US]
De-Chlor HD [US]
Detuss [US]
Dex PC [US]
Dicel™ DM [US]
Dihistine® DH [US]
DuraTan™ Forte [US]
Endal® HD [US]
Endal® HD Plus [US]
H-C Tussive [US]
Histex™ HC [US]
Histinex® HC [US]
Histinex® PV [US]
Histussin® HC [US]
hydrocodone, carbinoxamine, and
  pseudoephedrine
hydrocodone, phenylephrine, and
  diphenhydramine
Hydro DP [US]
Hydron CP [US]

Hydron PSC [US]
Hydro-PC II [US]
Hydro PC II Plus [US]
Hydro-Tussin™ HC [US]
Hyphed [US]
Kidkare Cough and Cold [US-OTC]
Maxi-Tuss HC® [US]
Maxi-Tuss HCX [US]
Mintuss HC [US]
Mintuss HD [US]
Mintuss MS [US]
P-V-Tussin® Syrup [US]
PediaCare® Multi-Symptom Cold [US-OTC]
PediaCare® NightRest Cough and Cold [US-OTC]
Pediatex™ HC [US]
Phenabid DM® [US]
phenylephrine, hydrocodone, and chlorpheniramine
phenylephrine, pyrilamine, and dextromethorphan
promethazine, phenylephrine, and codeine
pseudoephedrine, hydrocodone, and chlorpheniramine
Q-V Tussin [US]
ratio-Cotridin [Can]
Relacon-HC [US]
Rescon DM [US-OTC]
Rindal HD Plus [US]
Robitussin® Pediatric Night Relief [US-OTC]
Rondec®-DM [reformulation] [US]
Rynatuss® [US]
Rynatuss® Pediatric [US]
Tanafed DMX™ [US]
Tannate-V-DM [US]
Tetra Tannate Pediatric [US]
Triaminic® Cold and Cough [US-OTC]
Triaminic® Night Time Cough and Cold [US-OTC]
triprolidine, pseudoephedrine, and

codeine (Canada only)
Tri-Vent™ DPC [US]
Tri-Vent™ HC [US]
TussiNate™ [US]
Uni-Tricof HC [US]
Uni-Tuss HC [US]
Vasophrinic DH [Can]
Vicks® Children's NyQuil® [US-OTC]
Vicks® Pediatric 44®m [US-OTC]
Viravan®-DM [US]
XiraTuss [US]
Z-Cof HC [US]
Antitussive
AllanVan-DM [US]
Anextuss [US]
Atuss® HD [US]
Babee® Cof Syrup [US-OTC]
benzonatate
Carbaphen 12® [US]
Carbaphen 12 Ped® [US]
carbetapentane, phenylephrine, and chlorpheniramine
Certuss-D® [US]
Codal-DM [US-OTC]
codeine
Codeine Contin® [Can]
Codimal® DM [US-OTC]
Codituss DM [US-OTC]
Coldcough HC [US]
Cordron-HC [US]
Coughtuss [US]
Creomulsion® Cough [US-OTC]
Creomulsion® for Children [US-OTC]
Creo-Terpin® [US-OTC]
Cytuss HC [US]
Dacex-DM [US]
De-Chlor HC [US]
De-Chlor HD [US]
Delsym® [US-OTC]
Detuss [US]
Dexalone® [US-OTC]
Dexcon-DM [US]

Dexcon-PE [US]
dextromethorphan
Duraphen™ II DM [US]
Duraphen™ DM [US]
Duraphen™ Forte [US]
Dynatuss-EX [US]
ElixSure™ Cough [US-OTC]
Endal® HD [US]
Endal® HD Plus [US]
Giltuss® [US]
Giltuss Pediatric® [US]
Giltuss TR® [US]
Guaifen™ DM [US]
guaifenesin, dextromethorphan, and
    phenylephrine
H-C Tussive [US]
Histinex® HC [US]
Histinex® PV [US]
Histussin® HC [US]
Hold® DM [US-OTC]
Hycodan® [US]
Hycomine® Compound [US]
hydrocodone and homatropine
hydrocodone, chlorpheniramine,
    phenylephrine, acetaminophen,
    and caffeine
hydrocodone, phenylephrine, and
    diphenhydramine
Hydro DP [US]
Hydromet® [US]
Hydron CP [US]
Hydron PSC [US]
Hydro-PC II [US]
Hydro PC II Plus [US]
Hydro-Tussin™ HC [US]
Hyphed [US]
Maxiphen DM [US]
Maxi-Tuss HC® [US]
Maxi-Tuss HCX [US]
Mintuss HC [US]
Mintuss HD [US]
Mintuss MS [US]
P-V-Tussin® Syrup [US]
PediaCare® Children's Medicated

Freezer Pops Long Acting Cough
    [US-OTC]
PediaCare® Infants' Long-Acting
    Cough [US-OTC]
Pediatex™ HC [US]
phenylephrine, hydrocodone, and
    chlorpheniramine
phenylephrine, pyrilamine, and
    dextromethorphan
pseudoephedrine, hydrocodone, and
    chlorpheniramine
Q-V Tussin [US]
Relacon-HC [US]
Rindal HD Plus [US]
Robitussin® CoughGels™
    [US-OTC]
Robitussin® Honey Cough
    [US-OTC]
Robitussin® Maximum Strength
    Cough [US-OTC]
Robitussin® Pediatric Cough
    [US-OTC]
Scot-Tussin DM® Cough Chasers
    [US-OTC]
Silphen DM® [US-OTC]
Simply Cough® [US-OTC]
SINUtuss® DM [US]
Tannate-V-DM [US]
Tessalon® [US/Can]
Triaminic® Thin Strips™ Long
    Acting Cough [US-OTC]
TriTuss® [US]
TriTuss® ER [US]
Tussigon® [US]
TussiNate™ [US]
Uni-Tricof HC [US]
Uni-Tuss HC [US]
Vasophrinic DH [Can]
Vicks® 44® Cough Relief
    [US-OTC]
Viravan®-DM [US]
XiraTuss [US]
Z-Cof HC [US]
Antitussive/Decongestant

Balminil DM D [Can]
Benylin® DM-D [Can]
carbetapentane and pseudoephedrine
Dimetapp® Infant Decongestant
Plus Cough [US-OTC]
Koffex DM-D [Can]
Novahistex® DM Decongestant
[Can]
Novahistine® DM Decongestant
[Can]
Pediacare® Children's Long Acting
Cough Plus Cold [US-OTC]
Pediacare® Infants' Decongestant
& Cough [US-OTC]
Pedia Relief Cough and Cold
[US-OTC]
Pedia Relief Infants [US-OTC]
pseudoephedrine and
dextromethorphan
Respi-Tann™ [US]
Robitussin® Childrens Cough
& Cold [Can]
Robitussin® Maximum Strength
Cough & Cold [US-OTC]
Robitussin® Pediatric Cough & Cold
[US-OTC]
Sudafed® Children's Cold & Cough
[US-OTC]
SudoGest Children's [US-OTC]
Triaminic® Cough [US-OTC]
Triaminic® Cough & Nasal
Congestion [US-OTC]
Vicks® 44D Cough & Head
Congestion [US-OTC]
Antitussive/Decongestant/Expectorant
Benylin® 3.3 mg-D-E [Can]
Calmylin with Codeine [Can]
guaifenesin, pseudoephedrine, and
codeine
Guiatuss™ DAC® [US]
hydrocodone, pseudoephedrine, and
guaifenesin
Hydro-Tussin™ HD [US]
Hydro-Tussin™ XP [US]

Mytussin® DAC [US]
Su-Tuss®-HD [US]
Ztuss™ Tablet [US]
Antitussive/Expectorant
Allfen-DM [US]
Altarussin DM [US-OTC]
Amibid DM [US]
Atuss® HX [US]
Balminil DM E [Can]
Benylin® DM-E [Can]
Brontex® [US]
Cheracol® [US]
Cheracol® D [US-OTC]
Cheracol® Plus [US-OTC]
Cheratussin AC [US]
Codiclear® DH [US]
Coricidin HBP® Chest Congestion
and Cough [US-OTC]
Diabetic Tussin C® [US]
Diabetic Tussin® DM [US-OTC]
Diabetic Tussin® DM Maximum
Strength [US-OTC]
Drituss DM [US]
Duratuss® DM [US]
Gani-Tuss DM NR [US]
Gani-Tuss® NR [US]
Genatuss DM® [US-OTC]
Guaicon DM [US-OTC]
Guaifen-C [US]
Guaifenesin AC [US]
guaifenesin and codeine
guaifenesin and dextromethorphan
Guaifenex® DM [US]
Guaituss AC® [US]
Guia-D [US]
Guiacon DMS [US-OTC]
Guiatuss-DM® [US-OTC]
Hycotuss® [US]
hydrocodone and guaifenesin
Hydro-Tussin™ [US]
Hydro-Tussin™ DM [US]
Iophen-C NR [US]
Iophen DM NR [US]
Koffex DM-Expectorant [Can]

Kolephrin® #1 [US]
Kolephrin® GG/DM [US-OTC]
Kwelcof® [US]
Maxi-Tuss HCG [US]
Mintab DM [US]
Mucinex® DM [US-OTC]
Mytussin® AC [US]
Phanatuss® DM [US-OTC]
Pneumotussin® [US]
Q-Bid DM [US]
Q-Tussin DM [US-OTC]
Respa-DM® [US]
Robafen® AC [US]
Robafen DM [US-OTC]
Robitussin® Cough and Congestion
    [US-OTC]
Robitussin® DM [US-OTC/Can]
Robitussin® DM Infant [US-OTC]
Robitussin® Sugar Free Cough
    [US-OTC]
Romilar® AC [US]
Safe Tussin® [US-OTC]
Scot-Tussin® Senior [US-OTC]
Silexin® [US-OTC]
Siltussin DM [US-OTC]
Siltussin DM DAS [US-OTC]
Su-Tuss DM [US]
Touro® DM [US]
Tussi-Organidin® NR [US]
Tussi-Organidin® S-NR [US]
Vicks® 44E [US-OTC]
Vicks® Pediatric Formula 44E
    [US-OTC]
Vitussin [US]
Z-Cof LA™ [US]
Cough and Cold Combination
    Histussin D® [US]
    hydrocodone and pseudoephedrine
    P-V Tussin Tablet [US]
Cough Preparation
    AccuHist® PDX Drops [US]
    AllanHist PDX [US]
    Anaplex® DM [US]
    Anaplex® DMX [US]

Andehist DM NR [US]
Bromaline® DM [US-OTC]
Bromatane DX [US]
Bromaxefed DM RF [US]
Brometane DX [US]
Bromhist-DM [US]
Bromhist PDX [US]
Bromophed DX [US]
Bromphenex DM [US]
brompheniramine, pseudoephedrine,
    and dextromethorphan
Brotapp-DM [US]
Carbofed DM [US]
Cardec DM [US]
Dimaphen DM [US-OTC]
Dimetapp® DM Children's Cold and
    Cough [US-OTC]
EndaCof-DM [US]
EndaCof-PD [US]
Histacol DM Pediatric [US]
Myphetane DX [US]
PediaHist DM [US]
Q-Tapp DM [OTC]
Expectorant
    Allfen Jr [US]
    Balminil Expectorant [Can]
    Benylin® E Extra Strength [Can]
    Diabetic Tussin® EX [US-OTC]
    Ganidin NR [US]
    guaifenesin
    Guiatuss™ [US-OTC]
    Humibid® Maximum Strength [US]
    Iophen NR [US]
    Koffex Expectorant [Can]
    Mucinex® [US-OTC]
    Organ-1 NR [US]
    Organidin® NR [US]
    Phanasin [US-OTC]
    Phanasin® Diabetic Choice
        [US-OTC]
    Q-Tussin [US-OTC]
    Robitussin® [US-OTC/Can]
    Scot-Tussin® Expectorant [US-OTC]
    Siltussin DAS [US-OTC]

Siltussin SA [US-OTC]
Tussin [US-OTC]
Vicks® Casero™ [US-OTC]
XPECT™ [US-OTC]

CRYPTOCOCCOSIS
Antifungal Agent
    Abelcet® [US/Can]
    Amphocin® [US]
    Amphotec® [US/Can]
    amphotericin B cholesteryl sulfate
        complex
    amphotericin B (conventional)
    amphotericin B lipid complex
    Ancobon® [US/Can]
    Apo-Fluconazole® [Can]
    Diflucan® [US/Can]
    fluconazole
    Fluconazole Injection [Can]
    Fluconazole Omega [Can]
    flucytosine
    Fungizone® [Can]
    Gen-Fluconazole [Can]
    GMD-Fluconazole [Can]
    itraconazole
    Novo-Fluconazole [Can]
    Riva-Fluconazole [Can]
    Sporanox® [US/Can]
Antifungal Agent, Systemic
    AmBisome® [US/Can]
    amphotericin B liposomal

CYSTIC FIBROSIS
Enzyme
    dornase alfa
    Pulmozyme® [US/Can]

DUCTUS ARTERIOSUS (CLOSURE)
Nonsteroidal Antiinflammatory Drug
        (NSAID)
    Indocin® I.V. [US]
    indomethacin

Nu-Indo [Can]

DUCTUS ARTERIOSUS (TEMPORARY MAINTENANCE OF PATENCY)
Prostaglandin
    alprostadil
    Caverject® [US/Can]

EDEMA
Antihypertensive Agent, Combination
    Aldactazide® [US]
    Aldactazide 25® [Can]
    Aldactazide 50® [Can]
    Aldoril® [US]
    Apo-Methazide® [Can]
    Apo-Triazide® [Can]
    atenolol and chlorthalidone
    benazepril and hydrochlorothiazide
    Capozide® [US/Can]
    captopril and hydrochlorothiazide
    clonidine and chlorthalidone
    Clorpres® [US]
    Dyazide® [US]
    enalapril and hydrochlorothiazide
    hydralazine and hydrochlorothiazide
    hydrochlorothiazide and
        spironolactone
    hydrochlorothiazide and triamterene
    Hyzaar® [US/Can]
    Hyzaar® DS [Can]
    Inderide® [US]
    lisinopril and hydrochlorothiazide
    losartan and hydrochlorothiazide
    Lotensin® HCT [US]
    Maxzide® [US]
    Maxzide®-25 [US]
    methyldopa and hydrochlorothiazide
    Minizide® [US]
    Novo-Spirozine [Can]
    Novo-Triamzide [Can]
    Nu-Triazide [Can]

Penta-Triamterene HCTZ [Can]
prazosin and polythiazide
Prinzide® [US/Can]
propranolol and hydrochlorothiazide
Riva-Zide [Can]
Tenoretic® [US/Can]
Vaseretic® [US/Can]
Zestoretic® [US/Can]
Diuretic, Combination
amiloride and hydrochlorothiazide
Apo-Amilzide® [Can]
Gen-Amilazide [Can]
Moduret [Can]
Novamilor [Can]
Nu-Amilzide [Can]
Diuretic, Loop
Apo-Furosemide® [Can]
bumetanide
Bumex® [US/Can]
Burinex® [Can]
Demadex® [US]
Edecrin® [US/Can]
ethacrynic acid
furosemide
Furosemide Injection, USP [Can]
Furosemide Special [Can]
Lasix® [US/Can]
Lasix® Special [Can]
Novo-Semide [Can]
torsemide
Diuretic, Miscellaneous
Apo-Chlorthalidone③ [Can]
Apo-Indapamide® [Can]
chlorthalidone
Gen-Indapamide [Can]
indapamide
Lozide® [Can]
Lozol® [US/Can]
metolazone
Mykrox® [Can]
Novo-Indapamide [Can]
Nu-Indapamide [Can]
PMS-Indapamide [Can]
Thalitone® [US]

Zaroxolyn® [US/Can]
Diuretic, Osmotic
mannitol
Osmitrol® [US/Can]
Resectisol® [US]
Diuretic, Potassium Sparing
Aldactone® [US/Can]
amiloride
Apo-Amiloride® [Can]
Dyrenium® [US]
Novo-Spiroton [Can]
spironolactone
triamterene
Diuretic, Thiazide
Apo-Hydro® [Can]
Aquatensen® [Can]
chlorothiazide
Diuril® [US/Can]
Enduron® [Can]
hydrochlorothiazide
methyclothiazide
Microzide™ [US]
Novo-Hydrazide [Can]
PMS-Hydrochlorothiazide [Can]

EMBOLISM
Antiplatelet Agent
Apo-Dipyridamole FC® [Can]
Asaphen [Can]
Asaphen E.C. [Can]
Ascriptin® [US-OTC]
Ascriptin® Extra Strength [US-OTC]
Aspercin [US-OTC]
Aspercin Extra [US-OTC]
aspirin
Bayer® Aspirin [US-OTC]
Bayer® Aspirin Extra Strength [US-OTC]
Bayer® Aspirin Regimen Adult Low Strength [US-OTC]
Bayer® Aspirin Regimen Children's [US-OTC]
Bayer® Aspirin Regimen Regular Strength [US-OTC]

Bayer® Extra Strength Arthritis Pain
   Regimen [US-OTC]
Bayer® Plus Extra Strength
   [US-OTC]
Bayer® Women's Aspirin Plus
   Calcium [US-OTC]
Bufferin® [US-OTC]
Bufferin® Extra Strength [US-OTC]
Buffinol [US-OTC]
Buffinol Extra [US-OTC]
dipyridamole
Easprin® [US]
Ecotrin® [US-OTC]
Ecotrin® Low Strength [US-OTC]
Ecotrin® Maximum Strength
   [US-OTC]
Entrophen® [Can]
Halfprin® [US-OTC]
Novasen [Can]
Persantine® [US/Can]
St. Joseph® Adult Aspirin [US-OTC]
Sureprin 81™ [US-OTC]
ZORprin® [US]
Fibrinolytic Agent
   Activase® [US]
   Activase® rt-PA [Can]
   alteplase
   Cathflo™ Activase® [US/Can]
   Retavase® [US/Can]
   reteplase
   Streptase® [US/Can]
   streptokinase
Vasodilator
   Apo-Dipyridamole FC® [Can]
   dipyridamole
   Persantine® [US/Can]

EMPHYSEMA

Adrenergic Agonist Agent
   AccuNeb® [US]
   Adrenalin® [US/Can]
   Airomir [Can]
   albuterol
   Alti-Salbutamol [Can]

Alupent® [US]
Apo-Orciprenaline® [Can]
Apo-Salvent® [Can]
Apo-Salvent® CFC Free [Can]
Apo-Salvent® Respirator Solution
   [Can]
Apo-Salvent® Sterules [Can]
Brethine® [US]
Bricanyl® [Can]
ephedrine
epinephrine
Gen-Salbutamol [Can]
isoproterenol
Isuprel® [US]
metaproterenol
PMS-Salbutamol [Can]
Pretz-D® [US-OTC]
Primatene® Mist [US-OTC]
ProAir™ HFA [US]
Proventil® [US]
Proventil® HFA [US]
Raphon [US-OTC]
ratio-Inspra-Sal [Can]
Ratio-Orciprenaline® [Can]
ratio-Salbutamol [Can]
Rhoxal-salbutamol [Can]
S2® [US-OTC]
Salbu-2 [Can]
Salbu-4 [Can]
Tanta-Orciprenaline® [Can]
terbutaline
Twinject™ [US]
Ventolin® [Can]
Ventolin® Diskus [Can]
Ventolin® HFA [US/Can]
Ventrodisk [Can]
VoSpire ER® [US]
Anticholinergic Agent
   Alti-Ipratropium [Can]
   Apo-Ipravent® [Can]
   Atrovent® [US/Can]
   Atrovent® HFA [US/Can]
   Gen-Ipratropium [Can]
   ipratropium

Novo-Ipramide [Can]
Nu-Ipratropium [Can]
PMS-Ipratropium [Can]
Expectorant
Iosat™ [US-OTC]
Pima® [US]
potassium iodide
SSKI® [US]
ThyroSafe™ [US-OTC]
ThyroShield™ [US-OTC]
Mucolytic Agent
Acetadote® [US]
acetylcysteine
Acetylcysteine Solution [Can]
Mucomyst® [Can]
Parvolex® [Can]
Theophylline Derivative
aminophylline
Apo-Theo LA® [Can]
Dilor® [Can]
Dylix [US]
dyphylline
Elixophyllin® [US]
Elixophyllin-GG® [US]
Lufyllin® [US/Can]
Novo-Theophyl SR [Can]
Phyllocontin® [Can]
Phyllocontin®-350 [Can]
PMS-Theophylline [Can]
Pulmophylline [Can]
ratio-Theo-Bronc [Can]
Theo-24® [US]
TheoCap™ [US]
Theochron® [US]
Theochron® SR [Can]
Theolair™ [Can]
theophylline
theophylline and guaifenesin
Uniphyl® [US]
Uniphyl® SRT [Can]

ENDOCARDITIS TREATMENT

Aminoglycoside (Antibiotic)

AKTob® [US]
Alcomicin® [Can]
amikacin
Amikacin Sulfate Injection, USP [Can]
Amikin® [US/Can]
Diogent® [Can]
Garamycin® [Can]
Gentak® [US]
gentamicin
Gentamicin Injection, USP [Can]
PMS-Tobramycin [Can]
SAB-Gentamicin [Can]
Sandoz-Tobramycin [Can]
TOBI® [US/Can]
tobramycin
Tobramycin Injection, USP [Can]
Tobrex® [US/Can]
Antibiotic, Miscellaneous
Vancocin® [US/Can]
vancomycin
Antifungal Agent
Amphocin® [US]
amphotericin B (conventional)
Fungizone® [Can]
Cephalosporin (First Generation)
Ancef® [US]
cefazolin
cephalothin
Penicillin
ampicillin
Apo-Ampi® [Can]
nafcillin
Nallpen® [Can]
Novo-Ampicillin [Can]
Nu-Ampi [Can]
oxacillin
penicillin G (parenteral/aqueous)
Pfizerpen® [US/Can]
pivampicillin (Canada only)
Pondocillin® [Can]
Unipen® [Can]
Quinolone
Apo-Ciproflox® [Can]

Cipro® [US/Can]
Cipro® XL [Can]
ciprofloxacin
Cipro® XR [US]
CO Ciprofloxacin [Can]
Gen-Ciprofloxacin [Can]
Novo-Ciprofloxacin [Can]
PMS-Ciprofloxacin [Can]
Proquin® XR [US]
RAN™-Ciprofloxacin [Can]
ratio-Ciprofloxacin [Can]
Rhoxal-ciprofloxacin [Can]
Sandoz-Ciprofloxacin [Can]
Taro-Ciprofloxacin [Can]

FEBRILE NEUTROPENIA
Colony-Stimulating Factor
  Neulasta® [US/Can]
  pegfilgrastim
Quinolone
  Apo-Ciproflox® [Can]
  Cipro® [US/Can]
  Cipro® XL [Can]
  ciprofloxacin
  Cipro® XR [US]
  CO Ciprofloxacin [Can]
  Gen-Ciprofloxacin [Can]
  Novo-Ciprofloxacin [Can]
  PMS-Ciprofloxacin [Can]
  Proquin® XR [US]
  RAN™-Ciprofloxacin [Can]
  ratio-Ciprofloxacin [Can]
  Rhoxal-ciprofloxacin [Can]
  Sandoz-Ciprofloxacin [Can]
  Taro-Ciprofloxacin [Can]

FEVER
Antipyretic
  Abenol® [Can]
  Acephen™ [US-OTC]
  acetaminophen
  Advil® [US-OTC/Can]
  Advil® Children's [US-OTC]
  Advil® Infants' [US-OTC]

Advil® Junior [US-OTC]
Advil® Migraine [US-OTC]
Aleve® [US-OTC]
Amigesic® [US/Can]
Anaprox® [US/Can]
Anaprox® DS [US/Can]
Apo-Acetaminophen® [Can]
Apo-Ibuprofen® [Can]
Apo-Napro-Na® [Can]
Apo-Napro-Na DS® [Can]
Apo-Naproxen® [Can]
Apo-Naproxen EC® [Can]
Apo-Naproxen SR® [Can]
Apra Children's [US-OTC]
Asaphen [Can]
Asaphen E.C. [Can]
Ascriptin® [US-OTC]
Ascriptin® Extra Strength [US-OTC]
Aspercin [US-OTC]
Aspercin Extra [US-OTC]
aspirin
Aspirin Free Anacin® Maximum
  Strength [US-OTC]
Atasol® [Can]
Bayer® Aspirin [US-OTC]
Bayer® Aspirin Extra Strength
  [US-OTC]
Bayer® Aspirin Regimen Adult Low
  Strength [US-OTC]
Bayer® Aspirin Regimen Children's
  [US-OTC]
Bayer® Aspirin Regimen Regular
  Strength [US-OTC]
Bayer® Extra Strength Arthritis Pain
  Regimen [US-OTC]
Bayer® Plus Extra Strength
  [US-OTC]
Bayer® Women's Aspirin Plus
  Calcium [US-OTC]
Bufferin® [US-OTC]
Bufferin® Extra Strength [US-OTC]
Buffinol [US-OTC]
Buffinol Extra [US-OTC]
Cetafen® [US-OTC]

Cetafen Extra® [US-OTC]
Comtrex® Sore Throat Maximum
    Strength [US-OTC]
Easprin® [US]
EC-Naprosyn® [US]
Ecotrin® [US-OTC]
Ecotrin® Low Strength [US-OTC]
Ecotrin® Maximum Strength
    [US-OTC]
ElixSure™ IB [US-OTC]
Entrophen® [Can]
FeverAll® [US-OTC]
Genapap™ [US-OTC]
Genapap™ Children [US-OTC]
Genapap™ Extra Strength [US-OTC]
Genapap™ Infant [US-OTC]
Genebs [US-OTC]
Genebs Extra Strength [US-OTC]
Gen-Naproxen EC [Can]
Genpril® [US-OTC]
Halfprin® [US-OTC]
Ibu-200 [US-OTC]
ibuprofen
Infantaire [US-OTC]
I-Prin [US-OTC]
Mapap [US-OTC]
Mapap Children's [US-OTC]
Mapap Extra Strength [US-OTC]
Mapap Infants [US-OTC]
Midol® Cramp and Body Aches
    [US-OTC]
Midol® Extended Relief [US]
Motrin® [US]
Motrin® Children's [US-OTC/Can]
Motrin® IB [US-OTC/Can]
Motrin® Infants' [US-OTC]
Motrin® Junior Strength [US-OTC]
Naprelan® [US]
Naprosyn® [US/Can]
naproxen
Naxen® [Can]
Naxen® EC [Can]
NeoProfen®
Nortemp Children's [US-OTC]

Novasen [Can]
Novo-Gesic [Can]
Novo-Naproc EC [Can]
Novo-Naprox [Can]
Novo-Naprox Sodium [Can]
Novo-Naprox Sodium DS [Can]
Novo-Naprox SR [Can]
Novo-Profen [Can]
Nu-Ibuprofen [Can]
Nu-Naprox [Can]
Pain-Eze [US-OTC]
Pamprin® Maximum Strength All
    Day Relief [US-OTC]
Pediatrix [Can]
Proprinal [US-OTC]
Riva-Naproxen [Can]
Salflex® [Can]
salsalate
Silapap® Children's [US-OTC]
Silapap® Infants [US-OTC]
St. Joseph® Adult Aspirin [US-OTC]
Sureprin 81™ [US-OTC]
Tempra® [Can]
Tycolene [US-OTC]
Tycolene Maximum Strength
    [US-OTC]
Tylenol® [US-OTC/Can]
Tylenol® 8 Hour [US-OTC]
Tylenol® Arthritis Pain [US-OTC]
Tylenol® Children's [US-OTC]
Tylenol® Children's with Flavor
Creator [US-OTC]
Tylenol® Extra Strength [US-OTC]
Tylenol® Infants [US-OTC]
Tylenol® Junior [US-OTC]
Ultraprin [US-OTC]
Valorin [US-OTC]
Valorin Extra [US-OTC]
ZORprin® [US]

FIBROCYSTIC DISEASE
Vitamin, Fat Soluble
    Alph-E [US-OTC]
    Alph-E-Mixed [US-OTC]

Aquasol E® [US-OTC]
Aquavit-E® [US-OTC]
d-Alpha-Gems™ [US-OTC]
E-Gems® [US-OTC]
E-Gems Elite® [US-OTC]
E-Gems Plus® [US-OTC]
Ester-E™ [US-OTC]
Gamma E-Gems® [US-OTC]
Gamma-E Plus [US-OTC]
High Gamma Vitamin E Complete™
[US-OTC]
Key-E® [US-OTC]
Key-E® Kaps [US-OTC]
vitamin E

FIBROMYOSITIS
Antidepressant, Tricyclic (Tertiary
    Amine)
amitriptyline
Apo-Amitriptyline® [Can]
Levate® [Can]
Novo-Triptyn [Can]
PMS-Amitriptyline [Can]

GRAM-NEGATIVE INFECTION
Aminoglycoside (Antibiotic)
AKTob® [US]
Alcomicin® [Can]
amikacin
Amikacin Sulfate Injection,
    USP [Can]
Amikin® [US/Can]
Diogent® [Can]
Garamycin® [Can]
Gentak® [US]
gentamicin
Gentamicin Injection, USP [Can]
kanamycin
Kantrex® [US/Can]
PMS-Tobramycin [Can]
SAB-Gentamicin [Can]
Sandoz-Tobramycin [Can]

TOBI® [US/Can]
tobramycin
Tobramycin Injection, USP [Can]
Tobrex® [US/Can]
Antibiotic, Carbapenem
ertapenem
Invanz® [US/Can]
Antibiotic, Miscellaneous
Apo-Nitrofurantoin® [Can]
Azactam® [US/Can]
aztreonam
colistimethate
Coly-Mycin® M [US/Can]
Furadantin® [US]
Macrobid® [US/Can]
Macrodantin® [US/Can]
nitrofurantoin
Novo-Furantoin [Can]
Antibiotic, Quinolone
gatifloxacin
Iquix® [US]
Levaquin® [US/Can]
levofloxacin
Novo-Levofloxacin [Can]
Quixin™ [US]
Tequin® [Can]
Zymar™ [US/Can]
Carbapenem (Antibiotic)
imipenem and cilastatin
meropenem
Merrem® [Can]
Merrem® I.V. [US]
Primaxin® [US/Can]
Primaxin® I.V. [Can]
Cephalosporin (First Generation)
Ancef® [US]
Apo-Cefadroxil® [Can]
Apo-Cephalex® [Can]
Biocef® [US]
cefadroxil
cefazolin
cephalexin
cephalothin
Duricef® [US/Can]

Keflex® [US]
Keftab® [Can]
Novo-Cefadroxil [Can]
Novo-Lexin [Can]
Nu-Cephalex [Can]
Cephalosporin (Second Generation)
Apo-Cefaclor® [Can]
Apo-Cefuroxime® [Can]
Ceclor® [Can]
cefaclor
cefoxitin
cefpodoxime
cefprozil
Ceftin® [US/Can]
cefuroxime
Cefzil® [US/Can]
Mefoxin® [US]
Novo-Cefaclor [Can]
Nu-Cefaclor [Can]
PMS-Cefaclor [Can]
Raniclor™ [US]
ratio-Cefuroxime [Can]
Vantin® [US/Can]
Zinacef® [US/Can]
Cephalosporin (Third Generation)
Cedax® [US]
Cefizox® [US/Can]
cefotaxime
ceftazidime
ceftibuten
ceftizoxime
ceftriaxone
Claforan® [US/Can]
Fortaz® [US/Can]
Rocephin® [US/Can]
Tazicef® [US]
Cephalosporin (Fourth Generation)
cefepime
Maxipime® [US/Can]
Macrolide (Antibiotic)
Akne-Mycin® [US]
Apo-Azithromycin® [Can]
Apo-Erythro Base® [Can]
Apo-Erythro E-C® [Can]

Apo-Erythro-ES® [Can]
Apo-Erythro-S® [Can]
A/T/S® [US]
azithromycin
Biaxin® [US/Can]
Biaxin® XL [US/Can]
clarithromycin
CO Azithromycin [Can]
Diomycin® [Can]
E.E.S.® [US/Can]
Erybid™ [Can]
Eryc® [US/Can]
Eryderm® [US]
Erygel® [US]
EryPed® [US]
Ery-Tab® [US]
Erythrocin® [US]
erythromycin
erythromycin and sulfisoxazole
GMD-Azithromycin [Can]
Novo-Azithromycin [Can]
Novo-Rythro Estolate [Can]
Novo-Rythro Ethylsuccinate [Can]
Nu-Erythromycin-S [Can]
PCE® [US/Can]
Pediazole® [US/Can]
PMS-Azithromycin [Can]
PMS-Erythromycin [Can]
ratio-Azithromycin [Can]
ratio-Clarithromycin [Can]
Romycin® [US]
Sandoz-Azithromycin [Can]
Sans Acne® [Can]
Theramycin Z® [US]
Zithromax® [US/Can]
Zmax™ [US]
Penicillin
Alti-Amoxi-Clav [Can]
amoxicillin
amoxicillin and clavulanate
potassium
Amoxil® [US]
ampicillin
ampicillin and sulbactam

Apo-Amoxi® [Can]
Apo-Amoxi-Clav® [Can]
Apo-Ampi® [Can]
Apo-Pen VK® [Can]
Augmentin® [US/Can]
Augmentin ES-600® [US]
Augmentin XR™ [US]
Bicillin® L-A [US]
Bicillin® C-R [US]
Bicillin® C-R 900/300 [US]
carbenicillin
Clavulin® [Can]
Gen-Amoxicillin [Can]
Geocillin® [US]
Lin-Amox [Can]
Novamoxin® [Can]
Novo-Ampicillin [Can]
Novo-Clavamoxin [Can]
Novo-Pen-VK [Can]
Nu-Amoxi [Can]
Nu-Ampi [Can]
Nu-Pen-VK [Can]
penicillin V potassium
penicillin G benzathine
penicillin G benzathine and penicillin
   G procaine
penicillin G procaine
Pfizerpen-AS® [Can]
PHL-Amoxicillin [Can]
piperacillin
piperacillin and tazobactam sodium
Piperacillin for Injection, USP [Can]
pivampicillin (Canada only)
PMS-Amoxicillin [Can]
Pondocillin® [Can]
ratio-Aclavulanate [Can]
Tazocin® [Can]
Ticar® [US]
ticarcillin
ticarcillin and clavulanate potassium
Timentin® [US/Can]
Unasyn® [US/Can]
Veetids® [US]

Wycillin® [Can]
Zosyn® [US]
Quinolone
   Apo-Ciproflox® [Can]
   Apo-Norflox® [Can]
   Apo-Oflox® [Can]
   Apo-Ofloxacin® [Can]
   Ciloxan® [US/Can]
   Cipro® [US/Can]
   Cipro® XL [Can]
   ciprofloxacin
   Cipro® XR [US]
   CO Ciprofloxacin [Can]
   CO Norfloxacin [Can]
   Floxin® [US/Can]
   Gen-Ciprofloxacin [Can]
   norfloxacin
   Norfloxacine® [Can]
   Noroxin® [US/Can]
   Novo-Ciprofloxacin [Can]
   Novo-Norfloxacin [Can]
   Novo-Ofloxacin [Can]
   Ocuflox® [US/Can]
   ofloxacin
   PMS-Ciprofloxacin [Can]
   PMS-Norfloxacin [Can]
   PMS-Ofloxacin [Can]
   Proquin® XR [US]
   RAN™-Ciprofloxacin [Can]
   ratio-Ciprofloxacin [Can]
   Rhoxal-ciprofloxacin [Can]
   Riva-Norfloxacin [Can]
   Sandoz-Ciprofloxacin [Can]
   Taro-Ciprofloxacin [Can]
Sulfonamide
   Apo-Sulfatrim® [Can]
   Apo-Sulfatrim® DS [Can]
   Apo-Sulfatrim® Pediatric [Can]
   Bactrim™ [US]
   Bactrim™ DS [US]
   erythromycin and sulfisoxazole
   Gantrisin® [US]
   Novo-Soxazole [Can]

Novo-Trimel [Can]
Novo-Trimel D.S. [Can]
Nu-Cotrimox [Can]
Pediazole® [US/Can]
Septra® [US]
Septra® DS [US]
Septra® Injection [Can]
sulfadiazine
sulfamethoxazole and trimethoprim
sulfisoxazole
Sulfizole® [Can]
Tetracycline Derivative
Adoxa™ [US]
Alti-Minocycline [Can]
Apo-Doxy® [Can]
Apo-Doxy Tabs® [Can]
Apo-Minocycline® [Can]
Apo-Tetra® [Can]
Doryx® [US]
Doxy-100® [US]
Doxycin [Can]
doxycycline
Doxytec [Can]
Dynacin® [US]
Gen-Minocycline [Can]
Minocin® [US/Can]
minocycline
Monodox® [US]
myrac™ [US]
Novo-Doxylin [Can]
Novo-Minocycline [Can]
Nu-Doxycycline [Can]
Nu-Tetra [Can]
oxytetracycline
Periostat® [US/Can]
Rhoxal-minocycline [Can]
Sandoz-Minocycline [Can]
Solodyn™ [US]
Sumycin® [US]
Terramycin® [Can]
tetracycline
Vibramycin® [US]
Vibra-Tabs® [US/Can]

HEART BLOCK
Adrenergic Agonist Agent
Adrenalin® [US/Can]
epinephrine
isoproterenol
Isuprel® [US]

H. INFLUENZAE
Toxoid
diphtheria, tetanus toxoids, and
acellular pertussis vaccine and
Haemophilus influenzae
b conjugate vaccine
TriHIBit® [US]
Vaccine, Inactivated Bacteria
ActHIB® [US/Can]
diphtheria, tetanus toxoids, and
acellular pertussis vaccine and
Haemophilus influenzae
b conjugate vaccine
Haemophilus B conjugate vaccine
HibTITER® [US]
PedvaxHIB® [US/Can]
TriHIBit® [US]
Vaccine, Inactivated Virus
Comvax® [US]
Haemophilus B conjugate and
hepatitis B vaccine

HISTOPLASMOSIS
Antifungal Agent
Amphocin® [US]
amphotericin B (conventional)
Apo-Ketoconazole® [Can]
Fungizone® [Can]
itraconazole
ketoconazole
Ketoderm® [Can]
Nizoral® [US]
Nizoral® A-D [US-OTC]
Novo-Ketoconazole [Can]
Sporanox® [US/Can]

HYPER-CHOLESTEROLEMIA

Antihyperlipidemic Agent,
  Miscellaneous
  colesevelam
  Colestid® [US/Can]
  colestipol
  WelChol® [US/Can]
Antilipemic Agent, 2-Azetidinone
  ezetimibe
  ezetimibe and simvastatin
  Ezetrol® [Can]
  Vytorin™ [US]
  Zetia™ [US]
Antilipemic Agent, HMG-CoA
  Reductase Inhibitor
  amlodipine and atorvastatin
  Caduet® [US/Can]
Bile Acid Sequestrant
  cholestyramine resin
  colesevelam
  Novo-Cholamine [Can]
  Novo-Cholamine Light [Can]
  PMS-Cholestyramine [Can]
  Prevalite® [US]
  Questran® [US]
  Questran® Light [US]
  Questran® Light Sugar Free [Can]
  WelChol® [US/Can]
HMG-CoA Reductase Inhibitor
  Advicor® [US/Can]
  Altoprev® [US]
  Apo-Lovastatin® [Can]
  Apo-Pravastatin® [Can]
  Apo-Simvastatin® [Can]
  atorvastatin
  BCI-Simvastatin [Can]
  CO Lovastatin [Can]
  CO Pravastatin [Can]
  CO Simvastatin [Can]
  fluvastatin
  Gen-Lovastatin [Can]
  Gen-Simvastatin [Can]

Lescol® [US/Can]
Lescol® XL [US]
Lipitor® [US/Can]
lovastatin
Mevacor® [US/Can]
niacin and lovastatin
Novo-Lovastatin [Can]
Novo-Pravastatin [Can]
Novo-Simvastatin [Can]
Nu-Lovastatin [Can]
PMS-Lovastatin [Can]
PMS-Pravastatin [Can]
PMS-Simvastatin [Can]
Pravachol® [US/Can]
pravastatin
RAN™-Lovastatin [Can]
ratio-Lovastatin [Can]
ratio-Pravastatin [Can]
ratio-Simvastatin [Can]
Riva-Lovastatin [Can]
Riva-Pravastatin [Can]
Riva-Simvastatin [Can]
Sandoz-Lovastatin [Can]
Sandoz-Pravastatin [Can]
Sandoz-Simvastatin [Can]
simvastatin
Taro-Simvastatin [Can]
Zocor® [US/Can]

HYPERLIPIDEMIA

Antihyperlipidemic Agent,
  Miscellaneous
  Antara™ [US]
  Apo-Fenofibrate® [Can]
  Apo-Feno-Micro® [Can]
  Apo-Gemfibrozil® [Can]
  bezafibrate (Canada only)
  Bezalip® [Can]
  Colestid® [US/Can]
  colestipol
  Dom-Fenofibrate Supra [Can]
  fenofibrate
  gemfibrozil

Gen-Fenofibrate Micro [Can]
Gen-Gemfibrozil [Can]
GMD-Gemfibrozil [Can]
Lipidil EZ® [Can]
Lipidil Micro® [Can]
Lipidil Supra® [Can]
Lipofen™ [US]
Lofibra™ [US]
Lopid® [US/Can]
Novo-Fenofibrate [Can]
Novo-Gemfibrozil [Can]
Nu-Fenofibrate [Can]
Nu-Gemfibrozil [Can]
PHL-Fenofibrate Supra [Can]
PMS-Bezafibrate [Can]
PMS-Fenofibrate Micro [Can]
PMS-Fenofibrate Supra [Can]
PMS-Gemfibrozil [Can]
ratio-Fenofibrate MC [Can]
TriCor® [US/Can]
Triglide™ [US]
Antilipemic Agent, HMG-CoA
  Reductase Inhibitor
  Crestor® [US/Can]
  rosuvastatin
Bile Acid Sequestrant
  cholestyramine resin
  Novo-Cholamine [Can]
  Novo-Cholamine Light [Can]
  PMS-Cholestyramine [Can]
  Prevalite® [US]
  Questran® [US]
  Questran® Light [US]
  Questran® Light Sugar Free [Can]
HMG-CoA Reductase Inhibitor
  Advicor® [US/Can]
  niacin and lovastatin
Vitamin, Water Soluble
  Advicor® [US/Can]
  niacin
  niacin and lovastatin
  Niacor® [US]
  Niaspan® [US/Can]

Slo-Niacin® [US-OTC]

HYPERTENSION

Adrenergic Agonist Agent
  inamrinone
Alpha-Adrenergic Agonist
  Apo-Clonidine® [Can]
  Carapres® [Can]
  Catapres® [US]
  Catapres-TTS® [US]
  clonidine
  Dixarit® [Can]
  Duraclon™ [US]
  guanabenz
  guanfacine
  Novo-Clonidine [Can]
  Nu-Clonidine [Can]
  Tenex® [US/Can]
  Wytensin® [Can]
Alpha-Adrenergic Blocking Agent
  Alti-Doxazosin [Can]
  Alti-Terazosin [Can]
  Apo-Doxazosin® [Can]
  Apo-Methyldopa® [Can]
  Apo-Prazo® [Can]
  Apo-Terazosin® [Can]
  Cardura® [US]
  Cardura-1™ [Can]
  Cardura-2™ [Can]
  Cardura-4™ [Can]
  Cardura® XL [US]
  Dibenzyline® [US/Can]
  doxazosin
  Gen-Doxazosin [Can]
  Hytrin® [US/Can]
  methyldopa
  Minipress® [US/Can]
  Novo-Doxazosin [Can]
  Novo-Prazin [Can]
  Novo-Terazosin [Can]
  Nu-Medopa [Can]
  Nu-Prazo [Can]
  Nu-Terazosin [Can]

phenoxybenzamine
phentolamine
PMS-Terazosin [Can]
prazosin
Regitine® [Can]
Rogitine® [Can]
terazosin
Alpha-/Beta- Adrenergic Blocker
  Apo-Labetalol® [Can]
  labetalol
  Labetalol Hydrochloride Injection,
    USP [Can]
  Normodyne® [Can]
  Trandate® [US/Can]
Angiotensin II Antagonist Combination
  eprosartan and hydrochlorothiazide
  Teveten® HCT [US/Can]
  Teveten® Plus [Can]
Angiotensin II Receptor Antagonist
  Atacand® [US/Can]
  Avapro® [US/Can]
  Benicar® [US]
  Benicar HCT® [US]
  candesartan
  Cozaar® [US/Can]
  Diovan® [US/Can]
  eprosartan
  irbesartan
  losartan
  Micardis® [US/Can]
  olmesartan
  olmesartan and hydrochlorothiazide
  telmisartan
  Teveten® [US/Can]
  valsartan
Angiotensin-Converting Enzyme (ACE)
  Inhibitor
  Accupril® [US/Can]
  Altace® [US/Can]
  Alti-Captopril [Can]
  Apo-Benazepril® [Can]
  Apo-Capto® [Can]

  Apo-Fosinopril® [Can]
  Apo-Lisinopril® [Can]
  benazepril
  Capoten® [US/Can]
  captopril
  cilazapril (Canada only)
  enalapril
  fosinopril
  fosinopril and hydrochlorothiazide
  Gen-Captopril [Can]
  Inhibace® [Can]
  lisinopril
  Lotensin® [US/Can]
  Mavik® [US/Can]
  moexipril
  moexipril and hydrochlorothiazide
  Monopril® [US/Can]
  Monopril-HCT® [US/Can]
  Novo-Captopril [Can]
  Novo-Cilazapril [Can]
  Novo-Fosinopril [Can]
  Nu-Capto [Can]
  PMS-Captopril [Can]
  Prinivil® [US/Can]
  quinapril
  ramipril
  ratio-Fosinopril [Can]
  Riva-Rosinopril [Can]
  trandolapril
  Uniretic® [US/Can]
  Univasc® [US]
  Vasotec® [US/Can]
  Zestril® [US/Can]
Antihypertensive Agent
  diazoxide
  eplerenone
  Hyperstat® [US]
  Inspra™ [US]
  Proglycem® [US/Can]
Antihypertensive Agent, Combination
  Accuretic® [US/Can]
  Aldactazide® [US]

Aldactazide 25® [Can]
Aldactazide 50® [Can]
Aldoril® [US]
amlodipine and benazepril
Apo-Methazide® [Can]
Apo-Triazide® [Can]
Atacand HCT™ [US]
Atacand® Plus [Can]
atenolol and chlorthalidone
Avalide® [US/Can]
benazepril and hydrochlorothiazide
bisoprolol and hydrochlorothiazide
candesartan and hydrochlorothiazide
Capozide® [US/Can]
captopril and hydrochlorothiazide
clonidine and chlorthalidone
Clorpres® [US]
Diovan HCT® [US/Can]
Dyazide® [US]
enalapril and felodipine
enalapril and hydrochlorothiazide
eprosartan and hydrochlorothiazide
hydralazine and hydrochlorothiazide
hydrochlorothiazide and spironolac-
tone
hydrochlorothiazide and triamterene
Hyzaar® [US/Can]
Hyzaar® DS [Can]
Inderide® [US]
irbesartan and hydrochlorothiazide
Lexxel® [US/Can]
lisinopril and hydrochlorothiazide
losartan and hydrochlorothiazide
Lotensin® HCT [US]
Lotrel® [US]
Maxzide® [US]
Maxzide®-25 [US]
methyldopa and hydrochlorothiazide
Micardis® HCT [US]
Micardis® Plus [Can]
Minizide® [US]
Novo-Spirozine [Can]

Novo-Triamzide [Can]
Nu-Triazide [Can]
Penta-Triamterene HCTZ [Can]
prazosin and polythiazide
Prinzide® [US/Can]
propranolol and hydrochlorothiazide
quinapril and hydrochlorothiazide
Quinaretic [US]
Riva-Zide [Can]
Tarka® [US/Can]
telmisartan and hydrochlorothiazide
Tenoretic® [US/Can]
Teveten® HCT [US/Can]
Teveten® Plus [Can]
trandolapril and verapamil
valsartan and hydrochlorothiazide
Vaseretic® [US/Can]
Zestoretic® [US/Can]
Ziac® [US/Can]
Beta-Adrenergic Blocker
acebutolol
Alti-Nadolol [Can]
Alti-Timolol [Can]
Apo-Acebutolol® [Can]
Apo-Atenol® [Can]
Apo-Bisoprolol® [Can]
Apo-Carvedilol® [Can]
Apo-Metoprolol® [Can]
Apo-Nadol® [Can]
Apo-Pindol® [Can]
Apo-Propranolol® [Can]
Apo-Timol® [Can]
Apo-Timop® [Can]
atenolol
Betaloc® [Can]
Betaloc® Durules® [Can]
betaxolol
Betimol® [US]
Betoptic® S [US/Can]
bisoprolol
Blocadren® [US]
Brevibloc® [US/Can]

carteolol
Cartrol® [US/Can]
carvedilol
Coreg® [US/Can]
Corgard® [US/Can]
esmolol
Gen-Acebutolol [Can]
Gen-Atenolol [Can]
Gen-Pindolol [Can]
Gen-Timolol [Can]
Inderal® [US/Can]
Inderal® LA [US/Can]
InnoPran XL™ [US]
Istalol™ [US]
Kerlone® [US]
Lopressor® [US/Can]
metoprolol
Metoprolol Tartrate Injection,
    USP [Can]
Monitan® [Can]
Monocor® [Can]
nadolol
Novo-Acebutolol [Can]
Novo-Atenol [Can]
Novo-Bisoprolol [Can]
Novo-Carvedilol [Can]
Novo-Metoprolol [Can]
Novo-Nadolol [Can]
Novo-Pindol [Can]
Novo-Pranol [Can]
Nu-Acebutolol [Can]
Nu-Atenol [Can]
Nu-Metop [Can]
Nu-Pindol [Can]
Nu-Propranolol [Can]
Nu-Timolol [Can]
Ocupress® Ophthalmic [Can]
oxprenolol (Canada only)
Phoxal-timolol [Can]
pindolol
PMS-Atenolol [Can]
PMS-Carvedilol [Can]
PMS-Metoprolol [Can]

PMS-Pindolol [Can]
PMS-Timolol [Can]
propranolol
Propranolol Hydrochloride Injection,
    USP [Can]
RAN™-Carvedilol [Can]
ratio-Carvedilol [Can]
Rhotral [Can]
Rhoxal-acebutolol [Can]
Rhoxal-atenolol [Can]
Riva-Atenolol [Can]
Sandoz-Acebutolol [Can]
Sandoz-Atenolol [Can]
Sandoz-Betaxolol [Can]
Sandoz-Bisoprolol [Can]
Sandoz-Metoprolol [Can]
Sandoz-Timolol [Can]
Sectral® [US/Can]
Slow-Trasicor® [Can]
Tenolin [Can]
Tenormin® [US/Can]
Tim-AK [Can]
timolol
Timoptic® [US/Can]
Timoptic® in OcuDose® [US]
Timoptic-XE® [US/Can]
Toprol-XL® [US/Can]
Trasicor® [Can]
Visken® [Can]
Zebeta® [US/Can]
Beta Blocker, Beta1 Selective
    Lopressor HCT® [US]
    metoprolol and hydrochlorothiazide
Calcium Channel Blocker
    Adalat® XL® [Can]
    Adalat® CC [US]
    Afeditab™ CR [US]
    Alti-Verapamil [Can]
    amlodipine
    amlodipine and atorvastatin
    Apo-Nifed® [Can]
    Apo-Nifed PA® [Can]
    Apo-Verap® [Can]

Apo-Verap® SR [Can]
Caduet® [US/Can]
Calan® [US/Can]
Calan® SR [US]
Cardene® [US]
Cardene® I.V. [US]
Cardene® SR [US]
Chronovera® [Can]
Covera® [Can]
Covera-HS® [US/Can]
DynaCirc® [Can]
DynaCirc® CR [US]
felodipine
Gen-Verapamil [Can]
Gen-Verapamil SR [Can]
Isoptin® SR [US/Can]
isradipine
nicardipine
Nifediac™ CC [US]
Nifedical™ XL [US]
nifedipine
nisoldipine
Norvasc® [US/Can]
Novo-Nifedin [Can]
Novo-Veramil SR [Can]
Nu-Nifed [Can]
Nu-Verap [Can]
Plendil® [US/Can]
Procardia® [US/Can]
Procardia XL® [US]
Renedil® [Can]
Riva-Verapamil SR [Can]
Sular® [US]
verapamil
Verapamil Hydrochloride Injection, USP [Can]
Verelan® [US]
Verelan® PM [US]
Diagnostic Agent
  phentolamine
  Regitine® [Can]
  Rogitine® [Can]
Diuretic, Combination

amiloride and hydrochlorothiazide
Apo-Amilzide® [Can]
Gen-Amilazide [Can]
Moduret [Can]
Novamilor [Can]
Nu-Amilzide [Can]
Diuretic, Loop
  Apo-Furosemide® [Can]
  bumetanide
  Bumex® [US/Can]
  Burinex® [Can]
  Demadex® [US]
  Edecrin® [US/Can]
  ethacrynic acid
  furosemide
  Furosemide Injection, USP [Can]
  Furosemide Special [Can]
  Lasix® [US/Can]
  Lasix® Special [Can]
  Novo-Semide [Can]
  torsemide
Diuretic, Miscellaneous
  Apo-Chlorthalidone® [Can]
  Apo-Indapamide® [Can]
  chlorthalidone
  Gen-Indapamide [Can]
  indapamide
  Lozide® [Can]
  Lozol® [US/Can]
  metolazone
  Mykrox® [Can]
  Novo-Indapamide [Can]
  Nu-Indapamide [Can]
  PMS-Indapamide [Can]
  Thalitone® [US]
  Zaroxolyn® [US/Can]
Diuretic, Potassium Sparing
  Aldactone® [US/Can]
  Dyrenium® [US]
  Novo-Spiroton [Can]
  spironolactone
  triamterene
Diuretic, Thiazide

Apo-Hydro® [Can]
Aquatensen® [Can]
Benicar HCT® [US]
chlorothiazide
Diuril® [US/Can]
Enduron® [Can]
eprosartan and hydrochlorothiazide
hydrochlorothiazide
Lopressor HCT® [US]
methyclothiazide
metoprolol and hydrochlorothiazide
Microzide™ [US]
moexipril and hydrochlorothiazide
Novo-Hydrazide [Can]
olmesartan and hydrochlorothiazide
PMS-Hydrochlorothiazide [Can]
Teveten® HCT [US/Can]
Teveten® Plus [Can]
Uniretic® [US/Can]
Ganglionic Blocking Agent
　Inversine® [US/Can]
　mecamylamine
Miscellaneous Product
　Aceon® [US]
　Coversyl® [Can]
　Coversyl® Plus [Can]
　perindopril and indapamide (Canada only)
　perindopril erbumine
　Preterax® [Can]
Rauwolfia Alkaloid
　reserpine
Selective Aldosterone Blocker
　eplerenone
　Inspra™ [US]
Vasodilator
　Apo-Gain® [Can]
　Apo-Hydralazine® [Can]
　Apresoline® [Can]
　hydralazine
　Loniten® [US]
　Minox [Can]
　minoxidil

Nitropress® [US]
nitroprusside
Novo-Hylazin [Can]
Nu-Hydral [Can]
Rogaine® [Can]
Rogaine® Extra Strength for Men [US-OTC]
Rogaine® for Men [US-OTC]
Rogaine® for Women [US-OTC]

HYPERTENSION (ARTERIAL)
Beta-Adrenergic Blocker
　Levatol® [US/Can]
　penbutolol

HYPERTENSION (CEREBRAL)
Barbiturate
　Pentothal® [US/Can]
　thiopental
Diuretic, Osmotic
　Amino-Cerv™ [US]
　Aquacare® [US-OTC]
　Aquaphilic® With Carbamide [US-OTC]
　Carmol® 10 [US-OTC]
　Carmol® 20 [US-OTC]
　Carmol® 40 [US]
　Carmol® Deep Cleaning [US]
　Cerovel™ [US]
　DPM™ [US-OTC]
　Gormel® [US-OTC]
　Keralac™ [US]
　Keralac™ Nailstik [US]
　Lanaphilic® [US-OTC]
　mannitol
　Nutraplus® [US-OTC]
　Osmitrol® [US/Can]
　Rea-Lo® [US-OTC]
　Resectisol® [US]
　Ultra Mide® [US-OTC]

UltraMide 25™ [Can]
Umecta® [US]
urea
Ureacin® [US-OTC]
Uremol® [Can]
Urisec® [Can]
Vanamide™ [US]

HYPERTENSION (CORONARY)
Vasodilator
Gen-Nitro [Can]
Minitran™ [US/Can]
Nitrek® [US]
Nitro-Bid® [US]
Nitro-Dur® [US/Can]
nitroglycerin
Nitrol® [Can]
Nitrolingual® [US]
NitroQuick® [US]
Nitrostat® [US/Can]
NitroTime® [US]
Rho-Nitro [Can]
Transderm-Nitro® [Can]
Trinipatch® 0.2 [Can]
Trinipatch® 0.4 [Can]
Trinipatch® 0.6 [Can]

HYPERTENSION (EMERGENCY)
Antihypertensive Agent
Corlopam® [US/Can]
fenoldopam

HYPOTENSION
Adrenergic Agonist Agent
Adrenalin® [US/Can]
dopamine
ephedrine
epinephrine
isoproterenol
Isuprel® [US]

Levophed® [US/Can]
norepinephrine
Primatene® Mist [US-OTC]

HYPOTENSION (ORTHOSTATIC)
Adrenergic Agonist Agent
Altafrin [US]
ephedrine
Alpha-Adrenergic Agonist
Amatine® [Can]
Apo-Midodrine® [Can]
midodrine
Orvaten™ [US]
ProAmatine® [US]
Central Nervous System Stimulant,
Nonamphetamine
Apo-Methylphenidate® [Can]
Apo-Methylphenidate® SR [Can]
Biphentin® [Can]
Concerta® [US/Can]
Daytrana™ [US]
Metadate® CD [US]
Metadate® ER [US]
Methylin® [US]
Methylin® ER [US]
methylphenidate
PMS-Methylphenidate [Can]
Riphenidate [Can]
Ritalin® [US/Can]
Ritalin® LA [US]
Ritalin-SR® [US/Can]

HYPOXIC RESPIRATORY FAILURE
Vasodilator, Pulmonary
INOmax® [US/Can]
nitric oxide

IDIOPATHIC PULMONARY ARTERIAL HYPERTENSION
Prostaglandin

iloprost
Ventavis™ [US]

ISCHEMIA
Blood Viscosity Reducer Agent
  Albert® Pentoxifylline [Can]
  Apo-Pentoxifylline SR® [Can]
Nu-Pentoxifylline SR [Can]
  pentoxifylline
  Pentoxil® [US]
  ratio-Pentoxifylline [Can]
  Trental® [US/Can]
Platelet Aggregation Inhibitor
  abciximab
  ReoPro® [US/Can]
Vasodilator
  papaverine
  Para-Time S.R.® [US]

LUNG SURFACTANT
Lung Surfactant
  beractant
  Survanta® [US/Can]

MALIGNANT EFFUSION
Antineoplastic Agent
  thiotepa

MALIGNANT PLEURAL MESOTHELIOMA
Antineoplastic Agent, Antimetabolite
  Alimta® [US/Can]
  pemetrexed
Antineoplastic Agent, Antimetabolite
  (Antifolate)
  Alimta® [US/Can]
  pemetrexed

MITRAL VALVE PROLAPSE
Beta-Adrenergic Blocker
  Apo-Propranolol® [Can]
  Inderal® [US/Can]

Inderal® LA [US/Can]
InnoPran XL™ [US]
Novo-Pranol [Can]
Nu-Propranolol [Can]
propranolol
Propranolol Hydrochloride Injection,
USP [Can]

MYCOBACTERIUM AVIUM-INTRACELLULARE
Antibiotic, Aminoglycoside
  streptomycin
Antibiotic, Miscellaneous
  Mycobutin® [US/Can]
  rifabutin
  Rifadin® [US/Can]
  rifampin
  Rofact™ [Can]
Antimycobacterial Agent
  ethambutol
  Etibi® [Can]
  Myambutol® [US]
Antitubercular Agent
  streptomycin
Carbapenem (Antibiotic)
  imipenem and cilastatin
  meropenem
  Merrem® [Can]
  Merrem® I.V. [US]
  Primaxin® [US/Can]
  Primaxin® I.V. [Can]
Macrolide (Antibiotic)
  Apo-Azithromycin® [Can]
  azithromycin
  Biaxin® [US/Can]
  Biaxin® XL [US/Can]
  clarithromycin
  CO Azithromycin [Can]
  GMD-Azithromycin [Can]
  Novo-Azithromycin [Can]
  PMS-Azithromycin [Can]
  ratio-Azithromycin [Can]
  ratio-Clarithromycin [Can]

Sandoz-Azithromycin [Can]
Zithromax® [US/Can]
Zmax™ [US]
Quinolone
  Apo-Ciproflox® [Can]
  Ciloxan® [US/Can]
  Cipro® [US/Can]
  Cipro® XL [Can]
  ciprofloxacin
  Cipro® XR [US]
  CO Ciprofloxacin [Can]
  Gen-Ciprofloxacin [Can]
  Novo-Ciprofloxacin [Can]
  PMS-Ciprofloxacin [Can]
  Proquin® XR [US]
  RAN™-Ciprofloxacin [Can]
  ratio-Ciprofloxacin [Can]
  Rhoxal-ciprofloxacin [Can]
  Sandoz-Ciprofloxacin [Can]
  Taro-Ciprofloxacin [Can]

MYCOSIS (FUNGOIDES)

Psoralen
  methoxsalen
  8-MOP® [US/Can]
  Oxsoralen® [US/Can]
  Oxsoralen-Ultra® [US/Can]
  Ultramop™ [Can]
  Uvadex® [US/Can]

MYOCARDIAL INFARCTION

Antiarrhythmic Agent, Class II
  Apo-Propranolol® [Can]
  Inderal® [US/Can]
  Inderal® LA [US/Can]
  InnoPran XL™ [US]
  Novo-Pranol [Can]
  Nu-Propranolol [Can]
  propranolol
  Propranolol Hydrochloride Injection,
    USP [Can]

Anticoagulant (Other)
  Apo-Warfarin® [Can]
  Coumadin® [US/Can]
  enoxaparin
  Enoxaparin Injection [Can]
  Gen-Warfarin [Can]
  Hepalean® [Can]
  Hepalean® Leo [Can]
  Hepalean®-LOK [Can]
  heparin
  HepFlush®-10 [US]
  Hep-Lock® [US]
  Hep-Lock U/P [US]
  Jantoven™ [US]
  Lovenox® [US/Can]
  Lovenox® HP [Can]
  Novo-Warfarin [Can]
  Taro-Warfarin [Can]
  warfarin
Antiplatelet Agent
  Apo-Dipyridamole FC® [Can]
  Asaphen [Can]
  Asaphen E.C. [Can]
  Ascriptin® [US-OTC]
  Ascriptin® Extra Strength [US-OTC]
  Aspercin [US-OTC]
  Aspercin Extra [US-OTC]
  Aspergum® [US-OTC]
  aspirin
  Bayer® Aspirin [US-OTC]
  Bayer® Aspirin Extra Strength
    [US-OTC]
  Bayer® Aspirin Regimen Adult Low
    Strength [US-OTC]
  Bayer® Aspirin Regimen Children's
    [US-OTC]
  Bayer® Aspirin Regimen Regular
    Strength [US-OTC]
  Bayer® Extra Strength Arthritis Pain
    Regimen [US-OTC]
  Bayer® Plus Extra Strength
    [US-OTC]
  Bayer® Women's Aspirin

Plus Calcium [US-OTC]
Bufferin® [US-OTC]
Bufferin® Extra Strength [US-OTC]
Buffinol [US-OTC]
Buffinol Extra [US-OTC]
clopidogrel
dipyridamole
Easprin® [US]
Ecotrin® [US-OTC]
Ecotrin® Low Strength [US-OTC]
Ecotrin® Maximum Strength
    [US-OTC]
Entrophen® [Can]
Halfprin® [US-OTC]
Novasen [Can]
Persantine® [US/Can]
Plavix® [US/Can]
St. Joseph® Adult Aspirin [US-OTC]
Sureprin 81™ [US-OTC]
ZORprin® [US]
Beta-Adrenergic Blocker
Alti-Nadolol [Can]
Alti-Timolol [Can]
Apo-Atenol® [Can]
Apo-Metoprolol® [Can]
Apo-Nadol® [Can]
Apo-Propranolol® [Can]
Apo-Timol® [Can]
Apo-Timop® [Can]
atenolol
Betaloc® [Can]
Betaloc® Durules® [Can]
Betimol® [US]
Blocadren® [US]
Corgard® [US/Can]
Gen-Atenolol [Can]
Gen-Timolol [Can]
Inderal® [US/Can]
Inderal® LA [US/Can]
InnoPran XL™ [US]
Istalol™ [US]
Lopressor® [US/Can]
metoprolol

Metoprolol Tartrate Injection, USP
    [Can]
nadolol
Novo-Atenol [Can]
Novo-Metoprolol [Can]
Novo-Nadolol [Can]
Novo-Pranol [Can]
Nu-Atenol [Can]
Nu-Metop [Can]
Nu-Propranolol [Can]
Nu-Timolol [Can]
Phoxal-timolol [Can]
PMS-Atenolol [Can]
PMS-Metoprolol [Can]
PMS-Timolol [Can]
propranolol
Propranolol Hydrochloride Injection,
    USP [Can]
Rhoxal-atenolol [Can]
Riva-Atenolol [Can]
Sandoz-Atenolol [Can]
Sandoz-Metoprolol [Can]
Sandoz-Timolol [Can]
Tenolin [Can]
Tenormin® [US/Can]
Tim-AK [Can]
timolol
Timoptic® [US/Can]
Timoptic® in OcuDose® [US]
Timoptic-XE® [US/Can]
Toprol-XL® [US/Can]
Fibrinolytic Agent
Activase® [US]
Activase® rt-PA [Can]
alteplase
Cathflo™ Activase® [US/Can]
Retavase® [US/Can]
reteplase
Streptase® [US/Can]
streptokinase
Thrombolytic Agent
tenecteplase
TNKase™ [US/Can]

Vasodilator
  Apo-Dipyridamole FC® [Can]
  dipyridamole
  Persantine® [US/Can]

ORGAN REJECTION
Immunosuppressant Agent
  daclizumab
  Zenapax® [US/Can]

ORGAN TRANSPLANT
Immunosuppressant Agent
  basiliximab
  CellCept® [US/Can]
  cyclosporine
  Gengraf® [US]
  muromonab-CD3
  mycophenolate
  Myfortic® [US/Can]
  Neoral® [US/Can]
  Orthoclone OKT® 3 [US/Can]
  Prograf® [US/Can]
  Protopic® [US/Can]
  Rapamune® [US/Can]
  Restasis® [US]
  Rhoxal-cyclosporine [Can]
  Sandimmune® [US]
  Sandimmune® I.V. [Can]
  Sandoz-Cyclosporine [Can]
  Simulect® [US/Can]
  sirolimus
  tacrolimus

PAIN
Analgesic Combination (Narcotic)
  propoxyphene, aspirin, and caffeine
Analgesic Combination (Opioid)
  acetaminophen, caffeine, and
    dihydrocodeine
  Panlor® DC [US]
  Panlor® SS [US]
  pentazocine and acetaminophen

Talacen® [US]
ZerLor™ [US]
Analgesic, Miscellaneous
  acetaminophen and tramadol
  Tramacet [Can]
  Ultracet™ [US]
Analgesic, Narcotic
  acetaminophen and codeine
  Actiq® [US/Can]
  Alfenta® [US/Can]
  alfentanil
  Alfentanil Injection, USP [Can]
  Anexsia® [US]
  Apo-Butorphanol® [Can]
  Astramorph/PF™ [US]
  Avinza™ [US]
  Balacet 325™ [US]
  Bancap HC® [US]
  belladonna and opium
  B&O Supprettes® [US]
  Buprenex® [US/Can]
  buprenorphine
  butalbital, aspirin, caffeine, and
  codeine
  butorphanol
  Capital® and Codeine [US]
  Ceta-Plus® [US]
  codeine
  Codeine Contin® [Can]
  Co-Gesic® [US]
  Damason-P® [US]
  Darvocet A500™ [US]
  Darvocet-N® 50 [US/Can]
  Darvocet-N® 100 [US/Can]
  Darvon® [US]
  Darvon-N® [US/Can]
  Demerol® [US/Can]
  DepoDur™ [US]
  dihydrocodeine, aspirin, and caffeine
  Dilaudid® [US/Can]
  Dilaudid-HP® [US/Can]
  Dilaudid-HP-Plus® [Can]
  Dilaudid® Sterile Powder [Can]

Dilaudid-XP® [Can]
Dolophine® [US/Can]
Duragesic® [US/Can]
Duramorph® [US]
Endocet® [US/Can]
Endodan® [US/Can]
ETH-Oxydose™ [Can]
fentanyl
Fentanyl Citrate Injection, USP
[Can]
Fiorinal®-C 1/2 [Can]
Fiorinal®-C 1/4 [Can]
Fiorinal® With Codeine [US]
hycet™ [US]
hydrocodone and acetaminophen
hydrocodone and aspirin
hydrocodone and ibuprofen
Hydromorph Contin® [Can]
Hydromorph-IR® [Can]
hydromorphone
Hydromorphone HP [Can]
Hydromorphone HP® 10 [Can]
Hydromorphone HP® 20 [Can]
Hydromorphone HP® 50 [Can]
Hydromorphone HP® Forte [Can]
Hydromorphone Hydrochloride
Injection, USP [Can]
Infumorph® [US]
Ionsys™ [US]
Kadian® [US/Can]
Levo-Dromoran® [US]
levorphanol
Lorcet® 10/650 [US]
Lorcet® Plus [US]
Lortab® [US]
Margesic® H [US]
Maxidone™ [US]
meperidine
meperidine and promethazine
Meperitab® [US]
M-Eslon® [Can]
Metadol™ [Can]
methadone

Methadone Diskets® [US]
Methadone Intensol™ [US]
Methadose® [US/Can]
Morphine HP® [Can]
Morphine LP® Epidural [Can]
morphine sulfate
M.O.S.® 10 [Can]
M.O.S.® 20 [Can]
M.O.S.® 30 [Can]
M.O.S.-S.R.® [Can]
M.O.S.-Sulfate® [Can]
MS Contin® [US/Can]
MS-IR® [Can]
nalbuphine
Norco® [US]
Nubain® [US]
Numorphan® [US]
opium tincture
Oramorph SR® [US]
Oxycocet® [Can]
Oxycodan® [Can]
oxycodone
oxycodone and acetaminophen
oxycodone and aspirin
OxyContin® [US/Can]
OxyFast® [US]
Oxy.IR® [Can]
oxymorphone
paregoric
pentazocine
Percocet® [US/Can]
Percocet®-Demi [Can]
Percodan® [US/Can]
Phrenilin® With Caffeine and
Codeine [US]
PMS-Butorphanol [Can]
PMS-Hydromorphone [Can]
PMS-Morphine Sulfate SR [Can]
PMS-Oxycodone-Acetaminophen
[Can]
Pronap-100® [US]
propoxyphene
propoxyphene and acetaminophen

ratio-Emtec [Can]
ratio-Lenoltec [Can]
ratio-Morphine SR [Can]
remifentanil
Reprexain™ [US]
RMS® [US]
Roxanol™ [US]
Roxanol 100™ [US]
Roxicet™ [US]
Roxicet™ 5/500 [US]
Roxicodone® [US]
Stadol® [US]
Stagesic® [US]
Statex® [Can]
Sublimaze® [US]
Subutex® [US/Can]
Sufenta® [US/Can]
sufentanil
Supeudol® [Can]
Synalgos®-DC [US]
642® Tablet [Can]
Talwin® [US/Can]
Talwin® NX [US]
Tecnal C 1/2 [Can]
Tecnal C 1/4 [Can]
Triatec-8 [Can]
Triatec-8 Strong [Can]
Triatec-30 [Can]
Tylenol® Elixir with Codeine [Can]
Tylenol® No. 1 [Can]
Tylenol No. 1 Forte [Can]
Tylenol® No. 2 with Codeine [Can]
Tylenol® No. 3 with Codeine [Can]
Tylenol® No. 4 with Codeine [Can]
Tylenol® With Codeine [US]
Tylox® [US]
Ultiva® [US/Can]
Vicodin® [US]
Vicodin® ES [US]
Vicodin® HP [US]
Vicoprofen® [US/Can]
Zomorph® [Can]
Zydone® [US]

Analgesic, Nonnarcotic
Abenol® [Can]
Acephen™ [US-OTC]
Aceta-Gesic [US-OTC]
acetaminophen
acetaminophen and diphenhydramine
acetaminophen and
    phenyltoloxamine
acetaminophen and tramadol
acetaminophen, aspirin, and caffeine
Acular® [US/Can]
Acular LS™ [US/Can]
Acular® PF [US]
Advil® [US-OTC/Can]
Advil® Children's [US-OTC]
Advil® Infants' [US-OTC]
Advil® Junior [US-OTC]
Advil® Migraine [US-OTC]
Aleve® [US-OTC]
Alti-Flurbiprofen [Can]
Amigesic® [US/Can]
Anaprox® [US/Can]
Anaprox® DS [US/Can]
Ansaid® [Can]
Apo-Acetaminophen® [Can]
Apo-Diclo® [Can]
Apo-Diclo Rapide® [Can]
Apo-Diclo SR® [Can]
Apo-Diflunisal® [Can]
Apo-Etodolac® [Can]
Apo-Flurbiprofen® [Can]
Apo-Ibuprofen® [Can]
Apo-Indomethacin® [Can]
Apo-Keto® [Can]
Apo-Keto-E® [Can]
Apo-Ketorolac® [Can]
Apo-Ketorolac Injectable® [Can]
Apo-Keto SR® [Can]
Apo-Mefenamic® [Can]
Apo-Nabumetone® [Can]
Apo-Napro-Na® [Can]
Apo-Napro-Na DS® [Can]
Apo-Naproxen® [Can]

Apo-Naproxen EC® [Can]
Apo-Naproxen SR® [Can]
Apo-Oxaprozin® [Can]
Apo-Piroxicam® [Can]
Apo-Sulin® [Can]
Apra Children's [US-OTC]
Asaphen [Can]
Asaphen E.C. [Can]
Ascriptin® [US-OTC]
Ascriptin® Extra Strength [US-OTC]
Aspercin [US-OTC]
Aspercin Extra [US-OTC]
Aspergum® [US-OTC]
aspirin
Aspirin Free Anacin® Maximum
  Strength [US-OTC]
Atasol® [Can]
Bayer® Aspirin [US-OTC]
Bayer® Aspirin Extra Strength
  [US-OTC]
Bayer® Aspirin Regimen Adult
  Low Strength [US-OTC]
Bayer® Aspirin Regimen Children's
  [US-OTC]
Bayer® Aspirin Regimen Regular
  Strength [US-OTC]
Bayer® Extra Strength Arthritis Pain
  Regimen [US-OTC]
Bayer® Plus Extra Strength
  [US-OTC]
Bayer® Women's Aspirin Plus
Calcium [US-OTC]
Bufferin® [US-OTC]
Bufferin® Extra Strength [US-OTC]
Buffinol [US-OTC]
Buffinol Extra [US-OTC]
Cataflam® [US/Can]
Cetafen® [US-OTC]
Cetafen Extra® [US-OTC]
choline magnesium trisalicylate
Clinoril® [US]
Comtrex® Sore Throat Maximum
Strength [US-OTC]

Daypro® [US/Can]
diclofenac
diflunisal
Dologesic® [US]
Dom-Mefenamic Acid [Can]
Easprin® [US]
EC-Naprosyn® [US]
Ecotrin® [US-OTC]
Ecotrin® Low Strength [US-OTC]
Ecotrin® Maximum Strength
  [US-OTC]
ElixSure™ IB [US-OTC]
Entrophen® [Can]
etodolac
Excedrin® Extra Strength [US-OTC]
Excedrin® Migraine [US-OTC]
Excedrin® P.M. [US-OTC]
Feldene® [US]
Fem-Prin® [US-OTC]
fenoprofen
FeverAll® [US-OTC]
Flextra 650 [US]
Flextra-DS [US]
flurbiprofen
Froben® [Can]
Froben-SR® [Can]
Genaced™ [US-OTC]
Genapap™ [US-OTC]
Genapap™ Children [US-OTC]
Genapap™ Extra Strength [US-OTC]
Genapap™ Infant [US-OTC]
Genebs [US-OTC]
Genebs Extra Strength [US-OTC]
Genesec™ [US-OTC]
Gen-Nabumetone [Can]
Gen-Naproxen EC [Can]
Gen-Piroxicam [Can]
Genpril® [US-OTC]
Goody's® Extra Strength Headache
Powder [US-OTC]
Goody's® Extra Strength Pain Relief
  [US-OTC]
Goody's PM® [US-OTC]

Halfprin® [US-OTC]
Hyflex-DS® [US]
Ibu-200 [US-OTC]
ibuprofen
Indocid® P.D.A. [Can]
Indocin® [US/Can]
Indocin® SR [US]
Indo-Lemmon [Can]
indomethacin
Indotec [Can]
Infantaire [US-OTC]
I-Prin [US-OTC]
ketoprofen
ketorolac
Ketorolac Tromethamine Injection,
    USP [Can]
Legatrin PM® [US-OTC]
Lodine® [Can]
Mapap [US-OTC]
Mapap Children's [US-OTC]
Mapap Extra Strength [US-OTC]
Mapap Infants [US-OTC]
meclofenamate
Meclomen® [Can]
Mefenamic-250 [Can]
mefenamic acid
Midol® Cramp and Body Aches
    [US-OTC]
Midol® Extended Relief [US]
Motrin® [US]
Motrin® Children's [US-OTC/Can]
Motrin® IB [US-OTC/Can]
Motrin® Infants' [US-OTC]
Motrin® Junior Strength [US-OTC]
nabumetone
Nalfon® [US]
Naprelan® [US]
Naprosyn® [US/Can]
naproxen
Naxen® [Can]
Naxen® EC [Can]
NeoProfen®
Norgesic™ [Can]

Norgesic™ Forte [Can]
Nortemp Children's [US-OTC]
Novasen [Can]
Novo-Difenac [Can]
Novo-Difenac K [Can]
Novo-Difenac-SR [Can]
Novo-Diflunisal [Can]
Novo-Flurprofen [Can]
Novo-Gesic [Can]
Novo-Keto [Can]
Novo-Keto-EC [Can]
Novo-Ketorolac [Can]
Novo-Methacin [Can]
Novo-Nabumetone [Can]
Novo-Naproc EC [Can]
Novo-Naprox [Can]
Novo-Naprox Sodium [Can]
Novo-Naprox Sodium DS [Can]
Novo-Naprox SR [Can]
Novo-Pirocam [Can]
Novo-Profen [Can]
Novo-Sundac [Can]
Nu-Diclo [Can]
Nu-Diclo-SR [Can]
Nu-Diflunisal [Can]
Nu-Flurprofen [Can]
Nu-Ibuprofen [Can]
Nu-Indo [Can]
Nu-Ketoprofen [Can]
Nu-Ketoprofen-E [Can]
Nu-Mefenamic [Can]
Nu-Naprox [Can]
Nu-Pirox [Can]
Nu-Sundac [Can]
Ocufen® [US/Can]
orphenadrine, aspirin, and caffeine
Oruvail® [Can]
oxaprozin
Pain-Eze [US-OTC]
Pain-Off [US-OTC]
Pamprin® Maximum Strength All
    Day Relief [US-OTC]
Pediatrix [Can]

Pennsaid® [Can]
Percogesic® [US-OTC]
Percogesic® Extra Strength
  [US-OTC]
Pexicam® [Can]
Phenagesic [US-OTC]
Phenylgesic [US-OTC]
piroxicam
PMS-Diclofenac [Can]
PMS-Diclofenac SR [Can]
PMS-Mefenamic Acid [Can]
Ponstan® [Can]
Ponstel® [US]
Prialt® [US]
Proprinal [US-OTC]
ratio-Ketorolac [Can]
Relafen® [Can]
RhinoFlex™ [US]
RhinoFlex 650 [US]
Rhodacine® [Can]
Rhodis™ [Can]
Rhodis-EC™ [Can]
Rhodis SR™ [Can]
Rhoxal-nabumetone [Can]
Riva-Diclofenac [Can]
Riva-Diclofenac-K [Can]
Riva-Naproxen [Can]
Salflex® [Can]
salsalate
Sandoz-Nabumetone [Can]
Silapap® Children's [US-OTC]
Silapap® Infants [US-OTC]
Solaraze® [US]
Staflex [US]
St. Joseph® Adult Aspirin [US-OTC]
sulindac
Sureprin 81™ [US-OTC]
Tempra® [Can]
Tolectin® [US]
tolmetin
Toradol® [US/Can]
Toradol® IM [Can]
Tramacet [Can]

tramadol
Tycolene [US-OTC]
Tycolene Maximum Strength
  [US-OTC]
Tylenol® [US-OTC/Can]
Tylenol® 8 Hour [US-OTC]
Tylenol® Arthritis Pain [US-OTC]
Tylenol® Children's [US-OTC]
Tylenol® Children's with Flavor
  Creator [US-OTC]
Tylenol® Extra Strength [US-OTC]
Tylenol® Infants [US-OTC]
Tylenol® Junior [US-OTC]
Tylenol® PM [US-OTC]
Tylenol® Severe Allergy [US-OTC]
Ultracet™ [US]
Ultram® [US/Can]
Ultram® ER [US]
Ultraprin [US-OTC]
Utradol™ [Can]
Valorin [US-OTC]
Valorin Extra [US-OTC]
Vanquish® Extra Strength Pain
Reliever [US-OTC]
Voltaren® [US/Can]
Voltaren Ophtha® [Can]
Voltaren Ophthalmic® [US]
Voltaren Rapide® [Can]
Voltaren®-XR [US]
ziconotide
ZORprin® [US]
Analgesic, Opioid
  acetaminophen, codeine, and
    doxylamine (Canada Only)
  Mersyndol® With Codeine [Can]
Decongestant/Analgesic
  Advil® Cold, Children's [US-OTC]
  Advil® Cold & Sinus
    [US-OTC/Can]
  Children's Advil® Cold [Can]
  Dristan® Sinus [US-OTC]
  Motrin® Cold and Sinus [US-OTC]
  Motrin® Cold, Children's [US-OTC]

Proprinal® Cold and Sinus
[US-OTC]
pseudoephedrine and ibuprofen
Sudafed® Sinus Advance [Can]
Skeletal Muscle Relaxant
Norgesic™ [Can]
Norgesic™ Forte [Can]
orphenadrine, aspirin, and caffeine

PERCUTANEOUS TRANSLUMINAL CORONARY ANGIOPLASTY (PTCA)
Anticoagulant (Other)
Angiomax® [US/Can]
bivalirudin

PNEUMONIA
Aminoglycoside (Antibiotic)
AKTob® [US]
Alcomicin® [Can]
amikacin
Amikacin Sulfate Injection,
USP [Can]
Amikin® [US/Can]
Diogent® [Can]
Garamycin® [Can]
Gentak® [US]
gentamicin
Gentamicin Injection, USP [Can]
PMS-Tobramycin [Can]
SAB-Gentamicin [Can]
Sandoz-Tobramycin [Can]
TOBI® [US/Can]
tobramycin
Tobramycin Injection, USP [Can]
Tobrex® [US/Can]
Antibiotic, Carbapenem
ertapenem
Invanz® [US/Can]
Antibiotic, Ketolide
Ketek® [US/Can]

telithromycin
Antibiotic, Miscellaneous
Alti-Clindamycin [Can]
Apo-Clindamycin® [Can]
Azactam® [US/Can]
aztreonam
Cleocin® [US]
Cleocin HCl® [US]
Cleocin Pediatric® [US]
Cleocin Phosphate® [US]
Cleocin T® [US]
Clindagel® [US]
ClindaMax™ [US]
clindamycin
Clindamycin Injection, USP [Can]
Clindesse™ [US]
Clindets® [US]
Clindoxyl® [Can]
Dalacin® C [Can]
Dalacin® T [Can]
Dalacin® Vaginal [Can]
Evoclin™ [US]
Novo-Clindamycin [Can]
Taro-Clindamycin [Can]
Vancocin® [US/Can]
vancomycin
Antibiotic, Quinolone
Factive® [US]
gatifloxacin
gemifloxacin
Iquix® [US]
Levaquin® [US/Can]
levofloxacin
Novo-Levofloxacin [Can]
Quixin™ [US]
Tequin® [Can]
Zymar™ [US/Can]
Carbapenem (Antibiotic)
imipenem and cilastatin
meropenem
Merrem® [Can]
Merrem® I.V. [US]
Primaxin® [US/Can]

Primaxin® I.V. [Can]

Cephalosporin (First Generation)
Ancef® [US]
Apo-Cefadroxil® [Can]
Apo-Cephalex® [Can]
Biocef® [US]
cefadroxil
cefazolin
cephalexin
cephalothin
Duricef® [US/Can]
Keflex® [US]
Keftab® [Can]
Novo-Cefadroxil [Can]
Novo-Lexin [Can]
Nu-Cephalex [Can]

Cephalosporin (Second Generation)
Apo-Cefuroxime® [Can]
cefoxitin
cefpodoxime
cefprozil
Ceftin® [US/Can]
cefuroxime
Cefzil® [US/Can]
Mefoxin® [US]
ratio-Cefuroxime [Can]
Vantin® [US/Can]
Zinacef® [US/Can]

Cephalosporin (Third Generation)
cefdinir
Cefizox® [US/Can]
cefotaxime
ceftazidime
ceftizoxime
ceftriaxone
Claforan® [US/Can]
Fortaz® [US/Can]
Omnicef® [US/Can]
Rocephin® [US/Can]
Tazicef® [US]

Cephalosporin (Fourth Generation)
cefepime
Maxipime® [US/Can]

Macrolide (Antibiotic)
Akne-Mycin® [US]
Apo-Azithromycin® [Can]
Apo-Erythro Base® [Can]
Apo-Erythro E-C® [Can]
Apo-Erythro-ES® [Can]
Apo-Erythro-S® [Can]
A/T/S® [US]
azithromycin
Biaxin® [US/Can]
Biaxin® XL [US/Can]
clarithromycin
CO Azithromycin [Can]
Diomycin® [Can]
E.E.S.® [US/Can]
Erybid™ [Can]
Eryc® [US/Can]
Eryderm® [US]
Erygel® [US]
EryPed® [US]
Ery-Tab® [US]
Erythrocin® [US]
erythromycin
GMD-Azithromycin [Can]
Novo-Azithromycin [Can]
Novo-Rythro Estolate [Can]
Novo-Rythro Ethylsuccinate [Can]
Nu-Erythromycin-S [Can]
PCE® [US/Can]
PMS-Azithromycin [Can]
PMS-Erythromycin [Can]
ratio-Azithromycin [Can]
ratio-Clarithromycin [Can]
Romycin® [US]
Sandoz-Azithromycin [Can]
Sans Acne® [Can]
Theramycin Z® [US]
Zithromax® [US/Can]
Zmax™ [US]

Penicillin
Alti-Amoxi-Clav [Can]
amoxicillin
amoxicillin and clavulanate

potassium
Amoxil® [US]
ampicillin
ampicillin and sulbactam
Apo-Amoxi® [Can]
Apo-Amoxi-Clav® [Can]
Apo-Ampi® [Can]
Apo-Cloxi® [Can]
Apo-Pen VK® [Can]
Augmentin® [US/Can]
Augmentin ES-600® [US]
Augmentin XR™ [US]
Bicillin® L-A [US]
Bicillin® C-R [US]
Bicillin® C-R 900/300 [US]
carbenicillin
Clavulin® [Can]
cloxacillin
dicloxacillin
Dycill® [Can]
Gen-Amoxicillin [Can]
Geocillin® [US]
Lin-Amox [Can]
nafcillin
Nallpen® [Can]
Novamoxin® [Can]
Novo-Ampicillin [Can]
Novo-Clavamoxin [Can]
Novo-Cloxin [Can]
Novo-Pen-VK [Can]
Nu-Amoxi [Can]
Nu-Ampi [Can]
Nu-Cloxi [Can]
Nu-Pen-VK [Can]
oxacillin
Pathocil® [Can]
penicillin V potassium
penicillin G benzathine
penicillin G benzathine and penicillin
G procaine
penicillin G (parenteral/aqueous)
penicillin G procaine
Pfizerpen® [US/Can]

Pfizerpen-AS® [Can]
PHL-Amoxicillin [Can]
piperacillin
piperacillin and tazobactam sodium
Piperacillin for Injection, USP [Can]
pivampicillin (Canada only)
PMS-Amoxicillin [Can]
Pondocillin® [Can]
ratio-Aclavulanate [Can]
Riva-Cloxacillin [Can]
Tazocin® [Can]
Ticar® [US]
ticarcillin
ticarcillin and clavulanate potassium
Timentin® [US/Can]
Unasyn® [US/Can]
Unipen® [Can]
Veetids® [US]
Wycillin® [Can]
Zosyn® [US]
Quinolone
Apo-Ciproflox® [Can]
Apo-Oflox® [Can]
Apo-Ofloxacin® [Can]
Cipro® [US/Can]
Cipro® XL [Can]
ciprofloxacin
Cipro® XR [US]
CO Ciprofloxacin [Can]
Floxin® [US/Can]
Gen-Ciprofloxacin [Can]
Novo-Ciprofloxacin [Can]
Novo-Ofloxacin [Can]
Ocuflox® [US/Can]
ofloxacin
PMS-Ciprofloxacin [Can]
PMS-Ofloxacin [Can]
Proquin® XR [US]
RAN™-Ciprofloxacin [Can]
ratio-Ciprofloxacin [Can]
Rhoxal-ciprofloxacin [Can]
Sandoz-Ciprofloxacin [Can]
Taro-Ciprofloxacin [Can]

Sulfonamide
  Apo-Sulfatrim® [Can]
  Apo-Sulfatrim® DS [Can]
  Apo-Sulfatrim® Pediatric [Can]
  Bactrim™ [US]
  Bactrim™ DS [US]
  Novo-Trimel [Can]
  Novo-Trimel D.S. [Can]
  Nu-Cotrimox [Can]
  Septra® [US]
  Septra® DS [US]
  Septra® Injection [Can]
  sulfamethoxazole and trimethoprim
Vaccine
  pneumococcal conjugate
    vaccine (7-valent)
  Prevnar® [US/Can]
Vaccine, Inactivated Bacteria
  Pneumo 23™ [Can]
  pneumococcal polysaccharide
    vaccine (polyvalent)
  Pneumovax® 23 [US/Can]

PNEUMONIA, COMMUNITY-ACQUIRED

Antibiotic, Quinolone
  Avelox® [US/Can]
  Avelox® I.V. [US/Can]
  moxifloxacin
  Vigamox™ [US/Can]

PRIMARY PULMONARY HYPERTENSION (PPH)

Platelet Inhibitor
  epoprostenol
  Flolan® [US/Can]

PULMONARY ARTERY HYPERTENSION (PAH)

Endothelin Antagonist

  bosentan
  Tracleer® [US/Can]
Vasodilator
  Remodulin® [US/Can]
  treprostinil

PULMONARY EMBOLISM

Anticoagulant (Other)
  Apo-Warfarin® [Can]
  Coumadin® [US/Can]
  enoxaparin
  Enoxaparin Injection [Can]
  Gen-Warfarin [Can]
  Hepalean® [Can]
  Hepalean® Leo [Can]
  Hepalean®-LOK [Can]
  heparin
  HepFlush®-10 [US]
  Hep-Lock® [US]
  Hep-Lock U/P [US]
  Jantoven™ [US]
  Lovenox® [US/Can]
  Lovenox® HP [Can]
  Novo-Warfarin [Can]
  Taro-Warfarin [Can]
  warfarin
Fibrinolytic Agent
  Activase® [US]
  Activase® rt-PA [Can]
  alteplase
  Cathflo™ Activase® [US/Can]
  Streptase® [US/Can]
  streptokinase
Low Molecular Weight Heparin
  Fraxiparine™ [Can]
  Fraxiparine™ Forte [Can]
  nadroparin (Canada only)

PULMONARY TUBERCULOSIS

Antitubercular Agent
  Priftin® [US/Can]

rifapentine

RESPIRATORY DISTRESS SYNDROME (RDS)
Lung Surfactant
  beractant
  calfactant
  Curosurf® [US/Can]
  Infasurf® [US]
  poractant alfa
  Survanta® [US/Can]

RESPIRATORY SYNCYTIAL VIRUS (RSV)
Antiviral Agent
  Copegus® [US]
  Rebetol® [US]
  Ribasphere™ [US]
  ribavirin
  Virazole® [US/Can]
Monoclonal Antibody
  palivizumab
  Synagis® [US/Can]

SKELETAL MUSCLE RELAXANT (SURGICAL)
Skeletal Muscle Relaxant
  atracurium
  cisatracurium
  doxacurium
  Nimbex® [US/Can]
  Nuromax® [US]
  pancuronium
  Quelicin® [US/Can]
  rocuronium
  succinylcholine
  Tracrium® [US]
  vecuronium
  Zemuron® [US/Can]

SMOKING CESSATION

Antidepressant, Monoamine Oxidase Inhibitor
  Alti-Moclobemide [Can]
  Apo-Moclobemide® [Can]
  Manerix® [Can]
  moclobemide (Canada only)
  Novo-Moclobemide [Can]
  Nu-Moclobemide [Can]
  PMS-Moclobemide [Can]
Partial Nicotine Agonist
  Chantix™ [US]
  varenicline
Smoking Deterrent
  Commit® [US-OTC]
  Habitrol® [Can]
  Nicoderm® [Can]
  NicoDerm® CQ® [US-OTC]
  Nicorette® [US-OTC/Can]
  Nicorette® Plus [Can]
  nicotine
  Nicotrol® [Can]
  Nicotrol® Inhaler [US]
  Nicotrol® NS [US]
  Nicotrol® Patch [US-OTC]

STROKE
Antiplatelet Agent
  Alti-Ticlopidine [Can]
  Apo-Ticlopidine® [Can]
  Asaphen [Can]
  Asaphen E.C. [Can]
  Ascriptin® [US-OTC]
  Ascriptin® Extra Strength [US-OTC]
  Aspercin [US-OTC]
  Aspercin Extra [US-OTC]
  Aspergum® [US-OTC]
  aspirin
  Bayer® Aspirin [US-OTC]
  Bayer® Aspirin Extra Strength [US-OTC]
  Bayer® Aspirin Regimen Adult Low Strength [US-OTC]

Bayer® Aspirin Regimen Children's [US-OTC]
Bayer® Aspirin Regimen Regular Strength [US-OTC]
Bayer® Extra Strength Arthritis Pain Regimen [US-OTC]
Bayer® Plus Extra Strength [US-OTC]
Bayer® Women's Aspirin Plus Calcium [US-OTC]
Bufferin® [US-OTC]
Bufferin® Extra Strength [US-OTC]
Buffinol [US-OTC]
Buffinol Extra [US-OTC]
Easprin® [US]
Ecotrin® [US-OTC]
Ecotrin® Low Strength [US-OTC]
Ecotrin® Maximum Strength [US-OTC]
Entrophen® [Can]
Gen-Ticlopidine [Can]
Halfprin® [US-OTC]
Novasen [Can]
Novo-Ticlopidine [Can]
Nu-Ticlopidine [Can]
Rhoxal-ticlopidine [Can]
Sandoz-Ticlopidine [Can]
St. Joseph® Adult Aspirin [US-OTC]
Sureprin 81™ [US-OTC]
Ticlid® [US/Can]
ticlopidine
ZORprin® [US]
Fibrinolytic Agent
Activase® [US]
Activase® rt-PA [Can]
alteplase
Cathflo™ Activase® [US/Can]
Skeletal Muscle Relaxant
Dantrium® [US/Can]
dantrolene

SYNCOPE
Adrenergic Agonist Agent

Adrenalin® [US/Can]
epinephrine
isoproterenol
Isuprel® [US]
Respiratory Stimulant
ammonia spirit (aromatic)

THROMBOLYTIC THERAPY
Anticoagulant (Other)
Apo-Warfarin® [Can]
Coumadin® [US/Can]
dalteparin
enoxaparin
Enoxaparin Injection [Can]
Fragmin® [US/Can]
Gen-Warfarin [Can]
Hepalean® [Can]
Hepalean® Leo [Can]
Hepalean®-LOK [Can]
heparin
HepFlush®-10 [US]
Hep-Lock® [US]
Hep-Lock U/P [US]
Innohep® [US/Can]
Jantoven™ [US]
Lovenox® [US/Can]
Lovenox® HP [Can]
Novo-Warfarin [Can]
Taro-Warfarin [Can]
tinzaparin
warfarin
Fibrinolytic Agent
Activase® [US]
Activase® rt-PA [Can]
alteplase
Cathflo™ Activase® [US/Can]
Retavase® [US/Can]
reteplase
Streptase® [US/Can]
streptokinase